ESSENTIALS OF MENTAL HEALTH NURSING

SECOND EDITION

ABOUT THE AUTHORS

J. Sue Cook

is an associate professor of nursing at California State University, Stanislaus at Turlock. She completed her BSN and MSN at California State University, Fresno; in 1980 she completed work on her EdD at the University of San Francisco. As a member of the California Nurses' Association, she served on the board of directors from 1984 through 1986. Her five-year term as government relations commissioner extends through 1991. As a speaker at Recovery Resources in Ceres, California, she addressed the topic of nursing diagnosis in mental health nursing. For the Psychiatric Inpatient Program of Stanislaus County, she presented a program about the mental health nursing process. She has served as a legislative liaison for a California state assemblyman and senator. Other activities include working as a part-time staff nurse at Scenic General Hospital and serving as curriculum coordinator for the BSN program at California State University. In 1987 she received the Meritorious Performance and Professional Promise Award from California State University, Stanislaus.

Karen Lee Fontaine,

associate professor of nursing at Purdue University Calumet, received her BS from Valparaiso University and her RN from Lutheran Hospital School of Nursing, St. Louis. She completed work on her MSN at Rush University in Chicago. She is a certified sex therapist in private practice and has presented numerous national seminars on human sexuality. She has contributed chapters to several books on the topics of stress management, sexuality and aging, altered patterns of sexuality, and violence. She received the Outstanding Undergraduate Teacher Award, 1982–1983, from Purdue University Calumet. She was named the outstanding educator of 1984 by the Gamma Phi chapter of Sigma Theta Tau.

Editor's note: The order of the authors' names is purely alphabetical. Each has contributed equally to the creation of this text.

Essentials of Mental Health Nursing

SECOND EDITION

J. SUE COOK, RN, EdD

KAREN LEE FONTAINE, RN, MSN

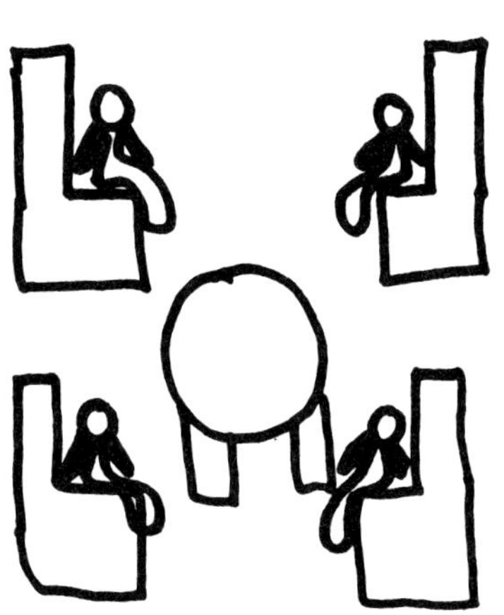

A Safe Place. *It is a place where everyone can share their problems, hurts, upsets, feelings, and emotions. It's a place where a person can be open about expressing their thoughts and know that they are kept safely confidential.*

Addison-Wesley Nursing

A Division of The Benjamin/Cummings Publishing Company, Inc.

Redwood City, California   Fort Collins, Colorado   Menlo Park, California
Reading, Massachusetts   New York   Don Mills, Ontario   Wokingham, U.K.
Amsterdam   Bonn   Sydney   Singapore   Tokyo   Madrid   San Juan

610.7368
C77
c.

This book is dedicated to:

The memory of Stephen M. Prewitt
Linda Hillman, who started this all

Managing Editor: Sally D. Elliott
Executive Editor: Debra Hunter
Sponsoring Editor: Mark McCormick
Editorial Assistant: Michèle Mangelli
Senior Production Supervisor: Bonnie B. Grover
Text Designer: Eleanor Mennick
Cover Designer: Rodolphe M. Zehntner, The Belmont Studio
Cover Illustrator: Joan Carol
Copyeditors: Toni Murray, Judith Johnstone, Stacey Post
Proofreaders: Judy Kennedy, Ruth S. Faur, RN, MS, Judith Johnstone
Indexer: Katherine Pitcoff
Compositor: G&S Typesetters, Inc.

The chapter opening art was created for this book as a project completely separate from writing of the manuscript. The clients' names and diagnoses are unknown to authors and publisher. The art has been placed throughout the book without attempting to make any correlation between a client's art and the chapter content.

Copyright © 1991 by Addison-Wesley Publishing Company, Inc. All rights reserved. No part of this publication may be reproduced, stored in a retrieval system, or transmitted in any form or by any means, electronic, mechanical, photocopying, recording, or otherwise, without the prior permission of the publisher. Printed in the United States of America. Published simultaneously in Canada.

Library of Congress Cataloging-in-Publication Data

Cook, J. Sue, 1946–
Essentials of mental health nursing / J. Sue Cook, Karen Lee Fontaine.—2nd ed.
p. cm.
Rev. ed. of: Essentials of mental health nursing / [editors] J. Sue Cook, Karen Lee Fontaine.
1. Psychiatric nursing. I. Fontaine, Karen Lee, 1943—
II. Title.
[DNLM: 1. Psychiatric Nursing. WY 160 C771e]
RC440.E82 1990
610.73′68—dc20 90-861
ISBN 0-201-12597-8 CIP
ABCDEFGHIJ-DO9543210

Addison-Wesley Nursing
A Division of The Benjamin/Cummings Publishing Company, Inc.
390 Bridge Parkway
Redwood City, California 94065

CONTRIBUTORS

Leslie Bonjean, RN, MSN
Coordinator for Associate Degree Nursing Program
Purdue University Calumet
Hammond, IN

Ellen Marie Bratt, RN, MSN
Associate Professor
Purdue University Calumet
Hammond, IN

Brenda Lewis Cleary, BSN, MSN, PhD
Assistant Professor, School of Nursing
Texas Tech University
Odessa, TX

Paula G. LeVeck, RN, PhD
Professor of Nursing
California State University, Stanislaus
Turlock, CA

Susan F. Miller, BSN, MSN
Staff Development Coordinator
JML Care Center
Falmouth, MA

Joseph E. Smith, MS, RN, CS
Senior Research Associate, Department of Psychiatry
University of Mississippi Medical Center
Jackson, MS

122512

Contents

Preface

In the first edition of *Essentials of Mental Health Nursing* our purpose was to provide students a text that contained all the necessary information about mental health nursing without overwhelming them with its size. The second edition continues in the same spirit. We have revised, reorganized, and added content based on our own use of the text, student input, and peer and reviewer comments. We believe that these changes make the second edition an even more "user friendly" and helpful text for nursing students.

Philosophical/Theoretical Frameworks

This text is based on the belief that the practice of mental health nursing means helping clients manage difficulties, solve problems, decrease emotional pain, and promote growth, while respecting clients' rights to their own values, beliefs, and decisions. To that end we encourage nursing students to engage in self-analysis in order to increase their own self-understanding and self-acceptance. This is important, because nurses who are able to clarify their own beliefs and values are less likely to be judgmental or to impose their own values and beliefs on clients. Furthermore, we view people holistically, in that we believe each person to be a set of interrelated systems continuously in the process of becoming, and possessing a unity and integration that incorporates body, mind, and spirit.

We have incorporated a variety of philosophies and theories to help students understand clients and their experiences. Philosophies of health, of suffering, and of nursing are explored for their impact on clients and nurses. Perspectives of personality—psychoanalytic, social-psychologic, behavioralistic, cognitive, developmental, humanistic, moral developmental, and feminist—are integrated throughout the text. Students are thereby encouraged to explore the many approaches to nursing care and practice. Additionally, throughout the text we examine the impact of sexism, racism, ageism, and homophobia on the mental health of the members of our society who suffer discrimination and prejudice.

Organization

The text is presented in two parts. Part One, Concepts in Mental health Nursing (Chapters 1 through 6), introduces students to philosophies, theories, nursing roles, and nurse-client relationships. In addition, the problem-solving method of the nursing process is applied to the beginning student, who is often fearful of interacting with psychiatric clients. This not only addresses a common student concern, but it also teaches students that they can apply the nursing process to themselves. There is a heavy emphasis on the development and assessment of effective and therapeutic communication skills. The student is also introduced to behavioral, affective, cognitive, and physical assessment skills as well as to the diagnosing, planning, implementing, and evaluating steps of the nursing process. Finally, Part One includes interdisciplinary treatment modalities, the interface of culture and mental health, and the management of crises throughout the lifespan.

Part Two, Nursing Care of Psychiatric Clients, consists of the remaining chapters, 7 through 17. Similarities and differences in disorders and treatment for children, adolescents, adults, and the elderly are presented in each chapter. All chapters are consistently organized, beginning with the knowledge base of behavioral, affective, cognitive, physiologic, and sociocultural characteristics and concluding with an overview of causative theories and medical treatment.

The Focused Nursing Assessment, highlighted in the text with a magnifying-glass logo, is then organized in the same pattern to help students correlate specific client responses with the general knowledge base. The repetitive categories reinforce learning and present a systematic way of assessing clients with a variety of disorders. Medications are presented in each of the disorders chapters to reinforce the medication information from Part One. Each chapter includes multiple nursing care plans using standard nursing diagnoses, goals, interventions, rationales, and outcome criteria. These extensive care plans enable students to avoid purchasing a separate text of psychiatric nursing care plans. Each of the chapters in Part Two includes listings of professional and self-help groups with addresses and phone numbers for client referral and students' personal use.

Pedagogy

We believe the nursing process is a critical learning activity in mental health nursing. The nursing process is introduced in Part One and is the organizing framework for Part Two. This type of consistency in organization is extremely important in helping students begin to assess and analyze systematically. The Focused Nursing Assessment tools follow the organizational pattern of the knowledge base. In many texts, students are given a general assessment tool and then left on their own to assess specific clients. We do not believe that beginning students have the skills to formulate the appropriate nursing assessment questions related to the client's medical diagnosis. Thus we developed Focused Nursing Assessment tools to aid students in learning the type and range of assessment questions to ask particular clients. The assessment questions are open-ended and reinforce the use of good communication skills. We chose to present the diagnosing, planning, and implementation phases of the nursing process in table format. Students do not have to search through pages of text material when writing nursing care plans for their clients. They are able to look for nursing diagnoses that are appropriate for their client and have the relevant material right at hand. The table format reinforces the importance of the nursing care plan as the foundation of client care—not simply busy work to be handed in to the instructor.

We have included many clinical examples to illustrate client behaviors, feelings, thinking patterns, and interaction in order that the material come alive in the students' mind and to avoid comprehension difficulty with abstract material. The material is reinforced at the end of each chapter with a more complete case example. New tables have been developed to highlight important text material and a new appendix includes the correct answers and rationales for the end-of-chapter review questions. Inclusion of rationales for incorrect responses is designed to assist the student in refining thinking and test-taking skills.

New and Revised Content

Two new chapters have been added to the second edition. Chapter 6, Consequences and Resolution of Developmental Crises, presents situational crises occurring at specific developmental stages across the lifespan. Topics covered are children of divorce, teenage parenthood, peer group formation, midlife crisis, generational conflict, ageism, and the losses of aging. These new topics reflect current issues in our culture that are placing the most stress on individuals and families and that are likely to result in people seeking mental health treatment. This chapter is additionally designed to help nurses anticipate and resolve their own personal crises.

Chapter 17, Issues Facing Mental Health Nursing, covers emotional and social nursing care for AIDS clients and their families and friends. This continues to be a critical care issue, as the more than 80,000 deaths in the United States thus far has equalled the losses from the Korean and Vietnam wars combined. The other current issue covered in chapter 17 is that of the homeless population. Antecedents to becoming homeless and the physical and mental health needs of this population are discussed with appropriate nursing interventions.

New information has been incorporated into a number of chapters. Moral developmental theories, crisis theory, crisis intervention, obesity, date rape, adult survivors of childhood sexual abuse, nurses and physicians who are drug dependent, co-dependency, adult children of alcoholics, and nurses who served in Vietnam all appear for the first time. We have also increased our coverage on communication, the grieving process, and living with a person suffering from mental illness.

New Features

New to the Second Edition is a glossary for the entire text. We decided this would be most helpful to students struggling to learn new terminology and concepts. The Appendices include a list of the American Nurses Association's Psychiatric Nursing Diagnoses for those faculty and students who prefer to use this classification system. In an effort to combat the rising toll of AIDS we have included "safer sex" guidelines in the appendix for client teaching and for students' personal use.

Instructor's Resource Manual

The Instructor's Resource Manual, which is available upon adoption of the text, consists of four sections in the Second Edition. The test bank has been revised and expanded from 240 questions in the first edition to 425 questions in the second. The questions are in the NCLEX format and review each step of the nursing process. Rationales are provided for the incorrect answers to help professors respond to students' questions about test items. The test bank is available on computer disks to decrease secretarial time in formatting exams.

The second section of the Instructor's Resource Manual contains additional class and lecture information for each chapter; it is designed to assist students in review and application of the text material. These handouts, which may be copied by the instructor, were created to help professors incorporate active learning within the classroom setting or with small-group work. The material may also be used to help students practice problem solving in mental health nursing practice and to help students who are having difficulty in grasping the material to learn the concepts through an additional teaching method. This material includes two case studies for each of the 11 chapters in Part Two of the text. These exercises have been tested and refined in the classroom setting.

The third section consists of transparency masters that are designed to assist professors in creating lecture presentations or for review of major concepts within each chapter. This section includes such items as a list of key words/concepts for every chapter, stages of grief, medications, distorted thinking processes, differentiation of depressive symptoms across the lifespan, family system models, and many other topics.

The fourth section consists of patient artwork created for the opening of each text chapter. We received more than we needed for the text and did not want to omit any of it. The artwork may be copied onto transparencies and used as additional classroom material. Some professors may wish to interpret the meaning of the work to help students begin to appreciate the inner world of their clients. Other professors may wish to ask students to share with each other their feeling and cognitive responses to each piece of art. No doubt some professors will find additional creative uses for the art and we hope they will share them with all of us.

Acknowledgments

There are many people we wish to thank for helping us refine our thinking in this second edition of *Essentials of Mental Health Nursing.* First we wish to thank our colleagues who contributed to this edition. Their names and affiliations are listed on page v. We also wish to thank Mary J. Roehrig and Shirley Sennhauser for their contributions to the first edition, which continue to influence this one. Special recognition is deserved for the extra efforts of Ruth Saddlemire Faur during the copyedit phase of production for this edition.

To our students: a very warm note of appreciation for your questions, comments, suggestions, and creativity. Special thanks to Tricia Dokupic,

Nola Isla, Carol Dillon, and Deanna Bilka, who willingly shared their extensive nursing care plans.

A special thank you goes to our reviewers, whose thoughtful comments greatly strengthened this edition: Joyce Adriance, Napa Valley College, Napa, California; Bridget Amore, Barry University, Miami Shores, Florida; Charles J. Beauchamp, Barry University, Miami Shores, Florida; Kate Burke, Delaware Technical and Community College, Georgetown, Delaware; Jeanne Gelman, Widener University, Chester, Pennsylvania; Brenda Lyon, Indiana University, Bloomington, Indiana; Veneda S. Martin, Kentucky State University, Frankfort, Kentucky; Louise Pitts, Valencia Community College, Orlando, Florida; and Bonnie Rickelman, University of Texas at Austin, Austin, Texas.

The staff of Ralph K. Davies Medical Center in San Francisco was invaluable in providing the clinical setting in which to validate the nursing diagnoses applicable to clients with AIDS. Harold Smith, Brian Christianson, Rick Childress, and Anne Owen willingly shared their professional expertise in dealing with the HIV-infected client. The AIDS clients who shared their perceptions on the focus of nursing assessments and plans of care influenced the final decisions on content, and to them we will be eternally grateful for sharing their world. From their insights, nurses may ease the pain of others in the future.

The professionals at Addison-Wesley have greatly assisted us in formulating our ideas into an improved learning tool. Armando Parces-Enriquez provided the opportunity for us to fine-tune an already successful product. Debra Hunter, executive editor, continues to heartily support our work. Mark McCormick, our sponsoring editor, has provided new insights and comfort and challenged us to be the best that we can be. Michèle Mangelli, editorial assistant, worked very hard in preparing our manuscript for production. Bonnie Grover, senior production supervisor, took that manuscript and made it into a fine text.

Last, and most important, to our families we say thank you for your unending support of this project. It is through your encouragement that we were able to stay on task.

Karen Lee Fontaine
J. Sue Cook

ABOUT THE CHAPTER OPENING ARTWORK

The artwork and commentary introducing each chapter were created by acute psychiatric patients at Stanford University Hospital in Palo Alto, California. The project grew naturally out of an existing expressive art program at Stanford, designed to help hospitalized people portray their private worlds—worlds often filled with despair, anxiety, confusion, anger, and apathy. Communication of these powerful feelings through writing and drawing helps decrease social isolation, as patients share common experiences with each other. Relief of inner tension is another frequent outcome, unmanageable emotions take form on paper, and containment of those emotions is achieved. In addition, caretakers' awareness about, and understanding of, their patients' inner realities is heightened, thus assisting them with treatment.

Participation in this project was voluntary. Written consent was required from both patient and psychiatrist, because of the highly revealing nature of the artwork. Patients who were flagrantly psychotic, disassociated, or paranoid were excluded, as a protective measure for them. Drawings and captions were contributed anonymously, to protect patients' rights to privacy.

Drawings were collected from an occupational therapy group at Stanford over a three month period. Minimal changes were made in group format and procedure to maintain continuity in the ongoing ward program. The group met weekly for about an hour, and was attended by an average of six patients. The first part of the session was devoted to quiet art activity. Self-expression and self-revelation were emphasized over artistic capability and pleasing results. Patients were informed that their work would be used in a textbook, to help educate nursing students about the feelings and thoughts of psychiatric patients. They were given specific guidelines for the publication about use of color, space, and content. Finally, they were asked to write brief descriptions of their pictures, to communicate intended meaning to readers. To stimulate expression and self-disclosure, patients were given a list of suggested topics:

- My Inner Self and My Outer Self
- A Safe Place
- How I See My Helpers
- How I See My Mental Illness
- What Helps Me Get Better
- Being in the Hospital

During the second half of group sessions, patients openly shared their drawings and commentary with therapists and other group members. People were invited, not required, to talk; privacy was respected. Those who participated were frequently surprised and reassured by the similarity of their feelings. As they explored delicate realms, patients experienced substantial support from each other and from staff.

To assess the impact of this project on patients, their comments and reactions were solicited at the end of the sessions. Since each picture was perceived as a contest entry, questions arose about how this would affect spontaneity and candor. It was a delight to discover the project was a therapeutic tool in itself. Comments reflected favorable attitudes: "It gave me a chance to achieve (something)," to "turn something negative (despair) into something positive," to "change from feeling like a loser to feeling like a winner," to "get a stroke at a time when you're feeling badly about yourself," and to "figure out how you felt—a picture is worth a thousand words!" The surprise of having one's creations valued stimulated multiple entries. One patient, whose drawings appeared in the first edition of this text, encouraged fellow patients to submit their artwork, proudly announcing he had "been published."

A psychiatric patient is usually submerged in a state of despondency, and carries with him or her a very wounded self-image. Treatment helps to alleviate this despair, to restore hope through psychotherapy, support, structure, medication, and the acquisition of improved coping strategies. Expressive artwork is one very effective tool; it helps channel overwhelming feelings into something constructive. In contributing to this textbook, patients experienced the opportunity to discover areas of personal strength, finding new avenues for individual expression along the way.

Vivian Banish

The art reproduced at the start of each chapter of the first edition of *Essentials of Mental Health Nursing* was a popular feature with both instructors and students. As this new edition took shape, it became clear that all of us at Addison-Wesley wanted to include new pieces of art drawn by clients of the mental health care system.

We were very pleased that the Department of Occupational Therapy at Stanford University's Medical Center was willing to participate in the art program; Vivian Banish could coordinate the effort; and that the doctors, nurses, and therapists who were involved in evaluating the art program and its appropriateness for their particular clients agreed to participate again. We especially thank the clients themselves who participated in the program. The drawings we received touched us and we share them with you in that spirit.

The legends that accompany each drawing are comments written by the artist. To set them into type, I have altered their words as little as possible, in order to retain the emphasis, the energy, and the poetry I found in the handwritten copy.

Space limitations prevent us from including all the art that was provided to us in this book. All the art not included here is printed in the Instructor's Resource Manual. Each piece, whether reproduced here or not, was equally valuable to us and to this art program.

Bonnie Grover
Senior Production Supervisor

Part One

CONCEPTS IN MENTAL HEALTH NURSING

CHAPTER 1

Nurses and Clients in Mental Health Care

KAREN LEE FONTAINE

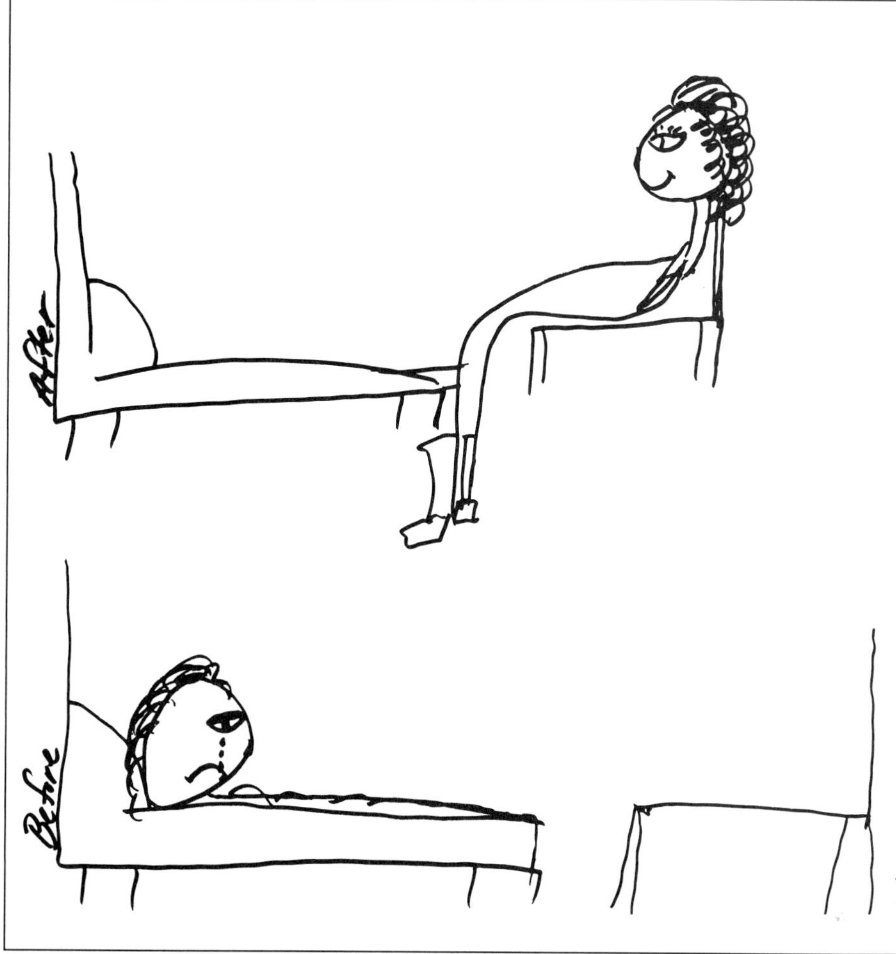

What Helps Me Get Better

When I first came into the Hospital in order for asking for help! *I had to first claim I had a Illness or some thing like that. At first I didn't have any kind of feelings or thoughts of my own. All I thought or felt was darkness and sadness.*

This Hospital that I went to really helped me out. I really thank my doctor but most of all I thank the Nurses for being so understanding warm and kind to under stand my sickness. I Thank you Medical people for learning and understanding Mental Illness.

■ *Objectives*

After reading this chapter the student will be able to

- Articulate personal philosophies of wellness and illness
- Define mental illness from a holistic perspective
- Explain how personal beliefs about suffering influence nursing practice
- Assess clients' behavioral, affective, cognitive, and sociocultural responses to illness
- Describe how the physical, emotional, and spiritual components of the nurse-client relationship function in unity
- Integrate characteristics of effective helpers into nursing practice
- Identify concerns about effectively communicating with clients
- Use a variety of nursing roles to implement the nursing care plan
- Use the problem-solving approach with clients
- Manage fears about clinical practice
- Use the evaluation process to improve nursing practice

■ *Chapter Outline*

Introduction

Clients and nurses and their interpersonal relationships are the core of nursing practice. The learning of interpersonal skills begins in the first nursing course, continues throughout the curriculum, and is refined and broadened during students' experiences with psychiatric clients. As the focus shifts from task and procedure functions to effective relationships, students begin to analyze themselves, their clients, and their relationships with them. With increased self-understanding comes increased understanding of others. Combining this understanding with a sound theoretical base and comprehensive client assessments immeasurably enhances the students' breadth and depth of diagnosis, planning, intervention, and evaluation.

Beginning with their early student experiences and continuing throughout their professional practice, nurses continually review a variety of philosophies. Personal and professional philosophies and values influence decisions and are fundamental to all nursing activities. Philosophies and values are consciously examined and clarified so that the nurse can approach each client situation with a clear, coherent, and helpful perspective.

Philosophy of Health

Individual definitions of wellness and illness reflect one's **philosophy of health** and influence the way in which health care is provided and received. These basic beliefs affect how clients are approached, the formulation of interventions, and the evaluation of the effectiveness of nursing care. Clients' beliefs determine when, if, and from whom health care is sought as well as which recommendations for improved health are heeded.

Wellness is neither a static state nor a concrete goal to be achieved; rather, it is a dynamic, lifelong process. Wellness differs from the mere absence of disease in that it is a growing toward potential, an inner feeling of aliveness. The person on the wellness side of the illness-wellness continuum has a sense of harmony and projects a general feeling of vitality. Wellness includes the ability to limit unnecessary stress, to maintain personal relationships, to like oneself, and to deal with organic problems.

Illness, on the other hand, is a person's subjective sense of disharmony, which may be within the self or between the self and the environment. Illness may be described as anxiety, guilt, suffering, dissatisfaction, or despair. A prolonged state of disharmony may result in disease.

Harmony, or congruency, with the self is reflected by more than simply a person's physiology and behavior. It is holistic, involving the entire person—body, mind, and spirit. Artificially separating these three dimensions can be confusing and misleading. This three-part model is a method of looking at and understanding the total person. Taking a **holistic view**, the nurse sees each person as a complexly interrelated and inseparable set of systems in process. In either wellness or illness, no part is separate. Each dimension relates to every other, with a unity and integration that transcends body, mind, and spirit.

It is not unusual for students to begin the study of psychiatric nursing believing many of society's myths and stereotypes about psychiatric clients. As students progress through the course they begin to understand there is no universally accepted definition of normal or abnormal behavior, affect, or thinking. Cultures often label as pathological any behavior, affect, or thinking that is unusual or not easily understood. Students study a variety of theories from which to understand clients and their experiences, and these theories are not altogether consistent with definitions of mental health and wellness. The **medical model** defines mental health as the absence of signs and symptoms of disability and uses diagnostic labeling to communicate what is meant by a cluster of abnormal behaviors. To facilitate communication with other disciplines, students need to know the terminology of diagnoses and what is specifically meant by these labels.

At the same time, it is possible to view mental health from other perspectives. Health can be seen as the ability to fulfill roles in life. Health can be assessed on the **adaptive model** by looking at environmental interactions and growth toward optimal functioning. Other models view the healthy person in the **process of becoming** and understanding the potential within (Leddy and Pepper, 1985). Within a **family context**, health is seen as an adaptive well-functioning family system. From a **spiritual perspective**, the mentally healthy person is one who feels connected with others and experiences a deep meaning in life. Holistic nursing is an integration of these theories and a reaching out beyond the labels to the person who is suffering.

Philosophy of Suffering

One's **philosophy of suffering**, that is, one's ideas about the cause and purpose of suffering in life, must be consciously assessed. Although some believe that illness and suffering are a natural part of human life and a way to further development of personhood, others may consider illness and suffering errors of the mind, a test of faith, a divine punishment, or an intrusion of evil (Pumphrey, 1977). The nurse's beliefs influence judgments made about the degree of suffering in others since suffering cannot be directly measured. These judgments influence how one intervenes with a client experiencing psychological discomfort or physical pain. If the nurse believes a client is suffering intensely, there may be more active involvement than with a client who appears in less distress. The desire to alleviate suffering is one of the major reasons that people give for choosing the nursing profession. It must be remembered that beliefs about suffering are, in fact, opinions, which if not personally identified by the nurse, have the potential for distorting client assessment (Davitz, Davitz, and Rubin, 1980).

Philosophy of suffering directly affects how nurses interact with clients. In Davitz, Davitz, and

Rubin's study (1980) it was found that nurses who believed in a higher level of client distress more often explained procedures, expressed empathy, stood closer and touched clients, and checked with other members of the health team when unable to answer questions. In contrast, nurses who inferred less distress tended neither to explain what they were doing nor to give clients rationales for tests. By responding briefly to client's questions or by changing the subject, they tended to be more distant and impersonal.

It is important that nurses review their own experiences with suffering to determine how these affect their nursing practice. Holm et al. (1989) found nursing assessment of clients' physical and emotional pain was influenced by the nurses' personal experiences with suffering. Effective nurses neither overreact to suffering nor ignore it.

Philosophy of Nursing

Having identified philosophies of health and suffering, nurses must analyze their **philosophy of nursing.** This will directly affect the people involved, clients and nurses alike.

The nursing process is based on knowledge, values, commitment, and action. Values and beliefs give direction and meaning to nursing practice within the interpersonal context.

The most important issue brought from the personal belief system to the professional role is caring. Not simply an emotion, caring is a value and a way of relating to others. It involves beliefs about the intrinsic worth of people and the ability to make an authentic commitment and a personal response to another person. In caring relationships, nurses are motivated to take actions for the sake of clients, and they are committed to assist clients in meeting needs and in growing toward potential (Holderby and McNulty, 1982; Watson, 1985).

Philosophies of health, suffering, and nursing determine how priorities are set and time is used, as well as the amount of energy expended and the degree of emotion involved. These values and beliefs contribute to nurses' positive self-regard, increased job satisfaction, and the development of a philosophy of life that has a personal and a professional impact (Holderby and McNulty, 1982; Watson, 1985).

Assessment

In assessing one's relationship with a client, three factors come into play:

- What the client brings to the relationship
- What the nurse brings to the relationship
- The physical, emotional, and spiritual dynamics that develop within the relationship itself

Self-Analysis

Self-analysis is a dynamic and ongoing process by which the nurse gains understanding of the physical, emotional, social, and spiritual aspects of the inner self. It is a process of examining, revising, rejecting, and reaffirming personal beliefs—a conscious reflection on one's life, through which one attempts to make sense of and give meaning to oneself. Through self-analysis, or introspection, the nurse clarifies personal values and reaches a deeper understanding of the self.

Since people do not live in isolation, self-analysis also means how one interacts with other people. Learning about oneself is not an easy process. It means looking beyond the ideal image of who one wants to be, to face the reality of who one is. It includes understanding the how and why of one's own behavior. Knowing oneself includes the identification of needs, such as the need to rescue others, the need to be strong, or the need to be liked by others. Identifying these personal needs increases the accuracy of behavioral analysis by helping nurses assume responsibility for their own behavior and the effect that behavior has on others.

With the greater understanding that self-analysis brings come other benefits for the nurse. Nurses learn to accept their strengths and limitations while continuing to struggle toward personal growth. They become able to take responsibility for their successes and their failures.

A person unaware of aspects of the self has a

tendency to rationalize as a defense or to project these traits onto someone else. Therefore one often dislikes in others those qualities one hates in oneself. Self-acceptance is, therefore, a prerequisite to acceptance of others.

Some nursing students will find themselves resisting self-analysis and growth. An unconscious fear of maturity may interfere with this process. Maturity means more independence and a higher level of responsibility for motivation and self-discipline. It means taking risks and being able to cope with disapproval. Some people resist maturation because they fear they or others will dislike what is discovered. Others become anxious when contemplating any type of change. An unconscious fear of success interferes with some people's growth. If one is successful, there is a higher standard to live up to and maintain. Success also implies that one supports, guides, or cares for those who are less successful in life, and this may feel overwhelming to some.

One's personal and professional self-concepts are closely intertwined. Nurses who feel good about themselves as persons are more likely to engage in responsible risk taking, which contributes to positive and productive professional self-concepts. Nurses who have negative personal self-concepts are less likely to take risks and have more difficulty functioning independently, which contributes to negative professional self-concepts. Both personal and professional self-concepts grow or stagnate together. To grow professionally means to grow personally (Leddy and Pepper, 1985).

Self-awareness is necessary if nurses are to collaborate with clients. To assist a client in solving a problem is difficult if the nurses themselves have not been able to resolve those particular concerns. Self-knowledge is vital in recognizing one's limitations in working with certain clients or issues.

Tim is a married 42-year-old nursing student. His wife has been an alcoholic for the past three years, and she refuses to acknowledge her problem. Through introspection and interaction with other nursing students and his instructor, Tim has become aware of his hurt and intense anger toward his wife. Knowing there is a strong possibility that he may unconsciously displace his feelings toward his wife onto alcoholic clients, which would interfere with the therapeutic process, he has requested that he not be assigned to an intensive relationship with an alcoholic client at this time.

All nurses at times experience feelings of anxiety, anger, or resentment toward some clients. The process of self-assessment assists nurses in understanding and professionally coping with these feelings and in responding more effectively in the clinical setting. Nurses who understand themselves well are able to plan, implement, and evaluate care in a more meaningful and holistic manner.

Analysis of Clients' Behavioral Responses to Illness

Effective nurses appreciate the complexity of their clients. Behavioral responses to illness have more than one cause and more than one purpose. Behavior often functions to protect clients' views of themselves. It is also an attempt to communicate with others and to meet needs. Behavior is not an isolated event; rather it is influenced by the past, present, and future and is logical according to the person's perception of reality.

People have a need for positive self-regard and positive regard from others. Behavior often functions in a way that meets this need. People who have a low level of self-acceptance often rely heavily on others to approve of them. Thus, much of their behavior centers around doing things to please others in an attempt to earn approval. Passive, overcompliant behavior or gift giving may be a seeking of approval from the nursing staff. Nonaccepting, complaining persons may be hypercritical of others to direct attention away from themselves, or they may blame others in an effort to feel better about themselves.

People who have a high level of self-acceptance are less fearful of being themselves and are more open to sharing with others. They view themselves as liked and accepted, capable and worthy, and they behave in ways that support this view. They accept responsibility for themselves and are less defensive toward and more accepting of others.

Behavior, then, reflects one's self-concept and is an attempt to protect and strengthen it. When people behave in ways that do not match their self-concept, they sometimes negate the behavior with statements such as "That really isn't like me to do that" or "That wasn't very nice of me." Thus, self-concept not only models behavior, it also judges and makes value statements about behavior.

Despite the level of self-acceptance, hospitalized people experience an increased dependence on staff and family. The severity of the illness determines the degree of the dependency. The hospital environment contributes to this loss of independence when people's clothes are taken away and they are asked to go to bed. Interacting with strangers while in bed and in pajamas certainly places clients in a less powerful position.

> *When Jane was admitted to a medical-surgical unit for a minor procedure she brought several jogging suits with her, which she wore during the day and evening. She said that she felt less vulnerable, less like a dependent patient, and more able to be assertive in her treatment plan when dressed in her own clothes.*

The hospital environment is highly structured and not individualized for clients. Routine and regulations dictate when one eats, sleeps, bathes, and receives visitors. Clients are not considered in the scheduling of treatments or diagnostic tests nor are they encouraged to take an active role in the treatment plan. Clients must accept strangers doing things to them and rely on strangers to meet their basic needs. This increased dependency, enforced by both the environment and the illness, leads to feelings of powerlessness. This may be accompanied by an unspoken fear that there will be a prolonged or lasting loss of independence. To minimize the loss of independence, nurses need to individualize routines as much as possible: favor alternative dress when practical, liberalize visiting hours, encourage clients who are able to visit the lobby and gift shop to do so, and in general provide options that enable clients to maintain as much autonomy as possible.

All the previously described behavior is meaningful in the context of how persons view their internal and external world, which then determines reality for each person. Reality is relative and is influenced by one's past experiences, present situation, and future expectations. Different perceptions of reality contribute to different behaviors in coping and adapting.

> *John, age 50, was admitted to coronary intensive care with his second myocardial infarction within 12 months. He and the staff remember each other, and relationships are quickly reestablished. John's family history has a high incidence of heart disease with no close male relatives living beyond the age of 55. His life pattern was one of a high-stress job, heavy smoking, and minimal exercise. He has always expected to die at a young age. Even before his first cardiac episode he put his affairs in order by writing a will and preparing his family as much as possible. He appears sad but calm and makes statements that indicate he is resigned to his fate.*

> *Betty, age 48, was admitted to coronary intensive care with her first myocardial infarction. She has never been hospitalized before and is overwhelmed by the equipment and the intense emotional tone of the unit. Hers is a family history of longevity with only one cousin having heart disease. Betty has consciously developed a healthy lifestyle in terms of nutrition, exercise, and stress-management techniques. She has always expected to live to an old age. Betty is now angry with both the staff and her family. She is bitter because she took care of herself and feels this "shouldn't have happened." Her anger interferes with her ability to cooperate with the treatment plan.*

Remembering that each person's response to illness is unique helps nurses understand the meaning of each person's behavior. One client may frequently use the call light because of a fear of dying and a need to know that the staff will prevent this by responding to the call for help. Another client, believing the nursing staff is inadequate or does not care what happens to clients, may frequently use the call light out of a sense of frustration. Still another client may be so lonely that the call light is used to achieve human contact. All behavior is an attempt to communicate, so nurses must be alert to cues about the meaning of the behavior to achieve an accurate client assessment.

Analysis of Clients' Affective Responses to Illness

There is a wide range of affective responses when people become ill and are hospitalized. The type of illness and the implications of a disease process are factors in how people respond. Nurses can expect the response to an acute, temporary illness to be different from the response to a chronic or terminal disease. Clients' expectations of what will occur in the hospital will affect their emotional responses to the experience. Past experiences influence current expectations. Some clients have had positive past experiences with nurses and physicians; they have found relief for pain or cure for disease. Other clients, finding no such relief or no such cure, have had negative past experiences. When expectations and reality match, clients experience less distress than when expectations are shattered by reality.

Illness and hospitalization are stressful events and place demands on clients' abilities to cope and adapt to the situation. Initially, people do not develop new coping behavior; rather, they rely on familiar patterns to cope with stress. These patterns may be exaggerated until either the stress disappears or more effective patterns are learned.

> *Susan's main coping behavior for work stress is to "intellectualize." When she is hospitalized, she seeks out information from all members of the health care team, reads about her medical diagnosis, asks for her family's opinion, and attempts to make informed decisions.*

> *Mike's main coping behavior for work stress is to become more dependent on his boss, letting her set the priorities for getting the work accomplished. When Mike is hospitalized, he relies on the nurse and the physician to make the decisions about the treatment plan. He becomes fearful if his family disagrees in any way with the professional staff.*

To assess the client's affective responses to illness and hospitalization, communication must allow both client and nurse to share their expectations of each other. The symbolic meaning of hospitalization, which influences the client's expectations, is formed by the client's past experiences of the hospital. These experiences may include pain, separation from loved ones, the death of others, or the shame of dependence. The client's past experiences and current expectations need to be taken into consideration when assessing affective responses to illness (Robinson, 1984).

Anxiety **Anxiety**, an emotion commonly felt during illness, occurs in response to the fear of being hurt or losing something valued. People become anxious when there is a threat to self-esteem, value systems, body image, or life itself. Anxiety alerts people to possible dangers and warns them of their vulnerability. It provides energy to remove or deal with the threat of hurt or loss. (See Chapter 8 for a more in-depth discussion of anxiety.)

Many clients are uncomfortable in sharing feelings of anxiety with nurses, dreading perhaps that they will be judged inadequate or childlike. When feelings of anxiety are not discussed, clients may try to deny the feeling or use other defenses to cope with it, such as somatic symptoms or demanding behavior. Anxiety is often accompanied by regressive behavior, including crying, constantly asking questions, misinterpreting information, or increased dependency (Robinson, 1984).

Helplessness and Hopelessness Closely related to the feeling of anxiety is the feeling of **helplessness**, which clients often experience. The emotional response of helplessness may be a coping response learned in the past or it may be an immediate response to a new situation. Hospitalized persons may feel helpless because of loss (of independence, income, job, self-esteem), change (in body image), or fear (of the disorder not being controlled). To intervene therapeutically, it is critical that nurses understand how clients perceive themselves and their situations. The feeling of **hopelessness** often accompanies helpless feelings. Clients experience hopelessness when they perceive no end to suffering, are presented with a chronic or terminal diagnosis, or are in the midst of a depressive reaction.

Guilt **Guilt** is another common affective response to illness. Nurses hear many statements relating to guilt such as "If I had only . . . " and "If I had only not. . . . " Much of this guilt is about past behaviors that clients believe have contributed to their disorder or disease. Behaviors such as smoking, drinking, drug usage, overeating, overworking, lack of exercise, or escalating conflict with family members are commonly bemoaned. The feeling of guilt may be related to the client's philosophy of suffering. If the person believes suffering is a punishment, there will be a search for wrongdoing. If the belief is that suffering is an intrusion of evil, the client may feel personally responsible and therefore guilty. Guilt may also arise from feelings of responsibility for other family members. Having the well partner assume added household responsibilities, alter work activities whether inside or outside the home, or deal with the financial burdens brought on by the illness can all cause a client to feel guilty. If there are children in the home, the client may feel guilty for relinquishing the parenting role. Unresolved guilt places clients at a higher risk for a depressive reaction.

Loneliness Still another common feeling that clients experience when hospitalized is **loneliness**. Clients are separated from their loved ones at a time when emotional support is most needed. The security of family is replaced with the uncertainty of strangers, and the shelter of the home is traded for the helter-skelter of the hospital. The familiar business of life is sacrificed to the unfamiliar routine of the institution. Many aspects of life that allow people to feel connected to one another are altered by hospitalization. An added burden occurs when clients fear expressing their loneliness and need for security to nurses. Adult clients may regard these as childish feelings and try to deny them. When this occurs, clients may make many requests of nurses to increase contact and feel reassured and safe. Other clients may fear expressing their needs for security because they believe nurses are too busy to have time to spend with them. These clients may become apathetic or seemingly indifferent to other people and the environment.

Anger Clients often experience **anger** when ill and hospitalized. The feeling of anger is a response to a threat, a hurt, or a loss. Thus, clients feel angry when they experience a sense of helplessness or powerlessness; when they are afraid; when their needs are not met; or when they are threatened with pain, loss of body parts, or death. Nurses recognize that anger, if it is not denied or suppressed, can motivate clients toward improvement or recovery. Nurses accept the client's right to be angry, create opportunities for verbalizing the feeling, and continue to care for and support the angry client (Robinson, 1984).

Hostility **Hostility** is different from anger in that it is destructive in intent. Often expressed to anyone who happens to be available, hostility may be acted out in a way harmful to both the hostile person and the recipient of the hostility. Nurses need to assess clients' possible sources of hostility. Some hostility arises out of a low self-esteem. If one does not like oneself, it is difficult to imagine others would have a different opinion. These persons, assuming others do not like them, then respond with hostile feelings. Hostility may be a response to a perceived threat from the environment. It may be a coping response to fear and anxiety, in that hostility can block these feelings from conscious awareness. Hostility may also be used as a defense to blame others for the situation rather than to accept painful responsibility. People fearful of revealing themselves to others may use hostility as a way of keeping them at a distance. To intervene appropriately, nurses must accurately assess the source and meaning of clients' hostility (Robinson, 1984).

Interpretation of Clients' Cognitive Responses to Illness

Cognitive responses to illness are influenced by self-concept, self-esteem, and self-acceptance. A person's **self-concept** is an organized set of thoughts about characteristics of the "I" or "me," that is, the person's self. Self-concept includes beliefs about the type of person one is (intrapersonal), how one relates to others (interpersonal), and one's significance in the family and the world at large (sociocultural). **Self-esteem**, the affective portion of the self, includes one's feelings and values of self, such as strength, courage, peacefulness, worth, and confidence. Each person also has an image of the ideal self, which is usually better than the perceived or actual self. **Self-acceptance** is the extent to which a person's self-concept is congruent with the ideal self. The larger the discrepancy between self-concept and ideal self, the less a person is able to accept or like oneself.

Illness and suffering affect self-concept, self-esteem, and self-acceptance. Hospitalization often makes clients vulnerable to thoughts of inadequacy and incompetency. They begin to doubt their worth, both to themselves and to others. The discrepancy between self-concept and ideal self increases with the decrease in self-acceptance.

Locus of Control The degree to which people believe that life events are under personal control is referred to as **locus of control.** People who have an **internal locus of control** assume responsibility for what occurs and believe outcomes are principally the results of their own actions. These people have a sense of being in control of their environments and lives. People who have an **external locus of control** are focused not on themselves but on others in the environment. They believe fate, luck, or more powerful people determine life events. People with an external locus of control feel helpless in assuming responsibility for change.

People tend to behave in ways that match their expectations. Clients with internal loci of control will be able to focus attention on themselves and the problems they face. They are able to use the problem-solving process. Clients with external loci of control identify the sources of their problems as being outside themselves. Potential solutions are thus also outside the client's control. Third-person pronouns such as *he* and *they* are used more frequently than the first-person pronoun *I*. In the face of their helplessness, it is more difficult for these people to use the problem-solving process.

Ambivalence Illness often results in **ambivalence**, or simultaneous conflicting attitudes. Initially, there may be ambivalence about seeking help from professionals: "I don't feel too sick, so maybe I will just wait it out. On the other hand, I could have something serious. Better treat it immediately." Or, "I really can't afford to go to the doctor. But if I really am sick, I could lose a lot of money if I can't work." And once health care is sought, many people are ambivalent about following the health care recommendations: "She said I have to take a week off from work. I'm so tired and that sounds great. But I have so much work to do, and it will simply pile up if I take a week off." Or: "I know I have to stop smoking. My breathing is never going to get better if I don't. But I enjoy smoking, and I can't face the thought of withdrawal."

Questioning **Questioning** is another cognitive response to illness. Clients often ask "Why me?" "What have I done to deserve this?" or "Why can't I get better?" Searching for meaning by examining the past is an attempt to gain control of the present and give direction to the future. Clients ask professionals if the medical diagnosis is incorrect and if the treatment plan is the best available option. Clients question family and friends about their commitment, love, and concern. The answers that clients give to themselves are closely related to their philosophy of suffering and their self-concept and self-acceptance (Musil and Abraham, 1986).

Denial Another cognitive response to illness is **denial**, a defense mechanism that decreases the immediate anxiety aroused when people become ill. A period of denial is often adaptive in that the person can conserve psychological and physical energy that would otherwise be spent in an anxiety reaction. When clients are unable to give up the defense of denial, serious problems may result that will interfere with movement toward health and wellness.

Respect For Clients' Spiritual Responses to Illness

Gaining **spirituality** is both an intrapersonal and interpersonal process. The individual component is the development of values and beliefs about the meaning and purpose of life, death, and what occurs after death. The interpersonal or relational component is the feeling of connectedness with others and with an external power often identified as God. Spirituality involves loving, trusting, and forgiving one's self and others as well as the ability to receive love, trust, and forgiveness from others and God. The result for many people is a sense of wholeness, integrity, and tranquillity.

Spiritual distress may occur during a time of illness. For some, this distress may be expressed as guilt over past behaviors or a feeling of injustice about their current situation. Others may focus on lack of fulfillment or an inability to find meaning and purpose in their lives. Feeling isolated and cut off from others is another source of spiritual distress for many people (Labun, 1988).

Recognition of Clients' Sociocultural Responses to Illness

In understanding clients' responses to illness, nurses assess the impact of illness on the family and the impact of the family on the member who is ill. Family interactions may be difficult for nurses to assess since each family uses specific behaviors in presenting themselves to others. These behaviors may be quite different from those the family uses when not being observed by outsiders. Only with the development of trust and rapport may nurses be allowed to view and assess the real family life.

Individual responses to illness are learned within a family and cultural context. It is within the family that the demands of the society and the family unit shape the person. Cultural norms are supported and modified by the family. Some families have an authoritarian structure with clear rules and regular time schedules. These families support traditions and do not publicly demonstrate feelings. Other families are more democratic, time schedules are modified more easily, change is more easily accepted, and the feelings of the members are more openly expressed. In still other families power is determined experimentally, and time schedules are irregular. These families encourage exploration and intuition, and feelings are passionately expressed.

Since most hospital structures are authoritarian, nurses could expect that clients who come from authoritarian families will adapt to hospitalization more readily than those who come from more democratic families. Regarding expression of feelings, the family and cultural norms are important for nurses to understand. Nurses should not consider clients inadequate when the cultural norm does not allow sharing feelings outside the family unit. Nor should nurses consider clients immature when they passionately share their feelings.

Illness and hospitalization of a family member is a crisis for the family unit. This disruption to the family can range from mild to severe and from temporary to permanent. Not only must the family continue with its day-to-day functioning, it must also handle the implications of the illness. Moreover, the family must tolerate and cope with the emotional responses of the member who is ill as well as with the responses of the other family members. Many stresses exist, such as the need to assume different roles; financial problems; and, if relatives move in to assist during the crisis, perhaps problems in adjusting to the new members. Some families, finding it difficult to share feelings about the experience, hesitate to ask for assistance from the nursing staff or social service department. Other families are more likely to seek answers and to request help in solving problems.

Understanding the sociocultural context will enable nurses to assess their clients more accurately and completely. When this is combined with behavioral, affective, and cognitive assessment, clients are assured of a holistic response from the nursing staff. The role of culture in nursing care is more fully discussed in Chapter 5.

Analysis of the Nurse-Client Relationship

The nurse-client relationship is the key factor throughout the nursing process. It is the means by which nurses are able to assess clients accurately, formulate nursing diagnoses, plan and implement nursing interventions, and evaluate the effectiveness of the nursing process. The therapeutic relationship is the primary instrument of change (Kasch, 1984). To facilitate change, nurses define and assess the nature of their relationships with clients from a holistic perspective.

The **physical component** of the nurse-client relationship includes all the procedures and technical skills that nurses do with or for clients. Cormack (1983) refers to the physical component as the high-visibility functions of nursing care. This technologic component of nursing education is easily defined and described for students. Successful students learn these skills and are well aware that omitting them can lead to a life-threatening state for clients. Students are praised and evaluated for tasks that can be observed, which reinforces the task orientation prevalent in the medical model of health care. Because more technologic knowledge is made available every day, it is vital that nurses continue to learn and practice their skills to ensure that the best possible physical care be provided.

The **emotional component** of the nurse-client relationship, which is as important as the physical component, involves the nurse responding to the client as one human being to another, rather than as health care provider and patient. Nurses should bring many qualities to these relationships: positive regard, a nonjudgmental attitude, acceptance, warmth, empathy, authenticity, congruity of verbal and nonverbal messages, and the ability to self-disclose. With the development of the emotional component, nurses encourage clients to share their thoughts on how they perceive the world, their past experiences and expectations, and their hopes and dreams for the future. Clients are also encouraged to share feelings such as fear, helplessness, hopelessness, guilt, loneliness, anger, joy, delight, or hopefulness. The emotional component of the nurse-client relationship Cormack (1983) calls low-visibility functions, which include such aptitudes as observing skills, analysis of psychodynamics, and verbal and nonverbal communication skills. To teach and learn these components of nursing care is more difficult because they are more abstract.

The **spiritual component** of the nurse-client relationship is the feeling of connectedness between the client and the nurse. It is that inner sense of being a part of something more than oneself. Nurses who are attuned to the spiritual component of the relationship respect clients' cultural values and religious views. They consider clients to be worthy and significant people and, when appropriate, help clients find meaning and purpose in life. When the spiritual component is neglected, clients and nurses alike can feel alienated, uninvolved, and isolated.

For the purpose of assessment, these three components are separated so that nurses can more accurately perceive their relationships with clients. In reality, all the components are interrelated and function as a unity. Nurses' physical care is not as effective if nurses and clients have no sense of being allied with each other or if there are restraints on the clients' thoughts and feelings. The essence of relationships is involvement. As summarized by Goldsborough (1969, p. 66): "Involvement essentially is caring deeply about what is happening and what might happen to a person, then doing something with and for that person. It is reaching out and touching and hearing the inner being of another."

The **power component** of the nurse-client relationship is related to the nurse's belief in locus of control. Nurses who reflect an external locus of control expect clients to give up control to the staff, who then do "to" and "for" clients with minimal client involvement. They allow clients to blame others for life's problems. These nurses may get trapped into feeling sorry for clients and will then commiserate with clients rather than focus on growth and change.

Nurses who believe in an internal locus of control redirect clients to devote energy and attention to themselves and their involvement in their problems. They do not regard clients as helpless, dependent people. They strongly emphasize clients' motivation and participation in developing more adaptive behaviors. The relationship is built around clients' needs to shape and control their own lives.

During the crisis of illness clients benefit from an internal locus of control that is balanced by a recognition that not everything is under personal control. The acknowledgment that some external force is involved enables many people to find meaning in life and utilize prayer or meditation for comfort and support (Moch, 1988).

With the consumer movement, clients are becoming more assertive of their right to self-determination. So, the client's status in the nurse-client relationship is changing from one of dependency to one of interdependency. The locus of control has shifted to the clients, with the nurses in supporting roles. This means that clients actively participate in the planning of their care and assume some responsibility for the outcomes of their treatment plans. The nursing process is done *with* them rather than *to* them. Nurses understand that clients have the ultimate power of accepting or rejecting proposed plans of care. This philosophy has led to the Patient's Bill of Rights, developed by the American Hospital Association in 1972. This bill of rights supports the internal locus of control in stating that clients have control over their bodies and the right to participate in any decision regarding their own care and treatment (Fenton, 1987).

In the past, nurses often made decisions for clients, based on the assumption that nurses knew what was best for clients. In reality, these decisions were often made to expedite functional nursing care. With the change in the nurse-client relationship to one of interdependency, nurses now present alternatives to clients and assist them with the problem-solving process. In assessing the nurse-client relationship, nurses determine how clients' rights are being maintained, how values are clarified, how information is given, and how decisions are supported. This active client role can only contribute to effective and sensitive nursing care.

Planning

As discussed earlier, caring is a way of relating to people that enables them to grow toward their full potential. Thus effective nursing interventions are implemented in a manner that recognizes the worth and dignity of people and considers the physical, emotional, social, and spiritual needs of clients.

Dealing with clients' needs can lead to feelings of discomfort or anxiety in nurses. Therefore both beginning and experienced nurses need support and supervision to maintain their effectiveness. Supervision is the process of having a teacher, head nurse, clinical specialist, or mentor evaluate one's clinical practice to increase one's knowledge and competency. It is an opportunity to share feelings about one's self and clients and to receive emotional support and guidance. Planning and implementation are more effective when clinical supervision is ongoing. Benfer (1985, p. 43) describes the need for supervision in this manner:

> A support system can best be provided through clinical supervision; the kind of clinical supervision that embraces an investigative approach toward understanding our interactions and behaviors in working with patients, as well as the human growth and development potential in each of us within our clinical work.

Characteristics of Effective Helpers

The ability to integrate the characteristics of effective helpers into nursing practice will increase growth and satisfaction for both clients and nurses. These several interpersonal qualities and skills are critical to the therapeutic relationship through which nursing interventions are implemented.

Positive Regard **Positive regard** is believing in the value and potential of the client. It is the affirmation of personhood and the process of dignifying and respecting the person (Rogers, 1967).

Some clients have minimal self-respect and great difficulty in valuing themselves. The nurse's positive regard is critical to reinforcing and strengthening the clients' self-worth.

In trying to understand behaviors that demonstrate positive regard it is helpful to first look at behaviors that deny it, such as arguing, mocking, or disagreeing with clients' feelings. These behaviors are an attempt to control or dominate clients. Denial of positive regard is also seen when nurses refuse to get involved with clients who have particular types of problems, thereby devaluing them by avoidance.

Many behaviors do communicate positive regard to clients, such as expressing concern for their feelings and protecting their self-esteem when it is threatened. Positive regard means focusing on clients' needs rather than on nurses' needs. It is faith in clients' abilities to solve problems and being considerate of and genuinely interested in them. It is expressing commitment to clients' growth and allowing them to grow in the direction they choose. Positive regard contributes to a safe, nonthreatening environment for clients.

Nonjudgmental Approach Another characteristic of effective nurses is a **nonjudgmental approach** to clients. It may be impossible for nurses to be completely nonjudgmental about clients. Cognitive judgments are made when nurses assess clients and formulate reasonable plans of care. Emotional judgments are evidenced by statements such as "I really like her" or "He frightens me." Clients are also judged within the social context of appropriate or inappropriate behavior. Spiritual judgments include moral approval or condemnation of another person.

A nonjudgmental approach to clients means that nurses are not harshly critical of them. To ensure this, nurses develop a keen sense of self-awareness to identify pejorative thoughts and feelings about particular clients. With this insight nurses can then avoid acting on negative judgments. Nonjudgmental nurses allow clients to talk about thoughts and feelings, and they respect clients as responsible people capable of making decisions and choices. It is a "being with" the client as described by Mayeroff in his book *On Caring* (1971, p. 43):

> When the other is with me, I feel I am not alone, I feel understood, not in some detached way but because I feel he knows what it is like to be me. I realize that he wants to see me as I am, *not in order to pass judgment on me, but to help me* [italics added]. I do not have to conceal myself by trying to appear better than I am; instead, I can open myself up for him, let him get close to me, and thereby make it easier for him to help me. Realizing that he is with me helps me to see myself and my world more truly, just as someone repeating my words may give me the opportunity really to listen to myself and have the meaning of my own words come home to me more completely.

Acceptance **Acceptance** of clients is another characteristic of effective nurses. Acceptance is an affirmation of persons as they are. Accepting nurses respect clients' thoughts and ideas and explore these to assist them in self-understanding. Acceptance is the recognition that clients have the right to free expression of feelings. As internal responses to one's perception of others and the environment, feelings are genuine and cannot be criticized, argued with, or denounced. To tell clients how they should or should not feel is to discount their past experiences, present state, and future potential. Often it is being uncomfortable with one's own feelings that leads to the discounting of others' feelings.

Unless it is detrimental to themselves or others, clients' behavior is accepted by effective nurses. Some behavior, such as masturbating in public, causes social embarrassment and discomfort to others and may later be a source of shame for the person. Clients are protected by being provided with private space and time for this normal human activity. Limits do need to be set on activities that will lead to the complete exhaustion of clients, and violence toward oneself or others can hardly be accepted.

In determining whether or not a behavior is acceptable, nurses must first assess the probable consequences of the behavior. If it is deemed to be detrimental to the client or others, a plan must be formulated for intervention. Remember that if a client is incapable of changing behavior or chooses not to change it, then physical force may be necessary. The following questions are asked in assessment: "Is this behavior detrimental, or is it rather just a source of irritation to me?" "Are the rules and regulations of the unit more important than the client's rights and dignity?" "Is this behavior dangerous enough to use physical force to stop it?" and "Am I willing and able to use physical force to change the behavior?" The following examples illustrate this process.

> *Maria is a nurse in the emergency department. She is assigned to a client, Tom, whom the police have picked up for drunk and disorderly behavior. He has been placed in a room that is designed to be safe for these types of clients. When Maria enters the room she finds Tom smoking a cigarette, which is against the rules of the department. When he ignores her requests to put out the cigarette, she attempts to take it away from him forcefully. Tom strikes out in anger, and Maria ends up with a facial cut needing sutures.*

> *Connie is a nurse on the psychiatric unit. She has been attempting to intervene with Roberta, a client who has become very angry with her roommate. When it is obvious that Roberta is getting out of control, Connie calls for help from other staff, and they quickly formulate a plan for intervention. As Roberta picks up a chair and threatens her roommate, three staff members surround her and firmly take the chair away from her. She is then escorted to the quiet room where two staff members remain with her until she has better control over her behavior.*

It is apparent that Maria attempted to enforce the rules of the department without asking herself the crucial questions. Since Tom was in a room by himself, there was no danger in his smoking a cigarette. Maria might have made the decision to remain with him while he finished his cigarette to prevent any accidents with the smoking material. But to use physical force to stop the behavior was inappropriate because the incident wasn't dangerous. If Maria was determined to stop Tom's behavior, she should have sought assistance and thought of a plan to accomplish this outcome. In contrast, Connie identified that Roberta's behavior was unacceptable because there was the danger of her roommate's being injured. A plan was formulated and implemented so that no one on the unit was injured, and Roberta was given the opportunity to talk about the feelings underlying her unacceptable behavior.

Warmth Another characteristic of effective nurses is **warmth**, the manner in which concern for and interest in clients is expressed. This does not mean that nurses should be effusive with clients or attempt to be their buddies. Warmth is primarily expressed nonverbally, by a positive demeanor, a friendly tone, or an engaging smile. Simply leaning forward and establishing eye contact is an expression of warmth, as is physical touch so long as this is acceptable and not frightening to the client.

Empathy Much has been written about **empathy** as a necessary characteristic of effective nursing. Empathy is the ability to see another's perception of the world. It is understanding how clients see themselves and the significance they give to life events. It is learning about their feelings, what they are striving to become, and what they need to grow and change. Throughout this process nurses must retain their own identities and remain objective. This means seeing clients' worlds but not experiencing the same reactions to these worlds. If nurses experience the same feelings they will be less effective in assisting clients toward growth. Nurses do not have to be angry to realize that clients are angry. They must, however, be able to explore feelings of anger with their clients.

Forsyth (1980) has described two conditions necessary for empathy to occur. The first of these is *consciousness* of oneself, of the client, and of the experiences of both. Nurses aware of their own values, attitudes, and reactions are less judgmental of clients and less likely to project their own attitudes and expectations onto them. The second condition is *temporality,* which refers to the ability to deal with clients' feelings immediately, not at nurses' leisure or when they feel more comfortable or secure. Empathy occurs where careful listening and responding occur.

Nurses must show they are trying to understand clients as well as possible. After careful consideration of the meaning of what clients are communicating and the feelings being expressed, nurses must validate this understanding with clients. Empathy occurs only *if nurses are able to communicate their understanding verbally so that clients are able to validate or correct nurses' perceptions.*

The accuracy of empathic interchanges must be evaluated by both nurses and clients if the relationships are to be effective. Accurate empathy can facilitate therapeutic collaboration and assist clients to experience and understand themselves more fully (Book, 1988; Marcia, 1987).

Authenticity Effective nursing care relies on nurses' **authenticity**, that is, on their being genuinely and naturally themselves in therapeutic relationships. When nurses make a commitment to clients they take on a professional role. This is different from "playing" the professional role, which makes a pretense of helping clients. When nurses are more concerned about how they appear than what they are and do, they erect a facade of helping and are incapable of being authentic with clients, peers, and supervisors.

Congruency Nurses are genuine when their verbal and nonverbal behavior indicates **congruency.** Clients can quickly sense when nurses are incongruent, or saying one thing verbally and another thing nonverbally. Congruency is necessary for clients to develop trust in nurses.

It is Steve's first day on the psychiatric unit as a nursing student. He is in the day room interacting with a group of clients and two other students. He appears tense with his upright body posture, clenched hands, and swinging foot. His voice is pitched higher than normal. One of the clients jokingly says to him, "What's the matter? Are you afraid of us crazies?" Steve quickly replies, "No, I'm not afraid. I like being here." The clients respond to him with looks of disbelief and change their focus to the other two students. Steve seeks out his instructor for assistance with this problem. The two of them discuss how his verbal and nonverbal communication did not match and the effect this had on the clients. Several weeks later, Steve finds himself becoming increasingly frustrated with a client who has consistently refused to participate in any unit activities. This time he is able to be congruent and express his frustration directly to the client rather than trying to cover up his feelings.

Patience It is vital that nurses have **patience** with clients to give them the opportunity to grow and develop. Patience is not a passive waiting but an active listening and responding to the client. Patience, which can allow clients to grow according to their timetables, not nurses' timetables, gives clients room to feel and think and plan what changes need to be made. Patience also allows clients to resolve uncertainties and deal with some of the discomfort that inevitably accompanies change and growth. Effective nurses are also patient with themselves. They look for opportunities to develop self-awareness and to gain new knowledge. Moreover, they recognize that professional competence is not simply a goal; it is a long-term process of learning and developing as a nurse.

Respect **Respect** for clients is another characteristic of effective nurses. Respect includes consideration for clients and confidence in their abilities to solve their own problems. Clients are referred to and called by the name they prefer, and it means the nurse-client relationship does not become a dependent, parent-child relationship.

Trustworthiness Still another characteristic of effective nurses, and one that all the preceding characteristics build toward, is **trustworthiness.** Nurses with good interpersonal skills help clients to attach emotionally to them, which in turn helps develop trust in them. This therapeutic attachment is facilitated through the nursing process (Mooney, 1976). Trustworthy nurses are dependable and responsible. They adhere to time commitments, keep promises, and are consistent in their attitudes. Clients learn that these nurses can be relied on. Trust is also built when nurses demonstrate their willingness to continue working with clients who show little progress.

Trustworthy nurses respect the confidentiality of the nurse-client relationship. Clients need to have their privacy protected since there continues to be a stigma to mental illness and psychiatric admission to the hospital. Nurses must reassure clients that information does not go beyond the health care team. Often, nurses and clients live in the same community, so clients fear that people outside the hospital will learn of their admission from the staff. To decrease this fear, nurses must stress the issue of confidentiality. In one survey on clients' views of confidentiality, "77% said that it was important to them that the hospital staff not tell anyone else what they revealed about themselves" and "80% said knowing that their communications would be kept confidential improved their relationship with the staff" (Schnid et al., 1983, p. 355).

Distrust may develop when clients do not have access to the information written about them in their charts. Clients have the right to read their records, which protects them by making sure that all viewpoints, including theirs, are represented. Sharing nursing notes can be beneficial in that further discussion can develop from the nurses' initial observations and interpretations.

Good interpersonal skills are the basis for a trusting relationship. As clients learn to trust nurses, they become more open to the opportunities to grow and develop. As summarized by Mayeroff (1971, p. 45): "If another person is to grow through my caring, he must trust me, for only then will he open himself to me and let me reach him. Without trust in me he will be defensive and closed."

Self-Disclosure Trust develops when nurses offer appropriate **self-disclosure**. Frequently, to create trust and openness, beginning students believe they should be no more than passive, nonjudgmental listeners. Trust and openness, however, cannot be achieved by nurses who withhold their thoughts and feelings. Only when relationships are mutual and active can real progress be made. Appropriate self-disclosure is always goal-directed and determined by clients', not nurses', needs. Nurses frequently ask clients to talk about their feelings as a therapeutic intervention. For clients who have minimal interpersonal skills, however, it is equally important to teach them how to perceive other people's feelings and to validate this perception. Through self-disclosure by nurses, clients can improve their interpersonal relationships. For clients, self-disclosure can lead to further self-exploration: Clients are often reassured that their feelings are real and human and are shared by others.

> *Berta, a nursing student, is in the termination phase of her relationship with Jim. Jim has been having difficulty in discussing his feelings about the impending separation. Berta uses self-disclosure as an intervention to help Jim articulate his feelings. She begins by saying, "You know, Jim, it is painful for me to say good-bye to you. We have worked very intensely together, and I have grown through this experience. I have learned how to listen more intently, and I am a better nurse from having worked with you. I feel sad when I have to say good-bye to someone I care about. I will miss our 2 o'clock time together." With Berta's self-disclosure, Jim is able to share his pain regarding the termination of the relationship.*

Humor **Humor** is a useful tool in effective nurse-client relationships. Some nurses erroneously consider humor to be "unprofessional." But healthful humor must be distinguished from harmful humor. Harmful humor ridicules other people; it laughs *at* them. This type of humor singles out and excludes persons from the group. Humor is potentially harmful if it is used to avoid resolving genuine problems. Healthful humor, on the other hand, is a way to elicit laughter between people. It occurs when one laughs *with* other people, and it does not exclude anyone. Healthful humor is appropriate to the situation and protects the person's dignity. A good sense of humor is a mature coping mechanism and can help people adapt in difficult situations (Osterlund, 1983).

Humor is a way to create and invite laughter. Vigorous laughing has healthful physiological effects on people. Laughter stimulates the respiratory system and increases blood oxygen levels, as well as increasing heart rate and improving circulation. A resulting increase in epinephrine levels contributes to a sense of well-being and alertness. Laughter stimulates the internal organs by "massaging" the abdomen. Muscular tension is decreased, as evidenced by the inability to carry a heavy object while boisterously laughing. All these changes have a euphoric effect on the person laughing (Merwin and Smith-Kurtz, 1988).

The psychological benefits of humor and laughter are many. Humor decreases anxiety and fear. It diffuses negative emotions, which the person cannot experience when laughing, and decreases stress and tension. In the highly structured hospital environment, humor offers some relief from the routine and lessens boredom. Humor may also be a safety valve for the energy generated by anger. Laughter helps regulate the intensity of emotion and decreases defensive behavior. If clients are able to look at an irritating situation and laugh rather than explode in anger, the energy is discharged in an adaptive manner. With the decrease in the intensity of the anger, clients can resolve the situation more effectively. Humor can also help change one's perspective. Objectivity is increased when people can look at themselves in a humorous manner. With the passage of time, a situation that was a source of pain can become a source of pleasure (Ferguson and Campinha-Bacote, 1989; Simon, 1988).

Humor and laughter affect the dynamics of a group of people. Since laughter is reciprocal, it increases the equality of nurse-client relationships. It is a way to establish bonds between nurses and clients, and it increases both participants' comfort in the relationship. Laughter is an invitation for people to come together. It forms bonds between people, increases interest in one another, decreases loneliness, and strengthens the cohesiveness of the group.

Clients' senses of humor may be a diagnostic cue for nurses. Changes in clients' patterns of laughter may indicate other difficulties in adaptation. Depressed clients retain a cognitive sense of humor, but they receive no pleasure and are unable to laugh. Manic clients find everything funny; however, because of lack of judgment, this can turn into sarcastic wit and be potentially harmful to others. Suspicious clients are unable to laugh about their situations and are so frightened that they view humor as evidence of a personal attack. When one tells a joke to obsessive-compulsive people, it is often taken as a serious remark. These people focus on the joke and try to explain it in great detail. The influence of alcohol, marijuana, or other drugs may decrease people's inhibitions so that nearly all stimuli in the environment appear funny. In assessing clients, it is appropriate to ask "What is your favorite joke?" Responses to this question give nurses an indication of clients' sense of humor. Nurses should also ask clients how frequently they laugh and if there has been any change in their laughter behavior. This assessment data will give nurses a more holistic view of clients.

Humor may also be used as a purposeful nursing intervention. Nurses can teach the benefits of laughter to clients, reminding them of the difference between healthful and harmful humor. Laughter groups can be started on hospital units where clients and staff bring jokes or watch funny videotapes together. Reruns of "Candid Camera" or Marx Brothers films are examples of material that has been used therapeutically (Cousins, 1983). Nurses could wear buttons imprinted with "Warning: Humor May Be Hazardous To Your Illness" as an invitation to clients to use the healing potential of humor.

Formal recreational activities and informal play are purposeful interventions that can encourage humor. Because noncompetitive play is fun and since it promotes social participation and interaction with others, it can strengthen clients' self-confidence and often improve contact with reality (Jack, 1987).

The skillful use of humor, formal recreation, and play as nursing interventions results in a more relaxed atmosphere and more flexible interactions with others. It may be a source of insight into conflicts and facilitate expression of feelings in a safe way. Humor is not the ultimate cure for emotional problems, but it often increases coping by enhancing insight, problem solving, and energy.

These characteristics of effective helpers—positive regard, nonjudgmental approach, acceptance, warmth, empathy, authenticity, congruency, patience, respect, trustworthiness, self-disclosure, humor—are part of the nursing process and facilitate the implementation of the plan of care. Only within the context of the nursing process are they conducive to clients' growth. Used in isolation from assessment, diagnosis, and planning, they become characteristics of a social rather than a professional relationship.

Communication

Communication is a key factor in the planning and implementation of nursing care. The purpose of communication is twofold: (1) to give and receive information and (2) to achieve interpersonal contact. To be effective, communication must be goal-directed. Communication skills include active listening, perceiving, verbal and nonverbal responding, validating, and problem solving.

To understand clients' experiences, nurses must listen to both overt and covert messages being given. **Overt messages** are conveyed by the words spoken and are heard in the context of clients' affective states. Voice intonation, body posture, and facial expression convey **covert messages.** An overt question like "What time are visiting hours?" may have different meanings depending on the covert messages that accompany it. It may be a simple request for information. If those words are said angrily in a loud tone of voice or if body posture is visibly tense, clients may be attempting to assume some degree of control in an environment in which they feel uncomfortably dependent. If those same words are said in a frightened tone of voice or if the eyes are dilated and the body quivering, clients may be terrified at being separated from loved ones and forced to interact with strangers. Problems may be caused not from a lack of technical communication skills but from an insensitivity to covert messages.

Nurses for whom listening and understanding are more important than verbalizing generally experience the most productive, satisfying interactions. A common concern of nursing students is "What am I going to say next, and what is the client going to say then?" Beginning students frequently focus on trying to say the "right thing" or use the "right technique" and so may appear either distant or oversupportive. More beneficial to clients is that students be themselves without pretense or falsification. As students become more comfortable with communication skills, saying the right thing becomes an issue secondary to listening and understanding.

Nurses must be aware of the pitfalls of being polite listeners. Often seen in social interactions, the pattern—in which polite listeners go through the motions of listening without truly hearing or understanding—can extend to nurse-client interactions. This may occur if students fear being regarded as inadequate or unintelligent. Polite listening happens when people are more interested in talking than in listening or when they are bored or impatient.

Nurses frequently assume that the majority of their communication has been listened to and understood by clients. Feelings such as anxiety or anger may interfere with clients' abilities to listen. The question "Has the client listened to and understood what I have said?" needs to be continually asked. When nurses suspect that clients have not understood what has been said, they can ask questions such as "Could you tell me what you heard me saying?" or "I'm not sure I said that very clearly. What did you hear?" to assess clients' comprehension.

Nurses are taught to ask many questions during the history taking and assessment process (see Chapter 2). When this continues into the implementation phase, difficulties will usually develop. The nurse and client become simply questioner and questionee. The relationship becomes unequal because the questioner has the power to determine the course of the interaction. There is the tacit understanding that the questioner is the authority figure and the questionee must be submissive. A clue that too many questions are being asked is when clients give short answers or seldom take the initiative during interactions.

One of the most difficult aspects of communication is periods of silence. Students often feel uncomfortable with silence because of a belief that they should always have something therapeutic to say. With silent clients, the tendency among anxious students is to be excessively verbal. Silence has many meanings. Among them are

- I am too tired to talk right now.
- I don't want to talk to you.
- I'm lost and don't know what to say next.
- I don't know where this discussion is going.
- I would like to think about what was just said.
- I'm comfortable just being with you and not talking.

To respond appropriately, the nurse must understand the client's silence. An observation such as "I've noticed that you have become very quiet. Could you tell me something about that quietness?" may encourage clients to share more.

Verbose clients may also pose problems for students. Students tend to be verbal with silent clients, but they tend to be passive with verbose ones. Students may be reluctant to interrupt either because they fear being thought disrespectful or because they feel inadequate in the face of such unrelenting talk. There may also be a sense of relief that at last clients are finally talking to them. Some students mistakenly interpret clients' incessant verbalizing as evidence that the interactions are therapeutic. The more experienced nurse will not remain passive with verbose clients. It is difficult to understand nonstop talk for more than 30 seconds. Moreover, interrupting a verbose client allows the nurse to focus on the concerns being expressed and to convey a sense of involvement with the client's problems. Helpful interruptions are

- "You are bringing up a number of concerns. Could we discuss them one at a time?"
- "Let me interrupt you for a minute to make certain I understand what you are saying."
- "I don't want to stop you, but I need you to slow down so that I can understand better."

Effective communication will produce more satisfying nurse-client interactions and relationships. (See Chapter 2 for a discussion of communication skills.) It is within the context of the relationship that planned nursing interventions are implemented with clients and changes are made toward a healthier, more adaptive life.

Nursing Roles

Roles are patterns of behavior appropriate to particular situations and people. Roles do not exist in isolation but rather take on meaning within an interpersonal context. Within the nursing process, multiple roles are used to help clients grow and change. The roles to use at any particular time are decided on the basis of the planned interventions. Within the variety of roles, nurses must strive for an overall consistency of behavior, which is especially helpful in promoting clients' growth.

> *Devin, a nursing student, has defined his relationship with Tania, a client, as a cooperative venture toward solving the problems that brought her into the hospital. During some of the interactions, they sit in the TV room on the couch, which defines an equal relationship. Other interactions take place in the unit's classroom where Devin sits behind the desk, which defines an unequal relationship. Devin is also inconsistent in that at times he tells Tania what problem they should work on, whereas at other times he has no goals in mind and expects Tania to make the decision. Because of these confused messages about Devin's role within the relationship, Tania's potential for growth is limited.*

> *Carlos, a nursing student, has defined his relationship with Marge, a client, as a cooperative venture toward her growth. Carlos makes certain they are always sitting facing each other with no physical obstacles between them. He consistently encourages Marge to take responsibility and initiative in deciding the topic for the interaction. He openly develops and shares his written plan of care with her, which they evaluate and modify together. Because his be-*

havior is congruent with his definition of his role within the relationship, Marge has a greater potential to realize change in her life.

Professional Role Within the nurse-client relationship, nurses must function in a **professional role** rather than in a social role with clients. Social roles are reciprocal in that both participants expect their individual needs to be met as fully as possible. The professional role, on the other hand, exists for clients, and the focus is on clients' needs. To decrease the potential for unhealthy dependency, nurses consciously attempt to not meet all needs. In the professional role, the nurse and client work together as a team; they form a therapeutic alliance, the goal of which is to assist clients' growth and adaptation.

Socializing Agent Nurses function as **socializing agents** with the client population. On a one-to-one basis, they focus on deficiencies clients may have in communicating thoughts and feelings to others. This social skill is then extended by individual clients to groups of peers on the unit. By participating in informal groups, nurses are able to evaluate clients' growth in social skills. Socializing helps to model appropriate group behavior. Informal conversations give clients the opportunity to discuss nonstressful topics and provide some relief from anxiety.

Teacher Another nursing role is that of **teacher.** A nurse teaches the client about relevant medical problems, the impact they have on the client's mental illness, and how the illness affects the medical problems. A great deal of teaching occurs in regard to the treatment plan. This teaching increases clients' control and decreases their fears by predicting what is likely to occur. Nurses explain the types of therapies available in the facility, what they are like, and the benefits derived from participating in them. Clients also need to be taught about the medications they are receiving. Specific information is given about the medication's purpose, its expected therapeutic effect, how long before the client will notice a change, and its usual side effects. Clients need to be told about any dietary or activity restrictions related to medications, as well as what to do if they forget to take a dose. Furthermore, nurses must instruct clients about any related blood work or situations in which the client should notify the physician immediately. In addition to oral instruction, written material must be provided as a reference.

Depending on client assessment, nurses may also be involved in teaching ADLs. Some clients may need to learn basic cooking, laundry, or shopping skills to be able to live independently. Those who have no diversions or hobbies may need assistance in selecting appropriate activities and in learning the skills associated with them.

Model Nurses can teach clients how to achieve the desired changes that have been identified. Not only do they teach more adaptive behavior directly but they also serve as **models** for clients. People learn by imitating attitudes, beliefs, and behavior. Modeling allows clients to observe and to experience alternative patterns of behavior. It assists clients in clarifying values and communicating openly and congruently. Nurses are powerful models for clients and as such need to be sensitive to their degree of influence. Sensitivity will help ensure that nurses do not impose their own value systems on impressionable clients.

Advocate Nurses also act as **advocates** for clients. Advocate responsibilities include adapting the environment to meet individual client needs such as privacy and social interaction. Nurse advocates support flexible routines for the client population. Another advocacy skill is the use of a variety of communication techniques to reach clients in ways they can understand and to which they can respond. Nurse advocates serve as links between clients and other members of the health team (Robinson, 1984). As community members, nurses serve as advocates for all recipients of mental health care by striving to remove the stigma of mental illness.

Taylor (1985, p. 13) defined advocacy in nursing as the situation in which a nurse helps clients to "authentically exercise their responsibilities to themselves and others." In this view of advocacy, clients are allowed to express feelings without censure or criticism. They are encouraged to be active in the treatment process and to become independent. In working toward planned goals, clients and nurses share perceptions. As client advocates, nurses teach responsible behavior of one client toward another, and they protect those clients temporarily unable to protect themselves.

Kohnke (1982, p. 2) writes that "the role of the advocate is to *inform* the client and then to *support* him in whatever decision he makes." Clients have a right to their own beliefs and values. They choose the direction in which they want to grow, and decide how best to achieve their goals. Nurses take care neither to undermine this process nor to rescue clients from the outcomes of their decisions. Because this view of advocacy is based on clients' rights to make decisions and clients' responsibilities for the consequences of those decisions, advocates respect the decisions even when they disagree with them.

Counselor Another nursing role is that of **counselor**. This role, based as it is on knowledge, skills, and values, is dependent on the caring and competency of nurses. The counseling role is most typically enacted during regularly scheduled one-to-one sessions. In the first phase of the counseling role, a trusting relationship is established to ensure accurate assessment. This is followed by the second phase, one of planning, implementing, and evaluating. The counseling interaction is directed toward specific goals and based on the plan of care developed by both the client and the nurse. Nurse-counselors create opportunities for clients to talk about thoughts, feelings, and behaviors that affect themselves and others. Effective verbal and nonverbal communication is both modeled and practiced during the interactions. This is the time that a variety of interventions are implemented, evaluated, and modified. Clients are encouraged to use the problem-solving process to cope more effectively with identified problem areas. The efficacy of counseling is seen when clients exhibit improved coping skills, increased self-esteem, and greater insight into and understanding of themselves.

Role Playing Another method of assisting clients to achieve their goals is through **role playing**, in which a specific past or future situation is recreated and enacted as if it were occurring in the present. Although a client usually assumes his or her own role, at times he or she may take on the role of another involved person. Nurses assume roles of persons significant to the situation; they may also coach clients in developing new responses and behaviors. Role playing is an active process in which proposed behavioral changes are actually tried out and practiced.

Juanita hopes to find a job as a secretary after she is discharged from the hospital. She and her nurse, Carla, have been planning the necessary steps in achieving this goal. Since interviewing for the job frightens Juanita the most, they decide to role-play the interview, with Carla playing the role of the prospective employer.

CARLA: Good afternoon. Won't you have a seat?

JUANITA: Thank you.

CARLA: I see you have filled out all the necessary forms. Tell me a little about yourself.

JUANITA: Carla, help! What am I supposed to say?

CARLA (*as herself*): Think for a moment about other jobs you have had, how well you did and what good characteristics you are bringing to this situation.

JUANITA: OK. Well, I have had three years experience after high school as a secretary for an insurance agent. I did filing, typed correspondence, and handled most of the office routine. I quit when I had my baby one year ago, and I am now ready to return to work. I can take shorthand and type 60 words a minute. I am a very hard and conscientious worker and would like the opportunity to work for you.

Juanita and Carla continue acting out the interview process. Afterward, they evaluate what occurred, how Juanita felt during the process, and what changes Juanita should make. They then make plans to do more role playing on the following day and use that activity as the basis of a shared evaluation.

As role players, nurses create situations in which new behaviors can be practiced in a nonthreatening environment. Role playing can increase clients' self-confidence in coping with problematic interactions, which in turn can increase their desire to implement what they have learned in real-life situations. Role playing can also help clients express themselves directly, clarify feelings, act out fears, or become more assertive.

All nursing roles are interrelated as strategies to plan and implement the nursing care plan. When a variety of skills are used, it is more likely that the planned behavioral, affective, and cognitive changes will occur.

Nursing Goals

Nursing goals in the context of this chapter are guidelines to assist students in focusing on their roles in the psychiatric unit and on the skills they bring to the clinical setting. These are by no means comprehensive but rather serve as a starting point for effective nurse-client relationships. Nursing goals ought not to be confused with client goals, which are measurable changes in client behavior. Obviously, however, nursing goals and client goals should be mutual in an effective nurse-client relationship.

Common nursing goals include

- Helping clients cope
- Teaching clients the problem-solving process
- Assisting clients to socialize

Helping Clients Cope One goal of mental health nursing is to assist clients in coping with present problems. The stress is on the present because change is only possible in the here and now. The past and future are also important, but as perspectives on the present. Meanings attached to past events influence present perceptions, as do expectations of the future. However, it is in the present that one evaluates the past, anticipates the future, and changes behavior. Clients who brood over past problems and hurts without attending to the present are in danger of accepting the problems as permanent, with no hope for change. Clients who have dire future expectations and ignore the present potential for change are likely to find their expectations fulfilled.

The second aspect of this nursing goal is the client's definition of present problems. If the focus is on nurses' definitions and objectives only, little progress will be made. Clients are not likely to work on difficulties they consider unimportant. Nurses may need to help clients describe and specify problems when these have been stated in vague and uncertain terms. This is done by asking specifically what the problem is and for whom it is a problem. When the client talks in generalities, the nurse cannot assume the specifics but rather helps the client be more explicit about what occurs and who is involved. The next step is to ask about the onset of the problem and what contributes to its continuation. This step helps clients explore the significance of the situation, as well as helping them describe values and beliefs influencing their definition of the problem. At the end of the process, nurses and clients should agree on a concrete problem definition and state it in such a way that possible solutions are implied. (See Table 1–1 for the steps in problem identification.)

Teaching Clients to Solve Problems After problems have been specified and client goals established, the next nursing goal is to teach clients the problem-solving process. It is important to focus on one problem at a time and to measure progress by small changes that occur. Each of the client's problems is connected, so changes in one problem will cause changes in the others. It is helpful to remind clients that in the past they have done their best to deal with problems and that now new solutions may be found. This gives recognition to past attempts while proposing a need for new skills. The nurse's role is to listen, observe, encourage,

Table 1–1 *Steps in Problem Identification*

Client definition
How would you describe the problem?
For whom is this a problem? You? Family members? Employer? Community?
Significance of the problem
When did this problem begin?
What are the factors that cause this problem to continue?
Past and future influence
What past events have influenced the current problem?
What are your future expectations and hopes concerning this problem?
What is the most you hope for when this problem is resolved?
What is the least you will settle for to resolve this problem?
Concrete problem definition
Is there more than one problem here?
Which part of the overall problem is most important to deal with first?

and evaluate. More effective coping behavior is the ultimate result of the problem-solving process.

Throughout the problem-solving process it is extremely helpful to have clients keep a written list of all the ideas generated. Items on the list can then be added to, modified, or deleted as time goes on.

The problem-solving process consists of

1. Determining the solutions that have been attempted
2. Listing alternative solutions
3. Predicting the probable consequences of each alternative
4. Choosing the alternative to implement
5. Implementing the chosen alternative in a real-life or practice situation
6. Evaluating outcomes

The first step is to find out what solutions have been attempted thus far. The specifics of the attempts, how the attempts were implemented, and what occurred as a result all must be clarified. Since the problem continues to exist, these attempts were not effective solutions, so they need to be either modified or discarded.

The second step is to have the client list alternative ways of solving the problem. Frequently, the client is able to suggest only one or two ideas. Nurses can propose brainstorming sessions to increase creativity in problem solving. This means that all possible solutions, even those unrealistic or absurd, are written down. Thinking of absurd solutions often opens the mind to other creative, realistic solutions to the problem. Finally, after clients have listed all of their ideas for solving the problem, nurses can add their own suggestions.

The third step is predicting the probable consequences of each of the alternatives. After thoroughly discussing this, the nurse and client move to the fourth step: choosing which alternative to implement. Nurses should take care not to make this decision for clients—doing so would undermine the process by placing clients in a childlike, dependent position. Using action-oriented terms, the solution selected should be further developed, as concretely and specifically as possible. At the same time, specific, measurable outcomes are formulated that will be used in evaluating the process.

The fifth step occurs when clients implement the proposed solution in either a practice or a real situation. Clients must be allowed to make mistakes during this step. If they are rescued from mistakes, they will receive the message that they are incapable of taking charge of their lives.

Evaluation is the sixth step in the problem-solving process. Outcomes are reviewed, and a determination is made about the success or failure in achieving them. Successfully achieving an outcome means that the solution was effective and that it can continue to be implemented. Failing to achieve an outcome means that clients and nurses need to analyze how and in what way the solution was ineffective. This is followed by a return to step 4, where either a new solution is selected or the old solution is modified. (See Table 1–2 for an outline of these steps.)

As clients experience the steps of problem solving, they increase their skills, which then can be applied to other problematic areas of life. With an improved ability to make and assume responsibility for decisions, an internal locus of control evolves, leading to feelings of competency and self-worth in clients.

Table 1–2 *Steps in the Problem-Solving Process*

List attempted solutions
- What have you done to try to solve the problem thus far?
- How exactly did you do this?
- What happened when you tried this?

List alternatives
- What other ideas do you think you could try?
- What might be some absurd solutions to this problem?
- What else might be effective?
- Have you thought about . . . ?

Predict consequences
- What might happen if you tried the first idea?
- Is there anything else that might happen?
- What might happen if you tried the second idea (etc.)?

Choose the best alternative
- Which alternative seems like the best decision at this time?
- What specific behaviors are you going to try with this alternative?
- Specifically, how will things be different if you are successful?

Implement the alternative
- With whom are you going to attempt this solution?
- When are you going to practice this new behavior?
- Is there anything you need from me to help you try this out?

Evaluation
- What was the result of your attempted solution?
- Were your expectations met successfully?
- Is there anything that needs to be modified?
- If you were not successful, what other alternative idea from the list could you try?

The following example illustrates the problem-solving process in action with a nursing student and an instructor. The process is the same between clients and nurses. When clients are acutely ill and unable to think logically, the problem-solving process is not an appropriate intervention.

Sue, a nursing student, has made an appointment to see her instructor, Ann, concerning her low test score on her first exam in the course. Sue states that she knows the material and just freezes up when she takes exams.

ANN: Since this is not a new problem for you, what have you tried in the past to decrease your test anxiety?

SUE: I've tried to tell myself not to worry, because I know the material.

ANN: Has this worked for you?

SUE: No. I still get scared before a test.

ANN: Have you tried anything else?

SUE: No, I just study hard and then do poorly on tests.

ANN: What else have you considered trying?

SUE: Well, I've thought about asking other students what they do if they get anxious.

ANN: Anything else?

SUE: No. I can't think what to do.

ANN: Let's brainstorm some ideas. This means even thinking of absurd and unrealistic solutions to your problems as well as practical solutions. (*in a humorous tone of voice*) For example, you could get sick before every exam and never have to have one again. Or you could quit school.

SUE: (*getting into the spirit of brainstorming*) Or I could get a terminal illness, and my instructors would feel sorry for me and not make me take any more exams. (*pause*) Seriously though, I seem to remember that the counseling service has some sort of program about test-taking skills.

ANN: You're right. They offer a free six-week course on improving test scores. I think the first part of it deals with test anxiety. (*pause*) What do you think will happen if you try any of these solutions?

SUE: Well, I'm not going to get sick or quit school! I want to continue in the program. Since my problem is anxiety and not lack of knowledge, it sounds like the counseling center is my best bet.

ANN: How will you know if that is the right solution to your problem?

SUE: Well, I guess if after I have learned the techniques, I can take the next exam without freezing up and improve my test score.

ANN: How are you going to go about trying this solution?

SUE: I'm going over to the counseling center when I leave your office and sign up. I'm kind of excited about doing something positive for a change.

ANN: Is there any other way I can help you at this time?

SUE: No, you have been a big help listening to me and getting me started.

ANN: After you have tried the course at the counseling center, I would like to get together with you again so we can evaluate if that solution worked for you. Would you make another appointment to see me in a couple of weeks?

SUE: Sure will.

Socializing Still another nursing goal is to assist clients in socializing behavior. All people need to believe they are valued by and significant to others within their environment. Some clients will need assistance in becoming socially integrated, in the hospital setting as well as in the community, whereas others will need only support to maintain their level of social integration. Nurses and clients work together to evaluate interpersonal and social competence. Direct questions are asked about clients' network systems of family and friends in the community. Appropriate questions probe for information on the size of the social network, frequency of contact with friends, reciprocity with family and friends, and the forms that social support takes for the individual client. Nurses should not assume all social networks are supportive, for some may be negative and draining (Powers, 1988).

Network size
- With how many family members do you maintain close contact?
- How many close friends would you say that you have?
- How many casual friends do you see when you are at home?

Frequency of contact
- How many times in the past month have you done something socially with your friends/family?
- How often do you visit, by phone or in person, with your friends/family?

Reciprocity
- Tell me about the people who you feel are a positive support system for you.
- In what ways are you able to be a positive support system for your friends/family?
- How many people contact you to make social plans?

Forms of social support
- What kind of material support do you receive from others?
- Who gives you advice when you need it?
- Who provides companionship for you?
- Who would you say you love, and who returns that love?

When deficits are uncovered in size, extent, support or reciprocity of the network, it is appropriate to use the problem-solving process to cultivate clients' social competency. The focus may be on improving their interactional skills, such as communication and assertive behavior, or it may be on enlarging their network in the community. Identifying resources such as support groups, self-help groups, and special-interest clubs may be particularly helpful for clients who have a limited network system (Gartner and Reissman, 1984). See Table 1–3 for a listing of community groups appropriate for some common types of psychiatric clients.

Implementation

Within the context of this chapter, implementation can refer to a client's or client's family's response to illness or the clinical setting, or a nurse's response to his or her own uncertainties.

Acutely Ill Clients and Their Families

In all clinical settings, nurses must be prepared to assess clients' affective, behavioral, cognitive, and sociocultural responses to illness. These skills, which are broadened during a psychiatric nursing course, are essential in all areas of nursing practice, including the medical-surgical setting. One example of how mental health concepts are integrated into nursing care for a physically ill client is in critical care nursing.

To intervene effectively with critically ill clients is a tremendous challenge for nurses. The nurse

Table 1–3 *Self-Help Groups in the Community*

Addiction
- Alcoholics Anonymous
- Al-Anon
- Alateen
- Adult Children of Alcoholics
- National Association of Recovered Alcoholics in the Professions
- Women for Sobriety
- Alternatives, Inc.
- Families Anonymous
- Narcotics Anonymous
- Gamblers Anonymous
- Cocaine Anonymous

Abuse
- Parents Anonymous
- Daughters and Sons United
- Abused Women's Aid in Crisis

Mental illness
- Depressives Anonymous
- Emotions Anonymous
- Manic-Depressives Anonymous
- Neurotics Anonymous
- Recovery, Inc.
- Schizophrenics Anonymous

Seniors
- SAGE: Senior Actualization and Growth Explorations

needs superior technical proficiency and the ability to function in high-stress situations. Critical care nursing also demands attending to the personhood of ill or injured persons and their families.

Clients who become suddenly ill face tremendous assaults on their emotional stability. Being well one moment and in danger of dying the next is extremely frightening. These persons are confronted with the reality of their own mortality and the threat of losing everything important in their lives. The panic that results is as significant as the physiological disruption, so clients are in desperate need of holistic nursing care. Norman Cousins (1983, p. 202) has said that "nothing is more essential in the treatment of serious disease than liberating the patient from panic and foreboding." Utter fear and panic lead to catecholamine flooding, constricted blood vessels, and destabilization of the heart at a critical time in the fight for survival (Cousins, 1983). Therefore, since panic is potentially fatal, it is essential that nurses assess for panic and intervene quickly.

Emergency treatment can intensify clients' panic. Being transported by an ambulance is frightening in itself, but the stress is frequently intensified by the piercing wail of the siren and a terrifying ride to the hospital. In emergency departments, clients are met by proficient professional staff whose immediate goal is to stabilize physiological status. Fear is heightened with separation from family, dependency on strangers, pain, loss of control, and the uncertainty of recovery. The environment in emergency departments and critical care units is a constant reminder of the threat to life and the real possibility of death. Even unconscious clients are often aware of what is being said around them and have reported feeling helpless and fearful that staff would prematurely end their lifesaving efforts (Finkelmeier, Kenwood, and Summers, 1984).

Almost all people who have been in an accident need to talk about the event. Resolution often depends on going over and over the situation and the accompanying feelings. Clients reliving and reexperiencing traumatic events need to be listened to and supported. To some extent, intervention is possible for all the emotional consequences of critical illness, thus improving the quality of the technical aspects of nursing care.

Family health is also threatened by the possibility of death to one of its members. Critical care nurses are so involved in the fight for survival of clients that families are often only a passing consideration in the treatment plan. Including families is crucial if nurses are to become a source of help rather than still another difficulty for families to deal with. Nurses assess family dynamics and each member's ability to cope with the traumatic event to ensure that interventions are specific to each family's problems. (See Table 1–4.)

Family responses are as varied as individual clients' responses to critical illness. Many families initially react with shock or denial and may appear numb or dazed. Denial, a defense used to cope with the overwhelming pain, is necessary to maintain stability when confronted with emotional overload. Some people will rely on emotional outbursts, such as crying or swearing, as a way to

Table 1–4 Nursing Care Plan During Acute Disruption of Health

Nursing Diagnosis: Anxiety related to unfamiliar surroundings.
Goal: Client will verbalize a decreasing level of anxiety.

Intervention	*Rationale*	*Expected Outcome*
Identify yourself by your name and position.	This will personalize interaction and provide specific information.	
Talk to client and explain what is happening.	Decrease fear of unknown; demonstrate respect, concern; interact.	Client verbalizes a brief understanding of where he or she is and what is occurring.
Acknowledge feelings of anxiety (eg, "It must be frightening to be in a new place").	Give recognition and worth to feelings.	
Explain equipment and personnel.	Familiarity with the environment will decrease anxiety.	
When transferring a client, inform him or her about the new unit. Answer questions honestly. Introduce client to new primary nurse.	Decreasing the newness of the unit will decrease the anxiety. Introductions facilitate transfer of relationships.	Client verbalizes an understanding of the new unit.

Nursing Diagnosis: Powerlessness related to being dependent on professional staff.
Goal: Client will verbally express an increased feeling of control.

Intervention	*Rationale*	*Expected Outcome*
Establish relationship as primary nurse.	Allows client to understand how he or she fits into the system.	
Acknowledge feelings (eg, "It must be frightening to feel like you have lost control over what is happening to you").	Helps client validate feelings of dependency in the unfamiliar situation.	Client verbalizes fears.
Before and during procedures and treatments, give client a clear explanation.	Repetition of explanations is necessary when anxiety is high and client's ability to comprehend is limited.	Client indicates verbally or behaviorally that teaching has been understood.
Give client as much control as possible over body and the environment.	Limited decision making increases client's feeling of control.	Client makes appropriate decisions.

Nursing Diagnosis: Impaired verbal communication related to state of unconsciousness.
Goal: Client will not be traumatized by verbal communication.

Intervention	*Rationale*	*Expected Outcome*
Do not discuss client's situation with other professionals unless far out of hearing range.	Client may have the capacity to hear and understand what is being said. This could lead to misinterpretation and fear.	Client does not hear inappropriate information from nurse or family.
Do not talk about other clients in this client's hearing.	Client may interpret what is overheard as information about his or her own case. Also, nurse appears less trustworthy.	
Talk as though client hears everything said (eg, inform as to what is occurring, enlist client strengths, propose plan of care).	Client is often able to hear and comprehend even when unable to respond.	

(Diagnosis continued)

Table 1–4 *(continued)*

Nursing Diagnosis *(continued)*: Impaired verbal communication related to state of unconsciousness.
Goal: Client will not be traumatized by verbal communication.

Intervention	*Rationale*	*Expected Outcome*
Explain to family that client may be able to hear and understand what is being said even if unconscious.	Family needs to be encouraged to talk to client and be careful of making frightening remarks that client may hear.	

Nursing Diagnosis: Fear related to being confronted with the possibility of death.
Goal: Client will use the energy of fear in the struggle for life.

Intervention	*Rationale*	*Expected Outcome*
Acknowledge and accept client's feelings.	Feelings are real, and client has a right to express feelings.	
Support coping behavior and defense mechanisms.	Defense mechanisms are used to maintain stability and must be supported to prevent emotional disorganization.	Client continues to use defense mechanisms to cope with the crisis.
Do not give false reassurance or take away all hope. Give negative information in a way that enables rather than devastates client. Identify the strengths and resources of the client.	Hope and positive beliefs can intensify medical treatment and increase client's chance of recovery. Those whose hope has been destroyed manage least well in dealing with illness (Cousins, 1983).	Client verbally or behaviorally demonstrates a will to live.
Propose a therapeutic alliance between staff and client by discussing what staff has to offer and what client has to offer in this struggle.	Determined partnership between client and staff will emphasize the plan to combat the problem and give client the feeling there is a chance.	

Nursing Diagnosis: Spiritual distress related to dying.
Goal: Client will experience as peaceful a death as possible.

Intervention	*Rationale*	*Expected Outcome*
Do not isolate client from family and staff.	Isolation increases any client's fears during the dying process.	Client verbally or behaviorally indicates a feeling of connectedness to others.
Use touch to communicate.	Touch is a powerful and comforting intervention.	
Use effective verbal communication skills.	This will reassure client that the nurse is present and involved.	
Ask family what religious needs/rites client has and make every effort to provide these before death.	Meeting of spiritual needs will ease the distress of client before death occurs.	

Nursing Diagnosis: Impaired verbal communication of family related to high anxiety from overwhelming stress.
Goal: Family will be able to communicate basic needs.

Intervention	*Rationale*	*Expected Outcome*
The same person interacts with family each time.	Consistency is necessary to establish a trusting relationship.	Family identifies professional contact person.

(Diagnosis continued)

Table 1–4 *(continued)*

Intervention	*Rationale*	*Expected Outcome*
Respond directly to family's feelings (eg, "I can understand how frightening this is for you" or "I hear you're angry at being separated from your husband right now").	The family needs to have feelings acknowledged and validated.	
If family member is in a panic state, use a firm, kind approach and a gentle restraint with touch (eg, taking the family member by the shoulders and making eye contact).	Since perceptual field is narrowed in panic, brief but firm communication is all that can be comprehended.	Panic level will decrease.
Some people will need structure to cope. Tell them clearly where to go and what to do next.	Many families have difficulty making decisions under conditions of stress.	Necessities will be accomplished.

Nursing Diagnosis: Knowledge deficit of family related to lack of information about condition of loved one.
Goal: Family will verbalize knowledge about condition of loved one.

Intervention	*Rationale*	*Expected Outcome*
"Contract" with family that assigned staff member will give current information every 30 minutes during the initial crisis period.	To decrease the fear and isolation experienced by family.	Family identifies professional contact person.
Repeat information as often as necessary. Don't assume they understood what was said.	Stress limits perceptual field and necessitates repetition of information.	Family repeats information accurately.
Assure family that client will be kept free from pain and as comfortable as possible.	Families often have fears and fantasies about client's condition.	Family verbalizes understanding of what is being done to help client.

Nursing Diagnosis: Spiritual distress related to death of a loved one.
Goal: Family will accept death according to philosophic and spiritual belief system.

Intervention	*Rationale*	*Expected Outcome*
Spouses should be allowed to be with client at the moment of death if they wish.	To continue sharing significant life experiences. Family will have fewer questions about the conditions surrounding the death.	
Provide privacy for family and remain with them.	To grieve without being exposed to strangers.	
When informing family of death, use specific words rather than vague euphemisms (eg, "Your wife has died" rather than "We've lost your wife").	When anxiety is high, clear and simple terms must be used to reduce misunderstanding.	Family verbalizes acceptance of the reality of the death.
Tell family what occurred and why.	To decrease fantasies family may have and fill in information gaps that may be present.	
Give them the opportunity and time to talk about and react to the loss.	Verbalization of grief is appropriate coping behavior. Nurse's willingness to listen reinforces this coping behavior.	

(Diagnosis continued)

Table 1–4 *(continued)*

Nursing Diagnosis *(continued)*: Spiritual distress related to death of a loved one.
Goal: Family will accept death according to philosophic and spiritual belief system.

Intervention	*Rationale*	*Expected Outcome*
Provide for religious needs to be met.	As a source of comfort to family. To fulfill religious rites.	Family verbalizes that spiritual needs are being met.
Offer the opportunity to see the body. Prepare them for the appearance of the body.	To present reality and begin the grieving process.	

Nursing Diagnosis: Ineffective family coping, compromised, related to sudden death of loved one.
Goal: Family will proceed through grieving process to point of acceptance.

Intervention	*Rationale*	*Expected Outcome*
Don't make family members feel inadequate if they can't function effectively. Be nonjudgmental and accepting.	Don't want to contribute to dysfunction by imposing own values. Responses to new experiences are unpredictable.	Family will get necessary support to make immediate plans.
If necessary, make phone calls for family.	Nurses must assume responsibility until a family member is able to assume responsibility.	
Assist with the concluding process by explaining what to do next, where the body will go, if there will be an autopsy, etc.	Families are often unfamiliar with the procedure and what responsibilities and legal requirements must be met.	
If necessary, help family find transportation home.	Strong emotions of moment make it unsafe for them to drive.	
Try to have someone waiting at home for the family.	Families need continued support after leaving the hospital.	
Give phone numbers of grieving groups in the area.	For continued support to prevent dysfunctional grieving.	Family will identify available services for further support.
Make a follow-up phone call to the family in a week.	Family members often need to review circumstances of death after the funeral. To fill in gaps of information regarding the death experience.	

discharge the energy of anxiety and fear. Some will attempt to cope by becoming dependent and in need of a great deal of reassurance. Others will act out their frustration by complaining, or they may even lash out in anger and accuse the staff of incompetence. Some families respond with feelings of "Why us?" and a sense of helplessness and hopelessness. Some will withdraw, whereas others will talk incessantly or laugh inappropriately in response to high anxiety.

Nurses also respond to the cognitive disruptions the family may be experiencing. Some families have unrealistic beliefs concerning the event, which will need to be corrected at some point in the treatment process if they are to adjust to the catastrophe. Family members are often unsure about the appropriateness of their response during the emergency and may even accuse themselves of negligence or look for evidence of their failure to have done the right thing. When anxiety is high, people are not able to make decisions and solve problems. Knowing this, nurses will intervene in a manner supportive of the family's inability to make decisions. Because the family may be confused or uncertain of what measures should be taken next, they need purposeful directions. When nurses diagnose, plan, and intervene, family members experience fewer symptoms of crisis and more adaptive responses to the traumatic event.

The nursing care plan (given in Table 1–4) is designed to meet the psychological and spiritual needs of clients and families involved in a critical disruption of health. This plan exemplifies how mental health concepts are used in medical-surgical nursing practice.

Fears About Clinical Practice: Management with Self-Care

At the onset of a course in mental health nursing, students often verbalize uncertainties and fears related both to themselves and to their clients. Students' personal fears often stem from being in an unfamiliar environment, not knowing what to talk about, believing they have nothing to offer, and thinking they will say the wrong thing. Students' fears of clients can be rooted in the stereotypes they have of people with mental illness; fear of rejection, of anger, and of being physically harmed by clients is not uncommon.

In an effort to provide students with information and specific help, the nursing student care plan shown in Table 1–5 has been developed. Applying the nursing process to oneself is an appropriate method of resolving problems of adaptation to the clinical unit.

Evaluation

In evaluating professional practice, nurses need to use the process of **self-evaluation.** Questions to be asked include

- What is my philosophy of illness and wellness?
- What role does suffering play in life?
- What is my philosophy of nursing?
- What characteristics have I brought to the relationship that have helped or hindered my clients' growth?
- What has been my primary focus—helping clients or needing to impress others with my skills?
- What characteristics do I need to maintain or modify to become a more effective helper?

Additional areas of self-evaluation are one's ability to learn from experiences and mistakes, capacity to care about and for clients, assumption of responsibility, and confidence in professional judgment.

In the evaluative process, nurses should also consider others' views. **Peer evaluation** is a rich source of information that supports professional growth. From peers nurses are able to determine the images they project and how they are viewed by others. Instructors and supervisors are able to suggest areas where more information or education is needed to improve professional practice. They can assist in the process of self-evaluation by sharing their perceptions of how the various roles have been enacted and by offering suggestions for change. To clarify any problem areas, instructors and supervisors may use role playing; to resolve any problems, they may use the problem-solving process.

Another source of information, which is often neglected, is the client population. To better understand their roles and behavior, nurses should also make use of **client evaluation.** Often clients are more certain than nurses in identifying helpful characteristics of nurses. Clients report that personal attributes such as warmth, acceptance, kindness, helpfulness, and friendliness are crucial to the development of a therapeutic alliance and relationship (Cormack, 1983).

Table 1–5 Care Plan for a Nursing Student

Nursing Diagnosis: Fear of being in an unfamiliar environment.
Goal: You will verbalize comfort on the unit by the third clinical day.

Intervention	*Rationale*	*Expected Outcome*
Think back to your first clinical day in nursing school. Identify what factors contributed to your fears at that time. Identify behaviors used to cope with your fears.	In new situations, one's fears tend to focus on the same personal issues (eg, inadequacy, interpersonal relationships, protection of self, etc). One tends to reuse coping behavior that has been successful in the past.	You identify and use past effective coping behavior.
Ask your instructor exactly what is expected of you the first week of clinical experience.	Understanding beginning role expectations and specific behaviors decreases anxiety.	You identify instructor's realistic expectations.
Ask your instructor about the norms of behavior for this particular clinical unit.	Understanding the formal and informal norms of the system eases integration into the health care team.	You use unit's norms to modify your own behavior.
Become acquainted with the physical environment.	Knowing where things are decreases anxiety.	You know where things are on the unit.
In the first postconference, discuss your expected fears and how those were either realized or not.	Processing expectations versus reality increases self-understanding and comfort in the new situation.	You distinguish between expectations and reality.

Nursing Diagnosis: Stereotypical fears about people with mental health problems.
Goal: You will verbalize a realistic understanding of people with mental health problems.

Intervention	*Rationale*	*Expected Outcome*
Identify your own cultural stereotypes about psychiatric clients.	Identifying stereotypes as the source of fears minimizes fears.	You distinguish between cultural stereotypes of clients and the reality of their behavior.
In your first preconference, discuss your expectations of clients' behaviors.	In sharing, similarities and differences arising from a variety of personal experiences become apparent.	You verbalize expectations.
Ask your instructor about the reality of clients' behavior on the unit.	Reassurance that most behavior is not out of the ordinary decreases anxiety.	
Identify specific fears of clients (eg, that they will be very bizarre or that they have better coping skills than you do).	Making fears specific rather than vague allows instructor to offer appropriate reassurance.	
Approach client as a person rather than as a diagnosis.	The medical diagnosis should not define the personhood of the client.	
Approach client as a person who has problems that can be solved.	This attitude decreases fears that client is a totally incapable person.	You approach clients as individuals who have both problems and strengths.
Identify healthy aspects and resources of client.	In many areas of life, client copes effectively and is no less capable than nonpsychiatric clients.	

(continued)

Table 1–5 *(continued)*

Nursing Diagnosis: Fear of not knowing what to talk about.
Goal: You will be able to talk comfortably on a variety of topics with clients.

Intervention	*Rationale*	*Expected Outcome*
When first meeting client population, introduce yourself and converse on a social level.	This creates the opportunity for both clients and students to become acquainted without the introduction of stressful topics.	You socialize therapeutically with clients.
Using the nursing care plan, follow client's lead in the topic to be discussed during the one-to-one interaction.	Deciding on a specific topic and goal keeps the interaction focused.	One-to-one interactions are goal-directed.
Give up the unrealistic self-expectation that you have to be absolutely right before you offer any observations to client.	A perfectionist approach to interactions will inhibit the process and contribute to client's retreating from the relationship.	You discuss fear of failure.
Risk sharing your perceptions with client and seek validation (eg, "It sounds as if you are angry" or "Am I hearing you correctly, that you are very frustrated over this situation?").	Even if perceptions are incorrect, sharing provides the necessary stimulation for client to express feelings.	You share perceptions with client.
You recognize own signs of increased anxiety and use measures to decrease anxiety.	Identifying and managing anxiety increases cognitive and oral skills.	

Nursing Diagnosis: Fear of having nothing to offer.
Goal: You will be able to describe professional strengths by the midterm of the course.

Intervention	*Rationale*	*Expected Outcome*
Identify your own fears of inadequacy by listening to your self-statements (eg, "How can I help this person when I don't know what's wrong with him?" or "These clients are too sick/well, so how can I help them?")	Making fears specific creates the opportunity for the instructor to identify solutions to the problem.	You describe specific fears.
If clients question your qualifications, simply state why you are here and what your role is on the unit.	Frequently clients' questions reflect a desire to get to know a student more personally or to understand what his or her purpose is.	You respond calmly to clients' questions.
Recognize that your knowledge and theory base will be increasing throughout the course.	Fears of inadequacy decrease as knowledge about psychiatric nursing and nursing skills increase.	You apply theory to clinical practice.
Identify the energy and enthusiasm you bring as a positive quality to be used therapeutically.	When energy is infused through the nursing process, creativity in the problem-solving process is increased.	You use energy creatively.
Recognize that a positive interpersonal relationship is therapeutic for client.	Positive contact with others may be the greatest lack in client's home environment. The experience of a positive relationship increases self-image and develops interactional skills for client.	You develop therapeutic relationships as you implement the nursing process.

(Diagnosis continued)

Table 1–5 *(continued)*

Nursing Diagnosis *(continued)*: Fear of having nothing to offer.
Goal: You will be able to describe professional strengths by the midterm of the course.

Intervention	*Rationale*	*Expected Outcome*
Recall characteristics of effective helpers.	Interpersonal qualities and relationship skills are more helpful in therapeutic change than technical aspects of effective communication.	You exhibit characteristics of effective helpers.
Involve client in the nursing process, and work together as a team toward specified goals.	Solutions to problems arise from working *with* client, not as the result of something done *to* client.	You use nurse-client team approach.

Nursing Diagnosis: Fear of hurting client by saying the wrong thing.
Goal: You will use more effective communication after the course.

Intervention	*Rationale*	*Expected Outcome*
Identify fantasies of saying the wrong thing and having destructive and irreversible consequences for client.	The quality of a caring relationship overcomes verbal mistakes. No student can destroy a client with a few ill-chosen words.	
Talk to other students who have been through this clinical experience.	Sharing helps a student look at fears realistically.	
Recognize that clinical experience is an opportunity to learn and that verbal mistakes will be made.	Opportunities for more appropriate interventions are seldom lost but, rather, postponed.	
If you have made a mistake, apologize to client and identify what would have been a more therapeutic response.	It is through the evaluative process that communication skills are refined.	You evaluate and modify verbal responses to clients.
Ask your instructor to use process recordings or audiotapes as a method to improve and increase your communication skills.	An instructor is a resource to assist in the evaluative process by providing objective feedback.	You use a variety of effective communication skills.

Nursing Diagnosis: Fear of rejection by the client.
Goal: You will effectively manage your feelings of rejection.

Intervention	*Rationale*	*Expected Outcome*
Identify what is the worst thing that will happen to you if client refuses to work with you.	Clients have a right to refuse a one-to-one relationship. If this occurs, a student has more opportunities to work with other clients.	You identify personal fears.
If client is exhibiting behavior that indicates unwillingness to work with you, validate this behavior with him or her.	The immediate behavior is the priority problem to be addressed.	You validate the meaning of client's behavior.
If client comments on your behavior, process these perceptions with your peers and instructor.	Analysis of one's own behavior decreases the potential of personalizing all client's comments as well as modifying one's behavior.	You do not personalize all client's behavior.
Do not let your fear of rejection prevent you from discussing sensitive problem areas with client.	Client may interpret fear as a lack of understanding of or commitment to solving client's problems.	You confront sensitive problem areas appropriately.

(continued)

Table 1–5 *(continued)*

Nursing Diagnosis: Fear of anger from client.
Goal: You will be able to tolerate verbal expression of anger from client.

Intervention	*Rationale*	*Expected Outcome*
Know and understand your own response to the feeling and expression of anger (eg, "Nice people don't get angry." "It's okay to feel angry, but it should always be talked about calmly." "I'm comfortable when people shout when they are angry.")	Identification of personal values prevents imposing one's own values on client.	You verbalize your own values about the feeling of anger.
Accept client's right to be angry.	Feelings are real and cannot be discounted or ignored.	You support client's right to express feelings.
Try to understand the meaning of client's anger.	Identification of how client feels hurt or threatened is the basis for resolving the anger.	
Ask client in what way you have contributed to anger.	Direct inquiry may prevent escalation of the anger. Assuming responsibility for one's own behavior is a positive role model for client.	You analyze your own contributing behavior.
Let client talk about the anger.	Talking about the feeling is necessary before the problem-solving approach is implemented to resolve the situation.	You remain with client who is angry.
Listen to client and react as calmly as possible.	The willingness to listen communicates care and concern.	
After the interaction is completed, take time to process your feelings and your responses to client with your peers and instructor.	Processing contributes to increased insight into one's own feelings. Analyzing responses is necessary to determine what needs to be modified or changed the next time client becomes angry.	You talk about your own feelings. You evaluate the interaction.

Nursing Diagnosis: Fear of physical harm from client.
Goal: You will not be physically harmed.

Intervention	*Rationale*	*Expected Outcome*
Ask instructor about the reality of these fears.	Physical violence very seldom occurs on the psychiatric unit.	
Recognize early signs of an impending violent outburst.	Early intervention prevents escalation of behavior.	You identify early signs of escalating behavior.
Seek help immediately from staff and instructor.	Professionals with experience are able to intervene effectively.	You alert staff to impending violent behavior.
If client begins to act out physically, stay out of staff members' way as they implement their plan of action.	Staff is prepared to intervene in a preplanned team approach. Students are *not* part of this team intervention unless given specific requests for assistance.	

SUMMARY

Philosophies

1. Wellness is a dynamic growth process toward one's potential and an inner feeling of vitality.
2. Illness is a feeling of disharmony or incongruence with one's body, mind, and spirit.
3. There are a variety of theories from which to understand mental health and illness. Holistic nursing is an integration of these theories and a reaching out beyond labels to the person who is suffering.
4. Personal beliefs about the role of suffering in life influence how nurses intervene with clients who are experiencing psychological discomfort or physical pain.
5. One's philosophy of nursing gives direction and meaning to nursing practice. A critical ingredient is caring, without which nurses could not make an authentic commitment or a personal response to clients.

Assessment

6. The process of self-analysis assists nurses in understanding and coping with their own feelings in a professional manner, thus allowing them to respond more effectively to clients.
7. Clients' behavioral responses to illness are determined by many factors and are an attempt to communicate and to meet needs. Behavior is influenced by the past, present, and future and is logical according to the client's perception of reality.
8. There is a wide range of affective responses when people become ill and are hospitalized. To intervene appropriately, nurses must accurately assess the source and meaning of the client's emotional response.
9. Illness and suffering influence clients' cognitive responses, particularly in terms of self-concept, self-esteem, self-acceptance, and locus of control.
10. Spiritual responses to illness include beliefs about the meaning of life and death as well as a feeling of connectedness with others and/or an external power.
11. Spiritual distress may be related to guilt; injustice; lack of fulfillment, meaning, or purpose of life; and detachment from others.
12. The practice of holistic nursing means that nurses must assess the impact of illness on the family as well as the impact of the family on the member who is ill.
13. The physical, emotional, and spiritual components of the nurse-client relationship are all interrelated and function in unity.
14. Both nurses' and clients' perceptions of locus of control within the nurse-client relationship determine the direction of nursing care and define the power within the relationship.

Planning and Implementation

15. Interpersonal qualities and relationship skills are critical to the nursing interventions implemented in the therapeutic relationship.
16. The ability to integrate characteristics of effective helpers into nursing practice will aid growth and increase satisfaction for both clients and nurses.
17. Effective communication is a key factor in the planning and implementation of nursing care.
18. There are a variety of interrelated nursing roles that serve as strategies for planning and implementing the nursing care plan.
19. Nursing goals are guidelines that assist in the planning of specific and individualized interventions.
20. Mental health concepts are used in all clinical areas of nursing practice.
21. Students can apply the nursing process to themselves to resolve problems of adaptation to the clinical unit.

CHAPTER REVIEW

1. You have assessed your client, Doug, as being on the wellness end of the continuum. Which one of the following statements best supports your assessment?
   (a) Doug has no evidence of any organic disease.
   (b) Doug says his life is boring but has little stress.
   (c) Doug is dissatisfied with his personal relationships.
   (d) Doug says he continues to grow daily and is satisfied with life.
2. It is important that nurses assess their personal philosophies of suffering because philosophy
   (a) Influences how nurses assess clients' suffering.
   (b) Is universally defined by nurses and clients.
   (c) Allows nurses to directly measure the degree of suffering.
   (d) Guarantees nurses from overreacting to suffering.
3. Sylvia is discussing problems she is having with her teenage sons. She states: "They don't respect me, they talk back to me, and they don't always tell me where they are going. I tried to be a good mother. The way they treat me just doesn't seem fair." Which one of the following is the most appropriate nursing diagnosis for Sylvia?

(a) Social isolation related to not being a major focus in her sons' lives.
(b) Spiritual distress related to a feeling of injustice in life.
(c) Anticipatory grieving related to sons growing up and leaving home.
(d) Decisional conflict related to how to parent teenagers.

4. Which one of the following situations best illustrates the positive process of introspection and self-analysis on the part of the nurse?
(a) Mary has elected not to work with battered women clients, since she continues to live with her violent husband.
(b) Tim has elected to work on the chemical dependency unit even though he severely abuses alcohol on weekends.
(c) Tanya wants to start a codependency group for partners of alcoholics in spite of her denial of her husband's alcoholism.
(d) Micha has elected to lead a grieving group since he has been unable to get over his wife's suicide a year ago.

5. Which one of the following examples best illustrates a client with an internal locus of control?
(a) Ed says his ulcer is due to too much stress from his job.
(b) Mary believes her accident was caused by her bad luck rather than by her drinking.
(c) Bob worries about catching every illness he is exposed to from others.
(d) Sue uses the problem-solving process to plan for her discharge.

REFERENCES

Benfer B: Clinical supervision as a support system for the care giver. In: *Psychiatric/Mental Health Nursing, Contemporary Readings,* 2nd ed. Backer B, et al. (editors). Wadsworth, 1985.

Book HE: Empathy. *Am J Psychiatry* 1988; 145(4):420–424.

Cormack D: *Psychiatric Nursing Described.* Churchill Livingstone, 1983.

Cousins N: *The Healing Heart.* Norton, 1983.

Davitz L, Davitz J, Rubin C: *Nurses' Responses to Patients' Suffering.* Springer, 1980.

Fenton MV: Development of the scale of humanistic nursing behaviors. *Nurs Research* 1987; 36(2):82–87.

Ferguson MS, Campinha-Bacote J: Humor in nursing. *J Psychosoc Nurs* 1989; 26(4):29–34.

Finkelmeier B, Kenwood N, Summers C: Psychological ramifications of survival from sudden cardiac death. *CCQ* 1984; 7(2):71.

Forsyth G: Analysis of the concept of empathy: Illustrations of one approach. *ANS* 1980; 2(2):33.

Gartner A, Reissman F: *The Self-Help Revolution.* Human Sciences Press, 1984.

Goldsborough J: Involvement. *Am J Nurs* 1969; 69(1):66.

Holderby R, McNulty E: *Teaching and Caring: A Human Approach to Patient Care.* Reston, 1982.

Holm K, et al.: Effect of personal pain experience on pain assessment. *Image* 1989; 21(2):72–75.

Jack LW: Using play in psychiatric rehabilitation. *J Psychosoc Nurs* 1987; 25(7):17.

Kasch C: Interpersonal competence and communication in the delivery of nursing care. *ANS* 1984; 6(2):71.

Kohnke MF: *Advocacy: Risk and Reality.* Mosby, 1982.

Labun E: Spiritual care: An element in nursing care planning. *J Adv Nurs* 1988; 13(3):314.

Leddy D, Pepper J: *Conceptual Bases of Professional Nursing.* Lippincott, 1985.

Marcia J: Empathy and psychotherapy. In: *Empathy and Its Development,* Eisenberg N, Strayer J (editors). Cambridge University Press, 1987.

Mayeroff M: *On Caring.* Harper & Row, 1971.

Merwin MR, Smith-Kurtz B: Healing of the whole person. In: *Post-Traumatic Therapy and Victims of Violence.* Ochberg FM (editor). Brunner/Mazel, 1988.

Moch SD: Towards a personal control/uncontrol balance. *J Adv Nurs* 1988; 13(1):119–123.

Mooney J: Attachment/separation in the nurse-patient relationship. *Nurs Forum* 1976; 15(3):259.

Musil CM, Abraham IL: Coping, thinking and mental health nursing. *Issues Ment Health* 1986; 8(3):191–201.

Osterlund H: Humor, a serious approach to patient care. *Nurs '83* 1983; 13(12):46.

Powers BA: Social networks, social support and elderly institutionalized people. *ANS* 1988; 10(2):40–58.

Pumphrey J: Recognizing your patient's spiritual needs. *Nurs '77* 1977; 7(12):64.

Robinson L: *Psychological Aspects of the Care of Hospitalized Patients,* 4th ed. Davis, 1984.

Rogers C, et al.: *Person to Person: The Problem of Being Human.* Lafayette, CA: Real People Press, 1967.

Schnid D, et al.: Confidentiality in psychiatry: A study of the patient's view. *Hosp Community Psychiatry* 1983; 34(4):353.

Simon JM: Therapeutic humor. *J Psychosoc Nurs* 1988; 26(4):8–12.

Taylor S: Rights and responsibilities: Nurse-patient relationships. *Image* 1985; 17(1):9.

Watson J: *Nursing: The Philosophy and Science of Care.* Colorado Ass. Press, 1985.

SUGGESTED READINGS

Eisenberg N, Strayer J (editors): *Empathy and its Development.* Cambridge University Press, 1987.

Forchuk C, Brown B: Establishing a nurse-client relationship. *J Psychosoc Nurs* 1989; 27(2):30–34.

Freud S: *Jokes and Their Relation to the Unconscious.* Norton, 1960. Originally published by Deuticke in 1905.

Henderson KJ: Dying, God & anger: Comforting through spiritual care. *J Psychosoc Nurs* 1989; 27(5):17–21.

Lane PL: Nurse-client perceptions: The double standard of touch. *Issues in Ment Health* 1989; 10(1):1–13.

McGhee PE: *Humor and Children's Development.* Haworth, 1989.

McMahon R: Partners in care. *Nurs Times* 1989; 85(8): 34–37.

Nagai-Jacobson MG, Burkhardt MA: Spirituality: Cornerstone of holistic nursing practice. *Holistic Nurs Pract* 1989; 3(3):18–26.

Neaves JJ: The relationship of locus of control to decision making in nursing students. *J Nurs Educ* 1989; 28(1): 12–17.

Newman, MA: The spirit of nursing. *Holistic Nurs Pract* 1989; 3(3):1–6.

Peterson EA, Nelson K: How to meet your clients' spiritual needs. *J Psychosoc Nurs* 1987; 25(5):34–39.

Porat F: *Self-Esteem.* R&E Publishers, 1988.

Rothenberg A: *The Creative Process of Psychotherapy.* Norton, 1988.

Stuart EM, Deckro JP, Mandle CL: Spirituality in health and healing: A clinical program. *Holistic Nurs Pract* 1989; 3(3):35–46.

CHAPTER 2

The Mental Health Nursing Process

J. SUE COOK

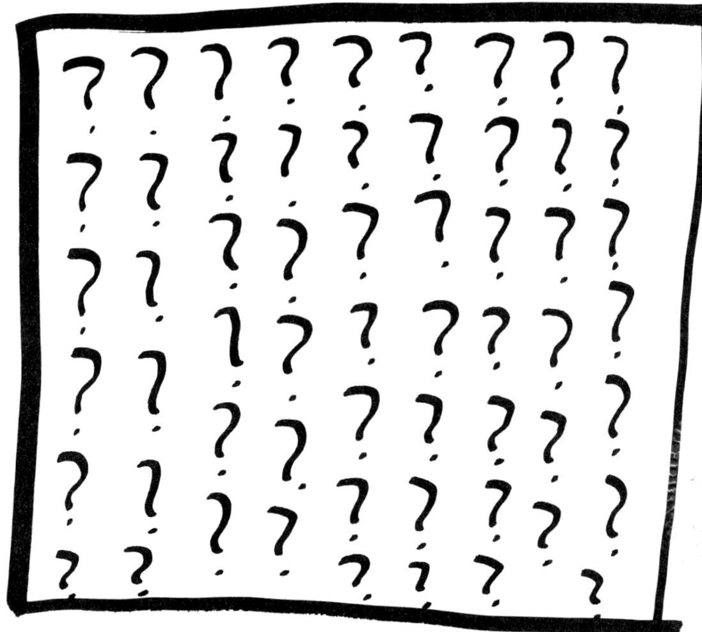

I feel trapped inside a body I don't wan't and I'm full of questions. Are things ever going to get better?

■ *Objectives*

After reading this chapter the student will be able to

- Discuss the philosophic and theoretic foundations of mental health nursing
- Explain six major theories underlying the development of mental health nursing concepts
- Discuss 11 nursing theorists who have developed models important to mental health nursing
- Compare the nursing process with the mental health nursing process
- Use therapeutic communication skills in the mental health setting
- Explain the ANA professional practice standards for mental health nursing
- Relate the types of assessment tools appropriate to the mental health setting
- List and use nursing diagnoses within the mental health setting
- Plan care for mentally ill clients
- Discuss three types of nursing interventions used in mental health nursing
- Explain evaluation of nursing care in the mental health setting
- Apply a self-evaluation checklist to nursing care given in the mental health setting

■ *Chapter Contents*

Introduction

Mental illness will touch the lives of almost all of us in some way. Nearly everybody knows, or knows of, someone who has had some type of mental problem. Yet, people still react to the concept of mental illness with anxiety, fear, shame, and guilt. If a family member has a heart attack, cancer, or other type of physical illness, the person receives flowers and sympathy. But change the diagnosis to mental illness, and the person receives avoidance, criticism, and ostracism.

Mental illness is one of the most common types of illnesses that occur in North American society. Many of the clients seen in family practice and the acute care hospital have psychiatric problems, which are often downplayed or ignored because of the ambivalent feelings even professionals have about mental illness. The attitudes of health care professionals can be changed only by increasing their knowledge base and understanding of the concepts of mental illness.

Philosophic Foundations of Mental Health Nursing

Nursing has evolved over many years. The American Nurses' Association's (ANA's) *Social Policy Statement* (1980), reflecting both historical and modern theory, defined **nursing** as

> the diagnosis and treatment of human responses to actual or potential health problems.

This definition provides a comprehensive view of nursing's contribution to health care. Because that health care system is complex, specialized disciplines have developed to meet the multiple needs of clients. One such specialized discipline is **mental health nursing**, which Evans et al. (1976) defined as

> a specialized area of nursing practice employing theories of human behavior as its science and purposeful use of self as its art. It is directed toward both preventive and corrective impacts upon mental disorders and their sequelae and is concerned with the promotion of optimal mental health for society.

Now that nursing and mental health nursing have been defined, an understanding of their philosophic foundations is essential to implement these practices.

Philosophy serves to identify, clarify, and justify nursing practice. The major justifications for practice are *theoretic, psychologic,* and *social.* Analysis of theory assists in clarifying the ideas related to mental health nursing practice. Psychologic justifications clarify the nature of the mind and the nature of humans. Social justifications relate to humans as social beings with social needs.

The foundations of mental health nursing stem from the very nature of human experience, that is, from the attitudes, values, feelings, and emotions of people. From these are formed thought patterns, which along with historical knowledge of culture and society, assist each person's internalization of human experience and behaviors. From this internal source are the decisions of daily life made (Strain, 1971).

The thought pattern presented in this text is humanism, in which a human is defined holistically as a dynamic pattern of physical, emotional, mental, and spiritual processes (Krieger, 1981). Lamont (1957) identified 10 central propositions of this person-centered theory, in which the individual is considered the center of the universe:

1. Nature is the totality of being and is a constantly changing system of matter and energy existing independently of any mind or consciousness.
2. People are an evolutionary product of nature, and humanism draws upon the laws and facts of science. A person's personality and body are inseparable, and there is no conscious survival after death.
3. There is ultimate faith in the person; a human being possesses the power to solve his or her own problems by using the scientific method.
4. Human beings possess genuine freedom of creative choice and action and are the masters of their own destinies.
5. Ethics or morality is the ground for all human values. Its highest goal is the worldly happiness, freedom, and progress of all humankind, irrespective of nation, race, or religion.
6. The individual attains "the good life" by harmoniously combining personal satisfactions and continuous self-development with significant work that contributes to the welfare of the community.
7. The widest possible development of art and the awareness of beauty arise from the belief that the aesthetic experience can become a reality in people's lives.
8. Social programs should be far-reaching and promote democracy, peace, and a high standard of living throughout the world.
9. All areas of economic, political, and cultural life should implement reason and the scientific method by using democratic procedures.
10. Basic assumptions and convictions should remain open to experimental testing, newly discovered facts, and more rigorous reasoning.

The nurse will use these beliefs and values when making nursing decisions. Recognizing and understanding one's own philosophy and comparing it to the premises of humanism are essential to good nursing care of the mentally ill client.

The ANA has developed guidelines for mental health nursing practice. These guidelines, called standards, form the historical cultural basis for the thought patterns related to mental health nursing practice, but their specific purpose is to maintain quality care for the mentally ill client. The ANA statements on the scope of psychiatric nursing practice and standards for mental health nursing practice stress the importance of the nursing process in prevention, intervention, and rehabilitation of the mentally ill.

In summary, then, mental health nursing is based on three main philosophic justifications: the theoretic focus on the concepts of the nursing process, the psychologic on the premises of humanism, and the social on the profession's accepted standards of mental health nursing practice.

Theoretic Foundations of Mental Health Nursing

In addition to understanding the philosophic base of mental health nursing, nurses need to understand theories from many disciplines. Theories help to predict the real world by systematically organizing statements that describe and explain that world. Theory can be described as the rationale for philosophic beliefs (Yura and Walsh, 1978).

The practice of mental health nursing has evolved over the years and has been influenced by advances in social change, science, and technology. However, the most important advance has come in the form of nursing theories practiced within the framework of the nursing process. The combination of basic theory, knowledge of the client, physical nursing skills, and communication skills assists nurses in meeting their clients' needs for emotional support.

To understand theories about mental health nursing, the nurse needs a general understanding of the theory-building process and nursing theorists. Several nurse-scientists have developed theories about the nature and science of nursing. These theories provide an organization for thinking, observing, and interpreting the nursing process.

Major Theories of Mental Health Nursing

A theory is the analysis of a set of facts and their relationships to one another. Several theories have affected the perception and development of nursing. Some were derived from the observation of nature; some were derived from the observation of humans in particular.

General Systems Theory Ludwig von Bertalanffy introduced **general systems theory** as a universal theory applicable to many disciplines. A **system** is a set of interacting elements that contribute to the overall goal of the system. Within systems are subsystems arranged in a hierarchy from the lowest level to the highest level.

Systems may be open or closed. **Open systems** are characterized by freedom of energy, matter, and information to move within the system's boundaries. **Closed systems** are theoretically the opposite of open systems; that is, there is no movement of energy, matter, and information within the system. However, no totally closed system is known to exist. In mental health, the family may be viewed as an example of both an open and a closed system. The family unit itself is closed because the movement of energy, matter, and information stays within the boundary of the family unit. However, the family unit interacts and exchanges with other systems, and these interactions have an effect on the interchanges within the family unit. Open systems maintain a steady state of dynamic equilibrium within the system. This balance has also been called homeostasis and homeodynamics. The mechanism of feedback is the manner in which the system maintains its steady state (Flynn and Heffron, 1984).

In mental health nursing, concepts from systems theory are used to understand client's behavior. The nurse and the client are part of both open and closed systems. A principal focus in the interactions between clients and nurses is feedback. The nurse uses feedback to assist the client in achieving homeostasis.

Adaptation Theory Theory applied to explain and understand how equilibrium is maintained to ensure the survival of open systems is called **adaptation theory**. Widely applied to biologic, physiologic, and psychologic responses of the person, adaptation theory is also the basis for many current medical therapies.

Our regulatory systems operate by a mechanism called compensation. Stressors disturb equilibrium by triggering the mechanism of compensation to help the body adjust to the stressor. Adaptation is the way the body responds to stressors. In the mental health setting, defense mechanisms are examples of adaptation (Leddy and Pepper, 1985).

Human Need Theory **Human need theory** is based on the concept that a need creates internal tension resulting from an alteration in the state of a system and the motivation necessary to meet that need. The fulfillment of needs organizes a person's behavior. To explain the priorities of human behavior, Abraham Maslow developed a hierarchy of needs: physiologic, safety, love and belonging, esteem, and self-actualization (see Figure 2–1).

Physiologic needs refer to maintaining physical well-being with adequate air, food, water, sleep, and so forth. Because these needs must be met before all others, they are the most influential. For some mental health clients, these needs may be overwhelming. For example, the schizophrenic client may not attend to physiologic needs, so the nurse intervenes and provides for them.

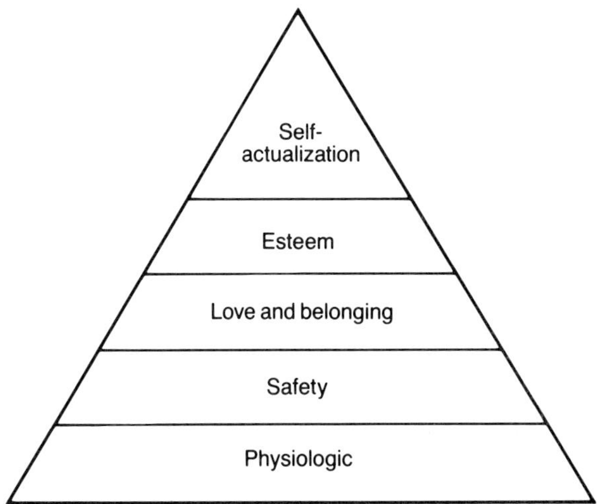

Figure 2–1 *Maslow's hierarchy of needs. Adapted from A. H. Maslow,* Psychological Review, 1943; 50:370–396. Reprinted with permission.

Safety needs—which relate to security, protection, and freedom from anxiety and fear—emerge once physical needs are gratified. For stable, peaceful, effective social systems, safety is necessary. The mental health client frequently needs assistance in meeting safety needs.

Love and belonging needs emerge when physiologic and safety needs are gratified. These needs arise through relationships with parents, spouses, children, friends, and colleagues. Love and belonging needs are met through affection, intimacy, togetherness, and respect. The mental health client often feels these needs have not been met.

Esteem needs, which emerge when love and belonging needs are met, are related to self-respect and respect for others. Esteem needs include a desire for strength, achievement, adequacy, mastery, and competence. Feelings of self-worth, confidence, and dignity are important factors in meeting esteem needs. Deprivation of esteem needs leads to compensatory and maladaptive behavior. Nurses assess these behaviors when caring for the mentally ill client.

Self-actualization is at the summit of the needs hierarchy, emerging only after physiologic, safety, love, and esteem needs have been satisfied. Even when all needs through the esteem level have been met, the client may feel restless unless doing what he or she is best suited for. This restlessness is the desire for self-actualization. The mental health nurse strives the help the client achieve it (Yura and Walsh, 1988).

Whether there are deficits in physical needs or esteem needs, feeling unloved and uncared for affects the client's responses to other needs and may result in the client's feeling helpless and inferior. There are many implications of human needs theory in mental health nursing.

Perception Theory To explain the system of behavior for fulfilling human needs, **perception**

theory was developed. Each person has a unique system of behavior for dealing with situations. The variables in studying perception are the physical environment, physiologic processes and interactions, and behavioral events. Contact with the environment is through energy-sensitive receptors.

The three types of receptor cells are exteroceptors, interoceptors, and proprioceptors. Exteroceptor cells are primarily sensory organ cells that receive energy from the external environment. Interoceptor cells are found within the organism and respond to changes in pressure, changes in temperature, and to pain. Proprioceptor cells respond to energy changes activated by movement and posture.

The development of perception is from simple to complex and is affected by meanings related to stimuli. These meanings are learned and affect perception the most when the stimulation occurs under ambiguous circumstances. The first perceptive processes learned are identification of objects. Once objects are identified, perception is further organized by manipulating and memorizing events, which assist the person in building many expectations about the environment. Feedback is the primary mechanism used to check the accuracy of one's perception.

Several suppositions support the relationship of experience to perception. First, generalization refers to the learning that takes place in one situation and is then applied to another situation involving the same type of schemata. To make an appropriate response, the person uses the memories of past experiences relevant to the current situation. The second supposition is that children and adults distinguish the constant qualities of a class of events or objects from chance variations occurring within the background. The final supposition is called verbal discrimination, which is necessary for naming, coding, and labeling experiences. The control of immediate perception and reasoning results from the use of verbal information (Allport, 1955; Day, 1966; Vernon, 1970; Yura and Walsh, 1978).

In mental health nursing, the perceptions developed by the client from early and current experiences interact with the perceptions of the nurse. Clarifying and validating perceptions form a focus of therapeutic communication between the client and the nurse.

Learning Theory A summary of writings about learning must cover many centuries. Englishman John Locke shaped a theory of learning that included the product of experience and the principles of association in acts of repetition as the basis for human learning. Ivan Pavlov, from Russia, developed the theory of classical conditioning from Locke's concepts. E. L. Thorndike of the United States complemented Pavlov's findings by building a theory about the associations formed between stimuli and responses. John B. Watson, another American, refined learning theory and postulated that behavior is determined by environmental conditions and that behavioral differences could be explained by environmental differences. In recent years, B. F. Skinner's works on reinforcers have added to the conceptualization of learning theory (Bevelas, 1978; Rohwer, Ammon, and Cramer, 1974).

A main principle of learning theory, called **stimulus-response (S-R) theory** in the literature, is operant conditioning. In *operant conditioning,* an organism emits a response to a stimulus; if that response is reinforced, the organism is likely to respond similarly in the presence of that stimulus in the future. Reinforcement can be positive or negative. Positive reinforcement presents a stimulus such as food or praise, whereas negative reinforcement consists of removal acts such as shock or scolding.

The concepts of stimulus, response, and reinforcement are the primary behavioral descriptions within learning theory. This is the basis for behaviorist theory, which has been useful in mental health nursing in planning token economies and conditioning more socially appropriate behaviors.

Communication Theory **Communication theory** focuses on the connections underlying interrelations and the interactions within or between systems. This theory is the basis of therapeutic communication between the nurse and the client. A communication system includes the source, transmitter, channel, receiver, and destination. The source of communication refers to formulation of meaning to a message. The transmitter transforms this message into information. During the process of transmission, channels can take several written messages and at the same time radio for audio messages. The receiver transforms the physical aspects of the information into a message. Finally, at the destination, a person's perceptual abilities interpret the message.

Feedback, an important factor in communication, is part of the two-way set of components that operates the communication system. Communication theory is the basis of problem-solving theories. The nurse uses problem solving to decode the communication between the nurse and client in the mental health setting.

Important Models of Mental Health Nursing

Since the beginning of nursing theory, nurses have been creating a theoretic system based on the assumption that each person is a unique blend of physical, cognitive, emotional, and spiritual factors that cannot be unblended. Nursing's emphasis on holistic viewing began as far back as Florence Nightingale. She challenged nursing to define itself and consistently pushed to do this herself.

In the years between Nightingale's work and the early 1950s, medical models of nursing, set forth primarily in procedural manuals, were developed. This procedural phase was important; it demonstrated that nursing was finally defining itself. After World War II, the focus and direction of nursing changed. The emphasis shifted from nursing action as tasks to nursing action as interpersonal processes. The increasing emphasis on interpersonal processes is evident in the following descriptions of the work of nurse-theorists.

Virginia Henderson Henderson's work, which first appeared in 1939, was greatly influenced by human need theory. A key concept proposed by Henderson was personhood. In personhood, mind and body were inseparable. Henderson saw that the unique function of the nurse was to assist a person in performing activities contributing to health. This assistance was needed when a client was sick or well and helped the client toward recovery or a peaceful death. The nurse helped the client develop the strength, will, or knowledge to gain independence as rapidly as possible. The components of Henderson's definition of nursing remain practicable today.

Henderson viewed the nursing process as individualized care based on patient needs. The care would be given according to a plan with a continual analysis of needs. It was Henderson who first wrote of patient-centered care and who proposed the nurse's independent role and function (Safier, 1977).

Hildegard Peplau In 1952, in *Interpersonal Relations in Nursing,* Hildegard Peplau analyzed nursing action by using an interpersonal framework. Communication theory, specifically the work of H. S. Sullivan, influenced Peplau's thinking.

Peplau defined nursing as an interpersonal process. The major concepts of her theory included growth, development, communication, and roles.

The therapeutic nurse-client relationship was the core of Peplau's theory. Communication was a problem-solving process that took place within the relationship—a collaborative process in which the nurse might assume many roles in helping clients meet needs and continue growth and development. Peplau believed that, as clients' conflicts and anxieties were resolved, their personalities were strengthened.

Like Henderson, Peplau viewed each person as an individual shaped by culture and biology. Peplau recognized four phases in the therapeutic relationship. During the first phase, orientation, the client decided that he or she needed help. Trust and rapport were then built between the nurse and the client so that accurate assessment and mutual goal setting could take place. During the second phase, identification, both the nurse's and the client's expectations were explored. The client began to trust the nurse and see him or her as someone who could help. Problems were identified during this phase, and initial solutions were discussed. During the third phase, exploration, the client might waver between dependence and independence. The nurse returned the client's trust by allowing him or her to explore and test solutions. Ideally, the client used all available resources to solve problems. During the fourth phase, resolution, a final battle between dependence and independence might occur. If the nurse had been successful and the relationship with the client effective, difficulties in terminating the relationship might occur. The strong nurse-client relationship, which had been built during the other phases, assisted the client in successfully meeting the challenge of resolution.

Far ahead of her own time in development of theory, Peplau set the groundwork for later theorists. Peplau remains a powerful force in developing mental health nursing theory and practice.

Ida Jean Orlando In 1961 Orlando presented a publication entitled *The Dynamic Nurse-Patient Relationship*. Orlando's work was greatly influenced by communication theory and drew from her own nursing notes. Orlando proposed that the nurse's responsibility was to see that the client's needs were met either by her own activity or by calling in the assistance of others. Orlando said that the nursing process was initiated by the client expressing the meaning of his or her behavior. To determine the nature of the client's distress and the help required to relieve it, the nurse had to explore the distress with the client. Orlando viewed the nursing process as a tool used to obtain an outcome through problem solving.

Dorothy Johnson Johnson defined the person as a bio-psycho-social being. Johnson's work was influenced by general systems theory and human needs theory. Johnson saw nursing care as a direct service to people and said that the achievement and maintenance of a stable state was nursing's contribution to client welfare. To Johnson, the primary purpose of nursing care was to assist the client to achieve and maintain this stability.

Johnson outlined four stages of the nursing process: first- and second-level assessment; diagnosis; intervention (restricting, defending, inhibiting, and facilitating); and evaluation (Johnson, 1980; 1961).

Imogene M. King King published *Toward a Theory for Nursing* in 1971. King's work was largely influenced by general systems theory. King, who thought of people as open systems, regarded nursing as a process of interactions between the nurse and client. In interaction, the nurse and client perceived each other and the situation, and through communication they achieved goals. King saw communication as the means by which goals were developed and explored as well as agreed on and achieved.

King viewed the nursing process as a human or interpersonal process. She defined it as action, reaction, interaction, and transaction between individuals and groups within social systems (King, 1981).

June Mellow Mellow introduced the second theoretic approach to psychiatric nursing five years after Peplau introduced her systematic framework for psychiatric nursing. Unlike other nursing theorists, Mellow based her work on psychoanalytic theory.

Mellow's concept of nursing and the nursing process was a result of her one-to-one work with schizophrenic patients. Mellow believed a symbiotic relationship developed between the patient and the nurse. Instead of investigating the developmental origins of the disorder, Mellow thought the nurse should attempt to provide corrective emotional experience. Through talking, listening, bathing, feeding, dressing, and providing recreation, Mellow believed nurses could develop emotional bonds with patients (Lego, 1975; Murry and Huelskoetter, 1983).

Dorothea E. Orem Orem developed the concepts of self-care, self-care deficits, and universal and health deviations. General systems theory influenced the development of Orem's work. Orem defined nursing as an effort toward designing, providing, and managing systems of therapeutic self-care. To Orem, the goal of nursing was to help individuals or groups when they needed help to achieve health.

Orem identified three steps to the nursing process: nursing diagnosis, design of a system of nursing, and actions of the nurse (Orem, 1980).

Martha Rogers Rogers contributed greatly to the nursing literature with her conception of humans as unitary and synergistic. General systems theory supported her work. Rogers stated that nursing was the attempt to promote symphonic interaction between humans and the environment. She believed that the coherence and integrity of humans and the direction and redirection of patterns of interaction between people and the environment assisted in realizing the potential for maximum health.

Recognizing the life process as the setting for nursing, Rogers saw the nursing process as nursing diagnosis, intervention, and evaluation of intervention (Rogers, 1970).

Joyce Travelbee Travelbee expanded the work of Orlando by writing on the unique nature of nursing practice in the interpersonal relationship. Travelbee saw nursing as an interpersonal process in which the nurse assisted the person or family to prevent or cope with the experience of illness and to find meaning in the experience.

Travelbee applied the nursing process to the development of nurse-client relationships. The phases Travelbee identified were the original encounter, emerging identities, empathy, sympathy, and rapport. Travelbee saw it was necessary to use observation, interpretation, decision making, action, and evaluation in developing nurse-client relationships (Travelbee, 1966).

Sister Callista Roy Roy developed the Roy Adaptation Model, which was based on the principles of adaptation theory. In Roy's model humans consisted of different elements linked together in a way that made the whole system susceptible to stresses from within the system or from the environment. Roy thought the recipient of nursing care was an adaptive system. She wrote that the system, in its simplest form, was a mechanism involving input, internal and feedback processes, and output. Nursing action, according to Roy, should promote patient adaptation.

The Roy Adaptation Model was based on eight assumptions that viewed humans as bio-psychosocial beings in constant interaction with a changing environment. Roy viewed health and illness as an inevitable dimension of life and believed people must be able to adapt to respond positively to life. She saw a person's ability to adapt as a function of his or her adaptation level, the condition of the client before adaptation, and the types and amounts of stimuli he or she was exposed to. Roy wrote that the adaptive level was the range of stimulation that led to a positive response. Roy believed a person could adapt according to physiologic needs, self-concept, role function, and interdependent relationships (Riehl and Roy, 1980).

Roy viewed nursing as a problem-solving process. She identified six steps in the nursing process: first-level assessment, second-level assessment, problem identification, goal setting, intervention or selection of approaches, and evaluation (Roy and Roberts, 1981).

Betty Neuman Neuman developed a nursing model for a total-person approach to client problems. Drawing significantly on Selye's General Adaptation Syndrome (GAS) theory, Neuman defined nursing as a unique profession primarily concerned with variables affecting the person's response to stressors.

Neuman developed an assessment-intervention tool for obtaining biographic client data; stressors perceived by the client; stressors perceived by the care givers; identification of intrapersonal, interpersonal, and extrapersonal factors; statement of the problem; summary of the goals; and intervention plan (Neuman, 1980).

Overview of the Mental Health Nursing Process

As has been stated, a philosophic base provides a foundation for nursing. The nurse enters the mental health setting with a set of beliefs and values underlying all the actions related to caring for clients. Similarly, each client has a set of beliefs and values that the nurse must try to understand. To help develop this understanding, the nurse applies theoretic concepts. The nursing process is the mechanism guiding the nurse's cognitive process in caring for clients.

Many authors have written about the nursing process. For instance, Yura and Walsh (1978) view the nursing process as the essence of nursing because it is central to all nursing actions. The structure of the nursing process provides a base from which systematic actions can proceed. Although there are variations among groups of nurses in the steps in the nursing process, the underlying theme is that the process is an organized, systematic, deliberate means of providing care to clients.

As the practice of nursing in general and mental health in particular has evolved, many changes have taken place. To better understand the present standards of practice, it is first necessary to review the historic perspectives of the nursing process.

Until the 1950s, nursing was viewed in functional terms. That is, nursing was described by the tasks and procedures performed by nurses. Peplau was the first to describe phases of a nurse-patient relationship. Later, Orlando, addressing the interpersonal aspects of the nurse-client relationship, stressed the need for deliberative rather than intuitive nursing action.

In the 1960s, nursing leaders began to write about nursing process as a scientific approach. Dorothy Johnson wrote about the necessity of systematic data collection with rigorous analysis (Johnson, 1961). In 1966, Kelly presented an article in *Nursing Research* that first described nursing diagnosis as determining the cause and alleviation of a symptom. Kelly saw the nursing assessment as incorporating not only data on the client's physical signs and symptoms but also on the client's social history and cultural background and on the physical and psychologic factors in the environment (Kelly, 1964; 1966).

In 1967, Yura and Walsh wrote the first major text describing four steps to the nursing process. By the 1970s, nursing was viewed by the profession as a scientific discipline. In 1973, the ANA adopted the *Standards of Nursing Practice.* These standards reflect a five-step nursing process.*

In 1982 the ANA adopted the *Standards of Psychiatric and Mental Health Nursing Practice* which also set forth a five-step nursing process. The steps were data collection, diagnosis, planning, treatment, and evaluation. (See Table 2–1 for a summary of these standards.) Like the nursing process, the mental health nursing process consists of five steps:

1. Assessment
2. Diagnosis
3. Planning
4. Intervention
5. Evaluation

(See Figure 2–2 for the interrelationships in this process and Table 2–2 for the five steps of the mental health nursing process.)

Assessment in Mental Health Nursing

Assessment involves reviewing the human condition from a data base in order to diagnose potential problems or affirm a state of wellness. In assessing, the nurse is able to confirm an illness state, identify prevailing problems, determine potential problems, and identify the wellness level of the client. Data collection, the basis of assessment, provides a comprehensive picture of the client. Accurate, systematic data collection leads to identification of client problems and nursing diagnoses. Therefore,

*Many states have revised their nursing practice to incorporate the nursing process. Most recently, the National State Board Test Pool (NCLEX) revised the examination format to include the five steps of the nursing process. Although the state board examination refers to the second step of the process as analysis, there has been a recent move toward calling this step diagnosis (Gordon, 1982).

Table 2–1 *Professional Practice Standards for Mental Health Nursing*

Standard I. Theory
The nurse applies appropriate theory that is scientifically sound as a basis for decisions regarding nursing practice

Standard II. Data Collection
The nurse continuously collects data that are comprehensive, accurate, and systematic

Standard III. Diagnosis
The nurse utilizes nursing diagnosis and/or standard classification of mental disorders to express conclusions supported by recorded assessment data and current scientific premises

Standard IV. Planning
The nurse develops a nursing care plan with specific goals and interventions delineating nursing actions unique to each client's needs

Standard V. Intervention
The nurse intervenes as guided by the nursing care plan to implement nursing actions that promote, maintain, or restore physical and mental health, prevent illness, and effect rehabilitation

Standard V-A. Intervention: Psychotherapeutic Interventions
The nurse uses psychotherapeutic interventions to assist clients in regaining or improving their previous coping abilities and to prevent further disability

Standard V-B. Intervention: Health Teaching
The nurse assists client, families, and groups to achieve satisfying and productive patterns of living through health teaching

Standard V-C. Intervention: Activities of Daily Living
The nurse uses the activities of daily living in a goal-directed way to foster adequate self-care and physical and mental well-being of clients

Standard V-D. Intervention: Somatic Therapies
The nurse uses knowledge of somatic therapies and applies related clinical skills in working with clients

Standard V-E. Intervention: Therapeutic Environment
The nurse provides, structures, and maintains a therapeutic environment in collaboration with the client and other health care providers

Standard V-F. Intervention: Psychotherapy
The nurse utilizes advanced clinical expertise in individual, group, and family psychotherapy, child psychotherapy, and other treatment modalities to function as a psychotherapist, and recognizes professional accountability for nursing practice

Standard VI. Evaluation
The nurse evaluates client responses to nursing actions in order to revise the data base, nursing diagnoses, and nursing care plan

Source: Adapted from E. Carter, *Standards of Psychiatric and Mental Health Nursing Practice* (American Nurses' Association, 1982). Reprinted with permission.

the plan and implementation of interventions rely on an accurate data base.

There are many sources of data, but the primary source is the client. The client's family and significant others are additional sources of data. Within the clinical setting are many sources of data: medical records, social records, results of diagnostic tests, nursing notes, change-of-shift reports, nursing care plans, and progress notes. When possible, a survey of the client's home and community provides still another source of data (Christensen, 1982B).

A primary function of the nurse in assessing the client is determining the extent to which human needs have been fulfilled. This provides a holistic approach to the care of the client. This approach fosters the individuality of the client by recognizing the variations in the person's patterns of interactions, the client's self-awareness, and the client's view of others. Along with recognizing the client's individuality, the nurse must also understand his or her own uniqueness. Each nurse has unique strengths, limitations, patterns of response, values, and attitudes that must be recognized before responding to those of the client. The nurse strives to be sensitive to the client's communication and understand its meaning within the client's frame of reference rather than the nurse's.

With a focus on assessing information related to the human needs of the client, it is important to include some general information about the client in the assessment. General factors about the client include age, gender, education, employment status, growth and development, cultural background, socioeconomic status, religious preference, physical

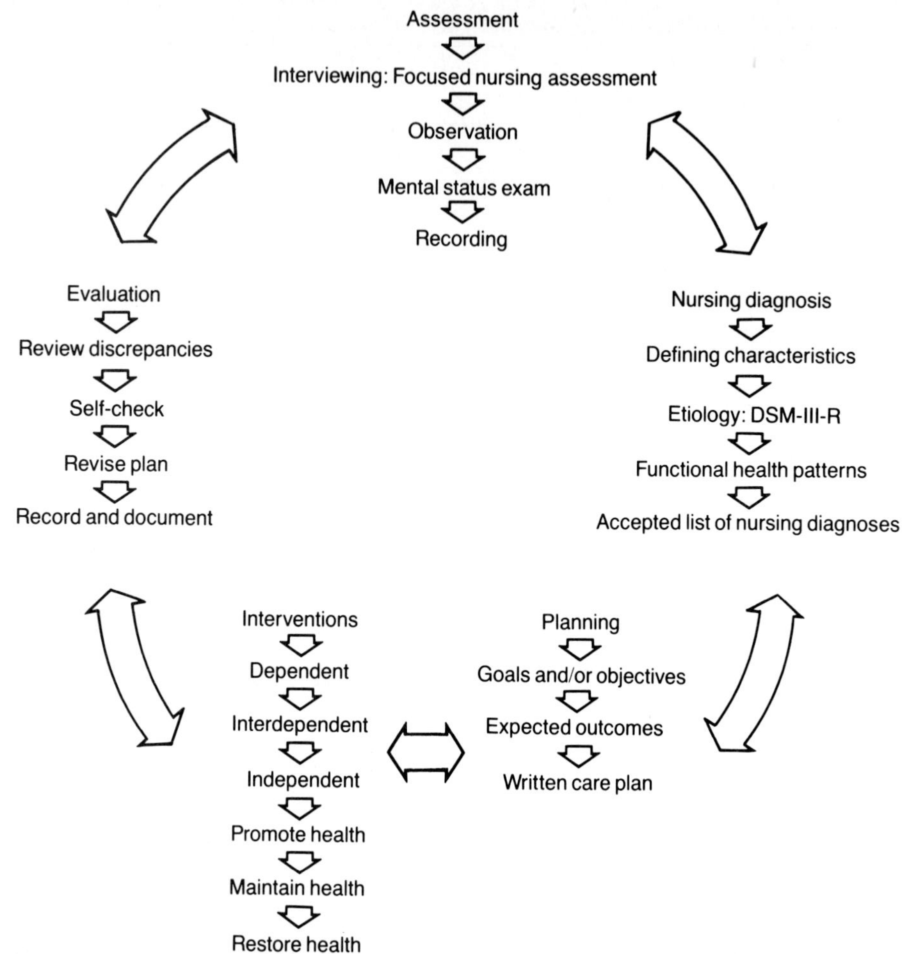

Figure 2–2 *The mental health nursing process.*

status, emotional status, coping patterns, lifestyle patterns, interaction patterns, and view of wellness-illness (Carpenito 1989A; Yura and Walsh, 1988).

The Nursing History

The nursing history is the main tool used in data collection. The nursing history is obtained through a planned interview with the client. The areas of data collection on a nursing history are based on a nursing model. For the purpose of this text, an eclectic model will be used. A sample nursing history follows. This tool—which incorporates biologic, social, cultural, and psychologic aspects of care—is designed for the initial assessment of all mental health clients. In each of the disorders chapters, nursing histories specific to the disorder are presented as Focused Nursing Assessments. They are suggested for use along with the basic model shown in this chapter.

Nursing History

General information

Biographical data

Name:

Address (number, city, state):

Table 2–2 *Five Steps of the Mental Health Nursing Process*

I. Assessment
  A. Systematic data collection
    1. Effective interviewing
    2. Observations of objective and subjective behaviors
  B. Recording of data
  C. Data review of documents available in the practice setting (ie, chart, medical histories, etc)

II. Nursing Diagnosis
  A. Standard nursing diagnoses
  B. Comparison of standard nursing diagnoses to diagnostic classification of mental disorders
  C. Recognition of actual or potential health problems within the scope of mental health nursing practice
  D. Opportunities for validation of diagnosis by peers in the practice setting

III. Planning
  A. Development of nursing care plan
    1. Specific client goals based on client needs
    2. Interventions unique to client needs
  B. Guide to therapeutic interventions
  C. Collaboration with others

IV. Intervention
  A. Nursing actions to promote, maintain, or restore physical and mental health
  B. Nursing actions to prevent illness
  C. Nursing actions to effect rehabilitation
  D. Interventions validated by client and peers
  E. Psychotherapeutic interventions
  F. Health-teaching interventions
  G. Activities of daily living interventions
  H. Somatic therapy interventions
  I. Therapeutic environment interventions

V. Evaluation
  A. Recording, communicating, and revising
  B. Evaluate client responses to nursing interventions
    1. Revise data base
    2. Revise nursing diagnosis
    3. Revise care plan
  C. Pursue validation, suggestions, and new information
  D. Document results of evaluation
  E. Evaluate self-performance on therapeutic interventions

(Nursing History continued)

Age:
Gender:
Ethnic origin:
Primary language spoken:
Birthplace:
Religious preference:
Marital status:
Occupation:
Educational background:
Employment status:
Health insurance:
Medical diagnosis (DSM-III-R):

Interview information
Date of admission:
Time of admission:
Date of interview:
Time of interview:
Interviewing nurse:
Others present for interview:

General observations made by the nurse

Appearance
Build and weight:
Describe what the client is wearing:
Is client attire appropriate for the environment:
Are there any particular nonverbal communications (ie, body language, eye contact, gestures, affect, etc):
Does client have steadiness of gait:
Is there any visible alteration in physical function:
Is there any visible alteration in mental function:
How does client move and speak:
Appearance of skin (eg, color, abrasions, lesions, rashes, reddened areas, etc):
Dentures:
Eyeglasses, contacts:
Prostheses, and if so, what kind:

Basic needs and activities for daily living
Air:
Observe client's breathing pattern for alterations and/or deficits:
Ask client to describe any difficulties in breathing:
Circulation:
Observe client's extremities for color, movement, and function:
Ask client to describe any difficulties in circulation:
Food/Fluid:
What foods do you eat?
Describe any dietary restrictions you have:
How many meals do you eat in a day?
Do you eat alone or with others?
Where do you eat your meals?
How often do you eat at home?
How often do you eat in restaurants?
What vitamins do you take, if any?
Have you had any recent changes in your diet or weight? If so, describe the changes:
Have you had any recent increases or decreases in your appetite? If so, describe the changes:
How many and what type of snacks do you eat each day?
Elimination:
How often do you urinate?
Describe the appearance of your urine:

Do you have burning when you urinate?
Describe the smell of your urine:
How often do you have bowel movements?
Describe the appearance of your bowel movements (eg, formed, loose, color, etc):
How often do you use laxatives to have a bowel movement?
How often do you use enemas to have a bowel movement?
What special foods do you eat to help you urinate or have bowel movements?

Neuro/Sensory:
Do you wear glasses to read? drive? other activities?
How long have you worn glasses?
Do you wear a hearing aid? If so, how long?
If you do not wear glasses or have a hearing aid, do you think you need them?
Do you have difficulty in identifying odors? If so, what odors?
Do you have difficulty tasting anything? If so, what?

Sleep/Rest:
In each 24 hours how much do you sleep and between what hours do you sleep?
How often do you take naps?
How do you feel with the amount of sleep you get (eg, rested, tired, etc)?
How often do you wake up in the night?
What helps you sleep (eg, back rubs, music, warm milk, sleeping pills, etc)?
What disturbs your sleep?
If you are disturbed, can you go back to sleep?
Do you sleep with a night-light?
Do you sleep with the window open or closed?
When do you rise?
Do you have difficulty sleeping in strange surroundings? If so, describe the difficulty:

Safety:
What household safety precautions do you take (eg, locking doors in the day or at night, bolting windows, keeping medicines clearly labeled, taking medicines as ordered by the doctor, etc)?
Describe how your usual environment is safe or unsafe:
What do you think is the best way to maintain safety?

Mobility:
What kind of physical activities do you do daily?
How long has it been since you've done physical exercise?
What kind of physical activity do you do at your job?
Are you satisfied with the amount of exercise you do? Why or why not?
Describe any physical limitations you have:

Comfort/Pain:
What type of pain do you most frequently experience?
What do you usually do for this pain?
Do you smoke? If so, how much?
Do you drink alcoholic beverages? If yes, how often? With whom do you drink? Do you drink alone?
Do you take tranquilizers? If so, which ones?
What other drugs do you take regularly?
How much coffee, tea, or cola do you drink a day?
Do you take drugs and alcohol at the same time? How often?
What foods are you allergic to?
What medications are you allergic to?
What other allergies do you have (eg, dust, animals, adhesive tape, etc)?
What type of treatment have you had for your allergies?
What major illnesses have you had?
What major surgeries have you had?
What impact have your illnesses or surgeries had on your current lifestyle?
What treatments are you currently receiving for your ailments?

Hygiene:
How often do you bathe or shower?
Do you prefer baths, showers, or sink baths?
What time of day do you prefer to bathe or shower?
What type of deodorants or colognes do you use?
How often do you brush your teeth? Floss your teeth?
When do you have dental checkups?

Sexuality:
How are your sexual needs being met (eg, intercourse, touching, fondling, masturbation, etc)?
Describe your needs in relation to your partner's needs?
Do they coincide? Conflict? How do you deal with your partner's needs?

Female clients:
Describe your menstrual cycles (eg, regularity, flow, etc):
When do you examine your breasts?
When do you have Pap smears?

Teaching/Learning:
What is your reason for coming in for treatment?
What do you expect to receive as a result of treatment?
How do you prefer to receive information (eg, printed materials, films, classes, etc)?
Describe any learning needs you feel you have:
What is the highest grade you attended in school?
How often do you read books? What kind of books or magazines do you like to read?
Are there any cultural beliefs or practices related to your illness that we should be aware of? If so, what are those beliefs (eg, evil spirits, healers, etc)?

Sociopsychologic:
What is your primary psychologic problem?
What do you think caused this problem?
What do you think is your major problem at this time?
How long have you had this problem?
What will help you get better?
Do you think you will get better? Why or why not?

Psychologic health

Coping patterns:
Who are the people significant to you?
Who do you talk to on a regular basis?
How much time do you spend alone?

How many people do you relate to each day?
How often do you see other people?
What do you do to handle stressful situations in your life (eg, eat, smoke, sleep, drink alcohol, have sex, withdraw, become angry, talk to someone, pray, read, listen to music, etc)?

Interaction patterns:
Who are the people in your immediate family?
How do you express your thoughts and feelings to others (eg, verbally, through hints, nonverbally)?
When do you voice your opinions to your family? Friends?
How do you feel about the way you interact with your family? Friends?

Cognitive patterns:
Did you have difficulty learning in school?
How often do you read? Do you like to read newspapers, books? What is the last book you read?
How difficult is it for you to learn new things?
How do you learn best (eg, listening, reading, watching)?
How do you function in your schoolwork or on the job?

Self-concept:
Are you at your desired weight? Why or why not?
What do you think about your appearance?
Have you had any physical alterations in your body?
How difficult was it to accept those changes?
Have those physical changes affected your relationships with family, friends, coworkers? If so, how?
Do you see yourself as better than, equal to, or less than equal to other people?
How do you express your thoughts and feelings to others?

Emotional patterns:
What type of mood are you usually in (eg, calm, depressed, pleasant, angry, excited, agitated, etc)?
Describe any mood changes you have had recently and how you expressed yourself during this period:
Are you satisfied with your usual mood? Why or why not?
What are your relationships with others when your moods change?
Are you satisfied with your behavior during mood changes? Why or why not?

Sociologic health

Family health:
Do you have any of these chronic illnesses in your family:
______ tuberculosis
______ diabetes
______ cancer
______ hypertension
______ depression
______ anxiety
______ heart disease
______ kidney disease
______ alcoholism
______ drug addiction
______ psychosis

Significant relationships:
Who are the most significant people in your life?
To whom do you feel closest? Why?
As a whole, how does your family get along?
What are the major conflicts in your family?
When your family members have concerns or need help, to whom do they go?
How do you feel your family supports your health-related concerns?

Family coping patterns:
How does your family handle stress?
How does your family make decisions? Who has the last word in decisions?
What happens if someone in the family disagrees with another?
Who is the caretaker if someone in the family gets sick?
What is your role in the family? Is this a role you are comfortable in? Why or why not?

Cultural patterns:
What social values were you reared with?
Of those values, which ones are important to you now?
What are your family traditions (eg, family gatherings, celebrations, head of home, foods, religious activities, health care practices, etc)?
In which of these traditions do you participate?

Recreation patterns:
What does your family do for fun?
How do you feel about leisure time (eg, dread it, look forward to it, etc)?
What are your hobbies? What hobbies do other members of your family have?
What interests do you have outside your work and family?
What resources does the family have for being involved in their interests (eg, materials, money, transportation, time, etc)?
When was the last time you and your family participated in leisure activities?

Environment:
Do you live in a multiple- or single-family dwelling?
Are you comfortable in the place you live? Why or why not?
What kind of personal space do you have?
Do you have pets? What kind?
Are there environmental problems of concern to you (eg, noises, sounds, odors, etc)?

Spiritual patterns:
What is your religious preference?
Are you practicing the same religion you were reared with? If not, do you feel any conflict about this?
Does your family practice your religion? If not, what do they think about your differences?
What are your primary religious practices (eg, meditation, prayer, bible study, church attendance, etc)?

Values:
What things are most important to you in life? Least important?
How do you incorporate these things into your lifestyle? If you do not, are you comfortable with this?

How do you feel about the morals you were brought up with?
Do your morals cause internal conflict or conflict with your family? If so, describe the conflict:
How do you fit into society?
Would you help someone you didn't know? Someone you did know? Why or why not?
Can you accept help from people you don't know? People you do know? Why or why not?
Self-evaluation:
Describe your major strengths:
Describe your major weaknesses:
Describe your special talents:
Rate yourself in comparison to others:
Summary of nonverbal observations
Emotional tone of the interview:
Client's attitude toward interview and interviewer:
Facial expressions, gestures, posturing, eye contact, tone of voice, movements, hand tremors, or other activities during the interview:
Topics avoided by client:
Interviewer's response to client:
Any characteristic speech patterns:
Client's grooming (eg, clean, no body odors, nails, hair, etc):
Pupil constriction or dilation:
Concentration on discussion (eg, attention span, quick movements, yawning, shifting in seat, eye contact, response time, understanding of spoken word, etc):

CASE EXAMPLE

Application of Nursing History to a Clinical Situation

Sharon S., a 35-year-old unemployed nurse assistant, was admitted to an orthopedic unit for chronic low-back pain. Sharon was allowed a seven-day admission to regulate her pain medication schedule and reduce her pain with pelvic traction. Sharon was discontent with the medication schedule ordered by the physician and became very hostile and demanding with the nursing staff. The staff found Sharon next to impossible to deal with and asked Sharon's physician for a mental health consult.

The following information was gathered by the nurse interviewing Sharon for a mental health consult.

Nursing History

General information
Biographical data
Name: Sharon S.
Address: 883 N. Millbrook, Apt. 3; Stockton, CA
Age: 35
Gender: Female
Ethnic origin: Caucasian
Primary language spoken: English
Birthplace: Bowling Green, Ohio
Religious preference: Protestant
Marital status: Divorced
Occupation: Nurse assistant
Educational background: High school graduate
Employment status: Unemployed
Health insurance: None
Medical diagnosis (DSM-III-R): Chronic low-back pain, no DSM-III-R diagnosis
Interview information
Date of admission: August 4, 1989
Time of admission: 9:00 A.M.
Date of interview: August 5, 1989
Time of interview: 8:00 P.M.
Interviewing nurse: Robert Silva, RN
Others present for interview: None

General observations made by the nurse
Appearance
Build and weight: A medium-frame female, approximately 5′4″ and 150 lb
Describe what the client is wearing: A black nylon gown and a blue flannel robe with black step-in slippers.
Is client attire appropriate for the environment: Since Sharon is in the acute hospital, the bed clothing is appropriate. However, the black nylon gown is very revealing and causes the client some difficulty in being taken in and out of pelvic traction.
Are there any particular nonverbal communications (eg, body language, eye contact, gestures, affect, etc): Sharon shuffles slowly when she walks and her shoulders roll forward. When Sharon sits, she shifts her weight to the right side. Sharon avoids looking the nurse in the eye. At times Sharon's eyes close and she grimaces in pain.
Does the client have steadiness of gait: Sharon is steady on her feet. However, she moves very slowly.
Is there any visible alteration in physical function: Sharon has no visible alterations in physical function.
Is there any visible alteration in mental function: Sharon responds slowly and is frequently interrupted by what she calls "stabbing pains" in her back.
How does the client move and speak: Sharon prefers to find a comfortable position before she begins to talk. Sharon speaks slowly. Sometimes she stops in midsentence because she has lost her train of thought. Sharon slurs some words when speaking in long sentences.
Appearance of skin (eg, color, abrasions, lesions, rashes, reddened areas, etc): Sharon is pale with dark circles under her eyes. She has reddened areas on her hips from the irritation of the pelvic traction belt. No bruises, abrasions, or lesions are noted.

Dentures: None

Eyeglasses, contacts: Sharon wears glasses for reading. She does not have contact lenses.

Prostheses: None

Basic needs and activities for daily living

Air: Sharon appears to have a normal breathing pattern. Sharon states that she usually has no difficulty in breathing except during acute episodes of pain when she may hyperventilate.

Circulation: Sharon's hands and feet are pale. Pulses are present in all extremities. Sharon is able to use her extremities normally. However, Sharon states that pain from her back radiates down her legs. Sharon states that she has no difficulty in circulation.

Food/Fluid: Sharon likes all types of food. However, she avoids milk products because of allergies. Sharon snacks through the day on nuts, cereal, or crackers and cheese and eats a regular meal at night. She usually eats alone while watching TV. Sharon often eats out at fast-food restaurants. She does not take vitamins. Sharon has noted a 15-pound weight gain over the past year.

Elimination: Sharon urinates about four times a day. Her urine is amber, she has no burning with urination, and no foul odors. Sharon has bowel movements every three days. Her BMs are hard and formed. Sharon uses milk of magnesia at least twice a month to have bowel movements. Sometimes Sharon uses packaged enemas to have bowel movements.

Neuro/Sensory: Sharon wears reading glasses. She has had glasses since she was in high school. Sharon states she does not have any hearing difficulties, difficulty identifying odors, or difficulty tasting anything.

Sleep/Rest: Sharon feels she has a problem getting enough sleep. She takes pain medicine every four hours, usually Empirin #4, and takes a muscle relaxant every six hours, usually Valium 10 mg. Sharon gets rests only between the times she takes the medicines. Usually she gets only about four hours of sleep at night. Sharon's sleep is easily disturbed if she moves suddenly, causing back pain. Sharon says one of the reasons she came to the hospital was to get some rest. She feels tired all the time.

Safety: Sharon feels her home environment is safe. She keeps her doors locked at night and tries to follow doctor's orders regarding the medications prescribed for her. Sharon keeps her medicines in a cabinet in the originally labeled containers.

Mobility: Sharon does no daily physical activity. Her pain is so severe that she is unable to do any exercise. Since Sharon has been incapacitated by pain, she has had to quit her job as a nurse assistant. Sharon feels her physical capacity is so diminished that it is an effort to get dressed in the morning.

Comfort/Pain: Sharon has been experiencing back pain for about six months, following a car accident. Sharon takes pain medication and muscle relaxants for the pain. Sharon smokes about one pack of cigarettes daily. She rarely drinks alcoholic beverages because of taking so much pain medication. Sharon drinks at least a pot of coffee a day and drinks three to four colas each day. Sharon is allergic to milk products and states she has allergies to Demerol, penicillin, Soma, and Flexiril. Sharon was not able to specify the reactions she has to food or drugs and has never been treated for allergies. Sharon has been basically healthy except for a hysterectomy at age 28 and an automobile accident three years ago. In the accident, Sharon fractured C-5, C-6, and strained the thoracic-lumbar region. Six months ago the lumbar area was reinjured in another automobile accident. Since the accident, Sharon had to quit working and has been on around-the-clock pain medications for the lumbar pain.

Hygiene: Sharon tries to take a shower daily in the evening. She uses deodorant and cologne because she feels the pain medications cause her to smell "funny." Sharon brushes her teeth in the morning and at night. She sees a dentist once a year when she can afford to go.

Sexuality: Sharon was not willing to give any details of her relationship with her boyfriend of the past two years. She stated that what they do is their personal business. Sharon has had a hysterectomy so has no periods. She does not check her breasts and does not wish to learn to check her breasts.

Teaching/Learning: Sharon stated she came in for treatment to get some sleep and rest. She felt that her pain medications at home were not helping her and she needed something stronger than Empirin #4 for her pain. Sharon is upset with her doctor because she was taken off her every six-hour Valium when morphine 8 mg was ordered every four hours around the clock. Sharon felt she was getting no pain relief after the first 24 hours in the hospital. The doctor refused to give her any more Valium or to increase her morphine dosage. Sharon stated that she had been real obnoxious to the nurses but they didn't seem to think she had real pain. Sharon didn't feel she had any learning needs. She was merely in the hospital to rest.

Sociopsychologic: Sharon became angry at the mention of the word *psychological*. She denied any psychological trouble and feels her problem is entirely physically based. Sharon wants to get better, but she doesn't think anything will help her now.

Psychologic health

Coping patterns: Sharon is estranged from her family. Her husband deserted her, taking their 6-year-old daughter when Sharon was recovering from her automobile accident three years ago. Sharon's parents have never been supportive and blame Sharon for the accident that destroyed her family. For the last two years Sharon has been dating a young man she met at a local bar. George, Sharon's boyfriend, has been her primary support system throughout the past two years. George has helped Sharon by keeping up her house and cooking for her since the accident six months ago. Sharon wanted him to move in, but he has not done so. Sharon doesn't see any other people besides George. Sharon says she handles stress by smoking. She notices that when she feels stressed, she smokes more cigarettes.

Interaction patterns: Sharon has no immediate family near her. She talks to her father occasionally on the telephone. Sharon says she is the strong one in her relationship with her boyfriend and has no problems verbally expressing her thoughts and feelings to him. Sharon feels she has a strong relationship with her boyfriend.

Cognitive patterns: Sharon did well in school. She states that she reads well and learns new things easily.

Self-concept: Sharon feels she is slightly overweight but is generally satisfied with her appearance. Sharon states that she has had no alterations to her body other than a hysterectomy and she is comfortable with the change in her body functions resulting from that surgery. Sharon states that she feels she is better than most people but tries not to let people know she feels that way. Sharon expresses her thoughts and feelings directly to others.

Emotional patterns: Sharon says she has been depressed since her automobile accident six months ago. She has stayed pretty much to herself while trying to get her back pain under control. Sharon says she sometimes doesn't get dressed all day and stays in her bed clothes. Sharon states that her boyfriend has helped her get through this trying period by cooking for her and encouraging her to go on with daily activities. Sharon says she wants to stop being depressed and get on with her life, without pain.

Sociologic health

Family health: Sharon denies any of the following diseases in her family history.

______ tuberculosis
______ diabetes
______ cancer
______ hypertension
______ depression
______ anxiety
______ heart disease
______ kidney disease
______ alcoholism
______ drug addiction
______ psychosis

Significant relationships: Sharon states that she feels closest to her boyfriend because he is there when she needs him. Sharon feels her family has drifted apart because of her parent's divorce several years ago. She denied any major conflicts in the family. Sharon states that her family does not like to hear about her illnesses. They quit coming to see her after her first automobile accident and change the subject when she talks about any of her physical problems.

Family coping patterns: Sharon stated that her family usually ignored stress and waited for it to go away. Sharon stated she couldn't remember much about family roles.

Cultural patterns: Sharon stated she was reared with Christian values and she still believes in those values. When asked to elaborate Sharon changed the subject.

Recreation patterns: Sharon says she has no hobbies and does not like leisure time. Sharon has spent most of her time recently focused on the pain she is experiencing and has not even felt like watching TV.

Environment: Sharon lives in an apartment and is satisfied with her living arrangements. She lives in an older neighborhood with few children. The neighborhood is quiet and most of the people are retired and stick to themselves. Sharon likes this arrangement because she is not forced to socialize with her neighbors.

Spiritual patterns: Sharon states she is Protestant and rarely goes to church. Sharon says religion is not a big part of her life.

Values: Sharon says regaining her pain-free state of health is most important to her right now. The least important thing to Sharon is getting remarried and having a family. Sharon says she is comfortable with her morals and changed the subject on attempts to explore this topic. Sharon did not feel comfortable being in a "charity" hospital and felt people were treating her with indifference because of her pay status. Sharon stated that she felt she would be treated better if she had insurance and was in a different hospital. She stated she doesn't like the superior attitude of the nurses taking care of her.

Self-evaluation: Sharon had difficulty stating her strengths and weaknesses. She stated that she could handle pain better than most because most people would have "gone off the deep end" by now with the kind of pain she had experienced.

Summary of nonverbal observations

Sharon seemed to be controlling her anger through most of the interview. She was trying to be polite but, at the same time, resented the interviewer. Sharon was cooperative and tried to answer the questions. At times, Sharon simply avoided the issue being discussed rather than confront the issue. At the beginning of the interview, Sharon stated that she resented the "psych crap" being used on her. She let the interviewer know that she would answer only what she felt like answering. As the interview progressed Sharon seemed more relaxed and less like she was being analyzed. At the beginning of the interview, Sharon would not make eye contact with the interviewer, but toward the middle of the interview, as Sharon began to relax more, she had eye contact with the interviewer. Sharon grimaced with pain several times during the interview. It is difficult to evaluate the genuineness of the pain because of the affect of the client. Sharon wanted the interviewer to think she was in excruciating pain during the interview. Yet, when the interview moved to a topic of interest, Sharon seemed to lose interest in expressing her pain. The client definitely avoided talking about family relationships and the relationship with her boyfriend. Sharon spoke slowly and at times slurred her speech. She had an injection of morphine before the interview. The interviewer had difficulty empathizing with Sharon because Sharon's attitude toward the interviewer and other nursing staff made it difficult to please this client. Sharon had a way of making the interviewer feel uncomfortable and put on the spot. Sharon was clean and had her brown hair pulled back and braided. She was in her own nightgown and bathrobe. Sharon had dark circles under her eyes and looked tired. Sharon's pupils were constricted and she seemed to have some trouble concentrating on the interview. Sharon asked to be excused after an hour, stating she needed to try to sleep because she was feeling more relaxed after getting some of her problems "off her chest."

Other Assessment Tools

The nursing history is only one of many assessment tools that a nurse should be able to use skillfully.

Observation Essential to the clinical practice of mental health nursing is **observation**, which pervades all client situations and involves watching and listening to clients' verbal and nonverbal communication. Observation requires the nurse, who needs to be sensitive to personal biases, to use all senses—vision, hearing, smell, taste, and touch.

Several techniques of communication assist the nurse in observation. First, the nurse gives some indication of understanding the client, that is, how the client views the world and the meaning the client attaches to experiences. Next, the nurse uses open-ended questions, which help in obtaining information needed to understand the client. With this technique, the nurse also validates and clarifies the client's intent in the communication. Third, and very important to observation of the client, is active listening, which involves interpreting the client's communications. The nurse responds to both verbal and nonverbal communication. Silence can be an effective active listening tool.

The nurse should validate or seek an understanding of the client's communication and perceptions. This feedback helps clients understand how their communication affects others. The nurse can also share observations with clients about their behavior, which also helps clients understand how others view them. A means the nurse can employ to encourage the client to expand and clarify communication is restating, in which the nurse repeats the client's thought. Finally, focusing is a way to enhance the client's ability to communicate. When the nurse observes a theme in the client's communication, the client can be encouraged to more thoroughly explore the topic (Hagerty, 1984; Wilson and Kneisl, 1988).

The Interview The primary communication tool used by the nurse in the mental health setting is the interview. A purposeful interaction between the nurse and the client, the mental health or psychiatric interview focuses on behavioral disturbances and on physical, emotional, and social histories; it also tests current mental status. The interview is a systematic attempt to gain a broad data base on which to plan nursing care.

The interview may be used to collect data, establish rapport with a client, provide help for a client, or assess client behaviors. Observations and data from interviews form the basis for the nursing diagnoses.

Hagerty (1984) presented some general guidelines about conducting interviews:

- Conduct the interview in a comfortable, quiet, and private room.
- Avoid interruptions.
- Set a good climate for the interview. Attitude is the nurse's principal tool.
- Allow between 30 and 60 minutes for the interview; the purpose or surrounding circumstances determine its length.
- Explain to the client at the outset that notes will be taken. If, for some reason, they are not taken during the interview, record data immediately after the session.

The Nurse-Client Relationship In mental health nursing, the nurse-client relationship is the primary vehicle by which the nurse applies the nursing process. By developing specific communication techniques, the nurse can improve his or her ability to get information from the client. By understanding how his or her own communication style is perceived, the nurse can enhance nurse-client rapport.

Communication Techniques. Verbal techniques that foster development of therapeutic communication have been written about for many years. (See Table 2–3 for a list of therapeutic techniques of communication and Table 2–4 for a list of nontherapeutic techniques of communication.) The most helpful therapeutic techniques are described in the following paragraphs.

Broad openings are also called open-ended statements and open-ended questions. The purpose of a broad opening is to acknowledge the client and to let the client know the nurse is listening and concerned about the client's interests.

Restating is also used to let the client know the nurse is listening. The nurse repeats the main thought or idea the client has expressed. All or part of the client's statement is repeated, depending on whether the nurse wishes to reinforce or focus on something important the client has stated. At first, the nurse may feel uneasy using this technique because it seems artificial. However, after several trials, the nurse will note how much the client responds when it becomes clear the nurse has heard what has been said.

Clarification is useful when the nurse is confused about the client's thoughts or ideas. Emotions are difficult for clients to express verbally, especially if the client is disturbed about the feelings being expressed. The nurse helps the client to clarify feelings, ideas, and perceptions as well as to correlate feelings and behaviors.

Reflection is more than restating, because it can relate to message content or feelings. Reflection allows the nurse to demonstrate to the client that what has been stated has been heard and understood. Reflection can be compared to paraphrasing, that is, to repeating the client's statement by emphasizing a key word. Reflecting feelings helps the client to focus on feelings and allows the nurse to demonstrate empathy for the client.

Focusing allows the client to stay with a specific problem and to analyze the problem without moving from topic to topic. This technique helps the client deal with reality. To learn to cope with problems, clients must first be able to identify their thoughts, feelings, and beliefs.

Sharing perceptions allows the nurse to have the client verify the nurse's understanding of the client's thoughts and feelings. This technique helps the nurse convey understanding of the client's problems. Confusion can be cleared up by using this technique.

Informing simply means giving information. As a technique used for health teaching, informing allows clients an opportunity to come to their own conclusions.

Suggesting consists of the nurse presenting alternative ideas so the client can solve problems more constructively. Giving advice should be differentiated from suggesting. Giving advice involves the nurse telling the client what to do. The nurse needs to avoid having the client remain dependent on advice, for the client may blame the nurse if the advice is unsuccessful in solving problems (Cook, 1981; Stuart and Sundeen, 1983; Travelbee, 1971).

Nonverbal techniques that foster development of therapeutic communication include several within the grasp of most nurses. These are described in the following paragraphs.

Active listening is crucial to all nurse-client relationships. To understand the client, the nurse must listen. But merely hearing the words spoken by the client is not enough. To use this technique successfully, the nurse needs to give complete attention to the client. Through active listening and being able to identify with the client's world, the nurse can develop empathy for the client. Active listening is the foundation of all other therapeutic techniques.

Silence is a technique used effectively with listening. It has the advantage of encouraging the client to continue to verbalize. Silence is a difficult technique to use since it makes the nurse uncomfortable and can be misperceived by the client. The technique can be used when the nurse is unsure of how to respond to the client. Eye contact and other nonverbal behavior can communicate the nurse's continued interest in and involvement with the client.

Table 2–3 *Therapeutic Communication Techniques*

Therapeutic Techniques	*Examples*
Using silence	No verbal response Sitting with client
Accepting	Yes. Uh hmm. I follow what you said. Nodding
Giving recognition	Good morning, Mr. Smith. You've tooled a leather wallet, how nice! I notice you've combed your hair.
Offering self	I'll sit with you awhile. I'll stay here with you. I'm interested in your comfort.
Giving broad openings	Is there something you'd like to talk about? What are you thinking? Where would you like to begin?
Offering general leads	Go on. And then? Tell me about it.
Placing the event in time or in sequence	What seemed to lead up to . . . ? Was this before or after . . . ? When did this happen?
Making observations	You appear tense. Are you uncomfortable when you . . . ? I notice you're biting your lips. It makes me uncomfortable when you . . .
Encouraging description of perceptions	Tell me when you feel anxious. What is happening? What does the voice seem to be saying?
Encouraging comparison	Was this something like . . . ? Have you had similar experiences?
Restating	CLIENT: I can't sleep. I stay awake at night. NURSE: You have difficulty sleeping?
Reflecting	CLIENT: Do you think I should tell the doctor . . . ? NURSE: You sound somewhat anxious about deciding whether to tell the doctor . . .
Focusing	This point seems worth looking at more closely.
Exploring	Tell me more about that. Would you describe it more fully? What kind of work?
Giving information	My name is Sue. Visiting hours are . . . My purpose in being here is . . . I'm taking you to the . . .
Seeking clarification	I'm not sure that I follow. What would you say is the main point of what you said?
Presenting reality	I see no one else in the room. That sound was a car backfiring. Your mother is not here; I am a nurse.
Voicing doubt	Isn't that unusual? Really? That's hard to believe.
Seeking consensual validation	Tell me whether my understanding of it agrees with yours. Are you using this word to convey the idea . . . ?
Verbalizing the implied	CLIENT: I can't talk to you or anyone. It's a waste of time. NURSE: Is your feeling that no one understands?
Encouraging validation	What are your feelings about . . . ? Does this contribute to your discomfort?
Attempting to translate into feelings	CLIENT: I'm dead. NURSE: Are you suggesting that you feel lifeless?
Suggesting collaboration	Perhaps you and I can discuss and discover what produces your anxiety.
Summarizing	Now, have I got this straight? You've said that . . . During the past hour you and I have discussed . . .
Encouraging formulation of a plan of action	What could you do to let your anger out harmlessly? Next time this comes up, what might you do to handle it?

Table 2–4 *Nontherapeutic Communication Techniques*

Nontherapeutic Techniques	*Examples*	*Nontherapeutic Techniques*	*Examples*
Reassuring	I wouldn't worry about . . . Everything will be all right. You're coming along fine.	Defending	This hospital has a fine reputation. No one here would lie to you. Dr. Barnes is a very able psychiatrist.
Giving approval	That's good. I'm glad that you . . .	Requesting an explanation	Why do you think that? Why do you feel this way?
Rejecting	Let's not discuss . . . I don't want to hear about . . .	Indicating the existence of an external source	Who told you that you are Jesus? Who or what made you do that?
Disapproving	That's bad. I'd rather you wouldn't . . .	Belittling feelings expressed	CLIENT: I have nothing to live for. I wish I were dead. NURSE: Everybody gets down in the dumps.
Agreeing	That's right. I agree.		
Disagreeing	That's wrong. I definitely disagree with . . . I don't believe that.	Making stereotypical comments	Nice weather we're having. I'm fine, how are you? Keep your chin up.
Advising	I don't think you should . . . Why don't you . . . ?	Giving literal responses	CLIENT: I'm an Easter egg. NURSE: What color Easter egg?
Probing	Now tell me about . . . Tell me your life history.	Using denial	CLIENT: I'm nothing. NURSE: Of course you're something. Everybody is somebody.
Challenging	But how can you be president of the United States?	Interpreting	What you really mean is . . . Unconsciously you're saying . . .
Testing	What day is this? Do you still have the idea that . . . ?	Introducing an unrelated topic	CLIENT: I'd like to die. NURSE: Did you have visitors this weekend?

Genuineness refers to the honesty and sincerity in a nurse-client relationship. In other words, the nurse does not think or feel one way and say or behave in another. Total self-disclosure is not needed to be genuine, but disclosing that part of the self that is real in a given situation is.

Respect is essential to nurse-client relationships. The nurse views the client as a person of worth. Respecting the client does not depend on the client's behavior, for the client is accepted as is. Respect is demonstrated in many ways: sitting silently with the client, apologizing to the client for an affront, sharing feelings about the client's behavior, and acknowledging the client for genuine responses.

Empathy refers to the nurse's ability to perceive feelings and meanings from the client's perspective. This technique should be a part of all nurse-client relationships. Because each person is unique, it is difficult to understand another human being completely. The more varied the nurse's experience, the more likely the nurse will be able to understand people.

Touch is a way for the nurse to personalize communication in emotional situations. However, the nurse needs to be aware of the client's feelings about touching and not infringe on the client's right not to be touched. Some clients are suspicious, have feelings of unworthiness, or are compulsive about germs and are made more anxious when touched. In therapeutic communication *touch* means placing an arm around a crying client or holding the hand of a client expressing remorse.

Facial expression and body movement are nonverbal techniques that cue the client to the nurse's responses. It is important that facial expressions and body movements correspond to the nurse's verbal statements (Cook, 1981; Stuart and Sundeen, 1983; Travelbee, 1971; Wilson and Kneisl, 1988).

Communication Channels. There are five major components to effective communication: sender, message, channel, receiver, and feedback. The sender is the person generating the message through a channel to the receiver, who reacts, or gives feedback about the message. Ideas, events, situations, emotions, attitudes, and knowledge can affect all components of communication. The nurse's responsibility is to recognize the interaction of these effects on the components of communication within the nurse-client relationship (Bradley and Edinberg, 1982). Table 2–5 gives an example of the components of communication with various affects.

When a receiver gives no feedback, or response, to the sender, the communication is called one-way communication. This type gives the sender the control. Examples of one-way communication are a television program, a lecture, a speech, and a written memo. This type of communication can cause difficulties in nurse-client interactions. If a client views the nurse as a person who gives information or is primarily responsible for sending messages, the client will assume little responsibility for changing his or her behavior. The client will not be actively involved in the relationship and will become dependent on the nurse to give directions.

Two-way communication is much more effective in the nurse-client interaction. In this type of communication the receiver becomes actively involved in the process of communication by receiving messages, responding, and giving feedback. As a result, nurses are better able to understand the needs of the client and facilitate the client's change

Table 2–5 *Components of Communication*

Interaction	*Analysis*
(Nurse walks briskly into the room, looking around quickly for a client needing medication.)	The nurse sets up a situation for an unplanned interaction and becomes the sender.
CLIENT: Why are you staring at me that way?	The client has just come from a group session after revealing a problem to the group. The client does not recall that the nurse was not present at the group session.
NURSE: (Firmly.) I'm not staring at you! I was looking for you.	The nurse did not realize she had sent a message to the client by briskly walking into the room. She gives the client feedback from the perspective of receiver rather than sender.
CLIENT: Well what do you want anyway? (Begins to cry.)	The client continues to react as a receiver in response to the nurse's attitude.
NURSE: Can't a person approach you without you crying?	The nurse continues to respond as the receiver and communication is disrupted.
CLIENT: It's just that you looked so mad. I didn't do anything.	The client takes the role of sender and reverses the message to the nurse.
NURSE: I think I understand your reaction. I was in a big hurry and you thought I was angry with you.	The nurse recognizes the confusion in the communication channel and clarifies her role to the client.

in behavior. Two-way communication is more time-consuming than one-way communication. However, it is the foundation of the nurse-client interaction.

Nurse-client interactions are people-oriented. This orientation is frequently in conflict with the other responsibilities the nurse may have in the clinical setting. Nurses generally have a number of physical tasks to complete at the same time they are engaged in a nurse-client interaction. Usually, it is the high-visibility tasks that are seen and measured; the low-visibility job of tending to psychological needs often goes unrecognized. Because the nursing system rewards nurses by giving promotions, pay raises, and performance evaluations based on the high-visibility tasks, nurse-client relationships can suffer. Establishing a sound nurse-client relationship is difficult to develop into a routine. It becomes very easy for nurses to fall into high-visibility tasks and to neglect developing the skills necessary to have quality nurse-client interactions.

With knowledge and understanding it is possible for the nurse to conduct low-visibility tasks while working on high-visibility tasks. For example, suppose the client is agitated and that medication has been ordered for periods of agitation. When the nurse approaches the client to give the injection, he takes the time to explain the procedure and reassure the client. The nurse's action in this instance does more than reduce the physical agitation; it also supports psychologic recovery.

The principles of communication and nurse-client relationships are applicable in a variety of settings and are most effective when attention is given to both high- and low-visibility tasks. Interactions should be structured to allow task completion while maintaining the client's sense of well-being. Good communication skills remain adaptable in many nursing settings.

The primary channels of communication are vision, audio, and kinesthesis. The visual channel involves seeing, observing, and perceiving. Observing body language, eye contact, posture, and appearance are importance aspects of the nurse-client relationship. One difficulty that arises in the nurse-client relationship is misinterpretation of what is seen. Recall the misinterpretation presented in Table 2–5. The nurse and and the client were perceiving the situation differently; thus, their relationship was disrupted. The auditory channel involves words, tone of voice, pitch of voice, and rhythm and speed of speech. These factors can influence the impact of the message on the receiver. The kinesthetic channel refers to physical affection, pain, emotional support, and physical support. There are cultural aspects to this channel of communication. In many cultures it is inappropriate to have physical contact of any kind with strangers. Nurses are strangers who are often cast into situations where touch is necessary. Touch can be the way to unleash the client's pent-up emotions, or it can be the way to drive a client into a rage. The effectiveness of using touch with the client is dependent upon how comfortable the nurse and the client are with this channel of communication.

Communication Style. The style in which one communicates is dependent upon the situation and the personalities in the nurse-client relationship. Several factors influence the nurse's communication style: openness, person-task orientation, self-disclosure, acceptance, defensiveness, and congruence.

Openness is a characteristic indicating that the individual is willing to listen, understand, and thereby modify the message within the communication process (Katz and Kahn, 1966). Openness can be affected by role. For example, one reacts differently to peers than to superiors or subordinates. At the other end of the spectrum, the individual may be closed, or unaccepting of any change in the intent of the message. Openness in nurse-client relationships involves giving and seeking information, praising, criticizing, asking questions, and giving suggestions.

Person-task orientation is another characteristic related to one's style of communication. Some people are totally task-oriented; others are people-oriented (Blake and Mouton, 1969). This factor affects the kind of information gathered and how the nurse relates in the nurse-client relationship.

Self-disclosure is a characteristic necessary to maintain a working nurse-client relationship. Self-disclosure involves being willing and able to talk about your feelings and perceptions honestly and directly (Jourard, 1971). Self-disclosure can range to extremes, from too much to none. In nurse-client relationships nurses must develop client sensitivity to develop timing and a sense of whether self-disclosure is appropriate. Trust is essential for the client to be able to self-disclose within the nurse-client relationship.

Acceptance of the client and one's self is a critical aspect of communication style. Acceptance only partially involves approving of another. More important to acceptance is an understanding of what the other believes or feels; the belief that he or she has the right to believe that way; and that no blame will accrue, even though behavior is wrong or needs change (Rogers, 1951). The term *nonjudgmental* has been used in conjunction with the concept of acceptance. Acceptance is sometimes not easy, especially in the face of conflict in attitudes and values. In a nurse-client relationship, both the nurse's and the client's feelings can be hurt. Hurt leads to frustration, disappointment, and anger. If acceptance is lacking, the fact should be recognized. Both parties must understand that nurse and client are doing their best at that point in time. Then they should continue to work on acceptance.

Defensiveness has overlapping meanings in the communication process. One interpretation maintains that defensiveness occurs when an individual responds as if he or she is being attacked. Another interpretation maintains that defensiveness is a mechanism against anxiety. In nurse-client relationships defensiveness is handled by recognizing and commenting on it. The nurse says, for example, "You seem angry, what's bothering you?" (Bradley and Edinberg, 1982).

Congruence is the final factor in communication style. Congruence refers to how well words, body language, and tone of voice fit together. The message sent should be consistent with the internal feelings and beliefs of the sender (Satir, 1976). In the nurse-client relationship congruence is important in creating a helping environment.

Each person, in the course of maturing and developing, has developed a unique style of communication. Table 2–6 presents the SELF Profile, which was developed to assist in developing a greater understanding of one's own communication style and that of others. The chart in Figure 2–3 is used to assign a category to the style of each test taker, and Table 2–7 lists the strengths and weaknesses of each category. Once a nurse has identified his or her predominant style, he or she can recognize the strengths and weaknesses of it and gain insight into reactions.

Mental Status Examination The mental status examination provides information about the client's current behavior and mental capabilities. It is useful when the client has demonstrated impaired thinking during the nursing history interview. Specifically, the mental status examination provides information about the client's general observations and behavior, speech, level of consciousness, emotional state, thought process or form, thought content, and cognitive functioning. The overall impression of the client's deficits, behavior, and performance provides the foundation for nursing diagnosis. (See Table 2–8 for an outline of the mental status examination.)

Further Testing Tests are an additional resource to help the nurse understand the client. Two types of psychologic tests are used: those that evaluate intellectual or cognitive functioning and those that describe personality functioning. Reasons for using these tests are (1) to determine mental deficiency, (2) to determine appropriate psychotherapy, (3) to assist in differential diagnosis, and (4) to assist in forensic psychiatry.

Many psychologic tests are available. The responsibility of the nurse is to be aware of the existence of tests and how these tools can add to the knowledge base of individual clients. The nurse also has the responsibility to collaborate with the psychologist for administration and interpretation of these tests (Stuart and Sundeen, 1983).

Recently laboratory tests have been added to diagnostic evaluation of the mentally ill client. Among these new diagnostic procedures are CAT (computerized axial tomographic) scanning, CT

Table 2–6 *SELF Profile*

Directions: For questions 1–14, place the number that describes you best in the blank at the end of each question.

Not at all like me	Somewhat like me	Occasionally like me	Usually like me	Very much like me
1	2	3	4	5

1. When in a group, I tend to speak and act as the representative of that group. ____
2. I am seldom quiet when I am with other people. ____
3. When faced with a leadership position, I tend to actively accept that role rather than diffusing it among others. ____
4. I would rather meet new people than read a good book. ____
5. Sometimes I ask more from my friends or family than they can accomplish. ____
6. I enjoy going out frequently. ____
7. It's important to me that people follow the advice that I give them. ____
8. I like to entertain guests. ____
9. When I am in charge of a situation, I am comfortable assigning others to specific tasks. ____
10. I often go out of my way to meet new people. ____
11. I often find myself playing the role of leader and taking charge of the situation. ____
12. I truly enjoy mixing in a crowd. ____
13. When I see that things aren't going smoothly in a group, I usually take the lead and try to bring some structure to the situation. ____
14. I make friends very easily. ____

For questions 15–20, write in the blank at the end of each question the letter that represents your response.

15. You are in a conversation with more than one person. Someone makes a statement that you know is incorrect; you are sure the others didn't catch it. Do you let others know? ____

    A. Yes
    B. No

16. After a hard day's work I prefer to ____

    A. Get together with a few friends and do something active
    B. Go home and unwind.

17. When planning a social outing with a small group, I am most likely to ____

    A. Be the first to suggest some plans and try to get the others to make a decision quickly
    B. Make sure everyone has a say in the planning and go along with what the group decides

18. You have just finished a three-month project for which you have sacrificed a great deal of your free time and energy. To celebrate, are you more likely to ____

    A. Invite some of your friends over and throw a party
    B. Spend a quiet, peaceful weekend doing whatever you wish, either by yourself or with a special friend

19. If I feel that I am underpaid for my work, I'm most likely to ____

    A. Confront the boss and demand a raise
    B. Do nothing and hope the situation improves

20. I think that those around me see me as primarily ____

    A. Gregarious and outgoing
    B. Introspective and thoughtful

Table 2–6 *(continued)*

To score your SELF Profile:
I. For items 15–20:
Give yourself 5 points for each A.
Give yourself 1 point for each B.

In the two columns of blanks that follow, enter the points you received for questions 15–20.

II. Now transfer each of the numbers you wrote for questions 1–14 to the appropriate blanks that follow.

III. Add the scores in each column.

1.	______	2.	______
3.	______	4.	______
5.	______	6.	______
7.	______	8.	______
9.	______	10.	______
11.	______	12.	______
13.	______	14.	______
15.	______	16.	______
17.	______	18.	______
19.	______	20.	______
Raw directive score	______	Raw affiliative score	______

Now, for each raw score, you will calculate a final score.

If you scored	Give yourself a
10–14	1
15–22	2
23–27	3
28–35	4
36–44	5

Final directive score ______ Final affiliative score ______

Enter your final directive score by placing a dot on the vertical line, the directive scale, in Figure 2–3. The directive scale shows your need and tendency to direct and control situations. If you score high on this scale, you tend to be comfortable supervising others and controlling situations. If you score low on this scale, you tend to be supportive and seek consensus from others.

Enter your final affiliative score by placing a dot on the horizontal line, the affiliative scale, in Figure 2–3. The affiliative scale measures your need and desire to be around others. If you score far to the left on this scale, you probably like it best when you're with people. If you score far to the right on this scale, you are probably self-contained, enjoy time alone or with a few close friends, and seek little interaction with others.

Connect the two dots by drawing a straight line. Shade the area between the line you drew and the intersection of the two scales. Note the label (S, E, L, or F) that is in the shaded quadrant of the figure. This label assigns you to a SELF type. Read about your type and other types in Table 2–7.

Do not reproduce. Copyright © 1988, National Press Publications. (Copies may be purchased at a minimal cost from National Press Publications, 6901 W. 63rd Street, Shawnee Mission, KS 66202-4007).

(computerized tomographic) scanning, MRI (magnetic resonance imaging) technique, PET (positron emission tomography) scanning, and neurochemical tests. EEG (electroencephalography) has been used for several years in looking at brain wave activity (Andreasen, 1984).

Nursing Diagnosis in Mental Health Nursing

As previously mentioned, the term *nursing diagnosis* first appeared in the literature in the 1960s. In 1973, the ANA included nursing diagnosis as part of

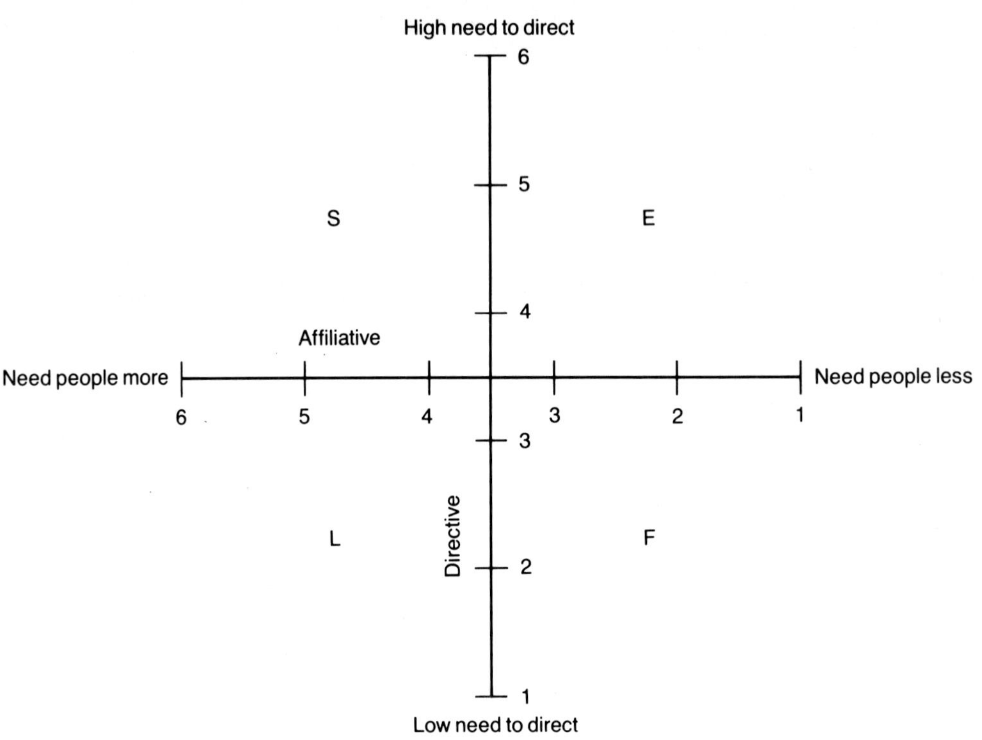

Figure 2–3 *Plotting your SELF results.*

Table 2–7 *SELF Characteristics by Type*

Type	*Strengths*	*Limitations*	*Type*	*Strengths*	*Limitations*
S	Persuasive	Pushy	L	Team-oriented	Too other-oriented
	Risk taker	Intimidating		Caring	Indecisive
	Competitive	Overbearing		Devoted	Impractical
	Pursues change	Restless		Enthusiastic	Vulnerable
	Confident	Impatient		Helpful	Hesitant
	Socially skilled	Manipulative		Accessible	Subjective
	Inspiring	Abrasive		Trusting	
	Open	Reactive		Sensitive	
	Direct	Dominating		Good listener	
	Outgoing			Good friend	
				Likes variety	
E	Practical	Dogmatic		Gregarious	
	Orderly	Stubborn		Peacemaker	
	Very direct	Rigid			
	Self-determined	Unapproachable	F	Exacting	Slow to get things done
	Organized	Distant		Thorough	Perfectionistic
	Traditional	Critical		Factual	Withdrawn
	Goal-oriented	Insensitive		Reserved	Dull
	Dependable			Meticulous	Sullen
	Economical			Practical	Shy
	Ambitious			Calm	Passive
				Has high standards	
				Risk avoider	

Do not reproduce. Copyright © 1988, National Press Publications. (Copies may be purchased at a minimal cost from National Press Publications, 6901 W. 63rd Street, Shawnee Mission, KS 66202-4007).

Table 2–8 *Mental Status Examination: General Observations and Behavior**

Appearance
- Dress (conservative, tasteful, inappropriate, meticulous):
- Grooming (clean, unkempt, disorderly):
- Facial expression (alert, vacant, sad, hostile, masklike):
- Eye contact:
- Motor behavior (mannerisms, agitated, statuelike):
- Posture (erect, slumped):
- Gait (steady, staggering, ataxic):
- General health (well nourished, undernourished, clear skin, circles under eyes):

Speech
- Pace (fast, slow):
- Interruptions (steady flow, skips from one topic to another, sudden interruption):
- Volume (loud, barely audible):
- Clarity (slurred, monosyllabic responses, pressured):
- Tone and modulation (altered, calm, hostile):

Level of consciousness
- Sensorium (altered, drowsy, confused, nonresponsive):
- General responsiveness to environment (distracted, able to sustain attention):
- Responds (answers questions, follows simple instructions):

Emotional state
- Mood (depressed, euphoric, anxious, sad, calm, frightened, apathetic, angry):
- Affect (intensity, appropriateness, lability, range of emotions):

Thought process (form)
- Forms of verbalization (rate of speech, clear, logical, organized, coherent):
- Signs of pathology:
  - Autistic thinking (individualized associations derived from within client):
  - Blocking (sudden stop in speech or train of thought):
  - Circumstantiality (tedious and irrelevant details causing indirect progression of thoughts):
  - Confabulation (imagined or fantasized experiences unconsciously filling in memory gaps):
  - Flight of ideas (rapid verbal skipping from one idea to the next without relationship to preceding content):
  - Fragmentation (disrupting of thoughts resulting in an incomplete idea):
  - Loose associations (disconnected associations between thoughts):
  - Neologism (making up new words that symbolize ideas, not understood by others):
  - Perseveration (repetition of some verbal or motor response involuntarily):
  - Tangentiality (thought digressions not related to preceding thoughts or ideas):
  - Word salad (a mix of words or phrases that lack meaning):

Thought content
- Theme:
  - Somatic (physical symptoms):
  - Rituals (repetitive thinking or behavior):
  - Destructive (violence, suicide, homicide):
  - Defensive (delusions, excessive ambivalence, distortions in perception, hallucinations):

Cognitive functioning
- Orientation (recognizes surroundings):
- Time (day, month, year):
- Place (knows location):
- Person (knows name):
- Situation (knows why seeking help or is hospitalized):
- Attention and concentration:
  - "Digit span" exercise. Have client repeat a series of three numbers forward and backward. Increase up to five or six numbers.
  - Simple arithmetic calculations
- Memory
  - Recent—have client report events of last 24 hours or recent news events
  - Remote—have client say birth date or list grades in school
- General intelligence (nonstandardized)
  - Attuned to environment
  - Relates recent news stories
  - Knows last five presidents
  - Other general questions: How many days in the week? What are the four seasons of the year? What is the nation's capital?
- Abstract thinking
  - Capacity to generalize
  - Finds meaning in symbols
  - Conceptualizes objects and events
- Insight and judgment:
  - How client relates problem (is the situation serious, does client feel treatment is necessary):
  - Judgment questions asking client to draw conclusions: What would you do if you found a wallet in the street? What would you do if you saw a child hit by a car?
- Perceptions and coordination:
  - Ask client to write name on a piece of paper (observe for ease, speed, coordination, correctness, tremors):
  - Ask client to draw common figures (circle, square, diamond, clock):

Summary
- Summarize all pathologic findings:

*Record general observations about the client. Observations that appear to be outstanding should be noted.

the nursing process in the *Standards of Nursing Practice.* In the same year, the National Conference Group for Classification of Nursing Diagnoses met formally to begin identification and development of nursing diagnoses. Marjory Gordon (1976), who chaired the first four national conferences, defines **nursing diagnoses** as follows.

> Nursing diagnoses, or clinical diagnoses made by professional nurses, describe actual or potential health problems which nurses by virtue of their education and experience are capable and licensed to treat.

Since the fifth conference on nursing diagnoses, more than 90 diagnostic categories have been accepted. (See Table 2–9 for the approved list of nursing diagnoses.) At the present, nursing diagnosis is the weakest link in the nursing process. This text attempts to strengthen the concept of nursing diagnosis in relation to mental health nursing practice.

To make the list of nursing diagnoses clearer and more usable, Marjory Gordon identified 11 functional health patterns:

Pattern 1: health perception–health management

Pattern 2: nutritional-metabolic

Pattern 3: elimination

Pattern 4: activity-exercise

Pattern 5: sleep-rest

Pattern 6: cognitive-perceptual

Pattern 7: self-perception

Pattern 8: role-relationship

Pattern 9: sexuality-reproductive

Pattern 10: coping–stress tolerance

Pattern 11: value-belief

The purpose of identifying functional health patterns is to alert the practitioner to potential nursing diagnoses when problems are assessed in one of these areas. (See Table 2–10 for a list of the nursing diagnoses applicable to each of the 11 functional health patterns.)

The structure of the nursing diagnosis assists the nurse develop clear and concise statements about the client's health status. The first step in developing a nursing diagnosis is to identify, by looking at the data base, the client's health status, concerns, or problems. Problems exist when the client is unable to meet a need. For example, if the client has a need for nutrition, this is not a nursing diagnosis. The nursing diagnosis is more specifically related to the problem created by the client's need for nutrition. The appropriately stated nursing diagnosis is nutrition, alteration: less than body requirements. This statement is precise and lends itself to nursing intervention.

To develop the nursing diagnosis clearly, it is necessary to consider the etiological factors underlying the problem or dysfunction. Certain risk factors may point to a specific etiology and predispose the client to a dysfunctional pattern. The cues to etiology are called **defining characteristics.** In this text, each chapter on specific mental disorders provides a knowledge base that includes the defining characteristics (behavioral, affective and cognitive, physiologic, and sociocultural) of problems likely to be seen in clients with that particular disorder. Those defining characteristics have been translated into etiologies. A two-part nursing diagnosis has been included in all the care plans for the disorders chapters. This text uses the nursing diagnosis and etiology underlying the diagnosis rather than nursing problems as the basis for the plan of care (Gordon, 1982; 1976; Lederer et al., 1990).

Psychiatric Nursing Diagnoses

In the mental health setting the **Diagnostic and Statistical Manual of Mental Disorders, Third Edition, (DSM-III-R)** has been the primary means of identifying psychiatric nursing diagnoses. However, this approach does not take into account the nurse's role in managing human responses to illness. As a result the ANA authorized a project that would re-

Table 2–9 *Nursing Diagnoses Approved by North American Nursing Diagnosis Association*

Pattern 1
Exchanging
Altered nutrition: more than body requirements
Altered nutrition: less than body requirements
Altered nutrition: potential for more than body requirements
Potential for infection
Potential altered body temperature
Hypothermia
Hyperthermia
Ineffective thermoregulation
Dysreflexia
Constipation
Perceived constipation
Colonic constipation
Diarrhea
Bowel incontinence
Altered patterns of urinary elimination
Stress incontinence
Reflex incontinence
Urge incontinence
Functional incontinence
Total incontinence
Urinary retention
Altered (specify type) tissue perfusion (renal, cerebral, cardiopulmonary, gastrointestinal, peripheral)
Fluid volume excess
Fluid volume deficit (1)
Fluid volume deficit (2)
Potential fluid volume deficit
Decreased cardiac output
Impaired gas exchange
Ineffective airway clearance
Ineffective breathing pattern
Potential for injury
Potential for suffocation
Potential for poisoning
Potential for trauma
Potential for aspiration
Potential for disuse syndrome
Impaired tissue integrity
Altered oral mucous membrane
Impaired skin integrity
Potential impaired skin integrity

Pattern 2
Communication
Impaired verbal communication

Pattern 3
Relating
Impaired social interaction
Social isolation
Altered role performance
Altered parenting
Potential altered parenting
Sexual dysfunction
Altered family processes
Parental role conflict
Altered sexuality patterns

Pattern 4
Valuing
Spiritual distress (distress of the human spirit)

Pattern 5
Choosing
Ineffective individual coping
Impaired adjustment
Defensive coping
Ineffective denial
Ineffective family coping: disabling
Ineffective family coping: compromised
Family coping: potential for growth
Noncompliance (specify)
Decisional conflict (specify)
Health-seeking behaviors (specify)

Pattern 6
Moving
Impaired physical mobility
Activity intolerance
Fatigue
Potential activity intolerance
Sleep pattern disturbance
Diversional activity deficit
Impaired home maintenance management
Altered health maintenance
Feeding self-care deficit
Impaired swallowing
Ineffective breastfeeding
Bathing/hygiene self-care deficit
Dressing/grooming self-care deficit
Toileting self-care deficit
Altered growth and development

Pattern 7
Perceiving
Body image disturbance
Self-esteem disturbance
Chronic low self-esteem
Situational low self-esteem
Personal identity disturbance
Sensory/perceptual alterations (specify) (visual, auditory, kinesthetic, gustatory, tactile, olfactory)
Unilateral neglect
Hopelessness
Powerlessness

Pattern 8
Knowing
Knowledge deficit (specify)
Altered thought processes

Pattern 9
Feeling
Pain
Chronic pain
Dysfunctional grieving
Anticipatory grieving
Potential for violence: self-directed or directed at others
Post-trauma response
Rape-trauma syndrome
Rape-trauma syndrome: compound reaction
Rape-trauma syndrome: silent reaction
Anxiety
Fear

Table 2–10 *Nursing Diagnoses Grouped by Functional Health Patterns*

Pattern	Nursing Diagnoses
Health perception–health management pattern	Growth and development, altered Health maintenance, altered Noncompliance (specify) Injury, potential for Breastfeeding, ineffective Health-seeking behaviors Potential for suffocation Potential for poisoning Potential for trauma
Nutritional-metabolic pattern	Body temperature, altered: potential Fluid volume deficit Fluid volume excess Hyperthermia Hypothermia Infection, potential for Nutrition, alteration in: less than body requirements Nutrition, alteration in: more than body requirements Swallowing, impaired Thermoregulation, ineffective Tissue integrity, impaired Oral mucous membrane, alteration in Skin integrity, impairment of
Elimination pattern	Bowel elimination, alteration Constipation Colonic constipation Perceived constipation Diarrhea Bowel incontinence Urinary elimination, alteration in patterns Urinary retention Total incontinence Functional incontinence Reflex incontinence Urge incontinence Stress incontinence
Activity-exercise pattern	Activity intolerance Cardiac output, decreased Disuse syndrome, potential for Diversional activity deficit Home maintenance management, impaired Mobility, impaired physical Respiratory function, potential alterations Ineffective airway clearance Ineffective breathing patterns Impaired gas exchange (Specify) self-care deficit: Feeding Bathing/hygiene Dressing/grooming Toileting Tissue perfusion, alteration in (specify) Cerebral Cardiopulmonary Renal Gastrointestinal Peripheral
Sleep-rest pattern	Sleep pattern disturbance
Cognitive-perceptual pattern	Comfort, altered Pain Chronic pain Decisional conflict Dysreflexia Knowledge deficit (specify) Potential for aspiration Sensory-perceptual alteration: (specify) visual auditory kinesthetic gustatory tactile olfactory Thought processes, altered Unilateral neglect
Self-perception pattern	Anxiety Fear Hopelessness Powerlessness Self-concept, disturbance in Fatigue Body image disturbance Personal identity disturbance Self-esteem disturbance Chronic low self-esteem Situational low self-esteem
Role-relationship pattern	Communication, impaired verbal Family processes, alteration in Grieving, anticipatory Grieving, dysfunctional Parenting, alteration in Parental role conflict Role performance, altered Social interaction, impaired Social isolation
Sexuality-reproductive pattern	Sexual dysfunction Sexuality patterns, altered
Coping–stress tolerance pattern	Adjustment, impaired Coping, ineffective individual Defensive coping Ineffective denial Coping, disabling or ineffective family Coping, potential for growth: Family Post-trauma response Rape-trauma syndrome Violence, potential for (specify)
Value-belief pattern	Spiritual distress

Source: Adapted from L. J. Carpenito, *Handbook of Nursing Diagnosis 1989–90.* (Lippincott, 1989). Reprinted with permission.

sult in identifying nursing diagnoses specific to the psychiatric client. The first classification system, **Psychiatric Nursing Diagnoses, First Edition (PND-I)**, was presented to nurses at the 1988 ANA convention (see Appendix B).

The ANA task force working on PND-I recognized the necessity of coordinating with the North American Nursing Diagnosis Association (NANDA) to develop a single comprehensive classification system. Thus work continues on the development of a joint classification system arising from PND-I. A discussion of the development of PND-I is beyond the scope of this text. A comparison of the accepted list of nursing diagnoses, psychiatric nursing diagnoses, and DSM-III-R is presented in Wilson and Kneisl (1988).

Application of the Nursing Diagnosis Process to a Clinical Situation

In reviewing the data base for Sharon S., several cues, or defining characteristics, point to specific etiologies underlying her problems. The functional health patterns with disruptions are nutritional-metabolic, elimination, activity-exercise, sleep-rest, cognitive-perceptual, self-perception, role-relationship, sexuality-reproductive, and coping–stress tolerance. (See Table 2–11 for the two-part nursing diagnoses identified from the data base for Sharon S.)

Table 2–11 *Nursing Diagnoses for Sharon S*

Nutritional-metabolic
- Nutrition, alteration in: more than body requirements related to weight 10% over ideal for height and frame

Elimination
- Bowel elimination, alteration in, potential for related to decreased activity level and side effects of pain medications

Activity-exercise
- Activity intolerance, unresolved related to avoidance of activity
- Mobility, impaired physical, disturbance in related to perceived inability to move due to pain

Sleep-rest
- Sleep pattern disturbance, unresolved related to pain, interrupted sleep

Cognitive-perceptual
- Comfort, alteration in: chronic pain related to preoccupation with pain

Self-perception
- Anxiety, potential for related to perceived threat to biologic integrity
- Hopelessness related to belief that it is impossible to change situation
- Self-concept, disturbance in body image, unresolved related to overconcern with somatic complaints

Role-relationship
- Communication, impaired: verbal, potential for related to withdrawal from interactions
- Role performance, altered related to employment status
- Social isolation, potential for related to preoccupation with somatic complaints
- Violence, potential for: directed at others related to hostile and threatening verbalizations

Sexuality-reproductive
- Sexual dysfunction, potential for related to loss of desire during episodes of pain

Coping-stress tolerance
- Coping, ineffective family: compromised related to disruptions in family structure
- Coping, ineffective, individual related to social withdrawal

Nursing Diagnosis Versus Medical Diagnosis in the Mental Health Setting

Diagnosis has long been accepted as part of medicine. Many classification systems and diagnostic labels have been developed over the years. The same may be said for psychiatry, a specialized branch of medicine. In psychiatry, mental disorders are classified in the *Diagnostic and Statistical Manual of Mental Disorders, Third Edition* (**DSM-III-R**). The protocol of the American Psychiatric Association, DSM-III-R has been in developmental stages since the 1970s. There are five client dimensions in DSM-III-R: mental disorders, personality and developmental disorders, physical disorders, severity of psychosocial stress, and global assessment of functioning (APA, 1987).

The dimensions are defined as axes. Clients may have diagnoses in one axis and no pathology in the other axes, or clients may present pathology in more than one axis. DSM-III-R is descriptive and leaves the analysis of etiology to the practitioner. In only a few disorders are the etiology and pathophysiology well established and included in the disorder's definition.

Nursing diagnosis can be compared to DSM-III-

R. The basis of both sets of diagnoses evolves from problem solving, which begins with data collection. Data collection involves reviewing signs and symptoms exhibited by the mentally ill client. With nursing diagnosis, those signs and symptoms are translated into defining characteristics, which become the basis for the etiology of the nursing diagnosis. With DSM-III-R, the signs and symptoms are translated into diagnostic criteria, including the essential and associated features of specific mental disorders. These features are considered with predisposing factors, and a differential diagnosis for the client ultimately results. Once the nursing diagnosis or DSM-III-R diagnosis is obtained, treatment plans are established for the client (Color, 1984).

In this text, DSM-III-R has been used as a means for organizing the knowledge base for a variety of mental disorders. The DSM-III-R diagnosis provides the base for defining characteristics of nursing diagnoses. That is not to say that nursing diagnosis in mental health nursing is based on DSM-III-R; rather, DSM-III-R is only one source of defining characteristics for consideration in refining the nursing diagnosis.

Nursing diagnosis and DSM-III-R are both products of the computer age. With these tools the mental health nurse has the opportunity to improve clinical practice by using a common classification for that practice. By consistently applying diagnostic labels to mental health clients, the nurse is able to plan more comprehensive services for the client, which greatly improves the client's care. A further description of DSM-II-R is presented in Chapter 4.

Planning Mental Health Nursing Care

Once the nursing diagnoses have been identified, the nurse proceeds to develop the plan of care. Planning a course of action is essential in assisting the client toward the goal of optimal wellness. **Planning** consists of (1) establishing nursing care priorities, (2) setting goals, and (3) identifying strategies for interventions. The basis of the planning step is assessment and the nursing diagnoses.

The judgment the nurse uses to establish priorities is based on theories, concepts, models, and principles. (Several theories related to nursing were reviewed at the beginning of the chapter.) In nursing literature, the model most commonly used to establish priorities is Maslow's hierarchy of needs (Christensen, 1986A). In using this theory, the nurse makes priority judgments. Basic needs for air, food, and water have priority over safety needs. Once basic needs are met, safety needs have priority over love needs, and so forth until all needs have been given attention. (See Table 2–12, which shows Sharon S.'s nursing diagnoses within the needs hierarchy.)

Once priorities have been established, the nurse and the client determine the goals for alleviating the problems. The nature of the goal will be determined by the nursing diagnosis. To increase the potential for attaining the goal, it should be set with the client's involvement. The nurse is responsible for providing the knowledge base to the client.

The goal should be broad and reflect the intended outcome. To meet these requirements, it is

Table 2–12 *Sharon S's Nursing Diagnoses in Priority by Need*

Physiologic needs
Nutrition, alteration in: more than body requirements
Bowel elimination, alteration in: constipation, potential for
Sleep pattern disturbance, unresolved
Safety needs
Activity intolerance, unresolved
Anxiety, potential for
Comfort, alteration in: chronic pain
Mobility, impaired physical, disturbance in
Love and belonging needs
Communication, impaired: verbal, potential for
Sexual dysfunction, potential for
Social isolation, potential for
Esteem needs
Self-concept, disturbance in body image, unresolved
Violence, potential for: directed at others
Coping, ineffective family: compromised
Coping, ineffective individual
Hopelessness
Role performance

necessary that goals be stated in terms specific enough to indicate the behaviors necessary to complete the goal. In some nursing schools, students are taught to develop objectives underlying the goals established in the plan of care. That activity is beyond the scope of this text, where the goal is written in measurable terms and expected outcomes in behavioral terms. This allows the student to consider the conditions and performance of the client in determining whether a goal is reached.

One way of making goals behavioral is to consider their three domains:

1. *Cognitive goals* deal with the client's intellectual capabilities, including knowledge and skills.
2. *Affective goals* deal with the client's emotions, attitudes, and values.
3. *Psychomotor goals* deal with the client's ability to perform motor skills.

Bloom, Krathwohl, Simpson, and others have described these three taxonomies in the educational literature (Popham, 1975). Their descriptions have been adapted to many disciplines, including nursing. Examples of behavioral indicators of each domain are (1) as an indicator of cognitive understanding the client "identifies," (2) as an indicator of affective appreciation the client "chooses" a value, and (3) as an indicator of psychomotor skill the client "executes."

Along with making the goals mutual and measurable, it is necessary to set deadlines for the attainment of goals. These deadlines then become part of the process of evaluating whether goals have been attained. As with the goals, the client and the nurse should mutually set the deadlines. It is the nurse's responsibility to help the client set reasonable deadlines.

To help the student establish a plan of care for clients with a variety of mental disorders, a format for expressing a nursing care plan has been developed. This format begins with the *nursing diagnosis* identified from the knowledge base presented. Next is the *goal* for the client, with the assumption that the nurse and client would mutually set it. Then comes the *intervention,* suggested planned actions specific to a variety of mental disorders defined within the DSM-III-R classification system. The *rationale* for planning the intervention is designed to assist the reader in applying concepts from the knowledge base to actions the nurse would take in actually caring for the client. Finally, the *expected outcome* is presented instead of an evaluation area. Although the expected outcomes could be used as a basis of evaluation, in this text they are listed to give the student cues to the indicators that goals have been attained. (See Table 2–13 for an example of the standard nursing care plan used in this text.)

Mental Health Nursing Interventions

The next step in the mental health nursing process is implementing the care plan by executing the **interventions**, those activities taken by the nurse to

Table 2–13 Standard Format for Nursing Care Plans

Nursing Diagnosis: The two-part diagnosis: approved diagnosis and etiology
Goal: Mutually established with the client and measurable

Intervention	*Rationale*	*Expected Outcome*
Planned interventions based on scientific rationale underlying the etiology	The scientific reason for completing the intervention	The behaviors demonstrated by the client, indicating goal attainment

affect the client's problem. Providing the rationale for nursing interventions is a very broad scientific knowledge base (theories, models, and principles in nursing; natural science; behavioral sciences; the humanities; and so on).

There are three basic types of interventions:

1. *Dependent interventions* are based on the client's medical diagnosis. These interventions are required by physician's orders and include administration of medications and treatments; they generally do not appear on the nursing care plan.

2. *Interdependent interventions* are based on clinical nursing problems collaboratively dealt with by physicians, social workers, and psychologists. An example of an interdependent intervention is discharge planning to a board and care home.

3. *Independent interventions** are based on nursing diagnosis. These interventions are stressed throughout this text.

(Table 2–14 shows how a care plan is implemented for one nursing diagnosis identified for Sharon S.)

As you have learned, the therapeutic relationship is the major independent intervention of the nurse in the mental health setting. The term *therapeutic relationship* is used rather than *social relationship* because the latter is characterized by superficiality; the therapeutic relationship is characterized by intimacy. In social relationships, there is limited self-disclosure because of minimum knowledge of the other participant; discussion is generally on neutral or general topics. In contrast, the therapeutic relationship is one of mutual acceptance, of safety and security. Mutual disclosure of perceptions, needs, desires, behaviors, and feelings is characteristic (Coad-Denton, 1978).

Therapeutic relationships take place in three phases: introductory, working, and termination. Often these phases overlap and are thought of as interlocking. The following paragraphs briefly describe the phases of the therapeutic relationship.

Introductory-Phase Therapeutic Relationships

The introductory (or getting-acquainted, or orientation) phase of the therapeutic relationship provides the time in which the nurse and client establish a mutually acceptable agreement or contract that serves as a guide to the relationship. The purpose of the relationship, the time limits for each visit, the place for interactions to occur, the limits of the relationship, and the confidentiality of the relationship should be established between the nurse and the client. The client should be advised of the termination process, and discharge planning should be initiated at this time. In this phase, the nurse becomes a significant other to the client, and the client develops trust in the nurse. Throughout the text, "establish a one-to-one relationship" or "establish a trusting relationship" will indicate the initial phase of a therapeutic relationship.

Usually the nurse initiates the therapeutic relationship with the client. The nurse begins by self-introduction, including his or her name and position. The nurse suggests working with the client to resolve the difficulties that have brought the client in for treatment. At this time, the meeting place is specified and the period for the interactions set. The nurse should ask how the client prefers to be addressed. It is essential that the nurse adhere to the mutually agreed on schedule to develop a sense of trust in the client.

Working-Phase Therapeutic Relationships

The second phase in a therapeutic relationship is the working (or maintenance) phase. It is difficult to characterize this phase because it is individ-

**Nursing orders* is a term seen in the nursing literature for interventions designed for the individual client stemming from a data base established about the client. *Nursing orders* has not been used in this text because the authors wish to emphasize the planned interventions stemming from the nursing diagnoses.

Table 2–14 Nursing Care Plan for One Nursing Diagnosis for Sharon S

Nursing Diagnosis: Alteration in comfort: pain related to preoccupation with somatic symptoms
Goal: Client will identify measures to control pain by the time of discharge

Intervention	*Rationale*	*Expected Outcome*
Assess pain measures that have been successful for client in the past	Will identify potential methods of pain control	States control methods that are successful and unsuccessful
Instruct client on nonpharmaceutical pain control methods: • position change • good posture and body alignment • immobilize the affected area • activity to distract from pain such as meditation • relaxation techniques • relaxing music • massage, heat, and cold pack if not contraindicated	Will provide alternative measures to alleviate pain and prevent overuse of pain medications	Uses new methods of pain control Reduced fatigue Verbalizes control over pain Sets realistic goals for pain control Uses referral resources
Provide a supportive environment: • reduce noise • eliminate excess traffic • clean linens • use measures to reduce pain	Will assist in reducing stress that increases pain	
Assist client in setting realistic goals for pain control	Will assist client in understanding the nature of pain and principles of pain control	
Assist client in planning lifestyle modifications: • review client's ability to implement changes in lifestyle • provide referral resources	Will assist client in incorporating lifestyle changes necessary to control chronic pain	

ualized to the nature of the client's problems. The following is a review of some nursing role guidelines applicable to this phase:

1. Strive to be sincerely interested and natural.
2. Allow the client to take the conversational lead. Encourage topics that are suggested by the client's comments or past demonstrated interests.
3. Avoid stating your opinion or holding forth about your personal interests.
4. Keep conversation open by merely restating the client's last words when he or she allows the conversation to lapse.
5. Say nothing if a response seems unnecessary or if no appropriate response suggests itself. Wait for the client to continue or say quietly, "Yes, go on."

6. Do not feel compelled to fill silences with chitchat. Wait a reasonable time for the client to continue.
7. To clarify a problem, question the client about a topic being discussed. In response to a client who is continually talking about moving to a distant state, one might comment, "If you leave this area, what plans do you have to find a new job and a place to live?"
8. Reflect the client's feelings or attitudes by restating his or her comments or implied attitudes.
9. Provide emotional support by remaining with the client when his or her feelings about the problem are acute.
10. Set limits to assist the client in gaining control of his or her behavior.

Termination-Phase Therapeutic Relationships

The third phase of the relationship is the termination (or concluding, or resolution) phase. The termination of the relationship should be included in the care plan from the introductory phase of the relationship. Termination can be a traumatic experience for the nurse and the client. It is not unusual for the client to act out feelings such as that of impending loss. The nurse needs to understand the client's sense of loss and help him or her express and cope with these feelings. Client's reactions may include gift giving, dependency, regression, anger, and so forth. In an effort to continue the relationship, the client may even introduce new material. The nurse may also sense feelings of loss and separation. A great deal of emotional energy goes into a therapeutic relationship. The primary goal of the termination phase is to help the client review what he or she has learned in the relationship and to transfer this learning to other interactions and relationships (Doona, 1979; Peplau, 1952; Taylor, 1982).

Table 2–15 *Sharon S and the Phases of Her Therapeutic Relationship*

Introductory phase	
NURSE:	Hello, Sharon, my name is Robert. I will be meeting with you today to obtain a nursing history.
CLIENT:	They did that already when I came in.
NURSE:	I realize that, Sharon, and I don't plan on repeating that history. I am from the mental health department, and I have come to get some more specific information.
CLIENT:	Great! Everyone thinks I'm a crazy!
Working phase	
CLIENT:	Like I told you yesterday, I haven't talked to my mother in years.
NURSE:	You said this doesn't bother you, yet you have told me about this two days in a row. Could it be bothering you unconsciously?
CLIENT:	I guess it could. I'd have to think about that one. I didn't realize it was bothering me that much until you mentioned it.
NURSE:	What about not seeing your mother bothers you the most?
Termination phase	
NURSE:	Sharon, today you will be going home, and I won't be seeing you again.
CLIENT:	The time sure went fast here. It's funny how I was so nasty to you the first day when I thought you were trying to pry into my personal life and use all that "psych crap" on me!
NURSE:	Yes, you did give me a bad time that day. But we have overcome that and I think looked at some of your basic problems. What do you think has helped you the most?
CLIENT:	I think knowing that someone accepted me for me and tried to understand my pain was what helped me look at what I've been doing for myself.

(See Table 2–15 for sample interactions between the nurse and Sharon S. during the course of their therapeutic relationship.)

Evaluation in Mental Health Nursing Care

The final step in the mental health nursing process is **evaluation**, and it is often the most neglected. In evaluation, the nurse compares actual progress with goals and examines his or her own performance.

Examination of Client's Progress

In the evaluation step, the nurse compares the client's health status after interventions to previously defined goals and expected outcomes. Ideally, an evaluation of outcomes should answer these questions:

- Were the planned interventions effective?
- Was the goal attained?
- Were the expected outcomes demonstrated?
- What changes took place in the client's behavior?
- Which nursing interventions were effective; which interventions need revision?
- Was the client satisfied with the nursing care?
- What plans need to be changed?
- Are new planned interventions necessary?
- Was behavior adequately recorded to plan changes in interventions?

Since the reader is not implementing the interventions outlined in each of the disorders chapters, expected outcomes have been devised as an evaluation step base. These outcomes, which focus on the changes in the client's behavior or health status, could be used to review discrepancies with actual outcomes in real client situations.

The nurse attempts to validate the results of the care plan by seeking client input and peer input and by self-evaluation. This validation takes place with recorded observations, discussion of insights, and review of the data base. It is important to document the results of the evaluation of nursing care.

Two additional criteria to be considered in evaluation are formative evaluations and summative evaluations. *Formative evaluation* is an ongoing process based on client responses to care. From the formative evaluation, the nurse reorders, modifies, or maintains the care plan. *Summative evaluation* is a terminal process and is used to determine whether the client has achieved the mutually set goals. Summative evaluations may be seen in the form of discharge summaries. (See Table 2–16 for an example of formative and summative evaluation documentation for Sharon S.)

Self-Evaluation

Because therapeutic use of self is crucial to working with the mental health client, it is important not only to evaluate client progress but also to evaluate oneself. Nurses who judiciously review their progress with clients and check their performance with peers can improve their clinical practice. A variety of methods of completing self-evaluation, such as process recording and performance checklists, are available. (See Table 2–17 for a performance checklist for self-evaluation.)

Table 2–16 *Examples of Formative and Summative Evaluation Documentation for Sharon S*

Formative Evaluation		**Summative Evaluation**	
Goal	*Evaluation documentation*	*Goal*	*Evaluation documentation*
Client will identify measures to control pain by the time of discharge.	On 8/6, Sharon took a warm bath in the whirlpool before being placed in traction. Sharon stated there was increased pain relief.	Client will identify measures to control pain by the time of discharge.	On 8/17, Sharon was discharged without pain medications on around-the-clock basis. Sharon planned to use pain medication only when the pain became unbearable and to call the physician should this occur. Sharon planned to be admitted to a pain control clinic.

Table 2–17 *Self-Evaluation Checklist*

Did I:	*Yes*	*No*	*Comments*	*Did I:*	*Yes*	*No*	*Comments*
1. Establish a therapeutic relationship with client?				14. Use open-ended statements?			
2. Accept client as a person?				15. Avoid talking too much?			
3. Accept client at his/her behavior level?				16. Use prompting to encourage initiative?			
4. Identify the purpose, times, and roles for the relationship?				17. Recognize my feelings and reactions to client?			
5. Clarify the confidentiality of the data?				18. Create a learning atmosphere for client?			
6. Stimulate initiative in client?				19. Pick up verbal leads and nonverbal cues?			
7. Allow client to make decisions?				20. Keep within the limits of my role?			
8. Actively listen to client?				21. Avoid giving my personal history and opinions?			
9. Use indirect approaches?				22. Use the data supplied by client in planning care?			
10. Focus on client and his/her concerns?				23. Maintain interest, attention, and support?			
11. Break silences?				24. Record data accurately without distortion?			
12. Avoid giving advice?				25. Help client connect and summarize?			
13. Avoid "why" and "how" questions?							

SUMMARY

Foundations of Mental Health Nursing

1. Most nurses feel uncomfortable when dealing with mentally ill clients. This text acquaints the reader with the foundations of mental health nursing practice.

2. The central propositions of humanism form the philosophic foundation for the text.

3. The theoretic base for the text is nursing process.

4. Mental health nursing borrows from other disciplines and theories to formulate its general concepts.

5. Nursing theorists use theories to develop models of nursing care. Hildegard Peplau, a nursing theorist, was one of the most powerful forces in the development of modern mental health nursing.

Nursing Process and Mental Health Nursing

6. Mental health nursing process is comparable to the nursing process used in all of nursing.

7. Five steps of the nursing process constitute the mental health nursing process.

8. ANA outlines the professional practice standards

for mental health nursing and incorporates the following steps into the process: assessment, diagnosis, planning, intervention, and evaluation.

Assessment in Mental Health Nursing

9. The nursing history is an essential tool in developing the assessment data base. It is from this information that the care plan is developed.

10. The basic nursing history tool in mental health nursing includes functional health patterns and sociocultural needs.

11. The mental health nurse uses observation, the interview, the nurse-client relationship, therapeutic communication techniques, the mental status examination, other tests, and the medical diagnosis to assist in formulating nursing diagnoses.

Nursing Diagnosis in Mental Health Nursing

12. Marjory Gordon's definition of nursing diagnosis and the approved list of nursing diagnoses apply to the mental health setting.

13. The etiology of the nursing diagnosis is derived from the data base obtained by the nursing history and other tools available to the mental health nurse.

14. Defining characteristics are observed as the data are collected and assist the mental health nurse in specifying the etiology underlying the nursing diagnosis.

15. DSM-III-R alerts the nurse to potential defining characteristics within specific mental disorder categories.

Planning in Mental Health Nursing

16. Once the nursing diagnoses are identified, it is important to establish priorities. Maslow's hierarchy of needs is one good way of establishing care priorities.

17. Goals are established to guide the planning phase. Including the client and establishing mutually acceptable goals are important to nursing care outcomes.

18. Goals are broad statements of what the client expects to accomplish with treatment and care.

19. Objectives, or expected outcomes, are necessary to spell out the behaviors the nurse will observe in the client to indicate that goals have been achieved.

Intervention in Mental Health Nursing

20. This phase has also been called implementation. Whatever the term, this is the phase in which the nursing care is given to the client.

21. The three basic types of mental health nursing interventions are dependent, interdependent, and independent.

22. A primary independent mental health nursing intervention is the therapeutic relationship between nurse and client. The three phases of the therapeutic relationship are introductory, working, and termination.

Evaluation in Mental Health Nursing

23. The final step of the mental health nursing process is evaluation.

24. The purposes of evaluation are determination of client progress, effectiveness of the nursing care plan, effectiveness of the interventions, determination of goal attainment, and provision of a new data base for changes in the plan of care.

25. Two criteria considered in evaluation are formative and summative evaluation. Formative is ongoing and summative is terminal evaluation.

26. Self-evaluation is an essential part of mental health nursing because of the nature of the use of self in independent nursing interventions.

CHAPTER REVIEW

The following questions refer to the case of Sharon S., the example in this chapter.

1. When completing the nursing history on Sharon, which one of the following best describes the assessment of her mobility?
   - (a) Sharon has limited mobility caused by low-back pain.
   - (b) Sharon is able to complete all activities of daily living.
   - (c) There are no limitations in Sharon's mobility.
   - (d) It is necessary for Sharon to remain on bedrest only.

2. Which of the following nursing diagnosis statements best relates to the assessment of Sharon's mobility?
   - (a) Self-care deficit: dressing
   - (b) Impaired physical mobility
   - (c) Diversional activity deficit
   - (d) Decreased cardiac output

3. A realistic goal in Sharon's care plan is best described by which one of the following?
   - (a) Client tends to activities of daily living.
   - (b) Client mobilizes with assistance.
   - (c) Client turns every 2 hours.
   - (d) Client accepts limitations in physical activity.

4. Which one of the following would be an appropriate intervention related to mobility?
   (a) Turn client every 2 hours.
   (b) Encourage correct body alignment.
   (c) Supervise all attempts to mobilize.
   (d) Teach client how to transfer from bed to wheelchair.

5. Which one of the following is the best example of evaluative data related to Sharon's mobility status?
   (a) Sharon requested a whirlpool bath.
   (b) Pain medication was given three times in one shift.
   (c) Sharon refused pain medication.
   (d) Sharon requested assistance in removing traction and going to the bathroom.

REFERENCES

Allport F: *Theories of Perception and the Concept of Structure.* Wiley, 1955.

American Nurses' Association, *Nursing: A Social Policy Statement.* Kansas City, Missouri, 1980.

Andreasen NC: *The Broken Brain.* Harper & Row, 1984.

Andrews PB: Nursing diagnosis. In: *Nursing Process.* Griffith JW, Christensen PJ (editors). Mosby, 1982.

Bevelas JB: *Personality: Current Theory and Research.* Brooks/Cole, 1978.

Blake RR, Mouton JS: *Building a Dynamic Organization Through Communication and Organization Development.* Addison-Wesley, 1969.

Bradley JC, Edinberg MA: *Communication in the Nursing Context.* Appleton-Century-Crofts, 1982.

Carpenito LJ: *Handbook of Nursing Diagnosis 1989–90.* Lippincott, 1989A.

Carpenito LJ: *Nursing Diagnosis: Application to Clinical Practice,* 3rd ed. Lippincott, 1989B.

Christensen PJ: Goals and objectives. In: *Nursing Process.* Griffith JW, Christensen PJ (editors). Mosby, 1986A.

Christensen PJ: Nursing assessment: Data collection of the individual client. In: *Nursing Process.* Griffith JW, Christensen PJ (editors). Mosby, 1986B.

Coad-Denton A: Therapeutic superficiality and intimacy. In: *Clinical Practice in Psychosocial Nursing.* Longe D, Williams R (editors). Appleton-Century-Crofts, 1978.

Color MS: I am nursing diagnosis . . . color me DSM III green. In: *Classification of Nursing Diagnosis: Proceedings of the Fifth Conference.* Mosby, 1984.

Cook JS: *A Mastery Learning Teaching Strategy for the Discrimination of Nurse-Patient Interaction Constructs in a Simulated Mental Health Clinical Setting.* (Dissertation.) University of San Francisco, 1981.

Day RH: *Perception.* St. Louis: William Brown, 1966.

Doona MB: *Travelbee's Intervention in Psychiatric Nursing,* 2nd ed. Davis, 1979.

Evans BL, et al.: *Statement on Psychiatric and Mental Health Nursing Practice.* American Nurses' Association, 1976.

Flynn JM, Heffron PB: *Nursing: From Concepts to Practice.* Bowie MD: Brady, 1984.

Gordon M: Nursing diagnosis and the diagnostic process. *Am J Nurs* (Aug) 1976; 76:1299.

Gordon M: *Nursing Diagnosis: Process and Application.* McGraw-Hill, 1982.

Hagerty BK: *Psychiatric–Mental Health Assessment.* Mosby, 1984.

Johnson DE: The significance of nursing care. *Am J Nurs* (Nov) 1961; 61:63–66.

Johnson DE: The behavioral system model for nursing. In: *Conceptual Models for Nursing Practice.* Riehl JP, Roy C (editors). Appleton-Century-Crofts, 1980.

Johnson DE: Professional practice in nursing. In: *The Shifting Scene: Directions for Practice.* National League for Nursing, 1967.

Jourard SM: *The Transparent Self.* Van Nostrand Reinhold, 1971.

Katz D, Kahn RL: *The Social Psychology of Organization.* Wiley, 1966.

Kelly K: Clinical inference in nursing, part I. *Nurs Res* 1964; 13:314–322.

Kelly K: Clinical inference in nursing, part II. *Nurs Res* 1966; 15:23.

King IM: *Toward a Theory for Nursing.* Wiley, 1971.

Krieger JP (editor): *Foundations for Holistic Health Nursing Practices.* Lippincott, 1981.

Lamont C: *The Philosophy of Humanism.* Philosophical Library, 1957.

Leddy S, Pepper JM: *Conceptual Bases of Professional Nursing.* Lippincott, 1985.

Lederer JR, et al.: *Care Planning Pocket Guide,* 3d ed. Addison-Wesley, 1990.

Lego S: The one-to-one nurse-patient relationship. In: *Psychiatric Nursing 1946–1974: A Report of the State of the Art.* Huey F (editor). American Journal of Nursing Co., 1975.

Maslow, AH: *Psychological Review,* 1943; 50:370–396.

Murry RB, Huelskoetter MMW: *Psychiatric/Mental Health Nursing: Giving Emotional Care.* Prentice-Hall, 1983.

Neuman B: The Betty Neuman health-care systems model:

A total person approach to patient problems. In: *Conceptual Models for Nursing Practice,* 2nd ed. Riehl JP, Roy C (editors). Appleton-Century-Crofts, 1980.

Orem DE: *Nursing: Concepts of Practice,* 2nd ed. McGraw-Hill, 1980.

Orlando IJ: *The Dynamic Nurse-Patient Relationship.* Putnam, 1961.

Peplau HE: *Interpersonal Relations in Nursing.* Putnam, 1952.

Popham WJ: *Educational Evaluation.* Prentice-Hall, 1975.

Rogers C: *Client Centered Therapy.* Houghton-Mifflin, 1951.

Rogers ME: *An Introduction to the Theoretical Basis of Nursing.* Davis, 1970.

Rohwer WD, Ammon PR, Cramer P: *Understanding Intellectual Development.* Hinsdale, IL: Dryden Press, 1974.

Romano C, McCormick KA, McNelly LD: Nursing documentation: A model for a computerized data base. *ANS* 1974; 4(2):43–56.

Roy C, Roberts SL: *Theory Construction in Nursing: An Adaptation Model.* Prentice-Hall, 1981.

Safier G: *Contemporary American Leaders in Nursing: An Oral History.* McGraw-Hill, 1977.

Satir V: *Making Contact.* Celestial Arts, 1976.

Strain JP (editor): *Modern Philosophies of Education.* Random House, 1971.

Stuart GW, Sundeen SJ: *Principles and Practices of Psychiatric Nursing,* 2nd ed. Mosby, 1983.

Taylor CM: *Mereness' Essentials of Psychiatric Nursing,* 11th ed. Mosby, 1982.

Travelbee J: *Interpersonal Aspects of Nursing.* Davis, 1966.

Travelbee J: *Interpersonal Aspects of Nursing,* 2nd ed. Davis, 1971.

Vernon M: *Perception Through Experience.* London: Methuen, 1970.

Wilson HS, Kneisl CR: *Psychiatric Nursing,* 2nd ed. Addison-Wesley, 1988.

Yura H, Walsh MB: *The Nursing Process.* Appleton-Century-Crofts, 1967.

Yura H, Walsh MB: *The Nursing Process,* 3rd ed. Appleton-Century-Crofts, 1978.

Yura H, Walsh MB: *The Nursing Process,* 5th ed. Appleton & Lange, 1988.

SUGGESTED READINGS

Bermosk LS, Mordan MJ: *Interviewing in Nursing.* Macmillan, 1976.

Carnevali DL: *Nursing Care Planning: Diagnosis and Management,* 3rd ed. Lippincott, 1983.

Collins M: *Communication in Health Care.* Mosby, 1977.

Duldt BW, Griffin K: *Theoretical Perspectives for Nursing.* Little, Brown, 1985.

Ellis JR, Nowlis EA: *Nursing: A Human Needs Approach.* Houghton Mifflin, 1977.

Enelow AJ, Swisher SN: *Interviewing and Patient Care.* Oxford, 1972.

Fitzpatrick JJ, et al.: Translating nursing diagnosis into ICD code. *AJN* (April) 1989; 89:493–495.

Goodwin JO, Edwards BS: Developing a computer program to assist the nursing process. *Nurs Res* 1975; 24(4):229.

Griffith JW: Nursing evaluation. In: *Nursing Process.* Griffith JW, Christensen PJ (editors). Mosby, 1982.

Guzzetta C, Dossey B: Nursing diagnosis: Framework, process, and problems. *Heart Lung* (May) 1983; 12:124.

Lamonica EL: *The Nursing Process: A Humanistic Approach.* Addison-Wesley, 1979.

Lewis GK: *Nurse-Patient Communication,* 2nd ed. St. Louis: William Brown, 1973.

Little DE, Carnevali DL: *Nursing Care Planning,* 2nd ed. Lippincott, 1976.

Mackinnon RA, Michele R: *The Psychiatric Interview in Clinical Practice.* Saunders, 1971.

O'Brien MJ: *Communications and Relationships in Nursing.* Mosby, 1974.

Okun BF: *Effective Helping,* 3rd ed. Brooks/Cole, 1987.

Pinnell NN, Meneses M: *Nursing Process.* Appleton-Century-Crofts, 1986.

Smitherman C: *Nursing Actions for Health Promotion.* Davis, 1981.

CHAPTER 3

Personality Theories and Mental Health

LESLIE BONJEAN

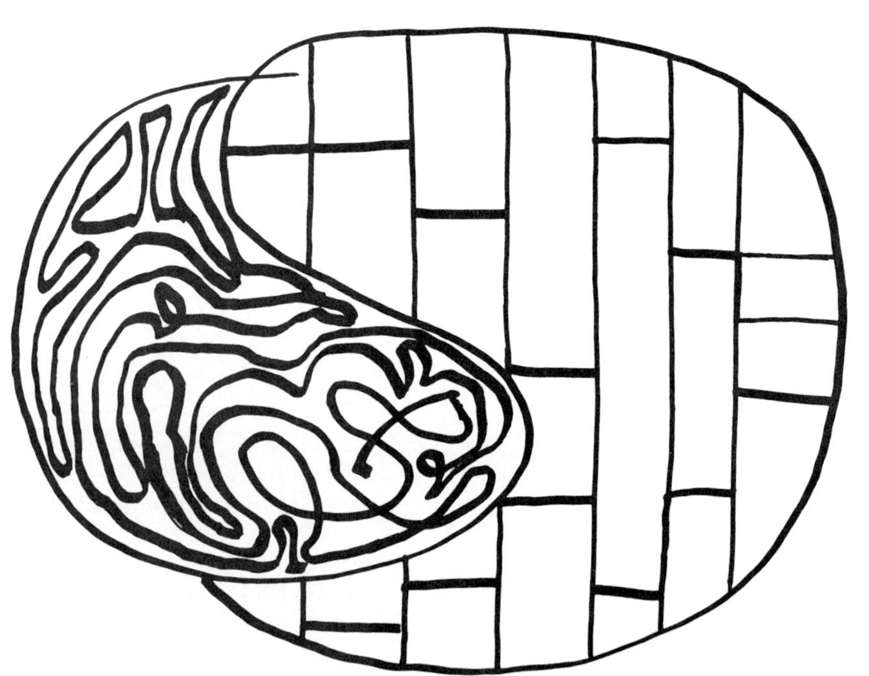

My inner world and outer world

My inner world feels entangled and confused. There are many different thoughts and feelings entwined into a maze. The lines appear to be flowing and integrated but in reality are separate pathways; some closed circuits and some spiraling dead end routes. Both traps of hopelessness and despair.

My outer world is very structured and orderly. The straight lines and open windows give me a sense of security and meaningful direction. I become fearful as the chaos of my inner being slowly encroaches on my orderly exterior existance.

▪ *Objectives*

After reading this chapter the student will be able to

- Discuss the value of theories and theoretic frameworks to nursing as a scientific discipline
- Explain the basic theoretic assumptions of psychoanalytic, social-psychologic, behavioristic, cognitive, developmental, humanistic, and moral development perspectives of personality development
- Analyze the theories presented in this chapter and their applicability to nursing practice
- Relate the theories presented in this chapter to clinical practice

▪ *Chapter Contents*

Introduction

The development of science and technology over the last century has led to the formulation of many different concepts and theories. Disciplines such as psychology, sociology, and philosophy, as well as the biologic and natural sciences have quested for knowledge through expansion of their theoretic bases. Since the days of Florence Nightingale, nursing has also sought to expand its science and wisdom through the development and application of theories. The profession has achieved this in two ways: (1) through research that has led to the development of nursing theories and (2) through the exploration, comprehension, and use of interdisciplinary theories.

Definitions of Theories

The major aim of science is to evolve theory. This is considered essential to a scientific discipline because theories draw together groups of concepts and interrelate them in such a way that meaning and understanding can be gleaned from them. These theories may then be used by practitioners to provide answers to questions and concerns. Because nursing is a practice discipline, theories are developed not only to name and explore concepts but also to offer a prescription for practice and an ability to predict outcomes of that practice.

The word *theory* comes from the Greek word *theorem,* which signifies a vision. Kerlinger (1973, p. 9) defines *theory* as "a set of interrelated constructs (concepts, definitions, and propositions) that present a systematic view of phenomena by specifying relationships among the variables, with the purpose of exploring and predicting phenomena." Stated more simply, Kim (1983, p. 10) defines *theory* as "a set of theoretical statements that specify relationships between two or more classes of phenomena (and therefore, concepts) in order to understand a problem or the nature of things."

Theories are developed and used as a means of

- Categorizing and organizing information
- Explaining why things occur
- Understanding the significance of past events
- Providing the ability to control events
- Providing the ability to predict future events

It is tempting to look at theories as abstract conceptualizations that have no practical value in the real world. Barbara Stevens (1979) suggests that practice is often equated with what is practical, and theory, at least by implication, is equated with the impractical. She believes this antiintellectual approach to theory interpretation and use stagnates the development of nursing and makes it nothing more than the passing on of folk wisdom from nurse to nurse. Certainly the development of theories is often an abstract process, but the end product is a practical guide. Referring to the Greek concept of theories as visions, it is indeed possible to see theories as a way to make visions of nursing a reality.

What is a vision for nursing? Certainly one goal is to provide scientifically based care. But consider whether this is the only requirement of good nursing. Knowing what to do and why to do it is extremely important, but it is not enough. A humanistic dimension must be added to the scientific knowledge. In other words, the vision for nursing is scientifically based humanistic care. This is what is meant by the term **holistic-humanistic nursing care**. Because the majority of theories used to guide nursing practice are based on conceptual interpretations rooted in a humanistic model of people, applying the theories can help nurses bring humanism to their profession. By its nature, the beginning phase of theory development forces researchers to conceptualize philosophies that clearly define their view of people and the universe. When that is done, relationships between the philosophy and the concepts must be compatible. The significance of this is that in addition to supplying a scientific road map for nursing practice, theories, with their built-in philosophies, provide a natural safeguard to assure humanistic practice.

The Articulation of Theories with the Nursing Process

As has been stated, theories provide scientific data to prescribe practice criteria. The nursing process is a way to organize that scientific data. It is the vehicle the nursing profession has chosen to divide abundant information into a workable system. Further, it is an intellectualization of the steps the nurse carries out, and it serves to organize and implement nursing actions. Theories, by their nature, provide a great deal of information that can be applied in many different situations. Theories are not meant to force practitioners into slots, but they are usually broad enough to allow for a great deal of creativity. Nurses are becoming more adept at using and applying theories creatively to particular practice situations. Although this opens up many possibilities for the care of clients, it makes the problem of organization even more complex.

A particular theory can guide practitioners in several ways. It can help them (1) to look at a particular situation in a specific way, (2) to predict what might happen in that situation, and (3) to see what actions have proven effective in the past. But it does not necessarily tell nurses how best to organize that information. The nursing process is structured to allow for systematic categorization of the data gathered by application of a theoretic framework to a practice situation. The nursing actions might well be prescribed by a particular theory. Speaking from a purely theoretic viewpoint, these actions belong solely to the nurse. The nursing process connects these actions to a particular client. It might be said, then, that the nursing process personalizes a theory to a client. This thought somehow has the power to make both theories and the nursing process less abstract.

Differing Philosophies

A wide variety of theories that may be applied to the practice of psychiatric and mental health nursing are presented in this chapter. Legitimate questions for beginning practitioners to ask include

- Which theories are the best?
- Which theories best fit a particular type of practice?
- Which theories are used most often?

There is, of course, no definitive answer to these questions. A survey of nurses practicing in the psychiatric and mental health areas would probably reveal as many different opinions as there are both theories and practitioners.

Although some nurses, particularly clinical specialists, might choose to base their practice on one particular theoretic framework, most employ a combination of theoretic frameworks. The beginner should learn to explore many approaches to care and practice working with all available theories. Through this exploration, students will begin to formulate their own answers to the preceding questions. The final decision is not nearly as important as the process one goes through to achieve it. Exploration and discovery make the decision of what theoretic framework to use a valid one.

Theories of Personality Development

Before attempting to learn about specific theories of personality development, it seems appropriate to look at the meaning of the term *personality*. Almost everyone has some familiarity with this term. In conversation it is often used to describe someone's degree of social comfort or skill. Often, people who are gregarious, humorous, fun, and entertaining are said to have "good" personalities whereas people who are uncomfortable and quiet around others are said to have "bad" personalities.

Another common way for people to describe someone's personality is by picking out the most remarkable thing about that person. For example, there is the aggressive personality, the generous personality, the mean personality, and the lazy personality. Personalities are described in literally hundreds of ways. Common sense dictates there is more to personality than the preceding descriptions suggest.

If one is seeking a comprehensive definition of the concept of personality, the literature provides little help. Many biosocial definitions are more similar to popular views than to biophysic definitions that account for organic influences. Other definitions attempt to define personality by describing adjustment behavior of people, and others attempt to combine biosocial, biophysic, and adjustment aspects. Obviously, scientists define personality in different ways, depending on the particular emphasis of their work. Hall and Lindzey (1970) write that no substantive definition of personality can be applied with any generality. Hall and Lindzey (p. 9) further submit that "personality is defined by the particular empirical concepts which are part of the theory of personality employed by the observer."

The Psychoanalytic Perspective of Personality

Psychoanalytic theory had its beginnings in the clinical practice of Sigmund Freud.

Sigmund Freud Sigmund Freud carried out the first systematic investigations to find how disorders of the mind and personality actually come about. Freud was a young physician who worked at the University of Vienna in the year 1885 as a lecturer in nervous disorders. He left his position at the university that same year to study under Jean Martin Charcot, a famous neurologist. Charcot was working with patients believed to have "hysterical disorders of the mind." These patients appeared to be blind or paralyzed, without a definitive physical diagnosis to explain their symptoms. Using hypnosis as his main therapeutic intervention, Charcot was attempting to work with these patients. During his work with Charcot, and later through an association with two other neurologists also using hypnosis with "hysterical" patients, Freud became convinced that the mental processes were much more complex than what one could observe through a person's consciousness. This started his lifelong commitment to the development of a comprehensive theory of personality development.

Aspects of Consciousness. Freud divided all aspects of consciousness into three categories:

- conscious
- preconscious
- unconscious

The first category, **conscious**, included all things that are easily remembered. Examples of this are addresses, phone numbers, anniversaries, special persons' birthdays, and the month in which spring break occurs. The second category, **preconscious** (sometimes called subconscious), contains all thoughts, feelings, and desires that have been forgotten but that can easily be recalled to consciousness. These might include old phone numbers or addresses, the feeling a woman had on her wedding day or during the birth of her first child, the name of a first girlfriend, or the animosity one felt toward his first boss. The third category, **unconscious**, encompasses thoughts, feelings, actions, experiences, and dreams that cannot be brought to conscious thought or remembered.

Id, Ego, and Superego. Freud theorized there were three components to the personality:

- id
- ego
- superego

Each of these has individualized functions, but the three are so closely interrelated that it is difficult to separate their individual effects on a person's behavior.

The biologic and psychologic drives with which a person is born constitute the **id.** Drives are inborn psychologic wishes that are represented as needs. Biologic hunger is described as a nutrition deficit, but in psychologic terms, it is a wish for food. The wish is the motivation factor that propels people to seek food. Therefore a person's drives serve to move behavior in a particular direction.

The id holds in reserve all psychic energy, which in turn furnishes the power for the operations of the ego and superego. The id has no knowledge of outside reality and functions totally within its own subjective reality. The id is completely self-centered, and its major concern is instant gratification of needs. Since the id cannot tolerate the tension that increases as needs are frustrated, it attempts to get those needs met as quickly as possible, without consideration of reality or morality. This principle of tension reduction is called the **pleasure principle**.

The id is capable of reflex action to reduce tension, such as blinking, sneezing, and sighing. This serves the immediate purpose of tension reduction in most basic need situations, but it does not usually produce the gratification needed in more complex instances. The id can also generate mental pictures and images in an attempt to remove tension. For example, a hungry person conjures up an image of food to release the tension brought about by the need for food. This is referred to as the **primary process.** Neither the reflex action nor the primary process is capable of completely reducing tension. The id is not capable of understanding the realistic action necessary for need gratification. At this point the ego system begins to work.

The **ego** is present because the drives of the id to get needs met must be mediated with objective reality. Consider the example of the person experiencing hunger. That person must learn to seek, prepare, and eat food before that need can be met. This means the person must differentiate between the mental image of food and the real meaning of food. In essence, the images are converted to perceptions that allow persons to meet their hunger needs. The basic purpose of this process is for the ego to meet id demands in a way that promotes well-being and survival. Whereas the id obeys the pleasure principle and operates according to the primary process, the ego obeys the reality principle and operates according to a secondary process.

The major function of the **reality principle** is to keep tension at some manageable level until an appropriate object can be found to meet the person's need or needs. The **secondary process** is simply thinking realistically. By means of this process, the ego can find ways to meet id needs and take some action to test if the plan will work. This is called **reality testing.** The ego is present to help the id meet its needs and will never knowingly frustrate them. The ego has little existence apart from the id and never becomes completely independent. The id-ego relationship is one of expediency, that is, it is there for a practical purpose and is necessary for survival of the species. The ego system does not concern itself with moral values or societal taboos. This function is reserved for the third component, the superego.

The **superego** is the accumulation of societal

rules and personal values as interpreted by individuals. These values are then passed to children through a process of reward and punishment. The emphasis of the superego is not reality but the ideal. It is the moral portion of the personality, and its goals are perfection as opposed to the id's pleasure or the ego's reality. For all practical purposes, it is what is referred to as "conscience" and is most concerned with right and wrong. As children are rewarded or punished for certain behaviors, they quickly learn what is acceptable, or "right," and what is unacceptable, or "wrong." When children are rewarded for good behavior, the experience is incorporated into their **ego-ideal**, which is a subsystem of the superego. The mechanism by which this process takes place is **introjection**, a form of identification that allows for the acceptance of the norms and values of others into one's self. Conversely, when children are punished for bad behavior, the experience is incorporated into their **consciences**. The dynamic for both these processes is that the ego-ideal rewards people by allowing them to feel good, and the conscience punishes people by making them feel bad. Without superego development, people are not capable of feeling good or bad about particular behaviors. Although these people are often thought to be immoral, it is probably more accurate to say they are amoral.

The superego, then, is a control system for the nonrational drives of the id and a propelling factor to help the ego system carry out its responsibility to the id by assisting it to choose objects of gratification not considered wrong or immoral. Freud saw the interplay between these components of the personality as having great significance in determining people's behavior. He also saw conflict arising when the three components strove to meet different goals. Freud believed the way in which people resolved these conflicts determined the status of their mental health.

Anxiety and Defense Mechanisms. The concept of anxiety is a thread that runs consistently through the psychoanalytic perspective of personality. From the Freudian point of reference, **anxiety** is defined as a feeling of tension, distress, and discomfort somewhat similar to fear but produced by a perceived or threatened loss of inner control rather than from external danger. The feelings brought about by anxiety are so uncomfortable that they force people to take some type of corrective action. The function of anxiety is to warn people of impending danger. It is a clear message to the ego that unless some palliative steps are taken, it is in danger of being overcome. The ego copes with anxiety by consistently applying rational measures to decrease these feelings of discomfort. This process is often successful in healthy persons, but there are times in the lives of all persons when the ego is unable to cope, and it resorts to less rational ways of handling anxiety. These processes are called the ego defense mechanisms.

Ego defense mechanisms alleviate the anxiety but do so by denying, misinterpreting, or distorting reality. This is true even with the use of defense mechanisms that Freud believed necessary and beneficial. Examples of this are *sublimation* and *displacement,* defense mechanisms that Freud considered necessary for social and personal motivation. Defense mechanisms themselves are a distortion of reality, and for the most part, their use creates a noncongruency between what the reality is and the person's perception of what the reality is. These processes, for the most part, operate at an unconscious level. (See Table 3–1 for a description of the major defense mechanisms.)

Psychosexual Development. The process by which personality develops from birth to adolescence is called **psychosexual development.** Each of the five stages identified by Freud is differentiated by characteristic ways of achieving libidinal, or sexual, pleasure. The psychosexual stages correspond to the maturational stages of the body and were identified by Freud as the (1) oral stage, (2) anal stage, (3) phallic stage, (4) latency stage, and (5) genital stage. Readiness to move through each of the psychosexual stages depends on how well the needs of the previous stage were met. For example, if a mother is warm and nurturing when feeding her children and gives them ample opportunity to meet their sucking needs, then the children learn to cope with

Table 3–1 *Ego Defense Mechanisms*

Defense Mechanism	*Example*	*Use*
Identification—An attempt to handle anxiety by imitating the behavior of someone feared or respected.	A student nurse imitates the nurturing behavior she observes one of her instructors using with clients.	Used to help people avoid self-devaluation.
Introjection—Form of identification that allows for the acceptance of others' norms and values into one's self, even when contrary to one's previous assumptions.	A 7-year-old tells his little sister, "Don't talk to strangers." He has introjected this value from the instructions of parents and teachers.	Used to help people avoid social retaliation and punishment. Particularly important for child's development of superego.
Projection—Process in which blame is attached to others or the environment for unacceptable desires, thoughts, shortcomings, and mistakes.	A mother is told her child must repeat a grade in school, and she blames this on the teacher's poor instruction. A husband forgets to pay a bill and blames his wife for not giving it to him earlier.	Allows people to deny the existence of shortcomings and mistakes. Protective of self-image.
Displacement—The transferring or discharging of emotional reactions from one object or person to another object or person.	A husband and wife are fighting, and the husband becomes so angry he hits a door instead of his wife. A student gets a C on a paper she worked hard on and goes home and yells at her family.	Allows for feelings to be expressed on or to less dangerous objects or people.
Rationalization—Justification of certain behaviors by faulty logic and ascription to it of motives that are socially acceptable but did not in fact inspire the behavior.	A mother spanks her toddler too hard and says it was all right because he couldn't feel it through the diapers anyway.	Helps people cope with the inability to meet goals or certain standards.
Denial—An attempt to screen or ignore unacceptable realities by refusing to acknowledge them.	A woman, though told her father has metastatic cancer, continues to plan a family reunion 18 months in advance.	Used as a temporary insulation from the full impact of a traumatic situation.
Repression—An unconscious mechanism where threatening thoughts, feelings, and desires are pushed down to keep them from becoming conscious. The repressed material is denied entry into consciousness.	A teenager, seeing his best friend killed in a car accident, becomes amnesic about the circumstances surrounding the accident.	Affords protection from traumatic experiences until a person has the resources to cope.
Reaction formation—A mechanism that allows persons to act oppositely to the way they feel.	An executive resents his bosses for calling in a consulting firm to make recommendations for change in his department but verbalizes complete support of the idea and is exceedingly polite and cooperative.	Aids in reinforcing repression by allowing feelings to be acted out in a more acceptable way.
Regression—Resorting to an earlier, more comfortable level of functioning that is characteristically less demanding and responsible.	An adult throws a temper tantrum when he does not get his own way. A critically ill client allows the nurse to bathe and feed him.	Allows people to return to a point in development when nurturing and dependency were needed and accepted with comfort.
Intellectualization—A mechanism by which an emotional response that normally would accompany an uncomfortable or painful incident is evaded by the use of rational explanations that remove from the incident any personal significance and personal feelings.	The hurt over a parent's sudden death is reduced by saying, "He wouldn't have wanted to live disabled."	Protects self-image from hurts and traumatic events.
Undoing—An action or words designed to annul some disapproved thoughts, impulses, or acts in which the person relieves guilt by making reparation.	A father spanks his child and the next evening brings home a present for him. A teacher wrote an exam that was far too easy, then constructed a grading curve that made it difficult to earn a high grade.	Allows people to appease guilty feelings and atone for mistakes.

(continued)

Table 3–1 *(continued)*

Defense Mechanism	*Example*	*Use*
Compensation—Covering up weaknesses by placing emphasis on a more desirable trait or by overachievement in a more comfortable area.	A high school student too small to play football becomes the star long-distance runner for the track team.	Allows people to overcome weaknesses and achieve success.
Sublimation—Displacement of energy associated with more primitive sexual or aggressive drives into socially acceptable activities.	A person with excessive, primitive sexual drives invests psychic energy into a well-defined religious value system.	Protects people from behaving in irrational, impulsive ways.
Substitution—A highly valued, unacceptable, or unavailable object is replaced by a less valuable, acceptable, or available object.	A woman wants to marry a man exactly like her dead father and settles for someone who looks a little bit like him.	Helps people achieve goals and keeps frustration and disappointment at a minimum.

the anxiety associated with oral activities and should be sufficiently developed to move to the next developmental stage. (See Table 3–2 for a summary of the defining characteristics of psychosexual development according to Freud.)

The Importance of the Psychoanalytic Perspective Psychoanalytic theory is one perspective by which clients may be assessed. This theory provides a systematic way of looking at how people develop in the early years of their lives and how they have learned to cope with the uncomfortable feelings of anxiety. Understanding psychoanalytic theory is beneficial for nurses because it provides a framework in which to assess behavior. For example, using Freud's theory makes it possible to distinguish malingering from regression and manipulation from denial. Anger directed at a nurse is much easier to excuse if projection is understood. Psychoanalytic theory gives a greater understanding of the mysterious workings of the mind and therefore brings nurses closer to clients.

As stated earlier, the nurse may creatively use the many theories available. After each major theory is discussed, a table gives examples of how the theory may be articulated with the assessment and diagnosis portions of the nursing process. The examples presented are in no way representative of all possibilities. (See Table 3–3 for applications of the psychoanalytic perspective.)

Table 3–2 *Stages of Psychosexual Development According to Freud*

Stage of Development	*Period*	*Defining Characteristics*
Oral	Birth–18 months	Principal source of pleasure from mouth, lips, and tongue. Dependent on mother for care so feelings of dependency are developed.
Anal	18 months–3 years	Focus on muscle control necessary to control urination and defecation. Expulsion of feces gives a sense of relief. Learns to postpone gratification by postponing the pleasure that comes from anal relief.
Phallic (oedipal)	3–6 years	Develops an awareness of the genital area. Sexual and aggressive feelings associated with functioning of the sexual organs are emphasized. Learns sexual identity during this stage. Masturbation and sexual fantasy are not unusual.
Latency	6–12 years	Sexual development dormant. Focus of energy on cognitive development and intellectual pursuits.
Genital	12 years–to early adulthood	Abundancy of sexual drive. Primary goal is to develop satisfying relationships with members of the opposite sex.

Table 3–3 *Assessment and Diagnosis Using Freud's Psychosexual Theory*

Assessment Data

1. What is the developmental stage of this client?
2. What tasks should this client be meeting?
3. Is there anything that is preventing achievement of tasks?
4. What are the biologic and psychologic threats to this client?
5. What needs of this client are not being met?
6. What are the client's perceptions of his or her personal situation?
7. Is there an obvious use of defense mechanisms?
8. What purpose are those defense mechanisms meeting for the client?
9. What signs of anxiety can be observed in this client?
10. Can the client's anxiety be validated?

Nursing Diagnosis

Developmental lag: Inability to meet sucking needs related to operative trauma to the mouth

Ineffective individual coping: Excessive use of regression post-MI related to fear of dying

The Social-Psychologic Perspective of Personality

The theories of Freud started a scientific revolution in the field of psychology. During the late nineteenth century other disciplines began to emerge and develop their own scientific bodies of knowledge. Sociologists and anthropologists started to believe that human development was more complex than previously thought. It was not long before these beliefs started filtering into the knowledge that had come primarily from the advances in psychology. Many disciples of Freud considered his vision single-minded because it ignored social and cultural influences. They started to reshape old thought and create new theories. This faction developed the **social-psychologic theory** of personality development.

Harry Stack Sullivan The work of Harry Stack Sullivan had its beginnings under the umbrella of the psychoanalytic perspective. But in the final analysis Sullivan created a developmental system markedly different from the Freudian perspective. His theory was the **interpersonal theory** of development.

Sullivan felt that personality was an abstraction that could not be observed apart from interpersonal relationships. Therefore, the unit of study for Sullivan was not the person alone but the person in the context of relationships. According to interpersonal theory, personality is manifested only in a person's interactions with another person or a group. Sullivan acknowledged heredity and maturation as a part of development but placed far more emphasis on the organism as a social rather than a biologic entity.

Although Sullivan saw personality more abstractly than Freud, he still viewed it as the axis of human dynamics in the interpersonal sphere. He identified three principal processes in this sphere: dynamisms, personifications, and cognitive processes.

Dynamisms. A **dynamism** in its simplest form can be defined as a long-standing pattern of behavior. One may think of a dynamism as a habit. Sullivan's conceptualization is open enough so that a person can even add new behaviors to a dynamism. As long as they do not change the pattern significantly, it is still considered the same dynamism.

In Sullivan's theory dynamisms highlight personality traits. For instance, a child who is mean can be said to have a dynamism of hostility. The important idea here is that any habitual reaction of one person to another or to a situation constitutes a dynamism. Sullivan viewed most dynamisms as meeting the basic human needs of an individual by reducing anxiety.

Sullivan believed that an infant first feels anxiety as it is transferred from his or her mother. As the person grows older, anxiety is felt as a response to a threat to his or her own security. Sullivan called the dynamism that develops to reduce anxiety the dynamism of the self, or **self system.** The self system is the protector of one's security.

Personifications. A **personification**, Sullivan theorized, is an image people have of themselves and others. Each individual has many such images, which are made up of attitudes, feelings, and perceptions that are formed from experiences. For example, a child develops a personification of a good teacher by having the experience of being taught by one. Any relationship that leads to a "good" experience results in a person having a favorable personification of the person involved in that relationship. Unfavorable personifications develop in response to "bad" experience.

Sullivan believed that personifications are formed in early life to allow people to cope with interpersonal relationships. As people grow older, however, very rigid personifications can interfere with interpersonal relationships.

Cognitive Processes. To Sullivan, **cognitive processes** were the third primary component of the interpersonal sphere. He believed that cognitive processes, like personifications, were functions of experiences. He believed these experiences could be classified as one of three types. The first is a *protaxic experience,* which he described as an unconnected experience that flows through consciousness. Examples of protaxic experiences are images, sensations, and feelings. Infants experience these most often, and protaxic experiences must occur before the other types. The *parataxic experience* happens when a person sees a causal relationship between events that occur at about the same time but are not logically related. Suppose, for example, that a child tells his mother he hates her and later she becomes ill. Parataxic thinking leads him to conclude that, every time he tells his mother he hates her, she will become ill. Sullivan contends that much of our thinking does not advance beyond the parataxic level. The third type of cognitive process Sullivan called the *syntaxic experience.* He saw the syntaxic experience as the highest level of thinking. This process of cognition concerns the validation of symbols, particularly verbal symbols. These symbols become validated when a group of people understands them and agrees on their meaning. This level gives a logical order to experiences and allows people to communicate. (See Table 3–4 for a summary of developmental stages according to Sullivan.)

Table 3–4 *Stages of Interpersonal Development According to Sullivan*

Stage of Development	*Period*	*Defining Characteristics*
Infancy	Birth–18 months	Oral zone is the main means by which baby interacts with environment. Breast feeding provides the first interpersonal experiences. Having needs met helps develop trust.
Childhood	18 months–6 years	Transition to this stage is achieved by child's learning to talk. Start to see integration of self-concept. Gender development during this time. Child is learning delayed gratification.
Juvenile	6–9 years	This is a time for becoming social. Child learns social subordination to authority figures. Social relationships give a sense of belonging.
Preadolescence	9–12 years	Need of close relationships with peers of same sex. Learns to collaborate. This stage marks the beginning of first genuine human relationships.
Early adolescence	12–14 years	Development of a pattern of heterosexual relationships. Searching for own identity. Ambiguity about dependence-independence issues.
Late adolescence	14–21 years	Prolonged introduction to society. The self-esteem system becomes more stabilized. Will learn to achieve love relationships while maintaining self-identity.

The Importance of the Social-Psychologic Perspective Social-psychologic theory provides yet another perspective from which the nurse can view human behavior. This theory conceptualizes development within a social context and allows the nurse to assess the influences of culture and social interaction on the behavior of clients. (See Table 3–5 for applications of the social-psychologic perspective.)

Table 3–5 *Assessment and Diagnosis Using Sullivan's Interpersonal Development Theory*

Assessment Data

1. At what stage of development, according to Sullivan, is this client?
2. What developmental tasks should this person be meeting?
3. Did achieving previous developmental tasks meet the interpersonal needs of this client?
4. If interpersonal needs were not met, what effect did this have on the client?
5. What is this client's personification of self? How does client describe self?
6. In what way does this client exhibit anxiety?
7. What are the client's coping mechanisms?
8. How does the client relate to other people?
9. In terms of people, what types of support systems does this client have?

Nursing Diagnosis

Anxiety: Change in interactional patterns related to increasing withdrawal from other people

Fear: Separation from usual support systems related to hospitalization

The Behavioristic Perspective of Personality

B. F. Skinner The **behavioristic theories,** particularly those of B. F. Skinner, had a major impact on the way in which scientists looked at personality development. Like the social-psychologic theorists, Skinner rejected many of the conceptualizations of Freud and his followers. In addition, he questioned the validity of ideas such as instinctual drives and personality structure—he felt these could not be observed and therefore could not be studied scientifically.

The major emphasis of Skinner's theory is functional analysis of behavior, which suggests looking at behavior pragmatically. It asks, What is causing a person to act in a particular way? and What entities in the environment reinforce that behavior? Behavioral theory is less concerned with understanding behavior in relation to past events than with the immediate need to predict a trend in behavior and to control it. Skinner did not attribute much importance to unconscious motivations, instincts, and feelings; he did attribute importance to a person's immediate actions.

Skinner thought a person's behavior could be controlled by rewards and punishments. All behavior, he thought, has specific consequences. Consequences that lead to an increase in the behavior he called **reinforcements**, or rewards, and consequences that lead to a decrease in the behavior he called **punishments.**

One of the assumptions of the behavioristic perspective is that behavior is orderly and capable of being controlled. Skinner believed people become who they are through a learning process and interaction with the environment. To carry this reasoning further is to say that problems and deficits in people are the result of faulty learning and therefore may be corrected with the provision of new learning experiences that reinforce different behavior. One of the major concepts within Skinner's system is the **principle of reinforcement** (sometimes referred to as operant reinforcement theory).

The ability to reinforce behavior is the ability to change the number of times a particular behavior occurs in the future. Skinner believed certain operations would decrease certain behaviors and increase other behaviors. According to the principle of reinforcement, conditioning behavioral change is most effective when a reinforcer follows the conditional response; in other words, a response is strengthened when reinforcement is given. Skinner referred to this as an *operant response,* that is, a response that works on the environment and changes it. An example of *operant conditioning* results when a nursing instructor teaches students it is all right to hand in papers late by always accepting late papers. However, handing in papers late can be decreased by the instructor's disallowing this behavior. Another way for the instructor to diminish the behavior is by handing out punishments for it; this is called a *punishing response.* Skinner believed we can predict, control, and explain behaviors by observing and understanding how the principle of reinforcement has been used to reinforce present behavior.

The theories of B. F. Skinner have been criticized by some and embraced by others. To some the idea of controlling people's behavior by a systematically applied reward-punishment system is abhorrent. One argument sometimes made in defense of the Skinnerian theory is that the use of punishment is not necessary to reinforce desirable behaviors. In other words, a systematic application of rewards is capable of reinforcing desirable behaviors, and the distribution of punishment is not necessarily part of the behavioral change.

The Importance of the Behavioristic Perspective Skinner's theories can be beneficial to the nurse in two major areas. The first area is client education. One of the ways people learn is through positive reinforcement of correct responses. One of Skinner's philosophies is that people do not usually fail to learn but that teachers fail to teach. If the client receives praise and nurturing feedback from the nurse-teacher, then, according to Skinner, success will be more likely. For this principle to work, goals must be clearly set forth so that success can be measured.

The second area in which Skinnerian principles of behavior might be applied is in the practice of mental health nursing. When a nurse or client or both wish to change behavior rather than value systems or personality traits. Behavioristic therapies are frequently used in psychiatric adolescent units, substance-abuse groups, and obesity and smoking clinics. Behavioristic theory helps both the nurse and the client understand more clearly what the client is gaining by acting in a certain way. (See Table 3–6 for applications of the behavioristic perspective in nursing.) Skinnerian theory has also been used by professionals who work with delinquents and criminals.

Table 3–6 *Assessment and Diagnosis Using Skinner's Behavioristic Theory*

Assessment Data

1. What specific behaviors of this client are identified as needing change?
2. What new behaviors are desired to replace the old ones?
3. Does the client agree that certain behaviors need to be changed?
4. How is the behavior that needs to be changed reinforced?
5. Who or what is doing the reinforcing?
6. What types of things are important to this client?
7. What types of rewards would reinforce the new, desired behaviors?
8. Is this client willing to do mutual goal setting?
9. Does this client clearly understand the goals?

Nursing Diagnosis

Noncompliance: Inability to set or attain mutual goals related to previous cultural influences

Knowledge deficit: Inadequate follow-through on instruction of colostomy care related to reinforcement of dependency by family

The Cognitive Perspective of Personality

The foremost contributor to the cognitive perspective of personality was Jean Piaget.

Jean Piaget Piaget felt that intelligence grows through the exposure of children to the world around them. He hypothesized that children's realities are confronted by ever changing environments and that it is during this process that children recognize discrepancies between their own reality and the environment. Resolving these discrepancies helps children learn new relationships between objects and therefore develop a more mature understanding.

According to Piaget's theory, the **cognitive theory** of personality, a child's ability to think matures through two processes. The first is **assimilation,** which refers to the incorporation of knowledge through the use of existing or familiar **schemes**, or patterns of recurring action. He identified three types of assimilation: biologic, mental, and social. *Biologic assimilation* occurs by taking food in the body and digesting it. *Mental assimilation* occurs by taking in information about the environment and giving it some perceptual meaning. Lastly, *social assimilation* occurs by learning the rules and regulations of society and fitting them into one's own personal value system. The purpose of assimilation is to allow people to fit the outside world with internal needs.

The second process is **accommodation**, which refers to the modification of existing schemes to incorporate new knowledge that does not fit into an old scheme. Piaget identified three types of accommodation: physical, mental, and social. *Physical accommodation* concerns postural change, for example, standing on toes to reach for an object on a high shelf. *Mental accommodation* refers to the intellectual adjustments people make in order to assimilate information. *Social accommodation* is the willingness to yield to pressure from the outside world to adhere to a particular value system. Accommodation involves changing responses to fit the realities of the outside world.

According to Piaget's theory, mental growth is achieved by a balance between assimilation and accommodation. He felt mental growth stagnates when one type of behavior predominates. For example, if children assimilate knowledge but are unable to accommodate it to the real world, Piaget suggested they will engage primarily in play and fantasy. If, on the other hand, children accommodate to everything and passively accept all in their surroundings, they will probably engage in imitation behavior rather than individualized learning.

Similar to Freud and Sullivan, Piaget constructed periods of intellectual development. He identified four major periods: (1) sensorimotor, (2) preoperational, (3) concrete operational, and (4) formal operational. Children develop new ways of thinking during each period, which are measurably different from one another. The speed by which a child moves through each period is variable, depending on genetic makeup and the environment. (See Table 3–7 for a summary of Piaget's periods of intellectual development.)

Table 3–7 *Phases of Cognitive Development According to Piaget*

Stage of Development	*Period*	*Defining Characteristics*
Sensorimotor	Birth–2 years	Infant is learning to get along with the world but does not think about it too much. Is beginning to learn to see objects as having their own existence. Behavior is goal-directed.
Preoperational thought	2–7 years	Understands that objects can be represented by symbols. Begins to acquire language. There is a belief that the child's opinion is the only one. Intelligence based more on intuition than logical reasoning. Can think about objects not directly in front of him or her. Imagination is active, and the child is learning to recognize relationships between things.
Concrete operations	7–11 years	Beginning of logical thinking. Reasoning is good for concrete events. Learns to classify things.
Formal operations	11–15 years	Can carry out systematic experiments to prove or disprove things. Ability to think in the abstract. Recognizes the value of own identity and is developing relationships with others.

The Importance of the Cognitive Perspective Piaget's theory of cognitive development, like other theories presented, provides a framework for assessment. This theory has obvious implications for pediatric nursing, but its principles may also be applied to adult learners. Because client education has become an extremely important part of professional nursing, it is vital for nurses to be proficient in the assessment of clients' learning readiness and cognitive capabilities. Cognitive developmental theory provides criteria on which to base these judgments. (See Table 3–8 for applications of the cognitive perspective.)

The Developmental Perspective of Personality

By expanding the psychoanalytic perspective, Erik Erikson, an American psychoanalyst, made major contributions to the theory of personality development.

Erik Erikson Erikson saw personality as developing through the entire life span rather than stopping at adolescence. He differed with Freud in

Table 3–8 *Examples of Assessment and Diagnosis Using Piaget's Theory of Cognitive Development*

Assessment Data

1. What is the age of the client?
2. In which Piaget period, according to the client's age, is this client?
3. Is the client able to perform the operations described in each period according to his or her age?
4. What specific characteristics of cognitive thinking does this client display?
5. If the client is an adult, does he or she display more tendency toward concrete operations, formal operations, or a combination of the two?
6. Is cognitive functioning affected by the client's illness?
7. What teaching strategies will be most effective within the client's ability to learn efficiently?
8. Does the client learn from the instruction and therefore meet learning objectives?

Nursing Diagnosis

Alteration in thought processes: Cognitive dissonance related to psychological conflicts

Anxiety: Inability to accommodate new knowledge related to change in health status

that he believed people could move backward to achieve developmental tasks they were unable, for whatever reason, to achieve before. Erikson's perspective, the **developmental theory** of personality, offered the hope of achieving a healthy development pattern sometime during a life span.

Although Erikson accepted the psychoanalytic perspective of the importance of basic needs and drives in children, he felt personality was shaped more by conflict between needs and culture than by conflict between the id, ego, and superego. He based this philosophy on the assumption that drives are much the same from one child to another, and cultures differ from one part of the world to another. He also felt cultures are capable of developing just as humans do.

Erikson believed the ego is much more important in determining personality than the id or superego. This idea stemmed from his view of culture. He believed that the ego is the mediating factor between the individual and society and that this relationship is at least as important as the influences of the basic drives. He also believed in the importance of relationships with social groups and felt this was evidenced by changes within the family and peer group. Erikson expanded the determinants of personality development from merely instinctual and biologic to social and cultural.

Another area where Erikson expanded psychoanalytic theories can be seen in his view of the future. Whereas Freud saw the most significance in past events, Erikson felt there was more significance in the future. He felt people's abilities to anticipate future events made a difference in the way they acted in the present. Many feel Erikson's theory is more hopeful and positive than Freud's. By expanding on the psychoanalytic perspective, Erikson acknowledged the chance to develop through the life span and to grow in a variety of ways.

According to Erikson each human being passes through eight developmental stages: (1) sensory, (2) muscular, (3) locomotor, (4) latency, (5) adolescent, (6) young adulthood, (7) adulthood, and (8) maturity. Each of the eight stages is characterized by conflicts and states a task that a person must achieve before moving on to the next developmental level. Erikson believed people had difficulty developing normally if they were unable to accomplish the tasks of the previous stage. (See Table 3–9 for a description of the eight stages of development according to Erikson.)

The Importance of the Developmental Perspective The developmental theories paint an ongoing picture of people and how they develop through the life span. This picture provides nurses with a framework from which they may carry out an assessment of relevant developmental criteria. It further assists nurses in making value judgments about the information received during the assessment process. It is much easier to analyze and understand people's behavior if one has a framework, such as the developmental theories, from which to work. (See Table 3–10 for applications of the developmental perspective.)

Table 3–9 *Stages of Social Growth and Development According to Erikson*

Stage of Development	*Period*	*Developmental Task*	*Defining Characteristics*
Sensory	Birth–18 months	Trust versus mistrust	Child learns to develop trusting relationships.
Muscular	1–3 years	Autonomy versus shame and doubt	Child starts the process of separation. Starts learning to live autonomously.
Locomotor	3–6 years	Initiative versus guilt	Learns about environmental influences. Becomes more aware of own identity.
Latency	6–12 years	Industry versus inferiority	Energy is directed at accomplishments, creative activities, and learning.
Adolescent	12–20 years	Identity versus role confusion	Transitional period. Movement toward adulthood. Starts incorporating beliefs and value systems that have been acquired previously.
Young adulthood	18–25 years	Intimacy versus isolation	Learns the ability to have intimate relationships.
Adulthood	24–45 years	Generativity versus stagnation	Emphasis on maintaining intimate relationships. Movement toward developing a family.
Maturity	45 years–death	Integrity versus despair	Acceptance of life as it has been. Acceptance of both good and bad aspects of past life. Maintaining a positive self-concept.

The Humanistic Perspective of Personality

Two psychologists pioneered the humanistic perspective of personality: Abraham Maslow and Carl Rogers.

Abraham Maslow Abraham Maslow wanted to create a "third force" in the field of psychology to present an alternative to psychoanalytic and behavioristic theories. His theories, which are comprised of the **humanistic theory** of personality, were unique and sometimes criticized because they were based on studies of highly creative and psychologically healthy people. Some researchers believed Maslow's methods were not scientific enough because his studies were conducted outside a laboratory and consisted only of observations and inferences.

Maslow identified two groups of human needs: basic needs and metaneeds. **Basic needs** are physiologic such as the need for food, water, and sleep. **Metaneeds** are growth-related and include such things as goodness, justice, and beauty. Under most circumstances, basic needs take precedence over metaneeds. A person who is hungry is going to be less concerned with truth and justice than a person who has met these basic needs. Maslow felt growth needs allow people to rise above an animal level of existence. People unable to meet their growth needs, Maslow postulated, are at risk for becoming psychologically disturbed.

In his humanistic theories, Maslow looked primarily at the healthy, strong side of human nature. He emphasized health rather than illness, success rather than failure. He even viewed basic physiologic needs and drives as healthy rather than as unhealthy urges to be controlled and tempered by reality. Maslow saw people as having an inborn nature that is essentially good or, at worst, neutral—a conceptualization different from many other theorists who felt inborn drives were bad or antisocial.

Carl Rogers Another psychologist closely related to the humanistic perspective of psychology is Carl Rogers. Like Maslow, Rogers believed people are motivated by the will to experience growth. His

Table 3–10 *Assessment and Diagnosis Using Erikson's Developmental Theory*

Assessment Data

1. What is the developmental stage of this client?
2. What tasks should this client be achieving?
3. Was the client successful in achieving the tasks of previous developmental stages?
4. During what stages did the client fail to achieve the developmental tasks?
5. What effect does this have on the client's psychosocial development?
6. How is this affecting the immediate problems confronting the client?
7. What are the environmental factors affecting this client and the client's present problems?
8. What social networks are available to this client?
9. How can these social networks affect outcomes of this present situation?
10. How might this client's culture affect the outcomes of the present situation?

Nursing Diagnosis

Social isolation: Absence of supportive significant others related to inability to engage in satisfying social relationships

Ineffective individual coping: Despair related to inability to maintain a positive self-concept during developmental stage of maturity

theories are an outgrowth of experiences and observations gathered from his practice of psychotherapy.

According to Rogers, people are not born with a self-concept but with an innate urge to become self-fulfilled. Maturity, he feels, comes when people have the ability to distinguish their body and thoughts from the outside world. As maturation occurs, people have expectations about their own ability and begin to develop value systems that enable them to make judgments about their own behavior. These values may stem from a person's own desires or be imposed from society. When a person's values are in conflict with society's values, problems arise.

Rogers believed the potential for people to become fully adjusted depends on their ability to symbolize or name experiences, the end result of which is that they are able to understand any part of their behavior. Rogers called these people **fully functioning.** Characteristics of this group include an awareness of both faults and weaknesses, high positive regard for self, and the ability to maintain sustaining relationships.

The Importance of the Humanistic Perspective The need for humanistic guidelines in nursing practice was discussed earlier in this chapter. Because the practice of nursing is based on humanistic conceptualizations of people, these theories fit nicely with many of the basic philosophies of the profession. Many nursing curricula have integrated Maslow's writings into their philosophic frameworks. Humanistic theories continue to be useful in establishing these guidelines because they present a positive, dynamic view of people and their environment. (See Table 3–11 for applications of the humanistic perspective.)

Table 3–11 *Assessment and Diagnosis Using Maslow's Humanistic Theories*

Assessment Data

1. Is this client meeting his or her basic needs?
2. How does this client describe these basic needs?
3. Other than basic needs, what other needs does the client consider important?
4. What is your description of the metaneeds being met by this client?
5. How does this client express self creatively?
6. What types of behaviors can be described that indicate this person is moving toward self-actualization?
7. How does this person describe his or her capabilities and resources?
8. What obvious needs are being frustrated at this time?
9. How does the client see these needs as being frustrated?

Nursing Diagnosis

Alteration in tissue perfusion: Unable to meet basic needs of oxygenation related to cardiopulmonary insufficiency

Disturbances in role performance: Inability to meet needs previously met by enactment of preillness role, related to change in physical capacity to resume previous roles

The Moral Development Perspective of Personality

What is virtue? What is morality, and how do people develop it? Philosophers have considered these questions through the ages. This section will focus on the work of two modern theorists of moral development, Lawrence Kohlberg and Carol Gilligan.

Lawrence Kohlberg Kohlberg is one of the few contemporary psychologists who sees morality as an ethical concept rather than a behavioral concept. He sees moral development and morality as coming from the principle of justice. For Kohlberg, justice is the balance between obligations and responsibilities, a principle that demands higher respect for persons than for laws. To him, justice is the end point of moral development; in other words, morally speaking, people develop toward the highest levels of justice.

Kohlberg identified six stages of moral development. As Table 3–12 shows, these six stages are grouped into three levels. Stage 6 reflects the highest level of moral reasoning; stage 1 reflects the lowest. Where people fall in Kohlberg's stages is based on how they solve specific moral dilemmas.

Kohlberg believed that at the less mature levels of moral development, where justice is not fully understood or differentiated, people can make unsophisticated moral judgments that are not im-

Table 3–12 *Six Stages of Moral Reasoning According to Kohlberg*

Stage of Development	*Period*	*Defining Characteristics*
Level I: Preconventional Emphasis on external control. The standards are those of others, and they are observed either to avoid punishment or to reap rewards.	4–10 years	Stage 1: *Punishment and obedience orientation.* "What will happen to me?" The child obeys the rules of others to avoid punishment. Stage 2: *Instrumental purpose and exchange.* "You scratch my back, I'll scratch yours." The child conforms to rules out of self-interest and consideration for what others can do in return.
Level II: Morality of conventional role conformity The child now wants to please other people and can decide whether some action is "good" by the standards of authority figures.	10–13 years	Stage 3: *Maintaining mutual relations, approval of others, the golden rule.* "Am I good? The child wants to please and help others, can judge the intentions of others, and develop his or her own ideas of what a good person is. Stage 4: *Social system and conscience.* "What if everybody did it?" The youngster is concerned with doing his or her duty, showing respect for higher authority, and maintaining the social order.
Level III: Morality of autonomous moral principles The attainment of true morality. For the first time, the individual acknowledges the possibility of conflict between two socially accepted standards and tries to decide between them. The control of conduct is now internal, both in the standards observed and in the reasoning about right and wrong. Stages 5 and 6 may be alternate methods of the highest level of reasoning.	13 years, young adulthood, or never	State 5: *Morality of contract, individual rights, and democratically accepted law.* The person thinks in rational terms, valuing the will of the majority and the welfare of society. He or she generally sees these values best supported by adherence to the law, though he or she recognizes that there are times when there is a conflict between human need and the law. Stage 6: *Morality of universal ethical principles.* The person does what he or she, as an individual, thinks right, regardless of legal restrictions or the opinions of others. Action is in accordance with internalized standards. The alternate to acting in accord with these standards would be self-condemnation.

moral. On the other hand, he believed that people ought to develop toward the higher stages. Kohlberg related the ability for personality development and cognitive development with the ability to move through the six stages of moral development. He believed all three types of development go hand in hand.

Another theorist, Carol Gilligan, maintained that Kohlberg's view of moral development was not uniformly applicable.

Carol Gilligan Feminism has propelled women toward exploring new and unique ways of looking at themselves. This search for self has resulted in the formulation of many questions and concerns. For Gilligan, one point of concern was the moral development of women.

In Kohlberg's theory and related theories of moral development, the model was the prototype for males. Men were seen as the norm, the orientation from which judgments were made. Gilligan looked at the discrepancies between how these theories portrayed the development of women and how she thought women really developed.

Gilligan noticed that when girls were given Kohlberg's moral dilemmas to solve, their answers usually placed them in a stage of moral development that was lower than that of boys of the same age. As a result, females were frequently accused of showing a lack of logic and an inability to think for themselves. Gilligan (1982, p. 28) postulated, however, that females do not see a world made up of people and situations standing alone, but of relationships and human connections: "She does not see the dilemma as a math problem with humans but a narrative of relationships over time." Gilligan believed that the perspective of females was as valid as that of males, and she called for reconsideration of Kohlberg's stages, which she thought were valid for only one portion of the population.

In her emerging theory Gilligan has attempted to differentiate between male and female experiences. She feels we must study more seriously the intrasexual experiences that differentiate behavior so that the unique experiences of both sexes can be identified more clearly. Gilligan feels that this is particularly vital to women, who have been viewed as developmental "failures" rather than having a unique developmental reality. (See Table 3–13 for applications of Gilligan's theory.)

Table 3–13 *Examples of Assessment and Diagnosis Using Gilligan's Theory*

Assessment Data

1. How does this person describe himself or herself?
2. How does this person describe his or her internal reality?
3. Have you as a "helper" evaluated your own values and attitudes concerning sexual stereotyping?
4. Is this person able to set goals for himself or herself?
5. Do the person's goals for self include an emphasis on change or adjustment?
6. Does this person have support systems in which to strengthen growth?
7. Does this client wish to be viewed differently by society?

Nursing Diagnosis

Powerlessness: Disturbance in self-esteem related to maturational crisis

Ineffective individual coping: Inability to meet basic needs related to continual unmet expectations

Juanita Williams Carol Gilligan was not the only researcher who raised questions as to the validity of existing theories as they related to the personality development of females. Juanita Williams, like Gilligan, proposed that, in most human development theories, the male was the standard from which all humanity was judged.

Williams viewed women as developing in a holistic bio-psycho-social context. In addition to moral development she explored learning, modeling, reinforcement, sex-role identification, sex typing and socialization, cognitive development, and competence. Williams (1977, p. 383) stated, "Human behavior emerges from the neonatal repertoire and becomes organized in a social context." She does not believe that women's behavior is more unusual than men's, only less understood because of a lack of research. She wrote, "Women as a class have in common certain attributes, conditions and experiences which differentiate them from men and require that they be studied separately if their behavior is to be understood."

The Importance of the Moral Development Perspective In the course of their profession, nurses frequently make moral judgments. Kohlberg, Gilligan, and Williams give a perspective on how moral judgments are made and a framework in which to make them.

As researchers ask more questions about development all nurses—men and women—must keep abreast of the research so that they can best meet the needs of the people they care for.

SUMMARY

Defining and Articulating Theories

1. Theories organize information, explain why things occur, assist in understanding the significance of past events, and provide the ability to predict and control events.
2. The nursing process is structured to allow for systematic categorization of the data gathered by applying a theoretic framework to a practice situation.

Theories of Personality Development

3. Freud defined three levels of consciousness: conscious, preconscious, and unconscious. The three components of personality are the id (the source of energy and drives), the ego (which provides reality testing and survival) and the superego (which provides rules and values).
4. The ego defense mechanisms alleviate anxiety by denying, misinterpreting, or distorting reality.
5. The Freudian psychoanalytic stages of development are oral, anal, phallic, latency, and genital.
6. Sullivan's interpersonal theory of development emphasizes interpersonal relationships. The stages of development in this theory are infancy, childhood, juvenile era, preadolescence, early adolescence, and late adolescence.
7. Behavioral theories of personality look at what causes people to act in particular ways and what entities in the environment reinforce that behavior.
8. According to Piaget's cognitive theory of development, mental growth is achieved by a balance between assimilation and accommodation. There are four periods of intellectual development: sensorimotor, preoperational, concrete operational, and formal operational.
9. Erikson's theory states that personality is shaped more by conflict between needs and culture than by conflict between the id, ego, and superego. It has a greater focus on the future than on the past.
10. Erikson's stages of development are sensory, muscular, locomotor, latency, adolescent, young adulthood, adulthood and maturity.
11. Humanistic theories emphasize health rather than illness and the potential for people to become self-fulfilled.
12. Gilligan has differentiated male and female development in that masculinity is defined through separation and femininity is defined through attachment.

CHAPTER REVIEW

Mr. Cohen is a 42-year-old male client two weeks post myocardial infarction. The nursing assessment describes Mr. Cohen as uncooperative and childlike. He is not retaining the information being taught to him in the client education program. His call light is on frequently but he is unable to communicate any specific need.

1. If applying the principles of the psychoanalytic theories of Freud, which of the following would be most true?
   - (a) Mr. Cohen is not adjusting because of a failure to assimilate this experience.
   - (b) Mr. Cohen would improve if the principles of behavior modification were employed.
   - (c) The unconscious use of ego defense mechanisms are being used by Mr. Cohen to protect against the uncomfortable feelings of anxiety.
   - (d) Mr. Cohen has failed to label his experience and therefore is not adapting well.
2. The primary nurse has assessed Mr. Cohen as showing symptoms of regression. Which of the following would be the best example of regression?
   - (a) A client who is critically ill allows the nurse to bathe and feed him.
   - (b) A student gets a C on a paper and goes home to yell at her family.
   - (c) A father spanks his child and the next morning brings home a present for him.
   - (d) A client feels very angry with his nurse and is overly friendly to her.

3. If the nurse was assessing Mr. Cohen's behavior within a behavioristic perspective, which one of the following questions would it be most appropriate to ask himself or herself?
   (a) What are the contextual stimuli confronting this client?
   (b) What is causing him to act this way and what factors in the environment support this behavior?
   (c) What type of basic human needs are not being met?
   (d) Which ego defense mechanisms are preventing Mr. Cohen from getting better?

4. In using Skinner's theory to plan intervention, the nurse would do which one of the following things?
   (a) Implement strategies that meet basic human needs.
   (b) Implement strategies to build trust and rapport.
   (c) Encourage Mr. Cohen to talk about past experiences with illness.
   (d) Reward the behaviors in Mr. Cohen that the nurse wishes to encourage.

5. If the nurse was assessing Mr. Cohen's behavior within a behavioristic perspective, which one of the following questions should the nurse ask himself or herself?
   (a) Other than basic needs, what other needs does the client consider important?
   (b) What is the developmental stage of this client?
   (c) Is there an obvious use of defense mechanisms?
   (d) How is the behavior that needs to be changed reinforced?

REFERENCES

Bevelas JB: *Personality: Current Theory and Research.* Brooks/Cole, 1978.

Gilligan C: *In a Different Voice: Psychological Theory and Women's Development.* Harvard University Press, 1982.

Hall CS, Lindzey G: *Theories of Personality,* 2nd ed. Wiley, 1970.

Kerlinger FH: *Foundations of Behavior Research,* 2nd ed. Holt, Rinehart, and Winston, 1973.

Kim HS: *The Nature of Theoretical Teaching in Nursing.* Appleton-Century-Crofts, 1983.

Kohlberg L: *Essays on Moral Development.* Harper & Row, 1981.

Miller JB: *Toward a New Psychology of Women.* Beacon Press, 1976.

Riehl J, Roy C: *Conceptual Models of Nursing Practice,* 2nd ed. Appleton-Century-Crofts, 1980.

Stevens B: *Nursing Theory: Analysis, Application and Evaluation.* Little, Brown, 1979.

Williams JH: *Psychology of Women.* Norton, 1977.

SUGGESTED READINGS

Briggs D: Social learning: A holistic approach. *J Holistic Nurs* 1988; 6(1):31–36.

Crockett MS: Self-reports on childhood peer relationships of psychiatric and nonpsychiatric subjects. *Issues Ment Health* 1988; 9(1):45–71.

Friedemann M: Closing the gap between grand theory and mental health practice with families. *Arch Psychiatr Nurs* 1989; 3(1):10–19.

Gordon VC, et al.: A 3-year follow-up of a cognitive-behavioral therapy intervention. *Arch Psychiatr Nurs* 1988; 2(4):218–226.

Johnson JE, et al.: Alternative explanations of coping with stressful experiences associated with physical illness. *ANS* 1989; 11(2):39–52.

Morath JM: Theory-based intervention: A case study using Sullivan's interpersonal theory of psychiatry. *Perspect Psychiatr Care* 1987; 24(1):12–19.

Omery A: Values, moral reasoning and ethics. *Nurs Clin North Am* 1989; 24(2):499–508.

Rosenstock IM, et al.: Social learning theory and the health belief model. *Health Educ Q* 1988; 15(2): 175–183.

CHAPTER 4

Psychiatric Treatment Modalities

SUSAN F. MILLER

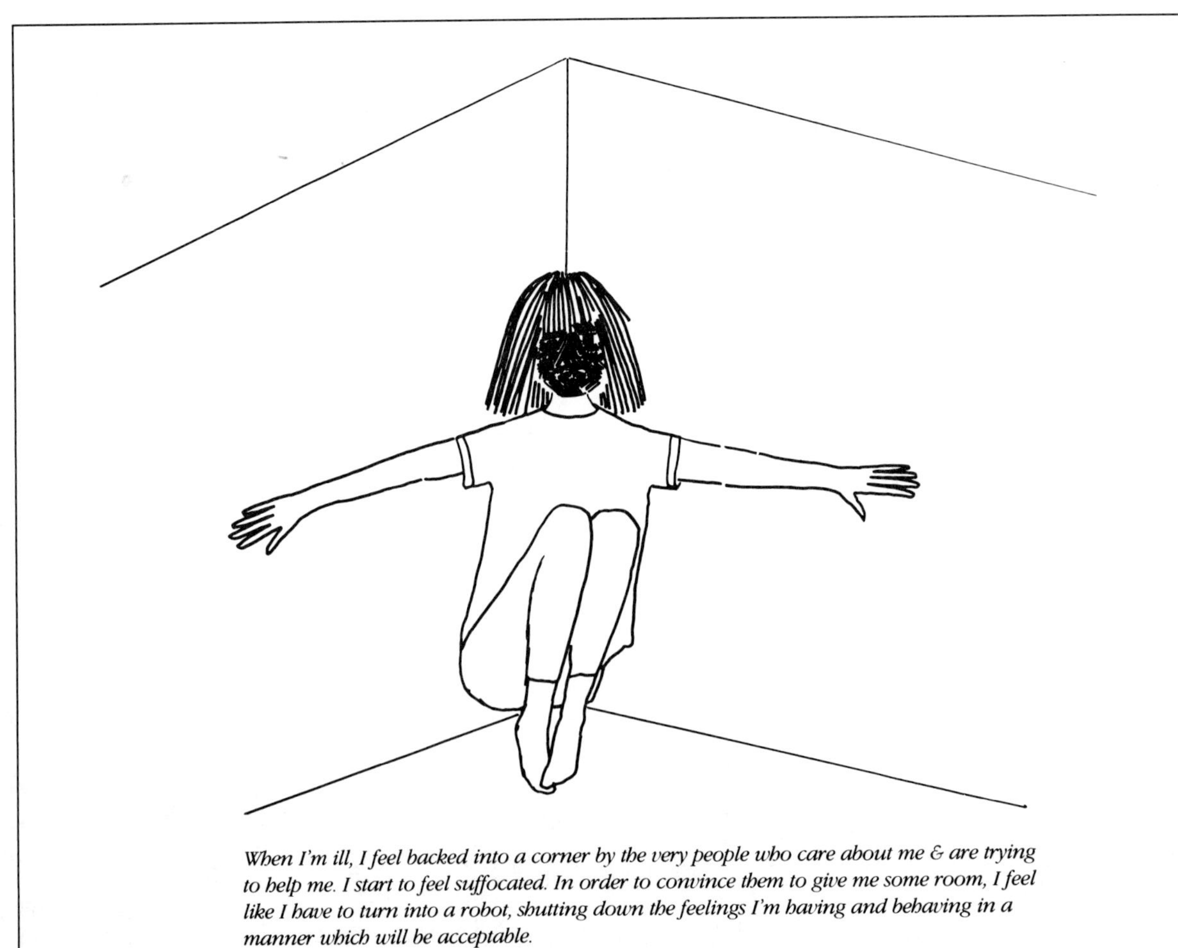

When I'm ill, I feel backed into a corner by the very people who care about me & are trying to help me. I start to feel suffocated. In order to convince them to give me some room, I feel like I have to turn into a robot, shutting down the feelings I'm having and behaving in a manner which will be acceptable.

■ *Objectives*

After reading this chapter, the student will be able to

- Identify conditions under which clients enter the mental health system
- Identify components of the community mental health system
- Describe the ethical principles used to resolve ethical dilemmas in mental health nursing
- Discuss primary, secondary, and tertiary prevention with implications for nursing practice
- Describe the implications of the Patients' Bill of Rights to mental health treatment
- Identify the major modalities used to intervene in mental health problems
- Describe the impact of DSM-III-R on mental health intervention
- Identify the role of laboratory tests in the diagnosis and treatment of mental disorders
- Discuss possible outcomes of current research on diagnosis and treatment of mental health problems

■ *Chapter Outline*

Introduction

A revolution in psychiatric treatment occurred in the 1960s, when the community mental health system was born. In 1967, Gerald Caplan defined the **community mental health model**, which was intended as a means for bringing mental health care to the total population by providing a series of comprehensive services in the community (Caplan, 1970). Since then, this model has been the publicly funded system for the treatment of mental health. Recently, however, dissatisfaction about the system has surfaced. Many psychiatrists have moved out of the system, leaving nonmedical professionals, including nurses, room to carve out autonomy within their own professional practices.

Problems in Community Mental Health Centers

Langsley (1985) has identified the major problems encountered by community mental health centers:

- Deinstitutionalization causing neglect of the chronically ill and leaving them with inadequate community support systems

- Inaccessibility of care for children, the elderly, rural populations, and minority groups
- In many instances, issues related to governance, particularly in regard to participation by those served, interpreted to mean community control of governance
- Financial problems created by the dual system of care: the community mental health programs causing shifts of funds from state hospitals to community agencies
- Staffing problems with shortages of mental health professionals
- Difficulties developing realistic catchment areas reflecting political boundaries, natural communities, and geographic regions
- Decline in the enthusiasm for primary prevention because of the inability to see effects of activities
- Moving away from a health model to a social services model
- Client's perception of lower quality of care being offered by paraprofessionals
- Low profile within the community with too few persons aware of available services

With these problems in mind, the mental health nursing student enters a new world set aside from the usual hospital environment. This chapter introduces the student to the vast array of treatment modalities available to the psychiatric/mental health client.

Client Entry into the Mental Health System

Entry into the mental health care system is based on assessment of a pattern of behavior manifested by suffering and impairment in intrapersonal, interpersonal, and environmental stimuli.

Once disruptive behavioral patterns have been identified and responses to physical and interpersonal stimuli altered, the person may decide to seek mental health care. In addition to self-referral, referral by significant others, mental health professionals, and societal agents are pathways to psychiatric treatment. (See Figure 4–1.) Entering the mental health care system through the emergency room of a tertiary care center is another available option.

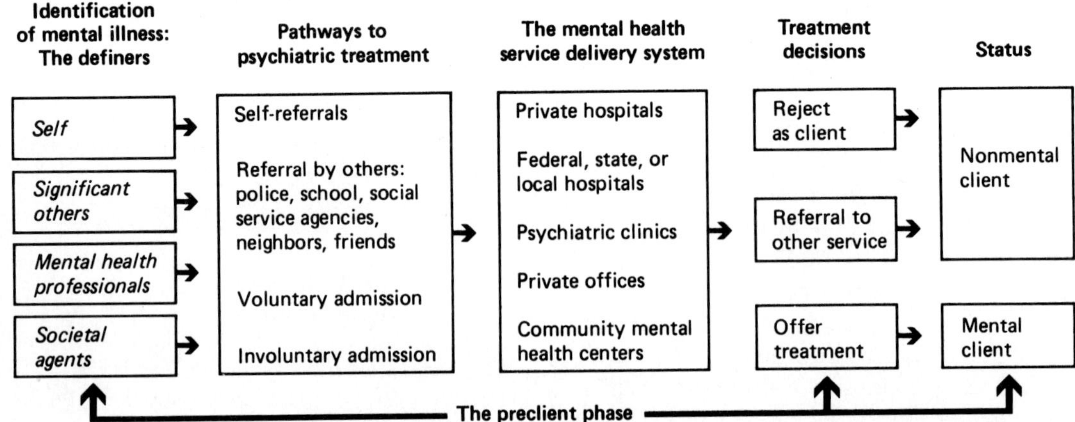

Figure 4–1 *The Process of becoming a client in the mental health care system. Reprinted from J. E. Ruffin, Sociocultural aspects of mental illness. In:* Comprehensive Psychiatric Nursing, *J. Haber et al. (editors). McGraw-Hill, 1978.*

Heather Arnold was seen in the emergency department for evaluation of grandiose, obtrusive, and hostile behavior in addition to a diminished physical state. As a technical writer for a large computer firm, the 28-year-old woman has been known to be a capable and congenial employee. Over the past two months, however, Heather has become increasingly aggressive in the office, demanding additional assignments and full of self-praise while belittling the work of colleagues. Erratic performance and incomplete projects have contributed to frequent absenteeism. Heather is belligerent when supervisors attempt to discuss her job performance. Creditors have been calling the company to seek payment for outstanding bills. Threatened with losing her job, Heather reluctantly agrees to talk with the company's nurse. Following an interview, she agrees to accompany the nurse to the emergency department for further evaluation.

Approaches to Mental Health Care

Mental health care services are provided through collaboration among representatives from several disciplines. Each discipline provides separate but not always distinct services to the client. (See Figure 4–2.) Regardless of the discipline, psychosocial intervention is an interpersonal process, and team members must understand their respective roles and functions. Failure to come to agreement on goals and approaches to care can lead to client dissatisfaction with fragmented care. Interdisciplinary development of the treatment plan and goals relating to the client's return to optimal functioning encourages client participation and compliance with the therapeutic regimen.

Clients who enter the mental health care system will participate in a psychiatric interview and mental status examination that will help identify the problem. Physical examination may suggest conditions that have behavioral manifestations. Following

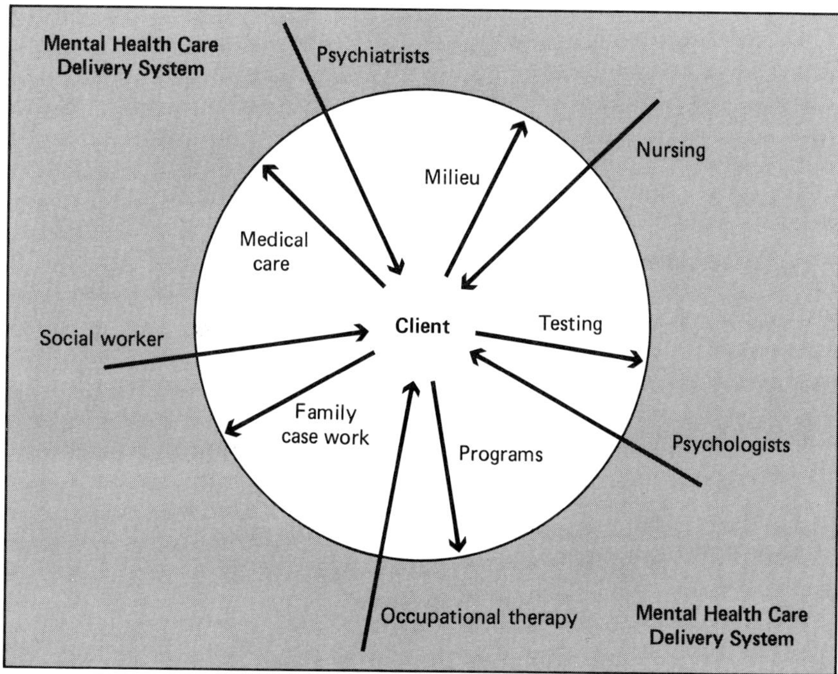

Figure 4-2 Client interaction with the mental health care system.

the analysis of data, formulating an understanding of the mental disorder occurs, and the treatment plan is developed.

The decision to recommend an outpatient setting or hospitalization requires

- Clarifying the client's problem(s)
- Assessing the client's ability to participate in the treatment plan
- Determining the amount and type of supervision necessary to monitor pharmacotherapy
- Identifying the degree of structure required to ensure safety and client participation in treatment modalities (milieu, occupational, individual, and group therapies)

The role of the nurse in the care of clients with mental health problems depends on the setting and levels of preparation. However, as Lang et al. (1980) discuss, a part of the nurse's role is invariably assessment and data collection, which enables

- Analysis of data
- Application of theory
- Application of knowledge of psychosocial and pathophysiologic principles integrated with nursing process
- Use of therapeutic techniques
- Evaluation of intervention
- Collaboration in research and use of research findings to transfer new knowledge and promote practice derived from scientific methods

Outpatient Services The emergency room is frequently viewed by the community as the entry point for mental health care. Of all clients seen in emergency departments of community and urban hospitals, 5 to 15 percent require psychiatric treatment or consultation. Moreover, emergency room client records indicate that psychosocial intervention is necessary in most situations (Yoder and Jones, 1982).

Emergency departments in private, state, or community hospitals provide evaluation and identification of mental disorders. Social workers, nurses, and psychiatrists serve in a liaison role by referring clients to appropriate treatment modalities. Crisis intervention by community-based mental health professionals can offer clients help in establishing equilibrium and returning to precrisis functioning.

Emergency care takes place in private psychiatric clinics, private therapists' offices, and community mental health centers. In 1980, mental health visits totaled 79 million: 50 percent were seen by psychiatrists and psychologists in private practice; 40 percent were seen by nonpsychiatrist physicians, nurses, and social workers; and 10 percent were seen in organized settings such as emergency departments, outpatient clinics, and mental health centers.

The probability of using mental health services varies with age, race, education, and income. The group with the greatest probability of having at least one outpatient visit consists of white females between the ages of 25 and 64, with 13 or more years of education and from all socioeconomic levels (Taube et al., 1984). Recent data indicate that people are using mental health services with increased frequency. Several reasons may explain this:

- The stigma associated with mental health problems is decreasing.
- There is more opportunity to receive adequate treatment in outpatient settings.
- Public awareness of available resources is increasing.
- Nonrestrictive settings decrease fear and instill hope for a return to optimal functioning.

Hospital Admittance State laws describe the conditions for voluntary and involuntary admission to hospitals for mental disorder. Voluntary admission occurs when the client initiates a written request for inpatient treatment. Involuntary admission is sought when the client has been determined to be a danger to self or to society.

Hospitalization may be indicated for several reasons:

- Failure of all other interventions, with an increase in symptoms or maladaptive behavior to a disabling level
- Failure to clarify diagnosis
- Failure of environment (therapist, family, work) to further tolerate client behavior
- Persistent reinforcement by the environment of maladaptive behavior
- Initiation of a new form of treatment that requires supervision
- Exacerbation of a chronic illness resulting from noncompliance with an outpatient treatment plan

The feasibility of short-term, partial, or long-term hospitalization depends on the time required to identify client problems, formulate and implement the plan, and evaluate the client's response and ability to participate and take control of the plan in a less restrictive setting. Focusing on the acuity of the mental health problem contributes to the client's and family's acceptance of short-term or partial hospitalization.

Characteristics of Clients in the Mental Health System

A general description of behavior includes the person's patterns of thinking, feeling, and responding to intrapersonal, interpersonal, and environmental experiences. Since alterations in behavior are defined in relation to a given culture, behavior that deviates from the cultural norm may indicate the need for mental health intervention.

Another view of behavior identifies those responses that interfere with the well-being of the person or group as maladaptive. The term *well-being* is used not only in the survival sense but also refers to the person's ability to actualize potential (Coleman et al., 1984). To initiate and maintain satisfactory interpersonal relationships, to do meaningful work, to face reality as it is defined by personal strengths and limitations, and to find meaning in life all contribute to personal growth and fulfillment.

Another perspective uses systems theory to explain characteristics contributing to psychosocial disorders. The mentally healthy person is capable of loving, setting goals, learning, regulating self, and responding to people and events in the environment and is therefore an open system with the ability to process information to and from the environment (Mamar, 1983). This person can receive, process, store, and respond to experiences. The interaction between the biologic system, physical environment, and community is a source of strength and stress.

Conflicts in any system cause a ripple in one or all of the others. These ripples, or stressors, are indicated by a functional interruption or impairment of thought process, affect, communication, and relationships.

Response to stressors is a dynamic process in which behaviors vary with conditioning factors, including client personality and environmental supports. Conditioning factors allow opportunities to solve problems before behavior becomes maladaptive and function is impaired. Significant dysfunctional behavioral or psychologic patterns move the client into the mental health care system. These characteristics are associated with a painful symptom or impairment in one or more areas of function (behavioral, physiologic, or psychologic); they are not limited to a conflict between the client and society.

An interactional model of mental disorder (Wallace, 1988) identifies the cause as the intersection of conditions rather than one specific etiology. Experiences are determined by the intersection of psychobiologic and other conditions in the environment. For example, according to Wallace a depressive disorder is not exclusively due to an external event such as the death of a spouse; neurochemical activity; or a set of perceptions, affect, and attitudes relating to the spouse. The cause of depression and resulting dysfunctional behavior is the intersection between the death, the client's neurochemistry, and affective and cognitive responses.

Martha Grey, a 75-year-old retired secretary, was brought to the physician's office by her granddaughter. Mrs. Grey had become progressively forgetful and withdrawn since the death of her husband six months previously. Refusing to eat or leave her home, Mrs. Grey speaks only of her husband. She is unable to recognize current friends and refers to her granddaughter by her daughter's name.

The demographics of clients in the mental health system is changing to reflect the changes in the U.S. population at large. The number of Americans over 65 years of age will double by the year 2030. Of that group those 85 years old and older make up the most rapidly growing population segment. Health care providers will treat the disorders that frequently afflict this segment—in particular, dementia, Alzheimer's type, and depression—more often as the number of those over 85 increases. The challenge to health care providers will be to assess, diagnose, and treat the problems effectively (Rubin, Zorumski, and Burke, 1988). The older client's ability to return to optimal self-care activities in a community setting will depend upon accurate diagnosis, treatment, and community support.

Older adults rarely take the initiative in seeking treatment for mental health problems. Inability to distinguish concerns from the normal aging process, fear of mental illness, or severe functional impairment are typical factors that delay treatment of elderly clients. Elders usually depend upon significant others in their support network to bring them to treatment. As in Mrs. Grey's case, the primary physician is usually the person to whom the client or family turns for help.

Changes in habits, cognitive function, general health, affect, and self-care activities are usually early indications of depression or dementia. In many cases depression and dementia are reversible. Therefore, all changes in mental status and functional performance should be evaluated (Reynolds et al., 1988).

Living with a Person Who Has Mental Illness

Living with a person who has a psychiatric disorder presents special challenges to family members or others with whom the client has significant relationships. These people must face the problems that beset healthy families as well as adjust lifestyle, communication, and responses to the ill person's behavior (Hyde, 1980).

The mentally ill person's behavior usually forces these families to cope with frequent disappointment. The family may have to cancel recreational and social activities in the family and community. Anxiety about the ill person's behavior may cause the family to avoid entertaining.

Tension described as a toxic atmosphere develops in the home. The toxic atmosphere is brought about by two major factors:

- Constant negative feelings, including anger, resentment, guilt, tension, anxiety, and depression
- Hectic, fast-paced home environment

Although Hyde's work refers to the effects of a toxic atmosphere upon clients with schizophrenia, the concepts can be applied to all family members.

In their efforts to avoid conflict, families tread carefully, supressing feelings of disappointment, anger, and frustration about the client's behavior. Without guidance, families tend to overprotect clients, tolerating inappropriate behavior for extended periods until an eruption of hurt, angry feelings occurs. Although achieving a period of calm for the short term, overprotection encourages the illusion that the client is more dependent than reality indicates. In fact, clients are extremely sensitive to the feelings of others, and the avoidance behavior of families may actually precipitate crisis. Table 4–1 is a summary of client behaviors and effective family responses.

Nurses and counselors can assist families in modifying behavior to exhibit more adaptive and

Table 4–1 *Summary of Client Behaviors and Effective Family Responses*

Client Behavior	*Family Response*
Game playing, which provokes anger, irritation, and frustration in family members	Expresses, honestly and clearly, feelings and expectations about client behavior.
	Provides client with appropriate social and recreational outlets.
Runaway behavior	Assists the client in planning for and attaining independent living within functional ability.
Emotional withdrawal and isolation	Examines and reduces overprotective behavior while providing a private space in the home.
Chemical/alcohol use and related behavior	Does not tolerate client's use in the home. May require structural residential rehabilitation program.
Frequent and prolonged periods of decompensation marked by self-care deficit and noncompliance with treatment	Expresses confidence in efforts to assist the client.
	Acknowledges powerlessness to change client's situation.
	Gradually lets the client go until opportunities to assist return.

functional responses. Opportunities to identify, discuss, and resolve behavior problems as they happen must be provided. Openness allows for the "detoxification" of the environment and facilitates accurate interpretation of feelings and responses (Walsh, 1985).

In addition to counseling services, the client and family can seek self-help support groups that enable families to cope more effectively with clients. Through sharing, families can express feelings in a supportive and empathic atmosphere while learning new coping strategies. The group provides a source of socialization for many care givers who rarely have a chance to get away from the home. While learning ways to cope with behavioral problems, group members exchange information about resources for financial and legal help, for rehabilitation and housing, and for information about psychiactric disorders and treatment (Bernheim, Lewine, and Beale, 1982).

Once the illness and related problems have been identified and accepted, the family must learn to live and respond to each other in a positive way. The treatment team is essential to the family's efforts to develop adaptive methods of living together and solving problems.

Legal and Ethical Issues in Psychiatric/Mental Health Nursing

Studies indicate that about one in seven persons will experience a mental disorder in any six-month period (Black, 1988). Mental disorder affects a person's capacity to make decisions about health and well-being, raising questions of ethics, law, and social policy.

Mental illness leaves the client vulnerable to manipulation by health care givers who overlook the ethical and legal dimensions of psychiatric treatment. The dilemma for care givers is how to maintain the client's personal control or liberty in situations where public welfare and the client's best interests can be rationalized (Garritson, 1988).

In psychiatric mental health nursing, as in other health care specialties, the professional nurse is called upon to evaluate and choose goals, set priorities among conflicting values, interpret and give meaning to actions, make judgments about right or wrong courses of action, and establish minimal expectations of conduct (Jameton, 1984). The nurse makes ethical judgments when deciding to use medication, restraint, or seclusion for the client. Not including the client in the decision-making process is also a substantive ethical issue.

A nurse practicing in the mental health setting is responsible for providing care consistent with the American Nurses' Association code of ethics (see Table 4–2). In addition, when deciding on a course of action, the nurse must systematically question and analyze choices in the context of his or her own values. Perhaps legislation protecting mental health clients is required because of the long history of disregard for the ethical implications of psychiatric intervention and the conflict between the rights of individuals and the rights of society.

The nurse must examine the principles of autonomy, beneficience, and justice to determine the correct intervention. *Autonomy* refers to respect for the client's capacity to participate in and agree to decisions affecting health and well-being. *Beneficience* is the nurse's duty not to harm the client and to relieve pain and suffering. *Justice* ensures that treatment and intervention are provided fairly. If justice prevails, then everyone receives the same treatment unless relevant ethical considerations support treating someone differently.

> *Ann P, an RN, is the only float working a busy evening shift on a Saturday night. A 25-year-old client, Mary, approaches Ann. Mary is depressed but wants to talk for the first time since her admission two days ago. The charge nurse informs Ann that another client, John, requires one-to-one supervision following a suicidal gesture. John has received medication.*
>
> *Ann is torn between her duty to comfort and support Mary and her duty to John, who requires intensive monitoring. The scarcity of*

Table 4–2 *ANA Nursing Code of Ethics*

Principles
1. The nurse provides services with respect for human dignity and the uniqueness of the client, unrestricted by considerations of social or economic status, personal attributes, or the nature of health problems.
2. The nurse safeguards the client's right to privacy by judiciously protecting information of a confidential nature.
3. The nurse acts to safeguard the client and the public when health care and safety are affected by the incompetent, unethical, or illegal practice of any person.
4. The nurse assumes responsibility and accountability for individual nursing judgments and actions.
5. The nurse maintains competence in nursing.
6. The nurse exercises informed judgment and uses individual competence and qualification as criteria in seeking consultation, accepting responsibilities, and delegating nursing activities to others.
7. The nurse participates in activities that contribute to the ongoing development of the profession's body of knowledge.
8. The nurse participates in the profession's efforts to implement and improve standards of nursing.
9. The nurse participates in the profession's efforts to establish and maintain conditions of employment conducive to high-quality nursing care.
10. The nurse participates in the profession's effort to protect the public from misinformation and misrepresentation to maintain the integrity of nursing.
11. The nurse collaborates with members of the health professions and other citizens in promoting community and national efforts to meet public health needs.

Source: Nursing Code of Ethics (American Nurses' Association, 1976). Reprinted with permission.

nurses requires that one client must wait for care. Ann must determine what relevant difference justifies her caring for one client over the other at this time. Therefore, in deciding who receives care, she must weigh the benefits and burdens to each client and select an action in this situation.

Hospitalization

Short-term hospitalization for diagnosis, rapid stabilization with medication, therapeutic activities that enhance functional capacity, and a rapid return to the community is the desired approach to episodes of psychiatric distress or decompensation. As a result of the deinstitutionalization movement of the 1970s, however, many clients with chronic psychiatric disorders have been unable to manage self-care activities and have become the homeless and exploited street people found in every community. These clients often require rehospitalization because they are not able to manage in the community. In some areas adequate housing and supervision in group living arrangements have been the successful alternative to hospitalization. Another proposed alternative is to maintain inpatient hospital beds to protect clients from the consequences of self-care deficits.

Commitment

Commitment, including voluntary admission, forces examination of significant issues:

- The needs and liberty of clients
- The needs and rights of staff, other clients, and the community

The nurse's duty to "do no harm" and to relieve pain and suffering requires a constant balance of ethical issues. Wherever possible, client autonomy and liberty must be ensured by a return to the least restrictive setting and avoidance of any treatment that limits autonomy and participation in treatment decisions. Such treatments include chemical restraint or medication, physical restraint or seclusion, mechanical restraint, assault, or confinement with special vests or other binders.

A recent approach to the needs of the chronically ill is called **outpatient commitment.** This alternative to hospitalization provides more structure than typical community placement. The client is released to a community agency and subject to conditions imposed by judicial order. The client must agree to treatment at a designated treatment center and to take medications as prescribed (Brooks, 1987). Preliminary data suggest that, for chronic and noncompliant clients with histories of decompensation due to noncompliance with medication therapy and frequent rehospitalization, outpatient commitment is an effective alternative to hospitalization.

A psychiatrist diagnosed Mary B as a paranoid schizophrenic. The diagnosis was made on the basis of general interviews in which Mary gave inappropriate and irrational responses to interview questions. Mary was delusional, heard voices, and feared the devil was "out to get her." The court established, on the basis of clear and convincing presenting evidence, that Mary had a mental disorder necessitating commitment for treatment.

Competence and Capacity

Competence is a legal determination that a client can make reasonable judgments and decisions about treatment and other significant areas of personal life. An adult, as defined by an individual state, is competent as long as a judge does not declare him or her incompetent following a hearing when witnesses present supporting information. When a court rules someone incompetent, it appoints a guardian or surrogate to make decisions on that person's behalf.

Competence is distinguished from the **capacity** to make decisions. The dictionary defines *capacity* as the power of receiving and holding knowledge and impressions, or mental ability. Competence refers to the long-term general ability to manage one's affairs. Capacity may refer to specific situations at different points in time. A client may be designated as incompetent to sign legal contracts for bank loans but may have the capacity to participate in treatment decisions.

> *A 30-year-old, James, was diagnosed as having schizophrenia five years ago. James is transferred to the Medical Center from the Community Mental Health Center. His family cannot be located. The client is suffering from kidney failure, and the physicians recommend renal dialysis. James refuses dialysis and begins to tell a story about a family member who had a long and painful course of treatment on dialysis. The physicians are left with the dilemma of what to do.*

Clients have a right to refuse treatment if they have the capacity to grant informed consent (Macklin, 1987). The question remains: Should a person, regardless of the presence of psychiatric disorder, be coerced into accepting life-preserving treatment of any kind?

Physicians and nurses tend to take the paternalistic approach to decision making by acting out of the client's best interest. However, the best interests must be weighed in terms of the benefits and burdens of the treatment. Acknowledgment by physicians and nurses that the client's best interest is ideally determined by the client is essential to the decision-making process. It is also important to weigh the client's right to participate in that process regardless of whether the treatment preserves life or modifies behavior. The decision to utilize lifesaving dialysis or behavior-modifying psychotropic medication must include a respect for the client's autonomy, including careful evaluation of the benefits and risks (Kazorowski, 1988).

Decision-making capacity can be determined according to the outcome of the decision. In James's case, refusing dialysis would result in certain death; therefore, his physicians determine that, because of a psychiatric disorder, James does not have the capacity to make this important decision. Another test of capacity involves examining the process by which the client makes decisions. This concept holds that, although the client may lack capacity for some decisions, he or she may be capable of making others. Therefore, the client's prior knowledge, experiences, and feelings must be considered in determination of capacity (Hastings Center, 1987).

Informed Consent

Laws identify that the client has a right to be free from intentional harm; therefore, where there is no consent or authorization, the health care provider is held responsible for battery or offensive touching according to law (Creighton, 1986). Again, the health care provider—usually the physician—is held to the standards of care to provide reasonable information according to the client's, not the health care worker's, needs. The information presented includes explanation of the psychosocial problem, nature and purpose of procedure, consequences of treatment, and alternative approaches. As in confinement, mental illness does not preclude the client's right to receive explanations about treatment and to authorize such treatment. Inherent in the right to consent is the right to refuse, which does not end after consent is given; at any time, the client may withdraw consent. The legal aspects of informed consent should be clearly understood because of the potential for negligence or malpractice litigation.

The ethical dimension of informed consent reinforces a belief in the client's autonomy and capacity to make choices and is dependent upon accurate and sufficient information with which to make those decisions. The dilemma comes in deciding what type and how much information is given to clients.

Clients have a right to know about their medications and the side effects of those medications. By clearly stating the actions of neuroleptic medications as well as the potential side effects, including tardive dyskinesia, the nurse takes the risk that the client might refuse to take the prescribed medications. The benefits and burdens to the client and community are considered when the nurse medicates clients against their will or chooses to respect the client's right to refuse. Table 4–3 cites an example of the client's right regarding medications. The example is drawn from the state of Massachusetts.

Table 4–3 *The Client's Rights Regarding Medications*

Massachusetts law protects the client's right—as an inpatient or outpatient of a mental health or mental retardation facility—to participate in decisions regarding medication. The law also defines, restrictively and specifically, those situations in which the client may be forcibly medicated. These protections have recently been reaffirmed by the Massachusetts Supreme Judicial Court in the case of *Rogers* v. *Commissioner of Mental Health,* 390 Mass. 489.

The client must be told and have the capacity to understand

- The nature and extent of illness
- The medication(s) prescribed and why
- The benefits to be derived
- The risks generally and special risks

Source: Adapted from *Your Rights Regarding Medication* (Mental Health Legal Advisors Committee, 1984). Used with permission.

Voluntary Admission

Voluntary admission occurs if the client, for the purposes of assessment and treatment of psychosocial problems, consents to confinement and signs a document indicating as much. Specific procedures are governed by individual states; generally, the document indicates a minimum confinement period, at which time the client must give notice of intention to leave the facility. This notification period provides the health care team with time to complete discharge arrangements or to seek authorization for longer confinement through the courts, should it be necessary, to ensure client and community safety.

Involuntary Commitment

As with voluntary admission, individual states establish procedures for **involuntary commitment.** However, establishing the presence of mental illness is only a preliminary procedure; it is not a sufficient condition for hospitalization (Malmquist, 1979). A licensed physician determines the likelihood of harm to self or others.

Commitment is for a limited time. The period varies by state statute. For example, in Arkansas, disposition is 45 days; in Idaho, it is three years. In Alaska, the District of Columbia, and Texas, the length of disposition is indeterminant. At the end of the confinement period, the health team must discharge the client or petition the court for continued hospitalization. The client may be offered the opportunity to sign a voluntary request for hospitalization after commitment. If signed, the voluntary admission rescinds the involuntary commitment. This approach encourages the client to participate in care.

Refusal of treatment following voluntary or involuntary confinement is an issue facing mental health care providers, and solutions have been sought in the judicial system. One position maintains that commitment to a treatment facility implies consent for treatment on the basis of questionable competence (Malmquist, 1979). However, as stated earlier, confinement and the presence of mental illness do not preclude the client's capacity to make decisions about treatment.

The use of psychotropic medications, a major component of treatment plans, is controversial because these medications have "mind altering" properties, which allegedly interfere with client civil rights. In 1975 seven clients from Boston State Hospital charged that they were given antipsychotic medications, a type of psychotropic medication, against their will. This group of voluntarily and involuntarily confined clients stated that this practice was a violation of the First Amendment (freedom of speech), Fourth Amendment (inviolability of person), Fifth and Fourteenth Amendments (rights to due process laws), Eighteenth Amendment (rights to freedom from cruel and unusual punishment), and the right to refuse treatment (Applebaum and Gutheil, 1980). The judge presiding decided in favor of the clients. This decision poses a serious question to mental health care providers: Is psychotropic medication essential and, in some cases, the exclusive treatment modality?

The client's refusal of such treatment contributes to confinement with an inadequate treatment plan, thereby delaying the client's return to the least restrictive setting. On the other hand, states have determined criteria for the administration of psychotropic medications without consent in emergency situations. These are acute eruptions of behavior contributing to the likelihood of serious harm to the client or others. Physicians must order the medication only for the duration of the emergency; the nurse monitors the client for side effects, provides support during this often frightening experience, and ceases administration when behavior has abated (Ayd, 1985).

Ensuring the client's safety and a treatment plan that facilitates return to self-care are objectives of hospitalization. The nurse must identify decisions to use medications and other forms of behavior control (such as isolation or aversive treatment) without client permission as restrictions of autonomy. Therefore, the benefits and burdens of such therapeutic intervention must be weighed in all treatment decisions. Proper support and monitoring of all treatment ensure that the standards of care are maintained and that treatment is appropriate to the client behavior (Kebbee, 1987).

Recent court decisions have been in accord with the rights-driven model of determining the client's right to refuse treatment (Applebaum, 1988). The rights-driven model supports autonomy and holds that competent persons have the right to control intrusions on their bodies. This approach extends informed consent to all committed clients.

The most desirable approach to treating hospitalized clients includes accurate assessment of competence. If the client is found to be incompetent, the judge acts in the client's best interest. The best interest is determined on the basis of "substituted judgment," or what the client would choose if competent and what a reasonable person would decide in a similar situation. After following the process, medication or other restraint intervention may be used if it is in the client's best interest. The key factor is that the emphasis is on the client's competence and not reported benefits and potential outcome of the intervention. Figure 4–3 illustrates the process of determining intervention without client consent.

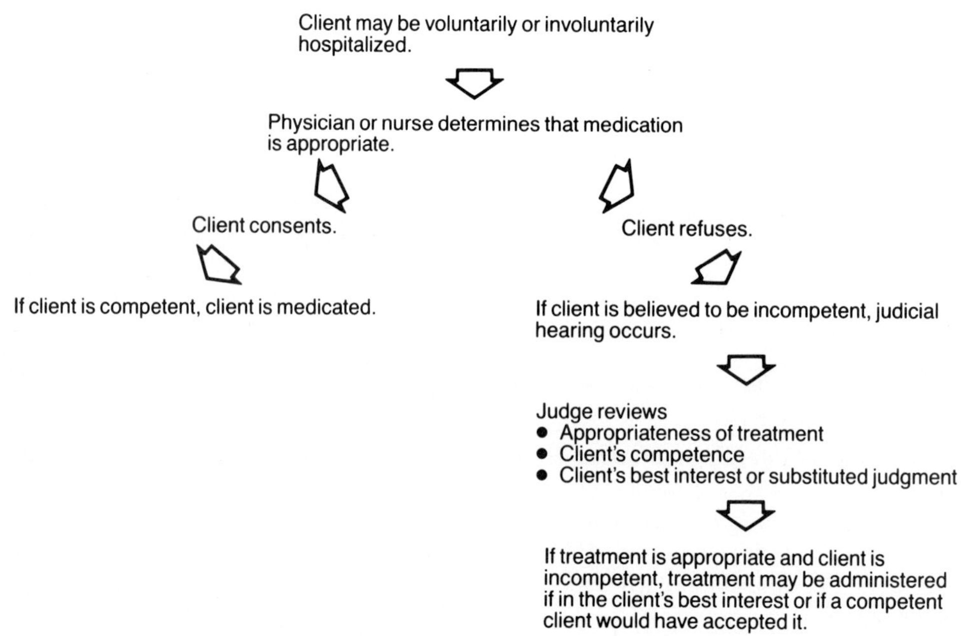

Figure 4–3 *Decision-making model: Administration of restraining therapy.*

Adapted from P. S. Applebaum, The right to refuse treatment with antipsychotic medications. *Am J Psychiatry* 1988; 145:416.

Implications for Nursing Practice

Nurses need to know the laws governing mental health intervention in their states and to provide care according to accepted standards of practice. All nursing decisions need to be based on sound ethical reasoning, which includes the notion that the client can make decisions about health and well-being, that intervention will avoid inflicting intentional harm, and that intervention will be in the client's best interest and contribute to his or her welfare. As a practical guide in decision making, the nurse can use the Patient's Bill of Rights (Table 4–4) in determining treatment. Finally, constitutional rights are unconditional in application and should prevail when the nurse is in doubt of specific civil rights.

Table 4–4 *Mentally Ill Patient's Bill of Rights*

The right to appropriate treatment in the least restrictive setting
The right to an individualized written treatment, or service, plan with periodic review and revision of the plan
The right to ongoing participation in the treatment plan
The right to refuse treatment
The right to not participate in experimentation in the absence of informed, voluntary consent
The right to freedom of restraint or seclusion other than as a mode of treatment
The right to humane treatment that includes reasonable protection from harm and privacy
The right to confidentiality of records
The right to have visitors and to communicate with others via phone or mail
The right to assert grievances with respect to infringement of rights
The right to referral to appropriate resources on discharge

Source: Adapted from: Mental Health Systems Act Report. *Amendment to Senate* Bill 1177 1980 (Sept 23). No. 96-980.

Major Treatment Modalities

Each age has experienced maladaptive behavior similar to the types that bring people to mental health care providers today. Techniques employed over the centuries to encourage desirable and adaptive behavior include degrees of exhortation, punishment, brainwashing, incentives and faith healing—all of which have enjoyed marginal success and much controversy (Coleman, 1984).

This section will describe the major treatment modalities in use today.

Psychoanalytic Psychotherapy

Assessment Individual verbal **psychotherapy** defines a method of intervention that attempts to facilitate client behavior or change, thereby making client self-actualization possible to

- Reduce client fears
- Restore higher-order thought processes
- Assist the client to face reality
- Reduce anxiety
- Improve interpersonal communication

Sigmund Freud, a Viennese physician, developed the phenomenon of the "Talking Cure." The field of psychotherapy, though controversial at times in its philosophy and technique, has built on Freud's basic premise that if the therapist can arrange a special set of conditions that encourage the client to talk about individual problems, behavior changes may be accomplished as the client discovers events from the unconscious.

Theories and techniques emerging from Freud's initial work were not always successful, and followers began to propose alternative theories emphasizing hereditary and environmental influences. Disagreeing with procedures, therapists—such as Adler, Jung, Park, Dollard, Miller, and Rogers—began to use various techniques that allowed them to be more active, reflective, and personal.

Psychoanalytic psychotherapy was a fresh approach of viewing human behavior; it used and built on careful observations of actual clients, and inductively developed theories about human behavior and strategies to intervene in maladaptive behavior (Ford and Urban, 1963).

Implementation Individual verbal psychotherapy has four elements:

- It involves two people. The interaction is confidential, and the client is required to discuss very personal aspects of life not discussed in other relationships; therefore, the interaction assumes that trust and respect between the client and therapist develop.
- The mode of interaction is verbal. The client talks of thoughts, feelings, experiences, and perceptions. The therapist listens, encourages, and clarifies. This interaction can be intensely emotional.
- The interaction is prolonged. Extensive and permanent behavior change by clients takes time. The client, making new discoveries about self and approaches to the world, attempts to incorporate this new knowledge. Time allows the client to incorporate knowledge and modify aspects of life, including the successful termination of the therapeutic relationship.
- The therapist-client relationship is a series of planned purposeful interactions that seek to change client behavior.

By convention, the psychotherapist is often called an analyst, and the therapy is often called analysis. The analyst's task is to discover the client's conflicts and determine a strategy that will bring about change in the client. Because of repression that keeps the client unaware of these factors, the client repeats maladaptive behaviors. Through analysis, the client reduces the conditions interfering with awareness of those factors. Discovering the painful events and talking about them enables the client to discharge emotion that has been associated with these events. Energy previously directed toward keeping painful memories out of conscious awareness is now used to think of a solution to the problems. This allows the client to choose a course of action not based on self-disapproval.

The Client. For psychoanalytic psychotherapy to be successful, the client must have the ability to form interpersonal relationships and the motivation to continue through an often prolonged process. Moreover, the client must be aware of reality and needs to report and think logically about events. Finally, the client is expected to keep regular appointments of three or more sessions per week (Ford and Urban, 1963).

The Analyst. The analyst must integrate a strong knowledge base in psychologic theory and the techniques of psychoanalysis. The analyst must also have a thorough understanding of personal behavior to avoid observations of the client that are distorted by the analyst's own behavior and views.

Through interpretation or explanation, the analyst provides the client with a set of alternative ways to view behavior. The analyst should be skillful in providing information to the client in a manner that allows the client to discover meaning.

The analyst-client relationship provides the client with a safe environment in which to talk about and solve painful conflicts. Therefore, the analyst maintains a neutral but attentive approach to the client.

The Process of Analysis. Analysis is an evolution of a *corrective emotional experience* for the client. The path to the goal may be painful, and the relationship is likely to experience periods of stress. When successfully worked through, these stressful periods indicate that the analysis is progressing. The client learns new methods of coping with old conflicts.

Free association is the manner in which subjective responses such as thoughts, memories, dreams, and feelings are reported in an unedited fashion.

Transference is a process whereby the client unconsciously displaces onto others patterns of behavior and emotional reactions that originated as reactions to significant people encountered during childhood. Since the analyst takes on a relatively passive and anonymous role, many of these emotions are transferred to the analyst. Only the unrealistic and childlike expectations of the client are transference reactions.

Transference is distinguished from the concept of *therapeutic alliance.* The alliance is between the analyst and the healthy, rational part of the client's personality, or ego.

Transference, which can be positive, consists of those attitudes or feelings that originated in childhood relationships but are inappropriate in the therapeutic relationship (McKinnon and Michelo, 1971).

Attributing omniscience to the analyst may encourage rapport and client confidence and thereby appear positive. However, if this continues, the client looks to the analyst for advice in a manner similar to that of a child and fails to initiate a course of action that leads to making independent decisions.

Generally, the analyst has either a sympathetic or an antagonistic response to clients (McKinnon and Michelo, 1971). The analyst unconsciously attributes qualities to the client that arise from the analyst's life. Countertransference reactions are inappropriate, and the analyst often seeks supervision from other analysts to ensure that these reactions do not interfere with the therapeutic process. Countertransference occurs when the analyst is unable to recognize the significance of personal behavior. The analyst may be alerted to countertransference reactions when feelings such as inattention, boredom, anger, and sympathy are experienced. These reactions are not bad, but the analyst has a professional responsibility to manage personal bias so that the therapeutic relationship is not impeded by the analyst's resistance.

Evaluation In time, the analyst interprets dependent behavior as a form of resistance used by the client to avoid the goals of analysis. To maintain an anxiety-free state, the client avoids facing conflicts. Resistance is manifested in a variety of communication patterns, including

- Silence
- Censoring or editing thoughts
- Overtalkative but superficial conversation
- Intellectualization
- Generalizations
- Concentrating on trivial details
- Affective display

Reluctance to participate in the analysis is also demonstrated by client behaviors, including

- Frequent requests to change appointments
- Many somatic complaints
- Late or forgotten appointments
- Second-guessing the analyst
- Seductive or manipulative behavior

Interpretation involves the analyst describing in detail the client's pattern of behavior, including defense mechanisms and resulting symptoms. Timing of interpretations is essential to the success of analysis because it entails removing client defenses. The client must be strong enough to function without the defenses and to use alternative healthy coping behaviors. Successful analysis leaves the client free to make choices about behavior and breaks the repetitive cycle of maladaptive behaviors.

Short-Term Psychotherapy

Traditional analysis is expensive, time-consuming, and impractical for clients who don't have the luxury of spending three to five years in three-day-per-week sessions. Modifications in traditional psychoanalytic procedures and goals have been made in response to the increased demand for affordable mental health care.

In **short-term psychotherapy**, the therapist assumes an active role. Emphasis on trust and empathy ensures rapport and facilitates the client's desire to work with the therapist on problem identification and solution. This is in sharp contrast to the passive role assumed by the psychoanalyst, where the goal is personality reconstruction through client understanding or insight into interpretations made by the analyst.

The therapeutic environment must be a positive one that enables the client to discard ineffective coping mechanisms, thereby reducing anxiety. The client is encouraged to develop strategies that will enhance productivity so that symptoms will be exchanged for healthy coping behaviors.

Usually, the length of short-term psychotherapy varies; however, a limit of around 20 sessions has been suggested (Aguilera and Messick, 1986). Throughout the series of planned purposeful interactions, problems of recent onset are more amenable to successful outcome, and acute disruptive emotional experiences such as major losses are treated through complete evaluation. Following this, pharmacotherapy, environmental manipulation, and adjunct therapies may be employed to ensure the client's early return to the preillness level of functioning.

Successful brief psychotherapy depends on a therapist-client relationship that contributes to client self-esteem, communication, and development of more adaptive behavior patterns.

Variations of brief psychotherapy are used by nurse clinicians, psychiatrists, psychologists, and social workers as a major treatment modality. The goals of this modality include (Lego et al., 1984):

- Removing or modifying existing painful feelings or symptoms
- Encouraging healthy or adaptive patterns of behavior
- Promoting client growth and personal development

Group Therapy

Assessment **Group therapy** is a treatment modality based on interpersonal learning. Clients experience conflicts of intrapersonal and interpersonal origin. Therefore the group experience allows individual clients to work through transference and derive a corrective emotional experience from personal and shared insights by using the group as a social microcosm in which to experiment with new patterns of behaviors (Yalom, 1984).

Through interaction over time, a group member fulfills a basic need to be related to others by winning approval, thereby correcting misperceptions of the self as an unrelated person.

Borrowing concepts from psychoanalytic psychotherapy, group members observe and describe through free association their own and each other's thoughts, feelings, and experiences. Therapist and clients engage in reflection, clarification, and interpretation. Therefore transference and countertransference reactions are multiple, diverse, and rich, providing an important basis on which the group discovers more satisfying modes of behavior.

Group psychotherapy is complex, but it provides many advantages when used by trained therapists with appropriately selected clients. As Yalom (1984) discusses, factors that contribute to the success of group therapy techniques include

- Installation of hope—Group members are often at different points in therapeutic progress; therefore, they may witness improvement in others—an experience that provides incentive to continue therapy.
- Universality—The client sees that his or her pain is not unique and that others share similar problems.
- Education—Therapists and group members may provide instruction in mental health, treatment regimen, and general problem-solving strategies.
- Altruism—In group therapy, members receive through sharing with others, thereby contributing to feelings of usefulness and increased self-esteem.
- Corrective primary family group experience—Clients entering therapy usually report less than satisfactory family experiences. The group resembles a family, and members assume a variety of roles that stimulate transference reactions. Working through interpersonal conflicts within the

group allows the clients to discover and understand how family relationships affect behavior, and it allows for the redefinition of those relationships on more satisfactory terms.

- Development of social skills—In the dynamics of the ongoing group process, members learn to be direct, to speak clearly, and to be kind and courteous. In addition, group therapy often involves role playing, which allows members to prepare for stressful social experiences such as job interviews, inviting a friend out, or reporting unsatisfactory service.
- Imitative behavior—Modeling behavior after that of the therapist or other group members occurs as a result of the intensity of the interpersonal process. When the client identifies a positive trait from another and incorporates this into personal behavior patterns, the client is experimenting with new behaviors.
- Corrective emotional experience—Group therapy exposes clients to unpleasant experiences under protected circumstances where maladaptive behavior is determined to be inappropriate and the work of selecting more satisfactory approaches to situations and conflicts takes place as a result of expression of strong emotion. This expression involves risk taking within a group supportive of the client's struggle. Feelings are shared and assumptions are validated, facilitating the client's ability to interact with others.
- Existential factors—These provide opportunity for clients to deal with the meaning of their existence and their place in the world.
- Interpersonal learning—Learning to expand the repertoire of skills necessary to participate in varied interpersonal exchanges helps the client decrease the chances of distorting interpersonal messages.
- Group cohesion—The client learns about the power of the group and the effect of the group's goals on the behavior of individual group members.

There are two types of group psychotherapy: education groups and supportive therapy groups. In an *education group,* the leader presents material on a variety of issues. These time-limited groups assemble for the purpose of sharing and discussing information or learning new skills. The leaders may be professionally trained, or they may be people who have experienced and successfully worked through a problem situation. Examples of these groups include medication groups, women's issue groups, parent effectiveness groups, and substance-abuse groups (Lego et al., 1984).

In a *supportive therapy group,* a leader facilitates members in efforts to work through conflicts and to encourage new patterns of behavior within a supportive atmosphere. Examples of these groups include substance-abuse groups, veteran's groups, and support groups for clients with cancer.

Implementation In most inpatient hospital settings, clients are assigned to participate in small groups as an important adjunct to milieu therapy. Outpatient groups are important in the treatment of many problems, and selection criteria depend only on the presence of a target behavior, for example, alcoholism, child abuse, phobias.

Selection of Group Members. Selection criteria depend on the structure, size, and goals of the group. Because of the interpersonal nature of this treatment modality, profoundly disturbed clients are excluded from groups until their behavior has modified to a point where it will not disrupt group activities. Selection criteria include

- Client motivation
- Social behavior traits acceptable to other group members
- Potential to derive therapeutic results from the experience

Homogeneity of group members enhances attraction to the group, but heterogeneous factors such as sex, cultural factors, ability to communicate, intelligence, and coping styles must be balanced to ensure that all members will participate and have the potential to benefit from the experience (Stuart and Sundeen, 1983; Sadock, 1985).

The goals and composition will contribute to whether the group is open or closed. An *open group* allows members to come into the group while the group is in progress. Open groups have the benefit of ensuring that the membership will be maintained, but its transient nature may interfere with group cohesiveness and continuity in issues discussed. A *closed group* limits membership to those who started in the group and does not seek replacements for those who leave.

Role of the Group Leader. As the group's creator and convener, the leader is responsible for the group. Stuart and Sundeen (1983) examine the role of the leader or coleader in terms of the developmental sequence of group therapy. A major part of the leader's role is determining the group's purpose and membership criteria. Selection of members is based on the criteria discussed earlier and the purposes of the group.

Initially, the members are strangers and the leader, as the unifying force, helps the members in their attempts to relate to one another. At first, the members share a relationship with the leader, but with time, the movement is derived from their relationship with one another. The group then builds a social network, and acceptable codes of behavior emerge. The group develops strategies to deal with tardiness, absenteeism, nonparticipation, and disruptive and unkind behavior.

Throughout the therapeutic process, the leader assumes two basic roles (Yalom, 1984):

- Technical expert. Using a variety of nondirective or directive approaches, the leader moves the group in a desirable direction. The leader may give explicit directions for conduct or imply suggestions.
- Model-setting participant. The leader shapes behavior by the example set in personal behavior within the group. The leader molds the group in a health-oriented direction by encouraging adaptive behavior. Through encouraging frank expression of feelings, the leader sets a model where responsibility and restraint temper honesty with concern for others' feelings and defenses. By modeling the leader's responses, the group members work toward improving interpersonal skills.

Qualifications of Group Leaders. The qualifications of group leaders include (Rosenfeld, 1984; Sadock, 1985):

- Theoretic preparation through lectures, readings, formal courses, and workshops
- Supervised practice in the role of coleader and leader
- Experience in the role of group therapy member

The American Group Psychotherapy Association is the principal accrediting organization for group therapy leaders. Membership is open to all professionals who have at least a master's degree in a mental health discipline.

Evaluation The number of sessions depends on the goals of the group. Education groups, which are task- and content-oriented, may accomplish the tasks in a limited number of sessions. Support groups, which are process-oriented with a less structured agenda, often continue until the clients or leader determines that the purposes of the group have been achieved.

Subjective evaluation by group members indicates satisfaction with the therapeutic experience when

- Personal needs and goals for therapy are met
- Satisfaction is derived from relationships with group members
- Satisfaction is derived from participation in group tasks

- Satisfaction is derived from application of skills learned in experiences outside the group

Evaluation of client outcomes is as essential as the therapeutic effort itself. A research orientation should be somewhat flexible but scientific in its approach to the study of client behavior. Tempered with humanism, the therapist must evaluate the degree of change, the nature of change, the mechanisms whereby group experience effected change, and the role of other environmental factors experienced by group members. Although traditional approaches to evaluation of therapeutic intervention are not applicable to group therapy, the clinician must remain open to new evidence that will provide a scientific basis on which group therapeutic outcomes can be measured (Yalom, 1984).

Family Therapy

The family, a complex system of interacting persons, provides for biologic and social survival of its members. The modern family also provides opportunity to evolve a personal identity and to attempt new experiences, patterning of sexual roles, training to assume social roles and acceptance of social responsibility, and the cultivation of learning and support for individual creativity (Ackerman, 1958). The configuration of the family determines the roles assumed by members. The process of role identification is not always clear and has caused much of the stress experienced by families in the 1980s.

Assessment Ackerman (1958), a pioneer in the field of family dynamics, makes an important analogy about the demands placed on modern families—an analogy that remains valid today:

> The family may be likened to a semipermeable membrane, a porous covering sac, which allows a selective interchange between the enclosed members and the outside world. Reality seeps through the pores of the sac selectively to affect the enclosed members in a way predetermined by the quality of the sac. The influence exerted by the family members on the outside world is also affected by the quality of the sac. Adverse conditions within the sac or in the surrounding environment may destroy it, in which case the members lose their protective envelope. Menacing external conditions may cause the pores of the sac to shrink, thereby contracting the sac and holding the members more tightly within it. A family sac thus constricted and isolated from the environment cannot carry out its functions normally or long survive. Favorable external conditions expand the sac and promote a more fluid interaction with the external world. Excess tension within the sac arising from a state of imbalance among the members may warp the sac. Unless balance is restored, the accumulated internal pressure will eventually burst it.

As described by the analogy, the distinction between mentally healthy and dysfunctional families is not always clear. The protective sac enables the family members to function in the outside environment while relationships within the family unit deteriorate. Adaptive capacity of families can be examined in terms of a continuum with healthy, adaptive function at one end and family disorganization at the other.

Balance can also be examined in terms of an inverse triangle, where realistic approaches to problem identification and solution are sought by members engaged through cooperation. (See Figure 4–4.) The point of the triangle struggles against the demands of family members and community expectations to maintain equilibrium.

A *genogram,* or pictorial representation, of the role structure, relationship structure, and demographic data of the family, emerges. (See Figure 4–5.) Family members not discussed are just as important as those described. The genogram provides information about relationships and indications of problem areas (Lego et al., 1984).

The therapist observes and collects data on family interactional patterns. As Stuart and Sundeen (1983) discuss, considerations guiding family assessment include

- Family assessment data
- Family structure (genogram)
- Description of home environment
- Health and related developmental factors

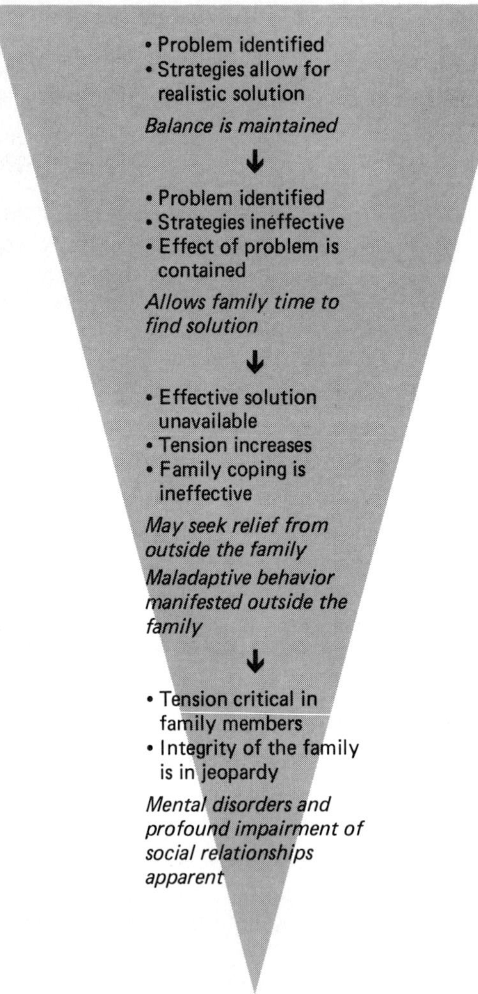

Figure 4–4 *Continuum of family adaptation.*

- Financial status
- Developmental stage in family circle
- Any maturational or situational crises
- Family role structure
- Sociocultural influences
- Strengths and weaknesses identified by family and therapist
- Problems identified

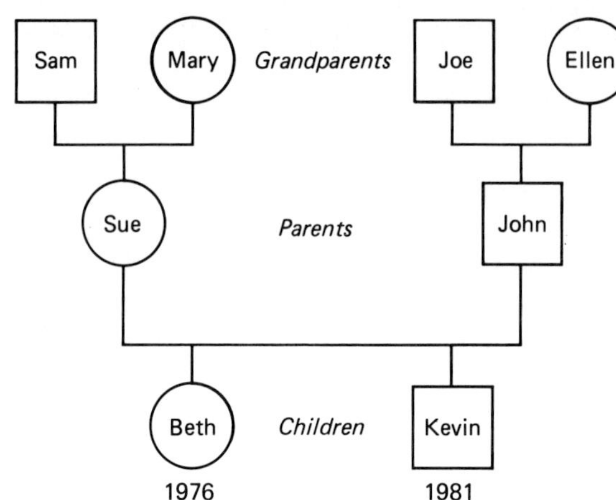

Figure 4–5 *Genogram for assessment of family relationships.*

The entire family participates in the assessment. Arrangements are made to determine the number of sessions, the members to include, and the location. Besides family group therapy, there may be the need for marital therapy and individual therapy for family members.

Family Intervention Family intervention is indicated when the therapist or family determines that the family system is impaired because of the presence of a psychosocial problem or mental disorder in one or more family members. Impairment of family functioning may be identified by schools, courts, or health care providers.

In cases where one member has been identified as the client, family intervention may be used to assist the family to cope with the client and to improve overall communication and interpersonal relationships among all family members.

Therapeutic approaches to family therapy may be modeled on psychoanalytic group therapy, where the family must examine conflicts from the point of each member achieving personality reconstruction. The more popular approach to family therapy views the family as a system and disorganization as the inability to communicate and appreciate roles. As goals are clarified, communication is improved, and the family learns new and healthy approaches to conflict resolution moving toward reorganization.

Family therapy takes place in the home or an office setting. Fagin (1967) identifies advantages of the home setting:

- Planning ensures presence of all members
- The therapist becomes a guest; therefore, a measure of control remains with the family
- Comfort with the setting encourages family members' participation

Once a setting has been determined, the therapeutic approach must be appropriate to the social and personal attributes of members (Caplan, 1970). A nondirective, passive psychoanalytic approach will confuse some families further, compromising their ability to communicate.

When an identifiable crisis brings a family into treatment, active, direct, and supportive intervention allows family members to solve problems through effective communication. This risk taking by family members restores confidence that control and conflict resolution can be achieved.

Identifying strengths within the family unit enhances self-esteem and control over behavior. Finding confidence to express feelings and needs, individual family members then recognize that other members have needs. Therefore improved communication may ensure fulfillment and satisfaction of the family as individuals and as a unit.

Evaluation Family therapy is practiced by many mental health disciplines and requires extensive knowledge of family dynamics, communication theory, and general therapeutic behaviors. This treatment modality is effective because the family is viewed as a unit; therefore, health needs are interdependent and improvement in the function of the total unit enhances that of the individual members of the family unit.

The end of the therapeutic experience may, in fact, be the beginning. Effective communication allows family members to become aware that individual pain is also an indication of family pain. Therapy provides members with skills necessary to become partners in the resolution of problems (Caplan, 1970).

Behavior Therapy

Behavior therapy is based on evidence that all behavior is learned, so undesirable or maladaptive behavior can be exchanged for desirable and adaptive behavior. The therapist uses a set of established principles to mobilize the client's expectation of hope and help for relief of anxiety to decrease the strength of maladaptive behavior while adaptive behavior becomes more prevalent (Wolpe, 1969).

Conditioning refers to the process by which the client learns to change behavior. There are three conditioning operations:

- *Reciprocal inhibition*—An anxiety-inhibiting response occurs in the presence of an anxiety-causing stimulus; when this occurs over time, the result is a weakened anxiety response. The client learns to take control of situations by responding in a manner that inhibits anxiety or other undesirable behavior.

  Harry becomes anxious before meals about contaminating his food with dirty hands. So, Harry washes his hands. Therefore, Harry's anxiety about dirty hands is decreased and he is able to eat his meal.

- *Positive reconditioning*—This is the replacement of undesirable behavior with desirable behavior. The desired behavior is rewarded each time it occurs, whereas undesirable behavior is either not rewarded or punished. To be rewarded, the client learns to respond with desirable behavior. Skinner (1953) identified the notion of reinforcement in *operant conditioning. Positive reinforcement* refers to behavior-maintaining consequences, and *negative reinforcement* refers to behavior-inhibiting consequences. Therefore reinforcers are specific and must be identified for each client.

Mary is a 16-year-old female with behavior suggestive of an eating disorder. Mary has gained five pounds in one week following institution of an operant conditioning program. Listening to her stereo cassette player is very important to Mary. Therefore for every meal completed, Mary is allowed to listen to one hour of music. Should Mary refuse to finish a meal, the stereo is removed until the next meal is eaten.

- *Experimental extinction*—This refers to the progressive weakening of behavior through repeated nonreinforcement of that behavior.

Assessment The behavioral therapist conducts a thorough assessment, which includes an exploration of maladaptive behaviors and the circumstances occurring before, during, and after responses. The therapist learns about the client's *stimulus-response pattern* for each painful behavior, for the relationship between these patterns becomes the focus of therapy. Correct identification of stimuli that precede painful behavior is essential to a therapeutic outcome.

Initial assessment includes history, mental status examination, and psychometric testing to provide sufficient data on which therapeutic goals and strategies are determined. The therapist assesses client problems and directs intervention toward behaviors having the most detrimental effect on client behavior.

Intervention Wolpe (1969) identifies general guidelines for behavioral therapy.

- The therapist approaches the client in an objective, nonjudgmental manner.
- The client is assured that painful reactions are reversible.
- Inaccurate information (for example, "That is the way I am") is corrected first.
- The client must be empowered to allow control of behavior.

The therapist regards the client in a holistic perspective, including physical conditioning factors and experiences that result in learned response patterns maintained over time. The therapist takes an active role in the therapeutic process, assisting the client to determine what behavior is learned. Maladaptive behavior may therefore be exchanged for adaptive approaches.

Techniques of Behavioral Therapy *Behavioral rehearsal* allows the client to act out unpleasant situations in the safety of the therapeutic environment. Techniques for language, phrasing, emphasis, and body language provide the client with confidence to attempt the desired response. The client "knows" how to behave in a manner that will elicit desired responses.

With *systematic desensitization* the client is first taught techniques to achieve a state of relaxation. The painful stimuli is introduced piecemeal, from least stressful to most stressful exposure. At each step, the client practices relaxation responses so that the situation becomes less threatening. Finally the client assumes total control over previously disabling behavior.

Overcoming fear by degrees empowers the client to assert control over other aspects of life. Systematic desensitization has been particularly useful in the treatment of phobic disorders. The therapist introduces images suggestive of the client's fear. These images and discussion of the painful event continue until a level of discomfort is reached by the client. With time, the client masters relaxation techniques and asserts control over how much stress is introduced. Finally, the client is able to confront and deal with the previously anxiety-causing situation by employing adaptive behaviors.

The behavioral therapist emphasizes mastering techniques that enable the client to solve problems by actually giving up maladaptive response patterns rather than by simply understanding the dynamics of the painful response.

Evaluation Behavioral therapies are effective when the dysfunctional behavior is limited and client strengths allow for mobilization of those resources when the maladaptive behavior is removed (Beck, Rawlins, and Williams, 1984). Behavioral therapy is based on established research principles and learning theory. Validated by statistical correlations, clinical criteria for therapeutic change include

- Decrease in maladaptive behavior
- Increase in work productivity
- Improved interpersonal relationships
- Improved ability to solve problems caused by environmental and situational stressors

Behavioral therapies have been effective in enhancing adaptive behavior for a variety of psychosocial problems regardless of the client's intellectual capacity and functional ability.

Electroconvulsive Therapy

Electroconvulsive therapy (ECT) was introduced in 1937 by Ugo Cerletti and Lucio Bini. On the basis of their clinical experience with epileptic clients who demonstrated an absence of schizophrenic behavior and operating on the theory that seizure activity prevented schizophrenic behavior, these physicians developed a method of inducing a grand mal seizure in schizophrenic clients. Later this modality was extended to people of all ages with various mental disorders (Beck, Rawlins, and Williams, 1984; Weiner, 1985).

ECT is the introduction of an electric current through one or two electrodes attached to the temples. Following preparation, moistened electrodes are held firmly in place and a tonic seizure of 5 to 15 seconds is produced following the introduction of a 70 to 130 volt current for 0.1 to 0.5 second (some sources say up to 1.0 seconds) (Beck, Rawlins, and Williams, 1984; Weiner, 1985). Bilateral application of electrodes has been replaced by a unilateral approach because of questions about efficacy of the bilateral method. Given the added risk for memory impairment following bilateral application, the unilateral placement is the method of choice, although there is some indication that more treatments may be required to produce the desired effect (Hahn, Barkin, and Oestreich, 1986).

The exact mechanism of action for ECT is unknown. Neurochemical and neurohumoral changes associated with the ictal activity appear to be important results. These changes produce alterations in mood and depressive symptoms. Other changes reported are neuroendocrine with the hypothalamic nuclei being affected by ECT (Weiner, 1985).

With the development of less invasive somatic therapies, such as psychotropic medications in the 1950s, there was a major reduction in the use of electroconvulsive therapy for treatment of schizophrenia, manic episodes, and depression (Weiner, 1985). As controversial today as it was 50 years ago, ECT, or electroshock therapy (EST), is restricted in its use and monitored for its effectiveness. Research has not verified the usefulness of ECT in schizophrenia, but Janicak (1985) reports on recent studies that confirm ECT as superior to placebo and tricyclic antidepressant medication in cases of life-threatening depression in elderly clients (Meyers, 1988). ECT may be a useful adjunct to the treatment plan and may be effective with highly agitated and disorganized clients while prescribed psychotropic medication is taking effect.

Assessment Assessment of the client's physical state and mental status is essential to determine indications or contraindications for ECT. Involvement by family and significant others is necessary to ensure that the client is prepared to consent to this intervention and has knowledge of the rationale, procedure, residual effects, and risks associated with ECT.

Serious depression that does not respond to other forms of therapy constitutes the outstanding indication for ECT. Indeed, a preoccupation with suicide has been observed to be dramatically reduced following ECT. Approximately 15 to 20 percent of clients with schizophrenia are treated with ECT.

Modern ECT is a safe procedure, and when adequate assessment is completed, it is useful to a variety of clients. However, it may be contraindicated when the following are present (Weiner, 1985):

- Recent evidence of myocardial infarction
- Evidence of increased intercranial pressure

- Severe underlying hypertension
- Presence of intracranial masses

Because ECT may cause transient elevation of cerebrospinal fluid pressure, neurologic examination must rule out space-occupying lesions or increased intercranial pressure. Alterations in cardiac output or recent history of myocardial infarction contraindicate ECT because of client susceptibility to arrhythmias induced by electric current.

Anesthesia is a necessary part of ECT because of the respiratory paralysis associated with muscular relaxation. Before induction of ECT, the client is anesthetized with short-acting barbiturates, so the client's overall risk for general anesthesia needs to be first determined.

Client psychologic readiness to undergo the procedure must be assessed, and maximum support is necessary throughout the experience.

Intervention ECT is usually administered in the morning, and the client is required to have had nothing by mouth after the preceding midnight. Approximately 30 minutes before the procedure, atropine (0.6–1.0 mg) is administered intramuscularly to block vagal stimulating effects of ECT and decrease oropharyngeal secretions. Extremely agitated or anxious clients may receive an antianxiety agent such as diazepam (Valium) within one hour of ECT.

The nurse should prepare the client by

- Explaining the procedure
- Assuring the client no pain will be experienced
- Avoiding the use of the word *shock,* and using the word *treatment* instead
- Staying with the client and stating that she or he will not be left alone
- Having the client void
- Having the client remove false teeth, hairpins, and jewelry

In the final check before the procedure, the nurse should validate that the client has been NPO since midnight, check the baseline vital signs, place emergency equipment in the treatment room, and have a signed consent on the chart.

Administration of a short-acting barbiturate such as methohexital (Brevital) or thiopental (Pentothal) intravenously induces anesthesia. Brevital is the usual drug because cardiac arrhythmias occur less frequently with this drug (Weiner, 1985).

Central nervous system seizure stimulation and not peripheral seizure movements is the measure of ECT effectiveness. Therefore the electric current is used in conjunction with a neuromuscular blocking agent such as succinylcholine (Anectine). This causes the desired central nervous system effect of ECT without the potential dangers that may be caused by peripheral seizure movements.

The client is preoxygenated with 95–100 percent oxygen before treatment (Shader, 1976). Once a state of complete muscle relaxation is achieved, the electrodes are applied with conduction jelly. For bilateral treatment, the electrodes are placed just above the bisection of a line that connects the outer corner of the eye and the beginning of the pinna of the ear. Unilateral treatment requires that the temporal electrode be placed on the nondominant side with the second electrode on the mid-forehead. A safety bite block is placed in the mouth following assessment of the mouth for loose or broken teeth and removal of dentures.

A tonic seizure of 5 to 15 seconds occurs immediately following electric stimulation. The peripheral clonic movements, however slight, then begin, lasting 10 to 60 seconds. The initial seizure in a series is often the longest, and oxygen is provided during the clonic phase and in the recovery phase. The client feels no pain during the seizure and recovers almost immediately following the seizure, because of the short action of the barbiturate and neuromuscular blocking agent administered.

Evaluation The recovery period requires close supervision and monitoring of neuromuscular, cardiac, respiratory, and mental status. The postictal confusion state experienced by many clients may be frightening, so the client may require additional reassurance. This postseizure agitation and confusion is markedly decreased following unilateral treatment. Still, the client should not be left alone until vital signs are stable.

ECT is administered in a series, but there are no absolute criteria for determining the number of treatments required. Generally, the treatments may be scheduled three days a week on alternate days and then tapered to twice and finally once a week at the end of the series.

Depressive reactions usually respond to 6 to 12 treatments where effectiveness is evidenced by improvement in client sleep patterns and personal hygiene. Psychopharmacology and group therapies may be introduced at this time to ensure continued improvement.

Adverse Effects of ECT The principal adverse effects of ECT are memory loss and confusion.

Memory Loss. The memory loss, which is disturbing to the client, involves short-term decrease in the ability to acquire new information and amnesia for recent events. Memory loss usually does not appear until the fourth treatment, and it usually returns within one to six months following treatment. When many treatments have been given, however, memory loss may be prolonged (Weiner, 1985).

Confusion. Impaired social functioning and disorientation tends to occur more often in elderly clients and is experienced in proportion to the number of treatments. Unilateral placement of electrodes significantly reduces the occurrence of confusional states.

Concerns raised by mental health care professionals (Kalayam and Steinhart, 1981; Sheridan, Patterson, and Gustafson, 1985) and society at large address the following issues:

- Memory loss
- Ethical issue of passing an electric current through the human brain
- Adverse cardiac effects
- Possibility of spontaneous seizures after treatment
- Brain damage from hemorrhage

Much of the frightening images of ECT are residual effects from earlier, unsophisticated technology. Today, clients are thoroughly assessed and prepared for the procedure. Anesthetics and muscle relaxants avoid many complications seen during the procedure of 50 years ago. Recent studies agree that ECT, properly administered and monitored, has been used consistently and with dramatic success, often as a lifesaving measure in clients experiencing depressive disorders.

Psychopharmacology

Behavior change is the desired outcome for each treatment modality described, but the manner in which change occurs has been the target of much debate. Research by neurophysiologists has yielded important information about the role of the central nervous system (CNS) and biochemical mechanisms in regulating consciousness, emotions, and behavior. Methods developed to measure and map these activities form the basis of the biologic theory of etiology of mental disorder.

All behavior is regulated by the interrelationship of chemical and structural parts of the CNS. Alteration in any part of the system may result in maladaptive behavior and mental disorders. Substances that can correct these imbalances may result in changes in client behavior.

A holistic view of mental illness requires that understanding and correcting biochemical problems are the basis of an interactional approach to treatment. Although medications alter biochemical reactions, psychotherapy can facilitate emotional display and sustain adaptive behavior patterns.

The functions of the CNS are dependent on the action of neurohormonal agents located in the brain and peripheral tissues. Neurohormones, or **neurotransmitters**, are a group of amino acids, chemical substances produced by the brain and stored in inactive forms in synaptic vesicles (Hahn, Barkin, and Oestreich, 1986). When stimulated, these substances are released in an active form and stimulate designated reactions.

Secreted by synaptic knobs contained on the dendrite and soma of neurons, neurotransmitters are necessary for messages to be transmitted across the synapse, the juncture between one neuron and another.

The neurotransmitters are released from the synaptic vesicles when the presynaptic neuron is activated. Engaging in inhibitory and excitatory activity regulated by the availability of the amino acids, the rate of neurotransmitter formation is kept in balance to meet body needs (Sheridan, Patterson, and Gustafson, 1985).

When released, the neurotransmitter diffuses across the synaptic cleft and attaches itself to a receptor on the postsynaptic cell, triggering the activities characteristic of that cell.

Inhibition of neurotransmitter action is due to enzymatic transformation to inactive substances, or reuptake. When adequate amounts of neurotransmitters are available, the amino acids are either excreted in the urine or stored in synaptic vesicles (reuptake). Pituitary and adrenal effects may also contribute to neurotransmitter inhibition and excitation. Medications that cause excess or deficiency in neurotransmitters will affect client behavior.

Though still nonspecific in therapeutic action, psychopharmacologic agents, or psychotropic medications, reduce disordered thinking, anxiety, delusions, withdrawal, manic and depressive states. Remarkable changes in behavior of state hospital clients following administration of chlorpromazine (Thorazine) in the 1950s contributed to the deinstitutionalization movement and enabled clients to participate in other therapeutic modalities.

Researchers are finding new evidence linking disturbances in availability of neurotransmitters to behavioral states. Of the more than 30 neurotransmitters identified, acetylcholine, dopamine, norepinephrine, and serotonin have been found to increase and decrease the rate of neuron stimulation, thereby regulating changes in mood states, thought processes, and psychomotor responses (Anognostakos and Tortora, 1984). (See Table 4–5 for a review of the relationship of anatomy and physiology of the CNS to behavior.)

Table 4–5 *The Relationship of Anatomy and Physiology of the CNS to Behavior*

Mental processes require functioning nervous system (brain, spinal cord, spinal nerves, organs).

Changes in cerebral blood flow affect behavior.

The neuron is the functional unit of the nervous system.

Neurotransmitters conduct impulses from neuron to neuron.

Neurotransmitters are excitatory—acetylcholine, norepinephrine, serotonin, dopamine—and inhibitory—gamma aminobutyric acid (GABA), dopamine.

Extrapyramidal pathway initiates voluntary motor movements to ensure smoothness of movement.

Sympathetic division of autonomic nervous system is involved in "fight or flight" responses.

Limbic system controls emotional experiences and behavior.

Hypothalamus controls autonomic nervous function and secretion of pituitary hormones.

Acetylcholine Acetylcholine is secreted by many areas of the brain. Reduction in this substance has been implicated as a cause of cognitive changes in healthy elderly clients as well as in the severity of dementia in certain clients (Creasey and Rapoport, 1985).

Dopamine Dopamine is secreted by neurons that originate in the midbrain. The sensitivity of receptor sites to dopamine has been offered as an explanation for psychotic behavior and is supported by indirect pharmacologic evidence. Antipsychotic medications that block the transmission of dopamine result in diminished disordered thinking and related signs (Hahn, Barkin, and Oestreich, 1986).

Norepinephrine Norepinephrine secreted by cell bodies in the reticular formation system of the brain stem and the hypothalamus, which is associated with feelings of rage and aggression, maintains sleep-wake patterns and directs the release of chemicals stimulating responses to emotional stimuli such as increased heart and respiratory rates in panic states. Low norepinephrine-to-epinephrine ratios have been documented in a study of clients reporting a history of suicidal behavior (Ostroff et al., 1985).

Serotonin Serotonin is secreted by areas of the nuclei of the brain, including the hypothalamus, pineal gland, midbrain, and spinal cord. Alterations in serotonin levels are associated with changes in behavior, and many drugs that inhibit serotonin induce changes in mood state.

Assessment As stated earlier, psychotropic medications do not represent a cure for mental disorders, but when taken by selected clients under controlled situations, they may alter behavior, facilitating participation in other treatments and ADLs.

Assessment should include the same attention to physiologic status observed in any situation where pharmacotherapy is indicated. Because of the incidence of adverse effects and the narrow therapeutic range of effectiveness, information about client reliability is necessary to ensure that medications are taken according to instructions. Family and other support people included in the assessment phase provide valuable information about the client's overall physical and mental health, experience with medications, and reliability.

Assessment of the client's usual daily patterns is useful when planning a schedule of administration that will not interfere with those activities. The time spent in assessing and planning for medication therapy will net benefits in client compliance and satisfaction with the treatment plan. Shader (1976) and Hahn, Barkin, and Oestreich (1986) discuss additional factors to be considered in assessment.

- The type and degree of behavior dsyfunction
- History of coping behavior
- Sleep problems
- Indications of possible drug dependence
- Past drug history
- Behavioral response to drugs
- Need for environmental control

Once the selection of medications has been determined, a teaching plan that includes information about rationale, administration schedule, adverse effects, and a plan for intervention in those effects must be implemented with client and family involvement. Monitoring for effectiveness is essential to ensure that dosage is increased or decreased appropriately.

When properly monitored, psychotropic medication contributes to change in client behavior, facilitates resumption of daily activities, and prevents hospitalization. Drugs modify behavior only as long as the client takes them, however. Recurrence of maladaptive behavior and return to inpatient settings is often related to nonuse or misuse of medications (Hahn, Barkin, and Oestreich, 1986). In addition, manipulation of the social environment and improvement in interpersonal skills is necessary to produce sustained change.

This chapter will discuss the four major classifications of psychotropic medications:

- Antipsychotic agents
- Antidepressant agents
- Antimanic agents
- Antianxiety agents

(See Table 4–6 for a list of these psychotropic medications.)

Antipsychotic Agents **Antipsychotics**, or neuroleptics, were the first group of drugs that caused significant change in behavior of clients with mental disorders. Discovered quite by accident, the rauwolfia alkaloids—primarily used to treat hypertension—were found to reduce disordered thinking in schizophrenic clients. Further study resulted in the identification of chlorpromazine hydrochloride (Thorazine) in 1951.

Primarily used to treat schizophrenia and related disorders, the antipsychotic medications are a group of related drugs that have similar effects on behavior but differ in chemical composition; therefore, potency, beneficial effects, and adverse effects vary.

These medications are nonaddicting, lipid soluble, and have a half-life of 2 to 30 hours, with 6 hours being the average in most clients. The anti-

Table 4–6 *Psychotropic Medications*

Class	*Generic Name*	*Trade Name*	*Usual Adult Dosage (mg)*
Antipsychotic agents			
Phenothiazines	Chlorpromazine HCl USP	Thorazine	25–800
	Triflupromazine HCl USP	Vesprin	100–150
	Fluphenazine decanoate	Prolixin Decanoate	5–20
	Fluphenazine enanthate	Prolixin Enanthate	12.5–100
	Fluphenazine HCl USP	Permitil, Prolixin	1–15
	Thioridazine HCl USP	Mellaril	100–300
Thioxanthenes	Thiothixene	Navane	4–30
Butyrophenone	Haloperidol USP	Haldol	1–15
Dibenzoxazepine	Loxapine succinate	Loxitane	20–250
Dihydroindolone	Molindone HCl	Moban	15–225
Antidepressant agents			
Tricyclic	Amitriptyline HCl USP	Elavil	75–100
		Asendin	200
	Amoxapine HCl USP	Asendin	150
	Desipramine HCl USP	Norpramin	150
	Doxepin HCl	Sinequan	75
	Imipramine HCl USP	Tofranil	150
	Nortriptyline HCl USP	Aventyl/Pamelor	150
	Protriptyline HCl	Vivactil	30
	Trimipramine malate	Surmontil	100
Tetracyclics	Maprotiline HCl	Ludiomil	150
Monoamine oxidase inhibitors	Isocarboxazid USP	Marplan	30
	Phenelzine sulfate USP	Nardil	30
New agents	Trazedone HCl	Desyrel	400
Antimanic agents			
	Lithium carbonate	Eskalith, Lithane	Dosage adjusted to maintain serum level 1.0–1.5 mEq/L
	Lithium citrate	Cibalith-S	
	Fluoxetine	Prolac	40–80
Antianxiety agents			
Benzodiazepines	Alprazolam	Xanax	0.75–4.0
	Chlordiazepoxide HCl USP	Librium	15–100
	Clorazepate Dipotassium	Tranxene	15–60
	Diazepam USP	Valium	6–40
	Lorazepam	Ativan	2–6
	Oxazepam	Serax	30–120
Miscellaneous agents	Doxepin HCl	Sinequan	75–150
	Hydroxyzine HCl USP	Atarax	200–400
	Hydroxyzine Pamoate USP	Vistaril	200–400
	Meprobaniate USP	Equinil, Miltown	1200–1600
	Buspirone	BuSpar	15–60 daily in divided doses

psychotics are almost completely absorbed by the gut, and the liver removes about 65 percent of the drug on the first pass. Although most of the medication is eliminated from the body, urinary metabolites have been found in the urine at 18 hours. Because of their affinity for fatty tissue, antipsychotic medications may be found in circulation 18 months after they are discontinued. This is an important feature to consider when these drugs are taken by elderly clients or anyone who has significant liver impairment.

Mechanism of Action. Since the exact mechanism of action is not clearly understood, the dopamine hypothesis is offered to explain the action of antipsychotic medications. Recall that dopamine has an excitatory effect and is present in high concentrations in the brain. In fact, dopamine affects autoinhibitory receptors, thereby interfering with reuptake mechanisms as well as affecting post-synaptic receptors in the limbic system and hypothalamus. Dopamine is also the transmitter used in a major neuronal pathway consisting of cell bodies in the upper brain stem and corpus striatum or basal ganglia, a region involved in the central control of movement, a mechanism that is defective in the presence of parkinsonism (Sheridan, Patterson, and Gustafson, 1985).

Antipsychotic medications have a high affinity for dopamine receptor sites and therefore inhibit binding of dopamine. The drugs antagonize or compete with dopamine for a place on receptor sites. In response to low levels of dopamine, increased synthesis may occur, but because its uptake is blocked, the substance is destroyed and eliminated.

Because of nonspecific action, antipsychotic medications reduce disorganized thinking, characterized by delusions, hallucinations, and thought disorder, while also causing motor deficits similar to those observed in Parkinson's states as well as alterations in temperature control, cholinergic activity, vasodilation, and seizure threshold.

Benefits of antipsychotic medications include:

- Diminished psychotic behavior
- A calming effect without oversedation
- Nonaddictive
- May be used for antihistamine, antiemetic, and analgesic properties

Adverse Effects. Because antipsychotic medications block dopamine uptake at receptor sites, the major side effects of these drugs are expected extrapyramidal symptoms caused by diminished dopaminergic activity in the basal ganglia at the corpus striatum.

Extrapyramidal effects or symptoms can occur after a single dose of phenothiazines or after long-term use of the drugs. The four major categories of extrapyramidal effects may be summarized as follows:

- *Pseudoparkinsonism*—most often occurs in older people and includes depressed activity, tremor, masklike expression, rigidity, drooling, loss of associated movements of the arms, restlessness, shuffling gait, and "pill-rolling" tremor
- *Dystonias*—seen in younger clients following parenteral administration with the client complaining of fatigue, muscle rigidity, perioral spasms, abnormal posturing, mandibular movements, dysphasia, dysphagia, oculogyric crisis, weakness of arms and legs, and prolonged abnormal tonic contractions of muscle groups
- *Akasthesia*—most often seen in middle-aged people and includes restlessness; increased motor activity, which may become exacerbated with client's attempts to control movement; fine hand tremor; jittery movements; facial tics; and insomnia
- *Dyskinesia*—sudden involuntary clonic-type muscular contractions resulting in torsion spasm, oculogyric crisis, drooping of head, protrusion of the tongue, inability to swallow, grimacing, and flailing of arms

Dyskinesia is the least common disturbance but probably the most frightening to client and nurse. Rapid parenteral administration of an antiparkinsonian agent will produce a dramatic and rapid reversal of symptoms. Trihexyphenidyl hydrochloride (Artane) or benztropine mesylate (Cogentin) have antihistominal and anticholinergic properties that depress synaptic transmission in cholinergic neurons, maintaining a balance with overall decrease in dopamine synthesis and resulting in reversal of the symptoms described. Tardive dyskinesia is a more pronounced and usually irreversible effect of long-term treatment with antipsychotic medications. The syndrome is characterized by rhythmical involuntary movements of the mouth, face, tongue, or jaw. Protrusion of the tongue, puffing of cheeks, puckering of mouth, and chewing movements may be associated with involuntary movements of extremities. Breathing disturbances, respiratory grunting, or alterations in speech pattern with head nodding and twisting movements of head and neck are also seen.

Other alterations in motor movements include swinging and stamping of feet or rocking from foot to foot sideways while standing. Finger movements may be exaggerated when the client walks (Cole and Gardos, 1976).

Although the syndrome varies with clients, altered finger and tongue movements are common early manifestations. It is therefore important for the nurse to assess carefully for disturbances in motor function. Table 4–7 lists abnormal involuntary movements.

Extrapyramidal signs of the acute type may respond readily to antiparkinsonian drugs, but this is not the case with tardive dyskinesia; in fact, these drugs may make the condition worse. Prolonged use of antipsychotic drugs may induce a supersensitivity of the postsynaptic neurons to dopamine, and sudden withdrawal of these drugs or addition of anti-Parkinson's agents may exacerbate symptoms (Itil et al., 1981). Maintaining clients on low doses of antipsychotic drugs has been somewhat useful in reducing signs of tardive dyskinesia.

In addition to the CNS effects described, auto-

Table 4–7 *Abnormal Involuntary Movements*

Involuntary Movements	*Assessment*
Facial and oral	Muscles of facial expression eg, movement of forehead, eyebrows, periorbital area, cheeks; includes frowning, blinking, smiling, grimacing
	Lips and perioral area eg, puckering, pouting, smacking
	Jaw eg, biting, clenching, chewing, mouth opening, lateral movement
	Tongue Rate only increase in movement both in and out of mouth, not inability to sustain movement
Extremity	Upper (arms, wrists, hands, fingers) Include choreic movements, (ie, rapid, objectively purposeless, irregular, spontaneous), athetoid movements (ie, slow, irregular, complex, serpentine). Do not include tremor (ie, repetitive, regular, rhythmic)
	Lower (legs, knees, ankles, toes) eg, lateral knee movement, foot tapping, heel dropping, foot squirming, inversion and eversion of foot
Trunk	Neck, shoulders, hips eg, rocking, twisting, squirming, pelvic gyrations

nomic nervous system effects require diligence in the assessment of clients taking antipsychotic medications.

Elderly clients are at greater risk for developing extrapyramidal symptoms because of diminished dopamine transmission with aging. Antipsychotic medications should be used in very low doses in elderly clients (Lohr, 1988), because of these age-related changes of normal aging:

- Reduced cardiac output
- Reduced glomerulfiltration rate
- Reduced activity of hepatic enzymes
- Reduced albumin/globulin ratio
- Increased relative fat content
- Increased neurotransmitter receptor sensitivity

Orthostatic hypotension is a common and potentially serious effect that compromises safety and leaves the client at risk for injury. Because of adrenergic blocking effect, the client is prone to circulatory collapse due to peripheral vasodilation. The client may complain of lightheadedness when standing, which is more pronounced on rising from bed in the morning. In response to hypotension, compensatory tachycardia occurs, contributing to subjective signs of palpitations, dizziness, faintness, and weakness. Tolerance usually develops in response to these signs, but safety should be stressed in the teaching plan.

Anticholinergic Effects. These effects are due to antipsychotic drugs blocking action of acetylcholine receptors at the synapse, between internal organs and nerve fibers. All antipsychotic medications cause some degree of anticholinergic effect, but the client often develops some tolerance over time. The symptoms are uncomfortable and interfere with client compliance. Client teaching should provide information about the reason for these effects, as well as strategies that may reduce discomfort.

Peripheral effects include dry mouth (decreased salivation), blurred vision (blocking of ciliary muscle nerves), constipation, decreased gastric secretion and motility, decreased sweating, nasal congestion, and urinary retention. Clients must be monitored for excess water intake because of the potential for water intoxication.

CNS effects—such as confusion, poor memory, disorientation, agitation, or delirium—may vary in severity and may be mistaken for deterioration in the client's mental status. When any of these effects occur, the antipsychotic medication dosage may be reduced or discontinued temporarily. If the client improves in the absence of the drug, it is verification that the behavior was drug-related. (See Table 4–8 for a list of additional adverse side effects of antipsychotic drugs.)

Neuroleptic Malignant Syndrome. A rare but often fatal toxic reaction to antipsychotic medication is Neuroleptic Malignant Syndrome (NMS). NMS is characterized by hyperthermia, muscle rigidity, and altered consciousness in the absence of an infectious process or other neuroleptic drug–induced extrapyramidal side effects (Caroff and Mann, 1988).

Research does not indicate a clear etiology for NMS, but previous history of NMS or symptoms associated with NMS along with high-dose (nontoxic)

Table 4–8 *Additional Adverse Effects of Antipsychotic Drugs*

Cholestatic jaundice (obstructive)
Allergic skin reactions including contact dermatitis (maculopapular, urticarial, petechial)
Photosensitivity (resembles severe sunburn)
Blood dyscrasias (agranulocytosis and leukopenia)
Abnormal pigmentation (grey-blue pigmentation on areas of skin exposed to sun)
Decreased seizure threshold
Impaired temperature regulation
Endocrine interference (women: amenorrhea, delayed ovulation, galactorrhea) (men: gynomastia, alycosuria, hyperglycemia, weight gain)
Teratogenicity (cross the placenta where metabolites have been found in fetal plasma)

neuroleptic treatment place the client at greater risk for developing the syndrome. Because of the lethality of the condition, nurses must assess and monitor all changes in consciousness, muscle rigidity, elevated temperature, and other autonomic changes in clients who are in the early phases of neuroleptic therapy (Gelenberg, 1988).

Treatment of NMS is a medical emergency requiring discontinuation of neuroleptic medication and intervening with supportive treatment for dehydration, hyperthermia, and cardiac dysrhythmias. In 1988 Caroff and Mann reported that 25 out of 256 cases of NMS, or 10 percent of cases reported between 1980 and 1987, ended in death. The relationship of NMS to the dopamine blockade reaction is the current focus for research in pharmacological intervention in NMS.

Antidepressant Agents **Antidepressants** affect behavior in clients who exhibit alterations in mood states, including

- Diminished self-concept
- Regressive, self-punitive behavior
- Withdrawal
- Alterations in sexual function, eating patterns, sleep-wake cycle, and constipation
- Alterations in activity level (agitation or motor retardation)

Antidepressant medications—and, to some extent, ECT—reverse these symptoms. Once the depression is relieved, the client has more energy and motivation to participate in other forms of psychotherapy. Improved appetite, elevation in mood, increased physical activity, and improved sleep patterns enable the client to participate in ADLs while manipulating the environment to allow more control over potential stressors (Cole, 1988).

Mechanism of Action. Current research offers the catecholamine hypothesis as a biologic model to explain the etiology of depression. Alterations in mood characterized by depression and other symptoms are affected by neurotransmitter action. Clinical and laboratory studies confirm that deficiency of serotonin and norepinephrine correlate with the presence of depression indicated by low levels of these neurotransmitters present in postmortem brain tissue studied from suicide victims. Clinical observations of clients treated with reserpine, a rauwolfia derivative, yielded data suggesting that depression was an adverse effect of that medication. Reserpine causes norepinephrine to be deactivated by the enzyme monoamine oxidase (MAO). Indeed, the earliest classification of antidepressant medications, MAO inhibitors (MAOI), relieve depression by inhibiting the synthesis of the enzyme monoamine oxidase, thereby decreasing intracellular norepinephrine and serotonin.

MAOI drugs relieve depressive symptoms, but widespread and nonspecific actions cause many adverse effects that make them a less likely selection by clinicians. These drugs are useful in the treatment of depressions that are not responsive to tricyclic therapy.

Rapidly absorbed by oral administration, the onset of antidepressant action varies from several days to a few months. However, the action of these drugs may be prolonged after discontinuation of therapy. The tricyclic antidepressants increase the level of neurotransmitters in the brain by reducing the reuptake of free norepinephrine and serotonin from the synaptic cleft so that more amine is available to allow for transmission of impulses. These antidepressants also exhibit strong anticholinergic effects, which cause the adverse effects of these medications.

The tricyclics are rapidly absorbed by the gastrointestinal tract and are metabolized by the liver. The tricyclics are bound to plasma and tissue proteins. The wide variety in plasma levels among people requires that dosage be titrated to achieve therapeutic effect. Technology provides a process that measures serum plasma levels of imipramine HCl (Tofranil) and desipramine HCl (Norpramine) and nortriptyline HCl (Aventyl/Pamelor) and uses 200 mg/ml as a therapeutic level for these drugs. The major disadvantage of tricyclic antidepressant drugs in the treatment of major depressive disorder is that onset of therapeutic effect takes up to four weeks, whereas adverse effects appear within hours of administration.

Adverse Effects. Major adverse effects of *tricyclic antidepressants* are due to anticholinergic action, and though not often requiring discontinuation of therapy, they are unpleasant and may affect the client's willingness to follow through with the treatment plan. Anticholinergic effects include dry mucous membranes of mouth and nose, blurred vision, constipation, urinary retention, and esophageal reflux due to reduction in esophageal sphincter tone. Elderly people are bothered most by anticholinergic effects.

Some incidence of cardiac arrhythmias including T-wave changes on electrocardiogram with tachycardia, palpitations, syncope hypertension, thrombophlebitis, and stroke have been reported in susceptible clients.

Endocrine effects may include decreased libido, impotence, breast engorgement in females, and gynomastia in males.

Tolerance usually develops to sedative and anticholinergic effects, but practice shows that administration of the largest dose at bedtime reduces perception of unpleasant effects while not interfering with therapeutic effects.

Tetracyclic antidepressants are chemically similar to the tricyclics. Besides affecting mood, these drugs also have antiaggression and weak anticholinergic properties. The major benefit of tetracyclic drugs in selected clients is that onset of therapeutic effect is evidenced within about two weeks of initial oral administration. The adverse effects are similar to those of tricyclic antidepressants, but decreased anticholinergic effects and more rapid onset of therapeutic action contribute to its use for selected clients. Adverse effects from MAOI include orthostatic hypotension, insomnia, fatigue, and weakness. Other anticholinergic signs as well as skin rashes may also occur. Because serious hepatotoxicity can occur, MAOI are contraindicated in clients with known liver dysfunction.

The greatest potential for adverse effects occurs with MAOI interaction with other substances. (See Table 4–9 for a list of foods and medications to avoid with MAOI therapy.) The interaction with other drugs may cause potentiation or altered action of those agents (McEvoy, 1988). Drugs that have catecholamine action in the presence of MAOI cause a pronounced vasopressor response resulting in marked hypertension. Hypertensive crisis is extremely frightening and dangerous to the client. It is characterized by hypertension, occipital headache, nausea, vomiting, fever, sweating, dilated pupils, and chest pain. Hypertensive crisis, which can progress to the point of intercranial bleeding and death, is the most serious toxic effect of MAOI.

Table 4–9 *Substances to Avoid with MAOI Therapy*

Food	*Medication*
Strong aged cheeses (Cheddar, sauterne, Camembert, Stilton, processed cheese)	Amphetamines
Sour cream	Over-the-counter cold, hayfever, or weight-reducing agents containing ephedrine and phenylpropanolamine
Wine (especially vermouth, Chianti, sherry, burgundy, riesling)	Meperidine HCl (Demerol)
Beer	MAOI may potentiate the effects of: CNS depressants, opiate analgesics, barbiturates, alcohol, sedatives
Canned figs	
Raisins	
Liver (especially chicken liver)	
Bananas	
Avocados	
Chocolate	
Soy sauce (more than one tablespoon per day)	
Yeast extracts	
Yogurt	
Papaya products	
Monosodium glutamate (MSG)	
Excessive caffeine	
Foods that require bacteria or molds in preparation	

The most important challenge that antidepressant drug therapy poses for nurses is that the delayed therapeutic effect of medication requires that supportive therapy and supervision of the client be maintained. Diligence in the evaluation of self-destructive tendencies must continue while therapeutic action results in elevation of mood and increased energy level. A severely depressed client may have diminished resources to follow through with a suicidal plan, but as the energy level increases and the original problem has not been resolved, the client is at greatest risk for self-destructive behavior. Monitoring the client's response to therapy is important to ensuring client safety. In cases of severe depression, short-term hospitalization may be indicated to monitor effectiveness of therapy and client safety.

Antimanic Agents Lithium carbonate, an **antimanic**, is a naturally occurring salt that is effective in the treatment of mania and in preventing recurrent cycles of depression in bipolar disorder. In about 80 percent of clients, lithium is successful in reducing the behaviors described in DSM-III-R, which include marked elevated mood for one week and/or three of the following behaviors:

- Hyperactivity
- Pressure of speech
- Flight of ideas
- Inflated self-esteem
- Decreased sleep
- Distractibility
- Excessive involvement in activities with possible painful consequences not recognized

Mechanism of Action. In the chemical group with sodium and potassium, lithium is hypothesized to inhibit the release of norepinephrine and serotonin to increase reuptake of norepinephrine and to increase synthesis and turnover rate of serotonin (Sheridan, Patterson, and Gustafson, 1985). By altering sodium transport in nerve and muscle fibers, it is theorized that lithium accelerates presynaptic destruction of catecholamines in opposition to MAOI, preventing transmitter release at the synapse, which decreases postsynaptic receptor sensitivity to correct manic behavior.

Manic and recurrent depressive states characterized by bipolar disorder respond to lithium treatment because of the effect on sodium metabolism and transport. During depression, cell sodium is high, and lithium facilitates sodium exit; conversely, in manic states, lithium causes sodium retention in the cell (Hahn, Barkin, and Oestreich, 1986).

Lithium is distributed evenly in body water, and absorption is rapid after oral administration. Plasma concentrations peak within 2 to 4 hours, but serum and intracellular balance is reached within six to eight days of the initiation of treatment. Important to note is that lithium crosses the placenta and fetal concentrations are similar to maternal lithium levels.

Lithium does not depress the CNS in therapeutic doses but relieves signs of excessive motor and mental activity. Serum levels are measured to monitor dosage and prevent adverse side effects (Klerman, 1981). Serum measurement is necessary because of the fine line between therapeutic and toxic levels. Levels necessary to control acute mania range from 1.0 mEq/L to 1.5 mEq/L (Rodman et al., 1985). Levels below 1.0 mEq/L may cause symptoms to recur, and toxic effects are more likely with dosages above 1.5 mEq/L. Once manic behavior has responded, dosage is adjusted to the point that 300 mg of lithium three or four times a day will maintain serum levels at 0.8–1.2 mEq/L.

Adverse Effects. Therapeutic doses of lithium cause little or no unpleasant side effects. Initial fatigue, muscle weakness, fine tremor, or nausea and vomiting subside shortly after initial doses. Thirst, polyuria, and fine tremor will persist.

CNS effects that include confusion, lethargy, slurred speech, and ataxia occur when serum levels reach 2.0 mEq/L and indicate the need for dosage reduction. Serious toxic reactions include convulsions, delirium, and coma. Hypothyroidism, sometimes irreversible, indicates the need for regular monitoring of thyroid function.

Lithium is excreted primarily by the kidneys; therefore, renal toxicity is a potential problem for all clients and particularly for those who already have renal dysfunction.

Intervention in lithium toxicity. Assessment of all systems and supportive intervention that maintains cardiovascular, neurologic, and renal function is indicated. The drug is discontinued and methods to promote lithium excretion are used to restore electrolyte and fluid balance. Intravenous administration of osmotic diuretics (Mannitol) and alkalinization of urine by administration of sodium bicarbonate force diuresis and increase excretion of lithium ion.

Lithium is contraindicated in clients with known renal or heart disease or who have depleted sodium levels with dehydration, brain damage, or pregnancy. Clients stabilized on lithium therapy should maintain normal intake of sodium in the diet, and fluids should be increased to about three quarts a day. With conditions that increase sodium excretion (perspiration, fever, diarrhea), the client should increase salt and fluid intake to prevent accumulation of toxic lithium levels.

Although identified by Cade in 1949, lithium was not approved for use in the United States until 1970. Since then, however, lithium has proved to be effective in the great majority of clients with manic behavior.

Antianxiety Agents The use of **antianxiety agents** for the treatment of anxiety disorders has come under scrutiny. Anxiety can be manifested in a single episode of panic or in chronic disabling tension states. Symptoms of anxiety vary in intensity and type, but subjective signs include inner feelings of tension and increased sympathetic nervous system responses such as tachycardia, hypertension, tremor, reduced salivation and gastric secretion, dilation of pupils, and excessive perspiration. The client is unable to concentrate, judgment is impaired, and decision making is altered or absent.

Pharmacotherapy, when indicated for the treatment of anxiety, is appropriate to decrease the crippling effects of anxiety so that the client can engage in other forms of therapy that will enhance coping ability and control over the anxiety-causing situation.

Benzodiazepines, the major group of antianxiety agents, act on the limbic, thalamic, and hypothalamic centers of the CNS. Theory identifies that the muscle relaxant, antianxiety, sedative, hypnotic, and anticonvulsant actions are due to inhibition of the neurotransmitter gamma aminobutyric acid (GABA). The benzodiazepines inhibit excitatory synaptic transmission resulting in skeletal muscle relaxation (Sheridan, Patterson, and Gustafson, 1985). The benefit of these drugs is that therapeutic effects occur without sedation that would interfere with ADLs. These medications are readily absorbed by the gastrointestinal tract, metabolized by the liver, and excreted in the urine.

A non-benzodiazepine anoxiolytic, buspirone, has been found to be comparable to benzodiazepines for the treatment of general anxiety disorder. This drug has a gradual onset and does not act on the GABA complex. Buspirone acts upon dopamine and serotonin receptors by inhibiting serotonin turnover and increasing dopamine turnover (Cole, 1988). Studies indicate that buspirone (BuSpar) does not contribute to abuse because it has not been shown to cause physical or psychological tolerance.

Adverse effects are usually dose-related and include drowsiness, fatigue, weakness, ataxia, and syncope. Elderly clients report these effects most often. Overdosage causes CNS depression, including somnolence, confusion, diminished reflexes, and coma. Usually associated with potentiation of other CNS depressants such as alcohol, toxic reactions are usually reversible and include attention to respiratory and cardiovascular support.

Therapy must include assessment of client tendency to drug dependence. Prolonged use of high doses of antianxiety agents causes tolerance and physical and psychologic dependence. Sudden withdrawal of the drug can result in severe CNS irritability (acute psychosis and grand mal seizures), anorexia, vomiting, and diarrhea. Withdrawal of the drug should be supervised to provide for close monitoring to ensure client safety.

The Role of the Nurse in Pharmacotherapy The success of psychopharmacology depends on identification of disordered behavior and accurate assessment of physical and mental status to ensure that client selection is appropriate. Therapy must be monitored and dosage constantly evaluated for therapeutic and adverse effect.

Elderly clients must be assessed to determine preexisting medical conditions and medications. Elderly clients experience greater sensitivity and variability in responses to psychopharmacologic agents because of normal physiological changes identified earlier in the chapter. Because of extended half-lives of medications, anticholinergic, cardiac, and other side effects, initial and maintenance doses tend to be lower than those appropriate for younger adults (Jenke, 1985).

It is important for the nurse to remember that medication is an adjunct to the treatment plan. Successful pharmacotherapy can facilitate the client's participation in other aspects of care that contribute to sustained adaptive behavior and satisfaction with life.

Beeber (1988) offers several caveats to the nurse administering psychotropic medications in general hospitals or psychiatric settings:

- Not all clients receiving psychotropic medications are psychotic.
- Refusal to take medication is not necessarily a sign of irrationality.
- The nurse needs to determine for whose benefit the medication is being given.
- Medication given as a form of chemical restraint is inappropriate.
- Systematic evaluation of abnormal involuntary movements must extend beyond the initial phase of pharmacotherapy.

Additional Treatment Modalities

In addition to the individual, group, and pharmacotherapies discussed, many alternative therapies have emerged as a result of changing views and knowledge about mental disorders. (See Table 4–10 for a summary of these alternative treatments.) Within the treatment setting, a variety of new roles that may be practiced by many members of the health care team have likewise emerged.

Table 4–10 *Alternative Treatment Therapies*

Treatment	*Expected Outcome*
Biofeedback	Clients will manipulate involuntary events, first with equipment then through self-regulation of involuntary responses.
Rational emotive therapy	Client will use self-analysis to correct distortions of the world to enhance satisfaction with life and self-fulfillment.
Transcendental meditation	Client will achieve rest, relaxation, and awareness to enhance potential.
Holistic counseling	Client will achieve growth of body, mind, and spirit through awareness and adaptation of healthy behavior.
Milieu therapy	Client will participate in activities in a therapeutic environment that improves communication, decision making, independence, and work performance.
Other behavioral therapies	Client will participate in identifying rewards to reinforce more socially acceptable behavior within the treatment setting.

Biofeedback The term *biofeedback* was coined in 1969, but the concept was derived from cybernetics during World War II. The two general types of biofeedback are *specific* and *nonspecific.* In the specific type, the client is provided feedback training for an actual condition such as hypertension. For the nonspecific type, the client is taught the general skill of relaxation. Biofeedback has been used for some of these conditions (Stroebel, 1985):

- Neuromuscular rehabilitation
- Fecal incontinence and enuresis
- Raynaud's syndrome
- Migraine headaches
- Tension headaches
- Cardiac arrhythmias

- Idiopathic hypertension and orthostatic hypotension
- Myofacial pain
- Grand mal epilepsy
- Asthma

Rational Emotive Therapy Rational emotive therapy (RET) was developed by Albert Ellis. The basic premise underlying this therapy is that people become neurotic because they are saturated with irrational ideas. RET assists the client in directing neurotic thoughts to logical, rational thinking (Ellis and Harper, 1975).

Transcendental Meditation Maharishi Mahesh Yogi developed transcendental meditation in 1958. The essence of Eastern thought was made relevant to a modern Western world. The full potential of the person is to be developed by a realization of pure consciousness, which is developed by transcending all experiences through meditation. The person should meditate for at least 20 minutes a day. It is felt that the longer the meditation takes place, the closer to a state of pure consciousness one becomes (Yogi, 1963).

Holistic Counseling Since holistic health is seen as predominantly a wellness model, the idea of holistic counseling is to help people move to high-level wellness. Stress-management practices emphasize several principles related to human beings:

- They move naturally toward a state of wellness or wholeness.
- They have an unlimited capacity for self-awareness.
- They are capable of taking responsibility for their healing and their health status.
- They have the ability to regulate the status of their own health.

Self-healing and the *therapeutic touch* with the intent to heal are methods holistic counseling uses to direct the mind's energy (Krieger, 1981).

Milieu Therapy Milieu therapy was developed by Maxwell Jones (1953). This therapy is based on a concept that the client's physical and interpersonal surroundings should be therapeutic 24 hours a day. This "therapeutic community" fosters self-respect, self-esteem, and self-confidence within the client. Clients are free to make personal decisions and assume responsibilities. Client government allows and encourages clients to take responsibility for and plan group activities. For example, in therapeutic community meetings, clients and personnel make plans, discuss mutual problems, and bring feelings into the open (Kyes and Hofling, 1980).

The professional nurse assumes several roles in psychotherapeutic management of the milieu to achieve balance between the client's need for protection and control with needs to achieve independence (Keltner, 1985). The role of the nurse in milieu management includes

- Individual client-nurse therapy
- Group facilitation
- Facilitation of milieu governance (i.e., community meetings)
- Nursing care provided through the nursing process and coordination of the medical plan of care
- Participation in the discharge planning process
- Participation in family intervention
- Leadership in the multidisciplinary team

Transactional Analysis Developed by Eric Berne (1964), Transactional Analysis is a form of group therapy that assists the client in focusing upon communication patterns. These patterns are analyzed to teach the client to be aware of the effects they have on themselves and others.

The unit of communication is a transaction. Two or more people exchange messages in the form of transaction stimulus and transaction responses. Each person communicates from three potential ego states:

- Parent
- Adult
- Child

The parent ego state is the parentlike part of the self sending messages with a parental tone by using *shoulds*, *don'ts*, *why nots*. The child ego state sends and receives messages based on childlike wishes and memories. Dependency needs, rebelliousness, and fearful and whiny messages are expressed through childlike transactions. Finally, the adult ego state collects data, makes assessments, and solves problems by using information from the parent and child ego states.

In *complementary transactions,* responses are appropriate and expected. Communication at this level tends to be noncontroversial and superficial, proceeding smoothly as long as transactions remain complementary.

Effective communication becomes blocked when transactions are crossed. *Crossed transactions* are complicated because one person relates from an ego state that was not expected. For example, an adult-to-adult transaction is, "Maybe we should talk about why you are staying away from home." The unexpected response avoids an adult-to-adult discussion: "You are always checking up on me and criticizing me." This response is from a child ego state. Additional barriers to effective communication include nonverbal, or hidden, communication on the part of sender or receiver.

In Transactional Analysis clients and significant others learn to identify their transactions or reduce negative communication and to enhance clear communication to and through the adult ego state. Through this process of mutual recognition and other forms of nonverbal and verbal stroking, or positive reinforcement, effective communication is achieved.

Other Behavioral Therapies Behavioral therapy developed in the 1960s and early 1970s. The systematic application of principles of learning to the treatment of disorders of behavior is the emphasis of behavioral therapy. Systematic desensitization is a method used to assist the client in overcoming maladaptive anxiety by approaching the feared situations gradually. The concepts of positive reinforcement and extinction have been used to shape client behaviors. Positive reinforcement such as food, avoidance of pain, or praise strengthens behavior. Extinction or no stimulus tends to weaken behavior and make the behavior occur less frequently.

A *token economy* was first developed by Ayllon and Azrin for chronic psychotic eating problems. Since that time, adaptations of the token economy—a system of reinforcements (rewards) for desired behaviors—have been used in many settings to obtain self-help behaviors from clients.

Behavioral therapy has also been used for teaching clients social skills. The chronic client often has social ineptness, so modeling of social behaviors is useful in returning the client to the community (Brady, 1985).

Psychiatric Assessment and Diagnosis

The principal assessment tools in modern psychiatry are classification, diagnostic testing, brain imaging, and neurochemical testing.

The DSM-III Revolution—Classifying Mental Disorders

First published in 1980, the third edition of the *Diagnostic and Statistical Manual of Mental Disorders* (DSM-III), and revised in 1987 (DSM-III-R), describes a nomenclature developed by physicians, psychologists, social workers, and nurses following clinical testing of diagnostic criteria.

DSM-III-R is unique in the use of a multiaxial system for problem identification. Providing a systematic and holistic approach to client problem identification, five axes describe five major function areas. The reliance on clinician descriptions of client behaviors based on agreed criteria (rather than on nonspecific theoretic formulations, as in the second edition) provides an objective basis for diagnosis and encourages the likelihood of agreement among health team members as well as accurate data on which treatment goals are determined in relation to prognosis. The multiaxial approach allows for balanced assessment of environmental, physiologic, and interpersonal stressors, including client strengths and weaknesses. Data are used to ensure collaboration in identification of client problems and intervention strategies.

Major clinical syndromes or patterns of behavior suggesting psychopathology are identified on Axis I. Usually limited to a single major problem, a second problem—for example, substance abuse—may contribute to the client's maladaptive behavior and is therefore listed.

Personality disorders (Axis II) describe specific personality types when no disorder exists, providing added insight into the client's coping style and reasons for seeking treatment when indication of a mental disorder is not apparent. Consideration of physical disorders or conditions is necessary to a holistic approach to the maladaptive behavior indicated on Axis I and Axis II.

A clear understanding of the physical conditions noted on Axis III is important to the overall management of the therapeutic plan, which is ensured through medical and nursing collaboration.

Axis IV and Axis V require assessment of the severity of psychosocial stressors and the highest level of adaptive functioning within the past year. This documentation explains in relative terms the degree of stress the client has experienced identifying adaptive capability in respect to areas of function in interpersonal relationships, occupational functioning, and use of leisure time.

Indicating a pattern of adaptation over time, Axis IV and Axis V are significant to predict client recovery to the preillness state and to determine realistic therapeutic goals by client and care givers. (See Tables 4–11 and 4–12 for examples of DSM-III-R evaluations.)

Table 4–11 *Multiaxial Categories of DSM-III-R*

Axis	*Example*
I: Clinical Syndromes	Alcohol abuse in remission
II: Personality Disorders Specific Developmental Disorders	Dependent personality
III: Physical Disorders and Conditions	Gastritis
IV: Severity of Psychosocial Stressors	Loss of spouse six months ago
V: Highest Level of Adaptive Functioning Past Year	Grossly impaired

Table 4–12 *Example of DSM-III-R Classification of Major Mental Disorder and Related Nursing Diagnosis for a Client*

Client	*DSM-III-R Diagnosis*	*Nursing Diagnosis*
Mrs Grey is a 75-year-old woman requiring maximum assistance to maintain nutritional hygiene and safety needs	Major Depression (Axis I)	Dysfunctional grieving Ineffective coping: disabling Inadequate nutrition: less than body requirements Impaired social relationships Potential for self-injury

Global Assessment of Functioning Scale (GAF Scale)

The Global Assessment of Functioning Scale (GAF Scale) is utilized to determine an overall judgment of the client's psychological, social, and occupational functioning (American Psychiatric Association, 1987). Clinicians rate the client for two time periods:

- Current period. The functional level at the time of initial assessment.
- Past year. The highest level of functioning for a few months during the past year.

Absent or minimal symptoms (eg, mild anxiety before an exam), good functioning in all areas, interested and involved in a wide range of activities, socially effective, generally satisfied with life, no more than everyday problems or concerns (eg, an occasional argument with family members).

If symptoms are present, they are transient and expectable reactions to psychosocial stressors (eg, difficulty concentrating after family argument); no more than slight impairment in social, occupational, or school functioning (eg, temporarily falling behind in schoolwork).

Some mild symptoms (eg, depressed mood and mild insomnia) OR some difficulty in social, occupational, or school functioning (eg, occasional truancy, or theft within the household), but generally functioning pretty well, has some meaningful interpersonal relationships.

Moderate symptoms (eg, flat affect and circumstantial speech, occasional panic attacks) OR moderate difficulty in social, occupational, or school functioning (eg, few friends, conflicts with coworkers).

Serious symptoms (eg, suicidal ideation, severe obsessional rituals, frequent shoplifting) OR any serious impairment in social, occupational, or school functioning (eg, no friends, unable to keep a job).

Some impairment in reality testing or communication (eg, speech is at times illogical, obscure, or irrelevant) OR major impairment in several areas, such as work or school, family relations, judgment, thinking, or mood (eg, depressed man avoids friends, neglects family, and is unable to work; child frequently beats up younger children, is defiant at home, and is failing at school).

Behavior is considerably influenced by delusions or hallucinations OR serious impairment in communication or judgment (eg, sometimes incoherent, acts grossly inappropriately, suicidal preoccupation) OR inability to function in almost all areas (eg, stays in bed all day; no job, home, or friends).

Some danger of hurting self or others (eg, suicide attempts without clear expectation of death, frequently violent, manic excitement) OR occasionally fails to maintain minimal personal hygiene (eg, smears feces) OR gross impairment in communication (eg, largely incoherent or mute).

Persistent danger of severely hurting self or others (eg, recurrent violence) OR persistent inability to maintain minimal personal hygiene OR serious suicidal act with clear expectation of death.

Toward a Search for Diagnostic Tests

Despite advances made through the development of a nomenclature that is useful to all mental health care providers, the search for empirical methods to verify diagnostic findings continues.

Described in its significance to the multiaxial evaluation of Axis III, physical examination identifies existing physical conditions that may be the source or contributing factor in emerging maladaptive behavior. Therefore, accurate physical assessment is necessary to determine the client's ability to tolerate somatic therapies, particularly psychopharmacology. Behavioral changes often precede clinical findings on physical examination, which reveal alterations in body systems.

High technology has been introduced to refine psychiatric diagnostic procedures, providing qualitative and quantitative evidence of mental disorders before clinical signs are evidenced. Through these methods, mental disorders may be prevented in susceptible persons.

Laboratory tests measuring serum medication and neurotransmitter levels will allow clinicians to fine-tune pharmacotherapy to yield optimal therapeutic effects while preventing toxic levels, adverse effects, and client dissatisfaction with the treatment plan.

Brain Imaging Electricity, magnetism, and radiation provide ways of assessing mental functioning.

Electroencephalography (EEG). Electrodes attached to areas of the client's scalp record a portion of the brain's electric activity, transmitting to a graph that records brain waves on a moving strip of paper. EEG is valuable in assessing seizure activity and neurologic disturbances.

Magnetic Resonance Imaging (MRI). MRI is being explored as a tool for the assessment of mental function. The part of the body to be studied is placed in a scanner, exposing nuclei in the hydrogen atoms of the body to a magnetic field. (Hydrogen atoms are selected for study because of the body's large water content.) The action of these atoms is studied in response to the magnetic field. Following the cutoff of the magnetic field, the energy absorbed by the nuclei becomes an electric charge, which is measured and analyzed by a computer. Images of diseased organs and absence of chemicals in organs indicate a disease state before onset of clinical signs (Kyba, Russell, and Rutledge, 1987).

Brain Electric Activity Mapping (BEAM). This noninvasive procedure measures and displays the electric activity of the brain on a television monitor and compares the image to a normal image. BEAM may be used to diagnose dyslexia, schizophrenia, depression, dementia, epilepsy, and tumors.

Positron Emission Tomography (PET). Positron emission tomography is being used to study the efficiency of the brain as a diagnostic tool in the detection of schizophrenia, bipolar disorder, and senile dementia. The client is injected with a soluble solution containing a radioisotope. As the radioisotope circulates in the body, it emits positively charged electrons called positrons. Positrons collide with negatively charged electrons in tissues, causing a release of gamma rays. The gamma rays are recorded, and a computer constructs a colored PET scan to show where the radioisotopes are being used by the body.

Computerized Axial Tomography (CAT). Radiographs are taken following the intravenous injection of contrast medium over 1 to 2 minutes. The injection is followed by another series of scans. The image is translated by a computer onto an oscilloscope representing cross-sectional images of the brain. Altered areas of density may enhance diagnosis by correlating clinical evidence and client history with abnormal findings on a CAT scan.

Computerized Electroencephalographic Mapping. The findings of standard EEG are entered into a computer. The computer converts EEG signals to numbers that can be analyzed and displayed as color graphics or maps to illustrate the location and magnitude of EEG impressions. As colors change, researchers can identify seizure activity or areas of the brain responsive to psychopharmacological agents.

Regional Cerebral Blood Flow Mapping (RCBF). RCBF allows superficial cerebral blood flow mapping. Future research may provide a method of diagnosing, confirming, and locating the pathology of schizophrenia as a prefrontal brain dysfunction (Sargent, 1988).

Single Photon Emission Computed Tomography (SPECT). SPECT offers a less expensive alternative to PET, permitting imaging of deep brain blood flow and neurotransmitter activity while clients perform selected tasks. Initial research has found that SPEC may be useful in identifying clients who can benefit from antidepressant medication. SPECT has also been used to identify muscarinic acetylcholine receptors, which are important to the potential diagnosis of Alzheimer's disease and related disorders (Sargent, 1988).

Neurochemical Tests Neuroendocrinologic tests have become a part of the evaluation of clients with depressive behavior features. The principal neurochemical test is the *dexamethasone suppression test* (*DST*). Clients who meet criteria consistent with DSM-III-R receive 1 mg dexamethasone orally, and plasma cortisol levels are drawn at 8 AM, 4 PM, and 11 PM. Plasma cortisol levels greater than or equal to 4μg/dl at 8 AM, 4 PM, or 11 PM define dexamethasone nonsuppression. Exogenous cortisol (dexamethasone) will cause cortisol suppression in nondepressed clients. The test identifies approximately 50 percent of clients who meet DSM-III-R criteria for depressive illness. Furthermore, the test qualitatively assesses adequacy of antidepressant medication because DST suppressors show a significant and clinically meaningful response to antidepressants compared with a placebo (Khan et al., 1988).

Planning for Psychiatric Treatment

The Joint Commission on Mental Illness and Health reported in 1961 on the strengths and weaknesses of the mental health services delivery system of that time. Remedies included strong emphasis on community-based services and the reduction in size and, in some cases, closing of large state hospitals, thereby upgrading the quality of care to ensure the client's rapid return to the community.

Legislation in the form of the *Mental Retardation Facilities and Community Mental Health Centers Act of 1963* provided funding to establish a network of publicly funded community mental health centers throughout the country. Reallocation of resources targeted for the development of an integrated system of care having roots in the community is the basis of the present mental health care delivery system.

Caplan (1961) identified a three-tiered approach to intervention in mental health problems:

1. Primary prevention
2. Secondary prevention
3. Tertiary prevention

Using this framework, nursing intervention at the *primary prevention* level is designed to identify population groups at risk for experiencing psychosocial problems. Guidance and support is designed to focus on client strengths, so the client's ability to find solutions to problems and to promote health and well-being is enhanced. Emphasis is on development of client potential rather than on intervention in pathology.

Axis IV and Axis V are relevant to the role of nursing in the assessment of environmental and psychologic stressors as well as to adaptation in social, occupational, and leisure activities. Appropriate environmental manipulation, health teaching, and counseling are used to enable the client to attain potential.

Secondary prevention includes early diagnosis and intervention in mental health problems and developing strategies that support the client's interpersonal and intrapersonal competence. Depending on the severity of functional impairment, a variety of assessment methods and treatment approaches may be used to reduce the duration of illness in inpatient or outpatient settings.

Emergency intervention may include short-term hospitalization to complete physical and psychiatric assessment, monitor client safety, and select appropriate intervention strategies. Discharge planning that includes identification of community supports enhances the client's ability to return to a precrisis level of functioning.

Brief hospitalization uses the therapeutic milieu to create an environment that supports the objectives of the treatment plan. The client joins with the mental health care team to develop strategies that will enhance function and satisfaction with life. Using a group setting to work out problems relating to daily life, the client actively evaluates progress. Jones (1978) identifies that the social environment of the hospital unit is used by clients to enhance their awareness of behavior as seen by others, which helps them learn more effective behavior patterns.

Crisis intervention is an intensive community-based effort to assess and diffuse volatile psychosocial situations rapidly. Aguilera and Messick (1986) describe a time-limited approach to problem identification designed to promote the client's return to a precrisis level of function within four to six weeks. Intervention is directed toward developing rapport with the client, clarifying the presenting problem, and enhancing the client's existing problem-solving ability.

Crisis intervention focuses on the immediate problem and seeks an answer to the question Why have you come for help now? A precipitating event of major consequence usually has occurred within 10 to 14 days before the client perceives and responds to the stress.

A thorough assessment of supports and previous coping behaviors includes an evaluation of the client's self-destructive feelings and behavior. If there is considerable threat to client safety, inpatient intervention may be necessary. A determination of the highest level of function is made, and alternative solutions are offered.

Throughout crisis intervention the clinician assumes an active, controlling approach that focuses upon the present. Environmental manipulation and positive reinforcement are used to assist the client in understanding factors that precipitated the event. Crisis is an opportunity to initiate changes in behavior that contribute to improved problem resolution, and the clinician points out these causal relationships to the client.

Emotional display of suppressed feelings in a protective setting is essential to reduce tension and promote problem recognition and problem-solving strategies. By appealing to the healthy and capable part of the client's personality, the clinician assists the client to use strengths to solve new problems. Additionally, the clinician facilitates the client's own healing ability as the client learns to modify the negative effects of stressors, assume control of personal decision making, and reduce the likelihood of dysfunctional responses to recurring crises.

Residential care settings have applied crisis intervention techniques to prevent or effectively manage critical mass. Critical mass refers to an environment that enables client behavior to escalate or the client to lose control, resulting in assaultive or other dangerous behavior that threatens the welfare of others and the stability of the milieu (see Table 4–13). A four-step strategy has been used to prevent, identify, or reduce a system's risk of reaching a critical mass (Rosenstock, 1982).

Aguilera and Messick (1986) describe a paradigm for understanding the relationship of stressful

Table 4–13 *Model for Prevention of Critical Mass*

Stage	*Strategy*
1. Dynamic homeostasis: an environment that encourages effective communication	• Daily staff meeting • Exchange of feelings and support from client to client and from client to staff • Changes in policy discussed with clients and staff • Clarification and reassurance offered during any change • Routine repairs and maintenance of the milieu • Client-to-staff ratio based upon acuity • Client participation in milieu governance • Milieu programs are adequate and varied • Ongoing evaluation of structure and program in the milieu
2. Alert for possible crisis: a transition stage where instability in one part of system can provoke a crisis state	• Destructive aggression by clients is recognized and promptly managed • Frequent staff and client meetings to identify and solve problems • Special activities to diffuse tension and isolate volatile clients
3. Crisis: assaultive, destructive behavior results by failing to recognize and respond effectively to stage 2	• Rapid assessment of crisis • Separate the leaders from the group • Increase use of positive reinforcers for nonassaultive clients • Specific therapeutic groups to process outcome • Remove damaged property and restore milieu quickly
4. Return to dynamic homeostasis: transition to stage 1 or period of alert to avoid another crisis	• Schedule activities that involve clients to retain sense of control and esteem • Community meeting to continue problem solving • Incorporate client's significant others in milieu activities • Staff adequately to strengthen morale and enhance staff communication between shifts

Source: Adapted from H. A. Rosenstock and M. McLaughlin, On the primary prevention of critical mass: A systems strategy for adolescent units. *NAPPH Journal* (Jan.) 1982; 13:9–11.

events to client behavior. The therapist facilitates resolution of crisis through identification of balancing factors that allow the client to perceive the event realistically, use situational supports, and use more effective coping behaviors.

Tertiary prevention is aimed at reducing the effects of a mental disorder. A rehabilitation framework provides opportunities for the client to return to a prehospitalization level of functioning. Correcting problems that interfere with functioning and prolong a return to the community is emphasized. Auditory and visual problems that may contribute to paranoid thinking or incontinence due to a physiologic cause are examples of such problems. Rehabilitation activities are designed to maintain independence in ADLs and increase potential for independent living.

Alternatives to hospitalization—such as outpatient commitment, day treatment programs, foster home placements, community residences, and psychiatric home care—provide supervision, support, and a therapeutic milieu. After-care programs decrease client isolation by providing involvement in social and work situations that will enhance a client's interpersonal skills. Supervision of clients in after-care programs provides frequent opportunities to evaluate the client's level of functioning and allows for rapid intervention to prevent further disabling effects of the mental disorder.

Psychiatric home care is a recent development in tertiary care. Clients who have a psychiatric disorder, are homebound, and who require the specialized knowledge and skills of a psychiatric mental health nurse, may receive outpatient services in the home. Home care requires support and involvement of family and significant others while enhancing client self-care, independence, and dignity. Pelletier (1988) describes the goals of a psychiatric home care program:

- Development of collaborative relationships with attending psychiatrists and community referral resources
- Care by highly qualified staff current with trends in psychiatric/mental health nursing
- Respect for the integrity of the patient/family client/psychiatrist dyad
- Assistance for the client to remain in the community provided by comprehensive care and drawing upon agency and community resources
- An easy transition from hospital to home
- Development of an educational resource to the client, family, and/or significant other on such issues as medication and diet regimen, interpersonal relations, and individual coping strategies
- Ongoing community education
- A resource to the medical community that defines the mental health needs of clients
- In cooperation with nursing schools, educational opportunities to future mental health professionals

Evaluation and Future Trends

Intervention in mental disorders as a scientific approach is still in its infancy, so one might anticipate controversy over nomenclature and therapeutic modalities. However, the current holistic emphasis on behavior and assessment of strengths is enhanced by the descriptive approach to mental disorders. This multidisciplinary approach, which emphasizes adaptation rather than cure, questions the validity of the medical model. Descriptions of client behavior leads to greater common ground, resulting in the testing of diagnostic labels and therapeutic modalities.

By increasing the specificity of assessment and intervention techniques, vulnerable people will be assisted to expand their cognitive, social, and problem-solving skills. People will be better able to meet their potential, use environmental supports, and reduce vulnerability toward disordered behavior. Perhaps the research into the neurochemical determinants of mental disorders, including genetic factors, will change the direction of the present mental health care delivery system so that the aim will not necessarily be to cure but rather to enhance the person's level of functioning and quality of life. Adaptation may be achieved through biochemical modifications, environmental manipulation, and social learning skills.

Nursing has already developed mechanisms to ensure the highest quality of practice. The competencies for practitioners are outlined in the ANA's *Standards of Psychiatric and Mental Health Nursing Practice* (Carter et al., 1982). The primary mechanisms are peer review, continuing education, and certification.

The challenge for mental health lies in the development and use of relevant theories related to the client's mental health problems. The concept of nursing diagnosis being developed by nurse theorists will be used along with DSM-III-R to communicate clearly and research client mental health problems.

Increasingly, technologic advances in the diagnosis and treatment of mental disorders are being used to ensure identification of people at risk for mental disorders. These new developments raise ethical concerns about a modality that can identify a mental disorder before behavior is manifested. Developing technology for prevention, early identification, and treatment of mental disorders—however beneficial to the consistency and accuracy of diagnostic formulation—requires that none of us lose sight of intervention that is client-centered and therapies that strengthen and support the intrapersonal, interpersonal, and environmental adaptation of the client.

The National Institute of Mental Health Task Force has mapped out an agenda for future innovation and refers directly to the role of psychiatric mental health nurse researchers (1987). The task force states that efforts to advance knowledge about therapeutic actions and to enhance the capabilities of individual clients and significant others to respond to actual and potential mental health problems should be the objective of clinical and research practice.

SUMMARY

1. The community mental health system came about in the 1960s and is based on a model by Gerald Caplan.

2. Although there are some problems related to the community mental health movement, it is the basic publicly funded system for the treatment of mental health today.

3. A client's entry into the mental health system is based on the client's responding to intrapersonal, interpersonal, and environmental stimuli in a manner not consistent with usual responses.

4. Two major approaches to acute mental health problems are hospitalization and outpatient services.

5. The major characteristics moving clients into the mental health system are a painful symptom and impairment in one or more areas of function (behavioral, physiologic, or psychologic); they are not limited to a conflict between the client and society.

Legal and Ethical Issues in Psychiatric/Mental Health Nursing

6. Clients enter the community hospital for treatment in much the same manner that they pursue relief of other health problems. The client is able to leave the facility by choice or by mutual agreement with the physician.

7. Commitment refers to detaining a client in a hospital setting because his or her behavior is a threat to the client or to society.

8. *Competence* refers to the determination that a client can make appropriate judgments and decisions about treatment and care.

9. Informed consent is a law that provides the client with a right to be free from intentional harm by providing reasonable information on the standards of care.

10. Voluntary commitment occurs when the client consents to confinement for the purposes of assessment and treatment of psychosocial problems and signs a document indicating as much.

11. Involuntary commitment is a set of established procedures that allows for confinement of clients for treatment in the mental health system. Each state sets its own procedures.

12. The rights for mental health clients include appropriate treatment; an individualized, written treatment plan; participation in the treatment plan; and the right to refuse treatment. In addition, a client does not have to

participate in experimentation without informed consent; is free to not be restrained or secluded as a mode of treatment; has reasonable protection from harm and privacy; has a right to confidentiality of records; may have visitors, can use the phone and mail; can assert grievances; and is referred to appropriate resources on discharge.

Major Treatment Modalities

13. Psychoanalytic psychotherapy was developed by Sigmund Freud and is one of the original approaches to therapy. This therapy is verbal and involves an individual client and therapist.

14. Since psychoanalytic psychotherapy is expensive and time-consuming, short-term psychotherapy has replaced much of psychoanalysis. Techniques vary, but the emphasis is on individual therapy.

15. Group therapy borrows from the concepts of psychoanalytic psychotherapy but is designed to deal with groups of clients. Group therapy is designed for a variety of purposes such as education and support.

16. Family therapy is geared to assist the family in identifying roles and stresses within the family structure.

17. Behavior therapy is based on the concept that behavior is learned, and therefore maladaptive behavior can be changed to desirable and adaptive behavior.

18. Two biologic treatment modalities are electroconvulsive therapy (ECT) and psychopharmacology.

19. Additional treatment modalities are biofeedback, rational emotive therapy, transcendental meditation, holistic counseling, milieu therapy, and other behavioral therapies.

Psychiatric Assessment and Diagnosis

20. The *Diagnostic and Statistical Manual of Mental Disorders*, third edition, Revised (DSM-III-R) is a nomenclature system of identifying the categories of mental illness.

21. The DSM-III-R is a multiaxial system with five axes: Axis I is usually limited to a single or major problem, Axis II describes specific personality types when a disorder exists, Axis III offers a clear understanding of the physical conditions noted in this axis, Axis IV and Axis V require assessment of the severity of psychosocial stressors and the highest level of adaptive functioning within the past year.

22. Advances have been made in diagnostic tests. Some of the diagnostic tests used are electroencephalography, magnetic resonance imaging, brain electric activity mapping, positron emission tomography, computerized axial tomography, regional cerebral blood flow mapping, single photon emission computed tomography, and neurochemical tests.

Planning for Psychiatric Treatment

23. Caplan proposes a three-tiered approach to intervention in mental health problems.

24. Primary prevention is designed to identify population groups at risk for experiencing psychosocial problems.

25. Secondary prevention includes early diagnosis and intervention in mental health problems, developing strategies that support the client's interpersonal and intrapersonal competence.

26. Tertiary prevention is aimed at reducing the effects of a mental disorder.

Evaluation and Future Trends

27. Current and future advances in diagnosis and treatment of mental disorders should join the art of the therapeutic relationship with technology to ensure identification of people at risk for mental disorders.

CHAPTER REVIEW

1. When clients enter the mental health system what tool(s) are used to help identify the problem?
   (a) Psychiatric interview and mental status examination
   (b) Physical examination and medical interview
   (c) Occupational therapy evaluation
   (d) Psychologic testing

2. A client may be hospitalized when a mental disorder occurs. Which one of the following is a reason for hospitalization?
   (a) No other intervention has been tried.
   (b) The family wants the treatment.
   (c) The treatment requires close supervision.
   (d) A change in environment is indicated so the client can observe others with maladaptive behavior.

3. Which of the following statements best describes the home environment of a family living with a person who has mental illness?
   (a) Positive significant relationships aid the client in recovery.
   (b) Constant negative feelings, which may include anger, resentment, guilt, and anxiety.
   (c) Embarrassment in social situations, due to client's reactions.

(d) Close family relationships to compensate for the ill member.

4. Which of the following ethical principles does commitment of a mentally ill client violate?
(a) Beneficience
(b) Justice
(c) Liberty
(d) Autonomy

5. When a therapist's response to a client is sympathetic or antagonistic because of qualities of the therapist's life, the relationship involves
(a) Therapeutic alliance
(b) Milieu
(c) Countertransference
(d) Empathy

6. Which one of the following is a qualification for a group therapy leader?
(a) Theoretic preparation
(b) Role model
(c) Ability to self-disclose
(d) Presence of clinical judgment

REFERENCES

Ackerman NW: *The Psychodynamics of Family Life.* Basic Books, 1958.

Aguilera D, Messick J: *Crisis Intervention Theory and Approach,* 4th ed. Mosby, 1986.

American Psychiatric Association: *Diagnostic and Statistical Manual of Mental Disorders, Third Edition, Revised.* American Psychiatric Association, 1987.

Anognostakos NP, Tortora GJ: *Principles of Anatomy and Physiology,* 4th ed. Saunders, 1984.

Applebaum PS: The right to refuse treatment with antipsychotic medications: Retrospect and prospect. *Am J Psychiatry* (Apr) 1988; 145:413–419.

Applebaum PS, Gutheil TG: The Boston State Hospital case: Involuntary mind control or the right to rot. *Am J Psychiatry* (June) 1980; 137:720–723.

Ayd FJ: Problems with orders for medication as needed. *Am J Psychiatry* (Aug) 1985; 142:939.

Ayllon, T, Azrin NH: *The Token Economy: A Motivational System for Therapy and Rehabilitation.* Appleton-Century-Crofts, 1968.

Beck CM, Rawlins RP, Williams SR: *Mental Health-Psychiatric Nursing.* Mosby, 1984.

Beeber LS: It's on the tip of the tongue: Tardive dyskinesia. *J Psychosoc Nurs* (Aug) 1988; 26:32–33.

Beis EB: *Mental Health and the Law.* Aspen Systems, 1984.

Berne E: *Games People Play.* Grove Press, 1964.

Bernheim KA, Lewine RR, Beale CC: *The Caring Family: Living with Chronic Mental Illness.* Random House, 1982.

Black OW: Communicating with patients who have psychiatric problems. AFP (Jan) 1988; 37:161–164.

Brady JP: Behavior therapy. In: *Comprehensive Textbook of Psychiatry,* 4th ed. Vol. II. Kaplan HI, Sadock BJ (editors). Williams and Wilkins, 1985.

Brekke JS: What do we really know about community support programs? Strategies for better monitoring. *Hosp Community Psychiatry* (Sept) 1988; 39:946–951.

Brooks AD: Outpatient commitment for the chronically mentally ill: Law and policy. In: *Improving Mental Health Services: What Social Science Can Tell Us.* Mechanic, O (editor). *New Directions for Mental Health Services* (37), Jossey-Bass, 1987.

Caplan G: *An Approach to Community Mental Health.* Grune & Stratton, 1961.

Caplan G: *Community Psychiatry.* Davis, 1970.

Caroff SN, Mann SC: Neuroleptic malignant syndrome. *Psychopharmacology Bulletin* (4) 1988; 24:25–29.

Carter E et al: *Standards of Psychiatric and Mental Health Nursing Practice.* American Nurses' Association, 1982.

Church OM: From custody to community in psychiatric nursing. *Nurs Res* (Jan/Feb) 1987; 36:48–55.

Coburn KL, Sullivan CH, and Hundley J: High-tech maps of the brain. *A J Nurs* (Nov) 1988; 1500–1501.

Cole J: The drug treatment of anxiety and depression. *Medical Clinics of North America* (July) 1988; 72:815.

Cole JO, Gardos G: Tardive dyskinesia. *Pharmacology Update* 1976; 151–163.

Coleman JC et al: *Abnormal Psychology and Modern Life,* 7th ed. Scott, Foresman, 1984.

Conklin C, Whall AL: Why a psychogeriatric unit? *J Psychosoc Nurs* (May) 1985; 23:23–27.

Creasey H, Rapoport SI: The aging human brain. *Ann Neurol* (Jan) 1985; 17:2–9.

Creighton H: *Law Every Nurse Should Know,* 5th ed. Saunders, 1986.

Ellis A, Harper RA: *A New Guide to Rational Living.* Prentice-Hall, 1975.

Fagin C: Psychotherapeutic nursing. *Am J Nurs* 1967; 67:298–304.

Ford DH, Urban HB: *Systems of Psychotherapy.* Wiley, 1963.

Garritson SH: Ethical decision making patterns. *J Psychosoc Nurs* (Apr) 1988; 26:22–29.

Gelenberg AJ: A prospective survey of neuroleptic malignant syndrome in a short-term psychiatric hospital. *Am J Psychiatry* (Apr) 1988; 145:517–518.

Hahn AB, Barkin RL, Oestreich SJ: *Pharmacology in Nursing,* 15th ed. Mosby, 1986.

Harris E: Psych drugs. *Am J Nurs* (Nov) 1988; 1507–1518.

Hastings Center: *Guidelines on the Termination of Life-Sustaining Treatment and the Care of the Dying,* pp. 23–31. Wolf SM (project director). Indiana University Press, 1987.

Hyde A: *Living with Schizophrenia.* Contemporary Basic Books, 1980.

Itil TM et al: Clinical profiles of tardive dyskinesia. *Comp Psychiatry* (May/June) 1981; 22:282–289.

Jameton A: *Nursing Practice: The Ethical Issues.* Prentice-Hall, 1984.

Janicak PG et al: Efficacy of ECT: A meta-analysis. *Am J Psychiatry* 1985; 42(3):297–302.

Jenke MA: *Handbook of Geriatric Psychopharmacology,* p. 52. Littleton: PSG Pub. Co., 1985.

Jones M: *The Therapeutic Community.* Basic Books, 1953.

Jones M: Nurses can change the social systems of hospitals. *Am J Nurs* (June) 1978; 78:1012–1014.

Kalayam B, Steinhart M: A survey of attitudes on the use of electroconvulsive therapy. *Hosp Community Psychiatry* (Mar) 1981; 32:185.

Kazorowski J: Refusing life sustaining treatment. *J Psychosoc Nurs* (Mar) 1988; 26:9–12.

Kebbee P: Methods of monitoring quality in a psychiatric setting. *J Quality Assurance in Nurs* (May) 1987; 64–70.

Keckich WA, Morgan HE: The diagnosis and treatment of behavioral disturbance in the elderly. *Connecticut Medicine* (Sept) 1985; 49:578–581.

Keltner N: Psychotherapeutic management: A model for nursing practice. *Perspect Psychiatr Care* (Apr) 1985; 23:125–129.

Khan et al: DST results in nonpsychotic depressed outpatients. *A J Psychiatry* (Sept) 1988; 145:1153–1156.

Klerman G: The spectrum of mania. *Comp Psychiatry* (Jan/Feb) 1981; 22:11.

Krieger D: *Foundations for Holistic Health Nursing Practices.* Lippincott, 1981.

Kyba FN, Russell LO, Rutledge JN: Imaging:The latest in diagnostic technology. *Nurs '87* (Jan) 1987; 13:45–47.

Kyes J, Hofling CK: *Basic Psychiatric Concepts in Nursing,* 4th ed. Lippincott, 1980.

Lamb HR: Deinstitutionalization at the crossroads. *Hosp Community Psychiatry* (Sept) 1988; 39:941–945.

Lang N et al: *Nursing: A Social Policy Statement.* American Nurses' Association, 1980.

Langsley DG: Community psychiatry. In: *Comprehensive Textbook of Psychiatry,* 4th ed. Kaplan HI, Sadock BJ (editors). Williams and Wilkins, 1985.

Lego S et al: *The American Handbook of Psychiatric Nursing.* Lippincott, 1984.

Leichman AM: Legal and ethical aspects of psychiatric nursing. In: *Psychiatric Mental Health Nursing,* 2nd ed. Bocher B et al (editors). Wadsworth, 1985.

Lohr JB, Bracha, HS: *Psychiatric Clinics of North America.* Association of Psychosis and Movement Disorders in the Elderly (March) 1988; 11:1:61–81.

Macklin R: Mortal choices: Ethical dilemmas in modern medicine. Houghton Mifflin, 1987.

Malmquist CP: Can the committed patient refuse chemotherapy? *Arch Gen Psychiatr* (Mar) 1979; 36:351.

Mamar J: Systems thinking in psychiatry: Some theoretical and clinical implications. *Am J Psychiatry* (July) 1983; 140:833.

McEnvoy GK (editor): *Drug Information '88.* American Society of Pharmacists, 1988.

McKinnon RA, Michelo R: *The Psychiatric Interview in Clinical Practice.* Saunders, 1971.

Meyers BS, Alexopoulos GS: Geriatric depression. *Medical Clinics of North America* (Jul) 1988; 72:847.

National Institute of Mental Health: *Report of the Task Force on Nursing.* National Institute of Mental Health, (Sept) 1987.

Ostroff RB et al: The norepinephrine to epinephrine ratio in patients with a history of suicide attempts. *Am J Psychiatry* 1985; 142(2):224–227.

Pelletier LR: Psychiatric Home Care. *J Psychosoc Nurs* (Mar) 1988; 26:22–27.

Reynolds, OF et al: Bedside differentiation of depressive pseudodemential from demention. *A J Psychiatry* (Sept) 1988; 145:1099–1103.

Rhodes AM, Miller, RD: *Nursing and the Law,* 4th ed. Aspen Systems, 1984.

Rodman MJ et al: *Pharmacology and Drug Therapy in Nursing,* 3rd ed. Lippincott, 1985.

Rosenfeld MS: Crisis intervention: The nuclear task approach. *Am J Occup Ther* 1984; 38(6):382–385.

Rosenstock HA, McLaughlin M: On the primary prevention of critical mass: A strategy for adolescent units. *NAPPH* (Jan) 1982; 13:9–1.

Rubin EH, Zorumski CF, Burke WJ: Overlapping symptoms of geriatric depression and Alzheimer-type dementia. *Hosp Community Psychiatry* (Oct) 1988; 39:1074–1078.

Sadock BJ: Group psychotherapy, combined individual and group psychotherapy, and psychodrama. In: *Comprehensive Textbook of Psychiatry,* 4th ed. Kaplan HI, Sadock BJ (editors). Williams and Wilkins, 1985.

Sargent M: Update on brain imaging. *Hosp Community Psychiatry* (Sept) 1988; 39:933–934.

Shader RI: *Manual of Psychiatric Therapeutics.* Little, Brown, 1976.

Sheridan E, Patterson HR, Gustafson EA: *Falconers's the Drug, the Nurse, the Patient,* 7th ed. Saunders, 1985.

Skinner BF: *Science and Human Behavior.* Macmillan, 1953.

Stroebel CF: Biofeedback and behavioral medicine. In: *Comprehensive Textbook of Psychiatry,* 4th ed. Kaplan HI, Sadock BJ (editors). Williams and Wilkins, 1985.

Stuart GW, Sundeen SJ: *Principles and Practices of Psychiatric Nursing,* 2nd ed. Mosby, 1983.

Taube et al: *Utilization and Expenditures for Ambulatory Mental Health Care During 1980.* USHHS Publication No. 84–200000. US Government Printing Office, 1984.

Teicher M: Biology of anxiety. *Medical Clinics of North America* (Jul) 1988; 72:791–814.

Wallace ER: What is the truth? Some philosophical contributions to psychiatric issues. *A J Psychiatry* (Feb) 1988; 145:137–142.

Walsh ME: *Schizophrenia: Straight Talk for Family and Friend.* Warner Books Inc, 1985.

Weiner RD: Convulsive therapies. In: *Comprehensive Textbook of Psychiatry,* 4th ed. Kaplan HI, Sadock BJ (editors). Williams and Wilkins, 1985.

Wing KW: *The Law and the Public's Health,* 2nd ed. Health Administration Press, 1985.

Wolpe J: *The Practice of Behavior Therapy.* Pergamon Press, 1969.

Yalom ID: *The Theory and Practice of Group Psychotherapy,* 2nd ed. Basic Books, 1984.

Yoder L, Jones SL: The emergency room nurse and the psychiatric patient. *J Psychosoc Nurs* (June) 1982; 20:22.

Yogi MM: *The Science of Being and the Art of Living.* Signet Books, 1963.

SUGGESTED READINGS

Andreasen NC: *The Broken Brain: The Biological Revolution in Psychiatry.* Harper and Row, 1984.

Ayllon T, Azrin NH: *The Token Economy: A Motivational System for Therapy and Rehabilitation.* Appleton-Century-Crofts, 1968.

Barofsky I, Budson RD (editors): *The Chronic Psychiatric Patient in the Community: Principles of Treatment.* S.P Medical and Scientific Books, 1983.

Beier DG, Valens EG: *People-Reading.* Stein and Day, 1975.

Bender B, Murphy D, Mark B: Caring for clients with legal charges on a voluntary psychiatric unit. *J Psychosoc Nurs* (Mar) 1989; 27:16–20.

Berne E: *Beyond Games and Scripts.* Grove Press, 1976.

Black K: *Short-term Counseling: A Humanistic Approach for the Helping Professions.* Addison-Wesley, 1983.

Bostrom A: Assessment scales for tardive dyskinesia. *J Psychosoc Nurs* (June) 1988; 26:8–12.

Breger L: *From Instinct to Identity.* Prentice-Hall, 1974.

Cappon D: *Coupling: Understanding the Chemistry of Close Relationships.* St. Martin's Press, 1981.

DeLuca A et al: Psychosocial changes in persistently psychotic schizophrenic patients after an 80% reduction of neuroleptic medication. *J Psychosoc Nurs* (Aug) 1988; 26:13–17.

DiBella GA et al: *Handbook of Partial Hospitalization.* Brunner/Mazel, 1982.

Donnelly J: The incidence of psychosurgery in the United States, 1971–1973. *Am J Psychiatry* 1978; 135:1476.

Ellis A: *Humanistic Psychotherapy: The Rational-Emotive Approach.* Julian Press, 1973.

Fast J: *Body Language.* Evans, 1970.

Fine R: *A History of Psychoanalysis.* Columbia University Press, 1979.

Finkel NJ: *Mental Illness and Health: Its Legacy, Tensions, and Changes.* Macmillan, 1976.

Goble FG: *The Third Force: The Psychology of Abraham Maslow.* Grossman, 1970.

Golton MA: *Your Brain at Work: A New View of Personality and Behavior.* Frank, 1983.

Gurman AS, Razin AM: *Effective Psychotherapy: A Handbook of Research.* Pergamon Press, 1977.

Krauss JB, Slavinsky AT: *The Chronically Ill Psychiatric Patient and the Community.* Blackwell, 1982.

Mattes JA: Optimal length of hospitalization for psychiatric patients: A review of the literature. *Hosp Community Psychiatry* 1982; 33:824.

May R: *The Meaning of Anxiety.* Norton, 1977.

Miller J: *States of Mind.* Pantheon Books, 1983.

Prim R: Water intoxication. *J Psychosoc Nurs* (Nov) 1988; 26:16–18.

Rhodes S, Wilson J: *Surviving Family Life.* Putnam, 1981.

Robinson L: *Psychological Aspects of the Care of Hospitalized Patients,* 3rd ed. Davis, 1976.

Rogers CR: *Client Centered Therapy.* Houghton Mifflin, 1951.

Roman M, Raley PE: *The Indelible Family.* Rawson, Wade, 1980.

Rubin TI: *One to One: Understanding Personal Relationships.* Viking Press, 1983.

Skinner BF: *Science and Human Behavior.* Free Press, 1953.

Skinner BF: *Beyond Freedom and Dignity.* Knopf, 1971.

Smith MI, Glass GV, Miller TI: *The Benefits of Psychotherapy.* Johns Hopkins University Press, 1980.

Snyder SH: *Biological Aspects of Mental Disorder.* Oxford University Press, 1980.

Sundberg ND: *Assessment of Persons.* Prentice-Hall, 1977.

Taylor GR: *The Natural History of the Mind.* Dutton, 1979.

Torrey EF: *The Death of Psychiatry.* Chilton, 1974.

Ullman M, Krippner S, Vaughan A: *Dream Telepathy.* Macmillan, 1973.

Willi J: *Dynamics of Couples Therapy.* Jason Aronson, 1984.

Wilson C: *New Pathways in Psychology: Maslow and the Post-Freudian Revolution.* Taplinger, 1972.

Wittrock MC et al: *The Human Brain.* Prentice-Hall, 1977.

CHAPTER 5

The Role of Culture in Mental Health and Illness

PAULA G. LEVECK

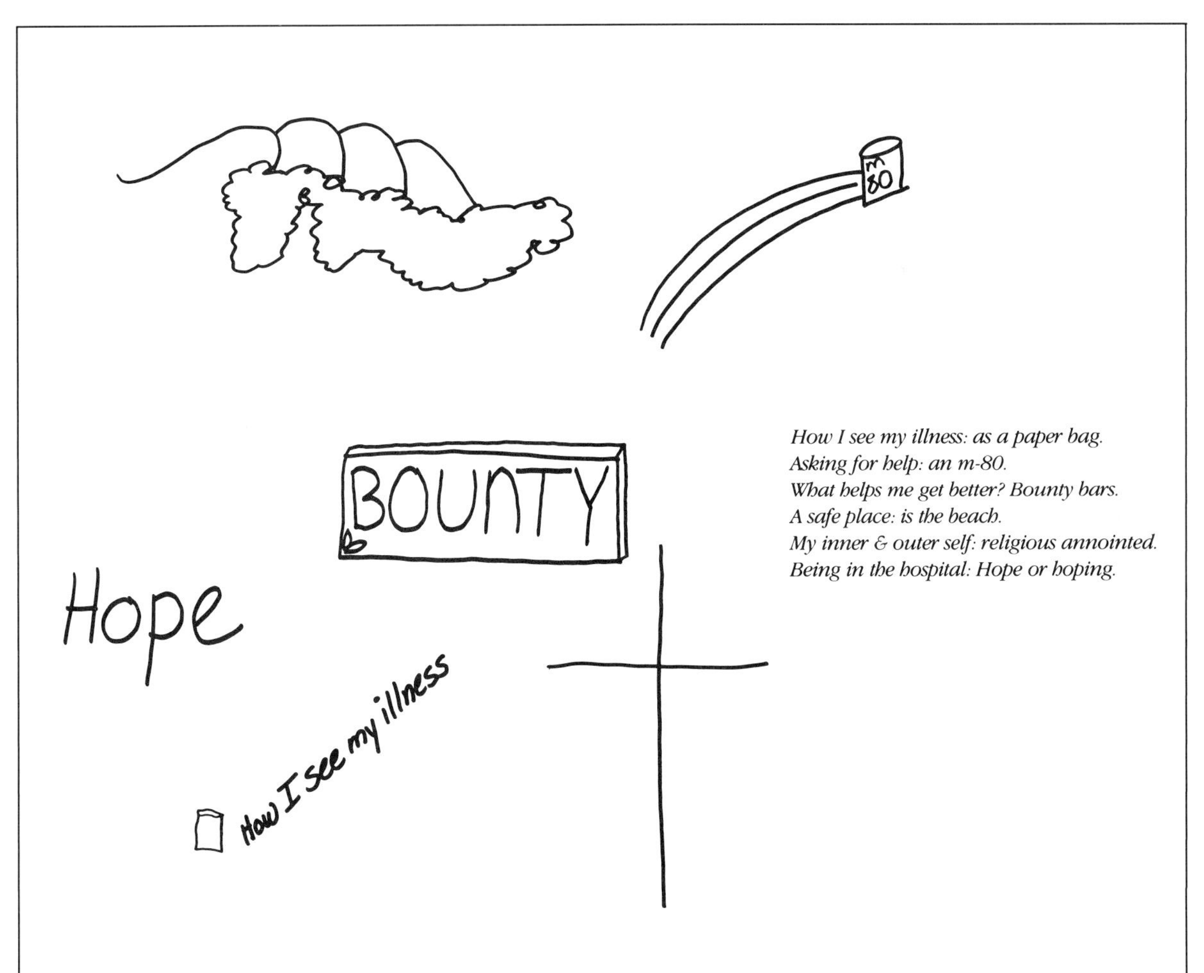

How I see my illness: as a paper bag.
Asking for help: an m-80.
What helps me get better? Bounty bars.
A safe place: is the beach.
My inner & outer self: religious annointed.
Being in the hospital: Hope or hoping.

■ *Objectives*

After reading this chapter the student will be able to

- Define the general concepts of culture, subculture, ethnicity, world view, ethnocentrism, enculturation, acculturation, assimilation, and pluralism
- Discuss the relationship of cultural and mental illness
- Identify the implications of culture to mental health nursing
- Recognize the importance of communication and culture
- Discuss cultural concepts, health beliefs, mental illness, and nursing care for five major cultural groups: Native American, African American, Asian American, Southeast Asian immigrants, and Hispanic American
- Recognize variations in American cultural structures
- Incorporate cultural concepts into nursing assessments

■ *Chapter Outline*

Introduction

Nursing, and especially psychiatric/mental health nursing, consists of encounters between individuals, and one of the things that influences those encounters is the cultural difference between people. This chapter focuses on the cultural concepts that are important for the nurse to know to provide sensitive, individualized mental health care to all clients. Examples from five American cultures are presented to show how nursing care can reflect sensitivity to cultural differences.

General Concepts

Culture is the pattern of all learned behavior and values shared by members of a particular group. It is transmitted by members of the group from one generation to the next. All individuals and groups have culture; it is one measure of our humanness. There are hundreds of cultures and subcultures, each with its own history and learned ways of feeling, thinking, and behaving. Through participation in cultural groups, human beings meet a variety of needs, from the biologic to the spiritual.

Societies can be stratified by socioeconomic classes as well as by geographic, racial, ethnic, religious, gender-related, and behavioral characteristics. These distinctions can cut across cultural lines, creating subgroups within cultures, or **subcultures.** Thus, further distinctions such as those between "high" and "low" culture and between formal and indigenous culture can emerge even within a particular cultural group.

Ethnicity refers to an individual's sense of belonging to a group that shares a unique cultural, social, and linguistic heritage. From a clinical viewpoint, however, more than a distinctiveness is defined by this heritage. It also involves conscious and unconscious choices related to a deep psychologic need for security, identity, and historical continuity. It is transmitted in an emotional language within the family and reinforced in the larger community. Ethnic identity provides an abiding connection with a group, a heritage that cannot be taken away (Giordano, 1973).

Culture and Values

Humans grow up into the culture that surrounds them. Children develop a clear idea of what cultural prescriptions they must follow, and these prescriptions strongly influence each individual's personality. Sometimes people become so attached to their own set of prescriptions and how personal needs are met that they stereotype, judge, and reject people who abide by other rules. This may be an inevitable, though unfortunate, outcome of cultural conditioning—each person believes his or her culture must be right or the individual could not conform to it. The cultural conflicts between differing ideas of what is right—between differing values—underlie much of the conflict between individuals, societies, and nations.

Part of how we construct a system of values within a culture is through the **world view**, the outlook on the universe characteristic of a particular people, that is, how they view self as separate from others; how they divide humans, nonhumans, and the supernatural; how they distinguish relationships among human beings and the natural environment; and how they perceive past, present, and future. Those living in both the Roman and the Chinese empires, for example, considered themselves to be the literal center of the universe, and all other peoples were deemed barbarians.

This tendency, called **ethnocentrism,** exists even when cultures have a more modern sense of geography. The tendency of all human beings to regard their own culture as the best can affect health care providers as well. Health care workers may see their own medical reality as the only true or valuable perspective and lose sight of the client's own experience. Viewing the client solely in the context of the medical environment can create barriers to clear communication, correct perception, and accurate clinical judgment because the client's own perspective, or world view, is not taken into account. This can be particularly troublesome in psychiatric settings, where the client's symptoms are primarily in the areas of thinking, feeling, perceiving, and behaving—all aspects of human experience profoundly governed by culture.

Cultural Conflict

Culture affects values and an individual's sense of reality. When a person from one culture lives in a place where another culture is dominant, mental and emotional conflict can occur. Understanding how this conflict can arise is important to understanding the experience of members of cultural minorities. The concepts of enculturation, acculturation, assimilation, and pluralism are important to this understanding.

Enculturation is the process of learning one's own culture and its world view. **Acculturation** is the process of learning a new culture, of changing the cultural patterns—beliefs, values, and behavior—that one follows to those of another group.

Acculturation is the complex interplay of a person's own desire to become part of the other culture, to assimilate, and the new culture's willingness to allow the person in. This concept is particularly relevant to the situation of immigrants in the United States.

There are two perspectives on the value of permanently exchanging one's own culture for that of another. The **assimilation**, or "melting pot," model expects minority group cultures to adopt the values and behavioral patterns of the majority. The **pluralism** model, on the other hand, suggests that ethnic minority cultures have unique strengths that should be preserved, and that they should be encouraged to maintain their traditions. The extinction of ethnic identity that results from total assimilation gives rise, say the pluralists, to several emotional conflicts within the person.

In fact, for many ethnic Americans, psychiatric symptoms are often linked to the stress and conflict of their experience of being in two cultures at once. Coming from cultures that may be less capitalistic, less sexually frank, or less individualistic, people from different ethnic backgrounds may well feel intense emotional and mental conflict. Sometimes the conflict surfaces within the family as a tension between generations; sometimes the conflict takes place within the person as he or she feels torn between two worlds.

Culture and Poverty

Added to the problems of discrimination and cultural conflict, the mental health of minority groups is also affected by poverty. When coupled with experiences and conditions of minority status, individuals and groups living in poverty suffer physical and emotional hardships that can adversely affect their mental health.

The epidemiologic study in Chicago by Favis and Dunham (1939) showed that first admission rates for most psychoses, including schizophrenia, were highest in the central slum section of the city and regularly decreased as one moved out toward more prosperous suburban areas. The famous Hollingshead and Redlich (1958) study of psychiatric disorders in New Haven, Connecticut, revealed two important findings: (1) The lower class was found to have 12 times the amount of schizophrenic illness found in the upper class, and (2) treatment was inequitably distributed among the classes. The Midtown Manhattan Study (Langer and Michael, 1963; Srole et al., 1962; Srole, 1975), using multiple research techniques, found a high prevalence of mental impairment throughout the population's three socioeconomic classes and the highest rates in the lower class.

Culture and Mental Illness

Mental health and mental illness are defined differently in different cultures. Each culture has different definitions for normal and abnormal, for good and bad, for healthy and unhealthy states and behaviors. The concept of **cultural relativity** acknowledges these differences in various cultures and thus the difficulty in assigning an absolute definition to mental health and illness with a culturally mixed population. For instance, the American values of competition, achievement, and autonomy would be deviant behaviors in societies that value nonaggression, cooperation, and allegiance to the community.

All cultures, however, seem to have an idea of mental and emotional disorder. The description of these disorders varies widely from one culture to another, and not all mental illness known to one society appears in others. There is always a relationship between the culture of a group and the kinds of mental illness suffered by members of that group. When there are features of an illness that differ from culture to culture, it is called a **culture-bound illness** or syndrome, an ethnic psychosis, a hysterical psychosis, or a culture-specific syndrome. Windigo psychosis among certain North American Indian tribes, susto among Hispanics, voodoo illness among African Americans and koro among Chinese males are a few examples (Leff, 1981).

Culture can also provide people with the means of dealing with stress and mental illness. These means may range from the use of confession as a cathartic therapy in some Native American tribes to extended healing ceremonies involving members of one's social circle to shamanism. Different cultures may assign the responsibility for dealing with mental disorder to the individual, to the family and community, or to a specially designated healer.

Just as different behaviors may denote mental illness, depending on the culture, the same behaviors may be perceived and evaluated in different ways, or they may occur with different frequency, depending on the culture. Homosexuality, for example, is viewed in different cultures as a natural expression of human sexuality, as a sin against divine law, as a crime against nature, as an amusing idiosyncrasy, or as an illness (Wallace, 1970). Suicide is another example. Among the Navaho, it is unacceptable because of the effect on family members, and cultures strongly influenced by Roman Catholicism view suicide as a sin. Among the Indochinese, on the other hand, suicide is a personal decision, may have acceptable motives, and may be considered an honorable solution to some dilemmas. Depression is experienced as heaviness on one's chest or as illness of the heart among the Chinese. Hallucinations may mark a person as a potential healer, a shaman, among traditional Native Americans and Southeast Asians. In the dominant U.S. culture, however, a hallucinating person would probably be diagnosed as a schizophrenic.

Implications for Mental Health Nurses

Nurses may often encounter clients with cultural backgrounds different from their own. Understanding specific cultural reactions and, particularly, culturally influenced expressions of mental health and illness, is important to providing effective mental health care. The nurse views mental health and illness from a holistic perspective, incorporates cultural factors into a comprehensive assessment, and takes into account the total context within which a person stays well or becomes sick.

Nurses need to realize that even clients from their own ethnic or cultural group may not fully embody "typical" characteristics thought to be representative of that group. Therefore individualized and comprehensive assessments are always prerequisites to planning. Even the DSM-III-R case handbook has inadequate information on clients' sociodemographic characteristics (Spitzer, 1981). In otherwise excellent case histories and presentations, social and cultural assessments are often lacking.

Barriers to Care Sometimes a client's behavior is misdiagnosed because of the nurse's lack of knowledge and understanding about what forms a normal reaction to situations within a particular cultural group. What may appear "abnormal" to the nurse would be an acceptable response within the client's reference group. For example, the Indian patient in *One Flew Over the Cuckoo's Nest* illustrates how Indians may be hospitalized as psychotic (catatonic schizophrenic) when exhibiting behaviors that may be normal for them.

Nurses need to be aware that ethnicity and socioeconomic class can affect how clients view their interactions with members of the mental health team and what their expectations of psychiatric treatment are. Research (Link and Dohrenwend, 1980) indicates that minority populations tend to underuse mental health services. When they do use these services, their symptoms tend to be more severe than those of the dominant population. People in lower socioeconomic classes, though more likely to be emotionally distressed, were less likely to seek treatment by mental health professionals. Based on studies of 17 community mental health centers, Sue (1977) has reported on mental health services that are unresponsive to persons other than whites. Many clinicians and researchers in social science and psychiatry have looked at possible correlations between poor client outcomes and the failure of white upper–middle class therapists to relate effectively to ethnics and the poor. White ethnics, especially those in the lower-middle class, may even avoid mental health services because of the stigma that the label "patient" carries with it.

When participation in treatment is used to measure the extent of mental illness in ethnic populations, all minorities, with the exception of African Americans, show lower rates of admission to mental health services than do Caucasian Americans. However, when subjective self-reports and psychiatric diagnoses are used, psychopathology appears more widespread than actual treatment statistics suggest. Many psychiatric symptoms are expressed as physical complaints and thus go unrecognized. The experience of stigma and shame also tends to encourage care giving at home. And, lastly, treatment by indigenous healers may be preferred to treatment in the mental health system. Hall and Bourne (1973), who surveyed root doctors, faith healers, and magic vendors in an African American ghetto in Atlanta's South Side, suggested that these indigenous therapists be used as community mental health workers. Lubdhansky, Egri, and Stokes (1970) studied Puerto Rican spiritualists and suggested incorporating them into the mental health system as paraprofessionals. Healing efforts may thus become more consistent and coherent for members of subcultures.

Clients from differing cultures may react to the physical design of a mental hospital or psychiatric unit. That is to say, the material environment, types and spatial arrangements of furniture, privacy versus crowding, and distance from nurse's station may all influence the ease or difficulty with which a client who is not white American will adjust to hospitalization and interact with personnel (Hall, 1979).

Another barrier to culturally appropriate and sensitive care is the use of stereotypes by nurses. A stereotype is a fixed perception or conventional belief about, for example, an ethnic or religious group or a race. Stereotypes prevent nurses from making accurate and individualized assessments of clients and profoundly influence the quality of nursing care given and received. Nurses need to be aware that assessments of clients as hostile, resistant, and uncooperative may be the result of the nurse's own unconscious stereotype projected in such a way that it has elicited negative and distancing responses from the client. Perceptive clients detect incongruent behaviors in the nurse and may respond with protective behaviors of their own.

Communication The nurse needs to communicate with family spokespeople and include their thoughts in the assessment process and their participation in the overall treatment plan. In many ethnic groups, family members expect to be near the hospitalized client as much as possible to give emotional support, look after medical treatment, and meet needs that the health care providers do not address, such as needs for special foods, ethnic meals, herbs, and the like. Some family members may want, or actually bring in, indigenous healers to complement the curing techniques of the established health care system. Even for economically secure clients or clients with access to many community resources, extended families remain important, often as the support system of choice.

Cultures vary in their patterns of verbal and nonverbal communication. The very way in which questions are asked during an assessment interview must be culturally tailored. Communication codes differ as to whether direct or indirect probes are preferred and at what point in an interaction they may appropriately occur. Some clients expect, even require, handshaking and smiling. Others prefer only the touching necessary for a physical examination and serious facial expressions. African Americans or Asians often look down or away from the nurse. Although this behavior may be labeled paranoid, suspicious, or evasive by nurses, it is a culturally normal means of relating to persons in positions of authority. Communication styles evolve as adaptive responses to encounters perceived as dangerous. Nurses need to sort out normative from symptomatic verbal and nonverbal responses.

If translators need to be used for non-English-speaking clients, the same interpreter should be used for each interview if at all possible. This helps to establish rapport, continuity, and consistency in understanding communication themes and patterns. If nurses are communicating through interpreters, three important variables can lead to distortions and affect the nurse's assessment of the client (Marcos, 1979):

- The interpreter's language competence and translation skills
- The interpreter's lack of psychiatric knowledge

- The interpreter's personal attitudes toward either the client or nurse

More research is needed on the relationships between language barriers and assessment of psychopathology.

Crucial to being able to communicate effectively in psychiatric nursing is empathy, which is all the more important when relating to people whose language, values, beliefs, appearance, and behavior differ from the nurse's own. A caring relationship can atone for many transcultural mistakes, but building the bridge across cultures in mental health nursing is the nurse's responsibility, not the client's.

Native Americans

> [During] a national meeting of mental health professionals and tribal leaders, one of the tribal leaders asked a young psychiatrist to describe the nature of the mental health problem among American Indians. The psychiatrist attempted to go into an in-depth analysis of how he saw the problem, and he soon became entangled in his own rhetoric. There followed a silence as he tried to collect his thoughts. After a length of time in which everybody was becoming quite uncomfortable, the chairman of the Miccousukee Tribe of Florida, Mr. Buffalo Tiger, stood up and said, "Let me explain it this way. . . . Today," he said, "Indians are like a man who got up early in the morning and looked out his door and saw something shining in the road a little way away. It was something he wanted and he walked over and picked it up and when he was done picking it up he saw something further along that he also wanted. He went and got that and it happened again and he kept walking down the road picking up things. Then, all of a sudden, he turned around and he couldn't find his way back home again." (Bergman, 1973, pp. 663–666)

The term *Native American* or *American Indian* can have a number of interpretations: a resident of a reservation, a person declaring a certain percentage of Indian blood, a caste, a sociocultural group, or a legal term. Reported numbers of tribes vary from 250 to more than 400; suffice it to say, they are numerous and diverse. Most Native Americans live on federal reservations and in small rural communities; about 40 percent are in urban centers at any given time. Among tribes in the United States, there are more than 300 different languages and dialects (Meketon, 1983). Native Americans comprise only 0.6 percent of the total U.S. population according to the 1980 census. They are a people, however, with a unique history and relationship with the dominant white culture.

Through the long history of colonization of North America by Europeans, violence and brutality have been common experiences for Native Americans. Assimilation has not been a primary issue for Native Americans, as it has been for immigrant groups. Neither the immigrants nor the Native Americans saw a solution to their conflict in integrating the latter into the society of the former. Normal separation of the two societies survives today, with the relegation of many Native Americans to reservations. Some may attempt to assimilate into the dominant culture, but they are often poorly equipped and subject to discrimination as they compete for jobs. Tribal values espouse cooperative rather than competitive living, a value that does not survive well in a capitalistic economy and culture.

Consequently, the self-concept of many Native Americans has suffered numerous and extreme attacks, and their levels of stress are high. Henderson and Primeaux (1981) state that 75 percent of Native American families have annual incomes below $4000 and that their unemployment is almost 10 times higher than the national average. They also state that almost 60 percent of the adult Native American population has less than an eighth-grade education. These data suggest poverty and alienation from mainstream society.

Cultural Concepts

Although values and norms among different Native American tribes may be quite divergent, sometimes even in opposition, many are quite similar. Henderson and Primeaux (1981) describe general characteristics that apply to many traditional Native Americans:

- An orientation to the present rather than the future

- A time consciousness that relates to what they are doing and to whom they are with at any given moment rather than to actual clock time
- Cooperation rather than competition
- Giving to others rather than keeping for oneself
- Respect for age rather than idealization of youth

Among traditional Native Americans, ties to family, both nuclear and extended, are very strong. Both economic and social support may be provided by the family. *Family* might refer either to relatives on both sides in a marriage or to an entire clan without blood ties. A Native American extended family may consist of several three generational households. Older females occupy an important position in many Native American tribal communities and may need to be involved in decision making regarding psychiatric treatment for members of their families.

Health Beliefs

Disease for Native Americans is tied to spiritual beliefs; medicine and religion are inseparable. The very word *medicine* means mystery to Native Americans. But to generalize about Native Americans loses the rich diversity of beliefs and practices that do actually exist, not to mention shifts that have taken place due to diffusion and acculturation. In the past, each tribe created its own coherent and intact health care system. However, access to formal education, Christianity, technologic developments, and relationships among tribes makes the survival of any pristine traditional healing systems doubtful. Depending on the nature, symptoms, and diagnoses of their conditions, many Native Americans even choose to rely on Western health care systems.

As nontechnologically oriented people do in general, Native Americans believe in the harmony between human beings and the earth, and between mind, body, and soul. The inextricable connection between the individual, social, and natural environments requires attending to the needs and welfare of the total. All living systems are interrelated. Thus, harmful acts or wrongdoing at one level will reverberate throughout, from the individual, to the social system, to the natural environment and universe that support human life. The etiology of disease—physical, emotional, or mental—is disharmony.

Disease symptoms are usually attributed, to some degree, to supernatural causes. Fear of witchcraft is prevalent among Native Americans, as is the belief that illness may be caused by witchcraft (Vogel, 1970). Other beliefs regarding the cause of sickness include violation of a taboo, intrusion of an object or spirit into the body, and loss of soul. Violations of the incest taboo are especially dangerous and may be punished by insanity (Kennedy, 1961). *Moth madness* appears to be a culture-specific disorder that still occurs among Navahos. It is thought to be caused by having incestuous thoughts, which then implant a moth embryo in the brain. When the moth grows and flaps its wings, the afflicted person is compelled to run or fall into a fire. Object intrusion, which may be the result of witchcraft, can be treated by sucking out the foreign objects. Spirit intrusion requires a healing ritual to exorcise the evil spirits. Mental illness due to loss of the soul requires the recovery of the soul, for the person is believed to be in danger of dying if it is not regained. A soul may be stolen by bad spirits or witches, and it is often lost during a dream. In each of these examples, disequilibrium is present. Once a balance within the person is restored, physical, emotional, and mental symptoms will subside.

Before entering the mental health system, it is not unusual for Native American clients to seek treatment from traditional indigenous healers if they are available. The most important person in Native American healing is the medicine man, who is often elevated to positions of extreme power and authority. Many of them are believed to be endowed with supernatural powers for intervention between human beings and the spirit world.

Medicine men (and women) are often quite diverse and stratified. Some are singers; others, diviner diagnosticians; some specialize in caring for souls; and others specialize in herbs, massage, or midwifery. The supernatural abilities of healers may be used only for healing by some and for both good and evil by others. Healers use therapeutic tools such as charms and fetishes to ward off evil, along with herbs and medicines known to have curative properties.

The great faith in the medicine man's capacity to intervene in the spirit world, combined with the participation of one's extended family and tribe during curing ceremonies, offer psychotherapeutic benefits lacking in the white man's mental health system. Carstairs (1969, p. 409) has written that spiritual healing

> may be based on quite ill-founded theories of the causation of disease, but it has two striking advantages over supposedly scientific reliance upon physical treatments: first, the patient is not exposed to the undesirable side effects of many of the newest psychotropic drugs; and second, spiritual healing requires the participation of other persons in addition to the patient and thus helps to reintegrate the mentally ill patient with the rest of the community from whom he has become estranged.

Most social scientists, especially anthropologists who have studied non-Western—that is, nonscientific—medicine, believe in the psychotherapeutic benefits of traditional healing practices. The interest of Western clinicians and researchers in public confession, social support systems, networks, and tribal therapy in the last 20 years attests to the discovery of a holistic, or systems, approach to symptoms manifested by and within a given person.

Mental Illness

Alcoholism is the most widespread and severe emotional and mental disorder in the Native American community in terms of both mortality and morbidity. The Indian Health Service has the responsibility of serving, and striving for optimal care of, Native Americans living on reservations in 25 states and Aleut and Eskimos living in Alaska. Government statistics, however, reflect an increasing death rate from alcoholism. "It seems that while illnesses that are germ-specific are being reduced or successfully contained, the symptoms of social 'unhealthiness' are increasing" (Joe, Gallerito, and Pino, 1976, p. 86).

High suicide and homicide rates along with deaths from alcoholism are four times higher than the rate for Americans as a whole (Bullough and Bullough, 1982). Often, Indians are killed while drunk in moving-vehicle accidents or by their friends, or ultimately, by cirrhosis of the liver. Sociologic and psychologic explanations for these accidental or violent deaths are widespread and tend to center on the multiple barriers to development of individual and ethnic identity and pride. Both historical and contemporary relationships between the white and Indian systems have fostered passivity, dependency, second-class citizenship, and low self-esteem.

The high suicide rates among youths are especially alarming. In 1980 through 1982 U.S. Indian and Alaska Native rates for ages 10 through 24 were 2.8 to 2.3 times as high as general U.S. rates. The suicide rate is much higher among males, who tend to use violent and highly lethal methods. Suicide occurs mainly in tribes with "loose social integration," which are the tribes undergoing rapid socioeconomic change (May, 1987).

In addition to violent behavior such as suicide and homicide, there is an increasing problem of domestic violence such as spouse and child abuse and rape (Pambrun, 1980). Adjustment to a technologically superior culture, which has control over Native Americans' welfare, has fostered aggression at one extreme and depression and self-depreciation at the other. Moreover, experiences of loss due to the high death rate are prevalent among Native Americans as a group. Even among children, multiple grieving experiences are not unusual.

Indians are often inhibited from using mental health services that are dominated and controlled by whites. Historically, Native Americans have been the recipients of disparaging attitudes and poorly organized care from white health care providers. They suffer discomfort when they come into contact with psychiatric personnel. Their culturally patterned response of silence and withdrawal from these stress-producing encounters may generate additional psychiatric labels such as *catatonic schizo-*

phrenia, hostility, paranoia, and *depression.* Donald P. Jewell (1979) provides an excellent account of a Navaho Indian man diagnosed for 18 months as a catatonic schizophrenic. In fact, during the author's investigation and interviewing of the patient, it became clear that the Navaho's reaction was normal given his culture and the situations to which he was responding.

Nursing Care

When a Native American is hospitalized, nurses on psychiatric units need to realize how important frequent visits by relatives may be. Nursing care plans should be designed with input from significant others, especially those occupying positions of authority in the Indian family systems. Family involvement is a necessary condition for restoration of health. Family, or even tribal, participation in therapeutic activities is probably, in some cases, a prerequisite to gaining rapport. Some clients are known to have been taken out of hospitals or to terminate treatment prematurely because family members, especially the elders, were not included.

Although nurses are unlikely to encounter Native Americans who do not speak English, both verbal and nonverbal interactional patterns will remain powerfully influenced by socialization practices within tribal cultures. Native American communication patterns may differ markedly from those of the dominant white society. Pacing of verbal exchanges is slower, the tone is lower, silences are longer, and observations are intense and penetrating. Silences are cherished to enable Native Americans to give thought to what they will say and to communicate proper values. At the same time, they are sensitive to the nonverbal communication of others. Some Native American clients may regard continuous eye contact during interviews by the nurse as insulting or disrespectful. Stares may be interpreted as attempts to control the client's spirit. In general, Native Americans are very sensitive to others' body language. To guarantee rapport building and therapeutic relationships, nurses need to be totally congruent in their verbal and nonverbal communication.

History taking and therapeutic interviews must be structured carefully and executed leisurely, allowing time for clients to respond to questions and statements. Generally, comments reflecting observations are more acceptable than direct questions, which may be considered impolite. Because of their preference for the oral tradition, Native Americans generally would rather that notes not be taken during interviews. Establishing the right pace is a key to developing rapport; active listening is a therapeutic imperative.

For Native Americans, stressors exist at every level: psychologic, socioeconomic, cultural, and spiritual. Entry into the mental health system should not exacerbate already existing conflicts between Native American and white cultures. The nurse, by respecting cultural relativity and questing for cross-cultural understanding, can play a large role in creating caring interactions that foster cure.

African Americans

Defining the category of African Americans is exceedingly complex in that, besides the descendants of slaves in this country, it also contains persons of African ancestry from Haiti, who speak French; from Cuba and Puerto Rico, who speak Spanish; from Brazil, who speak Portuguese; and from Jamaica, who speak English. Although they may all connect with African roots, African Americans differ in what they identify as their most recent country of origin, their first language, their spiritual beliefs—in short, their ethnicity. Therefore it is important to elicit national origin and its associated features when possible. Moreover, since many African Americans are economically and educationally disadvantaged compared to whites, attributes believed to be related to ethnicity or race are confounded by the added variable of social status. Social class membership, in many instances, may be a stronger measure of differences than cultural affiliation.

Single-parent, low-income African-American families increased from 31 to 45 percent between 1970 and 1980. Research on social support systems in these families with adolescent or preadolescent children has suggested that the families coping most successfully have networks where reciprocity exists in both emotional and instrumental support. Mothers in dysfunctional families reported unequal exchanges, that is, they gave more than they received (Lindblad-Goldberg and Dukes, 1985). These findings reinforce the hypothesis of many mental health clinicians that it is the quality of a social network, rather than the number of people composing it, that determines how effectively a family will function within the network. An adaptive response to poverty conditions exists when goods and services are swapped in a system of exchange.

The high level of participation in social support systems is thought to relate to the African-American tradition of doing for others, the need for economic support and the actual services provided, and the functional quality of the network of support systems. Therefore nurses need to inquire about friends in the community; about relatives such as grandparents, aunts and uncles, and godparents; and about the church and businesses. All these people and institutions may have strongly influenced the client's psychologic and social growth and development.

Cultural Concepts

Most African Americans are capable of formal "white" behavior when interacting with the dominant culture; they express informal "black" behavior within their own communities. African-American culture, which has evolved in the United States, is the result of the extinction of some Africanisms (West African traits) and the survival of others in the context of the slavery system identity and the dominant white culture. African-American culture has undergone several changes based on both historical and psychocultural forces. From the experience of slavery, during which African Americans were treated as pieces of property, through Reconstruction and Jim Crowism to the 1950s and 1960s and through the Black Power movement of the 1970s, African Americans have struggled to experience ethnic pride and a sense of individual self-identity. Nobles and Nobles (1976) assert that the uniqueness of African-American psychology stems from positive aspects of African philosophy—a system that centers on a oneness with nature, the survival of the tribe, a natural rhythm of time, and a sharing of experiences. Hill (1971) identified five strengths of African-American families:

- Male and female role flexibility in the African-American community
- Strong kinship bonds
- Orientation toward high achievement
- Orientation toward work
- Orientation toward religion

Because the church has been, and remains, a powerful influence determining the quality of psychologic life for many African Americans, it is essential to elicit religious affiliation from African-American clients. Religious organizations are second only to the extended family system in providing support, purpose, and nurturance to its members.

Although African Americans are affiliated with many religions, vast numbers belong to Protestant and Roman Catholic churches. Baptists and several fundamentalist Protestant churches often have largely African-American congregations, which reflect the unique stamp of African-American culture.

Within fundamentalist Protestantism, religious beliefs of many African Americans are influenced by African conceptions of the universe and the spiritual world along with the teachings of Christianity. Voodooism or faith healing are instrumental in their conceptions of the etiology of illnesses and appropriate care practices. Further, increasing numbers of African Americans are now practicing Muslims, and Islam requires a highly regulated and specific lifestyle that influences health and dietary practices.

African Americans speak both English and Black English, a dialect variously labeled and interpreted. At its simplest, it is a combination of English words and West African language patterns. The nurse's understanding of this speech helps to overcome some of the initial obstacles that may be present when nurses who are not African Americans interact with African-American clients. Contrary to many people's opinion, Black English is not an impoverished language nor does it suggest cognitive inferiority or limited ability to communicate. In Black English, there is a tendency to drop final consonants, to use double and multiple negatives, and to use the verb *to be* in a continuous present tense (Taylor, 1976). Like all languages, it is a standardized language, and it contains African language characteristics in addition to English dialect (Dillard, 1972).

Along with Black English is an orientation to the oral tradition. This implies a preference for spoken rather than written communication, a greater spontaneity in speaking, and a higher level of participation from the group or audience listening to the speaker. Nurses who strive to develop therapeutic communication with African-American clients need to become knowledgeable about Black English, about preferences for verbal interaction, and about the importance of verbal and nonverbal congruence.

Health Beliefs

Folk medicine thrives mainly in urban ghettos and the rural South. Folk practices range from the purely magical to the empirically or scientifically logical. Many poor African Americans experience the world as both natural and unnatural, and their illnesses can be divided in the same way. Maintenance of physical and mental health is desirable and requires a balance in the human and physical environments. To prevent illnesses, these African Americans must remain alert to the natural phenomena around them for guidance in correct behaviors and appropriate timing.

As in many other groups, disease can be the product of being out of harmony either with personal hygiene or with proper behavior, both of which would constitute natural explanations of disease. Unnaturally caused diseases, both physical and mental, are explained by magic and witchcraft. Several researchers have reported that mentally ill African-American clients frequently believe they are victims of a hex and view their symptoms as due to malign magic often perpetrated by a significant member in their family system or social network (Snow, 1983). Persons out of God's grace because of sinful behavior or wrongdoing are particularly vulnerable to demonic or evil forces. Sexual jealousy and envy are frequent reasons for being hexed.

"Among Blacks, witchcraft beliefs may be described as roots, rootwork, witchcraft, Voodoo or Hoodoo, a fix, or a mojo—an evil 'put on' or thrown at 'the victim'" (Snow, 1983). So great can the fear of witchcraft be that the ill or injured person must find the folk healer who has the specific powers required, or death might ensue. Successful curers, such as voodoo priests and root doctors, are those whose powers can counteract the bad work done by witches or conjurers. As Snow (1983) explains, these folk medical beliefs seem to reflect three major world view themes among lower-class African Americans:

- The world is a hostile and dangerous place.
- The person is liable to attack from external sources.
- The person is helpless, with no internal resources to combat such attack; he or she must depend on outside aid.

It is unlikely that people with mental or emotional symptoms caused by witchcraft would voluntarily enter the mental health system, but there are instances of successful collaboration between folk healers and psychiatrists in the treatment of a given client. Many African Americans appear to have a growing interest in sources of help that provide an alternative to the established health care system. They find explanations in astrology and positive support in mediums, prophets, readers, and others who participate in the occult world.

Mental Illness

African Americans are known to suffer the full range of mental, emotional, and behavioral disorders. All minorities, but African Americans in particular, are often evaluated on the basis of a "deficit" model of behavior; that is, the norm of middle-class whites is the norm against which African Americans are measured and judged. African Americans and their families, communities, and culture are viewed as negative and pathologic. Disproportionally high percentages of African Americans, then, are given psychiatric diagnoses.

Epidemiologic statistics on rates of mental illness among African Americans have been confusing and have been based primarily on hospitalization and many misdiagnoses, giving rise to the myth that African Americans have more mental illness than whites. Psychiatric epidemiology has generally suggested that manic depressive disorders rarely occur among African Americans (and among lower socioeconomic groups in general). However, recent research shows that manic depressive disorder and perhaps affective disorders do occur at a significant rate (Jones, Gray, and Parson, 1981). Somatic complaints occur more frequently in depressed African-American clients than they do in depressed white clients.

The paranoid response, given the history of race relationships in the United States, is a coping mechanism frequently employed by African Americans. Grier and Cobbs (1968), two psychiatrists who have written about the rage of African Americans, believe that African Americans, in order to survive, have developed adaptive personality traits. They suggest that African Americans suffer cultural paranoia as well as cultural depression, cultural masochism, and cultural antisocialism—that is, until proved otherwise, whites are to be distrusted. Thus clients, before entering the "professional" system, may have worked their way through a lay referral system consisting of family, friends, neighbors, and lay consultants. If these resources are considered inadequate, the client will seek help from formal mental health services. African Americans may postpone seeking health care because of either a fatalistic outlook or a reluctance to deal with the risk of discrimination in the predominantly "white" health care system.

Nursing Care

Potential barriers to empathy and therapeutic communication with African-American clients can stem from commonly held myths among white Americans about African Americans. Bradshaw (1978) explains that some of the most widespread myths are

- African slaves had no culture or civilization.
- The African-American family is pathologic, unlike the nuclear white family.
- Matriarchy is universal in African-American families.
- Slavery has produced total chaos in African-American families.
- Psychopathology is an inevitable consequence of one-parent, female-dominated households.
- The African-American male is either sexually inferior or sexually superior to the white male.
- African Americans rarely develop severe depression or commit suicide.

These myths have been evolving for several hundred years within the dominant white culture. Nurses need to explore their own beliefs and attitudes to make certain that these myths are not included as objective data in client assessments.

Even when nurses and clients come from similar ethnic or racial backgrounds, errors in nursing diagnoses are made. When there is a cultural (and often social) distance between the nurse and client, the probability of error increases. Research into psychiatric diagnoses and records of African-American versus white clients has shown significant discrepancies—for instance, more notes being written about white clients than about African-American clients (DeHoyos and DeHoyos, 1965). With essentially the same clinical symptoms, African Americans have been given the diagnosis of schizophrenia more often than whites, who have been given the diagnosis of psychotic depression or another affective illness (Raskin, Crook, and Herman, 1975; Simon et al., 1973). Explanations of these findings suggest that stereotypes of African-American psychopathology lead to errors in assessment by mental health personnel. Stereotypical views include the ideas that

African-Americans are too blissful a racial group to experience depression, too interpersonally deprived to suffer grief related to loss, too hostile to engage in therapeutic relationships, and too impulse ridden to engage in problem solving. Diagnostic tests, such as the Minnesota Multiphasic Personality Inventory, sometimes confirm stereotypes and clinical errors and should be used only with the utmost scrutiny and culturally sensitive interpretations.

A nurse can expect the minister of an African-American client's church to be viewed as a significant other and perhaps to collaborate with other persons in the client's support system and with the mental health team. Pastors and other church members might be helpful in providing data about the client's self-concept and interpersonal relationships.

To assess clients who exhibit a paranoid response, it is essential to separate a healthy, realistically based suspiciousness or "cultural paranoia" from that which is clearly a component in a delusional system. For example, an African-American male client who believes a white policeman may shoot him for the slightest wrong is not paranoid; such a feeling can be a sign of mental imbalance in a middle-class white man (Poussaint, 1980). Either way, nurses need to understand the context within which these thoughts, or thought disorders, were generated and to comprehend that the hostility may not be directed at them only, or at all (Spurlock, 1975). An earnest endeavor to sort out race-related psychologic and interpersonal issues from those issues that stem from the client's more immediate relationships and environment helps immensely in developing a therapeutic alliance. All communication must be open, unambiguous, and comprehensible to the client. Clients are under extreme stress and may experience high anxiety upon hospitalization. Cognition is limited and perception is distorted when anxiety is severe.

Differentiating between actual paranoia and "a healthy cultural suspiciousness, an adaptive response to the experience of racism" (Carter, 1974) may be a clinical ability difficult for nurses who are not African American to develop. To do so, nurses need to examine their own assumptions and possible misinterpretations of the behavior manifested by African-American clients.

The mental, emotional, and behavioral responses of African-American clients do reside within the person; that is, they are the client's reactions to life experiences. Nonetheless, nurses need to remind themselves that the actual problem might be low self-esteem, helplessness, loss, a somatic complaint, or thought and perceptual distortion. The problem might also be racism, which can be encountered in almost every facet of existence. Nursing intervention may involve strategies that focus on the social and environmental forces precipitating mental illness as well as on the psychologic and interpersonal dynamics.

A study of white and African-American male inpatients in a Veterans Administration psychiatric unit revealed less violence among African Americans, although discussions with nurses and ward physicians led the researchers to expect more (Lawson, Yesavage, and Werner, 1984). In another study of an acute inpatient unit, African Americans were disproportionately secluded, which was interpreted as a possible demonstration of the staff's racial bias (Soloff and Turner, 1981).

The Moos Ward Atmosphere Scale, administered to African-American and white inpatients in a Veterans Administration hospital, showed significant racial differences in perceptions of the ward's social environment, namely, a more negative perception among African Americans. The findings raise questions about whether treatment differences between African-American and white clients cause African Americans to develop a more negative perception or whether African Americans enter the unit with a more negative perception, which then causes the predominantly white staff to treat them differently, that is, to give them fewer privileges and more restrictions (Flaherty et al., 1981). The study certainly suggests a relation between the social structure and feelings of reduced spontaneity and autonomy among African-American clients and their greater tendency to terminate hospitalization against medical advice. Nurses and other staff members need to look at their mental health settings' policies, practices, and living conditions to assess sensitivity and responsiveness to the values and lifestyles of all cultural groups.

Asian Americans

Asian Americans, sometimes referred to as the model minority, are an incredibly heterogeneous population. Their parents, ancestors, or they themselves were born in the Philippines, China, Japan, Korea, Vietnam, Cambodia, Laos, or Thailand. White Americans' attitudes and thoughts about Asian people are complex combinations of reality, fantasy, and stereotyping and are rarely based on intimate knowledge of each culture. To Asians, however, belonging to particular national, ethnic, and religious groups is essential to their experience of a coherent identity. They do not appreciate mistaken assumptions by health care personnel regarding their ethnicity.

Filipinos, the largest population of Asian Americans in the western states, came from numerous islands in the Philippines and are, therefore, quite diverse in ethnicity, language, and socioeconomic and educational status. Most Filipinos arrived in one of two primary immigration waves: the wave of male laborers who immigrated from 1905 through 1935 or in the wave of educated professional urbanites who immigrated from 1966 to the present.

Chinese Americans came in large numbers to California after the gold rush in the mid-1800s. They suffered through various exclusionary and repressive legislation and experienced many instances of scapegoating, brutality, and persecution by white Americans.

Many Japanese-American families have been in the United States for four generations. They suffered through the Japanese Exclusion Act in 1924. The incarceration of more than 100,000 Japanese Americans in internment camps during World War II dealt a grave blow to a group that had, in fact, adopted the American way of life to a high degree.

Asian Americans make up about 2 percent of the U.S. population, but this percentage is increasing with recent waves of immigrants from Southeast Asia. The most recently arrived immigrants and refugees will manifest the purest expression of their particular culture. Individuals and families in the United States for two or three generations generally manifest some degree of acculturation to the dominant American culture. Thus, any generalizations about Asians tend to be useless; instead, specific assessments must be made. Asian Americans have experienced culture conflict and culture shock, social change, minority group status, and racism. Although many of them are strong in natural support systems, their resources through the mental health system have been weak. Substantial disagreements exist about the emotional and mental well-being of Asian Americans. Asian Americans are, generally, far more reluctant to use mental health services than white Americans are (Brown et al., 1973; Kitano, 1969; Sue and McKinney, 1975; Sue and Sue, 1974; Sue and Zane, 1987).

Cultural Concepts

The influence of Taoism, Confucianism, and Buddhism underlies cultural values, interpersonal and social behavior, and health care beliefs and practices throughout Asia. To achieve balance, Taoist philosophy requires a flow with nature, a moderation in all things. Confucianism has given rise to rules for correct conduct within the family and the community. Buddhism has produced a belief in the value of good deeds rather than accumulation of goods. Western insight-oriented psychotherapy is generally not acceptable for the less acculturated Asian Americans. This is due to traditional Chinese philosophy, which emphasizes harmonious interpersonal relationships, interdependence, and mutual moral obligation or loyalty to achieve a state of psychosocial homeostasis or peaceful coexistence with family and other fellow beings (Hsu, 1971).

The extended kinship family system is prevalent among Chinese and Japanese Americans. Even if they are not living within the same household or in proximity to one another, strong emotional bonds and carefully constructed rules regarding roles and accompanying obligations are present. The less acculturated the Asian-American family, the more male-dominated it tends to be, with rigidly prescribed functions for each gender, each generation, and each role relationship (parent-child, husband-wife, brother-sister). Deference to and respect for parental authority is taught early and thoroughly to Chinese and Japanese children. Even adult Asians who are capable of assertive behaviors outside the home may display (according to white Americans) extreme degrees of submissiveness to their elders. Women, except perhaps as mothers-in-law, may show even more exaggerated acts of obedience, suggesting inferiority and dependence.

Filial piety (*hsiao* in Chinese, *kōkō* in Japanese) is another concept indicating the social obligation of the young to the old, of the duty to care for one's parents and to reciprocate for what one has been given. Traditionally, this has meant that elders actually live in their children's homes. When this arrangement involves varying degrees of acculturation to the dominant culture's normative methods of treatment of the aged, the result can be a conflict-ridden situation. Asians who fail to fulfill family and social contracts often experience high degrees of guilt and shame.

Chinese and Japanese Americans have been well socialized to feel guilty when they behave unacceptably and, perhaps even more devastating, to feel shame. The guilt stems from failing to live up to expectations, and the shame from dishonoring one's family and community and from giving one's group a bad name. Traditionally, families have played a major role in caring for the physically and mentally ill. Sometimes, a psychotic family member has been maintained within the family fold for years to save face, before allowing intervention from outsiders or hospitalization.

The Asian situational orientation is one manifestation of key differences between Asians and Americans and has been described by many authors (Hsu, 1971; Kitano, 1969). Because of the emphasis on harmony among persons, Asians will take steps to avoid conflict when possible. Confrontations, direct questions, expression of negative feelings, even active participation when authority figures are present all violate codes of conduct that are hundreds of years old. Among Japanese, the *enryo* norm is a standard requiring behaviors that communicate humility, reserve, politeness, respect, nonassertiveness, and even self-effacement in social interactions. Chinese Americans may be guided by a desire to accommodate rather than to confront and to control feelings rather than to express feelings (Chen-Louie, 1983). Thus, individual and group therapies designed for catharsis and disclosure may be contraindicated for many Asian-American clients. Participation could create additional stresses and, from a cultural perspective, be inappropriate if not actually psychologically and socially destructive.

Health Beliefs

Chinese medicine, which is both a science and an art more than 5000 years old, permeates every healing system in Asia. Every Asian country has molded Chinese medicine to fit its particular geographic region, religious beliefs, availability of herbs and foods, and cultural idiosyncracies.

Yin and yang are viewed as primordial elements out of which the universe has evolved; they pervade all natural phenomena and are endowed with numerous qualities. As Foster (1978, p. 63) explains

> Yang represents heaven, sun, fire, heat, dryness, light, the male principle, the exterior, the right side, life, high, noble, good, beautiful, nature, order, joy, wealth—in short, all positive elements. Yin represents the opposite: earth, moon, water, cold, dampness, darkness, the female principle, the interior, the left side, death, low, ignoble, bad, ugly, vice, confusion, and poverty—in short, all the negative elements.

Body parts are endowed with yin or yang; yin is in the heart, lungs, liver, spleen, and kidneys, whereas yang is in the stomach, gall bladder, bladder, and small and large intestines. Within the individual and within the universe, a balance in the constant interaction between yin and yang must be maintained throughout life. When balance is not achieved at all, death occurs; when there are disruptions in balance, illness occurs. Techniques such as acupuncture and moxibustion (a wormwood poultice), meditation, or the ingestion of herbs help produce proper balance.

Traditional Chinese medicine is also based on a balance among five elements contained in the human body and the universe: earth, water, fire, metal, and wood. Many phenomena were thought to occur in fives, and an elaborate system of matching numbers has characterized Chinese medicine.

Belief in a humoral pathology, which in some fashion is now thought to be worldwide, also permeates many health beliefs and healing practices among Asian Americans. This explanatory system, believed to have its genesis in Greece and written about by Hippocrates, stated that four body humors must be in balance to have a healthy body: blood, which is hot and wet; phlegm, which is cold and dry; black bile, which is cold and dry; and yellow bile, which is hot and dry (Foster, 1978). From this early system, the belief in a dichotomy between hot and cold—a dichotomy used to judge diseases, foods, herbs, and therapeutic practices—has predominantly survived. Symptoms or diseases classified "hot" must be treated by a "cold" technique, and vice versa. No designation of cold or hot—whether for foods, drugs, disease conditions, or curing techniques—is constant for all cultures. When a client uses the hot-cold explanatory framework, the nurse needs to discover, for each client, what constitutes illnesses, substances, and practices that are cold and that are hot. For example, if a drug is seen as cold, it should be given with a beverage that is hot; if a symptom is interpreted as hot, cold food should be eaten.

More recent Asian immigrants to the United States may still be fully embedded in the hot-cold system. Others who appear quite Americanized may adhere to only a few substances and conditions to which the properties of hot or cold apply.

"The most central indigenous Filipino health concept is that of balance" (Anderson, 1983, p. 815). When an imbalance occurs—whether it be in the hot-cold balance of humors, foods, air, personal cleanliness, disorderliness, or irregularity—illness may occur. Negative emotions such as grief, anxiety, fear, stress, and low self-esteem, as well as unsettling experiences can also lead to disequilibrium. In the Filipino folk belief system, these imbalances may be due to natural causes or unnatural (personalistic) causes such as ghosts, sorcerers, or a deity. Among Filipinos, as is true among Asians in general, this primary theme of balance is lived out not only in self-care health behaviors but also in proper social interaction with people at all levels and in all spheres of one's life. Correct social conduct is highly valued and often involves a focus on the form of one's interpersonal behavior.

Mental Illness

Overall rates for mental and emotional illness among the Chinese are roughly equivalent to the reported rates from other cultures. All categories—including schizophrenia, affective psychoses, senile psychoses, and depression—have been cited. However, questions can be raised about the validity of statistics regarding the distribution of mental and emotional disorders among Asian Americans. Compared with all other populations, they tend to be more often diagnosed as psychotic, have high rates of diagnoses as neurotic, and low rates of behavior disorders (Sue, 1977). Analysis of behavioral patterns of Japanese and Filipino American clients diagnosed as paranoid schizophrenic in the Hawaii State Hospital showed that Japanese Americans expressed more depression, withdrawal, disturbance in thinking, and inhibition, whereas Filipino Americans expressed more delusions of persecution and overt signs of disturbed behavior (Enright and Jaeckle, 1963).

Depression illness has been of low prevalence partly due to the strong tendency to somatize, frequently producing physical symptoms. A finding among clinicians everywhere is that Asians and Asian Americans are more likely than Caucasians to display and communicate somatic complaints that are actually manifestations of underlying depression. Clients communicate symptoms of tenseness, headaches, pressure on the chest, weakness, and insomnia. Physical symptoms probably reflect the belief in the unity of mind and body, the prohibition against expression of self-disclosure or strong emotions, and the stigma attached to the diagnosis of a psychiatric illness (Sue and Morishima, 1982).

Cultural-specific syndromes do exist among

Asians, but their expression is rare among immigrants in the United States. A culturally conditioned anxiety state (or depersonalization syndrome according to some researchers) that occurs in Asians in Hong Kong and Southeast Asia and infrequently in the United States is called *koro.* A client with koro fears his penis will shrink and withdraw into his abdomen and possibly cause his death. Belief in the existence of this illness intensifies ordinary guilt and anxiety over actual or fancied sexual excess, especially masturbation. *Amok,* from which the American phrase *running amok* comes, is a condition found primarily in Indonesia, where a person, usually a young male, following a depression, has an overwhelming urge to murder. He randomly and frantically runs throughout the village, wielding a machete or other weapon. A low frustration tolerance to interpersonal stress appears to create a reaction of blind rage.

Asian Americans are generally thought to be underrepresented in the psychiatric health care system. Through their study of Chinese Americans, Tsai, Teng, and Sue (1980) suggested seven reasons for the underutilization of mental health services—reasons that may apply to Asian Americans in general:

- Stigma and shame
- Availability of alternative resources
- Cost
- Location and knowledge of facilities
- Hours of operation
- Belief systems about mental health
- Responsiveness of services

Stigma and shame, especially, directly relate to cultural values that require one to avoid behaviors and labels that would disgrace both the self and the family. Even white Americans attach a stigma to mental illness. Stigma, coupled with intense embarrassment, may prohibit a self-referral or family referral until severe symptoms are present. Asians may resist involvement in the mental health system because of the belief that mental illness is caused by organic or somatic factors and can be alleviated by willpower, avoidance of morbid thoughts, and concentration on pleasant thoughts. The self-disclosure and analysis of "morbid thoughts" that many Western approaches to mental health require would cause Asian Americans to seek treatment through medical, rather than psychiatric, systems or through indigenous practitioners, such as herbalists.

Nursing Care

The American value of being direct and expressing feelings is not embraced by all persons. Indeed, self-control and restraint are highly valued among Asian Americans whether it be feelings of anger or pain or interpersonal experiences of conflict and disagreement. When Asians do have outbursts of anger or aggression, especially women, there may be feelings later of shame or embarrassment because behavior of this sort violates their code of conduct. If, for instance, Chinese Americans were verbally or behaviorally to act on negative emotions, especially feelings of anger or resentment, they would be ostracized by their family and community. Even though the suppression or regression of emotion might lead to psychophysiologic or mental symptoms, these are considered less painful than being cut off from one's source of physical and psychologic support.

For Asian Americans, the psyche and soma are inseparable. Asian Americans understand and accept that stress in interpersonal relationships can cause depression or psychophysiologic symptoms. This does not mean, though, that clients will talk intimately or analytically about personal feelings or situations. But the desire for return to a harmonious state with the social order as it exists is so strong that people may stay in treatment for a long time. They will take medications to improve physical well-being and use introspection and meditation to improve emotional well-being. These techniques, consistent with Confucianism and Buddhism, are in stark contrast to some Western schools of psychotherapy and psychiatric treatment, which rely on verbal communication and interpretation of behaviors. Many Asians prefer structure, guidance, and direction to introspection, tough-feeling techniques, or high levels of verbal participation (Atkinson, Maruyama, and Matsui, 1978).

Social integration and self-control, not autonomy, are highly valued in Asian culture. Therefore therapeutic relationships between nurses and Asian American clients might produce goals antithetical to goals established for white, middle-class European Americans. Even second-generation (*nisei*) and third-generation (*sansei*) Japanese who appear highly assimilated retain close family and ethnic social group ties. They value the individual's responsibility to accommodate to, not to change or criticize, the social structure. Nurses need to use their knowledge of sociocultural variables as well as individualized assessments to elicit the client's unique attributes and the salient features of the cultural group with which the client identifies.

Asians often perceive the use of medication differently from Westerners. Many do not understand the need to take pills over a long period, especially if the symptoms for which they are being treated abate. Traditional herbalists often cure with one dosage, the belief being that it need be given only once if the medicine is correct. Many Asians also believe Western dosages are too strong for them, so they may adjust the amount of medication they take to a level they believe safe. The nurse needs to give thorough explanations about medications, their actions, side effects, and differing forms, and to tailor the explanations to the client's and family's level of understanding and cultural belief system.

In general, Asian Americans are less verbal than white Americans. Family members have well-defined nonverbal acts that convey caring for those who are sick. Including the family in nursing care is essential for the members to fulfill their responsibilities to the ill or hospitalized person. On top of the disequilibrium responsible for the psychiatric symptoms, hospitalization creates an imbalance that may exacerbate the symptoms.

If more than one Asian American is in the same treatment setting at one time, the nurse should consider therapeutic activities that enable them to relate to one another unless, of course, there are known to be antagonistic relationships or feelings between the individuals or the ethnic groups to which they belong. Formality, along with subtle and indirect questions and statements, is the preferred mode of interaction. Emphasis should be on concrete, behavior-oriented solutions to problems rather than on analysis or insight into the etiology of symptoms. Families—nuclear, extended, and three-generational—should be included in discussions and decisions and always treated with respect.

Culturally relevant and sensitive nursing care for Asians requires

- The elimination of racist attitudes and practices
- Availability of bilingual or bicultural personnel
- An understanding of the cultural backgrounds and experiences of Asian Americans
- Consciousness of one's own cultural biases
- A willingness to be taught by the client and his or her family

Southeast Asian Immigrants

The Hmong used to say that the world reached only so far as a man could walk.

But how do they explain away the fact that the Hmong's ancestral home was China? "We were slaves," one will say. "To escape, we make a big cloth—3,800 Hmong stood on it. A good spirit made a big wind and blew us out of China into Laos."

If the old timer is pressed, he will admit that they fled on foot.

However, the truth of it is that the "good" spirit was their feet, and the wind that motivated them was their desire for freedom. The Hmong people remind us that their name means "free men."

To achieve that noble state the Hmong spent centuries "runnin' and dyin'." That's all they have known.

In time of trouble, the Hmong reflect on their past. In troubled times before, they used to say: "There's always another mountain." But not anymore. They have run out of mountains. (*The Bilinguist,* June 1985, pp. 1–2)

In 1975, the Southeast Asian (or Indochinese) refugees admitted to the United States were, generally, young, well-educated Vietnamese urbanites. They were Catholic, in good health, and embedded in family groups. Beginning in 1979, a second wave of Southeast Asians—including but not limited to Vietnamese, Cambodians, Laotians, and Hmong—entered the United States. They are ethnically, nationally, and religiously diverse; range from rural to urban; and vary in language skills, literacy, and health. They are refugees, the boat people, who escaped their war-torn countries under abominable life-threatening conditions to come to a culture that is radically foreign from their own and that often seems not to welcome their presence. Many neither speak nor understand English, and they have not been taught how to use health care and other resources in the community.

Cultural Concepts

Most Vietnamese, Cambodians, and ethnic Laotians are Buddhists. Small percentages practice Islam; Christianity; Taoism; Confucianism; and animism, which is a belief in spirits. Among the Hmong, animism is prevalent.

Southeast Asian societies rest on the solid structure of the family. They are based on highly organized, multigenerational patrilineal systems with clearly specified role expectations in male-dominated households. Filial piety remains strong, as do rules to guide proper behavior in social interactions. Southeast Asians are private with their feelings of guilt, depression, and shame. Although they may experience extreme suffering, this is accepted as part of life. If help is needed, family and friends are the preferred sources.

Health Beliefs

The hill people, Hmong and Mien, have belief systems uniting religion and medicine through shamanistic helpers—physician-priests who negotiate with gods to alleviate disease. Lowland people espouse a more widespread belief system, that of natural medicine, which reflects the prime importance of maintaining balance in the hot-cold continuum and belief in the healing power of nature. The hot-cold theory may permeate beliefs about bathing, medicines, venipuncture, foods, dermabrasive procedures, and cutaneous hematomas. Because a relationship between body and spirit is believed in, psychosomatic illnesses are acceptable. When the body is diseased, the spirit is affected, and if the spirit is distressed, the body becomes afflicted. But behavior that clearly suggests a mental disorder brings shame on oneself and one's family. Prompt treatment with quick results is desired and expected. If the belief system centers on the supernatural—such as on evil spirits as the cause of mental aberrations—the refugee will use a tribal shaman to exorcise the intruding spirit. Buddhists may attribute mental disorders to past wrongdoings, which produced bad karma. Psychiatric illnesses, which are highly stigmatizing, are widespread among the recently arrived Southeast Asian immigrants (Owan, 1985).

Mental Illness

A 1976 study by the Mental Health Task Force for Indochinese Refugees (Robinson, 1980) identified the following sources of stress:

- Traumatic and violent uprooting from their homeland
- Shock of separation from family and friends
- Long and uncertain periods of waiting in refugee camps
- Cultural alienation
- Mixed reactions from Americans
- Future uncertainties
- Language difficulties
- Unavailability of jobs, particularly those commensurate with previous training and experience
- Inadequate living arrangements

- Conflict with sponsors
- Breakdown in traditional family structure caused by generational conflict

These stresses produced numerous psychosomatic symptoms, anxiety, depression, and conflicts between generations and between spouses. A posttraumatic stress disorder has developed among many Cambodian concentration camp survivors—a disorder sometimes lasting several years after the imprisonment. The most outstanding symptoms have been nightmares, intrusive thoughts, emotional numbness, avoidance, and hyperactive startle reactions (Boehnlein et al., 1985; Kinzie and Fleck, 1987; Kinzie et al., 1987; Mollica, Wyshak, and Lavelle, 1987).

The gamut of mental and emotional disorders may be manifested among Southeast Asians, but conditions with nonpsychotic symptoms may be contained within the kinship system. Anxiety and depression are the two most prevalent conditions in the nonpsychotic category for which Southeast Asians will most readily seek help (Tung, 1985). Depression, as is typical for Asians, will be masked by many physical complaints.

Survivor syndrome has been identified among refugees as a constellation of symptoms, including depression and guilt for having survived when beloved family members and others died. This reaction is often delayed, becoming apparent after all the immediate problems of relocation are resolved and the refugee has had time to reflect on the past (Ingall, 1984). Indeed, loss may emerge as the greatest single problem that refugees must cope with. Multiple losses—homeland, family, possessions, sense of security, self-esteem, identity—have produced unresolved and intense grieving. Many Southeast Asians in the mental health system may need guidance, permission, and support from the nurse to move through the grieving process.

One of the most serious and perplexing developments among apparently healthy Hmong Laotian young men has been more than 75 "nightmare" deaths. "All died during sleep, had been in good health, and suffered a remarkably similar and mystifying terminal agony, marked by labored respiration, a terminal groan, and tonic rigidity" (Ingall, 1984, p. 370). The exact cause of death is unknown, but theories suggest the psychic trauma of repeated nightmares resulting from war, poverty, and relocation may be the cause.

Nursing Care

There are no exact counterparts for mental health personnel or mental health services in Southeast Asia. Many Indochinese do not know how to act or what to expect in encounters with people from the mental health system. Many fear hospitals as places where one goes to die. Some treatment procedures violate Southeast Asian beliefs about the human body and what is safe to do to it; thus, reactions to routine tests may be quite strong and alarming.

It is not unusual for Southeast Asians to attribute an almost mystical status and omniscience to physicians (Jacobson, 1982). Nurses and other mental health workers, by virtue of their relationship to doctors, may also be expected to have awesome powers. Southeast Asians may respond with mistrust and anxiety if a nurse asks many or detailed questions—the nurse is expected to have answers without having to ask the client for them. Medications are expected and appreciated but apparent noncompliance sometimes occurs because they are to be taken only as long as one feels ill. Southeast Asians may also feel Western medicine is not appropriate for them because they are so different. The family—and for the Hmongs, perhaps the clan leader as well—is of paramount importance, so they must be involved in decision making about care.

Southeast Asians value the ability to control the expression of emotions and to avoid overt conflict. About personal matters or feelings, they seldom talk openly. They make every effort to save face and to maintain self-esteem, and they are reluctant to criticize or make negative statements. For refugees suffering posttraumatic stress disorder, the opportunity to ventilate about their remarkable and horrifying experiences has been one of the most successful aspects in some treatment programs designed especially for Southeast Asians (Kinzie,

1981). Whenever possible, nurses should try to avoid direct questions. Inquiries should be framed in such a way that Southeast Asian clients have latitude in responding and can choose among alternatives rather than have to answer yes or no. The aim is to keep communication open without the client's fearing that the nurse may be offended by his or her replies (Armour, Knudson, and Meeks, 1981).

The nurse needs to assess all behaviors for their cultural meaning and relevance. A client who sees or talks with a dead family member may not be hallucinating and may, therefore, not be psychotic. Beliefs in the ability to communicate with the dead are not abnormal for a people who live closely with the supernatural and with spirits. In some instances, indigenous healers and members of the mental health system can provide services to a client and to his or her family without canceling the unique contribution each makes to the recovery process.

Ishisaka, Nguyen, and Okimoto (1985) suggest that the primary therapist or nurse may want to consider the following areas for history taking:

- Family life and experiences during childhood
- Life experiences before becoming a refugee
- Reasons for escaping, the escape process, losses, and expectations
- Life in the camps, attitudes about camp life, problems of subsistence
- Sponsorship in the United States, expectations of life in the new land, experiences with culture conflict, survival problems, coping strategies
- Family life adjustments if the family has been in residence for several years
- Current concerns and expectations for the future
- Client's current understanding of adjustment difficulties

Southeast Asians have long and rich heritages that need to be honored and supported during their difficult periods of resettlement in the United States. Nurses will find the use of competent, trusted, and consistent interpreters helpful in overcoming any language barriers. The nurse needs to understand the extreme culture shock that has accompanied the whole refugee experience. This will enable the nurse to empathize with the client and to pace interactions slowly, gently, and purposefully.

Hispanic Americans

Hispanic Americans constitute a rapidly growing ethnic and—since Spanish is a first, or only, language for many—language minority. A heterogeneous population, Hispanic Americans differ markedly along a number of dimensions: country or locale of origin, length of residence in the United States, degree of acculturation or assimilation, fluency in English, employment and educational opportunities, socioeconomic status, political ideology, reasons for migration, and family structure (Torres-Matrullo, 1981).

Spanish-speaking people in the United States numbered well over 14 million by the early 1980s. So rapidly is this population growing that it may be equivalent to the number of African Americans by the year 2000. Hispanic Americans have arrived from Cuba, Puerto Rico, Mexico, and many countries in Central and South America. Within each of those countries exist various groups of people of Spanish, African, or Indian ancestry.

Cultural Concepts

Many Hispanic American clients are embedded in large extended family networks. Their kinship system is a strong and structured social unit from which their identity evolves. Besides a nuclear family, Hispanic Americans are tied to other relatives both collaterally and multigenerationally. Through the *compadre system,* they select godparents who also function as kin, as a second set of parents. These extended and godparent families function as social support systems for their individual members throughout life, especially in times of crisis, such as illness. When this support is not available, because of disruptions in family units caused by immigration, the Hispanic immigrant may experience a loss of personal and social identity.

Roles in traditional Hispanic American families tend to be clearly and rigidly defined. The head of the household is the man; he is to be respected and obeyed and is the dominant member, as are men in general. The strict differentiation in sex roles requires men to behave according to the *macho* norm. The woman is expected to fulfill the roles of mother, wife, and homemaker. The need to work outside the home for additional income, however, is creating a change in these traditional roles.

Hispanic American families tend to be child-centered. Much love is lavished on the children, who are socialized into roles that discourage competition and encourage cooperation, working and sharing together. Children may be raised by many adults in the extended family system. In less acculturated families, emphasis continues to be placed on macho behavior for men and passive, home-centered behavior for women.

The predominant religion among Hispanics is Catholicism. Some estimate that as many as 90 percent of Hispanic Americans are members of the Catholic Church although they may not all be actively practicing Catholicism. For those vitally involved in their Catholic beliefs, religion will be a powerful influence in many aspects of their lives. During illness or hospitalization, religion, along with families and friends, may provide strong support. Rituals are an integral part of religious practices for many Hispanic Americans, and the priest may be a significant source of reassurance during hospitalization. The client who views his or her problems as punishment from God must be allowed to participate in any services or ceremonies designed to reestablish a proper relationship with God.

Hispanic culture is often in direct conflict with Anglo-American culture. This conflict can be internalized and produce an ambivalence leading to emotional and mental symptoms. Anglo-American values of individualism and competition oppose the Hispanic values of group orientation and cooperation. Intergenerational problems abound among the Hispanic Americans themselves between assertive, even disrespectful, youth and elders who expect submission and obedience.

One of the cultural characteristics of many Hispanic Americans is a greater orientation to the present than to the future; indeed, there can be a total involvement in the here and now. Their relationship to time frames may be more casual than Anglo Americans', and they may be absorbed more by the quality of an interaction than by how much time has been allotted to an exchange. Nurses need to assess the client's primary orientation to time because this is a major factor in developing plans regarding nursing intervention and appropriate goals.

Health Beliefs

The folk medicine of Hispanic Americans is an elaborate system of beliefs and practices about the nature of health, the etiology of diseases, and the techniques for healing. It is made up of native American and Spanish folk beliefs plus components from classical medicine. Although beliefs vary widely from one country to another, even from one town to another, the attributes of hot and cold as a way of classifying foods, beverages, herbs, medicines, symptoms, and disease conditions are present everywhere (Foster and Anderson, 1978).

This explanatory theory, the hot-cold (*caliente-frio*) theory, is important to many Hispanic Americans as a framework that governs how they live their lives and how they determine the causes of, and treatment for, diseases. Interpersonal relationships must be balanced, as must self-care practices for the maintenance of health and a feeling of well-being. Nurses need to familiarize themselves with the particular application of this theory by each Hispanic American client to understand its relevance and the form it takes for that person.

Throughout Latin America a folk healing system called *curanderismo* also exists. Among many Mexicans and traditional Hispanic Americans, especially in the Southwest, curanderos (male folk healers) and curanderas (female folk healers) continue to be important sources for treatment when people have physical or mental illnesses. The extent to which these folk healers are used is arguable. Perhaps of greater importance to nurses who work with Hispanic American clients is understanding that even Hispanics who do not espouse or practice this system of healing may have been influenced by its beliefs about the causes of illnesses and how to cure them. Thus, they may bring to encounters with a nurse a set of expectations that will affect the nursing process and course of recovery. Maduro (1983, p. 868) has identified eight major philosophic premises that underlie the system of curanderismo:

> Disease or illness may follow 1) strong emotional states (such as rage, fear, envy or mourning of painful loss); 2) being out of balance or harmony with one's environment; 3) a patient is often the innocent victim of malevolent forces; 4) the soul may become separate from the body (loss of soul); 5) cure requires the participation of the entire family; 6) the natural world is not always distinguishable from the supernatural; 7) sickness often serves the social functions, through increased attention and rallying of the family around a patient, of reestablishing a sense of belonging (resocialization); and 8) Latinos respond better to an open interaction with their healer. These nuclear ideas or attitudes about health, illness and care are culturally patterned and are both conscious and unconscious (implicit).

Findings by Schepler-Hughes (1983, p. 844) suggest that time and acculturation have greatly eroded the belief in, and practice of, curanderismo in comparison to its strength and pervasiveness 20 to 30 years ago. However, she did find some aspects of curanderismo still supported by informants: "a strong religious interpretation of the meaning of sickness, a belief in the pathogenic nature of strong emotion, a tendency to attribute unexplained physical or emotional malaise to troublesome or malevolent interpersonal relations and a belief in the salutary effects of balance and moderation in behavior, feelings and human relations."

Treatment by curanderos usually consists of herbs, cleanings (*limpias*), and massages, any or all of which take place in a highly personalized relationship between the client and the healer. The curandero's perspective also reflects the world view of the client: the belief in equilibrium at all levels—physical, psychologic, social, and spiritual; the restoration of balance between hot and cold; and the interconnectedness of mind and body. When diseases relate to the spirit world, such as in soul loss caused by fright (*susto*), the curandero has the ability to return the soul to the body through intervention with the spirit.

In general, Hispanic Americans are more accepting of aberrant behavior than Anglo Americans tend to be. They often differentiate between nervous behavior and crazy behavior. Being *loco,* the latter behavior, is stigmatizing and may be seen as evil or dangerous. Among unacculturated Hispanic Americans, folk healers may be preferred for treatment of psychotic behavior.

Among Puerto Ricans, there prevails a system of *espiritismo,* which is an adaptive mechanism to deal with alien environments as well as a form of psychotherapy (Comas-Diaz, 1981). In this system, folk healers are called *espiritistas,* and they treat problems ranging from conflicts with significant others (primarily family members), psychophysiologic symptoms, sleeping disorders, hallucinations (both auditory and visual), and all kinds of nervous and psychotic behaviors. Espiritismo asserts that the visible world is surrounded by a world of invisible spirits, which may be inside (incarnate) or outside (nonincarnate) human beings. Communication between these two categories of spirits is through mediums, the espiritistas. Levels of spirits also exist, and progress through various levels is made by undergoing trials (*pruebas*) to achieve the highest level of spirituality. Espiritismo teaches that people comprise both matter and spirit. If illness results from physical causes, physicians are visited; if illness results from spiritual causes, an espiritista is the healer of choice. The diagnostic and treatment procedures are an elaborate collection of techniques and experiences aimed at overcoming the causes and achieving higher spiritual development.

Several Puerto Rican cultural beliefs support espiritismo: communication between the living and the dead, especially through dreams; the power of envy to cause misfortune to another or to one's family; the nonseparation of physical and psychologic health; and the stigma of mental illness and of needing to see a mental health professional. In espiritismo, the client is suffering from a cause (*causa*) but is not sick or blamed for the symptoms. Judgments are not made on the person. Several instances now exist of clients receiving simultaneous espiritismo and Anglo-American treatment with much success.

Even Puerto Rican clients who participate willingly in the Anglo-American psychiatric system may retain beliefs in espiritismo. If so, the nurse needs to understand and respect these clients and to determine the relevance of their beliefs to the nursing process. In this way, the nurse can make a connection between both systems. Beliefs in folk illnesses and folk healers will not necessarily keep Hispanics, or any minority population, from accepting conventional care, but they will influence expectations about treatment and the course of recovery.

Mental Illness

For Hispanic Americans, as with other ethnic groups, a full range of emotional and mental illnesses may be expressed, although cross-cultural incidences and prevalences vary. In a comparison study of Mexican-American and Anglo-American psychiatric clients, several differences were noted. Mexican-American women were more acutely and affectively disturbed and more likely to show catatonic symptomatology. Mexican-American men were more alcoholic and assaultive, manifesting an exaggeration of the macho pattern in their symptomatology. The women were more prone to crying spells, hyperactivity, irritability, depression, and temper tantrums. The men exhibited both chronic and occasional alcoholism as well as threats and attempts to hurt others (Meadow and Stoker, 1965). Arrendondo (1987) suggests that alcoholism may be the most serious health problem among male Mexican-Americans, especially since alcohol consumption has been supported by cultural and religious views.

For emotional experiences to precipitate physical and mental symptoms is common. Feelings such as shame, embarrassment, sorrow, anger, lust, fear, and rejection are considered potentially dangerous, and one can become sick from having them. Puerto Ricans, for example, value the suppression and repression of assertive or aggressive behavior and the capacity to remain outwardly calm and dignified. When they discuss feelings of nervousness, they are often describing situations in which they felt anger (and subsequent guilt). Puerto Rican clients often convey a basic depression and anxiety, but their symptoms would be physical: aches, inability to sleep, weakness, dizziness, loss of appetite, and heart palpitations. Among Hispanics, psychophysiologic disorders and, to a lesser degree, conversion reactions are not uncommon, partly because of the belief in the oneness of mind and body. Physical illnesses can be caused by upset nerves, and it is not unusual for Hispanic clients to refer to the connection between physical ailments and "*los nervios*." For many Hispanic men, sickness is interpreted as a weakness, physical or moral; they will not admit to it readily. If they do, physical symptoms are more acceptable than mental ones.

Mal puesto is a disease thought to be caused by a witch who has acted at the request of another person. The victimized person may be anorexic, show restlessness, and suspiciousness or paranoid thoughts. Beliefs in witchcraft suggest that an evil befalls a person because he or she has in some way offended God and is, therefore, susceptible to the evil, satanic powers of a sorcerer (*brujo*) or witch (*bruja*). Hexing can produce quite different symptoms, such as physical complaints, interpersonal or job difficulties, and mental illnesses. The utilization of witchcraft reflects conflict in the social network.

The folk illness *susto,* or magical fright, has been widely studied by anthropologists. Susto, in many cases, results from a traumatic experience that is usually unexpected, such as witnessing a death, being involved in an accident, or discovering that one's spouse is having an affair. Although there is some diversity in etiology and treatment, general beliefs underlying susto include loss of soul because the person afflicted is believed to have disturbed spirit guardians. Symptoms include insomnia, anxiety, loss of appetite, and palpitations. For persons suffering from susto, curanderos are the healers of choice, or they can be used in collaboration with the Anglo-American psychiatric health care system. Research has shown that curanderos are effective in bringing about recoveries from mental disorders (Madsen, 1964).

Generally, Hispanic Americans have been underrepresented in mental health facilities. Rather than reflecting a lesser incidence of mental illness, researchers suggest that complex social and cultural variables are barriers to the use of Anglo-American psychiatric systems. Language, prejudicial and discriminatory treatment by Anglo-American staffs, use of culturally inappropriate therapies, lack of mental health facilities within Hispanic-American communities, and use of alternative healing systems are all possible barriers (Karno and Edgerton, 1969).

Nursing Care

Hispanic Americans generally prefer more closeness, both physical and interpersonal, than Anglo Americans do. Therefore to facilitate building rapport, nurses might sit closer to a Hispanic client, and demonstrate warmness through shaking hands or touching shoulders. Hispanics appreciate being addressed by both their maternal and paternal last names; doing so will communicate respect and interest. Interviewing might also at times be preceded by "*la platica,*" or small talk, an exchange that is socially correct for Hispanics and that helps to pace interviews at a rate more familiar to them. A client who fails to maintain eye contact should not necessarily be interpreted as resistant or evasive. Sustained gazing may be viewed as disrespectful at times and thus avoided by Hispanic clients.

Many Hispanic Americans tend not to discuss personal and family matters with others, especially those outside the family system. Even though the nurse and other members of the mental health team are in helping roles, it may be some time, if ever, before more traditional clients will disclose highly private information in interviews and therapeutic relationships. On the other hand, because Hispanic Americans are so interpersonally and socially oriented, they may work well in individual and group verbal therapies if allowed to self-disclose at their own pace under safe conditions.

A behavioral model of therapy for Spanish-speaking clients can be successful when it involves a contractual agreement between the nurse and the client regarding goals and how to achieve them. The more flexible and culturally relevant the nursing intervention, the greater the potential for congruence with the client's values and perceptions of problems.

The Hispanic-American family plays a paramount role at every point in the illness experience. Responsibility for the health and welfare of family members is taken seriously. Families should be allowed to participate in nursing care planning and intervention to the extent judged therapeutic by both nurse and client.

For the psychiatric client who speaks only Spanish or for clients for whom English is a second language, interpreters may be required or desired. Especially when anxious, highly stressed, or panicked, Hispanic-American clients who speak English may prefer, or involuntarily fall back on, their native language to communicate fear and distress or confusion. Bilingual nurses are ideal therapists at these times; if not available, however, the nurse should work with an interpreter acceptable to both client and nurse.

Cultural and Nursing Assessment

Between all illnesses and human culture, there is an intimate and unavoidable link. All human groups develop theories, scientific or religious, about mental and emotional disorders—theories about their cause, diagnosis, prognosis, and treatment. These theoretic explanations may vary as much as individual cultures do. Human reactions to intrapersonal, interpersonal, and societal stress and conflict may also take many forms.

The United States is a culturally pluralistic society. An understanding of a client's culturally derived customs, values, and beliefs can provide nurses with explanations for behaviors they might otherwise feel confused about or judge. Out of a cultural assessment, nurses can generate culturally appropriate nursing diagnoses, which will enable the nurse to develop care plans and carry out culturally relevant interventions. This ensures a nursing process that uses both holistic and individualized care.

The nursing history found in Chapter 2 contains a well-organized and thorough outline to guide the nurse in making comprehensive assessments of psychiatric clients. The following questions highlight areas of inquiry in creating a data base that, along with the sociologic, psychologic, biologic, and spiritual assessments, ensures individualized cultural assessments.

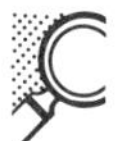

FOCUSED NURSING ASSESSMENT AND CULTURAL ASSESSMENT

With what ethnic or racial group do you identify?
What is your country of origin, and where have you lived?
What are reasons for the moves and relocations, and how have you experienced them?
What rituals and customs do you practice? Which of these do you have to observe while in the mental health setting?
What prohibitions are present that stem from your cultural or religious beliefs?
What restrictions regarding activities of daily living and communication patterns result from your cultural and religious values and sanctions?
To what extent are you cultural?
In what ways have you acculturated to the dominant white culture? In what ways not?
What language(s) do you speak, read, and write? To what degree of fluency?
If bilingual or multilingual, in what language do you primarily think?
What important characteristics of your language(s) and ways of communicating affect the interview process and nurse-client interactions?
What is your explanatory system for illness in general, and for emotional or mental illness in particular?
What are the appropriate roles and behaviors of your family members and significant others regarding your recovery?
What meaning does hospitalization or involvement in the mental health system have to you?
How does your religion relate to your beliefs about illness and treatment practices?
What religious or cultural influences are there on kinds of food permitted or preferred, on how food is prepared, and on how and when it is eaten?
How does your ethnic, racial, and cultural identity relate to your self-view and self-esteem?
What is your cultural patterning in response to stress and hospitalization?
What racial or anatomical features do you have that affect physical assessment and care and how you view yourself?
What physiologic characteristics do you have that relate to your cultural, ethnic, or racial heritage?

Variations in American Structures

During the last three decades remarkably significant changes have taken place in basic American structures. Due largely to the rise of the women's movement and the Gay Rights movement, the composition of the family unit and roles related to gender have undergone profound and controversial shifts.

Feminism

The women's movement is "possibly the most significant and consequential social phenomenon of the present era" (Kolbenschlag, 1981, p. ix). It has exploded the myth of wife, mother, and homemaker as the American dream for women and the traditional belief that the nuclear family is both natural and good (Deckard, 1975). It has enabled women, and society in general, to see that the middle-class ideal of companionate marriage has often produced overworked, stressed-out "superwomen" who have two jobs—one inside and one outside the home. The traditional service-oriented female roles and subsequent sex role conflict have led to large numbers of female psychiatric patients with depression as the most common emotional problem (Chesler, 1972).

In *Women's Reality* a psychotherapist writes clearly and succinctly about the White Male System as the American culture and the illusion that it represents all of reality (Schaef, 1985). She conceptualizes this system as the context within which all others—such as the Native American, Asian American, Black, Chicano and above all, the Female System—have had to develop their identities and behavior. From the male's point of view she describes the Perfect Marriage: the man parent and the woman child, an arrangement which has, of course, been severely criticized by the women's movement because it stultifies the woman's growth.

Feminism had led to unprecedented debate, literature, and social change that has impacted on males, children, and the family as well as on women. It has convinced vast numbers of people and groups that individual deviance from the customary structures of marriage and the family often reflects social pathology in the traditional structures, not psychologic pathology in the individual who deviates. Feminist leaders have continued to force the socioeconomic, educational, political, legal, religious, and medical establishments to reevaluate employment, abortion, rape, child care, the family, and medical self-care and self-help in terms of equal rights. Feminists demand full male participation in early child care and assert that parenting must supplant mothering. They suggest that the Pill, which allows a female to have control over her biologic self, was the first step toward real autonomy. They demand that stereotyped sex-linked roles must give way to fundamental changes in the socialization of girls and women and in their relationships with men, other women, and children. The converging of men and women's worlds—of logic and emotion, work and family, nurturance and discipline—may result. Although the women's movement has not been totally cohesive or coherent in thought or behavior, it has truly been transformational in striving for equality and ending men's power over women (Segal, 1987).

The Gay Rights Movement

In 1973, after long and acrimonious controversy about whether homosexuality was a disorder, the American Psychiatric Association (APA) put the matter to a vote of its members. Although the vote was not unanimous, the association decided to stop categorizing homosexuality as a disorder and to adopt a civil rights resolution on behalf of gay people (Bayer, 1981). Homosexuality as a category was dropped from the second edition of the *Diagnostic and Statistical Manual of Psychiatric Disorders.* This momentous event was one additional victory in the liberation of gay people and a sign of their increasing strength as a social and political force.

The APA decision about homosexuality was a sign that American society is moving toward greater social diversity in personal and family lifestyles, sexual identity, and expression. But this change is taking place alongside an intense and ongoing hatred and fear of homosexuality. The Moral Majority, in particular, speaks out that homosexuality is socially pathologic and religiously immoral and, therefore, a valid target for repressive and legal sanctions. Serious and sometimes violent conflicts arising from homosexuals' challenge of traditional stereotypes continue. However, there is growing recognition and acceptance of the large numbers of gay men and lesbian women and the wide diversity of homosexual relationship forms (Paul et al., 1982).

In regard to the relationship of children raised by single lesbians or gay couples, three areas of concern have emerged: (1) whether the children would grow up to be homosexual or develop an atypical gender-role orientation (2) whether there is a moral danger, and (3) whether children would suffer social isolation from significant others and peers because of society's stigmatization of homosexuality (Hart and Richardson, 1981). Thus far, there is no substantive evidence that a homosexual home environment is a potentially damaging one (Paul et al., 1982). What research there is suggests that commonly held assumptions and myths regarding homosexuality, based largely on antigay propaganda, are not valid. The belief that homosexual parents are "unfit" has not been confirmed. Some mental health professionals and researchers are suggesting that role modeling is more important than sexual orientation and activities, that how one behaves as a mother or father is more paramount than whether one is heterosexual or homosexual.

The first generation to grow up in openly gay homes will undoubtedly have wide-ranging feelings about their parents' homosexuality. In *Whose Child Cries,* Gantz (1983) presents 5 of the 23 families he spent over three years periodically living with and interviewing. His book consists of numerous candid discussions and descriptions of how children feel about their parents' homosexuality, the heavy responsibility of secrecy regarding parents' sexual orientation, isolation from peers, and poignant sensitivities to parents' and the community's reaction to homosexuality. He concludes that the basic issue is love, not sexual orientation.

Stepfamilies

Within the dominant U.S. culture there is widespread divorce, single parenting, remarriages, and stepfamilies. These relatively new structures have few traditions and models to guide their development. The traditional nuclear family has been touted tenaciously as the only viable family form. Therefore, alternative configurations—such as single parenting, parenting openly as a homosexual, and the variety of stepfamily arrangements now in existence—have been viewed as "culturally disadvantaged." These alternative forms carry negative connotations based on mythology and fairy tales—consider the stereotype of the wicked stepmother, for example (Visher and Visher, 1979). The reality is that the new family structures are present in large and growing numbers and that they are complex in their dynamics and challenging in their implications for individual and societal development.

It is estimated that over 35 million Americans live in stepfamilies, a situation in which at least one of the adults is a stepparent. The couple may or may not be married and one child or several children may live with or visit them. The transition from a former marriage or single-parenting system to a stepfamily arrangement requires tremendous changes. Because family members are often unprepared for this passage, crisis within the individual or the new family may occur. Counseling is frequently advisable, both before and after formation of the stepfamily.

In stepfamilies all individuals enter with a total or partial loss of a significant relationship. Work on the grieving process thus emerges as a basic task for all members to complete. Literature produced by researchers, counselors, and members of stepfamilies is strikingly uniform in findings and experience. The works report problems of role confusion, unrealistic expectations, guilt, and identity and loyalty conflicts (Capaldi and McRae, 1979). Stepparent-stepchildren disagreements, name confusion, lack of family unity, sexual issues (such as attraction for stepparents or stepsiblings), stepsister and stepbrother fights, and discipline difficulties also occur (Craven, 1982). Because stepchildren belong to two family units, boundaries of stepfamilies are permeable compared to the parameters of nuclear families. Multiple parents are at risk for forming conflicting alliances. The past plus present interpersonal bonds tax the formation of the bonds necessary to enable the stepfamily to feel a sense of wholeness and to function as a separate, but open system. Research to date does not suggest long-range negative effects simply due to stepchild status. Outcomes depend much more on how a stepfamily deals with the numerous challenges to growth and development with which it is confronted.

Dr. Lucille Duberman thinks that "eventually the dominant form of the American family will be the remarried family" (Visher and Visher, 1979, p. 207). Whether this prediction is realized remains to be seen. It is clear, however, that stepfamilies are increasing in numbers, complexity, and visibility. They contain the potential for developing new family patterns, for providing new models of family relationships, and for new experiences in building trust and love on foundations other than biology. Stepfamilies may represent "the next phase in the reorganization of the family system" (Einstein, 1985, p. 150). Societal institutions must recognize that what formerly constituted deviance is now a common form.

Single-Parent Families

The estimates of the number of single-parent families vary from 10 to 20 percent of all American families (Klein, 1973; Knight, 1980). Explanations as to causes also vary. The feminist movement, with its consciousness-raising discussions and support groups, increased desire for equality and careers outside the home and decreased satisfaction with the traditional role of the housewife and of living through others. This movement has certainly been a major influence in the high divorce rate and decisions to become pregnant outside of marriage. (Advances in birth control enabled women to separate marriage from parenthood.) Women, through their examination of gender roles, have moved out of household tasks and opted for companionship in an accepting and nurturing environment. Thus far, the effect of the single lifestyle on the psychologic development of children seems to relate to what kind of man or woman the single parent is, what kind of cultural climate surrounds the child, and variables within the child.

Although single parenting has gained social acceptance, American institutions have not yet developed adequate support structures for it. Parents Without Partners provides the most comprehensive information on resources for single parents and their children.

Feminists (both women and men), homosexuals, and other liberationists will persist in their pursuit of monumental change within American culture and society. Psychiatic nurses must be aware of these ongoing changes and understand that they constitute strong sociocultural forces within the dominant U.S. culture. The continuing transition will produce, at one end of the spectrum, psychiatric and social casualties as well as, at the other end, individuals, families, and groups that will evolve into higher levels of adaptation.

SUMMARY

1. Culture is a pattern of all learned behavior and values shared by a member of a particular group.

2. Subcultures are subgroups within cultures.

3. *Ethnicity* refers to our sense of belonging to a group that shares a unique cultural, social, and linguistic heritage.

4. World view is the outlook on the universe characteristic of a particular people.

5. Ethnocentrism is the tendency of all human beings to regard their own culture as the best.

6. Enculturation is the process of learning one's own culture and its world view.

7. Acculturation is the process of learning a new culture.

8. Assimilation is the expectation that minority group cultures will adopt the majority, or mainstream, values and behavioral patterns.

9. In a society that incorporates pluralism ethnic minority cultures are viewed as having unique strengths that should be preserved.

10. Because mental illness is defined differently in different cultures, it is difficult to assign an absolute definition to mental health and illness within a culturally mixed population.

11. Nurses may often encounter clients with cultural backgrounds different from their own.

12. Nurses should view mental health and illness from a holistic perspective and incorporate cultural factors into a comprehensive assessment of the client.

13. Barriers to care include misdiagnosis due to lack of knowledge and understanding about cultural norms, clients' views and expectations of psychiatric treatment, and cultural stereotypes.

14. Communication is especially important. Cultures vary in their patterns of verbal and nonverbal communication. Translators are important for non-English-speaking clients.

Native Americans

15. Most Native Americans live on federal reservations or in small rural communities.

16. General cultural concepts vary among tribes, but some of the common concepts include orientation to the present rather than the future, cooperation rather than competition, giving to others, and respect for age.

17. Ties to family, both nuclear and extended, are very strong.

18. Medicine and religion are inseparable. The harmonious relationships between human beings and the earth, and between mind, body, and soul are part of the health belief system of the Native American.

19. Alcoholism is the most widespread and severe problem in the Native American community. High suicide and homicide rates along with deaths from alcoholism are four times higher among Native Americans than among the general population.

20. Nursing care should include input from significant others. Family involvement is essential in gaining rapport

with the client. History taking should be leisurely and reflect observations.

African Americans

21. African Americans differ in their culture depending on their country of origin. African Americans come from Africa, Haiti, Cuba, Puerto Rico, Brazil, and Jamaica.

22. Religious affiliation is a powerful influence in African-American lives. Beliefs range from fundamentalist Protestantism to voodooism.

23. Folk medicine thrives in urban ghettos and in the rural South.

24. Disproportionately high percentages of African Americans are given psychiatric diagnoses.

25. Barriers to care in the African-American community are the nurse's own beliefs and attitudes toward the client, stereotypes of African-American psychopathology, and lack of understanding of "cultural paranoia" experienced by the African American.

Asian Americans

26. Asian Americans have been referred to as the model minority and include persons from the Philippines, China, Japan, Korea, and Southeast Asia.

27. Eastern philosophy emphasizes harmonious interpersonal relationships, interdependence, and mutual moral obligation or loyalty to achieve a state of psychosocial homeostasis.

28. The humoral pathology permeates many health beliefs and healing practices among Asian Americans.

29. Asian Americans are thought to be underrepresented in the mental health system because of the shame brought to the family of a client diagnosed as mentally ill.

30. Mental and emotional illness among Asian cultures is roughly equivalent to that reported from other cultures.

31. Culturally relevant nursing care requires sensitivity from the nurse. Asian Americans are generally less verbal than white Americans, and formality is the preferred mode of interaction.

Southeast Asian Immigrants

32. Recent Southeast Asian immigrants include Vietnamese, Cambodians, Laotians, and Hmong.

33. Buddhism is a strong religious element in these groups. Animism is prevalent among the Hmong.

34. Natural medicine and the hot-cold theory permeate beliefs regarding bathing, medicines, venipuncture, foods, dermabrasive procedures, and cutaneous hematomas.

35. Anxiety and depression are the conditions for which Southeast Asians will most readily seek help.

36. Nurses and other mental health workers are thought to have awesome powers. Nurses are expected to have answers without having to ask the client for them and are mistrusted if they do not possess this power.

Hispanic Americans

37. Hispanic-American clients are embedded in large extended family networks.

38. The male is the dominant member of the family, and there is a strict differentiation of family roles. Families tend to be child-centered.

39. Catholicism is the predominant religion among Hispanics.

40. Folk medicine is an elaborate system of beliefs and practices about the nature of health, the etiology of diseases, and the techniques for healing.

41. Hispanic Americans are treated for a full range of mental illnesses. Males are alcoholic and assaultive, and females are prone to hysteric behavior and depression.

42. Nurses should sit close to the Hispanic client and demonstrate warmness through handshaking and shoulder touching. These actions assist in building rapport in a culture that prefers closeness.

43. Families should be allowed to participate in the care of the ill client.

Variations in American Structures

44. The women's movement has resulted in major changes in the family unit in American families. It has changed the myth of wife, mother, and homemaker as the American Dream for women.

45. Feminism is embodied in the women's movement. Feminists have forced socioeconomic, educational, political, legal, religious, and medical establishments to look at major issues affecting women.

46. The Gay Rights movement is another major force to change American families. An accomplishment of this movement was to have homosexuality deleted as a category from the *Diagnostic and Statistical Manual of Mental Disorders* in 1973.

47. Stepfamilies have become dominant in American culture. This factor has given rise to the problem of dealing with the grieving process as divorce, remarriage, and stepfamilies emerge.

48. Single-parent families have resulted from the feminist movement. This family structure is gaining in accep-

tance, but society still lacks adequate support for the single-parent family.

CHAPTER REVIEW

1. Which of the following terms describes the pattern of all learned behavior and values shared by members of a particular group?
   (a) ethnicity
   (b) world view
   (c) culture
   (d) society
2. Which of the following is oriented to the present rather than the future, emphasizes cooperation rather than competition, and focuses on giving to others?
   (a) Native-American culture
   (b) Asian-American culture
   (c) Hispanic
   (d) African-American culture
3. Which culture includes descendants from Africa, French-speaking Haiti, Spanish-speaking Cuba and Puerto Rico, Portuguese-speaking Brazil, and English-speaking Jamaica?
   (a) Native American
   (b) Southeast Asian
   (c) Hispanic
   (d) African-American
4. Which is the ethnic group often described as the model minority?
   (a) Asian Americans
   (b) African Americans
   (c) Hispanics
   (d) Native Americans
5. Which of the following groups is a rapidly growing subculture in the United States, whose members are embedded in large extended family networks? Their kinship system, the compadre system, functions as a social support system for individuals throughout their life.
   (a) Native Americans
   (b) Southeast Asians
   (c) Hispanics
   (d) African Americans
6. A major change in American family units has been occurring over the past few decades. It is said that between 10 and 20 percent of American families are of this type:
   (a) nuclear
   (b) single-parent
   (c) extended
   (d) traditional

REFERENCES

Anderson JN: Health and illness in Filipino immigrants. *West J Med* (Dec) 1983; 139:811–819.

Armour M, Knudson P, Meeks J (editors): *The Indo-Chinese: New Americans.* Brigham Young University, 1981.

Arrendondo R, et al: Alcoholism in Mexican-Americans: Intervention and treatment. *Hosp Community Psychiatry* (Feb) 1987; 38:180–183.

Atkinson DR, Maruyama M, Matsui S: The effects of counselor race and counseling approach on Asian Americans' perceptions of counselor credibility and utility. *J Couns Psychol* (Jan) 1978; 25:76–83.

Atlas SL: *Single Parenting: A Practical Resource Guide.* Prentice-Hall, 1981.

Bayer R: *Homosexuality and American Psychiatry: The Politics of Diagnosis.* Basic Books, 1981.

Bergman R: A school for medicine men. *Am J Psychiatry* (June) 1973; 130:663–666.

Boehnlein JK, et al: One-year follow-up study of post-traumatic stress disorder among survivors of Cambodian concentration camps. *Am J Psychiatry* (Aug) 1985; 142:956–959.

Bradshaw WH: Training psychiatrists for working with blacks in basic residency programs. *Am J Psychiatry* (Dec) 1978; 135:1520–1524.

Brown TR et al: Mental illness and the role of mental health facilities in Chinatown. In: *Asian Americans: Psychological Perspectives.* Sue S, Wagner N (editors). Science and Behavior Books, 1973.

Bullough VL, Bullough B: *Health Care for the Other Americans.* Appleton-Century-Crofts, 1982.

Capaldi F, McRae B: *Step-families: A Cooperative Responsibility.* Franklin Watts, 1979.

Carstairs GM: Changing perception of neurotic illness. In: *Mental Health Research in Asia and the Pacific,* pp. 405–414. Caudill W, Lin T (editors). Honolulu: East-West Center Press, 1969.

Carter JH: Recognizing psychiatric symptoms in black Americans. *Geriatrics* (Nov) 1974; 29:95–99.

Chen-Louie T: Nursing care of Chinese American patients. In: *Ethnic Nursing Care.* Orque MS, Bloch B, Monrroy LA (editors). Mosby, 1983.

Chesler P: *Women and Madness.* Doubleday, 1972.

Comas-Diaz L: Puerto Rican espiritismo and psychotherapy. *Am J Orthopsych* (Oct) 1981; 51:636–645.

Craven L: *Stepfamilies: New Patterns in Harmony.* Julian Messner, 1982.

Deckard B: *The Women's Movement: Political, Socioeconomic and Psychological Issues.* Harper & Row, 1975.

DeHoyos A, DeHoyos G: Symptomatology differentials between Negro and white schizophrenics *Int J Soc Psychiatr* (Autumn) 1965; 11:245–255.

Dillard SL: *Black English: Its History and Usage in the United States.* Vintage Books, 1972.

Einstein E: *The Stepfamily: Living, Loving and Learning.* Random House, 1985.

Enright JB, Jaeckle WR: Psychiatric symptoms and diagnosis in two subcultures. *Int J Soc Psychiatr* (Winter) 1963; 9:12–17.

Favis REL, Dunham HW: *Mental Disorders in Urban Areas: An Ecological Study of Schizophrenia and Other Psychoses.* University of Chicago Press, 1939.

Flaherty JA et al: Racial differences in perception of ward atmosphere. *Am J Psychiatry* (June) 1981; 138:815–817.

Foster G, Anderson BG: *Medical Anthropology.* Wiley, 1978.

Gantz, J: *Whose Child Cries: Children of Gay Parents Talk About Their Lives.* Jalmar Press, 1983.

Giordano J: *Ethnicity and Mental Health Research and Recommendations.* National Project on Ethnic America of the American Jewish Committee, 1973.

Grier WH, Cobbs PM: *Black Rage.* Basic Books, 1968.

Hall AL, Bourne PG: Indigenous therapists in a southern black urban community. *Arch Gen Psychiatr* (Jan) 1973; 28:137–142.

Hall ET: Proxemics: The study of man's spatial relations. In: *Culture Curers and Contagion.* Klein N (editor). Chandler & Sharp, 1979.

Hart J, Richardson D: *The Theory and Practice of Homosexuality.* Routledge and Kegan Paul, 1981.

Henderson G, Primeaux H: *Transcultural Health Care.* Addison-Wesley, 1981.

Hill R: *The Strengths of the Black Family.* Emerson Hall Publishers, 1971.

History of Hmong people: Just runnin' and dyin'. *The Bilinguist* (June) 1985; 1:1–2.

Hollingshead A, Redlich F: *Social Class and Mental Illness.* Wiley, 1958.

Hsu FL: *The Challenge of the American Dream: The Chinese in the United States.* Wadsworth, 1971.

Ingall MA: Southeast Asian refugees of Rhode Island: Psychiatric problems, cultural factors, and nightmare death. *Rhode Island Med J* (Aug) 1984; 67:369–372.

Ishisaka HA, Nguyen QT, Okimoto JT: The role of culture: The mental health treatment of Indochinese refugees. In: *Southeast Asian Mental Health: Treatment, Prevention, Services, Training, and Research,* pp. 41–63. Owan TC (editor). DHHS Pub. No. (ADM) 85–1399. UDHHS, 1985.

Jacobson J: *A Provider's Guide for Southeast Asian Refugee Health Care.* Minnesota Dept. of Health, 1982.

Jewell DP: A case of a "psychotic" Navaho Indian male. In: *Culture Curers and Contagion,* pp. 155–165. Klein N (editor). Chandler & Sharp, 1979.

Joe J, Gallerito C, Pino J: Cultural health traditions: American Indian perspectives. In: *Providing Safe Nursing Care for Ethnic People of Color.* Branch MF, Paxton PP (editors). Appleton-Century-Crofts, 1976.

Jones BE, Gray BA, Parson EB: Manic-depressive illness among poor urban blacks. *Am J Psychiatry* (May) 1981; 138:654–657.

Karno M, Edgerton RB: Perception of mental illness in a Mexican-American community. *Arch Gen Psychiatr* (Feb) 1969; 20:233–238.

Kennedy DA: Key issues in the cross-cultural study of mental disorders. In: *Studying Personality Cross-Culturally.* Kaplan B (editor). Peterson, 1961.

Kinzie JD, et al: Posttraumatic stress disorder among survivors of Cambodian concentration camps. *Am J Psychiatry* (May) 1984; 141:645–650.

Kitano HHL: Japanese-American mental illness. In: *Changing Perspectives in Mental Illness.* Plog S, Edgerton R (editors). Holt, Rinehart and Winston, 1969.

Klein C: *The Single Parent Experience.* Avon Books, 1973.

Knight BM: *Enjoying Single Parenthood.* Van Nostrand Reinhold, 1980.

Kolbenschlag M: *Kiss Sleeping Beauty Goodbye: Breaking the Spell of Feminine Myths and Models.* Bantam, 1981.

Langner T, Michael S: *Life Stress and Mental Health.* Free Press, 1963.

Lawson WB, Yesavage JA, Werner PD: Race, violence, and psychopathology. *J Clin Psychiatr* (July) 1984; 45:7: 294–297.

Leff J: *Psychiatry Around the Globe.* Dekker, 1981.

Lindblad-Goldberg M, Dukes JL: Social support in black, low-income single-parent families. *Am J Orthopsych* (Jan) 1985; 55:1:42–58.

Link B, Dohrenwend BP: Formulation of hypotheses about the ratio of untreated to treated cases in the true prevalence studies of functional psychiatric disorders in adults in the United States. In: *Mental Illness in the United States: Epidemiological Estimates.* Dohrenwend BP et al (editors). Praeger, 1980.

Lubdhansky I, Egri G, Stokes J: Puerto Rican spiritualists view mental illness: The faith healer as a paraprofessional. *Am J Psychiatry* (Sept) 1970; 127:312–321.

Madsen W: *The Mexican-Americans of South Texas.* Holt, Rinehart and Winston, 1964.

Maduro R: Curanderismo and Latino views of disease and curing. *West J Med* (Dec) 1983; 139:6:868–874.

Marcos LR: Effects of interpreters on the evaluation of psychopathology in non-English speaking patients. *Am J Psychiatry* (Feb) 1979; 136:171–174.

May PA: Suicide among American Indian youth: A look at the issues. *Children Today* (July–Aug) 1987; 16: 22–25.

Mays VM: Identity development of Black Americans: The role of history and the importance of ethnicity. *Am J Psychother* (October) 1986; XL:582–593.

Meadow A, Stoker D: Symptomatic behavior of hospitalized patients. *Arch Gen Psychiatr* (March) 1965; 12:267–277.

Meketon MJ: Indian mental health: An orientation. *Am J Orthopsych* (Jan) 1983; 53:110–115.

Mollica RF, Wyshak G, Lavelle J: The psychosocial impact of war trauma and torture on Southeast Asian refugees. *Am J Psychiatry* (Dec) 1987; 144:1567–1572.

Nobles WW, Nobles GM: African roots in black families: The social-psychological dynamics of black family life and the implications for nursing care. In: *Black Awareness.* Luckraft D (editor). American Journal of Nursing Co., 1976.

Owan TC (editor): *Southeast Asian Mental Health: Treatment, Prevention, Services, Training, and Research.* DHHS Pub No (ADM) 85–1399. UDHHS, 1985.

Pambrun A: Birth to school age. In: *Life Cycle of the American Indian Family,* pp. 27–40. American Indian/Alaska Native Nurses Association Publishing Co., 1980.

Paul W et al (editors): *Homosexuality: Social, Psychological and Biological Issues.* Sage Publications, 1982.

Poussaint AF: Interracial Relations and Prejudice. In: *Comprehensive Textbook of Psychiatry,* Vol. III. Kaplan HI, Freedman AM, Sadock B (editors). Williams and Wilkins, 1980.

Raskin A, Crook TH, Herman KD: Psychiatric history and symptom difference in black and white depressed inpatients. *J Consult Clin Psychol* (Feb) 1975; 43:73–80.

Robinson C: Special report: Physical and emotional health care needs of Indochinese refugees. *Indochinese Refugee Action Center.* (March) 1980; 1–40.

Schaef AW: *Women's Reality: An Emerging Female System in a White Male Society.* Winston Press, 1985.

Schepler-Hughes N: Curanderismo in Taos County, New Mexico—A possible case of anthropological romanticism? *West J Med* (Dec) 1983; 139:875–884.

Segal L: *Is the Future Female? Troubled Thoughts on Contemporary Feminism.* Peter Bedrick Books, 1987.

Simon RJ et al: Depression and schizophrenia in hospitalized black and white mental patients. *Arch Gen Psychiatr* (April) 1973; 28:509–512.

Snow LF: Traditional health beliefs and practices among lower class black Americans. *West J Med* (Dec) 1983; 139:800–828.

Soloff PH, Turner SM: Patterns of seclusion: A prospective study. *J Nerv Ment Dis* (Jan) 1981; 169:37–44.

Spitzer RL et al: *DSM-III Casebook.* American Psychiatric Association, 1981.

Spurlock J: Psychiatric States. In: *Textbook of Blaçk Related Diseases.* Williams RA (editor). McGraw-Hill, 1975.

Srole L: Measurement and classification in socio-psychiatric epidemiology: Midtown Manhattan study (1954) and midtown Manhattan restudy (1974). *J Health Soc Behav* (Dec) 1975; 16:347–364.

Srole L et al: *Mental Health in the Metropolis: The Midtown Manhattan Study,* Vol. 1. McGraw-Hill, 1962.

Sue S: Community mental health services to minority groups. Some optimism, some pessimism. *Am Psychol* (Aug) 1977; 32:616–624.

Sue S, McKinney H: Asian Americans in the community mental health care system. *Am J Orthopsych* (Jan) 1975; 45:111–118.

Sue S, Morishima JK: *The Mental Health of Asian Americans.* Jossey-Bass, 1982.

Sue S, Sue DW: MMPI comparisons between Asian American and non-Asian American students utilizing a student health psychiatric clinic. *J Couns Psychol* 1974; 21:423–427.

Sue S, Zane, N: The Role of Culture and Cultural Techniques in Psychotherapy. *Am Psychol* (Jan) 1987; 42: 37–45.

Taylor C: Soul talk: A key to black cultural attitudes. In: *Black Awareness.* Luckraft D (editor). American Journal of Nursing Co., 1976.

Torres-Matrullo C: Mainland Puerto Rican communities: A psychosocial overview. In: *Institutional Racism and Community Competence.* Barbarin OA et al (editors). (ADM) 81–907. USDHEW, 1981.

Tsai M, Teng LN, Sue S: Mental status of Chinese in the United States. In: *Normal and Deviant Behavior in Chinese Culture.* Kleinman A, Lin TY (editors). Reidel, 1980.

Tung TM: Psychiatric care for southeast Asians: How different is different? In: *Southeast Asian Mental Health: Treatment, Prevention, Services, Training, and Research.* Owan TC (editor). USDHHS (ADM) 85–1399, 1985.

Visher EB, Visher JS: *Step-Families: A Guide to Working with Stepparents and Stepchildren.* Brunnel/Mazel Publishers, 1979.

Vogel VJ: *American Indian Medicine.* University of Oklahoma Press, 1970.

Wallace AFC: *Culture and Personality,* 2nd ed. Random House, 1970.

SUGGESTED READINGS

Abad V, Boyce E: Issues in psychiatric evaluations of Puerto Ricans: A sociocultural perspective. *J Oper Psychiatr* 1979; 10:28–39.

Adelbimpe VR: Overview: White norms and psychiatric diagnosis of black patients. *Am J Psychiatry* (March) 1981; 138:279–285.

Adelbimpe VR et al: Symptomatology of depression in black and white patients. *J Nat Med Asso* (Feb) 1982; 74:185–190.

Barbarin OA et al (editors): *Institutional Racism and Community Competence.* USDHEW (ADM) 81–907, 1981.

Barnouw V: *Culture and Personality,* revised ed. Dorsey, 1973.

Berkman LF, Syme SL: Social networks, host resistance and mortality: A nine-year follow-up study of Alameda County residents. *Am J Epid* (Feb) 1979; 109:186–204.

Boehnlein JK: Culture and society in posttraumatic stress disorder: Implications for psychotherapy. *Am J Psychother* (Oct) 1987; XLI:519–530.

Bowser BP: Racism and Mental Health: An Exploration of the Racist's Illness and the Victim's Health. Chapter 11 in: *Institutional Racism and Community Competence.* USDHEW (ADM) 81–907, 1981.

Branch MF, Paxton PP: *Providing Safe Nursing Care For Ethnic People of Color.* Appleton-Century-Crofts, 1976.

Bush MT, Ullom JA, Osborne OH: The meaning of mental health: A report of two ethnoscientific studies. *Nurs Res* 1975; 24(2):130–138.

Carkuff RR, Pierce R: Differential effects of therapist's race and social class upon patient depth of self exploration in the initial interview. *J Couns Psychol* 1970; 3:632–634.

Cassel J: The contribution of the social environment to host resistance. *Am J Epid* (Aug) 1976; 104:107–123.

Clark MM: *Health in the Mexican-American Culture.* University of California Press, 1959.

Cobb CW: Community mental health services and the lower socioeconomic classes: A summary of research literature on outpatient treatment (1963–1969). *Am J Orthopsych* (April) 1972; 42:404–414.

Cohen R: Principles of preventive mental health programs for ethnic minority populations. *Am J Psychiatry* 1972; 128(12):79–83.

Cumpinha-Bacote J: Culturological assessment: An important factor in psychiatric consultation-liaison nursing. *Arch Psychiatr Nurs* (Aug) 1988; II:244–250.

Elling RH: *Socio-Cultural Influences on Health and Health Care.* Springer, 1977.

Fernando S: Racism as a cause of depression. *Int J Soc Psychiatr* (Spring) 1984; 30:1 and 2:41–49.

Flaskerud JH: A proposed protocol for culturally relevant nursing psychotherapy. *Clinical Nurs Specialist* (Winter) 1987; 1:150–157.

Hallowell A: Values, acculturation and mental health. *Am J Orthopsych* 1950; 20:732–743.

Hecker M: *Ethnic American 1970–1977.* Dobbs Ferry, NY: Oceana Publications, 1979.

Henderson G, Primeaux MH (editors): *Transcultural Health Care.* Addison-Wesley, 1981.

Horwitz A: The pathways into psychiatric treatment: Some differences between men and women. *J Health Soc Behav* (June) 1977; 18:169–178.

Kendrick EA, McMillan MF, Pinderhughes CA: A racial minority: Black Americans and mental health care. *Am J Soc Psychiatr* (Spring) 1983; 111:11–18.

Kiev A: *Curanderismo: Mexican-American Folk Psychiatry.* Free Press, 1968.

Kinzie JD: Evaluation and psychotherapy of Indochinese refugee patients. *Am J Psychother* (Apr) 1981; XXXV: 251–261.

Kinzie JD et al: An Indochinese refugee psychiatric clinic: Culturally accepted treatment approaches. *Am Psychiatry* (Nov) 1980; 137:1429–1432.

Kitano HHL: *Japanese-Americans: The Evolution of a Subculture,* 2nd ed. Prentice-Hall, 1976.

Kluckhohn C, Murray HA: Personality formation: The determinants. In: *Personality in Nature, Society, and Culture.* Kluckhohn C (editor). Knopf, 1956.

Kulka RA, Veroff J, Douvan E: Social class and the use of professional help for personal problems, 1957 and 1976. *J Health Soc Behav* (Mar) 1979; 20:2–17.

Landy D (editor): *Culture, Disease and Healing: Studies in Medical Anthropology.* Macmillan, 1977.

Laval RA, Gomez EA, Ruiz P: A language minority: Hispanic Americans and mental health care. *Am J Soc Psychiatr* (Spring) 1983; III:42–49.

Leff J: The cross cultural study of emotions. *Culture, Med Psychiatr* 1977; 1(3):317–350.

Leininger M: *Transcultural Nursing Concepts, Theories, and Practices.* Wiley, 1978.

Leininger M: Witchcraft practices and psychocultural therapy with urban U.S. families. In: *Transcultural Nursing Concepts, Theories, and Practices.* Leininger M (editor). Wiley, 1978.

LeVine ES, Padilla AM: *Crossing Cultures in Therapy: Pluralistic Counseling for the Hispanic.* Brooks/Cole, 1980.

LeVine RA: *Culture, Behavior, and Personality.* Chicago: Aldine, 1973.

Long KA: The experience of repeated and traumatic loss among Crow Indian children: Response patterns and intervention strategies. *Am J Orthopsych* (June) 1983; 116–126.

Louie KB: Cultural issues in psychiatric nursing. In: *The American Handbook of Psychiatric Nursing.* Lego S (editor). Lippincott, 1984.

Lynch LR (editor): *The Cross-Cultural Approach to Health Behavior.* Fairleigh Dickenson University Press, 1969.

Manson SM, Walker RD, Kivlahan DR: Psychiatric assessment and treatment of American Indians and Alaska natives. *Hosp Community Psychiatry* (Feb) 1987; 28: 165–173.

Marsella AB, Pedersens PB (editors): *Cross Cultural Counseling and Psychotherapy.* Pergamon, 1981.

McGoldrick M, Pearce JK, Giordano J: *Ethnicity and Family Therapy.* Guilford Press, 1982.

Milio N: Values, social class, and community health services. *Nurs Res* 1967; 16(1):26–31.

Mollica RF, Blum JD, Redlich FC: Equity and psychiatric care of the black patient, 1950 to 1975. *J Nerv Ment Dis* (May) 1980; 168:279–286.

Muecke M: In search of healers—Southeast Asian refugees in the American health care system. *West J Med* (Dec) 1983; 139:835–840.

Murillo N: The Mexican American family. In: *Chicanos Social and Psychological Perspectives.* Mosby, 1971.

Murillo N: The Mexican-American family. In: *Hispanic Culture and Health Care.* Martinez RA (editor). Mosby, 1978.

Orque MS, Bloch B, Monrroy LA: *Ethnic Nursing Care.* Mosby, 1983.

Overfield T: *Biological Variation in Health and Illness.* Addison-Wesley, 1985.

President's Commission on Mental Health. *Report to the President.* US Government Printing Office, 1978.

Primeaux MH: American Indian health care practices. *Nurs Clin N Am* 1977; 12(1):55–65.

Primeaux, MH: Caring for the American Indian patient. *Am J Nurs* 1977; 77(1):91–94.

Reinert BR: The health care beliefs and values of Mexican-Americans. *Home Health Care Nurse* 1986; 4:23–31.

Rogler LH: What do culturally sensitive mental health services mean? The case of Hispanics. *Am Psychol* (June) 1987; 42:565–570.

Rothenberg A: Puerto Rico and aggression. *Am J Psychiatry* (April) 1964; 120:962–970.

Rubel AJ: The epidemiology of a folk illness: Susto in Hispanic America. *Ethnology* 1964; 3:268–283.

Sinclair L: Native adolescents in crisis. *Canad Nurs* (Sept) 1987; 8:28–9.

Siskind JA: Cross-cultural issues in mental health: Minority perspectives. In: *Institutional Racism and Community Competence.* (ADM) 81–907, USDHEW, 1981.

Skinner BF: *Beyond Freedom and Dignity.* Knopf, 1972.

Spector RE: *Cultural Diversity in Health and Illness,* 2nd ed. Appleton-Century-Crofts, 1985.

Stenger-Castro EM: The Mexican-American: How his culture affects his mental health. In: *Hispanic Culture and Health Care.* Martinez RA (editor). Mosby, 1978.

Sullivan HS: *The Interpersonal Theory of Psychiatry.* Norton, 1953.

USDHEW: *Indian Health Trends and Services.* Public Health Service, Indian Health Service. (HSA) 78–12009, US Government Printing Office, 1978B.

Yap PM: The culture-bound reactive syndromes. In: *Culture, Disease, and Healing.* Landy D (editor). Macmillan, 1977.

CHAPTER 6

Consequences and Resolution of Developmental Crises

ELLEN MARIE BRATT
KAREN LEE FONTAINE

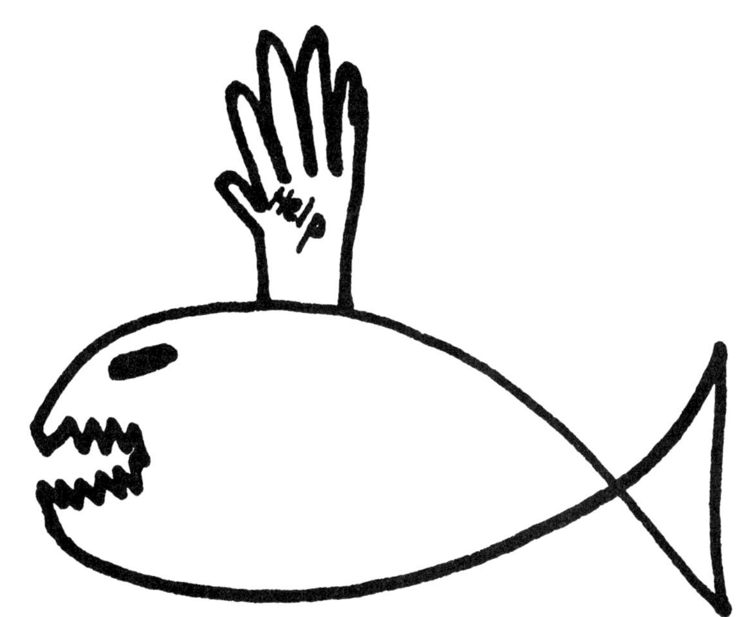

Asking for Help

A child passing thru the leviathan's jaws
Swallowed to fill perverted appetite
Satisfied with stolen innocence.
I cry, feeling the guilt that is theirs
I want my own tears of agony
But nothing is mine any more
All my tears are insignificant
in their sea of guilt. Their lies float unnoticed—
Secrets safe behind the wide eyes
of a child's dulled innocence.
But my hand is out. I'm so scared.
Hold it before they see it, or I pull
it in again

▪ *Objectives*

After reading this chapter the student will be able to

- Describe how nursing interfaces with developmental crises
- Explain the basic theories of adult development
- Apply crisis theory to unexpected events occurring throughout the life span
- Identify behavioral, affective, cognitive, and psychosocial characteristics of developmental crises
- Identify consequences of unexpected crises throughout the life span
- Assess client's coping skills
- Apply the nursing process when intervening with clients experiencing developmental crises
- Distinguish between adaptive and maladaptive resolutions to developmental crises

▪ *Chapter Outline*

Introduction

The process of human development is a continuous and dynamic force that brings to each person a unique expression of the individuality of that person. Different challenges, events, and choices arise in each stage of life. Throughout history, great authors have explored this journey through life. Some depict this journey from an optimistic perspective with joy, wonder, wisdom, humor, and hope as the final outcome. Some writers view the journey with bitterness, despair, and pessimism. Regardless of the approach taken, each stage brings a different set of circumstances that evoke thought-provoking questions: "Who am I?" "Where have I been?" "Where am I going?" These questions can be answered spiritually, philosophically, or concretely—depending on one's personal frame of reference.

This chapter views human development from the perspective of **life span developmental psychology**, which studies development from birth through death and is concerned with describing, explaining, and at times modifying the changes occurring over the entire life span (Baltes, Reese, and Lipsitt, 1980). A Biblical quotation (Ecclesiastes 3:1–2) summarizes this view of human development: "To everything there is a season, and a time for every purpose under the heaven: A time to be born, and a time to die; a time to plant, and a time to pluck up that which is planted. . . . "

Crisis States

Throughout life, people experience events to which they must respond. Many of these events are **expected life changes** that are anticipated at particular ages—changes such as graduation, employment, marriage, and parenthood. Depending on individual circumstances, expected life changes may evoke **maturational crises**. Because of individual differences, not all people choose or have the opportunity to experience all the expected life changes. **Unexpected life changes**—such as divorce, serious illness, or death—may occur at the same time individuals are struggling with expected transitions. The addition of unexpected events may contribute to a **situational crisis**. Resolving a maturational or situational crisis in an adaptive manner leads to growth and development. Maladaptive resolution of the crisis stunts growth and development and often has negative consequences for the individual, family, and community.

There are many definitions of *crisis,* most of which concur that a **crisis** is a turning point in a person's life—a point at which usual resources and coping skills are no longer effective. Two symbols in the Chinese language communicate the meaning of *crisis:* the symbol for *danger* and the symbol for *opportunity.* This text views the developmental crisis as both a danger and an opportunity (Johnson, 1986).

All people experience psychologic trauma at some point in their lives. Neither stress nor emergency situations necessarily constitute a crisis. It is only when the expected or unexpected event is perceived subjectively as a threat to need fulfillment, safety, or a meaningful existence that the person enters a maturational or situational crisis state. The inability to maintain emotional equilibrium is an important feature of a crisis. This state of disequilibrium usually lasts four to six weeks. Typically, the high level of anxiety during this short period forces the individual to

- Adapt and return to the previous level of functioning
- Develop more constructive coping skills
- Decompensate to a lower level of functioning

It is important to recognize that it is during the four to six weeks of disequilibrium that the individual in crisis is most open and receptive to professional intervention. Since the individual is viewed as essentially healthy and capable of growth, behavioral, affective, cognitive, and psychosocial changes may be made in a short period by focusing on the stressor and applying the problem-solving process. The crisis state confronts the individual with personal choices, and nurses actively participate with the client in restoring emotional equilibrium by using effective coping skills. The minimum goal of nursing intervention is to help the client adapt and return to the precrisis level of functioning. The maximum goal of nursing intervention is to help the client develop more constructive coping skills and move on to a higher level of functioning.

The life span perspective of this chapter studies unexpected events at various developmental stages. Situational or maturational crises may develop in response to these life events. The concepts of dependency and self-concept are two organizing themes for understanding these events.

Dependency exists within a relationship in which one person is sustained by or relies on another person. The implication is that one who is highly dependent is not able to exist alone. Dependence also exists where someone requires assistance with one or more activities of daily living (ADLs) because of mental or physical infirmity. ADLs may be basic activities (such as bathing, feeding, dressing, toileting, and ambulating) or instrumental activities (such as meal preparation, grocery shopping, housekeeping, medication administration, transportation, and financial management). Although infants and elderly persons are frequently seen as dependent, dependency is a common theme throughout the life span. Dependency issues involve how well a person is able to individuate; assume responsibility for self; and balance dependence, independence, and interdependence.

A **self-concept** is an organized set of thoughts or cognitions about characteristics of the "I" or "me," that is, the person's self. Self-concept includes beliefs about the type of person one is (intrapersonal), how one relates to others (interpersonal), and one's significance in the family and the world at large (sociocultural). **Self-esteem**, the affective portion of self-concept, includes one's feelings and values of self, such as strength, courage, worth, and confidence.

An unexpected life event that may lead to a situational crisis during childhood is the divorce of one's parents. In the past 20 years there has been a significant increase in the divorce rate and in the total number of people involved. If the rates continue to rise, it is predicted that 50 percent of all first marriages will end in divorce. In 1985 there were 1.2 million divorces involving more than a million children. Considering that it may take several years for a child to adapt to divorce, at any given time millions of children are struggling with dependency and self-concept issues. Children of divorce often experience the loss of *dependency* on one parent and a fear of abandonment by the other parent. Since divorce frequently involves lifestyle changes, children may be rapidly expected to assume more family responsibility and therefore become more independent. *Self-concept* may be threatened by feelings of guilt for the divorce, beliefs of unworthiness, and fears for one's own married future (DeV.Peters and McMahon, 1988).

One of the tasks of adolescence is letting go of *dependencies* on the family so that the adolescent can begin functioning as a young adult. Peer groups become the primary source of identification and support. Within this context, most adolescents learn age-appropriate social skills. It is estimated that 12 to 50 percent of adolescents experience shyness and social anxiety with their peer group. For some, this is mild and transient; others are unable to adapt and never become a part of a peer group. They suffer from loneliness and skill deficits and go on to develop isolated lifestyles as adults. A few adolescents become involved in gangs, which foster high dependency on and minimal individuation from the gang and thus delay normal growth and development. The medical diagnosis for adolescents who join gangs is conduct disorder, group type. It is estimated that 9 percent of boys and 2 percent of girls under the age of 18 have this disorder. Maturational crises may develop in response to either peer group isolation or gang involvement (DSM-III-R, 1987; Kelly and Hansen, 1987).

Parenthood is an event typically expected to occur at an age later than adolescence. Adolescence is a critical time for solidying one's identity and *self-concept.* When the roles and identity of parenthood are superimposed on this struggle, a crisis may develop. The United States is the only developed nation where the teenage pregnancy rate has been increasing in recent years. Young African-American women continue to have a higher rate of teen pregnancies than young white women, but recent trends show birth rates decreasing for African-American teens and increasing for white teens. By the age of 20, 19 percent of white women and 41 percent of African-American women are mothers. The United States also leads all developed countries in the rate of abortions for teenagers. Of all abortions in this country, 25 to 28 percent are performed on teenagers (Greenberg, 1989).

To be free of dependents is a common desire for individuals during their midlife years. A situational crisis may develop when middle-aged people find themselves with adult children who continue to live at home or the need to care for elderly parents. They may feel *trapped by dependents,* both the older and younger generations, at a time when increased freedom was the expectation. In addition, a maturational *self-concept* crisis during midlife is not uncommon. Individuals must cope with changes in bodily function and appearance as well as social role changes. They need to define themselves according to who they are now and their significance to family, friends, employer, and community.

Fear of dependency and loss of control are dominant themes during late life. It is estimated that 20 percent of the elderly population requires some assistance with one or more basic ADLs and that almost 40 percent require assistance with one or more instrumental ADLs (National Center for Health Statistics, 1983). The frail elderly thus experience a forced dependency on family or institutions—a dependency that may evoke a situational crisis. Mandatory retirement for the vigorous elderly may threaten their sense of interdependency and create a struggle with social meaning in old age. Ageism contributes to *self-concept* issues for the elderly. In a society that places a premium on youth, older people may feel useless, unimportant, and incapable. The older person's self-definition involves searching for the meaning of life (one's own and human existence as a whole) and the meaning of death. Adaptive resolution of this maturational crisis contributes to spiritual well-being in late life.

Significance to Nursing

In all types of clinical practice settings and as community members, nurses encounter people experiencing expected and unexpected events. To provide holistic care, children with physical illnesses must be treated within the context of their family situation. Pediatric nurses must understand the need for regression and help children manage their anger and fear when parental divorce coincides with physical illness. The maternal/child nurse understands the need to adapt nursing care according to the developmental level of the teenage parent. Without specific age-appropriate interventions, the outcome of teenage pregnancy may be tragic. With the rapid expansion of adolescent admissions to psychiatric facilities, mental health nurses must be prepared to intervene with the developmental crises of the teen years. On adult medical-surgical units, clients' physical disruptions of health may compound transitional stages, with the combination resulting in a crisis state. For example, a person struggling with midlife self-concept issues may have difficulty coping when cardiac problems are added. Recovery from surgery may be delayed when individuals must return home to shoulder the responsibility of caring for elderly parents. Providing holistic care in the geriatric setting means nurses must assist elderly clients in resolving dependency issues and facilitate their search for the meaning of life and death.

In addition to professional responsibilities, nurses must often manage these same events in their own lives. Nurses marry and divorce, their teenagers may unexpectedly become parents, and they may have adolescents with anxiety and conduct disorders. During the midlife years nurses may be caring for older and younger generations in the family as well as experiencing their own midlife crisis. As nurses age, they must manage the crises of their own later life.

This chapter is designed to help nurses anticipate and resolve personal crises as well as plan and intervene with clients experiencing crises. To improve the level of wellness, nurses must be involved in prevention and treatment of events and crises during developmental stages. To do this, they must understand how some people can adapt to crisis and experience growth and how others cannot. Through knowledge of characteristics, nurses can identify and intervene with those individuals at higher risk for maladaption. Applying the nursing process at this stage may contribute to improved future mental health. Through community education and support of appropriate public policy, nurses also have a role in preventing some events from occurring.

Theories of Human Development

To become knowledgeable about the intricacies of human life span development, a theoretic approach is needed to help illuminate stability and change over time. Sigmund Freud's psychoanalytic theory, Erik Erikson's psychosocial theory, and Jean Piaget's theory of cognitive development have made significant contributions, especially in the area of child development. (See Chapter 3 for detailed discussion of these theories.)

Developmental theories can be divided into stage and nonstage categories. **Stage theories** view development as progressing in stagelike sequence. Accordingly, development is divided into age-related periods where people are faced with particular problems and have specific abilities. Progression from stage to stage generally occurs along with new strategies developed from skills learned in previous stages. Each person passes through each stage, without skipping a stage, and enters and leaves a stage at a particular time. It is important to remember that stage theorists do not equate exact chronological age with stage development.

Nonstage theories can be useful for understanding tasks and crises throughout the life span.

These theories view development as a process and focus on ways people learn and grow.

One nonstage theory, **information processing theory**, looks at the way people take in information, process it, and act on it. This process is analogous to the way a computer works; input, process, and output are basic computer concepts. Information processing theory investigates the perception, attention, representation, memory, and retrieval of information throughout the life span. This approach to development gives a detailed view of cognitive abilities and the importance of feedback (Sternberg, 1985).

The **behavioral approach** to development is evident in the work of John Watson and B. F. Skinner. The importance of environment is critical to this view of development. It is thought that environment determines behavior, and if environment changes, behavior is altered. Classical and operant conditioning are instrumental to the process of learning behavior (see Chapter 3). Criticism of behavioralist theory focuses on the premise that its view of human development is too mechanical—that development is not as predictable as behavioralists believe (Rogers, 1980).

The third nonstage theory focuses on observation and imitation as a way to learn and develop. **Social-learning theory** investigates the process of imitation. Social-learning theorists believe that a person learns by observing others and imitating their behavior throughout development. Critics of this theory say that imitative behavior does not take into account the effect of maturation and the differences between imitative behavior of a child or an older adult (Bandura, 1986; Thomas, 1970).

Development Theories about Adults

For many years psychologists were unconcerned with adult development; building a theoretic framework to assist in understanding the adult was not viewed as important. The work of G. Stanley Hall (1922) is one of the few examples of adult development theory from the past.

Today the media has popularized the "older generation" in movies and television. Best-sellers such as Gail Sheehy's *Pathfinders* and *Passages* view adults as worthy of acknowledgment and research in greater depth. Terms such as *yuppie, baby-boomer,* and *midlife crisis* have become household words.

Part of this increased interest in adulthood can be explained on the basis of demography. The older adult is the fastest-growing portion of the population. In 1981, there were approximately 25 million people 65 years or older, or 11 percent of the population. By the year 2000, there will be 35 million Americans over age 65. It is thought that this population segment will almost double by the year 2030, when the projected population of seniors will be 64.3 million (Allan and Brotman, 1981; Guillford, 1988; Kubey, 1988).

Two factors have most likely contributed to the current interest in adult development: increased longevity and the fact that society is better educated. Developmentalists now realize that there is life and development after adolescence. Prior to the current interest, only Erikson's psychosocial theory addressed the life span perspective through the adult years.

The newer theories of development that emphasize adulthood are those of Peck, Vaillant, Levinson, Gould, and Neugarten. These theorists stress the commonalities in adulthood, and their theories were the first attempts at designing a framework for studying adults. Criticism of these theories focused on the idea that they were not truly life span theories.

Robert Peck (1968) elaborated on Erikson's theory of psychosocial adjustment. He found Erikson's theory about middle and late adulthood too vague. Peck's theory of adult development emphasized challenges and tasks (see Table 6–1).

George Vaillant expanded on Erikson's theory with his work with men in the Grant Study. His research indicated that men experience upheaval in their thirties and again in their fifties. In their thirties, men are concerned with moving up the "career ladder" and become conforming and materialistic. By their forties, men become less compulsive about work and take an introspective approach to the self. A reexamination of values and talents occurs at about the same age, and the result can be internal conflict. This conflict is often called

Table 6–1 *Peck's Theory of Adult Development*

Middle Age

Challenges	*Tasks*
Socializing rather than sexualizing in relationships	Finding meaningful and deep interpersonal relationships that are not sexual in nature
Valuing wisdom over physical powers	Learning to overcome the obvious physical decline seen in middle age and valuing the wisdom learned throughout life
Mental flexibility rather than rigidity	Learning to be spontaneous and open to new ideas rather than rigid in adherence to past thoughts and actions
Flexibility in social relationships rather than social impoverishment	Learning to expand social relationships in a meaningful way rather than dwelling on the inevitabilities of children leaving home and the aging process occurring in parents

Old Age

Challenges	*Tasks*
Ego differentiation rather than work-role preoccupation	Learning to value life beyond working and parenting and finding satisfying leisure activities
Body transcendence rather than body preoccupation	Learning to continue with a happy life despite the physical limitations and chronic illnesses associated with aging
Ego transcendence rather than ego preoccupation	Learning to come to terms with the inevitability of mortality by negotiating the contributions and accomplishments that have been made by the individual and his or her children

the midlife crisis. Another transition point for men occurs in their fifties, when men become more relaxed and accepting of both success and failure (Kaplan, 1988).

The book *The Seasons of a Man's Life,* by Levinson (1978), had a great influence on thoughts about adulthood. Levinson's theory emphasized four eras of life (see Table 6–2). Roger Gould (1980) expanded on the previous theories by including women in his studies. He identified seven phases of adulthood pertinent to women and men (see Table 6–3). Bernice Neugarten (1968) wrote extensively

Table 6–2 *Levinson's Eras of Adult Life*

Preadulthood Era: birth to age 22
A period of rapid growth in every area of life.

Early adulthood: 22 to 45 years
A period stressing personal identity and family raising. Occupational advancement is at its height. Love, sexuality, family, and job status predominate, although problems in all areas are seen. This is an era marked by many personal choices.

Middle adulthood: 45 to 60 years
A period of great transition, reevaluation, and coping with decreased physical abilities. This period is viewed as one where meaning in life and generosity to others is important.

Late adulthood: 60 to 85 years
A period of confronting the aging process and deciding that domination is no longer a goal. Coping with the changing relationship between the self and society and finding a balance of inner resources is important.

Table 6–3 *Gould's Phases of Adulthood*

Age	*Events*
16–18	The formation of identity, independence, and escape from parental control.
18–22	The young adult leaves home and is open to new ideas about life.
22–28	The importance of autonomy and goal attainment is seen. Self-confidence and commitment to family is important.
29–34	Marriages and goals are questioned and reevaluated. Dissatisfaction with lifestyle and economic problems are seen. Confusion and self-evaluation are inevitable.
35–43	Values are questioned and time becomes important in terms of mortality. An urgency to attain life goals becomes apparent.
44–53	This period is marked by relative stability and increased marital satisfaction. Thoughts regarding personal health become important.
54–64	This period is marked by mellowing of the self and the search for meaning and purpose in life.

about middle age and aging and emphasized the importance of culture, history, and "social clocks." Her thoughts reflected a sense of timing—that the self may progress too quickly or slowly in terms of the events in society.

Crisis Theory

Neither stress nor emergency situations necessarily constitute a crisis. A number of variables determine a person's risk for entering a crisis state. These variables are known as **balancing factors** and include

- How the person perceives the event
- What experience the person has had in coping with stress
- The person's usual coping abilities
- The support systems available to the person

The ability to balance these factors is essential for avoiding the crisis state. A crisis occurs when a person encounters a stressful situation that disrupts the equilibrium. This state of disequilibrium continues because of the absence of one of the balancing factors. In some cases, the person has a distorted perception of the event. Or the person may lack support or adequate coping mechanisms. The crisis develops as the problem remains unresolved and the disequilibrium continues. A crisis state is avoided when balance occurs in response to stressful events. In this situation the person has a realistic perception of the event, adequate coping mechanisms, and support sufficient to resolve the problem and regain equilibrium (Aguilera and Messick, 1978).

To understand the development of a crisis state, nurses must be knowledgeable about the phases of a crisis. Initially, people experience increased anxiety to the traumatic event, and their usual coping mechanisms become ineffective. As their ability to cope decreases, their anxiety increases to high levels. With this increased anxiety, they recognize the need to reach out for assistance. When both inner resources and external support systems are inadequate, these individuals enter an active crisis state. During this time they typically have a short attention span and are unproductive and impulsive. They experience distress in their search for meaning of the traumatic event. As the crisis state continues, there is deterioration of interpersonal relationships. As confusion and disorientation continue, individuals in crisis look to others to solve the problem, since they are consumed with feelings of "going crazy" or "losing their minds" (Johnson, 1986).

Adaptive Tasks and Coping Skills

Effective coping skills often prevent a crisis state in the face of traumatic events. Once in a crisis state there are behavioral, affective, cognitive, and psychosocial skills that people can draw on or learn so they can adapt to an unexpected event. The relative importance of these skills varies with each person and each crisis. Most likely, they are used in various combinations, with the effectiveness of specific skills depending on the specific event.

Behavioral skills involve seeking information as the first step in the problem-solving process. The person with behavioral skills identifies alternative ways of resolving the crisis and predicts probable consequences for each of the alternatives. The next step is choosing an alternative and taking concrete action. The final step is an evaluation of the consequences and, if necessary, a return to finding solutions (See Chapter 1 for more detail on the problem-solving process.) Other behavioral skills involve finding new sources to meet dependency needs, practicing independent behaviors, and learning social skills necessary for mature interdependence. To support self-esteem, individuals may develop new interests and activities or may even become active in helping others who are dealing with similar crises.

Affective skills focus on managing the feelings provoked by the event and maintaining a reasonable balance. Venting feelings by talking, crying, or even screaming allows for emotional discharge of anger, despair, and frustration. The ability to identify and discuss one's feelings is an adaptive skill. To be able to tolerate ambiguity and maintain some hope is very helpful during a crisis period.

Cognitive skills help the individual find meaning in and understand the personal significance of an unexpected event. Finding meaning is an ongoing issue during and after the crisis period. The result of the search is dependent on the individual's spirituality or philosophy of life. Some people may find this by living for causes beyond themselves. Others believe in divine purpose, which they find a great source of consolation. A cognitive skill that may be temporarily effective is denial. To prevent feeling overwhelmed, individuals may deny the unexpected event or its possible consequences. Another cognitive skill is the ability to redefine the unexpected event. In this instance, the person accepts the basic reality of the event but reshapes the situation into something favorable. For example, the individual might focus on the potential positive outcomes or compare himself or herself with those less fortunate. The goal of adaptive cognitive skills is to maintain a satisfactory self-image and a sense of competence and mastery.

Psychosocial skills enable a person in crisis to maintain relationships with family and friends throughout and after the crisis period. The person must be open to accepting the comfort and support offered by others. Family and friends may be sources of information that will enable the person to make wise decisions. Not to be overlooked are community resources such as hot lines, mental health centers, support groups, and self-help groups (Moos and Schaefer, 1986).

In addition to behavioral, affective, cognitive, and psychosocial skills, there are other factors influencing the outcome of unexpected events. Demographic and personal factors influence how a person defines and resolves these crises. These factors include age, gender, ethnicity, economic resources, spiritual resources, and past experiences. Factors specific to the unexpected event also influence the outcome. Tasks and coping skills vary between biologic, psychologic, environmental, and social crisis events. The more control a person has over these factors, the more adaptive they are likely to be. Successful resolution of crisis leads to growth and an increased ability to cope in the future. Failure to resolve the issues contributes to decreased adaptation and—perhaps—problems in the future.

Childhood

The rearing and socialization of children is one of the most important functions of the family. Thus the major significance of divorce is not that husbands and wives break up but that parents break up.

Self-Concept and Dependency Crisis: Children of Divorce

The current term for a divorced family is *binuclear family,* the two households formed after divorce that still compose one family system (Ahrons and Rodgers, 1987).

Separation and divorce may be the child's first significant loss. It is a loss quite different than loss through the illness or death of a parent. When a parent is hospitalized, the child maintains hope and confidence that the parent will soon return. With the death of a parent, grieving rituals aid the child in accepting the loss and the finality of the separation. When parents divorce, children fluctuate between hopefulness and hopelessness. Traditionally there have been no rituals to help the child grieve the loss of the familiar family structure (Kaslow and Schwartz, 1987).

Children's adaptation to divorce varies on a continuum from healthy to unhealthy. At the onset of separation it is difficult to predict what, if any, long-lasting changes will occur. Change from a nuclear to a binuclear family produces situational stress. Initially, the custodial parent may experience role overload and be unable to meet the emotional needs of the children. The out-of-home parent may struggle with ways to stay involved in child care. This situational stress often results in temporary emotional distress in the children. Typically these issues are resolved within one year, and the children return to the previous or an improved level of functioning.

Behavioral Characteristics The response of infants under one year of age is correlated with the custodial parent's response to the divorce. If the parent is frequently upset and anxious, the infant may respond by becoming fussy and irritable. If the parent is depressed, the infant may become listless and less responsive to environmental stimuli. Similarly, 1- and 2-year-old children may respond to the parent's emotional state. Not infrequently, they exhibit clinging and whining behavior until they feel more secure in the new family structure.

Temporary regression in response to anxiety is often displayed by 3- to 5-year-old children. This may be a return to baby talk, incontinence, or an earlier level of play and social behavior. Possessiveness over toys may be an attempt to gain some control and prevent further losses. For those children who believe their "bad" behavior was the cause of the divorce, a change to overly compliant behavior is not unusual. Anger may be expressed by overly aggressive behavior with other children and adults. Sleep disturbances and somatic symptoms may be indicative of anxiety or depression in response to the separation.

In school-age children, anxiety or depression may be manifested in new academic problems. Some use the energy of anxiety to excel in academics or extracurricular activities. In a hope for family unification, behavior is often geared toward bringing the parents together. Preadolescents may attempt to intervene directly with parental conflict or to be a source of comfort for one or both parents. Unhealthy adaptation occurs when generational lines are crossed and children are forced to take care of parents. Other children avoid conflict at home by withdrawing to their rooms or staying away from home as much as possible. A healthy adaptation to ongoing parental conflict is disengagement from the conflict and the resumption of former interests and activities. Children who feel betrayed and angry may attempt to manipulate their parents by playing one parent against the other. Many children of divorce are expected to become more responsible in household chores. When these responsibilities are age-appropriate it is a positive consequence. A negative consequence may occur when older children are required to become "parents" to younger siblings (Kaslow and Schwartz, 1987; Peck, 1989; Schuster and Ashburn, 1986).

Affective Characteristics Multiple fears are not uncommon among children of divorce. They may feel rejected and abandoned by the noncustodial parent and live in fear that the custodial parent may also reject and abandon them. Among siblings there may be fears of being split up between the binuclear homes. Not uncommonly, fears of the future arise regarding issues of living arrangements, holidays, financial problems, vacations, and so forth. Multiple fears contribute to a general feeling of confusion and insecurity.

Anger may be a dominant affective response. The anger may be directed at the parent whom the child has identified as being responsible for the separation and divorce. Some children direct anger at both parents. In some situations children feel responsible for the divorce, blame themselves, and experience a great deal of self-anger. When anger at the self is not resolved, guilt may be the dominant feeling. Even though the guilt is inappropriate, it may be more comfortable than the anxiety that would occur if they acknowledged their powerlessness to control conditions (Hutchinson and Spangler-Hirsch, 1989).

Children of divorce must grieve multiple losses. There is partial or total loss of one parent. A disruption may occur in contact with extended families. There may be the loss of a familiar home, school, and friends. Familiar routines change, and lifestyle changes may be abrupt and severe. Holidays heighten feelings of loss and separation at a time when other homes appear most bonded and joyful. Healthy adaptation means being able to manage these intense feelings as well as grieve and resolve the many losses (Kaslow and Schwartz, 1987; Wallerstein, 1986).

Cognitive Characteristics Children often blame themselves for parental separation and divorce. Preschoolers are very egocentric and have difficulty in viewing events as not being directly related to themselves. Young school-age children also tend to feel responsible for the divorce. They often view their behavior, especially "bad" behavior, as contributing to their parents' conflict. They believe that if somehow they could be "good" all the time, their parents would not fight and therefore would stay together. Older school-age children often try to understand the situation but experience thoughts of "being caught in the middle." Many children have hopes and fantasies about their parents reconciling and reestablishing the family unit.

Initially, children may be very concerned about who will care for them, whether they will have to move, if there will be enough money to survive, if the noncustodial parent will continue to parent and if their entire lives will be different. The reality of having one parent leave the home contributes to thoughts of losing the other parent through abandonment or death. Holidays emphasize families, and children of divorce may find them difficult times. When children are with one parent, they may worry about the other parent being all alone. They may be envious of their friends who celebrate holidays in an intact family unit. Some children are able to cognitively restructure their expectations and think of their situation as an opportunity to celebrate holidays twice and receive many more gifts.

In response to the anxiety of separation, children may identify with the absent parent, as if recreating the absent parent within themselves lessens the feeling of abandonment. Some children will make one parent the villain and the other the hero, perhaps in an effort to feel less responsible and guilty for the divorce. When this occurs, the stability of the binuclear family is threatened. Children of divorce may think of adults as unreliable, and they may question their parents' moral worth and even condemn them for "childish" behavior.

One cognitive task for children of divorce is the acknowledgment of the reality and permanence of the divorce. This is a gradual process that typically resolves by the end of the first year of the separation. During this time denial may be used to manage the many fears. Fantasies of undoing the divorce and reuniting the parents may help the children regain feelings of power and control during this vulnerable period.

Achieving a realistic hope for one's own future relationships is another cognitive task for a child of divorce. This process most typically occurs during the preadolescent and adolescent years. Not uncommonly, such a child fears marital failure in his or her own life. If this fear is not resolved so that the child's self-concept defines him or her as a person capable of loving and being loved, the result may be chronic loss of self-esteem and, due to fear of failure, avoidance of relationships (Kaslow and Schwartz, 1987; Wallerstein, 1986).

Psychosocial Characteristics Following the decision to divorce, parents must resolve a great many issues. Of primary importance is when and how to tell the children about the decision to separate. The most appropriate time is when the decision has finally been made. If possible, both parents should bring all the children together and give them the information. From both parents children need continual reassurance that they are responsible neither for the divorce nor for getting the parents back together. Providing repeated assurance that both parents will continue to love and take care of them is of utmost importance.

Managing the extended family is another issue in divorce. Relatives may be approving, solicitous, and anxious to help, or they may be critical and condemning if they believe divorce is a disgrace or an immoral act. Some extended families may be of help in providing a temporary place to stay, financial support, or child care. Other extended family members may fear they will never see the children in the future. Parents need to remember that grandparents, aunts, uncles, and cousins are a support system for their children and that it is helpful to encourage and reinforce these bonds.

For the sake of the healthy binuclear family, parents are advised to hire lawyers who are sensitive to the impact of divorce on the entire family system. When material possessions, custody, and financial support are contested, the associated distress has a negative impact on the children of divorce.

In the United States prior to the 1920s, paternal custody was the norm. Typically, when parents separated or divorced, the mother left and the father's female relatives assisted in raising the children. From the 1920s through the 1960s, maternal custody was the norm; the majority of children of divorce were raised in households headed by single mothers. In the late 1960s, society and the legal system began to look at the best interest of the child in determining custody. Currently, children over the age of 6 are asked questions about custody. They are not asked to choose one parent over the other; rather, they are asked their thoughts about their relationship and the pros and cons of living with each parent. This information is taken into consideration when custody is being determined by the courts (Guerin, 1987; Kaslow and Schwartz, 1987).

Resolution and Consequences The formation of binuclear families demands psychologic, social, and economic reorganization by all family members. The picture they once had of the future is gone, and a new future must be designed. If parental conflict was high prior to the divorce, the children may experience relief from stress with the new family structure. Children of divorce have rights to adequate child care and nuturing; parents divorce one another, not their children, and remain obligated to fulfill children's rights and needs. Children's adjustment to the binuclear family is correlated to the parents' adjustment. When parents cope well by living in the present and designing a new future, children are able to adapt and cope better. Additional support for children may be found in age-specific support groups found in many schools and religious congregations. These groups decrease children's sense of abandonment and isolation and help them manage feelings aroused by the divorce.

A minority of children suffer long-lasting negative consequences as a result of their parents' divorce. Most typically this occurs when the parents themselves are unable to adapt and continue with a conflicted relationship. Some parents pump the children for information about the life and relationships of the other parent, and the child feels like a spy in the enemy camp. One or both parents may criticize and blame the other in front of the children, in an effort to force the children to take sides in an unending dispute. Continuing with this level of anger results in children who feel less free and comfortable in the relationship with each parent. Children may become pawns and weapons when one parent uses them to punish the other. When one has control of the children and the other has control of the money, visitation rights and support payments may be used in retaliation. This is extremely distressing to the children, who feel caught in the middle between the feuding parents. When noncustodial parents completely distance themselves and become uninvolved and unsupportive of their children, the children suffer from intense feelings of rejection.

The self-concept of the few children who suffer long-lasting negative consequences of divorce may be one of inadequacy, failure, and worthlessness. Fear and a need to protect oneself from future pain may contribute to superficial relationships throughout life. Some children are overprotected by parents and develop a lifestyle of extreme dependency. Others are forced by circumstances or parents into premature maturity and develop a lifestyle of extreme independence. It may be difficult for these individuals to find an appropriate balance between dependence, independence, and interdependence (Walsh and Stolberg, 1989).

The negative consequences of divorce can be modified by parents who are able to adapt and cope. When both parents are able to continue their parenting in an atmosphere of support and a spirit of cooperation, the stress on the children is lessened. Children are able to cope better when each parent supports and encourages the children's relationship with the other parent. The more involved in parenting both adults remain, the less drastic the sense of loss for the children. This means easy and friendly access to both parents. Schedules planned in a cooperative manner contribute to a child's feeling of security. Key decisions about the children must be made together to prevent an escalation of old parental conflicts. Children adapt best when their parents are able to let go of their blame, hurt, and anger; live in the present; and plan for the future. This means developing new family roles, patterns, and rituals to help decrease the disorientation children feel after a divorce. Holidays, celebrations, and major life events require special negotiations in the best interest of the children.

Most children suffer no long-lasting effects when their parents divorce. By the end of the first year, most have returned to and resumed their normal levels of growth and development. Their self-concept is one of capability, adaptability, and goodness. Relationships with others demonstrate an appropriate balance between dependence, independence, and interdependence. However, some children seem to adjust and then experience a delayed reaction at adolescence. As children of divorce, these adolescents struggle with fears of betrayal, abandonment, and failure when entering relationships (Hutchinson and Spangler-Hirsch, 1989).

Adolescence

One of the major tasks of adolescence is individuation and separation from the family. Adolescents must give up their dependency on their parents, develop more independence, and form interdependent relationships with their peer group.

Dependency Crisis: Peer Group Formation

The peer group becomes the source of learning and evaluating the behavioral, affective, cognitive, and social skills necessary for responsible interpersonal adult behavior. The peer group is the means of promoting the adolescent's adjustment to the adult world. As such it is a necessity—not a luxury—of the teen years. Peers become idealized and serve as replacements for the formerly idealized parents. As the number of acquaintances increases during early adolescence, teens become aware of the importance of belonging to a group. New people and new events expand their worlds, and peer interactions help them test their self-concepts, values, and social identities. They develop the social skills necessary to manage competition and aggression within the group. Adolescents certainly do participate in the larger society, but the peer subculture is extremely influential in determining behavior, beliefs, and values.

The majority of adolescents work through this maturational crisis and develop into mature young adults. A small percentage of teens are unable to develop meaningful peer relationships and become isolated and lonely young adults. Another small percentage find their peer group within the gang structure and exchange the dependency on the family for the dependency on the gang. Remaining in the gang prevents growth toward social responsibility apart from the peer group (Kelly and Hansen, 1987; VanHasselt, 1987).

Behavioral Characteristics The majority of adolescents spend more free time with peers than with their parents or in being alone. Most of this time is spent in talking, and they describe themselves as being most happy when interacting with their friends. Adolescents who do not develop relationships within a peer group are deprived of this source of pleasurable interaction and spend much time alone. Exposure to new social situations demands new skills and different expectations of behavior. Loner adolescents do not have the opportunity to develop conversational skills—the skills needed to initiate conversations, state views, and make appropriate self-disclosures. With minimal skills their chances for social acceptance decrease, and they avoid interactions. Lack of social skills contributes to infrequent dating. Learning assertive skills such as making and refusing requests, giving feedback to others, and standing up for personal rights is very difficult outside a peer group. Loner adolescents have little opportunity to observe how their peers manage anger and to learn to manage their own aggressive impulses in peer interactions. They have difficulty learning the process of give and take in interpersonal situations. Lack of a peer group usually means limited participation in social and extracurricular activities. Loner adolescents often describe themselves as very lonely (Beck, 1987; Kelly and Hansen, 1987).

The most common reason for adolescents to be referred to mental health facilities is conduct disorder, which occurs more frequently in boys than girls and with a higher incidence in the disadvantaged population. Group type conduct disorder is diagnosed when the problem behavior occurs mainly as a group activity with peers. Some impressionable adolescents may get into serious delinquency during the period of normal adolescent rebellion. Gangs, as do other peer groups, determine rules of behavior for their members. Susceptible adolescents learn delinquent behavior from other gang members, and their deviant behavior is reinforced by the group. They develop a pattern of hostile, defiant, and socially inappropriate behavior, creating problems in homes, schools, and communities. Rights of nongang members are violated as well as the norms of society. With no concern for the feelings or well-being of others, gang members use physical aggression to meet needs and wants. Not infrequently, gang members are suspended from school for their deviant behavior. Substance abuse often occurs as a gang activity, and the gang turns to stealing and robbing to purchase drugs. High gang loyalty leads to rival gang behavior, and gang members are frequently injured in fights and may even be killed in a gang war. Violent offenses are strongly associated with gang membership (Dembo, 1988; Fulmer, 1988; McMahon and Forehand, 1988).

Affective Characteristics Loner teens are unable to form the intense and extensive friendships that other teens do. Some are fearful of intimate relationships, some experience anxiety in social situations, and some are too depressed to interact with others. There is limited opportunity for loners to experience their emotions and express them to others who are in a similar developmental stage. Empathy, the ability to take the perspective of another person and communicate an understanding of it, is learned through social interaction. Thus, adolescents with minimal interactions often have difficulty in being empathic with others. This lack of empathy contributes to further distance in peer relationships. Lack of peer group interaction during adolescence often results in young adults who are unable to establish caring and satisfying relationships with other young women and men.

Adolescents who join gangs are often very angry people whose delinquency is rooted in frustration and protest. They have a low frustration tolerance and impulsively act on their immediate feelings. Frustrated in their ability to achieve status by legitimate means, they protest against the standards of the middle class. Underneath the anger and frustration it is not unusual to find symptoms of anxiety and depression. To the gang members, the feelings of cohesiveness and loyalty to the gang are extremely intense. In socioeconomically deprived areas gangs represent an important source of affiliation. Fear may prevent adolescents who think of leaving the gang from doing so. One fear may be retaliation for their attempt to drop out of the group. And, since they have been unable to individuate and establish their own independence, they may fear a lack of personal identity apart from the gang (Dembo, 1988).

Cognitive Characteristics Adolescents who are unable to become part of a peer group often find it difficult to establish positive patterns of self-appraisal. Their self-image defines them as incompetent in social interactions. This negative perspective interferes with relationships, and the lack of relationships then contributes to further failure with peers. Teens without peers have limited opportunities to explore and enhance their increasing cognitive and problem-solving abilities with others of the same age. With lack of peer feedback, they may consider themselves less smart than their peers or have an inflated sense of their cognitive abilities. Continuing dependence on their families fosters a self-concept of incompetence and failure in relationships apart from the family. Since acceptance by peers is an important aspect of self-esteem, loner adolescents may have difficulty in seeing themselves as attractive and desirable people. Projection of this negative self-concept creates further distance and lack of intimacy in peer relationships (Kelly and Hansen, 1987).

Adolescents who belong to gangs develop a high level of solidarity in values and beliefs. Loyal gang members have a similar orientation to social behavior, school, and achievement in life. They value loyalty to the gang and disrespect the rights of all others. To drop out of or be suspended from school is not unusual. They place a high value on having money through whatever means possible. In spite of their projected image of toughness, many of these adolescents have low self-esteem. Since they have moved from a dependent relationship with the family to a dependent relationship with the gang, they have difficulty viewing themselves as independent, self-sufficient people. They identify with those whom they perceive as successful models; in deprived areas gang members may be the most visibly prosperous. It is not unusual for gang members to make self-defeating decisions. In some cases the decisions are self-destructive and even life threatening (Carter and McGoldrick, 1988).

Psychosocial Characteristics It may be difficult for a loner adolescent to find a place within the larger society. To become independent and confident adults, adolescents must learn how to interact with a variety of individuals and groups in diverse settings. This includes learning how to balance personal rights and group rights. Adolescents who have not developed these skills with peer groups may have difficulty as adults. Without group affiliation, adolescents find it difficult to gain independence from their parents. Conversely, when they have few or no peer friendships, these adolescents are forced to be dependent on their families for emotional and social support. The consequences may be young adults who struggle with interdependence and find the extremes of dependence or independence to be the most comfortable (VanHasselt, 1987).

Loyalty to the gang and group cohesion are necessary for gang existence. Individuals demonstrate loyalty by engaging in conflict and heeding the "call to arms." They value toughness and smartness as proof of a masculine identity, and the gang offers a form of social protection. The gang subculture most frequently develops in deprived areas where adolescents are blocked in their ambitions for a higher socioeconomic lifestyle. When legitimate means to successful goals are blocked by society, some adolescents seek opportunities for money and success by illegitimate means. It must be remembered that, in the face of frustration, delinquent behavior is only one adaptation. Many other adolescents in deprived areas make other choices and do not exhibit deviant behavior (Dembo, 1988).

Resolution and Consequences Nursing intervention is very appropriate with undersocialized and loner adolescents. Nurses can help these teens improve their social skills through role playing and problem solving. They need help in expanding their networks through extended family, extracurricular activities such as sports or hobbies, and involvement in community clubs and other social groups. This will give them opportunities to practice balancing personal rights and group responsibilities. They must be encouraged to conform enough to prevent rejection by their peers. Nurses can help dependent adolescents separate from their families by helping them to test their own ideas. Questioning family beliefs and values helps adolescents formulate more personal and meaningful value systems.

Successful resolution of peer group problems helps these adolescents to become more productive adults who are capable of forming satisfying adult relationships. Learning to use the problem-solving process will aid them in finding solutions for interpersonal problems. As their ability to anticipate potential consequences of interpersonal behavior increases, their self-confidence and self-concept will improve. Increased social competence is likely to prevent social maladjustment as adults.

The behavior of adolescents who remain on the periphery of gangs and exhibit mild forms of conduct disorder often improves over time. The more severe forms of conduct disorder tend to be chronic, and those suffering from them are likely to continue with maladaptive behaviors into adulthood. These people engage in antisocial and criminal behavior, often have a low educational level, and experience poor occupational adjustment and marital and family problems (McMahon and Forehand, 1988).

Not to be ignored in this context is the two-tier approach to troubled adolescents in America. White adolescents who act out with delinquent behavior are often referred to counseling and processed through the mental health system. African-American and Hispanic youths exhibiting the same behavior are most typically charged with delinquent offenses and processed through the criminal justice system. This is especially true for low-income families who cannot afford to send teens to private mental health facilities or hire lawyers to defend them. The outcome of this discrimination is the denial of mental health services to African-American and Hispanic adolescents and a perpetuation of gangs within the community (Dembo, 1988).

Self-Concept Crisis: Teenage Parenthood

Many adolescents are sexually active, but few are sexually responsible in preventing pregnancy. Teenage pregnancies are typically unplanned and often unwanted. Teens are unprepared for the behavioral, affective, cognitive, and psychosocial demands of parenthood. When children have children there are profound consequences for the teen mothers, their babies, and their families. The research on teen fathers is limited but at present seems to contradict the stereotype of uninvolvement or abandonment.

Both the experiences of being an adolescent and becoming a parent are maturational crises or expected life changes. However, when they occur at the same time with an unexpected pregnancy during adolescence, there are special needs and concerns to be managed. Adolescence is a critical time for struggling with one's personal development and solidifying one's identity and self-concept. When the roles and identity of parenthood are superimposed on this struggle, a crisis may develop, leading to a shaky passage to adulthood.

Behavioral Characteristics Adolescents reach biologic maturity before they have the behavioral skills of adulthood. Becoming a parent while still a teen contributes to many unexpected changes in one's life. With the decreasing stigma, many teens no longer marry when a pregnancy occurs. If the decision is made not to terminate the pregnancy, the chances are very high that the teen mother, as a single parent, will keep and raise the baby. Fewer than 5 percent of adolescent girls give their babies up for adoption (Byer, Shainberg, and Jones, 1988).

It is often difficult for a pregnant girl or teen mother to stay in school. Often, dropping out of school has the long-term consequence of unemployment or underemployment (most typically in low-paying jobs). Some teen mothers may find themselves forced to apply for public assistance to survive. After leaving their school peer group, some young mothers find themselves socially isolated at a time when peer group influence is highly important (Gilchrist and Schinke, 1987).

Teen fathers, often overlooked by the community and professionals, suffer from a negative stereotype. It has been assumed that teen fathers disappear and avoid involvement and responsibility. There is now an increased interest in this group, and research findings are beginning to appear in the literature. Many teen fathers are concerned and eager to be involved in parenting. Not infrequently they view responsible fatherhood as a part of their masculine identities. Many of them assume the role of provider for their children. If a teen father leaves school to support his child, he often ends up in low-paying jobs with minimal opportunities for advancement. Within the African-American community teen fathers are expected to participate in physical and financial care of their children. Those who do not lose respect within their neighborhood (Connor, 1988; Panzarine and Elster, 1986).

The primary factor determining the amount of the teen father's involvement is the teen mother's parents' willingness to include him. When teen fathers are given the opportunity and encouragement to be involved, many of them accept their new responsibilities (Fulmer, 1988). Barret and Robinson's (1986) study of 400 teen fathers involved in a program of vocational assistance, counseling, and parenting classes showed significant responsibility on the part of these young men. At the end of two years 82 percent had contact with their children on a daily basis and 74 percent were providing financial support. Ninety percent continued the relationship with the mothers of their children.

Teen parents need assistance in preparing for the baby. They will need to find food, clothing, and other needed supplies. They may need to find a place to live. They may need guidance in developing positive patterns of interaction with their children. Parenting classes help adolescents learn about the children's physical and emotional needs. Understanding normal growth and development will help these adolescents in coping and parenting more effectively (White-Traut and Pabst, 1987).

Affective Characteristics Teen mothers must learn to manage all the typical emotions of both adolescence and parenthood as well as emotions arising out of their particular situation. For some teens who were not nurtured well as children, the opportunity to nurture and mother a baby may be a compensation for feelings of emptiness. Teens who have dropped out of school and become socially isolated from their peer group may experience feelings of being trapped, which may contribute to feelings of depression. Most adolescent girls experience anticipatory anxiety over the process of labor and delivery. They are concerned about pain and how well they will manage during the process. After delivery they may need support to help them bond with their new children (Fulmer, 1988; Gilchrist and Schinke, 1987).

A teen father who has been excluded usually feels alienated and helpless. A teen father who is included usually describes his relationship with the mother and child as close and caring. Even when they decide not to marry, the father often has strong emotional ties to his girlfriend during and after pregnancy. Contrary to the stereotype, many teen fathers love the mother and child and desire to be active fathers (Barret and Robinson, 1986).

Cognitive Characteristics Initially, teen mothers and fathers may find the pregnancy exciting and glamorous. Not uncommonly, the pregnancy is proof of their sexuality, and they are elevated to an adult status. The sudden promotion to womanhood or manhood is self-affirming for some teens; others experience ambivalence toward the new role. Some see the child as giving a new meaning and purpose to life. Teen parents are forced to reorganize their self-concept and formulate new identities to accompany their new roles. They need to gain knowledge about pregnancy, labor, and delivery to ensure the best possible outcome. Since many teens have immature and unrealistic ideas about babies, they must change their thinking to match the reality of parenting. The more active the teen parents are in the decision-making process, the more active they are during and after the pregnancy (Barret and Robinson, 1986; Byer, Shainberg, and Jones, 1988).

Psychosocial Characteristics Teenage parenthood has consequences for individuals, families, and communities. Pretending the crisis does not exist or wanting it to go away only perpetuates and exaggerates the problem. Denial of adolescent sexual behavior contributes to the increasing rate of teen pregnancy. Denial of the reality of a pregnancy or fear of telling parents contributes to poor prenatal care and more complications for the high-risk pregnancy group. Denial of the need for a new family structure causes increased conflict between parents and teens. Community denial means lack of educational opportunities, inadequate child care, and many families living in poverty.

When teens become parents, they give up their carefree adolescence. Only one third of teen mothers marry the fathers of their children, and compared to other marriages those marriages are three times as likely to end in divorce. A new family identity must be formed in those families in which the teen mother and new baby remain in the home. Decisions about who is to parent and how parenting will be done need to be negotiated. Role conflict may occur when the parents have difficulty recognizing their adolescent daughter as a responsible parent. The most valuable asset to a teen mother is parents who are able to provide the necessary emotional and social support. Those who are able to continue their education and implement career goals fare better later in life. Lack of resources often means families being headed by young mothers.

These families are seven times more likely than other families to be living below the poverty level. Adolescent parenthood is a major cause of low-income family units in the United States. With a higher rate of teenage pregnancy among siblings and children of adolescent parents, the community problems continue to expand (Gilchrist and Schinke, 1987; Stark, 1988).

Resolution and Consequences Teen parents need support from peers, family, professionals, and the community. Nurses in a variety of clinical settings interact with teen parents and their children. As community members nurses may establish programs for the prevention of pregnancy as well as programs to support the family unit. On a national level, nurses can voice their support for public policies affecting high-risk families.

Assessing parent-child interaction is a nursing responsibility. Those who are at risk for parenting problems must be identified so cycles of frustration, occupational instability, poverty, and child neglect or abuse can be broken. In schools, churches, hospitals, clinics, and community centers, nurses can establish programs to educate young parents and improve their parenting skills. When severe parenting problems are identified, nurses should refer the young family to the appropriate social or mental health agencies.

At the community level there must be more of an effort to prevent teen pregnancy. Beginning in grade school and continuing on, children must be taught about reproduction, contraception, values clarification, responsible decision making, interpersonal communication, and the development of mature relationships. This type of educational program is done within the context of adolescent development. Decisions about sexual behavior and contraception require a perspective of the future. Many adolescents need guidance to begin to project long-term consequences of present behavior. Sophisticated communication skills are necessary for adolescents to refuse unwanted sexual attention, to resolve conflicts, and to establish responsible intimate relationships. Adolescent women and men must learn assertive skills to advocate for, obtain, and use contraceptives. Adolescent behavior is often inconsistent, since adolescents are not always able to convert knowledge and plans into action. Denying adolescent sexual behavior will not make teen pregnancy go away. Those developed countries with the most liberal attitudes toward sex, the most accessible contraceptive services, and the most complete sex education programs have the lowest rate of teen pregnancy, teen abortion, and teen childbearing (Connor, 1988; Gilchrist and Schinke, 1987; Murray and Park, 1988).

High schools must make efforts to accommodate young parents as they finish their educations and find acceptable jobs. With this support the teens are more likely to succeed financially. Low-cost child care facilities near the school are most helpful in allowing teens to continue in school. Teen parenting programs can be established in or near the school to allow teens to participate in nutrition and birthing classes, learn about growth and development, and be educated about and referred to appropriate medical care. Nurses must continue to design and implement creative approaches for supporting teen parents and their children.

Middle Adulthood

To most people, age 40 has a special significance because it connotes passage to middle age. "Over the hill" birthday parties frequently acknowledge, in a joking manner, that youth is lost. In many media portrayals the idea is presented that change occurs at or around this age. A popular game, Can You Survive Your Midlife Crisis?, summarizes some thoughts about this period. The object of this game is to get through the middle years "with more money, less stress, fewer divorce points, or to declare a midlife crisis in which you go broke, get divorced or crack up" (Gameworks, Inc. 1982, p. 2).

The middle adulthood period presents unique challenges to each person. Generally, the middle-aged adult is considered to be at the apex of life and expected to achieve maturity during this time. This is the period when one is to be most productive in the work setting. This peak of life frequently stimulates a period of self-assessment. The person begins to recognize the limits of physical and psychologic abilities and realizes that achievement of life goals may not be possible. Career assessment and the meaning of successes and failures are explored (Kaplan, 1988). Through introspection, the middle adult frequently struggles with the following questions: Is this *all* I am going to do? Is there enough *time* left to accomplish everything I need to do and want to do?

Middle adulthood is also a time for expanding relationships with adolescent children. The younger generation brings fresh, new ideas to situations, and parents are constantly reminded of their children's youth.

Many people in middle age have achieved status and power in influencing the decisions of others. Both maturity and experience become useful tools in shaping the younger and older generations. Through social support, financial support, or experiential support, the middle adult guides other generations.

Self-Concept Crisis: Midlife Crisis

The middle-aged person is faced with many circumstances, expected events, and unexpected events that challenge normal coping patterns. The term *midlife crisis,* which has become common in the English language, can be applied to this developmental crisis. A **midlife crisis** is a perceived state of psychologic and physical distress that results when a person's internal resources and external social support systems are overwhelmed by developmental tasks that require new adaptive methods (Kaplan, 1988).

As in any crisis, it should be recognized that a midlife crisis can be an opportunity for personal growth. People are faced with many tasks involving a variety of behavioral, affective, cognitive, and psychosocial characteristics. When usual coping mechanisms employed in resolving earlier conflicts become ineffective because of unexpected events during this transition period, a crisis may occur.

Behavioral Characteristics The literature supports the premise that at or around 40 years of age the middle adult becomes more aware of the distance between the self and the younger adult (Neugarten, 1968). For the first time, there is a realization of the effects of the aging process and the inevitability of one's mortality. This can be reflected in the behavior of the person. The inevitability of mortality may institute a change in the perspective about time. "In the time that is left" may become a dominant phrase. Time may be used more wisely in all areas of daily living.

Gould (1978) describes the midlife crisis as an opportunity for growth and calls this period the "crisis of urgency." Behavior reflects a "second adolescence," and much turbulence is demonstrated. Running out of time encourages the person to make an energetic attempt at achieving life goals and propels him or her toward growth.

The response to the physiologic limitations and health risks associated with the aging process may bring about behavior that demonstrates alterations regarding body strength. A realistic appraisal of physical performance takes place. The person no longer has the physical endurance of the younger adult and must adapt to a decrease in activity level, a decreased metabolic rate, and obvious physical changes within the body. The effects of dietary practices, smoking, alcohol consumption, and other lifestyle habits are explored. Attempts at altering certain "unhealthy" behaviors may occur.

A maladaptive response to physical decline may include behaviors that demonstrate depression, irritability, and anxiety about body image. Some middle adults may believe that their bodies will not change, and that the physical strength will continue as it was 20 years earlier. When asked to participate in a strenuous endeavor such as basketball or high-impact aerobics, they continue beyond the point of exhaustion. (Although some adults are in excellent physical shape and perform these feats in a way that competes with the younger generation, theirs is not the normal pattern.) In addition, the middle-aged person may become obsessed with youth and being young. Inappropriate youthfulness may be displayed in dress, choice of hairstyle, cosmetics, and overall appearance. Furthermore, there may be a general disdain for the aging body. Refusal to comply with health care prescriptions and protocols may take place as the person is unable to admit obvious physical changes.

Career development behaviors may change during a midlife crisis. New career goals may develop as success, high aspirations, and the importance of achievement take on new meaning. At this time the person may change jobs frequently or develop a new career path. "Doing what I always wanted to do" may become a frequent refrain. Or, the person may recognize the inability to advance in his or her career according to the standards set at an earlier age, and he or she may not be comfortable with this realization. Job promotions, which were once highly desired, may not always bring the anticipated rewards. Some persons do advance in their careers and experience financial and emotional rewards as they fulfill their potential goals. Others may never recover from the recognition that their careers were far from "successful."

Some middle adults display behaviors that demonstrate wanting more out of life. They may quit a job, move to a new location, divorce their spouse of many years, or engage in extramarital relationships. Building a new life is often a difficult endeavor, and the outcome is variable. Some people may be disappointed with the results; others may be pleased (Levinson, 1978).

"Second adolescence" behavior may be demonstrated by the person absorbed in fulfilling personal needs. During middle adulthood, **generativity**, which emphasizes meeting the needs of others, is the general expectation. The person going through second adolescence resorts to providing self-comforts and takes on the behavior and tasks of the young adult.

Leisure behavior may be modified. New hobbies, creative projects, and new uses for free time become important. The idea that play is a poor use of time is reevaluated. The person may realize the interplay between physical and intellectual endeavors. If so, sports activities may take on important new meaning. A differentiation between compulsive work and play and healthy work and play may take place.

Maladaptive behavioral responses to the midlife crisis may describe a person who is withdrawn, resigned, or isolated. Creativity and spontaneity may be lost and denial may occur through compulsive work. Drug and alcohol use may increase to a dangerous level. Overcompensation through repeated sexual conquests or decompensation through self-destructive behaviors may be seen.

Affective Characteristics A crisis period is a time of great concern with and awareness of one's self. It is difficult to be this self-conscious and feel at ease at the same time. To feel cheerful and happy when thinking about bodily changes, time running out, and death is almost impossible. Some people feel dissatisfied and trapped by their lives. Others experience shame and rage when confronted with their physical reality as compared to the unrealistic cultural ideals. It is not unusual for individuals in midlife crisis to feel jealous and resentful of their own children's youth. It is easy for the middle adult to be filled with despair when he or she can see only problems and no future potential. A pervasive feeling of boredom can lead to a sense of indifference about life and people. Boredom may also lead to the desire to break the monotony by change, finding new thrills, or some activity that will put a little fun back in life.

Not infrequently, middle adults experience problems in either maintaining or establishing intimate relationships. They often say their marriages are "empty" or that they feel alienated from their spouses. They complain about not feeling truly loving or loved. They are bored with sex, because it has become routine and is no longer the novel experience it once was.

In spite of all these negative feelings, there are also periods of hope and joy. Thus, one of the most difficult aspects of midlife crisis is the management of conflicting emotions. It is a period of ambivalence as one struggles with disappointment and satisfaction, hopelessness and hope, anger and love, hostility and cheerfulness, rage and excitement, and self-hate and self-love. The final outcome of the crisis depends on how one resolves these conflicting feelings.

Cognitive Characteristics The psychologist Klaus Riegal (1973) has described midlife as the stage in which the highest level of cognitive functioning occurs. Self-confrontation becomes a critical task for successful adaptation. This assists in placing life in perspective. All aspects of life are cognitively viewed. Awareness of mortality may initiate a reorganization of the value system or a reevaluation of one's spiritual purpose. Recognizing the significance of life, reflecting on the past, and setting new goals for the future become cognitive tasks of midlife.

The challenges facing the middle adult in the areas of work, family, and physical alterations may call for a redefinition of what is important. Philosophies of life and values toward career achievement, family, and the self may call for frequent self-reflection. Skepticism about things that were always accepted at face value often occurs. The person may adopt a different point of view that combines old beliefs and new revelations.

The ability to accept physical changes, acknowledge reality, find meaning in work, develop a positive identity, and place life in perspective fosters a higher level of functioning following the crisis period. When coping mechanisms are unsuccessful, maladaptive cognitive development may occur.

Psychosocial Characteristics The psychological tasks of midlife are the recognition and reassessment of important interpersonal relationships. The amount of time spent with children, spouse, aging parents, relatives, and friends is reassessed in terms of time and effort. Measures to reestablish the previous level of intimacy in the marital relationship may occur. Acknowledgment of one's own contribution to marital problems as well as acceptance of the partner's shortcomings is an adaptive response. Other adaptive psychosocial responses include achieving goals for the family and community; collaborating with others; demonstrating a love for others; valuing human relationships; and becoming active in religious, social, community, cultural, professional, and political endeavors.

Maladaptive psychosocial characteristics may demonstrate insecurity in social interactions. Becoming isolated, self-absorbed, or unresponsive to the needs of others is not unusual. Unavailability to children, spouse, parents, or friends reflects an inability to fulfill social responsibilities.

During this period social relationships are extremely important. A correlation between social fulfillment and stress has been statistically proved. The most socially active demonstrate less stress and more self-esteem than isolated adults. Those with deficits in social fulfillment demonstrate decreased self-esteem and distant behavior (Moos and Schaefer 1986).

Resolution and Consequences The midlife period is a time of self-reflection and self-assessment. A person enters this period with a unique personality, a variety of coping mechanisms, and different internal and external resources. The resolution of the midlife crisis reflects mastery of a number of tasks.

Adaptation involves acceptance of mortality, achieving a sense of identity and individuation, integrating creative and destructive forces, attaining a sense of community, and integrating components of the personality successfully.

Learning to channel one's emotional drive appropriately without losing spontaneity, vigor, humor, enthusiasm, and initiative are important characteristics for crisis resolution. If the middle adult can make choices based on appreciation of the past and anticipation of the future, he or she may be able to cope with personal upheavals during this period, without losing equilibrium.

The individual who cannot adapt becomes stagnant. This individual demonstrates little interest in life's activities and is frequently categorized as dull. Inability to cope with the physical limitations, social responsibilities, and reflective assessments that are needed describes a person who displays disequilibrium in many facets of life.

The generative middle adult uses appropriate coping mechanisms to deal with stressors and is a guide for future generations. His or her behavior demonstrates flexibility and a true sense of purpose. This person has successfully resolved events that were once perceived as a threat.

The nurse with well-developed problem-solving and communication skills can assist in making this period a positive experience. It is not unusual for anxiety or affective disorders to be superimposed on a midlife crisis. Through accurate assessment, diagnosis, planning, implementation, and evaluation, the nurse can provide the expertise that people need at this point in their life span development.

Dependency Crisis: Two-Generation Conflict

An unexpected event related to family structure may precipitate another crisis during middle adulthood. The literature supports the premises that "generation gaps" exist and that they have the ability to cause conflict within the family structure. **Generation gaps** occur because of differences in experience between various age groups. Not only are there differences in developmental tasks, but there are differences in all components of lifestyle. Typically, the middle adult's perception of appropriate dress, music, diet, sexual practices, decision making, and daily living differs from the adolescent's. With frequent confrontation and conflict between generations, the children's adolescence may be the most stressful time in parents' lives (Field and Widmayer 1982; Mead, 1970).

Generation gaps may in part be understood by examining the major life events of each generation. The middle adults of today were born during the late 1920s, the 1930s, and the early 1940s and probably experienced the effects of the Great Depression. Many learned that economic security was important and that material possessions may be lost for reasons beyond personal control. Their values and behavior were greatly influenced by inadequate material resources. World War II brought rapid social and technologic changes in their lifestyle. In contrast, the adolescents of today have grown up with the threat of total nuclear destruction and exposure to the affluence of the past 20 years. Increased family income has given many middle-class adolescents abundant material possessions. For economically deprived adolescents, being surrounded by prosperity may be a frustrating experience. The explosion of the technologic age and the availability of drugs have made current adolescent experiences far different than those of the middle adult's teen years.

The middle adult may also be in the "middle" in other ways. Gerontologic research indicates that family restructuring associated with aging parents may occur. Ten percent of parents over 65 live with their middle-aged children, and 25 percent of 18- to 25-year-olds live with their middle-aged parents. In 8 percent of families, three generations are living in the home. As the number of older adults rises, a crisis in care giving is predictable. There will be more elderly needing care and too few family care givers to provide it. The need to care for dependent parents can create a crisis for the middle adult (Grau, 1989; Troll, 1989).

At a time when they expected greater independence and more social mobility, middle adults may find that their dependent parents restrict their leisure time. Although most older adults wish to be independent of their adult children, it is primarily their offspring to whom they turn in the time of need. Elderly parents generally live in proximity to at least one adult child; maintain close contact with adult children; and receive physical, emotional, or financial assistance—especially from female adult children (Moos and Schaefer, 1986).

The middle adult may become sandwiched between the older and the younger generations. Assisting growing children; supporting children who have returned to the household because of divorce, finances, or other reasons; and providing care for aging parents can result in crisis for the middle adult who feels responsible for "everyone." Three generation gaps in the same household may increase the level of family conflict.

Behavioral Characteristics Filial responsibility is a feeling of personal responsibility toward parents. It emphasizes duty, protection, physical and emotional care, and financial support. The degree to which filial responsibility interrupts or enriches lifestyle depends on personalities, types of relationships, resources, and cultural or ethnic beliefs. Dependency of children and aging parents may cause disruption in ADLs and the behaviors of all three generations may need to adapt to accommodate it (Murray, 1989).

The decision to bring the dependent adult into the home is, for many people, difficult. Typically, the responsibility falls on the oldest daughter of the family. Social and recreational behaviors may need to be altered. Conflict may occur because of competing demands from other family members. Some middle adults may have difficulty in setting priorities with these multiple demands on time and energy. Adaptive behavior includes finding time for leisure activities. Relaxing time alone and with one's spouse is necessary even when privacy is reduced.

Role conflict often occurs between elderly parents and adult children. No matter how old, how successful, or how well established adult children are, they always remain a "child" in the eyes of the parent. This can lead to frequent power struggles within the family. Role reversal may occur, in which the adult child parents his or her own parents. Role reversal can be very unsettling because the elderly parents are no longer available as a resource and support for their adult children.

The care-giver role may present financial hardships. Middle adults who are planning for their own retirements may find the financial problems overwhelming. Home health services or day care programs for elderly parents may be economically out of reach. At the same time there may be demands from adolescent or young adult children for financial support for food, shelter, or schooling. Adaptive coping may include trial-and-error behavior and making the best of a necessary situation. Cooperation and learning to get along by all three generations contributes to family adaptation.

Affective Characteristics The middle adult may verbalize a wide range of feelings in two-generation conflicts. Emotional changes include feelings of frustration, anxiety, helplessness, depression, and lowered morale. He or she may experience sadness as the aging parent declines in physical or mental capacities. To feel guilty when it is recognized that institutionalization is the only alternative is a common affective response (Murray, 1989).

Many middle adults experience feelings of close emotional attachment to parents during this time in their lives. When the middle adult feels "down," it may be the parent to whom he or she turns for emotional support. The wisdom and knowledge gained through years of life experience is acknowledged and sought. These positive feelings may be seen more readily if the aging parent is still active and self-sufficient. Reminiscing about the shared good and bad times becomes important.

Conversely, the middle adult may describe the aging parent in cold, uncharitable terms. To give complete care to demanding aging parents may cause anxiety, hostility, and frequent mood swings in the care giver. Emotional exhaustion may be seen as restrictions of time and freedom increase. Abuse of the elderly may occur due to the frustration and anger at being the responsible care giver.

Simultaneously, middle adults may experience anger that their adult children have not left or have returned to the home. Lack of privacy and the need to continue financial support often contribute to increased conflict within the family. The frustration of being responsible for both the older and the younger generation may reach high levels in the middle adult who was anticipating a time of increased freedom.

Cognitive Characteristics Adolescence, middle age, and late adulthood are periods of evaluation and reevaluation. All three generations question the value of life from a philosophical, spiritual, and social perspective. Conflicts often develop as each generation expresses personal views. Sometimes an alliance occurs between grandchildren and grandparents, and the middle adult feels alienated. Understanding developmental issues and the needs of each generation contributes to adaptive response.

Psychosocial Characteristics Psychosocial adaptation in two-generation conflict situations includes maintaining sexual and emotional intimacy with one's partner; keeping in contact with grown children and their families, aging parents, siblings, and friends; and involvement in community activities beyond the family.

Understanding the stress involved in care-giving relationships is essential. As the dependence of the aged parent increases, both the older adult and middle adult may enter into greater conflict in interpersonal relationships. The loss of privacy and freedom on the part of the aged parent and the care giver can further increase stress.

The parent who is able to resolve conflict with the adolescent has learned to accept the adolescent's increasing need for independence. A realistic balance of dependence, independence, and interdependence is an adaptive response. Conflict decreases when parents are able to accept that an adolescent needs to be his or her "own person" with personal values, dreams, and opportunities.

Consequences and Resolution The middle adult's life experiences and earlier crisis resolutions are important in determining successful resolution of two-generation conflict. Defining whether the situation is a problem, a serious stressor, an annoyance, or a real joy is important to the outcome. All people do not see the same events as stressful. In managing the stress middle adults may utilize earlier coping behavior to develop creative resolutions.

Meeting needs in new ways that make life satisfying for all three generations is necessary. Adaptation involves letting go of parental authority in some situations, finding new sources of satisfaction for the self, and adjusting to care-giving demands. With the trend toward earlier hospital discharge and increase in home care, more adult children are becoming involved in caring for dependents in the home. An awareness of the stressors and active involvement of significant others is important for resolving crises.

Two-generation conflict can be a crisis that challenges the middle adult. Both stability and change are components of this period. The concept of generativity should instill excitement in the middle adult if successful resolution is to occur.

Late Adulthood

A person begins to age from the moment of conception. It is not until one approaches midlife and late life that the effects of aging are generally brought into awareness.

Self-Concept Crisis: Aging and Ageism

To understand aging and the developmental crisis that can occur in late life, it is necessary to define aging from several perspectives. **Biologic age** refers to the inherent biologic changes in an individual over time, ending with death. **Social age** refers to a person's roles, habits, and capacity to behave in a specific society when compared to others in the society who are the same age. **Psychologic age** refers to the adaptive responses a person makes to changing environmental demands (Burnside, 1988). These aspects of aging assist in understanding that growing old is not simply a matter of adding a number each time a birthday occurs. Biologic, social, and psychologic influences of aging must be considered when viewing the consequences of aging in late life. The many bodily changes, social encounters, and psychologic influences that occur can serve as catalysts for a self-concept crisis as one attempts to adapt to both expected and unexpected events in late adulthood.

The person in late adulthood has adaptations to make and issues to resolve. These include adapting to decreased physical ability, accepting and managing chronic illnesses, losing friends and family, and recognizing one's mortality. Added stress occurs when the elderly become victims of ageism. **Ageism** is a process of systematic stereotyping of and discriminating against old people simply because they are old. It occurs whenever an attitude or action discriminates solely on the basis of age. Ageist attitudes regarding older adults are not a new phenomenon in the United States. Throughout U.S. history the elderly have been categorized as unnecessary and burdensome. Ageism can be compared to racism and sexism by persons seeking an understanding of its causes and impact. It is perpetuated whenever older persons have decreased social status and decreased contact with younger individuals (Murray, 1989).

Behavioral Characteristics In the United States old age is often portrayed solely as a time of dependence and disease. Movies, books, magazines, television, and jokes often contribute to negative beliefs and attitudes about an aged person's behavior. Society's general fear of aging is projected onto all aging individuals. The young person, who considers time a priceless commodity, may demonstrate anger and frustration when driving behind an elderly person or moving through a grocery store behind an elderly person who moves more slowly. A lack of understanding about physiologic changes may contribute to the young person's frustration. All members of society must correct these negative attitudes if older adults are to successfully adapt to the aging process.

Older persons usually prefer to maintain households separate from their adult children or other relatives. However, disease and disability may require the individual to modify or accept assistance with ADLs. Learning to balance dependence, independence, and interdependence becomes essential at this time of life (Matteson and McConnell, 1988).

The income of the elderly can affect lifestyle and behavior patterns. The elderly are disproportionately represented in the low-income brackets. Their median income is approximately one-half that of younger groups. Over 80 percent of the elderly receive social security benefits, but many still have incomes below the poverty level. The problem of elderly poverty is especially acute for women and minorities, the fastest-growing segments of the aged population. Only 12 percent of white elderly are below the poverty level as compared to 22 percent of Hispanic, 32 percent of Native-American, and 35 percent of African-American elderly. Learning to adjust to decreased income or relying on significant others for financial assistance may become necessary. Even if the person has participated in financial planning for retirement, the death of a spouse, unexpected hospitalizations, and decreased insurance coverage can account for financial stressors during this period (Dychtwald and Flower, 1989; Grau, 1989; Matteson and McConnell, 1988).

Most older adults maintain activity levels and behavior in the later years that are similar to behavior in earlier life. Adaptation in old age is associated with maintaining as many activities as possible and finding new leisure and social activities. Many begin new creative endeavors, develop new art talents, and participate in special activities such as Senior Olympics and Elder Hostel.

Affective Characteristics One of the major affective tasks in old age is to review life accomplishments. When the elderly feel positive about the majority of life events, a sense of satisfaction or ego integrity is achieved. These people talk about happiness, a sense of hope, and an anticipation of the remaining future. If the individual views life as missed opportunities and failures, a sense of despair occurs. This despair is associated with feelings of frustration and bitterness.

Myths and stereotypes associated with aging are culturally determined. Ageism includes viewing the older adult as asexual, unemployable, unintelligent, and socially inept. When elderly people share in and believe these stereotypes, they find themselves feeling helpless, hopeless, and depressed. Table 6–4 includes some of the myths that have been perpetuated through the years.

Cognitive Characteristics Negative stereotyping is prevalent in the area of intellectual functioning of the older adult. Stereotypes include the beliefs that, with age, thinking and problem-solving abilities become rigid, judgment is impaired, learning capacity is reduced, memory lapses are frequent, and severe mental confusion is inevitable. These stereotypes may be an accurate portrayal of the cognitive functioning of only 10 to 15 percent of the older population. Although cognitive performance seems to peak during middle adulthood, at ap-

Table 6–4 *Ageism: Fiction or Fact?*

Fiction:	Most older people are placed in institutions.
Fact:	Only 5% are in institutions; 67% live in a family setting and 30% live alone.
Fiction:	Old age brings senility and feeblemindedness.
Fact:	Only 5% show serious mental impairment; only 10% suffer from mild to moderate memory loss.
Fiction:	Old people cannot learn.
Fact:	Learning is not impaired, though a longer period of time may be needed to respond to stimuli.
Fiction:	All old people are similar.
Fact:	There is a great deal of diversity in personalities, motivations, physical abilities, lifestyles, and economics among older people.
Fiction:	The next generation of older adults will be the same as the present generation.
Fact:	The next generation will have more formal education and healthier lifestyle habits, be more youthful in appearance, have access to more technology, and be more assertive in their communication style.

Adapted from: Dychtwald, 1986; Guillford, 1988; Murray, 1989.

proximately 50 years of age, there is much controversy about the course of cognitive development in the later years. Declines in later life may be smaller in magnitude than previously thought (Schuster and Ashburn, 1986).

Cognitive tasks of the aged include coming to terms with the inevitability of mortality, learning to continue to live a happy life despite physical limitations and chronic illness, and learning to value life beyond parenting and working roles. Those who are unable to adapt develop a rigid, narrow life perspective as well as a negative and unaccepting cognitive focus.

Spirituality may be heightened during late adulthood. Expanding spiritual involvement can be helpful as the older adult further refines a philosophy of life and experiences a sense of worth. Successful adaptation includes balancing a personal spiritual philosophy with appropriate altruistic activities. Together they can increase acceptance, worth, and self-esteem.

Psychosocial Characteristics Some elderly only need to modify their lifestyles; others are forced to make drastic changes. Activities must be altered according to physical limitations and declining physical strength. Elderly persons and their families are faced with the decision of where and how the elderly will live their remaining years. This may include searching the community for satisfactory living arrangements. For those with limited income, the standard of living may need adjustment. When work roles have been a major aspect of life, the older person needs to find other meaningful activities after retirement. Often there is a need to redefine roles and responsibilities. Some maintain or increase their involvement in community activities. Some pursue new interests, such as volunteer work, to feel needed. It is important that the elderly establish affiliations with their own age group as well as maintaining relationships with children, grandchildren, siblings, relatives, and friends. If they do not, they will become isolated within the community.

Consequences and Resolution Positive resolution occurs when the developmental tasks and issues with which the older adult is presented are balanced successfully. This resolution is dependent on adaptation to the many physical, emotional, and social challenges associated with aging and ageism. Hope and acceptance of this life stage occurs when previously used coping skills or new strategies are used to prevent or resolve a crisis. Maladaptive responses occur when tasks and challenges are not resolved. Those with maladaptive responses may live in the past, be unable to take pleasure and joy in the present, and exhibit depression and a sense of hopelessness.

Nurses in all clinical settings are encouraged to combat subtle and overt ageism. An awareness of the scope of the problem of ageism in health care settings is the beginning step in eradicating it. Ageism influences the attitudes of health care professionals and decision makers regarding aggressiveness of care for the elderly. Using chronologic age as a determinant for the type of care received and viewing treatment on the basis of an elderly person's perceived contribution to society are ageist practices. When older people themselves believe the stereotypes, their behavior may conform; they become victims of self-fulfilling prophecies. Ageism has the effect of robbing society of the contributions of its older members and denying these members fulfillment of their human potential.

Nurses have a professional and societal responsibility to confront ageism and help both younger and older people modify their expectations, attitudes, beliefs, and feelings toward the aged in our culture. This can be done by providing information on the aging process and providing contact with successful older adult role models. Nurses can be vital instruments in assisting an elderly person in the last stage of life to live it to the fullest extent.

Dependency Crisis: Dealing with Multiple Losses

Along with the self-concept crisis associated with aging and ageism is yet another crisis situation. Philosophers and poets have written extensively about the later years as the "season of loss." Loss of work roles with retirement, loss of body image, and loss associated with mortality are both expected and unexpected events for the older adult. Dealing with immortality and death is perhaps the most significant psychosocial stressor of late adulthood. Losing significant others can result in feelings of powerlessness and isolation. On the Life-Events Stress Scale developed by Holmes and Rahe (1967), death of a spouse receives a score of 100 and is considered the most stressful situation.

Another profound stressor facing the older adult is dealing with his or her own imminent death. Death is frequently viewed as the ultimate loss. It involves not only the loss of all significant relationships but also the loss of oneself. The older adult is more likely to think about death, more likely to discuss death, but less likely to show a fear of death (Wass and Myers, 1982). Death is not unique to the aged, but the chances of it occurring are greater for them than for any other age group. People are socialized to understand that aging and death are related. The dying process is seen by many persons as the final developmental step in the human life span.

Usually death is not a sudden, unexpected event. Generally the dying person and the family have had time before death to gradually accept the consequences associated with the impending loss. Unexpected deaths may have a greater potential for crisis because adaptive mechanisms have not been developed.

The elderly constantly face loss. For many people death is the ultimate loss because it is the loss of consciousness. Loss of significant others can occur not only by death, but also by relocation. Placing a loved one in a nursing home or having children move away can leave a void in the elderly person's life. Other losses include loss of control and competence, loss of some life experiences, loss of material possessions, and loss of dreams. The goal for the older adult who has confronted loss is to use adaptive mechanisms to understand and accept the inevitability of those losses and live the remaining years to the maximum potential.

Parkes and Brown (1972, p. 5) said that "the pain of grief is just as much a part of life as the joy of love. It is, perhaps, the price we pay for love, the cost of commitment." Grieving is a necessary process for effective functioning. Worden (1982) outlined four tasks that need to be accomplished to move past the grief process. The first task for the grieving person is accepting the reality of the loss. Denying the death or even denying the meaning of the death can lead to prolonged maladaptive grief.

The second task for the grieving person is accepting that grief is painful. Maladaptive ways of avoiding pain include use of alcohol or drugs, avoidance of angry feelings, remorse and sadness, and excessive work and sex.

The third task is adjusting to an environment that no longer includes the person who has died. New skills may need to be acquired. Doing things alone to remain as independent as possible is an adaptive response. The grieving person accomplishes the fourth task with the passage of time. He or she must withdraw much of the emotional energy invested in the deceased person and reinvest it in other relationships.

Stages of grief have frequently been cited in the literature. Many people have applied Elisabeth

Kubler-Ross's five stages of dying to the process of grieving. The first stage is denial, when people refuse to believe the reality of impending death. The second stage is anger and rage about the injustice and unfairness of life's ending. Bargaining, the third stage, occurs when dying people try to make a deal with God or fate in exchange for a longer life. Depression, preparatory grief for the end of life, is the fourth stage of dying. The final stage is acceptance, which includes disengagement from life and a quiet expectation of death.

Behavioral Characteristics When one becomes widowed, there are drastic life changes. Women are more likely than men to be widowed. Between the ages of 65 and 74, 40 percent of women and only 10 percent of men are widowed. In the over-75 age group, 70 percent of women and 30 percent of men are widowed (Allan and Brotman, 1981). In the past, widows were incorporated into the extended family structure and were considered a family responsibility. In today's society many women value independent living and choose to remain in their own homes—a response that is often a positive adaptation. However, if the single older woman becomes isolated from her family and friends, maladaption may occur in the areas of physical, psychologic, social, and financial well-being.

Personal loss brought about through widowhood is often extreme. Research indicates that widows have a higher rate of mortality and suicide and report poorer physical health. Most widows live alone, and many find this to be a problem. Because they feel uncomfortable or unaccepted alone, widows often curtail social activities. Research indicates that most widows eventually regain their equilibrium, but one in five never recovers from the grief (Kaplan, 1988).

Each phase of the grief process requires certain adaptations and behavior alterations. Physical symptoms of anxiety may appear. Weakness; shortness of breath; hyperventilation; anorexia; diarrhea; nausea; tightness in the chest; oversensitivity to noise; and feelings of helplessness, disbelief, and confusion occur in the **shock phase**. This period can last from a few minutes to several days. In the second stage, the **defensive retreat phase**, withdrawal and isolating the self from emotions occurs. This period may last from hours to days. Denial may be used to cope with intense anxiety as well as the feelings of helplessness and confusion.

With the **acknowledgment phase** admission of the loss begins. Anger and intermittent periods of denial are seen first. As time passes, the person grieving the loss becomes preoccupied with it. Physical symptoms in all body systems may occur, and experiencing symptoms similar to those of the deceased is not uncommon. This unconscious physical identification may be related to anger at the deceased for dying—anger that is then experienced as guilt. Depression and self-hate may exhaust the person if the guilt is not resolved. The next phases of grieving are the **idealization phase** and the **identification phase**. During these phases there is a conscious adoption of some characteristics of the deceased. After identification takes place, normal behavior patterns return and the **resolution phase**, the last phase, occurs (Gioiella and Bevil, 1985).

A number of factors influence the length of the process, its intensity, and the final outcome for each individual. Some of these factors are the degree of dependency, past experience with loss, the number of recent losses, present level of health, and the feelings of guilt and anger directed toward the deceased.

Affective Characteristics The affective characteristics of the grieving process are so closely intertwined with behavior that they are presented together in the previous section. Feelings of anger, guilt, depression, hopelessness, powerlessness, and feelings of wanting to regress to past experiences occur at different intensities. The losses associated with body image changes and work roles may produce similar feelings.

According to Erikson, ego integrity is the final task for the older adult, and success involves the blending of all facets of the previous phases of the life cycle. The successful older adult has found the ability to resolve the losses of aging and is able to integrate ongoing losses with a sense of hope and acceptance of an uncertain future.

Without a sense of ego integrity the older adult feels a sense of despair and disgust. When issues are not resolved there may be a continual desire to relive past experiences. There is an inability to find pleasure in the present and a sense of hopelessness presides.

Cognitive Characteristics Preparing for death is an important cognitive task for the older adult. This is accomplished in several ways. Most important is the performance of the life review. The life review involves talking about past opportunities, relationships, mistakes, and successes. This process fills a need and permits the older adult to make peace and accept death. The life review may include finalizing a long-awaited goal, resolving interpersonal conflict, or saying good-bye to significant others. The older adult who is able to place value on past experiences is more likely to face death with the least difficulty. This person finds meaning and understanding in life's final developmental task.

Psychosocial Characteristics The American culture is a death-denying culture in which talking openly about death is often considered taboo. This cultural attitude greatly influences the older adult's acceptance of the dying process. To fear death leads to the institutionalization of this final stage of growth. It is not uncommon for older Americans to spend their final days in hospitals and nursing homes. In general, people no longer die in the home, surrounded by family and friends. Family and professionals avoid talking openly with the dying person. Thus, many people experience the dying process alone. The cultural value of denial of death hinders the older adult's acceptance of death, and this natural process of life evolves into a crisis situation (Hoff, 1989).

Consequences and Resolution Living with the losses associated with aging and facing imminent death are potential stressors for the older adult. When coping with these stressors he or she may respond in an adaptive or maladaptive way. Some continually focus on what did not occur in life and are filled with a sense of despair. In the face of this overwhelming negativism, family and friends often avoid the despairing older adult. Many older adults are able to focus on positive achievements and review their lives with a sense of humor and high self-esteem. Family and friends find delight in sharing this positive process. As Plato stated in *The Republic:* "It gives me great pleasure to converse with the aged. They have been over the road that all of us must travel, and know where it is rough and difficult and where it is level and easy."

Some nurses have difficulty dealing with loss and death since they view the essence of caring as supporting life processes. To accept death as a process of life enables other nurses to support people through this final stage of growth. To be effective care givers, nurses must be willing to talk openly about death as well as accept their own mortality. As Hoff (1989, p. 418) states: "A healthy attitude toward our own death is our most powerful asset in assisting the dying through this final life passage and comforting their survivors."

Assessment

Assessment of potential developmental crises includes an accurate perception of the crisis from the client's viewpoint. The information elicited in the client history and physical examination should be specifically directed at gathering appropriate data. The following Focused Nursing Assessment for Clients in Crisis suggests guidelines for data gathering.

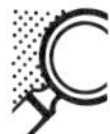

FOCUSED NURSING ASSESSMENT *for Clients in Crisis*

Individual Assessment

What is the most significant stress/problem occurring in your life right now?

For whom is this a problem? You? Family members? Employer? Community?

How long has this been a problem?

Is this a temporary or permanent problem?

What does this problem mean to you?
What are the factors that cause this problem to continue?
Have you had similar stresses/problems in the past?
What past events have influenced the current problem?
What other stresses do you have in your life?
How are you managing your usual life roles (spouse, parent, homemaker, worker, student, etc)?
In what way has your lifestyle changed as a result of this problem?
Describe how you have managed problems in the past.
What have you done to try and solve the problem so far?
What happened when you tried this?
Describe possible resources (eg, family, friends, employer, teacher, financial, religious).
What are your expectations and hopes concerning this problem?
What is the most you hope for when this problem is resolved?
What is the least you will settle for to resolve this problem?
Which part of the overall problem is most important to deal with first?

Family Assessment
How do you perceive the current problem?
In what way has the problem affected your roles in the family?
How has your lifestyle changed since this problem began?
Describe communication within the family before this current problem.
Describe communication within the family since the problem began.
How does the family typically manage problems?
What has the family done to try and solve the problem so far?
What happened when you tried this?
How well do you believe the family is coping at this time?
Describe possible resources (eg, extended family, friends, financial).
What are your expectations and hopes concerning this problem?
Which part of the overall problem is most important to deal with first?

Community Assessment
What are the special demands of the client's community?
What are the living conditions of the neighborhood?
How adequate or supportive is the school system?
Are recreational centers available?
Is there a community mental health center?
What support groups are available in the community?

It should be noted that anxiety and depression are the two most common presenting symptoms of poor coping and potential maladaptive resolution to the crisis. In the ideal situation clients recognize their own psychologic discomfort and actively participate with nurses in crisis resolution. If distortion or a lost sense of reality render the client unaware of maladaptive responses and unable to participate in resolution, psychiatric consultation may be advised.

Nursing Diagnosis and Planning

The planning phase should be based on developing nursing diagnoses and defining realistic and measurable goals generated from the assessment data. (See Tables 6–5 through 6–12 for lists of possible nursing diagnoses.) Planning involves developing creative strategies for crisis resolution. Including the family and significant others is essential if a workable plan is to be achieved. Effective communication between all participants is essential. New coping strategies may be initiated along with strategies the client has defined as helpful in past crisis situations.

Table 6–5 *Nursing Diagnoses for Children of Divorce*

Hopelessness related to loss of familiar family structure
Altered growth and development, regression, related to adapting to new family structure
Impaired social interaction related to acting out anger resulting from family disruption
Anxiety related to separation from out-of-home parent
Ineffective family coping, compromised, related to custodial parent experiencing role overload
Fear related to thoughts that custodial parent may abandon them
Fear related to thoughts that siblings may be separated
Fear related to thoughts of marital failure in own future adult lives
Family coping, potential for growth, related to healthy adaptation of binuclear family

Table 6–6 *Nursing Diagnoses for Socially Isolated Teens*

Impaired social interaction related to lack of conversational skills
Impaired social interaction related to anxiety in social situations
Impaired social interaction related to lack of empathy with others
Self-esteem disturbance related to incompetence in social situations
Self-esteem disturbance related to continued dependence on family

Table 6–7 *Nursing Diagnoses for Teens Involved in Gangs*

Impaired social interaction related to socially inappropriate behavior
Impaired adjustment related to delinquent behavior
Potential for violence, directed at others, related to disrespect for others' rights
Potential for violence, directed at others, related to fights with rival gangs
Fear related to inability to leave gang and establish own identity
Self-esteem disturbance related to highly dependent relationship with gang
Altered role performance related to using illegitimate means to achieve money and status

Table 6–8 *Nursing Diagnoses for Teen Parents*

Ineffective individual coping related to lack of education, which contributes to underemployment or unemployment
Social isolation related to leaving the school peer group
Ineffective family coping, compromised, related to girl's parents refusal to include teen father in parenting
Powerlessness related to feeling trapped by early parenthood
Anxiety related to anticipated labor and delivery process
Altered role performance related to sudden elevation to adult status and responsibilities
Ineffective denial related to fear of telling parents, which results in poor prenatal care
Ineffective family coping, compromised, related to increased conflict between parents and teen
Altered role performance related to parents' difficulty recognizing their adolescent daughter as a responsible parent
Family coping, potential for growth, related to involvement of teen father
Family coping, potential for growth, related to teen parents' participation in parenting classes
Family coping, potential for growth, related to teen parents' ability to complete education and find occupation

Table 6–9 *Nursing Diagnoses for Adults in Midlife Crisis*

Impaired social interaction related to inability in finding satisfaction with spouse
Altered role performance related to unsuccessful attempts at career achievement
Sexual dysfunction related to altered body image
Altered sexuality patterns related to inability to reestablish intimacy
Spiritual distress related to inability to find meaning and purpose in life
Ineffective individual coping related to inability to adapt to physical changes of middle age
Impaired adjustment related to a change in life goals and ambitions
Defensive coping related to continuation of youthful appearance and behaviors
Ineffective family coping, disabling, related to inability to balance work with other roles
Noncompliance related to lack of acceptance of decreased strength and endurance
Altered growth and development related to inability to accept challenges of the future
Altered growth and development related to personal dissatisfaction with life choices
Health-seeking behaviors related to reappraisal of lifestyle practices
Family coping, potential for growth, related to realistic use of time, interest, and energy
Family coping, potential for growth, related to finding pleasure in generativity
Body image disturbance related to inability to accept changes of aging
Self-esteem disturbance related to blocked career advancement
Anxiety related to recognition of own mortality
Anxiety related to unsuccessful attempts at using leisure time creatively
Anxiety related to inability to establish healthful living practices
Fear related to growing old
Fear related to unsuccessful attempts to form a philosophy of life

There are three basic **crisis intervention models** that provide a framework for intervention strategies. These are the equilibrium model, the cognitive model, and the psychosocial transition model.

The *equilibrium model* describes crisis as a state of psychologic or emotional disequilibrium, in which usual coping mechanisms and problem-solving abilities fail. The goal of this model is to help people reach a state of precrisis equilibrium. This model is useful as an early intervention when the person is out of control and unable to make ap-

Table 6–10 *Nursing Diagnoses for Two-Generation Conflict*

Impaired verbal communication related to youth's seeking independence
Potential altered parenting related to inability for open communication
Altered family processes related to conflicting lifestyle choices
Decisional conflict related to generational differences in values
Anxiety related to noncompliant adolescent behavior
Family coping, potential for growth, related to parents assisting youth in becoming responsible, independent adult
Social isolation related to acceptance of care giver role
Impaired social interaction related to lack of privacy within the home
Altered role performance related to role reversal of adult child and aging parent
Fatigue related to physical and emotional demands of the aging parent
Sleep pattern disturbance related to acceptance of care giver responsibilities
Diversional activity deficit related to restriction in time and freedom
Helplessness related to inability to find acceptable solutions for the care of the dependent parent
Anxiety related to increased parental-care responsibilities
Anxiety related to financial burden of caring for dependents of two generations
Potential for violence, directed at others, related to demands of the dependent adult
Ineffective family coping, disabling, related to conflicting demands for time
Social isolation related to lack of time for social or leisure activities
Family coping, potential for growth, related to seeing strength in intergenerational ties
Family coping, potential for growth, related to acknowledging wisdom and insight of the elderly

propriate choices. Stabilizing the individual until some coping abilities are regained is the major focus. For example, before identifying underlying factors for suicidal ideation, an individual considering suicide must be stabilized to the point of recognizing that life is worth living.

The *cognitive model* of crisis intervention describes crises in terms of faulty thinking about the events or situations that surround the crisis. The goal of this model is to assist people in becoming aware of and to change their beliefs and perceptions about the crisis event or situation. According to this model, people can gain control of crisis situations in their lives by changing their thinking. Removing the irrational portions of their thoughts

Table 6–11 *Nursing Diagnoses for the Aging Adult*

Alteration in nutrition, more than body requirements, related to decreased metabolic demand
Constipation related to immobility
Impaired social interaction related to altered living arrangements as a result of role change
Spiritual distress related to inability to find meaning in life
Impaired adjustment related to retirement from active work responsibilities
Social isolation related to unsatisfactory living arrangements
Altered role performance related to decreased strength and health changes
Altered sexuality patterns related to nonacceptance of body image
Ineffective individual coping related to unsuccessful attempts at forming a philosophy of life
Family coping, potential for growth, related to acceptance of wisdom and insight of the elderly
Family coping, potential for growth, related to finding satisfactory relationships with children and grandchildren
Noncompliance related to inability to recognize the aging process and its health care prescriptions
Self-esteem disturbance related to lack of acceptance of retirement role
Powerlessness related to inadequate finances and economic burdens
Hopelessness related to isolation from significant others
Anxiety related to inability to associate with own age group

Table 6–12 *Nursing Diagnoses for Older Adults with Multiple Losses*

Impaired verbal communication related to unsuccessful resolution of grieving process
Social isolation related to sudden occurrence of widowhood
Spiritual distress related to hopelessness and despair in life review
Ineffective individual coping related to multiple losses occurring during the same period
Impaired adjustment related to nonsupportive relationships from significant others
Defensive coping related to excessive guilt and anger in grieving process
Ineffective denial related to inability to complete the grieving process
Altered family processes related to inability to find appropriate social relationships after the death of significant other
Body image disturbance related to multiple physiologic losses
Self-esteem deficit related to continuous feelings of despair
Powerlessness related to inadequate societal provisions for the elderly
Altered thought process related to inability to work through the stages of grief
Fear related to inevitability of mortality
Dysfunctional grieving related to preoccupations with the deceased beyond normal grief process
Family coping, potential for growth, related to successful resolution of ego integrity

and retaining the rational components is the primary focus of interventions. Crisis intervention involves rehearsing positive statements about the situation until the negative disabling thoughts are removed. This model may be most appropriate after the client has been stabilized and returned to a state of precrisis equilibrium.

The *psychosocial transition model* views people as being made up of hereditary components plus learning that has occurred from exposure to social environments. A crisis state is related to psychologic, social, or environmental difficulties. In this model, crisis intervention takes on a collaborative role, helping the client assess internal and external difficulties and choose workable alternatives to the current behavior, attitudes, and use of environmental resources. The psychosocial transition model is most appropriate after the client has been stabilized (Gilliland and James, 1988).

The primary goal of crisis intervention is to assist the client who faces a stressful situation to resolve the immediate problem and regain emotional equilibrium. Assisting the client in the problem-solving process will, hopefully, lead to better use of coping mechanisms when dealing with future stressful life events.

The role of the nurse in crisis intervention is one of active participation in solving the problem. It is important to point out that the nurse does not take over and make decisions for clients unless they are suicidal or homicidal. The primary point of crisis intervention is self-help on the part of the client, with assistance from the nurse.

As a crisis intervener the nurse demonstrates caring, nurturing, listening, and willingness to help. The client and nurse reexamine any feelings or thoughts blocking effective coping. The nurse also assists the client in communicating directly with significant others to avoid feelings of isolation and withdrawn behavior. Persons who are highly independent may need to recognize the importance of interdependence; they may need to be taught to ask for help.

As an intervener the nurse assists in teaching and helping the client develop adaptive coping skills. During the crisis state the client is more receptive to trying a variety of coping behaviors to decrease anxiety. Examples of coping mechanisms that may be appropriate include open communication of feelings, relaxation techniques, and physical exercise.

The nurse keeps the client focused on the specific problem and specific goals leading to crisis resolution. With increased anxiety the client may have difficulty focusing on the specific task and may need direction to avoid fragmentation. The nurse must remember to continually reinforce the client's strengths by reviewing the crisis event, the coping effectiveness, and new methods of problem solving that have been learned.

In some crisis situations a team approach may be used. This is true in many short-term inpatient psychiatric treatment facilities. Generally the team is composed of a group of clinicians of different educational backgrounds. A psychiatrist, psychiatric mental health nurse, psychologist, social worker, minister, and student may make up the team. Leadership rotates with each team meeting, and one person assumes the role of primary person responsible for the management of the client. Continuity of care and adherence to goals must be reinforced when the team approach is used.

Nurses intervening in a crisis environment should possess professional characteristics that aid in resolving the crisis and restoring equilibrium. Effective nurse interveners

- Display calmness, poise, and control in an environment that is often out of control
- Possess ability to utilize therapeutic communication skills
- Display congruence between thinking, feeling, and acting
- Have accurate assessment skills
- Possess ability to diagnose, analyze, and synthesize assessment data
- Demonstrate ability to explore alternative solutions to problems
- Practice assertive communication, relaxation and stress reduction skills, and other helpful techniques

Consistency is an important aspect of intervention. Once the plan has been established, the need for consistency must be communicated to all people involved. Consistency is important in helping the client regain adaptive functioning patterns and avoiding maladaptive behaviors.

Evaluation

Evaluating the outcome of the specified interventions is the final stage of crisis intervention. It is also an ongoing process that begins in the planning stage and continues throughout the implementation stage. When clients are not meeting outcome criteria based on evaluation, the nurse returns to the assessment phase and modifies the plan as necessary. Through recognition of the dynamics of each potential crisis situation and conscientious use of the nursing process for critical problem solving, the nurse assists in making each stage of the life span a positive and meaningful experience.

SUMMARY

1. Maturational crises are expected events occurring at transition periods in normal growth and development. Expected life changes are those which are anticipated at particular ages. However, not all people choose or have the opportunity to experience all the expected life changes.

2. Situational crises are unavoidable and often unexpected traumatic events. Unexpected life changes refer to experiences one never expected to have or experiences one expected to occur at a different stage in life.

3. Developmental crises often occur when unexpected life changes happen at the same time individuals are struggling with expected transitions.

4. At the end of a crisis period, the individual will either adapt and return to a previous level of functioning, develop more constructive coping skills, or decompensate to a lower level of functioning.

Knowledge Base

5. Stage theories view development as progressing in stagelike sequence.

6. Information processing theory looks at the way people take in information, process it, and act on it.

7. The behavioral approach to development maintains that environment determines behavior and if environment changes, behavior is altered.

8. Social-learning theory believes that people learn by observing others and imitating their behavior throughout development.

9. Crises occur when stress disrupts equilibrium and there is a deficiency in problem-solving and effective coping.

10. The phases of crisis are traumatic event and ineffective coping, increased anxiety, needing to reach out for assistance, inadequate internal and external support systems, unproductive and impulsive behavior, deterioration of relationships, looking to others to solve the problem, feelings of "going crazy."

11. Behavioral coping skills include the use of the problem-solving process.

12. Affective coping skills emphasize managing the feelings provoked by the event.

13. Cognitive coping skills help the person find meaning in and understand the personal significance of the event.

14. Psychosocial skills enable the individual to maintain relationships with family and friends throughout and after the crisis period.

15. Separation and divorce may be the child's first significant loss. It is not uncommon for children to experience regression, anxiety, depression, and anger. Some children inappropriately blame themselves and worry about who will care for them. Adaptive resolution is partly dependent on the parents' abilities to function as a binuclear family.

16. Peer groups function to promote adolescents' adjustment to the adult world. Some teens are unable to develop meaningful peer relationships and become isolated and lonely young adults. They do not have the opportunity to develop social skills, experience intimate relationships, or develop a positive self-concept.

17. Some teens find their peer group within the gang structure. Their hostile, defiant, and socially inappropriate behavior creates multiple problems. Their anger is rooted in frustration and protest. They develop a high level of solidarity with the values and beliefs of the gang. The two-tier approach to troubled adolescents most typically results in white teens being processed through the mental health system and African-American and Hispanic youth being processed through the criminal justice system.

18. The United States leads all developed countries in

the pregnancy and abortion rates among adolescent women. There are profound consequences as a result of teen parenthood. Many choose to be single parents, often drop out of school, and are forced to reorganize their self-concept in formulating an identity as a parent. Many teen fathers are concerned and eager to be involved in parenting. Adolescent parenthood is a major cause of low-income family units in this country.

19. Midlife crisis is a period of acknowledging physical changes, focusing on career achievement, and further developing a philosophy of life. The ability to accept physical changes, acknowledge reality, find meaning in work, develop a positive identity, and place life in perspective fosters a higher level of functioning following the crisis period.

20. At a time when middle adults expect greater independence, they may find both their parents and young adult children dependent on them. All three generations may be living in the same home. Assisting children and providing care for aging parents may result in a crisis as lifestyles change, role conflict occurs, and financial burdens increase.

21. Ageism is a process of stereotyping and discriminating against older people on the basis of age.

22. Older adults may experience self-concept crises as they attempt to maintain their previous lifestyles. Maladaptive responses result in people who live in the past, take no joy in the present, and feel hopeless about all of life. Adaptive responses result in people who find meaning and understanding in the past and live in the present with a sense of joy and hope.

23. Older adults are faced with grieving multiple losses and dealing with their own imminent deaths. The phases of the grieving process are shock, defensive retreat, acknowledgment, idealization, identification, and resolution. The four tasks of grieving are accepting the reality of the loss, accepting grief as painful, adjusting to a new environment, and reinvestment in other relationships.

Assessment

24. For assessment to be accurate, the nurse must comprehend the crisis situation from the client's point of view.

25. Anxiety and depression are often cues of a potential maladaption to a crisis.

26. The assessment process includes the individual, the family, and the community in which they live.

Diagnosis and Planning

27. Including the family and significant others is essential if a workable intervention plan is to be achieved.

28. The goal of crisis intervention is to assist the person and family in distress by resolving the immediate problem and returning the people involved to a state of emotional equilibrium.

29. The nurse formulates appropriate nursing diagnoses and outcome criteria from the assessment data.

30. Three basic models provide a framework for interventions: the equilibrium model, the cognitive model, and the psychosocial transition model.

31. Nurses actively participate during crisis intervention. They help clients communicate, assist in the development of adaptive coping skills, and keep clients focused on the specific problem and specific goals.

Evaluation

32. Evaluation is based on the achievement or nonachievement of outcome criteria. Nonachievement demands a return to further assessment followed by modification of the plan of care.

CHAPTER REVIEW

Maria and Joe, both age 42, have begun marital counseling with a nurse psychotherapist. Maria states that Joe has been very "unsettled" for the past six months and alternately irritable and depressed for the past three weeks. The result has been strain on their marital relationship. They have been married 15 years and have no children. Joe is a vice-president of a successful small business, and Maria is a lawyer in private practice.

Joe has been worrying lately about "time running out" and concerned about achieving his long-term goal of owning his own business. He has been talking often about quitting his job and starting a business, but he has been unable to come to a definite decision. Sometimes he fantasizes about quitting the "whole thing" and running off someplace to "start a new life."

Maria is very suspicious that Joe is having an extramarital affair. Her suspicions are based on Joe's behavior during the last six months. He suddenly became concerned about his body and physical condition, joined a health club, and lost 15 pounds. He purchased an entire new wardrobe in an attempt to project a "younger" image. He has had more late evening business meetings and responds with anger when Maria questions him when he returns home.

1. According to developmental theories for adults, Joe is facing the challenge of

(a) Autonomy and commitment to family
(b) Urgency to attain life goals

(c) Finding meaning and purpose in past life
(d) Formation of identity and independence

2. Based on initial assessment data the nurse has determined that Joe is experiencing a maturational crisis. Before beginning crisis intervention it is important that the nurse ask Joe which one of the following questions:
(a) "Which part of the overall problem is most important to deal with first?"
(b) "It is important to know if you are having an affair. Is Maria correct about this?"
(c) "Are you having thoughts about hurting or killing yourself?"
(d) "In what ways does the need to make perfect decisions hinder your life?"

3. In assessing Maria and Joe as a couple, it is important that the nurse ask them which of the following questions:
(a) "Do you think Joe's affair is related to sexual problems in your relationship?"
(b) "Are the two of you jealous of one another's career opportunities?"
(c) "What have you done to try and solve the problems so far?"
(d) "Joe, if you quit your job do you expect Maria to support you?"

4. Which one of the following nursing diagnoses is most appropriate for Joe?
(a) Spiritual distress related to inability to find meaning and purpose in life
(b) Defensive coping related to continuance of youthful appearance and behaviors
(c) Ineffective family coping, disabling, related to inability to balance work and home roles
(d) Anxiety related to unsuccessful attempts at using leisure time creatively

5. The goal of crisis intervention is to
(a) Resolve all the problems that have occurred in the client's life
(b) Continue long-term therapy until the individual demonstrates improved coping
(c) Help the person understand how childhood crises have contributed to the current problem
(d) Resolve the immediate problem and return the person to the previous level of functioning or a higher level

6. The most important therapeutic tool the nurse utilizes in crisis intervention is
(a) The problem-solving process
(b) Client advocacy
(c) Client teaching
(d) A socializing agent

REFERENCES

Aguilera DC, Messick JM: *Crisis Intervention: Theory and Methodology,* 4th ed. Mosby, 1978.

Ahrons CR, Rodgers RH: *Divorced Families.* Norton, 1987.

Allan C, Brotman H: *Chartbook on Aging in America.* Prepared for 1981 White House Conference on Aging: Government Printing Office.

American Psychiatric Association: *Diagnostic and Statistical Manual of Mental Disorders,* 3rd ed., revised. Washington DC: American Psychiatric Association, 1987.

Baltes P, Willis S: "Toward Psychological Theories of Aging and Development." In: *Handbook of the Psychology of Aging.* Birren JE, Shaie KW (editors). Van Nostrand Reinhold, 1977.

Bandura A: *Social Foundations of Thought and Action: A Social Cognitive Theory.* Prentice-Hall, 1986.

Barret RL, Robinson BE: Adolescent fathers: Often forgotten parents. *Ped Nurs* 1986; 12(4):273–277.

Beck S: Research issues. In: *Handbook of Adolescent Psychology.* VanHasselt VB, Hersen M (editors). Pergamon Press, 1987; 227–241.

Beck SH, Beck RW: The formation of extended households during middle age. *J Marr and Fam* 1984; 46:277–286.

Burnside IM: *Nursing and the Aged: A Self-Care Approach.* McGraw-Hill, 1988.

Byer C, Shainberg LW, Jones KL: *Dimensions of Human Sexuality.* St. Louis: William Brown, 1988.

Carter B, McGoldrick M (editors): *The Changing Family Life Cycle,* 2nd ed. Gardner Press, 1988.

Connor ME: Teenage fatherhood: Issues confronting young black males. In: *Young, Black and Male in America.* Gibbs JT, et al. (editors). Auburn House, 1988; 188–218.

Country Beautiful: The life of man. *Country Beautiful,* 1973.

Dembo R: Delinquency among black male youth. In: *Young, Black and Male in America.* Gibbs JT, et al. (editors). Auburn House, 1988; 129–165.

DeV.Peters R, McMahon RJ (editors): *Social Learning and Systems Approaches to Marriage and the Family.* Brunner/Mazel, 1988.

Dychtwald K: Wellness and Health Promotion for the Elderly. Aspen Publications, 1986.

Dychtwald K, Flower J: *Age Wave.* Tarcher, 1989.

Field TM, Widmayer SM: Marriage and the family. In: *Handbook of the Psychology of Aging.* Wolfman BB (editor). Prentice-Hall, 1982.

Fulmer RH: Lower-income and professional families. In:

The Changing Family Life Cycle, 2nd ed. Carter B, McGoldrick M (editors). Gardner Press, 1988; 545–578.

Gameworks, Inc.: Instructions accompanying the game Can You Survive Your Midlife Crisis? 1982.

Gilchrist LD, Schinke SP: Adolescent Pregnancy and Marriage. In: *Handbook of Adolescent Psychology.* VanHasselt VB, Hersen M (editors). Pergamon Press, 1987; 424–441.

Gilliland BE, James RK: *Crisis Intervention Strategies.* Brooks/Cole, 1988.

Gioiella EC, Bevil CW: *Nursing Care of the Aging Client—Promoting Healthy Adaptation.* Appleton-Century-Crofts, 1985.

Gould R: *Transformations: Growth and Changes in Adult Life.* Simon & Schuster, 1978.

Grau L, Susser I: *Women in the Later Years.* Haworth Press, 1989.

Greenberg JS, et al.: *Sexuality: Insights and Issues.* St. Louis: William Brown 1989.

Guerin S, et al.: *The Evaluation and Treatment of Marital Conflict.* Basic Books, 1987.

Guillford DM: *The Aging Population in the Twenty-First Century.* National Academy Press, 1988.

Hall GS: In: *Developmental Psychology.* Moshman D, Glover J, Bruning RH (editors). Little, Brown, 1987.

Hoff LA: *People in Crisis,* 3rd ed. Addison-Wesley, 1989.

Holmes T, Rahe I: "The Social Readjustment Rating Scale." *J Psychosom Res* 1967; 11(2):213–218.

Hutchinson RL, Spangler-Hirsch SL: Children of divorced & single-parent lifestyles. In: *Children of Divorce.* Everett C (editor). Haworth Press, 1989; 5–24.

Johnson BS: *Psychiatric-Mental Health Nursing Adaptation and Growth.* Lippincott, 1986.

Kalish RA: *Death, Grief, and Caring Relationships,* 2nd ed. Brooks/Cole, 1985.

Kaplan PS: *The Human Odyssey-Life Span Development.* West, 1988.

Kaslow FW, Schwartz LL: *The Dynamics of Divorce.* Brunner/Mazel, 1987.

Kelly JA, Hansen DJ: Social interactions and adjustment. In: *Handbook of Adolescent Psychology.* VanHasselt VB, Hersen M (editors). Pergamon Press, 1987; 131–146.

Kingson ER, Hirshorn BA, Cornman JM: *Ties That Bind: The Interdependence of Generations.* Seven Lock Press, 1986.

Kubey R: The aging of aquarius. *The Chicago Tribune Magazine,* October 23, 1988.

Levinson DJ: *The Seasons of a Man's Life.* Ballantine, 1978.

Lowy L: *Social Work with the Aging.* Longman, 1985.

Matteson MA, McConnell ES: *Gerontological Nursing Concepts and Practices.* Saunders, 1988.

McMahon RJ, Forehand R: Conduct disorders. In: *Behavioral Assessment of Childhood Disorders,* 2nd ed. Mash EJ, Terdal LG (editors). Guilford Press, 1988; 105–153.

Mead M: *Culture and Commitment: A Study of the Generation Gap.* Doubleday, 1970.

Moos RH, Schaefer JA: *Coping with Life Crisis: An Integrated Approach.* Plenum, 1986.

Moos RH, Schaefer JA: Life transitions and crisis. In: *Coping with Life Crisis.* Moos RH (editor). 1986; 3–28.

Murray J, Park B: New study of teenage pregnancy. In: *Human Sexuality 88/89.* Pocs O (editor). Dushkin Publishing, 1988; 78–79.

Murray RB, Zentner JP: *Nursing Assessment & Health Promotion Strategies Through the Life Span,* 4th ed. Appleton & Lange, 1989.

National Center for Health Statistics, Feller B: Americans Needing Help to Function at Home. Advance data from *Vital Health Statistics,* No. 92, Washington, DC, D.H.H.S. Pub. No. (PHS) 83–1250, 1983.

Neugarten BL: *Middle Age and Aging.* University of Chicago, 1968.

Panzarine S, Elster A: Coping in a group of expectant adolescent fathers. In: *Coping with Life Crisis.* Moos RH (editor). 1986; 87–95.

Parkes CM, Brown R: Health after Bereavement: A Controlled Study of Young Boston Widows & Widowers. *Psychosom Med* 1972; 34:449–461.

Peck RC: Psychological development in the second half of life. In: *Middle Age and Aging.* Neugarten BL (editor). University of Chicago Press, 1968.

Peck JS: The impact of divorce on children at various stages of the family life cycle. In: *Children of Divorce.* Everett C (editor). Haworth Press, 1989; 81–106.

Riegal KF: Dialectic operations: The final period of cognitive development. *Human Development* 1973; 16: 346–370.

Rogers CR: *A Way of Being.* Houghton Mifflin, 1980.

Schuster CS, Ashburn SS: *The Process of Human Development,* 2nd ed. Little, Brown, 1986.

Stark E: Young, innocent and pregnant. In: *Human Sexuality 88/89.* Pocs O (editor). Dushkin Publishing, 1988; 80–83.

Sternberg RJ: What is an information-processing approach to human abilities? In: *Human Abilities: An Information Approach.* Sternberg RJ (editor). Freeman, 1985.

Thomas A, et al.: The origins of personality. *Scientific American* (Aug) 1970; 223:102–109.

Troll LE: Myths of midlife intergenerational relationships. In: *Midlife Myths.* Hunter S, Sandel M (editors). Sage, 1989; 210–231.

VanHasselt VB, Hersen M (editors): *Handbook of Adolescent Psychology.* Pergamon Press, 1987.

Wallerstein JS: Children of divorce. In: *Coping with Life Crisis.* Moos RH (editor). 1986; 35–48.

Walsh PE, Stolberg AL: Parental and environmental determinants of children's behavioral, affective and cognitive adjustment to divorce. In: *Children of Divorce.* Everett C (editor). Haworth Press, 1989; 265–282.

Wass H, Myers JE: Psychosocial aspects of death among the elderly: A review of the literature. *Personnel and Guidance Journal* 1982; 61:131–137.

White-Traut RC, Pabst MK: Parenting of hospitalized infants by adolescent mothers. *Ped Nurs* 1987; 13(2):97–100.

Worden JW: *Grief Counseling & Grief Therapy.* Springer, 1982.

SUGGESTED READINGS

Barry PD: *Psychological Nursing Assessment and Intervention.* Lippincott, 1984.

Bauer BB, Hill SS: *Essentials of Mental Health Care Planning and Interventions.* Saunders, 1986.

Bradshaw MJ: *Nursing of the Family in Health and Illness.* Appleton & Lange, 1988.

Breitung JC: *Caring For Older Adults.* Saunders, 1987.

Erikson EH: *Childhood and Society.* Norton, 1950.

Hurrelmann K, Engel U: *The Social Work of Adolescents: International Perspectives.* Walter de Gruyter, 1989.

Kermis MD: *Mental Health in Late Life: The Adaptive Process.* Jones & Bartlett, 1986.

Pinkston EM, Linsk NL: *Care of the Elderly: A Family Approach.* Pergamon, 1984.

Sheehy G: *Predictable Crisis of Adult Life.* Dutton, 1976.

Sundeen SJ, et al.: *Nurse Client Interaction—Implementing the Nursing Process.* Mosby, 1989.

Yurick AG, et al.: *The Aged Person and the Nursing Process.* Appleton-Century-Crofts, 1984.

Part Two

NURSING CARE OF PSYCHIATRIC CLIENTS

CHAPTER 7

Psychologic Influences on Physical Condition

J. SUE COOK
LESLIE BONJEAN

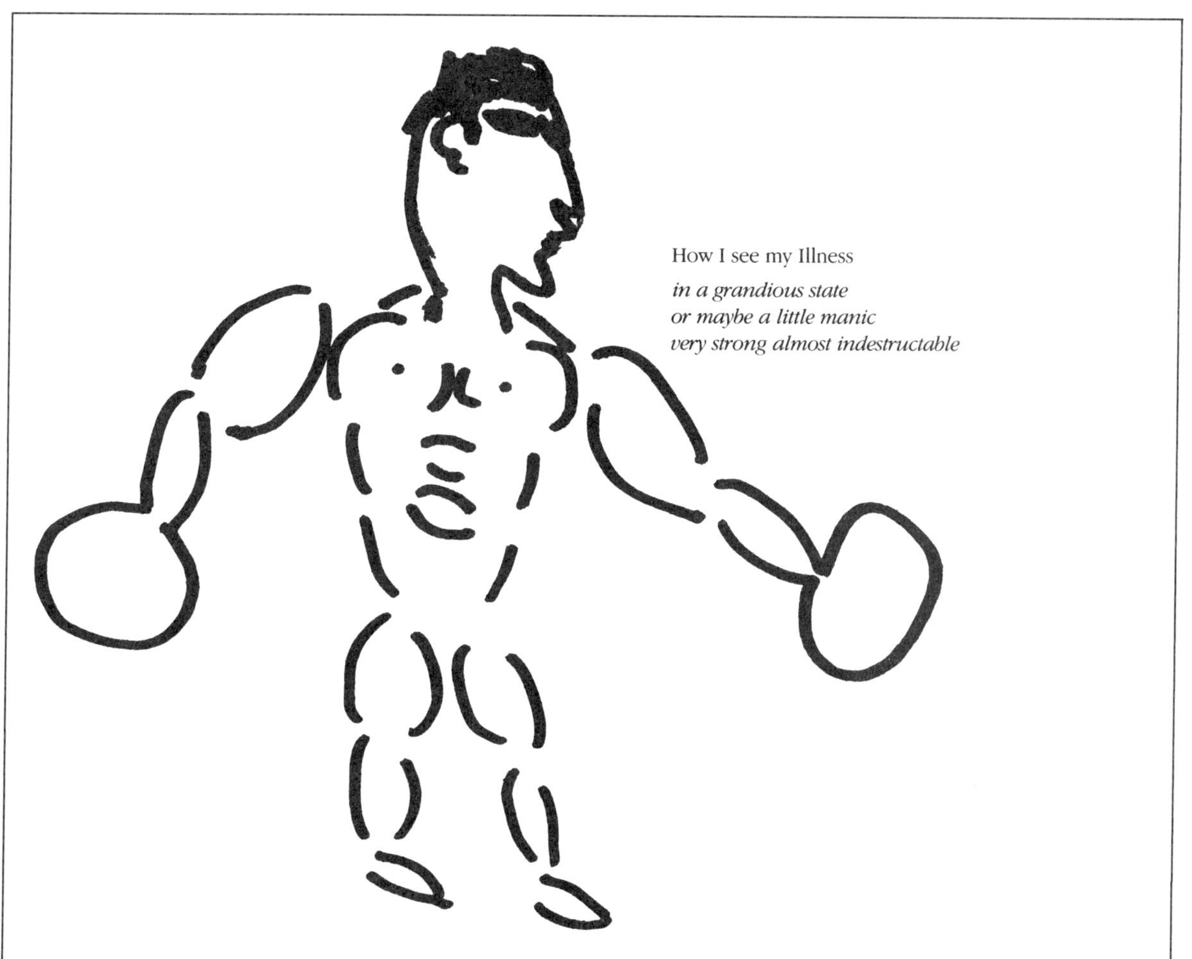

■ *Objectives*

After reading this chapter, the student will be able to

- Explain the concept of psychophysiologic disorders.
- Discuss the theory of stress.
- Describe the concept of crisis.
- Discuss current theory on psychophysiologic illness.
- Apply a nursing history tool to clients with coronary heart disease, cancer, respiratory disorders, gastrointestinal disorders, and other psychophysiologic disorders.
- Relate abnormal findings from the physical assessment of clients with various psychophysiologic disorders.
- Identify nursing diagnoses appropriate to clients with various psychophysiologic disorders.
- Prepare nursing care plans for clients with CHD, cancer, respiratory disorders, and gastrointestinal disorders.
- Discuss the evaluation of nursing care of the client with a psychophysiologic disorder.
- Apply the five steps of the nursing process to clinical situations involving clients with psychophysiologic disorders.

■ *Chapter Outline*

Introduction

The cases described in this chapter will sound like cases one would expect to see in a medical-surgical setting, rather than a psychiatric one. In fact they are, because the disorders depicted are psychophysiologic. Once classified as psychosomatic disorders, these types of problems are now included in DSM-III-R as "Psychological Factors Affecting Physical Condition." The presenting disorder is usually a physical disorder and, in some instances, may be a single physical symptom such as vomiting. Examples of physical conditions to which this category applies commonly include: obesity, tension headache, migraine headache, angina pectoris, painful menstruation, sacroiliac pain, neurodermatitis, acne, rheumatoid arthritis, asthma, tachycardia, arrhythmia, gastric ulcer, duodenal ulcer, cardiospasm, pylorospasm, nausea and vomiting, regional enteritis, ulcerative colitis, and urinary frequency. The diagnostic criteria for psychologic factors affecting physical condition include the following (American Psychiatric Association, 1987):

1. Psychologically meaningful environmental stimuli are related to the initiation or exacerbation of a specific physical symptom, condition, or disorder.
2. The physical condition involves organic pathology or an identifiable pathophysiologic process.
3. The criteria for a somatoform disorder are not present.

The term **psychophysiologic disorder** refers to the physical conditions in which psychologically meaningful events have been closely related to physical symptoms in a body organ system. In the field of nursing the concept of holism—the interaction between mind, body and the environment—has been recognized for a long time. The profession has identified the effects that individual experiences, thoughts, and perceptions can have on a person's life. In psychophysiologic disorders, manifestation of people's problems is through their bodies. For example, a person who has never learned to do adequate problem solving may be more prone to the development of an ulcer.

Disorders commonly referred to as psychophysiologic are cardiovascular disorders, specifically coronary heart disease (CHD) and hypertension (HTN); cancer; headaches; respiratory disorders, specifically asthma and allergies; gastrointestinal disorders, specifically peptic ulcers, ulcerative colitis, and irritable bowel syndrome; skin disorders, specifically dermatitis; and arthritis. This chapter will present disorders most likely to be found in the general hospital setting.

Theories of Stress

Since World War II much research has been done on the interaction between the mind and the body. Through the years numerous theories have been developed to explain the effects that psychological suffering can have on the body. The following section will describe those theories that seem most relevant to nursing. As with all theories, they are meant to give the nurse a scientific basis for understanding the person and his or her disease process. It is important to keep in mind that current research suggests that psychophysiologic disorders may be manifested for a number of reasons, rather than from a single cause. In other words, nurses may need to utilize multiple theories to gain an understanding of their patients in a holistic sense.

Selye's Model Hans Selye, considered the father of stress theory, conducted his initial studies of stress in the late 1930s, and in 1950 he published his famous treatise on the subject. Selye (1956) defined **stress** as "the nonspecific response of the body to any demand made upon it." That is, stimuli such as physical injury, infection, psychologic tension, and so forth can be considered **stressors** and produce a nonspecific response in the body.

Selye named the stress syndrome the **General Adaptation Syndrome (GAS)**. His studies suggested that adaptive hormones were released during stress creating common symptoms such as weight loss, fatigue, aches, malaise, and gastrointestinal upsets. According to Selye's theory, GAS appears whenever the body is subjected to continued stress. Manifestations of GAS include

- Stimulation of adrenal glands with hormone release
- Development of gastrointestinal ulceration
- Shrinkage of lymphatic tissues

Hypothesizing that GAS is an integral part of pathologic disease process, Selye considered faulty adaptation as the cause of disease. For example, if the body overdefends itself and produces too many proinflammatory hormones, diseases like arthritis, allergy, or asthma may develop (Selye, 1976, 1974).

Lazarus' Model Lazarus developed the cognitive-phenomenological approach to the study of stress. This approach notes that neither the stimulus theory nor the response theory of stress considers individual differences. The Lazarus model recognizes that environmental demands and pressures produce stress in large numbers of people. However the emphasis of the model is that people and groups differ in their vulnerability, interpretations, and reactions to certain types of events. The factors the Lazarus model takes into account are the cognitive processes that intervene between the stressful event and the reaction. Selye focuses on physiologic responses whereas Lazarus introduces mental and psychologic responses to stress (Lazarus, 1968; Coyne and Lazarus, 1980).

The concept of **cognitive appraisal** is a central component of the Lazarus model. The individual continually reevaluates judgments about the demands and constraints of the transactions within the environment. It is this evaluation process that determines the individual's reaction to stress, the emotions experienced, and the adaptational outcomes. *Primary appraisal* is a cognitive process in which the individual evaluates the significance of an encounter and its relationship to his or her well-being. The judgments one makes in primary appraisal are: (1) irrelevant, or has no personal significance and can be ignored; (2) benign-positive, or the state of affairs is beneficial or desirable; and (3) stressful, or there is harm-loss, threat, or challenge. *Secondary appraisal* is another cognitive process that involves ongoing judgments concerning coping resources, options, and constraints. Determinants of secondary appraisal include the person's previous experiences with such situations, beliefs about self and environment, and the availability of resources such as one's morale, health, energy, problem-solving skills, social support, and material resources (Coyne and Lazarus, 1980; Lazarus and Folkman, 1984).

Cognitive appraisals are not static, but shift in response to changes in internal and external conditions. Reappraisal occurs as the individual's evaluative judgments change. Reappraisal is considered a feedback process and has two phases. First is assessing new information or forming new insights about the environment and its relationship to the individual's well-being. The second is called defensive reappraisal, and consists of cognitive maneuvering to reduce stress. Coping is a process through which people manage the environmental and internal demands and conflicts that tax or exceed their resources. Coping serves two main functions: the alteration of the ongoing relationship between the person and the environment and the control of stressful emotions (Coyne and Lazarus, 1980; Lazarus and Folkman, 1984).

The Lazarus model suggests that psychophysiologic illness may depend on specific reactions to specific stressors. This specificity depends on several factors related to the nature and severity of the stress disorder: first, the characteristics of the environment; second, the nature of the individual facing the demands and the quality of the emotional response generated by the demands; and finally, the processes of coping that are mobilized must be considered (Monat and Lazarus, 1977).

Pathophysiology of Stress Using Selye's definition of stress, the following can be classified as sources of stress causing a disruption of cellular homeostasis:

- *Mechanical injury*—caused by force or pressure (eg, fracture, laceration, or contusion)

- *Physical agent injury*—caused by abnormal environmental conditions (eg, exposure to electricity or radiation)
- *Chemical agent injury*—caused by exposure to or intake of toxic chemicals (eg, alcohol, poisons, or drugs)
- *Physiologic deficit injury*—caused by inadequate supply of critical substances (eg, oxygen or glucose)
- *Injury by infection*—caused by invasion of host organism by pathogens (eg, influenza or pneumonia)

These sources of stress cause a series of nonadaptive cellular changes termed **degenerative changes**; they are characterized by an accumulation of water and fat within the cell. Degenerative changes lead to **necrosis**, or cellular death.

Compensatory Mechanisms and Stress

Cells do not always react to stress in a nonadaptive manner. Sometimes there are compensation patterns for disruptions in equilibrium. The mechanisms of adaptation are structural cell changes, inflammation and repair response, and immune response.

Almost all body cells are able to accommodate environmental demands by two primary mechanisms: cell hypertrophy and cell hyperplasia. **Cell hypertrophy** refers to an increase in size of an individual cell. A good example of this compensatory mechanism is the enlarged biceps of a weight lifter. Cellular enlargement can occur in specific organs when increased productivity is needed. This response can be seen in the heart and kidney. **Cell hyperplasia** refers to the increase in the number of individual cells. A good example of this compensatory mechanism is protective calluses on the skin responding to mechanical stress.

The inflammatory response is a series of physiologic responses to cellular injury. Even though this reaction is accompanied by redness, warmth, and pain, it is not naturally a pathologic process. Rather, the goal of this process is to re-establish equilibrium by paving the way to repair damaged tissue.

The immune response is a protective and adaptive mechanism. Its function is to inactivate potentially toxic substances within the body. An **antigen**, or foreign body, mobilizes this response.

Concept of Crisis

Crisis, though related to stress, is more sporadic. Stress is a part of our daily life, whereas crisis accentuates our life more dramatically. Gerald Caplan (1961) defined crisis as "when a person faces an obstacle so important to life goals, that for a time [it] is unsurmountable through the utilization of customary methods of problem solving." Examples of crises are sudden death of a family member, loss of a job, rape, severe family discord, and loss of a limb.

Caplan (1964) describes four developmental phases to a crisis:

1. The person faced with a serious problem or threat becomes tense and attempts to employ usual problem-solving techniques.
2. The person's coping mechanisms fail, causing further upset and disequilibrium.
3. The person mobilizes all possible internal and external resources to attack the problem as tension continues to build.
4. When the problem is not resolved, pressures continue to build and the person falls into a state of disorganization, immobilization, anxiety, or depression.

In modern psychiatry, we recognize that the body systems are not separate from the mind; instead, body systems are considered to be closely interrelated. Although only one organ or system may be affected, the entire body and psyche respond to disruptions.

As was pointed out in the past section, stress is a major factor in the development of disease. It is clear that the effects of stress are capable of playing havoc with the body's internal systems. This is not a simple cause-and-effect relationship and many other factors must be considered. The next three sections explore some of the basic biologic, sociocultural and psychologic theories that further explain the mediation between mind and body.

Biologic Theories

When discussing the biologic theories we are really talking about the person's "internal environment." This internal environment is made up of cells, body parts that have structure and function in a particular sort of way, and body systems that control actions, functions, and perceptions. The interaction among all of these things is what determines whether a person remains healthy or experiences an interruption in health.

Some theorists feel that the way the body is affected has been predetermined by that person's genetic make-up. They feel that everyone has a genetic pool that gives them unique biologic strengths and weaknesses. What organs or functions will be affected is thus determined by each person's genetic blueprint. In other words, certain organs will be more vulnerable to stressors and therefore be affected first. This theory suggests that this will be different for everyone.

Psychoimmunology has studied the interaction of the brain in modulating immunologic systems. These studies suggest that a relationship exists that elicits alpha and beta adrenergic responses, cholinergic responses, and autonomic innervation of the thymus and other lymphoid tissues. Although research has not revealed all the reasons these responses occur, it is known that perception plays a major role. People receive stimuli from their internal or external environments through their perceptual system and transmit them to the brain for interpretation. Any situation to which the person has a strong emotional response will bring about a physiologic response. It is important to remember that all people perceive stresses in different ways depending on their genetic make-up, life experiences, and earlier socializations. The potential for specific physiologic responses is different for everyone.

The information received by the person's perceptual system and transmitted to the brain for interpretation is then sent to the limbic system either directly or indirectly. This determines the physiologic response that will be triggered in the body. Physiologic responses will come from the autonomic nervous system, the immune system, and the endocrine system. The symptomatology that results reveals how this person manages stress. Clarifying examples are given later in the chapter when specific psychophysiologic disorders are discussed (Beare and Myers, 1990; Thompson et al., 1989).

Sociocultural Theories

Human beings are influenced by their social milieu. Throughout their lives all humans are subjected to a wide variety of experiences, and they cope in different ways. People who have had opportunities for loving relationships, appropriate expressions of anger, experiences in problem solving, and the building of a strong ego, seem able to stay within a comfort zone of healthy adaptation. Those whose experiences have not provided these opportunities do not fare as well. It appears that their ability to adapt becomes depleted.

Several factors seem to relate to the potential development of a psychophysiologic disorder. One is the influence of families on people's learned coping behavior. Issues such as dependency vs. independency, separation anxiety, open communication patterns, and attention-gaining behaviors are just a few that can impact a person's ability to adapt. Dysfunctional families seem unable to give the support necessary to cope adequately in later life. Skills needed to keep one's life on a manageable gradient are frequently not present. The problems that result may be psychologic or psychophysiologic in nature.

The external social environment also plays a role in the ways people learn to adapt to the stressors in their lives. In a society where the quality of life is good and the rules, roles, and customs are defined, people are usually better able to adapt to the normal stresses and crises of life. When the society offers support systems that help people realize their potential there seems to be less vulnerability to stress-related disorders. We know major changes in the social environment that cause people to feel unsafe or insecure create a much greater need for physiologic and/or psychologic adaptation. Those people who have well-integrated coping mechanisms find healthy adaptation possible, but those without adequate coping mechanisms will show a negative or maladaptive response.

A prominent sociologic theory linking psychosocial changes to physical illness grew out of Holmes and Rahe's studies of major life events. Their early studies used a questionnaire called the Schedule of Recent Experience (SRE) that has since been developed into the Social Readjustment Rating Scale (SRRS). (See Table 7–1 for the Social Readjustment Rating Scale.) This scale presents major life events in terms of Life Change Units, the varying values related to the amount of stress caused by the event. Through these studies it was discovered that the higher the individual's score in Life Change Units the more likely the person was to develop an illness (Holmes and Rahe, 1967). (See Table 7-2.)

The work of Holmes and Rahe has consistently shown a relationship between stressful life changes and illness and their findings have been under

Table 7–1 *Holmes and Rahe Social Readjustment Rating Scale*

Life change units	*Major life events*	*Life change units*	*Major life events*
100	Death of a spouse	29	Change in responsibilities at work
73	Divorce	29	Son or daughter leaving home
65	Marital Separation	29	Trouble with in-laws
63	Detention in jail or institution	28	Outstanding personal achievement
63	Death of a close family member	26	Began or ceased formal schooling
53	Personal injury or illness	25	Change in living conditions
50	Marriage	24	Revision of personal habits
47	Fired at work	23	Trouble with boss
45	Marital reconciliation	20	Change in residence
45	Retirement	20	Change in schools
44	Change in health behavior of family member	19	Change in recreation
40	Pregnancy	19	Change in church activities
39	Sexual difficulties	18	Change in social activities
39	Business readjustment	17	Mortgage or loan less than $10,000
38	Change in financial state	16	Change in sleeping habits
37	Death of close friend	15	Change in number of family get-togethers
36	Change to a different line of work	15	Change in eating habits
53	Change in number of arguments with spouse	13	Vacation
31	Mortgage or loan over $10,000	12	Christmas
30	Foreclosure of mortgage or loan	11	Minor violations of the law

Source: From Holmes TH and Rahe RH: The Social Readjustment Rating Scale. *J Psychosom Res,* 1967; 2:214. Reprinted by permission.

Table 7–2 *Life Events Units as Related to Physical Illness*

Life Events Units Range of Scores	*Relationship to the Development of Physical Illness*
1–149	No significant life change
150–199	33% chance of illness—mild life change
200–299	50% chance of illness—moderate life change
300+	80% chance of illness—major life change

Source: Adapted from Holmes TH and Rahe RH: The Social Readjustment Rating Scale. *J Psychosom Res,* 1967; 2:214. Used with permission.

scrutiny by other researchers. These researchers have found that individual differences in illness susceptibility due to biochemical agents, psychological coping factors, and social supports may be more pertinent than major life changes. Researchers such as Lazarus have moved the orientation of the study of stress toward the role of cognitive processes (Dohrenwend and Dohrenwend, 1974; Sarason, de Monchaux, and Hunt, 1975; Lazarus, 1966).

Another example of a sociologic theory related to psychophysiologic disorders is the proposal of **Type A** and **Type B** behavior. Friedman and Rosenman (1974) described the following characteristics of a Type A person:

- Talking explosively and rapidly
- Moving rapidly (eg, walking, eating)
- Becoming unduly irritated at delay (eg, waiting at a stop light)
- Trying to schedule more and more in less time
- Feeling guilty when relaxing
- Trying to do two things at once
- Described by others as a "workaholic"

Type B persons, on the other hand, did not demonstrate the same behavior pattern.

Culture plays a major role in the development or lack of development of a person's coping abilities. Definitions of health and illness and the ways in which a person is taught to deal with problems can be culture-specific. What may be perceived as stressful in one culture may not be perceived that way in another. Many of the stress disorders such as ulcers, hypertension, coronary heart disease, tension headaches, and anorexia nervosa do not occur in nonindustrialized societies. But as societies are exposed to change, these disorders begin to appear. A good example of this phenomenon is Japan, where the incidence of hypertension and coronary heart disease has increased since World War II. (See chapter 5 for more information on culture.)

Psychologic Theories

Researchers have attempted to identify personality factors associated with psychophysiologic disorders. Some of the factors studied were rigidity, high sensitivity to threat, and hostility. Though it is known that personality plays a role in the development of psychophysiologic disorders, it is unclear why some people who share specific personality characteristics develop disorders and others do not.

The potential for the development of disease is increased when individuals feel unable to cope. The source of this inability is a complicated array of previous experiences, personality traits, and learned behaviors. Many individuals whose coping mechanisms prevent healthy adaptation to stressful experiences report feelings of helplessness, hopelessness, and worthlessness.

Interpersonal relationships have also been studied as a cause of psychophysiologic disorders. These studies have centered on the effects of marital unhappiness, absence of positive human relationships, and dysfunctional family patterns. Given extreme feelings of lack of control over life combined with poor interpersonal relationships, it is understandable that an individual would have the potential to develop a stress-related disease.

Theorists postulate that, much like the psychologic regression seen as a response to illness or stress, psychophysiologic disorders represent physiologic regression as an attempt to resolve psychological issues. The physiologic regression is viewed as a failure of ordinary defense mechanisms to maintain homeostasis.

Learning experiences also affect how individuals perceive a particular situation or event. Past events have particular potential to distort the present. This can happen in two ways. First, the memory of traumatic experiences can cause so much fear and anxiety that the person is unable to utilize any known or affective defense mechanisms that work, and this leads to the psychologic stress being expressed through a body organ. Second are phenomena known as secondary gain. It may be that an individual derives certain benefits from experiencing a particular illness. The illness is not consciously chosen, as one might think; rather the defense was learned early in life as a way to get needs met. In many instances it has become the only way in which that child or adult can get needs met. An example would be a child who has an asthmatic condition and, consistently unable to get needs met through healthy channels, learns that having an asthma attack gets the attention needed. The secondary gain is the need fulfillment arising out of the asthmatic attacks.

The psychodynamics of behavior that help us understand the development of psychophysiologic disorders are many and varied. Like the biologic and sociocultural theories, the psychological theories are a combination of many ideas. There is rarely a single cause for any human behavior. That is why the theories discussed here lend themselves to multicausational interpretations.

Knowledge Base: Cardiovascular Disorders

The group of disorders linking psychologic and cardiac function and creating pathologic conditions in the heart and blood vessels are called **cardiovascular disorders**. Cardiovascular disorders are the leading cause of death in the United States. There are two major cardiovascular disorders, coronary heart disease (CHD) and hypertension (HTN). Coronary Heart Disease (CHD) continues to be the leading cause of death and disability in the United States. Approximately 1.5 million people will have a heart attack this year; 500,000 of these people will be under the age of 65. Only 65% of them will return to work. At least 550,000 Americans will die from heart attacks this year, and the cost of CHD to the United States this year is estimated at over $84 billion (Beare and Myers, 1990; Thompson et al., 1989).

Other factors which precipitate the onset of CHD are: a genetic predisposition in which there is a history of CHD in the family; type A personality traits; high levels of personal and professional stress. Other variables such as heavy cigarette smoking, sedentary life style, high-caloric/high-fat diet, high level of hostility, and emotional tension are contributing factors.

There are three forms of CHD: (1) **angina pectoris** results in periodic chest pains caused by an insufficient oxygen-rich blood supply to the heart; (2) **atherosclerosis** is a build-up of plaque in arteries and is related to an insufficient blood supply; and (3) **myocardial infarction**, also related to insufficient blood supply, is complete blocking of the heart's blood supply.

Behavioral Characteristics

Some individuals obviously display the anxiety and tensions they feel; others do not. It is important to remember this, because individuals with obvious Type A behaviors will usually leave no doubt as to their thoughts and feelings and it becomes obvious what is driving the person's behavior. Other people appear more low key, but that behavior is only a shell that covers more significant inner conflicts. It is necessary to make a distinction between important inward behaviors and outward behaviors. Some of the newer research suggests that it is the low-key person who may be most prone to coronary heart disease.

Other psychomotor behaviors associated with people prone to CHD are facial tightness, rapid eye blinking, knee jiggling, finger tapping, speaking rapidly, walking fast, eating fast, and being unable to sit with nothing to do.

Affective Characteristics

A great deal of research has been done on the anxiety and stress experienced by people prone to CHD. One thought is that the CHD-prone individual, though hard-driving, is never totally satisfied. Such people never experience complete satisfaction and always feel they have another goal to meet. This chronic dissatisfaction with self is many times linked with a personal life that predisposes the person to added stress. The mounting stress eventually makes these individuals susceptible to illness. The general perception is that, affectively, persons who are prone to the development of CHD feel more inner tension, worry, and anxiety than those who are not.

Complaints of anxiety occur in 10% to 14% of cardiology practices (Hackett, Rosenbaum, and Cassem, 1985). Panic symptoms of chest pain, palpitation, dyspnea, weakness, fatigue, dizziness, syncope and anxiety often bring clients to the cardiologist. The American Heart Association has identified the risk factors, classified as modifiable and immodifiable, in CHD. (See Table 7–3 for a list of these risk factors.)

Table 7–3 *Coronary Heart Disease Risk Factors*

Modifiable	*Unmodifiable*
Obesity	Age
Sedentary lifestyle	Gender (males have higher rate than females until after age 60)
Stressful lifestyle	Ethnicity (Caucasians have higher rates than blacks)
Hypertension	Genetic predisposition
Cigarette smoking	Family history of heart disease
Elevated serum lipids	
Diabetes mellitus	

Source: From *Heartbook,* American Heart Association. Reprinted with permission.

Cognitive Characteristics

Adaptation to the stresses of everyday life takes a certain amount of well-integrated planning. To remain healthy, individuals must be able to do certain things such as plan their time well, balance work with recreation, eat the right foods, and plan an exercise routine. To achieve this, these people must be able to think clearly and work out a plan in their minds. When stressors begin to increase in either intensity or number, it is sometimes more difficult to concentrate and focus cognitively. Because high stress is frequently linked to anxiety, nurses might expect to observe decreased cognitive functioning as levels of stress and anxiety rise.

Physiologic Characteristics

The major cause of CHD is atherosclerosis, that is, fatty deposits and cholesterol deposits on the arterial wall. There are three stages to the development of atherosclerosis including streaks of lipids in smooth muscle cells, progressive changes in the arterial wall and, finally, a lesion on the arterial wall. The lesions harden and cause rigidity of the artery (Beare and Myers, 1990; Luckman and Sorensen, 1987).

Sociocultural Characteristics

Genetic predisposition is a factor in CHD; however, the mechanism is unclear. It is felt that congenital defects are present in coronary artery walls causing a predisposition to the formation of plaques.

Studies demonstrate that hardworking, competitive parents help form similar traits and values in offspring. Still other evidence indicates that parents and classroom teachers groom children at an early age to be achievers and competitors. Parents of high-achieving children are likely to tell their children, especially sons, to keep trying in the face of failure while berating them for their unsuccessful efforts. Many children's books emphasize achievement.

Religious background also relates to the incidence of heart disease. Protestant religions emphasize independence and achievement, and Jewish families encourage achievement. The greatest incidence of heart disease is found in Protestants, then in Jews; least is found in Catholics (Arehart-Treichel, 1980). Friedman and Rosenman (1974) discovered that heart disease was more frequently seen in persons whose need for personal power took precedence over their religious faith than in persons whose faith took precedence over power.

Persons prone to angina share common characteristics with the person prone to heart attack or hypertension. These people tend to mask their dependency needs, insecurity, and fear of failure with an aggressive front; instead of expressing their inner psychological conflicts openly they produce angina pain (Arehart and Treichel, 1980).

Causative Theories

The experience of emotion is both physical and psychologic. Emotional responses are more extensive than physical responses and resemble the effects of physical stress on the cardiovascular system. Those effects include tachycardia, increased blood pressure, myocardial oxygen consumption, peripheral resistance, decreased muscle blood flow, and decreased renal circulation. The effect of emotion is considered more harmful to the heart than exercise primarily because of the lack of muscular activity associated with emotion. Emotional stress and stressful life events frequently precede cardiac problems (Hackett, Rosenbaum, and Cassem, 1985).

Medical Treatment

Medical treatments specific to atherosclerosis, hypertension, and angina pectoris may be found in medical-surgical texts. The focus of medical treatment in this text is prevention. The first step in prevention is identifying high-risk clients. This is done with a nursing history tool. Aside from the medical-surgical treatments referred to earlier, mild tranquilizers are given to reduce emotional tension. Most recently, biofeedback has been used to help teach people to relax. Secondly, preventive measures should be taken once the high-risk person is identified. The nurse's health teaching plays a major role in motivating the client to change high-risk behaviors.

Pharmacologic agents restricting lipid production or increasing lipoprotein removal have become available for persons who have not had success with diet control but who have stopped smoking. Niacin, clofibrate (Atromid) and probucol (Lorelco) restrict lipoprotein production, whereas cholestyramine (Questran), colestipol hydrochloride (Colestid) and genfibrazil (Lopid) increase lipoprotein removal (Gerald and O'Bannon, 1988).

Assessment

Nursing History Assessment of the client with CHD begins with data collection. The nurse may encounter the client for the first time in a general hospital setting or in a crisis intervention setting. To assist in determining the client's state of wellness, the nurse begins with a general history, which allows time for developing rapport with the client while conveying interest and support. Table 7–4 provides a general history for clients with psychological factors affecting physical condition. The focus of the nursing history tool for clients with CHD is to identify high-risk persons as well as specific cardiac problems. In addition to the general history tool for clients with psychological factors affecting physical condition, the nurse should add the following questions:

- Are you able to say no to requests from others?
- What is your perception of time? Do you have enough time to get things done?
- Do you wear a watch?
- How many appointments or activities do you schedule for one work hour?
- Do you usually feel rushed?
- What reaction do you have to waiting in lines? At stop lights?

(continued on p 244, col 1)

Table 7–4 *Nursing History Tool for Clients with Psychological Factors Affecting Physical Condition*

Social and Behavioral History

What is your usual pattern for activities of daily living?
How has your illness affected your usual level of functioning? In work? In household activities? In leisure activities?
Do any activities cause you discomfort? Which cause the least discomfort? The most discomfort?

What are your leisure activities?

Describe your relationships with other people.
When do you prefer to be alone? To be with others?
What makes you reach out to others?
What causes you to be upset with others?
Do you hold your feelings in when you are upset with others?
How do you resolve conflict with others?
How do people react to your diagnosis?
Has your behavioral pattern changed since your diagnosis?
What was your initial reaction to your diagnosis? Has it changed? Describe.
Would you describe yourself as timid? Shy?
How frequent is your contact with your parents? Other family members? Are you closer to your mother? Father?

Emotional History

What is your usual emotional reaction to stressful situations?
When you are under stress, describe any conflicting emotions you experience.
What kinds of situations cause you to be anxious? Angry?
How are you affected by anxiety?
How do you express anger?

What do you do to reduce emotionally stressful situations?
How many cigarettes do you smoke a day?
How much alcohol do you ingest a day?
Do you overeat or undereat?
What is your activity level?
What situations trigger stress for you?
What stressors do you avoid? Environmental factors?

Who are the people you consider most significant in your life?
Are these people effective support systems?
Do you consider your family members friends?
How many close friends do you have now? Have you had?
When do you turn to friends? When stressed?
What has been your most successful coping pattern?
What is your usual time frame for coping with stressful events?

What is your usual mood?
How has your diagnosis affected your usual mood?
When do you feel depressed? What precipitates your depression?
Have you felt more depressed since learning of your diagnosis?
Would you describe yourself as moody? Having fluctuations in mood?
How do your moods differ at work versus at home?
How frequently do you take the blame if something doesn't go right at home? At work?
Would you describe yourself as emotionally sensitive?
Would you describe yourself as aggressive? Competitive?
Would you describe yourself as a negative or positive person? Why?

(continued)

Table 7–4 *(continued)*

Cognitive and Perceptual History

Would you describe yourself as intellectual?
  Are you brighter than most people? Less bright?
  Would you describe yourself as being able to learn as well, less well, or better than others? Has your diagnosis influenced this ability?
  Would you describe yourself as decisive? Explain.
  Do you tend to make decisions quickly? Slowly? When?
  What decisions do you find easiest to make? Most difficult to make?
  Has your diagnosis influenced your ability to make decisions?
  Do you rely on your family members or significant others to make your decisions?
  Do you make more decisions than your colleagues? Fewer?

Would you describe yourself as a perfectionist? At work? At home?
  How much time do you spend at work versus leisure?
  Are you more conscientious about your work than your colleagues?
  Do you produce better work than your colleagues? More work?
  How do you respond to criticism of your work?
  How fastidious are you about your appearance?
  How does disorderliness or messiness affect your stress level?

Have your perceptions changed since your diagnosis?
  What fears have resulted from your diagnosis? How have attitudes of those around you changed?
  Would you consider yourself independent? Dependent? Why?

Physical and Motor History

What physical symptoms worry you?
  What physical symptoms brought you in for diagnosis?
  What do you do for (other symptoms listed by client)?

What medications are you taking?
  What do these medications do for you? Are they helpful?
  What are the side effects of the medications you take?

What are your eating patterns? Usual foods?
  How many meals do you eat a day? Snacks?
  How much and what kind of fluid do you take each day?
  Have you recently gained or lost weight? How much?
  Have you changed your eating patterns since your diagnosis?
  Do you usually take meals with your family? Colleagues?
  How often do you eat alone?
  Do you rush your meals?

What is your usual sleeping pattern?
  What disturbs your sleep?
  How do you feel after sleeping?
  Do you sleep more or less than your family? Friends?
  How many pillows do you use?

How do you feel after activity?
  Has your pattern of activities changed since your diagnosis?
  What activities do you enjoy most? Least?
  What activities do you find most difficult? Least difficult?
  How often do you engage in sexual activity?
  Has your diagnosis changed your pattern of sexual activity?
  Is your lifestyle sedentary, moderately active, or active?
  Do you exercise regularly?

(continued)

Table 7–4 *(continued)*

Physical and Motor History (continued)
Does pain affect your daily activities?
Would you describe your tolerance to pain as high or low?
How does pain affect your general sense of well-being?
Do you use medication to reduce pain? How often? Any side effects?
Besides medication, what do you do to reduce pain?
How is your general health?
Has your general health deteriorated or improved since your diagnosis?
What are your general health concerns?
What are your usual vital signs?
Have you noticed any edema (swelling) of your hands or feet?
Have you had problems with constipation? What do you do for it?
Have you experienced dizzy spells when you first get up?
How is your health compared to your family members? Colleagues?
Do you experience nausea? What do you do about it?

- What do you do for your physical symptoms? Headaches? Tightness in chest? Pain in chest? Muscle pains? Indigestion?

The nurse should plan enough time to complete this history.

Physical Assessment The aim of cardiac assessment is to determine the presence of any distress or pain. The presence of palpitations, dyspnea, orthopnea, edema, and cyanosis should also be determined. Inspection, palpation, percussion, and auscultation are the cardiac assessment modalities. **Inspection** includes observing for symmetry of the chest contour. **Palpation** identifies the apical pulse. **Percussion** is used to estimate the approximate borders of the heart within the chest cavity; also, changes of resonance to dullness are noted by using percussion. **Auscultation** allows the examiner to assess heart sounds.

The nurse must be alert to clinical manifestations of the major cardiac disorders. (See Table 7–5 for a summary of the manifestations of hypertension, angina pectoris, and myocardial infarction.) In physically assessing the client with cardiac disease, it is important to examine the pulses bilaterally to determine equalness. The nurse should note the fullness and the rate when checking pulses. Blood pressure should be taken on both arms, and orthostatic pressures may be indicated. The jugular veins should be observed for pulsations.

Nursing Diagnosis and Planning

Nursing diagnoses for clients with CHD are complex. Many of the diagnoses are based on the clinical manifestations of the primary disorder. The focus of the nursing diagnoses for CHD clients in this text is on the emotional and behavioral manifestations of CHD. The nurse must be sensitive to the client's emotional and physical needs. (See Table 7–6 for a summary of the nursing diagnoses for the client with CHD.)

The plan of care for the CHD client is based on individually identified nursing diagnoses. Mutual goal setting is extremely important in the CHD client; otherwise, compliance and changes in lifestyle may be compromised. The nurse selects interventions based on these mutually identified goals. (See Table 7–7 for the care plan for the client with CHD.)

Evaluation

The nurse evaluates the care of the CHD client by comparing the client's status to the goals set in the nursing care plan. (See Table 7–8 for an evaluation of the care of a client with CHD.) There are several expected outcomes commonly observed in clients

Table 7–5 *Clinical Manifestations of Major Cardiac Disorders*

Hypertension
Headache appearing in the morning but disappearing as the day goes by
Easily fatigued
Dizziness
Palpitations
Blurred vision
Epistaxis
Angina Pectoris
Chest pain or discomfort
Severe indigestion
Apprehension
Dyspnea
Diaphoresis
Nausea
Belching
Myocardial Infarction
Apprehension
Nausea and vomiting
Dyspnea
Diaphoresis
Extreme fatigue
Chest pain followed by dizziness or faintness

with CHD. These outcomes may be stated behaviorally as the client will:

- Experience freedom from pain and the ability to rest comfortably.
- Have vital signs within normal limits.
- Feel physical and emotional comfort and a sense of well-being.
- Show no evidence of fatigue from minimal expenditures of energy during periods of exacerbation of physical symptoms.

Table 7–6 *Nursing Diagnoses in the Client with Coronary Heart Disease*

Activity intolerance, potential
Anxiety
Comfort, alteration in (pain)
Communication, impaired verbal
Coping, ineffective individual
Diversional activity, deficit
Family process, alteration in
Fear, potential
Health maintenance, alteration in
Knowledge deficit, potential
Noncompliance, potential
Self-concept, disturbance in (body image, self-esteem, role performance, personal identity), potential
Spiritual distress, potential

- Demonstrate knowledge of what caused the symptoms, what to do about future symptoms, recommended changes in lifestyle, and appropriate activity levels.
- Talk about anticipated changes in lifestyle.

CASE EXAMPLE

A Client with Coronary Heart Disease

Rob Mello is a 40-year-old male working his way up the management ladder in a computer firm. His work is his primary world. Rob works long hours, and it is not unusual for him to eat his evening meal at his desk. Rob spends his few leisure hours with friends talking shop. One evening Rob was seized with chest pains while leaving his office at 10:00 PM. After being taken to the emergency room, Rob was treated in a coronary care unit and then placed on a telemetry floor for cardiac monitoring.

Nursing History

Location: Telemetry Floor
Client's name: Rob Mello Age: 40
Admitting diagnosis: Angina Pectoris, R/O MI
T=98.7. P=100, R=20, BP=130/90

(continued on p 251, col 1)

Table 7–7 Nursing Care Plan for the Client with CHD

Nursing Diagnosis: Potential activity intolerance related to cardiovascular response to activity.
Goal: During the course of treatment client will plan for a rest/activity pattern that will support increased tolerance of activity.

Intervention	*Rationale*	*Expected Outcome*
Place on bed rest until cardiovascular system can tolerate activity Provide rest periods between treatments Keep articles needed by client in easy reach (eg, water, tissues)	Will provide minimal expenditure of energy while cardiac muscle rests and heals	Absence of weakness after an active period No symptoms of cardiac distress during activity
Monitor the number of visitors	Will decrease excitability of client	
Encourage client compliance to cardiac rehabilitation program	METs (Metabolic Equivalents of Tasks) and stress testing under supervision assist client in increasing performance of activities while healing takes place	Participation in rehabilitation activities

Nursing Diagnosis: Anxiety related to cardiac clinical manifestations.
Goal: During the course of treatment client will learn new coping strategies for anxiety.

Intervention	*Rationale*	*Expected Outcome*
Assess level of anxiety: • mild • moderate • severe • panic	Will assist in determining the interventions necessary to reduce anxiety	Reduced anxiety
Stay with client during episodes of severe pain	Will prevent escalation of anxiety to panic level and offer reassurance to client	
Teach client new coping strategies for anxiety (eg, relaxation techniques) Assist client in using support systems (eg, family members)	Will assist in reducing and/or resolving anxiety	Demonstration of new coping strategies
Encourage client to verbalize concerns	Will increase client's insight into reasons for anxiety	Verbalizes insight into causes for anxiety
Administer antianxiety agents as needed	Will assist client in regaining control over anxiety	
Take steps to reduce anxiety. Extreme anxiety: • provide comfort measures (eg, warm bath, back rub) • use short, simple sentences with a firm, calm voice Mild to moderate anxiety: • encourage client to state when anxiety is present • encourage client to verbalize and explore apprehensions	Will reduce anxiety by providing a calming effect	Anxiety response correlates with events

(continued)

Table 7–7 *(continued)*

Nursing Diagnosis: Alteration in comfort: pain related to physical changes in arteries.
Goal: During the course of treatment client will participate in measures that eliminate and/or control pain.

Intervention	*Rationale*	*Expected Outcome*
Assess client's level of pain: • alertness • restlessness • elevated blood pressure • increased heart rate • arrhythmias • bounding or thready pulse • increased and shallow respirations • size, equality, and reactivity of pupils • muscles, tense or flaccid • color, moisture and temperature of skin • body movement (eg, guarding, favoring, posturing, alignment)	Will assist in determining the type of nursing intervention necessary Physiological changes occur as the body responds to pain	No angina attacks reported
Encourage bed rest and provide comfort measures: • decrease noise • decrease light • position comfortably	Will decrease intensity of pain	
Explain the importance of reporting pain	Early detection of pain will assist in maintaining better control	Client states comfort at least every half hour
Offer therapy as necessary for painful episodes: • administer analgesics as ordered • administer oxygen as ordered	Will assist in controlling pain	Pain eliminated and/or controlled
Obtain a 12-lead EKG, and monitor vital signs during painful episodes	Aids in documenting ischemia during a chest pain episode	
Stay with client during periods of intense pain	Will reduce client's apprehension and promote client's sense of well-being	

Nursing Diagnosis: Impaired verbal communication related to personality characteristics, ie, Type A character.
Goal: During the course of treatment client will develop alternative strategies for dealing with "bottled-up" emotions.

Intervention	*Rationale*	*Expected Outcome*
Initiate a one-to-one relationship with client	Will assist the client in learning to directly express feelings	Communicates stresses Control over angina attacks
Client teaching for: • appropriate communication techniques • assertive communication skills • stress reduction techniques	Will assist in resolving client's communication difficulties	Uses effective communication techniques
Encourage client to verbalize stress and frustration	Will assist in learning new skills	Reports feeling satisfied with communication
Encourage client to develop a support system (eg, family members)	Provides a setting in which new communication skills can be practiced	

(continued)

Table 7–7 *(continued)*

Nursing Diagnosis: Ineffective individual coping related to inability to deal with stress effectively.
Goal: During the course of treatment client will develop new coping responses to emotional reactions.

Intervention	*Rationale*	*Expected Outcome*
Initiate a one-to-one relationship with client	Will serve as a foundation for client to try out new coping responses	Client recognizes sources of stress Identifies skills, knowledge, and abilities to cope with stress
Client teaching on: • assertive communication • realistic goal setting • relaxation techniques • time management	Knowledge will increase client's attainment of new coping skills	Sets realistic goals No evidence of self-destructive behavior
Assist client in setting reasonable lifestyle goals	Will aid in improving client's choices about lifestyle	Productive lifestyle
Encourage client to develop changes in lifestyle (eg, proper diet, exercise)	Will assist client in developing new coping skills	

Nursing Diagnosis: Diversional activity deficit related to no and/or irregular pattern of leisure activities.
Goal: During the course of treatment client will identify a satisfactory leisure activity.

Intervention	*Rationale*	*Expected Outcome*
Have client describe usual pattern of diversional activities	Will provide information for planning future activities	States has free time without obligations
Assess client's perception of present situation	Client may not perceive usual pattern as a problem	
Assist client in identifying new diversional activities	Diversional activities must be personally meaningful	Lists diversions in which plans to participate
Support client in choosing new leisure activities	Will encourage client to participate in new activity	Plans to fit activity into daily routine

Nursing Diagnosis: Alteration in family process related to unmet emotional needs of its members.
Goal: During the course of treatment client will recognize alterations in family process.

Intervention	*Rationale*	*Expected Outcome*
Assess family structure	Will aid in understanding of role relationships	Effective communication to meet emotional needs
Encourage client to verbalize perceptions of family functions	Will assist in assessing interdependence of family members	Demonstration of mutual respect
Client teaching on: • communication techniques • stress reduction • problem-solving techniques	Will assist client in learning to relate more effectively with family members and reduce secondary gain received from illness	Verbalizes perceptions of family support
Encourage client to identify stressors within the family structure	Will assist client in determining the family's ability to adapt	
Provide opportunities for client to use new communication techniques with family members	Will give client an opportunity to evaluate new communication skills	

(continued)

Table 7–7 *(continued)*

Nursing Diagnosis: Potential fear related to life-threatening symptoms.
Goal: During the course of treatment client will express reduced and/or no fear.

Intervention	*Rationale*	*Expected Outcome*
Observe client for signs of fear: • panic • pupil dilation • increased agitation • increased pulse, respirations, blood pressure • diaphoresis	Early recognition of fear reaction assists in reducing the reaction	Absence of fear Reduction of fear Verbalization of fears related to perception of life-threatening symptoms
Share your observations of physical symptoms with client	Client's recognition of symptoms will assist in identifying fear reactions vs. pain episode	
Stay with client during periods of fear	Demonstrates understanding and support	
Assist client in identifying source of fear	Will assist in reducing the reaction	
Explain all procedures	Client will be able to more effectively reduce fear if understands the reaction	

Nursing Diagnosis: Alteration in health maintenance related to inadequate coping skills.
Goal: By time of discharge client will alter coping strategies for more effective lifestyle.

Intervention	*Rationale*	*Expected Outcome*
Health teaching on: • personal health practices • risk factors for heart disease	With increased knowledge client will assume greater responsibility for personal health	Attempts to maintain health Controls maladaptive behavior Uses health maintenance resources Uses social support systems Uses new coping skills (eg, relaxation techniques)
Use behavior modification techniques: • self-monitoring • guided practice and reinforcement • contracting	Will assist client in establishing environmental control over health practices	
Refer to therapy for cognitive restructuring techniques: • relaxation training • biofeedback • meditation • imagery		
Provide information on community resources and support groups	Use of support systems decreases high-risk status	

Nursing Diagnosis: Potential knowledge deficit related to cardiac risk factors.
Goal: During course of treatment client will gain knowledge of cardiac risk factors.

Intervention	*Rationale*	*Expected Outcome*
Assess client's understanding of cardiac risk factors	Will assist in determining learning needs	Client explains plans for health care actions
Give client information on cardiac risk factors	Will increase client's knowledge base and increase compliance	Client monitors body and mind for signs of illness

(Diagnosis continued)

Table 7–7 *(continued)*

Nursing Diagnosis *(continued)*: Potential knowledge deficit related to cardiac risk factors.
Goal: During course of treatment client will gain knowledge of cardiac risk factors.

Intervention	*Rationale*	*Expected Outcome*
Client health teaching on: • positive health actions (eg, stop smoking, reduce dietary salt intake) • techniques for gaining control over illness		Completes self-care and makes positive health care actions

Nursing Diagnosis: Potential noncompliance related to denial.
Goal: By the end of the course of treatment client will recognize the seriousness of condition.

Intervention	*Rationale*	*Expected Outcome*
Confront client with nurse's observations of behavior	Will assist in reducing denial	Performance of positive health practices
Discuss concept of secondary gain with client	Will encourage client to find more direct ways of meeting needs	Increases coping ability Participates in therapeutic treatment regimen
Assist client in clarifying values: • use reminders • use prompts • encourage self-monitoring • encourage behavioral analysis	Will assist in altering client's perceptions about illness	

Nursing Diagnosis: Potential disturbance in self-concept related to negative body image, feelings of inadequacy, and changes in self-perception.
Goal: While completing lifestyle changes client will maintain positive self-esteem.

Intervention	*Rationale*	*Expected Outcome*
Assess client's perceptions: • body image • feelings of self-worth • role performance • personal identity	Will assist in identifying disruptions in client's self-concept	States realistic body image Positive expression of physical limitations States self-worth
Give positive reinforcement when client attempts to improve personal appearance	Will enhance a positive body image and increase self-esteem	Appropriate communication skills
Communicate nurse's acceptance of client as worthwhile human being	Will assist in maintaining a constructive level of self-esteem	
Assist client in changing roles: • role clarification • role modeling • role rehearsal • role play • role taking	Will assist client in taking on newly acquired healthful roles	
Encourage client to verbalize concerns about personal identity	Will assist client in developing a positive self-concept	Positive acceptance of self

(continued)

Table 7–7 *(continued)*

Nursing Diagnosis: Potential spiritual distress related to life-threatening nature of symptoms.
Goal: During course of treatment client will express feelings that a spiritual being will assist in relieving suffering.

Intervention	*Rationale*	*Expected Outcome*
Listen to client's spiritual concerns	Will assist in relieving feelings of loneliness and separation from spiritual ties	Displays religious articles at bedside Shares sense of spiritual comfort
Assist client in clarifying spiritual values: • encourage prayer or meditation • offer to secure a spiritual advisor		Discusses death without undue anxiety
Assist client in finding meaning in illness: • offer religious or other readings • offer religious articles • prepare client for receiving spiritual advisor	Will assist client in increasing relationship with a spiritual being	
Offer to stay while client prays • touch client's hand if mutually comfortable • sit by client's side	Will help client endure suffering from pain and reduce fear of death	

Table 7–8 *Example of Evaluation of Nursing Care of a Client with CHD*

Plan	*Evaluation*
1. The client will remain on bed rest for 24 hours.	On 3/10 client became restless and attempted to get out of bed to use the urinal.
2. The client will demonstrate relaxation techniques at least once in 24 hours.	On 3/11 client used relaxation tapes to go to sleep.
3. The client will inform the nurse of all episodes of chest pain.	On 3/11 client had one episode of chest pain relieved in 10 minutes with one NTG under the tongue.

Health history
Height: 5′10″
Weight: 195 lbs
Eats two meals with snacks each day
Sleeps four to six hours at night
Smokes two packs of cigarettes a day
Drinks two to three beers a day

Social history
Divorced from spouse eight years
Lives alone in an apartment when not traveling
No children from previous marriage
Spends many hours traveling for job

Clinical data
EKG shows ST elevations
LDH: 600 IU
SGOT: 150 IU
CPK: 60 mU/ml
Chest x ray indicates slight enlargement of the heart
Telemetry indicates NSR with occasional PVCs

Nursing observations
In the initial telemetry floor admission interview, Mr. Mello is very concerned about getting out of the hospital as soon as possible because he is leaving for the Middle East in one week. Mr. Mello explains to you that his life centers around his work. In fact, it is all that is important to him. When he is in the home office, he works long hours preparing for his overseas trips. He frequently takes his meals at the office. He generally has little time for leisure.

Analysis/Synthesis of Data

Concerns	*Nursing diagnoses*
Pain	Anxiety
Anxiety	Impaired verbal communication
Lifestyle changes needed	Ineffective individual coping
No support system	Alteration in health maintenance
	Potential for noncompliance

Suggested Care Planning Activities

1. Determine the priorities for Mr. Mello's care.
2. Determine the support systems available to Mr. Mello.
3. Describe the significance of the laboratory findings.
4. Determine the developmental aspects to be considered in the care of Mr. Mello.
5. Identify nursing goals for Mr. Mello.
6. Describe the client teaching necessary to assist Mr. Mello toward recovery.
7. List and provide a rationale for nursing interventions in the care of Mr. Mello.

Knowledge Base: Cancer

Cancer is not a single entity; rather, it is a group of more than 100 diseases that have in common the unregulated growth of cells. Cancer is a major health problem in the United States and ranks as the second leading cause of death. One in four Americans can expect to develop cancer at some time during their lives (Beare and Meyers, 1990; Brunner and Suddarth, 1988). Cancer can affect any organ in the body, but it does not necessarily cause death.

Behavioral Characteristics

LeShan (1977), in a 21-year study of people who had cancer, identified their shared behavioral characteristics. They included poor self-image, an inability to express emotions (particularly anger and hostility), seeing themselves as victims and behaving that way, having a tendency toward self-pity, and difficulty developing and maintaining long-term relationships.

People prone to cancer often act as if they do not have any problems in their lives. They are cooperative and willing to please—the typical "nice guy." Other studies join LeShan in suggesting that the fear of conflict that underlies nice-guy behavior is related to self-alienation, poor self-image, and the inability to value one's own accomplishments. Other identified behavioral characteristics that are common include conscientiousness, commitment, and religiosity.

Affective Characteristics

LeShan (1977) also identified several affective characteristics in his study of cancer patients. He found these individuals to have feelings of helplessness, hopelessness, and depression. They frequently reported feelings of despair and disappointment. Feelings of resentment were prevalent but were skillfully covered up by a pleasing, compliant personality. Issues of loss, loneliness, and desertion were also common themes.

Cognitive Characteristics

The cognitive characteristics of greatest significance to people with cancer are those that help them fight the effects of the disease process. For instance, the ability to be creative, be receptive to new ideas, grow intellectually, seek out new experiences, and the motivation to seek out the "best" medical care have all been identified as characteristics that increase remission rates.

Physiologic Characteristics

As has been stated, cancer is a group of many diseases; however, there are two major pathologies present in the development of cancer: (1) dysfunction in cellular growth (proliferation) and (2) dysfunction in cell maturity (differentiation).

Dysfunction in cellular growth originates in the stem cell and begins when cells enter the cell cycle. Although the rate of cell growth differs in various body tissues, all cancer cells grow indiscriminately and haphazardly. **Dysfunction of cell maturity** results in cancer cells morphologically different from the cells from which they develop. These cells have been called undifferentiated and appear immature (Beare and Myers, 1990; Luckman and Sorensen, 1987).

Sociocultural Characteristics

A traumatic childhood has been demonstrated in cancer victims; often cancer victims report a lack of closeness to their parents. Birth order has also been demonstrated as significant in cancer susceptibility. Only children seem to be protected from cancer, and first-born children seem to fit into the category of only children. The length of time a person remains the youngest child may relate to susceptibility. There also seems to be a relationship between cancer development and the person's perception of loss of parental love and affection as a traumatic event.

Cancer affects people of all ages and races, but the incidence of cancer and death rate for cancer is higher in African-Americans (especially males) than in whites; environmental and social factors appear related to this (Kneisl and Ames, 1986).

Causative Theories

The two primary causative theories of cancer development are genetic origin and nongenetic origin. The physiological mechanisms were explained above. In **genetic origin**, which is related to the dysfunction of cellular profusion, a mutation occurs in the stem-cell DNA, or virus-induced genetic material is added to the stem-cell DNA. In **nongenetic origin**, which is related to dysfunction in cellular differentiation, there is altered cell synthesis or cell function with DNA left intact (Luckman and Sorensen, 1987).

Medical Treatment

Prevention, early detection, and prompt treatment are the cornerstones in the medical treatment of cancer. The nurse plays a vital role in educating and motivating the public to change various unhealthful behaviors. A moderate lifestyle of consistent periods of rest and sleep, proper diet, exercise, leisure time, and ability to cope with or reduce stress all promote health. The public should be made aware of all suspected carcinogens. Females should learn to self-examine their breasts, and males to self-examine their testicles. And the warning signs of cancer should be widely disseminated. (See Table 7–9 for the seven warning signs of cancer.)

Table 7–9 *American Cancer Society Seven Warning Signs of Cancer*

C hange in bowel or bladder habits.
A sore that does not heal.
U nusual bleeding or discharge from any body orifice.
T hickening or a lump in the breast or elsewhere.
I ndigestion or difficulty in swallowing.
O bvious change in a wart or mole.
N agging cough or hoarseness.

Reprinted with permission from the American Cancer Society.

The primary goals of cancer treatment are cure, control, or palliation. Cure involves treatment with a follow-up phase and no return of cancer. Control involves retreatment of the cancer with the cancer under control for long periods of time. Palliation is the relief of symptoms with as high a quality of life as possible.

The primary treatment modalities for cancer are surgery, radiation, chemotherapy, and immunotherapy. Surgery is generally used along with other therapies to cure and control cancer. Radiation, the most frequently used treatment, changes the physical and chemical make-up of the cells. Chemotherapy is used as a treatment for solid tumors and for control of cancer cells. Immunotherapy is used as an adjunct therapy with the other types of treatment (Beare and Myers, 1990; Luckman and Sorensen, 1987).

Assessment

Nursing History Assessment of the client with cancer begins with data collection. The nurse should incorporate questions about lifestyle to serve as a basis for client teaching and prevention. A diagnosis of cancer is usually accompanied by fear; indeed, the mere mention of the word *cancer* may paralyze the client with fear and hinder the client's progress. To decrease this fear, the nurse should use a low-key manner. Assessment begins with a general history to assist the nurse in determining the client's present health status. (See Table 7–4 for a general history for clients with psychological factors affecting physical condition.) The focus of the history tool for clients with cancer is to identify high-risk behaviors and the primary concerns related to the cancer. In addition to utilizing the general history tool of Table 7–4, the nurse should ask the following questions:

- How do people react to your diagnosis?
- Have you felt more depressed since learning your diagnosis?
- What are your concerns about disfigurement?
- Have you heard of the seven warning signs of cancer?
- Do you experience anorexia? What do you do for it?
- Has your sense of taste altered?
- What high-protein foods do you eat?

The nurse should plan enough time to complete this history.

Physical Assessment The aim of physical assessment in the cancer client is to identify potential problems caused by treatment or by the symptoms themselves. For example, pancreatic cancer may cause constipation and decreased desire to eat. Vital signs are taken to establish a baseline of normal limits for the client. This baseline is especially important if the client is receiving special procedures. A general systems assessment begins with observation of the skin. Alopecia (loss of hair) occurs as a side effect of some chemotherapeutic agents and radiation, and necrosis of tissue results from other chemotherapeutic agents. Any reddening or other changes in the skin should be noted.

In examining the chest, the nurse should note any complaints of chest wall irritation or symptoms of heart failure. Pericarditis, myocarditis, and cardiotoxicity are complications of cancer treatment. Fever, dry cough, and dyspnea on exertion may be indicative of pneumonitis. The client may also be susceptible to respiratory infection.

The gastrointestinal system may present problems for the cancer client. Chemotherapy and radiation can alter normal gastrointestinal function. There may be dryness of the mucous membranes in the mouth. Stomatitis accompanied by esophagitis is not uncommon. Nausea and vomiting may be noted as a result of destruction of the epithelial lining of the gastrointestinal tract, and diarrhea may occur as a result of the denuding of the epithelial lining of the small intestine. Constipation may occur as a result of dysfunction of the autonomic nervous system or as a side effect to pain medications.

The nervous system may be affected by radiation resulting in increased intracranial pressure. Some peripheral neuropathy may be noted after chemotherapy.

The genitourinary system may be affected by nephrotoxicity resulting from accumulation of chemotherapeutic agents. Cystitis may be observed as a result of destruction of the epithelial lining of the bladder. The nurse will observe urgency, frequency, and hematuria. Sexual function may be disrupted either because of therapeutic destruction of sexual cells or because of accumulation of symptoms from therapy such as fatigue, diarrhea, nausea and vomiting, pain, anxiety, or fear (Luckman and Sorensen, 1987; Brunner and Suddarth, 1988).

Nursing Diagnosis and Planning

There are many nursing diagnoses for clients with cancer. The physical aspects of cancer alone support many diagnoses. Although important, these diagnoses are deemphasized in this text to accentuate the psychosocial diagnoses. Optimum quality of life is of major concern to the nurse in caring for the client with a medical diagnosis of cancer. A positive approach to the client assists in affecting the client's quality of life and improving the attitudes of caretakers, family members, and the client. (See Table 7–10 for a summary of the nursing diagnoses for the client with cancer.)

The plan of care for the cancer client is based on individually assessed nursing diagnoses. The primary goal of the care is physical and emotional support. Although the nurse should attempt to set goals for client diagnoses with the client, the nature of the client's illness may leave the client in protracted periods of denial making it necessary for the nurse to set goals. Of major consideration in developing an adequate plan of care is the client's

Table 7–10 *Nursing Diagnoses for the Client with Cancer*

Activity intolerance
Anxiety
Comfort, alteration in (pain)
Communication, impaired verbal, potential
Coping, ineffective individual, potential
Family process, alteration in, potential
Fear
Grieving, anticipatory
Powerlessness, potential
Self-concept, disturbance in (body image, self-esteem, role performance, personal identity)
Sexual dysfunction
Social isolation
Spiritual distress, potential

family or support system. Cancer is a disease having ramifications for the entire family unit. Nursing interventions are based on the goals identified for client care. (See Table 7–11 for the care plan for the cancer client.)

Evaluation

The evaluation of the care of the client with cancer is based on the goals identified in the care plan. (See Table 7–12 for evaluation of the care of a client with cancer.) In general, the expected outcomes for the client with cancer may be behaviorally stated as the client will:

- Be able to cope with stressful life events.
- Have continued personal contacts offering comfort and reassurance.
- Be able to express feelings and concerns about illness and dying.
- Be able to discuss the impact of the disruptions in body image.
- Be able to act out feelings of rage, fear, despondency, pain, and so forth.
- Have confidence in the treatment team.
- Live as fully as possible within physical limitations.
- Have reduced discomfort with minimal distress.

CASE EXAMPLE

A Client with Cancer of the Colon

Gary Miller, a 26-year-old male, lost his father when he was six. He had a lonely childhood and felt he had come into his own in high school when he discovered friends with his interest in architecture. Since Gary had to help support his mother, he took a job as an apprentice contractor instead of pursuing a college degree in architecture. As he became more and more lonely, he lost interest in life. Gary was admitted to the hospital with acute rectal bleeding. His diagnosis was confirmed as cancer of the colon.

Nursing History

Location: General Hospital, Oncology Unit
Client's name: Gary Miller Age: 26
Admitting diagnosis: Colon Cancer
T=97.6, P=90, R=18, B/P=110/60

Health history
Height: 6′0″
Weight: 150 lbs
Eats three meals a day
Sleeps six to eight hours at night
Denies ever smoking
Drinks occasional beer or wine

Social history
Never married
Lives with mother
Has no special interests or hobbies

Clinical data
Stools hematest positive
Hgb 9.0
Hct 29

Nursing observations
On initial interview Gary appeared detached. He responded only when asked direct questions. He answered with minimal responses even when asked to elaborate. Gary appeared in a state of shock and would change the subject abruptly when the term *cancer* was mentioned.

(continued on p 263, col 2)

Table 7–11 Nursing Care Plan for the Client with Cancer

Nursing Diagnosis: Activity intolerance related to physiologic state created by treatment.
Goal: During the course of treatment client will maintain optimal level of mobility.

Intervention	*Rationale*	*Expected Outcome*
Encourage activities within client's physical limitations (eg, walking, self-care activities)	Will assist in supporting client's tolerance for activity	Optimal mobility Completes self-care activities Participates in activities
Adjust treatment schedule to allow for adequate rest		
Encourage visitors	Visitors and family increase self-esteem	Receives visitors
Include client and client's family in planning daily activities	Assists in gaining acceptance of disabilities	
Encourage client to express feelings about limitations		
Client teaching on monitoring activity: • when signs and symptoms of anoxia present • when feels fatigue		

Nursing Diagnosis: Anxiety related to life-threatening nature of medical diagnosis.
Goal: Before discharge client will be able to express concerns about death and dying.

Intervention	*Rationale*	*Expected Outcome*
Assess stage of grief (eg, denial, anger, depression, bargaining, acceptance)	Will assist in identification of predictable stage of client's grief reaction to diagnosis	
Recognize many day-to-day complaints are related to anxiety (eg, palpitation, nausea, diarrhea, irritability)	Fight or flight response is related to specific physical reactions	
Maintain a calm, nonstimulating environment	Will assist in reducing anxiety	
Assist client in diversional activities when physical condition permits: • grooming • walking • self-care activities	Will assist in reducing anxiety	Reduction of anxiety
Recognize presence of anxiety (eg, ask client "are you uncomfortable now?")	Will assist in gaining insight into anxiety	Ability to recognize anxiety
Client teaching on coping strategies: • reduce negative expectations • problem solving • assertive communication skills • muscle relaxation techniques • simple concrete tasks • talking to someone • therapeutic humor, e.g., watch funny television shows, laugh out loud	Will assist client in developing new coping strategies	Development of coping strategies for anxiety

(continued)

Table 7–11 *(continued)*

Nursing Diagnosis: Alteration in comfort (pain) related to growth of cancer cells.
Goal: During the course of treatment client will state reduction and/or alleviation of pain.

Intervention	*Rationale*	*Expected Outcome*
Assess the nature of client's pain: • location • characteristics (sharp, radiating, shooting, deep, superficial, etc) • onset • frequency (eg, constant, intermittent) • intensity (eg, severe, moderate)	Will assist in identifying needed comfort measures	
Assess client's physiologic reactions to pain: • alertness • restlessness • elevated blood pressure • increased heart rate • increased respirations • size, equality, and reactivity of pupils	Physiologic changes occur as the body responds to pain	Vital signs within normal limits
Comfort measures for various sites and types of pain: Abdominal cramping: • decrease fatty food intake • bland foods • small feedings • apply heat to abdomen • sitting position • check bowel sounds • monitor bowel movements Rectal pain: • position comfortably • sitz bath • warm, moist compress to rectal area • increase fluid intake • high bulk foods Bone pain: • handle gently • position comfortably • change positions slowly • support affected body parts • whirlpool bath Headache: • elevate head • apply cold, moist compress • gentle massage • decrease room lighting • make environment quiet	Will increase client's comfort	Pain eliminated and/or controlled
Encourage client mobility	Maximum activity level reduces pain	
Administer appropriate medications based on evaluation of pain	Many medications are used for pain control (sedative hypnotics, local anesthetics, ataractics, muscle relaxants, tranquilizers, analgesics, and narcotics)	Client states relief from pain medications

(continued)

Table 7–11 *(continued)*

Nursing Diagnosis: Potential impaired verbal communication related to client's reaction to cancer diagnosis or physical complications of the disease process.
Goal: During the course of treatment client will be able to reduce and/or resolve impaired communication.

Intervention	*Rationale*	*Expected Outcome*
Initiate a one-to-one relationship with client	Will encourage client to make an effort to communicate	Uses effective communication techniques
Be available to client to discuss concerns (eg, sit with client for intervals)	The presence of the nurse communicates concern and encourages communication	Reports accurate perceptions Oriented to time, place, and person
Be accepting of client if avoids talking about death or abruptly changes topic when death is mentioned	The client needs time to reach acceptance	
Use therapeutic techniques of communication: • open-ended statements • focusing • stating observations • exploring • silence • providing feedback • reflecting	Will assist client in resolving impaired communication	Appropriately expresses feelings
Encourage client to discuss fears (eg, death)	Will help client to move toward acceptance	
Provide alternative means of communication when client is verbally impaired (eg, sign language, pencil and paper)	Will assist client in effectively communicating needs	

Nursing Diagnosis: Potential individual ineffective coping related to inability of self to cope with the threat, usually denial, and other reactions to diagnosis of cancer.
Goal: During the course of treatment client will develop an accurate awareness of the illness.

Intervention	*Rationale*	*Expected Outcome*
Initiate a one-to-one relationship with client	Will assist in being able to assess client's understanding of diagnosis	Accurately states diagnosis Sets realistic goals
Assess client's emotional responses to cancer diagnosis	Will assist in planning effective nursing interventions	Uses skills to reduce anxiety and fear Absence of denial
Encourage client to explain understanding of cancer diagnosis (eg, where problem is, prognosis, etc)		Objectivity in problem solving States feelings of hope
Encourage client to discuss treatment expectations (eg, include in mutual goal setting)	Client involvement in planning increases goal attainment	
Teach client new skills as needed: • problem solving • decision making • goal setting • evaluation skills • relaxation techniques	Will assist client in accepting and living with diagnosis of cancer	

(Diagnosis continued)

Table 7–11 *(continued)*

Intervention	*Rationale*	*Expected Outcome*
Assist client in identifying possible coping responses: • diversional activities • constructive outlets for anger • ways to gain self-control • recognizing stages of grief • developing attitude of hope	Will assist client in dealing with emotional reactions to illness	
If terminal, assist client in being able to complete unfinished business	Will give the client comfort and a sense of well-being	

Nursing Diagnosis: Potential alteration in family process related to family's inability to deal constructively with a traumatic experience.
Goal: During the course of treatment client will recognize and work toward family's adaptation to the consequences of the diagnosis.

Intervention	*Rationale*	*Expected Outcome*
Assess family reactions to this situational crisis	Will assist in planning actions to reduce and/or resolve the crisis	Reduction of crisis Resolution of crisis
Discuss with client the impact of the crisis (diagnosis of cancer) on family members: • negative reactions • ability to adapt • expectations of family members • role adjustments • anticipatory grief	Will assist client in understanding that bereavement begins when family members realize the loss of client is inevitable and many emotions are exhibited	Effective family problem solving Participation in family counseling
If necessary, refer family members to supportive therapy, spiritual counseling, etc. Present a variety of alternatives, and include family in making choices	Will offer additional support to family members in a time of crisis	Client and family openly discuss problems and concerns
Encourage client to discuss feelings about coping skills with family	Will assist family in feeling involved in resolution of their crisis	

Nursing Diagnosis: Fear related to life-threatening nature of cancer diagnosis.
Goal: During the course of treatment client will express reduced fear.

Intervention	*Rationale*	*Expected Outcome*
Observe client for signs of fear: • pupil dilation • increased pulse, respirations, blood pressure • diaphoresis • agitation	Early recognition of fear assists in reducing the reaction	Absence of fear Reduction of fear Verbalization of fears related to death

(continued)

Table 7–11 *(continued)*

Nursing Diagnosis *(continued)*: Fear related to life-threatening nature of cancer diagnosis.
Goal: During the course of treatment client will express reduced fear.

Intervention	*Rationale*	*Expected Outcome*
Listen actively to fears: • be open • answer questions honestly • be caring • stay with client • use open-ended questions	Presence of an open, caring nurse may prevent fear and allow client to gain insight into fear reactions	
Encourage client to verbalize when timing appropriate on: • feelings about death • perceptions of danger • perceptions of ability to cope • questions about progress • questions about prognosis	Will assist client in identifying the source of fear and response pattern related to that fear	

Nursing Diagnosis: Anticipatory grieving related to potential loss of client to cancer.
Goal: Through the course of treatment client will be able to work through grieving process.

Intervention	*Rationale*	*Expected Outcome*
Assess client's phase of grief	The normal phases of the grieving process are denial, anger, bargaining, depression, and acceptance	Grief resolved Statements related to acceptance
Assist client in resolving denial: • caring manner • soft tone of voice • empathy • be realistic about loss • explain grief response • give client a reasonable period of time for denial	Nurses understanding each phase of grief will allow for more effective nursing interventions	No evidence of dysfunctional grieving
Assisting client through anger: • be tolerant • show understanding • do not take anger personally • offer ways to constructively express anger • encourage client expression of conflicts		Constructive relationships with others Absence of distorted emotional reactions
Assisting client through bargaining and depression: • use active listening • encourage expression of thoughts and feelings • point out reality, but do not argue • observe for suicidal actions or thoughts		

(Diagnosis continued)

Table 7–11 *(continued)*

Intervention	*Rationale*	*Expected Outcome*
Assisting client toward acceptance: • correct any misinformation about the nature of the disease • encourage use of coping kills • support expression of feelings (eg, crying) • observe for signs of depression • encourage discussion of both positive and negative aspects of diagnosis • encourage social interaction • encourage spiritual support		

Nursing Diagnosis: Potential powerlessness related to client verbalizations of no control over outcomes of cancer diagnosis.
Goal: During the course of treatment client will state perceptions of influence on outcomes.

Intervention	*Rationale*	*Expected Outcome*
Assess client's knowledge and perception of treatment	Will assist in planning for reduction of client's feelings of powerlessness	
Be accepting of client: • listen to statements about feelings of hopelessness • avoid being judgmental about reactions • allow expression of anger, guilt, and rage	Will facilitate client's feeling of self-worth and importance	
Assist client in controlling as much of the environment as possible: • provide privacy • have client wear own clothes • encourage independent behavior • involve client in decision making • put personal articles, call light, and telephone within reach • have client participate as much as possible in self-care activities • maintain client's sense of dignity	Will reduce feelings of powerlessness by giving client some control over the situation	
Assist client in reducing feelings of powerlessness: • have client describe powerlessness • identify uncontrollable events • identify controllable events • mutual goal setting • problem solving • review improvements in condition • provide any information that is needed • encourage questions • involve client in planning care • build a trusting relationship		Verbalizes a sense of control States feelings of adequacy Participates in decision making States feelings of hope Seeks appropriate assistance from others

(continued)

Table 7–11 *(continued)*

Nursing Diagnosis: Disturbance in self-concept (body-image, self-esteem, role performance) related to preoccupation with grief and loss.
Goal: By time of discharge client will begin accepting body image changes and develop a positive self-concept.

Intervention	*Rationale*	*Expected Outcome*
Initiate a one-to-one relationship with client	Will enhance client's self-esteem	Positive expressions of self-acceptance
Assess client's perception of body image	Will assist in planning appropriate nursing interventions	Participation in treatment
Encourage client to verbalize concerns about body image: • anger • anxiety • loss • fear	Will assist in moving client toward acceptance of changes within body	Demonstration of self-respect Demonstration of self-confidence
Accept client as a worthwhile human being: • spend time with client • avoid judgmental attitudes • offer supportive comments • be genuine • maintain a therapeutic environment	Will assist client in maintaining and improving positive self-esteem	
Encourage client to discuss feelings about the sick role	Will assist client in identifying the impact of the cancer diagnosis	

Nursing Diagnosis: Sexual dysfunction related to painful effects of disease and/or treatment.
Goal: As long as possible client will have adequate pain control to allow participation in sexual activities.

Intervention	*Rationale*	*Expected Outcome*
Administer necessary agents to reduce pain	Will assist client toward more comfortable sexual relations	Client reports satisfaction with sexual contact
Provide privacy for sexual contact	Will encourage client's expression of sexual desires	
Assist client in maintaining good personal hygiene	Clean, unsoiled environment without odors increases desire	
Provide articles for aesthetically comfortable environment		

Nursing Diagnosis: Social isolation related to client's doubts about ability to survive.
Goal: During the course of treatment client will maintain social contact with others.

Intervention	*Rationale*	*Expected Outcome*
Assess social history	Will assist in understanding client's current reactions	Reduction in social isolation Verbalizes feelings of loneliness
Assist client in identifying barriers to relationships with others (eg, stigma of diagnosis)	Will increase client's understanding of others' reactions	Participates in visits by family and friends

(Diagnosis continued)

Table 7–11 *(continued)*

Intervention	*Rationale*	*Expected Outcome*
Encourage visitors	Will provide client with opportunity for socializing	
Offer support for client's experience of loss: • recognize detachment as part of acceptance • help family understand detachment • sit silently with client • encourage family to sit with client, perhaps holding hand	Will assist client in accepting personal loss	

Nursing Diagnosis: Potential spiritual distress related to a lack of reconciliation with a spiritual being before death.
Goal: During course of treatment client will be able to complete any unfinished spiritual business.

Intervention	*Rationale*	*Expected Outcome*
Listen actively for client's: • allusion to spiritual distress • stated spiritual needs • search for meaning of illness	Will assist client in alleviating spiritual concerns	States spiritual comfort Requests religious articles and readings Requests spiritual counselor
Assist client in enduring suffering: • stay with client, hold hand • encourage prayer • encourage meditation • provide religious articles • call chaplain at client's request • provide religious or other readings	Will assist client in finding purpose in the illness	

Table 7–12 *Example of Evaluation of Nursing Care of a Client with Cancer*

Plan	*Evaluation*
1. The client will be able to express concerns about death and dying before discharge.	On 5/22 client began weeping when nurse went in to restart her IV. Client stated "I wish I could just die and get it over with!"
2. The client will state relief from pain at least every 4 hours.	On 5/23 client was medicated four times during a 24-hour period. Client stated that relief was obtained by the dose given.
3. The client will be able to work through the grieving process during current admission.	On 5/23 client told the nurse that she wanted to live only until June, when her son graduated from college. Then it would be okay to die.

Analysis/Synthesis of Data

Concerns	*Nursing diagnoses*
Fear of disfigurement, dependency	Alteration in comfort; pain
Inadequate support system	Impaired verbal communication
Dealing with grief	Ineffective individual coping
Pain	Fear
Change in body image	Anticipatory grieving
	Potential for powerlessness
	Disturbance in self-concept; body image, self-esteem, role performance, personal identity
	Social isolation

Suggested Care Planning Activities

1. Determine the priorities for Gary's care.
2. Determine the support systems available to Gary.
3. Describe the stage of grief Gary is most likely exhibiting.

4. Consider the type of reaction to be expected from Gary's family.
5. Consider the type of family support to be anticipated.
6. Describe the significance of the laboratory findings.
7. Determine the developmental aspects to be considered in Gary's care.
8. Identify nursing goals for Gary.
9. Describe the client teaching necessary to assist Gary toward recovery.
10. List and provide a rationale for the nursing interventions in Gary's care.

Knowledge Base: Respiratory Disorders

Many diseases are related to respiration. Changes in the rate, regularity, and depth of respiration correlate with many emotional and behavioral states. For example, a pain-stricken person gasps, a bored person yawns, a person in love or in deep sorrow sighs, and a person anxious or fearful hyperventilates. Moreover, many idioms allude to the relationship of emotion and respiration: "We're waiting with bated breath," "She takes your breath away," "We hold our breath in fear," and "His nose is out of joint."

One of the most common of the respiratory disorders, asthma, will be the focus of this text's discussion. The student is encouraged to review hyperventilation syndrome and allergies for their psychophysiologic bases. According to the National Institute of Allergy and Infectious Disease, 8.9 million Americans are affected by **asthma,** which is characterized by spasm of the bronchial tubes, swelling of the bronchial mucous membranes, and paroxysmal dyspnea. Five percent of children under 15 years of age are affected by asthma. In childhood, boys with asthma outnumber girls by a 2–3:1 ratio. However, in adolescence, this ratio drops to 1:1. Then after age 45, the proportion of men to women again increases. It is estimated that approximately 17% of all Americans have had asthma sometime during their life (Thompson et al., 1989; Weiner, 1985).

Behavioral Characteristics

The client with asthma has periodic attacks of wheezing and breathing difficulties. These attacks can be frightening and may even lead to death by suffocation. Two thousand people die of asthma each year in the United States (Kneisl and Ames, 1986). Asthma occurs early in life but may arise again in adulthood.

For most children, fear of separation is profound, and this seems to be particularly true with asthma-prone children. Mixed with immature coping mechanisms, this fear sometimes leads to feelings of helplessness and depression (Weiner, 1985). The regressive behavior sometimes seen in asthmatic children, which arises partly out of normal developmental issues and partly from some special psychologic and physical needs, creates a situation where the comforting that is given due to the illness can become a psychologic necessity. It is perfectly understandable that a child becomes attached to the comforting behaviors that resulted when he became sick. It is also understandable that parents become extremely fearful about their child's well being and sometimes life, and can easily fall into this pattern of overcompensating for their child's needs. This can, of course, create a new set of problems to solve.

Loneliness and varying degrees of dissatisfaction with interpersonal and social relationships are common in asthma clients. The loss of a mother figure or other adverse life events can trigger an asthma attack. The asthma-prone person may feel hopelessness about life, especially in the face of stressful events.

Affective Characteristics

Asthmatics experience the same emotions as other people. However, research shows them to be somewhat more sensitive to high emotion, which seems to predispose them to more serious physical effects. It is recognized that emotion has a bearing on the occurrence of asthmatic attacks. When asthmatic people feel anger, anxiety, fear, guilt, or jealousy, they become more vulnerable to an asthmatic attack.

Cognitive Characteristics

It is difficult to determine if patterns of thinking precede the onset of the disease or if they are a result of living with asthma. Many childhood asthmatics verbalize a strong desire for parental protection and want to remain in a dependent relationship. They may exhibit immature defense mechanisms or ineffective coping behaviors.

Physiologic Characteristics

The primary physical factors precipitating an asthmatic attack are respiratory tract infection, intolerance to certain drugs such as aspirin, cold weather or sudden changes in barometric pressure, exercise, and air pollutants.

The physical mechanism of an asthma attack is centered in the autonomic nerves, which when stimulated or irritated, become hypersensitive. These nerves, failing to cause smooth muscle relaxation, cause contraction. This, in turn, causes failure to decrease secretion of mucus and produces mucosal edema.

Antigen-antibody reactions also occur in the asthmatic person. When exposed to certain allergens, the asthmatic forms large amounts of immunoglobulin (IgE), which fixes to the cells of bronchial mucosa causing them to degranulate and release chemical mediators, primarily histamine (Groër and Shekleton, 1979).

In all lung volumes, there is an increased resistance to airflow, as is shown by prolonged respiration. The vital capacity of the lung is decreased, and the residual volume of air is increased. The lung is overinflated because of closure of the airways, and blood does not uniformly perfuse the lung. The respiratory rate may be markedly increased because of hypoxemia and acidosis. The CO_2 retained produces adverse effects on psychologic function, leading to delirium, stupor, and sometimes death.

Sociocultural Characteristics

Certain studies suggest that the development of asthma is a combination of environmental factors. Social and family relationships, infections, allergens, and occupational and industrial pollutants play major roles in the onset of asthma. These things combined with a genetic predisposition make some people very vulnerable to asthma.

Knapp (1985) found that moving to a new environment also seems to play a major role in the development of asthma. The forced adaptation to new substances and stressful changes may combine to make the person more vulnerable to attacks.

Causative Theories

Asthma is categorized for causation by three types: extrinsic (allergic), intrinsic (idiopathic or nonallergic), or mixed (both allergic and nonallergic).

Extrinsic asthma has its onset in childhood or adolescence. There is a family history of atopic (allergic) illness. The disease is seasonal with environmental changes and often clears after childhood. Attacks are precipitated by exposure to allergens like pollen, dust, and foods. **Intrinsic asthma** has its onset after age 35. There is no specific family history for atopic illness. The attacks are unpredictable, chronic, and severe and are precipitated by weather changes, infection, certain drugs, emotion, and exercise. **Mixed asthma** causes most suffering from this condition. The physiologic mechanisms underlying its causation were discussed above.

Medical Treatment

Medical treatment for asthma centers on diagnosis, treatment for acute attacks, and treatment for chronic asthma. Diagnosis is preceded by a history and physical examination. As part of the physical examination, various tests are conducted such as pulmonary function studies, chest x ray, arterial blood gases, allergy and skin testing, sputum specimen for gram-stain, culture and eosinophils, and blood levels of eosinophils.

The treatment for acute asthma attacks consists of administration of oxygen by nasal cannula. Medications most commonly administered are intravenous aminophylline, subcutaneous terbutalene or epinephrine, and intravenous corticosteroids. Respiratory therapy treatments and postural drainage are also used. Finally, at least 3 liters of fluids per day are forced.

The treatment for chronic asthma includes elimination of causative agents and, if indicated, desensitization. Several medications, either oral or inhaled, are used. Common oral compounds are theophylline, beta-adrenergics, and corticosteroids. Corticosteroids may be contraindicated in children because they affect growth. Common inhalants are beta-adrenergics, chromolyn sodium, and beclomethasone. The client may be taught postural drainage and come in for regular respiratory therapy sessions.

Assessment

Nursing History Assessment of the client with asthma begins with data collection that focuses on stressors precipitating the attacks. The principal reason for the nursing history is to help prepare long-term management goals for dealing with chronic asthma attacks. To determine the client's general state of function, the nurse begins with a general history. The nurse should develop rapport and provide a relaxed atmosphere when conducting interviews with the asthmatic client. (See Table 7–4 for a general history for clients with psychological factors affecting physical condition.) In addition to the general history tool of Table 7–4, the nurse should ask the following questions of the asthmatic client:

- How frequent is your contact with your parents?
- Would you say you are closer to your mother? Father?
- Are you able to say no to requests from others?
- What are your attacks like?
- How long have you had asthma attacks?
- Are your attacks seasonal?
- Do you know what precipitates the attacks?
- Do you follow a nonallergenic diet?
- What foods do you avoid?

Physical Assessment Physical assessment in this section is related to only the adult asthma client. The objective of respiratory assessment in the adult asthmatic is to ascertain the quality of ventilation. By observing the general shape of the chest and the respiratory pattern, the nurse begins the assessment. The chest is normally symmetrical, and respirations normally range from 12 to 20 per minute. The chest should move symmetrically with no intercostal bulging, retractions, or use of accessory muscles for breathing when observing a normal pattern. Tachypnea and prolonged expiration may be present in asthma.

Wheezes, high-pitched sounds noted (often only by using a stethoscope) on inspiration and expiration, are auscultated in asthma victims. The sounds result from a narrowed airway causing partial bronchial obstruction. Rales and rhonchi may also be present. **Rales** are crackling or bubbling sounds produced by air movement through fluid-filled alveoli. **Rhonchi** are low-pitched sounds that are usually heard on inspiration. Other sources say rhonchi are audible during inspiration, expiration, or both (Brunner and Suddarth, 1988). Sometimes the sounds decrease or even disappear after the client coughs. These sounds result from partial bronchial obstruction, usually from secretions. Pain from respirations, dyspnea, cough, sputum, and hemoptysis should also be assessed. A chest x ray should be obtained.

Nursing Diagnosis and Planning

As with medical diagnosis, nursing diagnoses for asthma may be grouped into diagnostic (identification of disorder), acute episodes, and chronic management. The focus of this text is on chronic management with emphasis on emotionally related

Table 7–13 *Nursing Diagnoses in the Client with Asthma*

Activity intolerance, potential
Anxiety
Coping, ineffective individual
Fear
Gas exchange, impaired
Health maintenance, alteration in
Knowledge deficit, potential
Parenting, alteration in
Self-concept, disturbance in (body image, self-esteem, role performance, personal identity)
Sexual dysfunction
Sleep pattern disturbance, potential

diagnoses. (See Table 7–13 for a summary of the nursing diagnoses for the client with asthma.)

The nursing care plan is developed around individually identified nursing diagnoses. Mutual goal setting is essential to restore and maintain adequate ventilation for the client. The nurse's primary concern is health promotion and maintenance to prevent attacks. The nurse must also teach the client how to manage acute attacks.

The nurse should recognize the panic felt by the client during attacks and help the client learn to relax. (See Table 7–14 for the care plan for the client with asthma.)

Evaluation

Evaluation of the care of the asthmatic client is completed by comparing the client's behavior to the mutually planned goals. (See Table 7–15 for an evaluation of the care of a client with asthma.) In general, the expected outcomes for the asthmatic client can be behaviorally stated as the client will:

- Not experience dyspnea.
- Express feelings of calmness.
- Have the energy to complete self-care activities.
- Appear relaxed.
- Be able to identify stressors that precipitate attacks.
- State ways to avoid infections.
- Plan for general health management.

CASE EXAMPLE

A Client with Asthma

Casey Edwards was 10 years old when he had his first asthmatic attack during a neighborhood game of football. Casey's mother had kept him extremely dependent on her for his safety, and to make sure he was taken care of properly, had always made him stay close to home. Even as an adult of 25, Casey still must listen to his mother's complaints that his wife cares for him improperly. One night Casey experienced a "smothering attack" at home. Casey's wife became alarmed and brought him to the emergency room. From there he was admitted to the medical floor during the evening shift.

Nursing History

Location: General Hospital, Medical Floor
Client's name: Casey Edwards Age: 25
Admitting diagnosis: Acute Bronchial Asthma
T=97.6, P=100, R=40, B/P=150/80

Health history
Height: 5′ 11″
Weight: 185 lb
Eats three meals a day, maintains a nonallergenic diet
Sleeps six to eight hours at night
Does not smoke
Does not take alcohol

Social history
Married for one year
Wife is expecting a baby
Spends leisure time doing odd jobs for his mother

Clinical data
Skin tests positive
Elevated serum IgE
Elevated eosinophils
ABG
pH 7.28
pCO_2 36

(continued on p 273, col 1)

Table 7–14 Nursing Care Plan for the Client with Asthma

Nursing Diagnosis: Potential activity intolerance related to dyspnea.
Goal: During the course of treatment client will participate in activities that maintain physiologic well-being.

Intervention	*Rationale*	*Expected Outcome*
Encourage client to assess physical limitations on activity Encourage client to identify factors that reduce tolerance for activity (eg, treatments, medications, environmental conditions, etc)	Will assist in identifying appropriate activities	Optimal mobility No SOB Engages in self-care activities Changes activities to account for physical limitations
Adapt self-care to meet client needs: • provide assistance only when client is in acute distress • provide nonstrenuous leisure activities • encourage client to increase activity within therapeutic limits • provide passive exercise	Will assist client in developing an activity pattern	

Nursing Diagnosis: Anxiety related to apprehensive response to threat of disrupted respirations.
Goal: During the course of treatment client will be able to reduce anxiety.

Intervention	*Rationale*	*Expected Outcome*
Encourage client to learn to recognize the presence of anxiety: • discuss thoughts and feelings before anxiety • discuss expectations related to anxiety • clarify the nature of the threat	Will assist client in appropriately using adaptive coping strategies	Reduction of anxiety Recognition of anxiety in self
Teach client coping strategies: • slow, deep breathing • use of bronchodilating drugs • recognition of secondary gains from maladaptive strategies • muscle relaxation techniques	Increasing client's knowledge base will assist in developing insight into anxiety	Use of new coping strategies

Nursing Diagnosis: Ineffective breathing pattern related to anxiety.
Goal: Throughout the course of treatment client will maintain adequate ventilation.

Intervention	*Rationale*	*Expected Outcome*
Assess breathing pattern: • rate of respirations • rhythm of respirations • depth of respirations • chest expansion • presence of distress (ie, SOB) • nasal flaring • use of accessory muscles • prolonged expiration	Will assist in determining client's ability to adequately ventilate	Adequate ventilation Effortless breathing Normal respiratory rate

(Diagnosis continued)

Table 7–14 *(continued)*

Intervention	*Rationale*	*Expected Outcome*
Place client in position of comfort (eg, sitting upright, leaning over bedside table)	Will assist client in attaining adequate ventilation	No use of accessory muscles for breathing
Identify allergens: • ask client about environmental allergens • eliminate dust • place allergen-free covers on pillows	Allergens exacerbate ineffective breathing patterns	
Ausculate lungs	Will assist in identifying abnormal breath sounds (eg, wheezes, rales, rhonchi)	No SOB
Monitor ABGs	Will ensure adequate ventilation	ABG within normal limits: pH: 7.35–7.45 po_2: 80–95 mm HG pco_2: 35–45 mm HG O_2 saturation: 95–99%
Administer medications as ordered	Bronchodilators, antihistamines, anti-infectives, expectorants, and corticosteroids assist in reducing physical symptoms	

Nursing Diagnosis: Ineffective individual coping related to impairment of adaptive behaviors for meeting life's demands.
Goal: During the course of treatment client will develop plans for alternative strategies for dealing with stress.

Intervention	*Rationale*	*Expected Outcome*
Assist client in identifying stressors: • environmental allergens • stressful changes in lifestyle • events causing unresolved anger	Recognizing stressors will assist client toward resolution	Recognition of sources of stress
Assist client in identifying stress-related health behaviors	Recognition of body responses to stress will assist client toward developing new coping strategies	Sets realistic goals for stress reduction
Client teaching for: • goal setting • assertive communication • relaxation techniques	Will assist client in developing new coping strategies	Uses new coping skills to reduce stress Develops support systems

Nursing Diagnosis: Fear related to an emotional response to the danger of being unable to get adequate oxygen.
Goal: At the initiation of respiratory treatments client will experience reduction in fear.

Intervention	*Rationale*	*Expected Outcome*
Assess client's basic response to fear (eg, fight or flight)	Will assist in planning fear reduction strategies	Verbalizes no fear Appears relaxed
When appropriate, encourage verbalization about: • feelings • perception of danger • ability to cope	Will assist in resolving fear response	No SOB

(Diagnosis continued)

Table 7–14 *(continued)*

Nursing Diagnosis *(continued)*: Fear related to an emotional response to the danger of being unable to get adequate oxygen.
Goal: At the initiation of respiratory treatments client will experience reduction in fear.

Intervention	*Rationale*	*Expected Outcome*
Assist client in coping with present fear: • remain calm • administer treatments promptly as ordered • stay with client during episodes of SOB • encourage slow, deep breathing • remove extraneous stimuli from environment		

Nursing Diagnosis: Impaired gas exchange related to prolonged expiratory phase trapping CO_2 and causing changes in sensorium.
Goal: During the course of treatment client will maintain adequate ventilation.

Intervention	*Rationale*	*Expected Outcome*
Ausculate lungs	Will assist in assessing breath patterns	Full lung expansion
Administer humidified oxygen as ordered	Will give client adequate blood-oxygen saturation	No wheezes, rales, or rhonchi
Encourage coughing and deep breathing	Will allow for full lung expansion	
Place client in position of comfort: • high Fowler's • sitting up in chair • leaning over bedside table		
Assess skin and nail color	Cyanosis will be in lips and nail beds if oxygen exchange is inadequate	Adequate ventilation
Monitor ABGs	Decreases in pco_2 and po_2 of more than 10 mm HG indicate poor perfusion and should be reported	ABGs within normal limits

Nursing Diagnosis: Alteration in health maintenance related to ineffective family coping.
Goal: Before discharge client will begin developing support systems for more effective health maintenance.

Intervention	*Rationale*	*Expected Outcome*
Assess client's present support system	Will assist in identifying health maintenance needs	Demonstrates health maintenance practices
Use behavior modification: • self monitoring • contracting • guided practice with reinforcement	Will assist client in developing more appropriate health maintenance skills	Reduced asthma attacks
Assist client in identifying support systems (eg, provide information on community resources)	Will encourage client to use available resources	Uses community resources

(Diagnosis continued)

Table 7–14 *(continued)*

Intervention	*Rationale*	*Expected Outcome*
Client teaching on: • problem solving • assertive communication • establishing personal health goals	Will assist client in assuming responsibility for health maintenance	

Nursing Diagnosis: Potential knowledge deficit related to living with asthma and functioning below level of potential well-being.
Goal: Before discharge client will learn preventive measures for asthma attacks.

Intervention	*Rationale*	*Expected Outcome*
Client teaching on: • theories about illness • nature of diagnosis • physical aspects of care • importance of recognizing stressors • removing environmental allergens • importance of adequate rest • importance of avoiding secondary infections • side effects of medications used for treatment	Increased knowledge base is related to greater client compliance	Client explains plans for preventive measures Describes benefits of preventive measures Monitors emotional state for signs of stress Monitors physical state for signs of respiratory infection States effects and side effects of medical treatments

Nursing Diagnosis: Potential alteration in parenting related to overprotection of nurturing figure.
Goal: By time of discharge client will recognize the relationship of altered parenting and disease condition.

Intervention	*Rationale*	*Expected Outcome*
Initiate a one-to-one relationship built on trust	Will encourage discussion of self-concept and self-esteem	Identifies childhood experiences affecting current condition
Actively listen	Will assist in identifying parental conflict	
Encourage client to discuss relationship with parent or nurturing figure	Will assist in resolving the conflicts felt by client	States feelings related to conflicts with parent(s)
Health teaching for family on what to do for client during asthma attacks	Will assist family in developing a supportive role to client	

Nursing Diagnosis: Disturbance in self-concept (body-image, self-esteem, role performance, personal identity) related to somatic expression of emotions.
Goal: During the course of treatment client will learn to accept more positive physical self.

Intervention	*Rationale*	*Expected Outcome*
Initiate a one-to-one relationship with client	Will indicate nurse is accepting of client as an individual	Decrease in number of asthmatic attacks
Assess client's perception of body: • is it pleasing? • not pleasing? • past experience with significant others? • value of physical self	Will assist client in developing a realistic body image	Demonstrates assertive communication Uses strengths

Table 7–14 *(continued)*

Nursing Diagnosis *(continued)*: Disturbance in self-concept (body-image, self-esteem, role performance, personal identity) related to somatic expression of emotions.
Goal: During the course of treatment client will learn to accept more positive physical self.

Intervention	Rationale	Expected Outcome
Avoid concentrating on physical symptoms (eg, give client a short time to discuss physical complaints and reduce time each session)	Will encourage client to develop new interpersonal skills to replace somatic complaints	
Client teaching on assertive skills: • use of "I" messages • offering clear expectations of others • use of negotiation • having posture, facial expression, and tone of voice congruent	Will assist client in developing more positive interpersonal skills	
Explore the benefits client receives from illness (eg, concept of secondary gain)	Client understanding of benefits of illness will assist in reducing physical symptoms	

Nursing Diagnosis: Sexual dysfunction related to preoccupation with somatic symptoms.
Goal: Before discharge client will recognize the impact of asthma on sexual functioning.

Intervention	*Rationale*	*Expected Outcome*
Client teaching on: • physical illness • process of illness • effect of treatments • side effect of medications • behavior changes necessary	Will increase client's understanding and assist toward changing maladaptive behaviors	Reduction of psychological conflicts
Counseling on: • realistic expectations of self • realistic expectations of others • dependency issues in partnership • sexual techniques	Will assist client in developing better sexual function	Verbalized understanding of relationship of disease process to sexual functioning

Nursing Diagnosis: Potential sleep pattern disturbance related to breathing pattern interrupting sleep.
Goal: In order to sleep in intervals of at least six to eight hours during the course of treatment client will participate in therapeutic regimen to reduce breathing difficulties.

Intervention	*Rationale*	*Expected Outcome*
Monitor environmental stressors: • allergens • place allergen-free pillow slip • noise level • comfortable temperature • plan treatments around rest periods • limit excessive number of staff • level of lighting lowered	Will assist client in obtaining satisfactory sleep Provide treatments to encourage sleep: • place in position of comfort (eg, semi-Fowler's) • use two or more pillows • give respiratory treatments before sleep • administer medications as ordered (eg, bronchodilators, corticosteroids, theophylline)	Sleeps six to eight hours States satisfaction with sleep States feels rested

Table 7–15 *Example of Evaluation of Nursing Care of a Client with Asthma*

Plan	*Evaluation*
1. The client will be able to maintain adequate ventilation during the course of treatment.	On 4/12 the client had respiratory treatments q 3 h and O_2 was maintained at 4 liters per nasal cannula. The client's respiratory rate ranged 20–24 and no SOB was noted. There were no wheezes, rales, or rhonchi auscultated.
2. The client will sleep for at least 6 hours in a 24-hour period.	On 4/12 the client had a respiratory treatment at 11 PM. On 4/13 the client slept until 4 AM.
3. The client will be able to reduce anxiety during the course of treatment.	On 4/12 the client pushed the nurse's call light and requested a Valium. The client stated, "I feel a little anxious."

Nursing observations

Casey was experiencing dyspnea and unable to complete an initial interview. After starting on IV aminophylline and nasal O_2, Casey was better able to respond to questions by the nurse. Casey is concerned about his wife who is seven months pregnant. He is afraid his mother will be critical of how they care for the child. Casey feels his asthma attack was a direct result of the emotional conflict over the upcoming birth of his child.

Analysis/Synthesis of Data

Concerns	*Nursing diagnoses*
Inadequate ventilation	Anxiety
Emotional conflict	Ineffective breathing pattern
Anxiety	Ineffective individual coping
Immature coping	Impaired gas exchange
Fatigue	Actual alteration in parenting
Disrupted sleep	Disturbance in self-concept: body image, self-esteem, role identity, personal identity
	Sleep pattern disturbance

Suggested Care Planning Activities

1. Determine the priorities for Casey's care.
2. Determine the support systems available to Casey.
3. Describe the significance of the laboratory findings.
4. Determine the developmental aspects to be considered in Casey's care.
5. Consider the stressors that Casey should be able to identify.
6. Identify nursing goals for Casey.
7. Describe the client teaching necessary to assist Casey toward recovery.
8. List and provide a rationale for nursing interventions in Casey's care.

Knowledge Base: Gastrointestinal Disorders

The gastrointestinal tract has a complex interaction with the psyche. The earliest phases of human development are labeled oral and anal. Innumerable everyday expressions refer to this relationship: "You're so sweet, I could eat you up"; "Spit it out"; "I'm fed up"; "I felt my stomach churning"; "My stomach was in my throat"; and "It's enough to make you vomit."

There are many behaviors connected to gastrointestinal functions. Changes in appetite, food intake, digestive functions, and elimination occur almost daily in relation to emotional stress. Disturbances relate primarily to two functions of the gastrointestinal tract that are under voluntary control: eating and defecation.

Since the gastrointestinal tract is complex and has many psychophysiologic disorders, one primary disorder, ulcerative colitis, will be discussed in this section of the text. The following is a listing of gastrointestinal disorders thought to be psychophysiologic:

1. *Esophageal disorders*—esophageal reflux, achalasia, esophageal spasm, and peptic ulcer of the esophagus
2. *Stomach disorders*—hyperacidity, and peptic ulcer disease
3. *Intestinal disorders*—chronic diarrhea, constipation, irritable bowel syndrome, spastic colon, and ulcerative colitis

As stated above, this chapter focuses on the intestinal disorder of ulcerative colitis. It should be noted that people with gastrointestinal disorders share a number of traits; therefore, much of the information about ulcerative colitis is also applicable to other gastrointestinal disorders.

Ulcerative colitis is a condition in which the colon and rectum are inflamed and ulcerated. Although ulcerative colitis can occur at any age, it is found most frequently in people between 15 and 40. The condition affects both sexes with a slightly higher incidence in females. Ulcerative colitis has its highest incidence in Jews, and its lowest incidence in African-Americans (Arehart-Treichel, 1980; Thompson et al., 1989; Brunner and Suddarth, 1988).

Behavioral Characteristics

Terms used to describe the behavior of clients with ulcerative colitis include immature and dependent. Often they are obsessed with perfection, orderliness, neatness, and punctuality. Behaviors may be manifested in different ways during the disease process. Some clients are ingratiating, submissive, and placating, whereas others are querulous and demanding. Some clients experience severe headaches before attacks, but during these periods clients have been noted to behave in ways quite different from how they behave during an attack. They may be more decisive, active, aggressive, and feel in control. These feelings, however, are accompanied by guilt and may contribute to the factors that precipitate an attack (Oken, 1985).

Affective Characteristics

People prone to ulcerative colitis have been described as emotionally sensitive with an excessive need for affection and love. Often they have had difficulty in identifying and expressing feelings and tend to repress negative emotions. They experience deep feelings of hurt when others suggest their lives are less than perfect and may respond with a great deal of hostility. They are at risk for developing depression.

Cognitive Characteristics

People with ulcerative colitis set extremely high, perfectionistic standards for themselves and are self-critical when they fail to reach these unattainable expectations. They are very sensitive to criticism. They may be egocentric, narcissistic, and grandiose about themselves.

Physiologic Characteristics

The primary physiologic characteristic of ulcerative colitis is diffuse inflammation of the mucosa and submucosa spreading distally up the colon. The disease begins in the rectum and sigmoid and eventually involves the entire colon. The mucosa becomes hyperemic, edematous, and bleeds with minimal trauma. Abscesses develop in the crypts of Lieberkuhn. Some of these abscesses heal, others form scar tissue, and the colon can become denuded in some areas (Brunner and Suddarth, 1988).

Sociocultural Characteristics

Almost all experts agree that sufferers of ulcerative colitis have had a traumatic childhood leading to excessive dependency on others. The typical situation is a dominating mother, a passive father, and an emotionally repressed home atmosphere. Some studies indicate that clients reflect the personality traits of their mothers: strict, domineering, perfectionistic, over-demanding, over-protective, emotionally suppressed, sexually prim, excessively concerned with neatness, obedient, and conforming.

Situations that may trigger attacks of ulcerative colitis are rape, birth of a deformed child, an operation, moving, divorce, changing jobs, death of a significant other, and school exams (Arehart-Treichel, 1980; Oken, 1985).

Causative Theories

The exact cause of ulcerative colitis is unknown. Some theories suggest an autoimmune reaction, viral infection, allergies, excessive enzymes, and emotional stress. Emotional responses do alter the blood supply to the colon mucosa, but it is unclear whether stress is the cause or the effect of the disease process. There appears to be a familial tendency in the development of ulcerative colitis (Brunner and Suddarth, 1988).

Medical Treatment

Medical treatments center on resting the bowel, reducing inflammation, eliminating infection, correcting malnutrition, and alleviating stress. Numerous pharmacologic agents are used to treat ulcerative colitis. Anticholinergics such as Banthine and Pro-Banthine are used to decrease gastrointestinal motility and secretions and to reduce smooth muscle spasms. Sedatives and antianxiety agents such as Dalmane and Valium are used to quiet the central nervous system. Antidiarrheals such as Lomotil are used to decrease gastrointestinal motility. Antimicrobials such as Azulfidine and Salazopyrin are used either to prevent or to treat secondary infections. Steroids such as cortisone or prednisone are used as anti-inflammatory agents. Immunosuppressives such as Imuran are used to suppress the immune response. Hematinics such as Imferon are used to correct iron deficiency anemia.

Dietary measures are also an important part of treatment. During acute attacks the client may be NPO and receive parenteral hyperalimentation. In remissions, a high-caloric, high-protein, and low-residue diet is indicated (Beare and Myers, 1990; Brunner and Suddarth, 1988).

Assessment

Nursing History When assessing the client with ulcerative colitis, an accurate data base is essential. Obviously, the client is the primary source of the data, but family members should also be observed. The nursing history focuses on the stresses that precipitate attacks. It is important that the nurse plan a quiet, calm, private atmosphere in which to conduct the interview. Table 7–4 provides a general history for clients with psychological factors affecting physical condition.

In addition to the questions on the general history tool of Table 7–4, the nurse should add the following questions:

- Would you say that you feel closer to your mother? Father?
- Was emotional expression encouraged in your household?
- What were the consequences of expressing emotions?
- What are your ulcerative colitis attacks like?
- Do other members of your family have ulcerative colitis?
- What do you think causes your attacks of ulcerative colitis?
- What is your usual diet?
- Are there any foods you avoid?

Physical Assessment The physical assessment of the ulcerative colitis client is focused on ruling out other problems such as cancer or diverticulitis. Because the effects of the disease are debilitating, a general systems assessment should be conducted. Problems that may be found are skin ulcers, malnutrition, anemia, abscesses, strictures or fistulas in the rectum, and electrolyte imbalance.

The modalities of assessment include inspection, percussion, auscultation, and palpation. Hyperactive bowel sounds may be auscultated in attacks of ulcerative colitis. The nurse should proceed with a head-to-toe general systems assessment (Brunner and Suddarth, 1988).

Nursing Diagnosis and Planning

For the client with ulcerative colitis, the goal of nursing intervention is supportive therapy. Nursing diagnoses developed from client data serve as the basis for establishing therapeutic goals. (See Table 7–16 for a summary of nursing diagnoses for clients with ulcerative colitis.)

The nurse plans care on the basis of individually identified nursing diagnoses. To establish a

Table 7–16 *Nursing Diagnoses for Clients with Ulcerative Colitis*

Activity intolerance, potential
Anxiety
Bowel elimination, alteration in (diarrhea)
Coping, ineffective individual
Family process, alteration in
Nutrition, alteration in (less than body requirements)
Self-concept, disturbance in (body image, self-esteem, role performance, personal identity)
Sexual dysfunction
Social isolation

supportive treatment plan, the client should agree with the goals set. The nurse is empathetic to the sensitive nature of the client with ulcerative colitis. (See Table 7–17 for the nursing care plan for the client with ulcerative colitis.)

Evaluation

In evaluating the care of the client with ulcerative colitis, the nurse compares the client's progress to the established goals. (See Table 7–18 for an evaluation of the care of a client with ulcerative colitis.) In general, the expected outcomes for the client with ulcerative colitis can be stated behaviorally as the client will:

- Experience a decrease in or absence of loose stools.
- Experience normal bowel sounds.
- Achieve a normal elimination pattern.
- Intake adequate nutrition.
- Maintain a normal body weight.
- Show no evidence of skin breakdown.
- Develop healthier coping mechanisms.

CASE EXAMPLE

A Client with Ulcerative Colitis

Delores Stubard, age 38, can be described as passive, compliant, timid, and dependent. Delores remembers that her mother was very demanding and that her father spent long hours at his menial job. Delores had ulcerative colitis as a teenager and, until the recent death of her father, had kept her condition under control. Since the funeral, Delores has been hospitalized three times. For this hospitalization she has been placed on hyperalimentation.

Nursing History

Location: General Hospital, Medical Floor
Client's name: Delores Stubard Age: 38
Admitting diagnosis: Ulcerative Colitis
T=99.8, P=110, R=20, B/P=100/60

Health history
Height: 5′5″
Weight: 110 lbs
Usually has three meals a day; but has been unable to eat for past two weeks
Sleeps five to six hours at night
Smokes occasionally
Drinks wine occasionally

Social history
Married for 12 years
Has two children, a boy 5 and a girl 7
Employed part time as a bank teller

Clinical data
Barium enema revealed strictures in the bowel
Bloody diarrhea; 15–20 stools per day for three days
Hgb 9.2
Hct 27
K^+ 3.2

Nursing observations
Mrs. Stubard is very quiet and timid. She apologizes profusely for the "foul odor" she has. Mrs. Stubard tells you her father died about six weeks ago, and she thought she had handled the situation well. She had not had an episode of colitis since the birth of her second child five years ago. Mrs. Stubard states she has lost 15 pounds in the last three weeks.

Analysis/Synthesis of Data

Concerns	*Nursing diagnoses*
Diarrhea	Anxiety
Anorexia	Alteration in bowel elimination; diarrhea
Bowel inflammation	

(continued on p 280, col 2)

Table 7–17 Nursing Care Plan for the Client with Ulcerative Colitis

Nursing Diagnosis: Potential activity intolerance related to verbal reports of weakness from excessive stools.
Goal: Throughout the course of treatment client will develop an activity/rest pattern allowing increased activity.

Intervention	*Rationale*	*Expected Outcome*
Assist client in identifying factors that reduce activity tolerance: • treatments • energy expended on bowel movements • stress in the environment	Will aid in planning more appropriate interventions	
Modify client's environment to allow for increased activity: • use of bedside commode • use of bedpan if extremely weak • call light, tissue, personal articles within reach • passive exercise • assist with self-care • adjust schedule to space self-care activities	Will assist in increasing client's energy level for physical activities	Absence of weakness during activity Improved mobility Participation in self-care

Nursing Diagnosis: Anxiety related to stressful life events.
Goal: During the course of treatment client will learn new coping strategies for stress reduction.

Intervention	*Rationale*	*Expected Outcome*
Assist client in exploring perceptions related to the cause of anxiety (eg, use of role play)	Will assist the client in developing insight into life events creating stress	Reduced anxiety
Encourage client to recognize the presence of anxiety: • discuss thoughts and feelings before anxiety • discuss expectations related to anxiety • clarify the nature of the perceived threat	Will assist client in recognizing maladaptive coping mechanisms	
Take steps to reduce anxiety Extreme anxiety: • comfort measures (eg, warm bath) • reduce lighting • reduce noise and distractions • use short, simple phrases • administer sedatives, tranquilizers, and other drugs as ordered	Will assist client in regaining self-control	Demonstration of new coping strategies
Mild to moderate anxiety: • remain calm • engage client in diversional activities • encourage client to vent feelings • use relaxation techniques	Will offer new coping strategies to client	
Client teaching on: • assertive communication • relaxation techniques • problem solving • development of new interests, hobbies		

(continued)

Table 7–17 *(continued)*

Nursing Diagnosis: Alteration in bowel elimination (diarrhea) related to inflammation of the bowel.
Goal: During the course of treatment client will achieve relief from loose stools.

Intervention	*Rationale*	*Expected Outcome*
Assess bowel movements: • frequency • appearance • presence of blood	Will assist in planning for nursing interventions	Decrease in the number of episodes of diarrhea. No more than three bowel movements a day Formed stool
Client teaching on: • use of antidiarrhea medications • diet modifications • perirectal skin care • personal hygiene (eg, handwashing)	Will assist client in relieving symptoms	
Monitor: • I and O • body weight	Will assist in assessing fluid volume deficits and electrolyte imbalance. Diarrhea causes loss of electrolytes (eg, K^+)	Stabilized body weight
Provide for client comfort: • keep bedpan or commode near • keep toilet tissue near • provide privacy for bowel movements • use room deodorizer • offer warm, soapy water after bowel movements (may use peri-bottle if area is tender)	Will relieve symptoms created by excessive number of loose stools	

Nursing Diagnosis: Ineffective individual coping related to inability to interpret threat correctly.
Goal: During the course of treatment client will develop awareness of emotional reactions to stress.

Intervention	*Rationale*	*Expected Outcome*
Encourage client to assess: • fears • situations causing anger • how feelings are expressed • how thoughts are related to feelings	Will assist client in gaining insight into stress reactions	States sources of stress Sets realistic goals
Client teaching on: • warning signs of stress • ways to gain self-control • ways to express anger • decision making • outlets for hostility	Will assist client in developing coping responses to stress	Demonstration of coping skills

Nursing Diagnosis: Alteration in family process related to a family system unable to meet emotional needs of its members.
Goal: During the course of treatment client will recognize alterations in family process as part of illness.

Intervention	*Rationale*	*Expected Outcome*
Assess family background	Will assist in identifying family relationships and history of bowel disease	Reduction of alterations in family process

(Diagnosis continued)

Table 7–17 *(continued)*

Intervention	*Rationale*	*Expected Outcome*
Allow family members to express feelings about illness and expected outcomes	Will assist family in gaining insight into disease condition	Demonstrations of mutual support
Assist client and family in learning to support each other	Will assist in learning to live with a chronic disease	
Encourage client and family to set goals for meeting each other's needs		

Nursing Diagnosis: Alteration in nutrition (less than body requirement) related to excessive number of bowel movements.
Goal: During the course of treatment client will modify diet to meet nutritional needs.

Intervention	*Rationale*	*Expected Outcome*
Assess nutritional status	Will assist in determining nutritional needs	Good skin turgor No more than three stools per day Weight gain Absence of fatigue
Identify foods irritating to bowel	Will assist client in retaining nutrients	
Provide nutritional supplements		
Monitor: • anemia • electrolyte imbalance • daily weight	Will assist in early detection of nutritional deficits	
Medicate as ordered for nausea before meals		
Provide foods in appropriate form for client: • soft • bland • TPN (total parenteral nutrition) as ordered	Will assist in client obtaining proper nutrients	

Nursing Diagnosis: Disturbance in self-concept (body image, self-esteem, role performance, personal identity) related to being dissatisfied with role performance.
Goal: During the course of treatment client will learn to accept body.

Intervention	*Rationale*	*Expected Outcome*
Encourage client to express feelings (eg, fear, anger, anxiety, etc) related to body changes	Will assist client in developing body image and self-concept	Positive expression of body image
Encourage client to verbalize concerns about performing hygiene tasks related to bowel function	Will assist client to be more self-accepting	Able to manage tasks related to bowel functions
Encourage client to engage in activities as normally as possible	Will improve client's self-esteem	Describes impact of body function on daily living

(continued)

Table 7–17 *(continued)*

Nursing Diagnosis: Sexual dysfunction related to disease state.
Goal: During the course of treatment client will be able to reduce stress over sexual concerns.

Intervention	*Rationale*	*Expected Outcome*
Assess client's sexual history	Client may avoid sex because of pain during intercourse	Client and partner discuss sexual concerns
Provide client and partner with an opportunity to discuss feelings, fears, etc about sexual activity	Will resolve concerns about sexual performance	States realistic expectations about sexual function

Nursing Diagnosis: Social isolation related to embarrassing nature of the disease.
Goal: During the course of treatment client will be able to reduce social isolation by developing feelings of social acceptability.

Intervention	*Rationale*	*Expected Outcome*
Assess social history	Will assist in determining the extent of social isolation	Lists at least two new planned activities
Assist client in identifying barriers to forming social relationships	Will assist client in developing insight into reasons for social isolation	Plans participation in new activities
Assist client in identifying potential social outlets within physical limitations	Will assist client in planning for social contact	Talks to others besides staff
Encourage involvement in social activities that do not focus on physical impairments		Participates in routine activities

Table 7–18 *Example of Evaluation of Nursing Care of a Client with Ulcerative Colitis*

Plan	*Evaluation*
1. The client will achieve relief from loose stools within 24 hours.	On 11/23 the client had seven loose stools. On 11/24 the client had three loose stools.
2. The client will develop an awareness of emotional reactions to stress before discharge.	On 11/25 the client stated "It's probably best that I'm in the hospital right now because my daughter is coming home with her three-year-old for Thanksgiving."
3. The client will modify diet to meet nutritional needs for 72 hours.	On 11/24 TPN was maintained at 83 cc per hour. The client demonstrated no untoward effects from the solution.

Inadequate rest	Alteration in family process
Poor coping mechanisms	Alteration in nutrition: less than body requirements
Weight loss	Social isolation

Suggested Care Planning Activities

1. Determine the priorities for Mrs. Stubard's care.
2. Determine the primary stresses in Mrs. Stubard's life.
3. Describe the significance of the laboratory findings.
4. Determine the support systems available to Mrs. Stubard.
5. Determine the developmental aspects to be considered in Mrs. Stubard's care.
6. Identify nursing goals for Mrs. Stubard.
7. Describe the client teaching necessary to assist Mrs. Stubard toward recovery.

8. Identify the needs special to Mrs. Stubard's rehabilitation.
9. List and provide a rationale for nursing interventions in Mrs. Stubard's care.

Other Biophysiologic Disorders

Over the past few years we have learned a great deal about negative behaviors leading to physical illnesses. It is impossible in one chapter to review all behaviors having an effect on physical illness, so a few have been dealt with in depth. The last few—migraine headaches, rheumatoid arthritis, eczema, and peptic ulcer—will be summarized briefly.

Migraine Headaches

The migraine headaches, also called vascular headaches, from which clients suffer are precipitated by emotional conflict or psychologic stress. Females are affected more than males. Migraine headaches are associated with high achievers who suppress aggression and hostility. The client has a strong conscience, a compulsion to do what is right, achieve perfection, and do one's duty. Frequently negative emotions are repressed or are expressed in immature displays of jealousy and rage which lead to frustration. Self-righteous behavior and being overcritical of others makes some migraine-prone people unpleasant company. Migraine sufferers are usually tense, worried, and humorless, and they tend to express their emotions in dramatic, vain, selfish, or demanding ways. If a particularly stressful life event occurs, a migraine occurs. Physical phenomena that accompany migraines are sensory dysfunction, motor dysfunction, dizziness, confusion, occasional loss of consciousness, gastrointestinal upset, and changes in fluid balance (Arehart-Treichel, 1980; Luckman and Sorensen, 1987).

Rheumatoid Arthritis

Clients suffering rheumatoid arthritis may have one parent who is punitive, rejecting, harsh and interested in his or her children only for ego enhancement and another parent who is gentle and compliant but ineffectual in the face of the dominant partner. Usually these clients are only children or first-born children or youngest children. Unfavorable childhood experiences such as divorce are common to those with rheumatoid arthritis. Victims of this illness, though often yearning to act like clinging vines, mask their desire with bossy or tyrannical behavior. They frequently dominate their own children and have weak egos (Arehart-Treichel, 1980).

Eczema

Clients who suffer eczema sometimes have parents who encourage dependency and sickness. These clients tend to repress negative emotions. They also tend to be timid and emotionally sensitive, especially in situations where they perceive the loss of approval or love. Eczema strikes people in their late 20s and subsides in later years (Arehart-Treichel, 1980; Engels, 1985).

Peptic Ulcer

Clients with ulcers are ambivalent about whether they want to be dependent or independent. In addition to this conflict, these people tend to secrete excessive acid, a characteristic that some studies say is inherited. These clients tend to be hardworking, meticulous, ambitious, self-centered, and sensitive to stress. Many ulcer victims experience traumatic life stresses, such as the threat of being deprived of the person on whom they are dependent (Arehart-Treichel, 1980; Oken, 1985).

SUMMARY

Perspectives on Psychophysiologic Illness

1. Many physical disorders are thought to be an expression of anxiety through physiologic processes rather than symbolically through coping mechanisms.
2. Some disorders thought to have a psychophysiologic base are coronary heart disease, cancer, headaches, asthma, ulcerative colitis, dermatitis, and arthritis.

3. Selye identified the general adaptation syndrome (GAS) as the body's adaptive response to continued stress.

4. GAS assists in understanding the psychophysiologic manifestations presented by various disease processes.

Cardiovascular Disorders

5. Cardiovascular disorders are the leading cause of death in the United States.

6. The two major disorders are coronary heart disease (CHD) and hypertension (HTN).

7. Risk factors for CHD include obesity, age, sedentary lifestyle, stressful lifestyle, hypertension, gender, cigarette smoking, ethnicity, and genetic predisposition.

8. Changes in lifestyle are essential in the nursing care of the client with CHD.

Cancer

9. The second leading cause of death in the United States is cancer.

10. The warning signs of cancer are change in bowel or bladder habits, sores that do not heal, unusual bleeding or discharge from any body orifice, thickening or a lump in the breast or elsewhere, obvious change in a wart or mole, and nagging cough or hoarseness.

11. The nurse works toward either cure, control, or palliation of symptoms.

Respiratory Disorders

12. There are many respiratory disorders thought to be related to emotional stress; one of the most common is asthma.

13. The increased resistance to airflow causes the asthma victim to panic when respirations are interrupted.

14. Factors precipitating an asthmatic attack are respiratory tract infection, intolerance to certain drugs such as aspirin, cold, exercise, and air pollutants.

15. The nurse is responsible for supporting the client when asthmatic attacks occur and assisting the client in learning to avoid precipitating factors.

Gastrointestinal Disorders

16. The gastrointestinal system is complex and has many psychophysiologic disorders related to it. One common disorder seen with increasing frequency is ulcerative colitis.

17. Ulcerative colitis is a condition in which the colon and rectum are inflamed and ulcerated.

18. The cause of ulcerative colitis is unknown but there is an overlay of physical symptoms and psychologic stress. Some researchers have proposed that emotional responses alter the blood supply to the colonic mucosa.

19. The primary nursing goal for the client with ulcerative colitis is supportive therapy.

Psychophysiologic Disorders a Challenge

20. Psychophysiologic disorders are complex and offer the mental health nurse a challenge.

21. The nurse must recognize that many of these clients have great dependency needs and require support from a caring individual.

CHAPTER REVIEW

1. Physical conditions in which psychologically meaningful events have been closely related to physical symptoms in a body organ system are called:
   (a) psychophysiologic disorders
   (b) psychopathic disease
   (c) pathophysiological phenomena
   (d) biopsychosocial dysfunctions

2. When a person faces an obstacle so important to life goals that for a time the problem is unsurmountable through customary methods of problem solving, which one of the following is he or she experiencing:
   (a) stress
   (b) anxiety
   (c) crisis
   (d) tension

3. The psychologic complaint most likely to be seen in the cardiac client is:
   (a) dyspnea
   (b) anxiety
   (c) fatigue
   (d) syncope

4. One of the major goals of treatment in the client with cancer is to relieve symptoms so that the client's quality of life may be as high as possible. Which of the following is the term used to describe this goal:
   (a) cure
   (b) control
   (c) recurrence
   (d) palliation

5. For a client with asthma, the goal is that the client develop alternate strategies for dealing with stress. Which of the following diagnoses is most related to this goal:
   (a) fear
   (b) ineffective individual coping
   (c) ineffective breathing pattern
   (d) alteration in health maintenance

6. An intestinal disorder that is thought to be psychophysiologic is:
   (a) obesity
   (b) esophageal reflux
   (c) ulcerative colitis
   (d) anorexia nervosa

REFERENCES

American Psychiatric Association: *Diagnostic and Statistical Manual of Mental Disorders,* 3rd ed. Revised. Washington DC, 1987.

Arehart-Treichel J: *Biotypes.* New York Times Book Co., 1980.

Beare PG, Myers JL: *Principles and Practice of Adult Health Nursing.* Mosby, 1990.

Brunner LS, Suddarth DS: *The Lippincott Manual of Nursing Practice,* 4th ed. Lippincott, 1988.

Caplan G: *An Approach to Community Mental Health,* Grune & Stratton, 1961.

Caplan G: *Principle of Preventive Psychiatry.* Basic Books, 1964.

Coyne JC, Lazarus RS: Cognitive style, stress perception, and coping. In: *Handbook on Stress and Anxiety,* Kutash IL et al. Jossey-Bass, 1980.

Dohrenwend BS, Dohrenwend BP (editors): *Stressful Life Events: Their Nature and Effects.* John Wiley, 1974.

Engels WD: Skin disorders. In: *Comprehensive Textbook of Psychiatry,* 4th ed. Kaplan HI, Sadock BJ (editors), Williams & Wilkins, 1985.

Friedman M, Rosenman RH: *Type A Behavior and Your Heart.* Knopf, 1974.

Gerald MC, O'Bannon FV: *Nursing Pharmacology and Therapeutics,* 2nd ed. Appleton & Lange, 1988.

Groer ME, Shekleton ME: *Basic Pathophysiology: A Conceptual Approach.* Mosby, 1979.

Hackett TP, Rosenbaum JF, Cassem NH: Cardiovascular disorders. In: *Comprehensive Textbook of Psychiatry,* 4th ed. Kaplan HI, Sadock BJ (editors). Williams & Wilkins, 1985.

Holmes TH, Rahe RH: The social readjustment rating scale. *J Psychosom Res* 1967; 11:213.

Knapp PH: Current theoretical concepts in psychosomatic medicine. In: *Comprehensive Textbook of Psychiatry,* 4th ed. Kaplan HI, Sadock BJ (editors). Williams & Wilkins, 1985.

Kneisl CR, Ames SW: *Adult Health Nursing.* Addison-Wesley, 1986.

Lazarus RS: *Psychological Stress and the Coping Process.* McGraw-Hill, 1966.

Lazarus, RS: Emotions and adaptation: Conceptual and empirical relations. In: *Nebraska Symposium on Motivation,* Arnold WJ (editor). University of Nebraska Press, 1968.

Lazarus RS, Folkman S: *Stress, Appraisal, and Coping.* Springer, 1984.

LeShan L: *You Can Fight for Your Life.* M Evan, 1977.

Luckman J, Sorensen KC: *Medical-Surgical Nursing: A Psychophysiological Approach.* Saunders, 1987.

Monat A and Lazarus RS (editors): *Stress and Coping.* Columbia University Press, 1977.

Oken D: Gastrointestinal disorders. In: *Comprehensive Textbook of Psychiatry,* 4th ed. Kaplan HI, Sadock BJ (editors). Williams & Wilkins, 1985.

Sarason IG, de Monchaux C, Hunt T: Methodological issues in the assessment of life stress. In: *Emotions: Their Parameters and Measurement.* Levi L (editor). Raven, 1975.

Selye H: *The Physiology and Pathology of Exposure to Stress: A Treatise Based on the Concepts of the General Adaptation Syndrome and the Diseases of Adaptation.* Acta, 1956.

Selye H: *Stress Without Distress.* Lippincott, 1974.

Selye H: *Stress in Health and Disease.* Butterworth, 1976.

Thompson JM, et al.: *Mosby's Manual of Clinical Nursing,* 2nd ed. Mosby, 1989.

Weiner H: Respiratory disorders. In: *Comprehensive Textbook of Psychiatry,* 4th ed. Kaplan HI, Sadock BJ (editors). Williams & Wilkins, 1985.

SUGGESTED READINGS

Bartal GM, et al: The connotative meaning of the term psychosomatic. (research review) *J Prof Nurs* (Nov-Dec) 1989:4(5):453–457.

Bayless TM, et al: Help your IBD patient help himself: The effects of Inflammatory Bowel Disease. *Patient Care* (October 15) 1988:22(16):139–148.

Essoka GS: Diabetes and stress across the life span. *J Adv Medical-Surgical Nurs* (September) 1989:1(4):44–54.

Johnson JE, et al: Alternative explanations of coping with stressful experiences associated with physical illness. *ANS* (January) 1989:11(2):39–52.

Thomas SP: Is there a disease prone personality? Synthesis and evaluation of the empirical literature. *Issues Ment Health* 1989:9(4):339–351.

CHAPTER 8

Psychologic Responses to Anxiety

KAREN LEE FONTAINE

How I see my Illness

I see my Illness as having a wall that surrounds me and separates me from the outside living world. Not only is there a wall around me but also I'm over a pit that will further take me away from the outside world. The outside world is where I want to live.

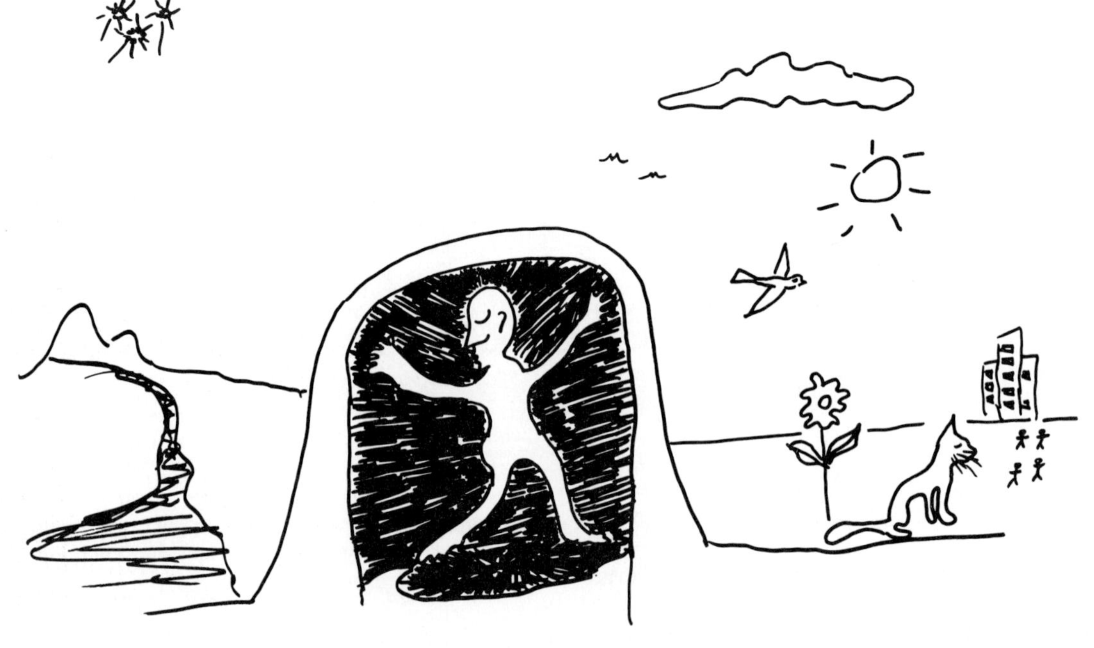

■ *Objectives*

After reading this chapter the student will be able to

- Describe the levels of anxiety
- Formulate examples of the conscious and unconscious attempts to manage anxiety
- Distinguish between the characteristics of the anxiety disorders
- Differentiate concomitant disorders from the anxiety disorders
- Analyze sociocultural characteristics that contribute to the anxiety disorders
- Apply the nursing process when intervening with clients experiencing anxiety disorders

■ *Chapter Outline*

Introduction

Anxiety is an uncomfortable feeling that occurs in response to the fear of being hurt or losing something valued. Some authors distinguish between the feelings of fear and anxiety. When this distinction is made, fear is a feeling that arises from a concrete, real danger, whereas anxiety is a feeling that arises from an ambiguous, unspecific cause or that is disproportionate to the danger. Other authors, as in this text, believing it makes no difference if the fear is real or not, use the words interchangeably, for the sensations are equally unpleasant (Barlow and Cerny, 1988).

John is a 20-year-old male who has just been admitted to the psychiatric unit. He complains about feeling "shaky and nervous" and says he is "very worried about the future" and "feels guilty for failing his parents." He also says he is having difficulty sleeping and has been losing some weight. After completing high school, John lived at home with his parents and one brother while attending the local junior college. Four weeks ago, John enlisted in the navy, after finishing his second year of college. He says he started missing his parents by the third day of his enlistment and became fearful of being away from home "in a strange place with strange people." He also says boot camp wasn't what he expected and that the navy was "just too strenuous." He began to experience nightmares about fighting and war. After two weeks of basic training, he began to experience panic attacks and then refused to participate in any more training. He was admitted to the psychiatric unit for evaluation where the navy physician stated that navy life was too stressful for him and that he could not cope with it. He was then given a medical discharge and returned to his parent's home. When John continued to exhibit symptoms of anxiety, his parents took him to a psychiatrist, who then admitted him. John says his father and mother expect him to do well in life, but he has not been able to do so up to now. He says he would like to feel better so he can get a job where he can help people rather than destroy them.

Anxiety alerts people to possible dangers and warns them of their vulnerability. The feeling provides energy to remove or deal with the threat of hurt or loss. Because it alerts the person to the need for action and is the driving force for most adaptations, anxiety can be viewed as the first step in the problem-solving process.

Simone, a nursing student, experiences moderate anxiety when required to do any public speaking. As a course requirement, she must do a class presentation on an ethical issue in nursing. Her anxiety about the presentation motivates her to practice it in front of her family for feedback and support. This helps her become comfortable with the topic, and she begins to view herself as knowledgeable and capable of speaking before her classmates. This problem-solving behavior reduces Simone's anxiety to a mild level, and her class presentation is successful.

Anxiety is not always detectable; often it is assessed by the person's own disclosure of the experience. It can be described as normal or abnormal, depending on the reality or the nonexistence of the threat or loss. Anxiety can also be described according to the duration of the feeling: For some people it is acute and short-lived; for others, persistent and chronic. The intensity of anxiety is described along a four-point scale: absence of anxiety, mild anxiety, moderate anxiety, severe anxiety or panic. (See Table 8–1 for the behavioral, affective, and cognitive characteristics that accompany the levels of anxiety.)

Coping Mechanisms and Defense Mechanisms

Consciously and unconsciously, people attempt to protect themselves from the emotional pain of anxiety. Conscious attempts are referred to as **coping mechanisms.** Physical activity, such as walking, jogging, competitive sports, swimming, or strenuous housecleaning, may be employed to burn off the tension associated with anxiety. Cognitive coping behavior includes realistically reviewing strengths and limitations, determining short- and long-term goals (both individual and family), and formulating a plan of action to confront the anxiety-producing situation. Affective coping behavior may include expressing emotions (laughter, words, tears) or seeking support from family, friends, or professionals. Stress-reduction techniques may also be used, such as meditation, progressive relaxation, visualization, and biofeedback. Effective coping mechanisms contribute to a person's sense of competence and positive self-esteem.

Unconscious attempts to manage anxiety are referred to as **defense mechanisms**. These often prevent people from being sensitive to anxiety and therefore interfere with self-awareness. When they allow for need gratification in acceptable ways, defense mechanisms may be adaptive; however, when the anxiety is not reduced to manageable levels, the defenses become maladaptive. (See Chapter 3 for examples of defense mechanisms.) Consistently using particular defenses leads to the development of personality traits and characteristic behaviors. How a person manages anxiety and which defense mechanisms are used is more behaviorally formative than the source of the anxiety. Consider the basic human need to be loved and cared for by another person. The anxiety produced when there is a fear of the loss of love may result in a variety of behaviors. One person may be driven to constantly look for love and affirmation and thus engage in

Table 8–1 *Characteristics According to Levels of Anxiety*

Level of Anxiety	*Behavioral*	*Affective*	*Cognitive*
Mild, or minimal	Sitting calmly, relaxed Content of conversation is appropriate and at normal rate, voice calm Can carry out well-known skills, non-competitive games	Unconcerned Feels comfortable, safe	Perceptual field is broad May have daydreams, fantasies
Moderate	Fine tremors of hands may occur Some difficulty sitting still Increased verbal output; rate, pitch, and volume of speech is heightened Often occurs during competitive games	Concerned about what may occur Feels nervous, shy, timid May enjoy the feeling of challenge	Perceptual field narrows Uses problem-solving behavior Increased concentration Optimal level for learning
Severe	Jerky movements with noticeable shaking of hands Body position changed frequently Overtalkative with increased rate, pitch, and volume of speech; speech unclear at times Difficulty sleeping may occur	Fears what may occur Feels need to respond Feels inadequate, ineffectual, insecure	Perceptual field narrows further Decreased self-evaluation and thoughts of inadequacy Decreased concentration, forgetfulness Difficulty making decisions Anticipates the worst
Panic	Gross body tremors interfere with ability to perform tasks Nonpurposeful and primitive behavior Constant talking that is difficult to understand Voice shrill and at shouting level May withdraw or strike out at others	Fears of not surviving the experience Fears of impending doom Feels dismayed, trapped, threatened, abandoned Feels terror and helplessness	Perceptual field extremely limited Concrete thinking Rambling thoughts, blocking of thoughts Confusion Poor judgment Unable to solve problems

frequent one-night sexual encounters. Another person may seek out and develop a warm, intimate relationship. A third person may be so frightened of not finding love and fearful of rejection that relationships are consistently avoided in an effort to decrease the anxiety. At times the management of defenses becomes so time-consuming that little energy remains for other facets of living. The consistent use of particular and fixed responses to anxiety leads to the development of the anxiety disorders presented in this chapter. The following is the list of the medical diagnoses, as described in DSM-III-R:

1. Anxiety disorders
   A. Anxiety states
      300.01 Panic disorder without agoraphobia
      300.21 Panic disorder with agoraphobia
      300.02 Generalized anxiety disorder
      300.30 Obsessive-compulsive disorder
      309.89 Posttraumatic stress disorder
   B. Phobic disorders
      300.22 Agoraphobia without panic disorder
      300.23 Social phobia
      300.29 Simple phobia
2. Dissociative disorders
      300.12 Psychogenic amnesia
      300.13 Psychogenic fugue
      300.14 Multiple personality

Understanding Anxiety

It is important that nurses understand the meaning of anxiety as well as the process, characteristics, and defenses of anxiety. Knowing this is necessary for nurses to intervene effectively with their own and other people's anxiety. Nurses, like other people, become anxious over many facets of their personal lives. What is more, they may experience anxiety in their professional roles, particularly when feeling insecure and inadequate in that role. Student nurses who are beginning their clinical experience in mental health nursing are often anxious. They are skeptical of their ability to intervene with the clients and are uncertain about what is expected of them in this role. As their skills increase and the role becomes more comfortable, the level of anxiety and the use of habitual defense mechanisms decrease.

It is estimated that 13 million adults, or 8 percent of the American population, suffer from anxiety disorders. Currently, anxiety disorders are the single largest mental health problem in the United States. Only 25 percent of those suffering from anxiety disorders receive psychiatric intervention; the remaining 75 percent utilize other health care facilities. Clients with varying levels of anxiety may be found in all types of clinical settings from community services to medical-surgical settings, to intensive care units. With the added stress and anxiety of an acute or chronic physical illness, the anxiety disorder may be especially pronounced. Therefore, all nurses must be prepared to intervene with clients experiencing generalized anxiety and with clients suffering from any of the anxiety disorders (Barlow, 1988; Dubovsky, 1987).

Anxiety in Childhood and Adolescence

It is not uncommon for children to experience anxiety or fear. This experience is usually temporary and requires no professional intervention. Very young children fear strangers, being left alone, and the dark; preschool children fear imaginary creatures, animals, and the dark. Anxieties over physical safety and storms are common among young school-age children. During the middle-school years the focus of anxiety changes to academic, social, and health-related issues. This focus continues as children grow. Older school children may fear war or nuclear threat (Barrios, 1988). (See Chapter 6 for developmental crises of childhood and adolescence.)

Anxiety disorders in childhood are fairly rare, short-lived, and characterized by multiple fears, sleep disturbances, some phobias, travel anxiety, and school refusal. Anxiety is classified as a disorder when it disrupts normal development or the child's or family's functioning. (See Table 8–2 for a comparison of disorders.)

A mild form of separation anxiety is fairly common in young children. Fear of losing parents is experienced by most children. **Separation anxiety disorders** may develop at any age. The schoolage child may develop school phobia or refusal when it becomes necessary to separate from parents, though not all school refusal is due to separation anxiety. Children who do suffer from separation anxiety generally come from a close-knit, caring family where they are subjected to solicitous, overconcerned parents. An eagerness to please and to conform are richly rewarded by the parents.

> *When Manuel was born, his mother was very ill. Frequent hospitalization for Manuel's*

Table 8–2 *Comparison of Anxiety Disorders in Children and Adolescents*

Characteristics	*Separation Anxiety Disorder*	*Avoidant Disorder*	*Overanxious Disorder*
Onset	Infancy to adolescence	2½ years and older	3 years and older
Duration	More than 1 month	Longer than 3 months	3 months or more
Stressors	Separation from significant person, other losses	Pressure to participate in social activity or group	Excessive pressure to perform, loss of self-esteem
Relationships with peers	Able to develop peer relationships but becomes fearful away from home	Reluctant to form interpersonal relationships; inhibited, shy, tearful in social situations	Eager to please, dependent
Physiologic expressions	Many somatic complaints: nausea, vomiting, stomachache, headache, palpitations, dizziness	Vasodilation (blushing), muscle tension	Respiratory distress, GI distress, sore throat, palpitations, headaches, dizziness, body aches, and pains
Essential features	Unusual stress at separation from home, parents, familiar surroundings	Avoids social activities, meeting new people; may have imaginary companions	Excessive worrying not associated with recent stress or specific situation
	Morbid fear that self or family will be harmed	Motor activity may be inhibited	Motor restlessness; nail biting, thumb sucking, hair pulling
	Animal, monster phobias	Perfectionism	Perfectionism and self-doubt
	Nightmares, sleep difficulties	Speech difficulties (without physiologic cause); often whispers	Talkativeness

mother brought him a series of babysitters. Manuel has always clung to his mother, as most children do, but now that he is about to enter school, he seems to cling even more to his mother's side. Manuel has had several accidents in the past two weeks and complains of headaches and stomachaches. Manuel is brought to the clinic because of his recent falls and complaints.

More prominent in girls, **avoidant disorder** is characterized by shyness and an abnormal reluctance to meet new people. Although relationships with family members may be warm and natural, the child can also become demanding and dictatorial. Pressure to join in school activities may bring about tears and timidity. Whispering, blushing, and difficulty speaking are common. Competitive pursuits are avoided, though the child may secretly fantasize about greatness in athletic, creative, or social activities. Perfectionism is frequently seen but probably in response to disparaging self-appraisal.

Overanxious disorder is also more common in girls, and it is characterized by an intense need to succeed. Typically, the child is the firstborn of a family in an upper socioeconomic level. Excessive worry, which cannot be traced to a stressful event or specific object, is experienced. Worrying about future events and social acceptance are common preoccupations.

Adolescence is frequently referred to as the age of anxiety. Developmentally it is the time to enhance one's ability to cope with frustration and manage stress. Common issues creating anxiety for adolescents are peer-group competitiveness, physical changes, fear of regression to dependency, absence of extended network of extraparental adults, confrontation with the reality of death, and threat of nuclear warfare and widespread unemployment or underemployment. Adolescents suffering from anxiety disorders may exhibit characteristics of childhood disorders or characteristics of adult disorders.

Identity disorder is characterized by impaired social or school functioning and many uncertainties about life goals, friendships, sexual orientation and behavior, religious and moral value systems, and group loyalties. Most adolescents ask, "Who am I?"; for the adolescent with identity disorder, who goes beyond the normal questioning of this developmental stage, the question has no answers. The self is an obscure mystery.

When other adolescents are beginning to make career choices or long-term goals, this teen is struggling to define who he or she is. The isolation and inner emptiness are crippling. Because the adolescent has been unable to define who he or she is, sustaining intimacy in a relationship is impossible. These adolescents have no values and loyalties of their own. So absorbed can they become in not knowing who they are and what they believe that they are unable to work and enjoy life. In short, they

- Struggle with self-identity.
- Are unable to choose a life pattern—to choose material success or service to humankind, for example.
- Cannot decide on a career.
- Are in conflict over friendship patterns and do not know who they want as friends. For example, they may join drug-oriented groups or cults because they can more easily lose themselves in a group.

Adolescent adjustment disorder is characterized by overwhelming stress that taxes the adolescent's ability to cope. The stressor is an expectation to assume a more independent adult role. To the expectations the adolescent responds with regressive behaviors: anxiety, depression, eating and sleeping disturbances, increased dependence on parents, somatic complaints, and impulsive acting out. This disorder is diagnosed in the absence of other mental disorders. Support from parents and teachers is essential in helping the adolescent make the transition from adjustment disorder to adulthood.

Knowledge Base

This section will describe various disorders that develop in response to anxiety. Included are discussions of relevant behavioral, affective, and cognitive characteristics.

Generalized Anxiety Disorder

Generalized anxiety disorder (GAD) is a chronic disorder affecting more than 5 percent of the population. It usually begins in late teens to early twenties with a female-to-male ratio of 2:1. GAD is manifested by the behavioral, affective, cognitive, and physiologic characteristics of the moderate level of anxiety (refer to Tables 8–1 and 8–3). These symptoms are continually present, with the most notable feature being chronic pathologic "worrying" that usually focuses on family, money, and work. Individuals with GAD may develop panic attacks, agoraphobia, or depression as a result of their persistant and uncontrollable symptoms (Barlow, 1988).

Table 8–3 *Comparison of Anxiety Disorders*

Disorder	*Sensations of Anxiety*	*Stimulus of Anxiety*
GAD	Experienced	Somatic events
Panic	Experienced	Somatic events
OCD	Avoided	Internal cognitive stimuli
Phobias		
Simple	Avoided	External objects/events
Social	Avoided	Social scrutiny/criticism
Agoraphobia	Experienced	Anxiety itself—fear of fear
PTSD	Experienced	Environmental cues
Dissociative disorders	Avoided	Traumatic events/recall

Panic Disorder

Some studies suggest occasional panic attacks occur in 35 percent of the population. Most frequently these episodes are associated with public speaking, interpersonal conflict, exams, or other situations of high stress. In addition, panic attacks may accompany a wide variety of affective and anxiety disorders (Barlow and Cerny 1988).

Panic disorder, with or without agoraphobia, usually develops between the ages of 25 and 45. Not uncommonly, the panic attacks are unexpected and last a few minutes to an hour. The behavioral, affective, cognitive, and physiologic characteristics are described in Tables 8–1 and 8–3. Some victims suffer only from nocturnal panic. These attacks awaken the person and usually occur within one to four hours after sleep, usually during non-REM sleep. No one knows the cause of nocturnal panic, although some believe it may be related to sleep apnea. Further discussion of panic is presented with agoraphobia since the two disorders often occur together (Barlow and Cerny, 1988).

> *Marta is a 32-year-old woman who has recently become overwhelmed with anxiety. She has a constant inexplicable fear of "doom and gloom," which came on suddenly. The only recent change in her life is a need for a breast biopsy. Both her mother and sister have a history of cancer of the uterus; both are physically well. Marta has experienced several panic attacks, and she fears they will recur. She is not sleeping well, fears being alone, and fears she is "going crazy."*

Obsessive-Compulsive Disorders

Obsessions are unwanted, repetitive thoughts, and **compulsions** are unwanted, repetitive actions. Obsessive-compulsive behavior is quite common in the general population: Of people with the specific behavior, 80 percent experience both obsessions and compulsions as a response to anxiety; the remaining 20 percent experience only obsessive thoughts. When obsessive-compulsive thoughts and behavior dominate a person's life, the person is described as having an **obsessive-compulsive disorder (OCD)**. This disorder affects approximately 2 percent of the population, or 1 million adolescents and 3 million adults. Onset usually occurs during a person's early twenties, but it may occur as late as age 50 and as early as age 5. An equal percentage of women and men are affected (Barlow, 1988; Emmelkamp, 1982; Hafner, 1988; Rapoport, 1989).

The term *obsessive-compulsive disorder* describes a heterogeneous group of disorders with a variety of precipitating factors. Characteristics of OCD may overlap with those of other anxiety disorders. In the past it was thought that OCD was a more severe form of obsessive-compulsive personality disorder. (See Chapter 10 for a discussion of personality disorders.) Most recent research indicates distinct differences between the disorders, with only 20 percent of people with OCD exhibiting characteristics of the personality disorder. Briefly, those with the personality disorder develop rigid patterns of behavior, restricted affect, and an excessive passion for productivity. The personality disorder is ego-syntonic since the person does not feel tormented or view the behavior as a problem (Rapoport, 1989).

The degree of interference in the lives of victims of OCD can range from slight to incapacitating. Rapoport (1989) describes the severity in terms of time involved in the compulsive behavior:

- *Mild*—less than one hour a day
- *Moderate*—one to three hours a day
- *Severe*—three to eight hours a day
- *Extreme*—involvement is nearly constant

Behavioral Characteristics Almost all people have experienced a mild form of obsessive-compulsive behavior called ***folie du doute,*** which consists of thoughts of uncertainty and compulsions to check a previous behavior. Some common forms of this are setting the alarm clock and checking it before being able to sleep, turning off an appliance and then returning to make certain it was indeed turned off, or locking the door and then checking to be sure it is locked. People are bothered by uncertainty and thoughts such as "Are you sure you locked the door?" There is a feeling of subjective compulsion: "You better check to make sure you locked the door." But there is often a resistance to the compulsion: "You don't have to check the door because you know you locked it." The obsessive thoughts continue and anxiety increases until the compulsive behavior is performed.

ShaRhonda's mother had frequently warned her of the danger of setting the house on fire if she forgot to unplug her curling iron. Now, as a young adult, ShaRhonda checks her curling iron twice in the morning before leaving home. She experiences obsessive thoughts directing her to check the curling iron even though she knows it is turned off. If she refuses to perform the compulsion, her anxiety mounts until she does check the curling iron. After checking, her anxiety decreases, and she can focus on other thoughts and behaviors. Some days ShaRhonda tries not to check the curling iron before leaving home, which then leaves her with a sense of anxiety throughout the day. Only when she returns home and checks the curling iron does her anxiety decrease.

Rituals, where the action is a specific or stereotypical pattern of behavior, are a type of compulsion. In a mild form, rituals are common. Because they are repetitive acts and are always the same, they decrease any need to make decisions, which provides a person with a sense of security and a feeling of having control over oneself and the environment.

When Marcus wakes up in the morning, he follows the same routine day after day. He plugs in the coffeepot, urinates, showers, shaves, dresses, and then reads the paper while drinking his coffee before leaving for work. One morning Marcus oversleeps and has only a few minutes to get ready for work. Skipping his morning shower, he quickly shaves, dresses, and leaves for work. The remainder of the day he experiences a feeling of mild anxiety, which he describes as "getting off on the wrong foot this morning."

Rituals are prevalent in religious orders, fraternal organizations, schools, and the military. There are also rituals on nursing units—rituals relating to report format, rounds, drug administration times, bathing and linen change times, and treatment routines. There are even greeting rituals between client and nurse. Because nurses are constantly confronted with human suffering, rituals develop to protect the nurse from being overwhelmed by the anxiety this stimulates (Chapman, 1983). Students beginning to practice in mental health nursing are frequently anxious, which is partly due to not knowing the routine and having to make many conscious decisions regarding their own behavior. As their experience increases, their anxiety usually decreases.

The anxiety of a person with OCD, however, is not lessened when the person gains confidence. In addition, people suffering from OCD often display consuming, and at times bizarre behavior. Cross-cultural comparisons of OCD victims throughout the world reveal behavior that is remarkably similar. The OCD sufferers describe their behavior as being forced from within. They say, "I have to. I don't *want* to, but I *have* to." Of the victims who are women, 90 percent are compulsive cleaners who have an unreasonable fear of contamination and avoid contact with anything thought to be unclean. They may spend many hours each day washing themselves and cleaning their environment. Cleaning rituals and avoidance of contamination decrease their anxiety and reestablish some sense of safety and control. With increased public awareness of AIDS, one third of people with OCD now cite fear of AIDS to explain their washing behavior.

Male victims are more likely to experience compulsive checking behavior, which is often associated with "magical" thinking. These individuals hope to prevent an imagined future disaster by their checking behavior, even though they recognize this is irrational. Children with OCD may appear to have learning disabilities when the compelling need to count or check interferes with homework and testing. Other obsessive behavior involves arranging and rearranging objects or repeating activities such as going in and out of a doorway (Barlow, 1988; Hand, 1988; Rapoport, 1989).

Since the onset of her OCD, Sylvia's ability to function has declined. She had to quit her job because her rituals for getting dressed in the morning stretched to six hours. Every day she spends eight hours cleaning her one-bedroom apartment. All her clothing must be washed three times and stored in plastic bags in her closet to prevent contamination. Her hands and arms are raw and scabbed as a result of washing with a strong disinfectant 50 to 60 times a day.

Affective Characteristics Obsessive-compulsive people often experience a great deal of shame about their uncontrollable and irrational behavior. Therefore, they may try to hide their behavior from others. They may be consumed with fears of being discovered. OCD sufferers respond to anxiety by feeling tense, inadequate, and ineffectual. To alleviate the anxiety caused by helplessness and powerlessness, control is all-important. They fear that, if they do not act on their compulsion, something terrible will happen. Thus, in most cases, compulsions serve to temporarily reduce anxiety. However, it is not uncommon for the behavior itself to create further anxiety. The affective distress may range from being mildly anxious to being anxious about thoughts and behaviors nearly constantly. The obsessive-compulsive person may also develop phobias when faced with situations in which they can no longer maintain control (Atwood, 1987; Rapoport, 1989).

To control her obsessive-compulsive behavior, Jeanine has developed a phobic avoidance of driving her car. In the past, whenever she hit a bump in the road, she obsessed that she may have hit someone. She felt forced to stop, get out, and check under and behind the car. The compulsive behavior became so severe that she would get in and out of the car, checking 20 times before she could continue driving. Her phobia of driving the car has developed in response to lack of control.

Cognitive Characteristics Obsessive-compulsive disorder is ego-dystonic, since victims feel tormented by their symptoms. There is a recognition of the senselessness of much of their behavior and a desire to resist it and obsessive thoughts. The drive to engage in the behavior is overpowering, however, and OCD victims often feel extreme distress about their actions.

The most common preoccupations involve dirt; safety; or violent, sexual, or blasphemous thoughts. OCD sufferers are consumed with constant doubts, which leads to concentration problems and mental exhaustion. They doubt everything related to their particular compulsion and cannot be reassured by what they see, feel, smell, touch, or taste. They say, "No matter how hard I try, I cannot get these thoughts out of my mind."

Yvette is a 27-year-old mechanical engineer. Her obsessive-compulsive behavior has been increasing during the past five years, and she is now in danger of losing her job because of decreased productivity. She checks and rechecks every project she is assigned to such a degree that she is unable to complete any project. She is able to identify when a project is completed, but her fear of making a mistake drives her to continue to recheck her work and avoid handing it in to her supervisor. She recognizes her behavior is unrealistic and will likely result in the loss of her job.

Phobic Disorders

Like obsessive-compulsive disorders, **phobic disorders** are behavioral patterns that develop as a defense against anxiety. Other features common to both disorders include fear of loss of control, fear of appearing inadequate, defense against threats to self-esteem, and perfectionistic standards of behavior (Salzman, 1982).

Almost all people try to avoid physical dangers. If this avoidance is generalized to situations other than realistic danger, it is called a phobia. It is estimated that 20 to 45 percent of the general population have some mild form of phobic behavior. However, phobic disorders are seen only in 5 to 15 percent of the population. As Goodwin (1983) and Maxmen (1986) point out, there are many phobic disorders, but they all have four features in common:

- They are an *unreasonable* behavioral response, both to sufferer and to observers.
- The fears are *persistent*.
- The sufferer demonstrates *avoidance behavior*.
- This behavior eventually becomes *disabling* to the sufferer.

Although the feared object or situation may or may not be symbolic of the underlying anxiety, in all phobic disorders there is the primary fear of losing control.

A simple phobia is a fear of only one object or situation and can arise after a single unpleasant experience. The most common phobias concern ancient dangers such as closed spaces, heights, snakes, or spiders. Very seldom are people phobic about modern dangers such as guns, knives, or cars. Phobias usually begin early in life and are experienced as often by men as by women. People with simple phobias experience anticipatory anxiety, that is, they become anxious even thinking about the feared object or situation. This disorder is not disabling unless the feared object or situation cannot be avoided (Rapoport, 1989).

Bill has a simple phobia of snakes. Since he lives in a large urban area with minimal likelihood of encountering a snake, he is not disabled by his phobia.

Janelle has a simple phobia of being in an elevator with other people. Her phobia is mildly disabling because she must use the stairway almost all the time. Her vocational opportunities are somewhat limited because she is unable to work on the upper floors of a high-rise office building.

Social phobias are fears of social situations. These may take many forms, such as stage fright, fears of public speaking, using public bathrooms, eating in public, being observed at work, or being in crowds of people. All these fears center around the loss of control, which may result in being embarrassed or ridiculed by others. The degree to which the person is disabled depends on how easily the social situation can be avoided (Barlow and Cerny, 1988).

Asela has a social phobia about using a public bathroom when others are present in the facility. As a result, her trips outside her home are limited in time to the extent of her bladder capacity.

Agoraphobia, the most pervasive and serious phobic disorder, is a fear of being away from home and of being unaided in public places when assistance might be needed. A person with agoraphobia will avoid groups of people, whether they be on busy streets or in crowded stores, on public transportation or at town beaches, at concerts or in movie houses. Places where the person might become trapped, such as in tunnels or on elevators, are also sometimes avoided.

Of diagnosed agoraphobics, 70 to 85 percent are women. Three theories have tried to explain the high incidence of agoraphobia in women. One theory suggests that men and women have agoraphobia in equal numbers. The agoraphobia is undetectable in most men, however, because socialization discourages males from expressing anxious feelings and teaches them to cope with anxiety through other means, such as alcohol. Another theory says that the statistics reflect a real difference between the sexes—that socialization has taught men to "tough out" their fears and women to avoid their fears. The third theory suggests that endocrine changes in women make them more susceptible than men to panic attacks.

Agoraphobia is often triggered by severe stress.

Moving, changing jobs, relationship problems, or the death of a loved one may precipitate it. The two peak times for the onset are between the ages of 15 and 20 and then again between the ages of 30 and 40. Some people may experience a brief period of agoraphobia, which then disappears, never to recur. If the agoraphobia persists for more than a year, the disorder tends to be chronic, with periods of partial remissions and relapses (Barlow and Cerny, 1988; Brehony, 1983).

To estimate the incidence of phobias in the general population is difficult, since many people are embarrassed by their fears and therefore secretive about any disorder they are experiencing. In addition, the diagnosis of agoraphobia without panic attacks is controversial. Therapists believe panic is an essential feature of agoraphobia; epidemiologists, however, report that there are individuals who do not experience panic. At this time the reason for this discrepancy is unclear (Barlow and Cerny, 1988).

In the past 20 years there has been an increase in the reporting of agoraphobia. The incidence ranges from 3 to 6 percent of the population, which means from 7 1o 12 million people suffer from this disabling disorder. The average victim suffers for 10 years before entering a specialized treatment program (Barlow, 1988; Hafner, 1988).

Behavioral Characteristics The dominant behavioral characteristic of phobic persons is avoidance. Fearing loss of control, these people avoid the phobic object or situation that increases their level of anxiety. If the person demonstrates minor rechecking or ritualistic behavior, avoidance may take on an obsessive-compulsive flavor. Even though these people know their fears are irrational, they still try to avoid the object or situation; if it cannot be easily avoided, the behavior may interfere with overall functioning and even their lifestyle.

Maureen has a phobic fear of dirt, germs, and contamination. This so dominates her life that whenever anyone enters her home from the outside she immediately scrubs the floor where they have walked, because "you can't tell where they have been or what dirt or germs they are bringing in on their shoes."

People who suffer from disabling agoraphobia are excessively dependent because their avoidance behavior dominates all activities. They may even be so panic-stricken outside the home that they become housebound.

Edith, who lives in a large urban area, developed agoraphobia 10 years ago during a time of severe marital distress. In the beginning she merely avoided large crowds of people. She then began to fear leaving her neighborhood. Five years ago she became housebound and experienced panic attacks if she attempted to leave her home. Two years ago her phobia progressed to the point that she cannot leave her living room couch; thus, she needs a great deal of assistance in activities of daily living. Her husband and a cleaning woman provide for her basic needs. She is alert and continues to manage all the household finances and any other activities that can be accomplished from her couch.

Affective Characteristics For persons suffering from phobic disorders, fear predominates. Mainly, there is fear of the object or situation. Further fears are of being exposed, which could result in being laughed at and humiliated, and of being abandoned during a phobic episode.

When confronted with the feared object or situation, phobic persons feel panic, which may include a feeling of impending doom. Panic in itself is often accompanied by additional fears, such as losing control, causing a scene, collapsing, having a heart attack, dying, losing one's memory, or going crazy. Having once experienced an unexpected attack of panic, phobic people begin to fear the attack will happen again. Because these attacks are so terrifying, the fear of another attack becomes the major stress in these people's lives. This fear of fear, which is extreme anticipatory anxiety, may become the dominant affective experience, particularly for people with agoraphobia (Hafner, 1988).

Cognitive Characteristics The behavioral and affective characteristics of people with phobic disorders are ego-dystonic. Although sufferers recognize their responses are unreasonable and their thoughts irrational, they are unable to explain them or to rid themselves of them. They are consumed with thoughts of anticipatory anxiety and have negative expectations of the future. Phobic persons develop a low self-esteem and describe themselves as inadequate and as failures. They believe they are in great need of support and encouragement from others. They begin to define themselves as helpless and dependent and often despair of ever getting better. They may even begin to believe they are mentally ill and fear ending up in an institution for the rest of their lives.

In an attempt to localize anxiety phobic persons often use defenses that allow them to remain relatively free of anxiety as long as the feared object or situation is avoided. Defenses—such as repression, displacement, symbolization, and avoidance—can also keep the original source of anxiety out of conscious awareness. In agoraphobia, however, defense mechanisms are not adequate to keep anxiety out of conscious awareness. Agoraphobics live in terror of future panic attacks, and anticipatory anxiety is a constant state. They may have difficulty assuming responsibility for their symptoms and tend to blame significant others for their problems.

> *Juanita has developed a fear of eating in public places, and it is at the point now that she must eat by herself in her bedroom. Six months after she was married, her husband threatened a divorce during a particularly nasty argument in a restaurant, which led to considerable social embarrassment. The anxiety caused by the fear of losing her husband was too painful to confront, so repression was used to force the fear out of conscious awareness. Since repression is never completely successful by itself, the anxiety became displaced from the relationship and was transferred to public eating places. Public eating places then became symbolic of all of her anxiety and fear, which she could then manage by avoiding eating in public. Unconsciously, this was a safer situation than directly confronting the problems in the marriage. A secondary gain of the phobic disorder was that, as long as she was helpless and dependent, her husband would not be likely to leave her.*

Posttraumatic Stress Disorder

People exposed to dangerous and life-threatening situations may develop a **posttraumatic stress disorder (PTSD)**. This disorder is described as acute when the symptoms begin shortly after the trauma and as chronic when the symptoms appear months or years later. Any time a trauma occurs, there is a potential for the victim to develop PTSD. Typically, it occurs after military combat, natural disasters, hostage situations, rape, assault, or extreme abuse. PTSD is less severe after a natural disaster, such as an earthquake or a flood, than it is after an unnatural disaster, such as a war or a kidnapping. It is important to understand that the victims of PTSD are normal people who have suffered abnormal events. The disorder involves recurrent experiencing of the trauma, with varied and complex changes in behavioral, affective, and cognitive processes (Ochberg, 1988).

War is one of the most traumatic events in life. It is estimated that 500,000 Vietnam veterans are currently suffering from PTSD. Often neglected in media coverage of PTSD are the nurses who served in Vietnam between 1964 and 1975. Fifty percent of them report ongoing symptoms of PTSD. These nurses worked six days a week, with a minimum shift of 12 hours that often extended to 24 hours. As Rogers and Nickolaus (1987, pp. 13–14) report, nurses who served in Vietnam are vulnerable because they

> hold themselves responsible for the death of patients. They feel guilty about not knowing enough, not being good enough, and not being efficient. They believe that they should have overcome the adversities and performed superhuman deeds.

Recent research is now focusing on the incidence of PTSD among rescue workers. Nurses, firefighters, police officers, paramedics, and physicians may be at risk for this disorder. According to current estimates, 4 out of 5 rescue workers experience significant stress symptoms, and 1 out of 25 eventually develop PTSD (Spitzer and Franklin, 1988).

Traumatic events may result in two categories of symptoms: undercontrol and overcontrol. Those with undercontrol relive the event and are diagnosed as having PTSD. Those with overcontrol experience denial and amnesia and are diagnosed as having one of the dissociative disorders. Thus, PTSD and the dissociative disorders have similar precipitating causes (Brende, 1984).

Behavioral Characteristics People with PTSD often exhibit hyperalertness, which results from their need to constantly search the environment for danger. Increasing anxiety can result in unpredictably aggressive or bizarre behavior. PTSD victims may resort to abusing drugs or alcohol in an effort to decrease this anticipatory anxiety. They may also behave as if the original trauma were actually recurring. Thus, they may try to defend themselves against an enemy in the past that is perceived to be in the present. Many of these people develop a phobic avoidance of activities or situations that remind them of the original trauma. This phobic avoidance may become so all-encompassing that a socially isolated lifestyle develops (Karl, 1989; Ochberg, 1988; Solomon, 1987).

Becky was raped 10 years ago, when she was 15. The rapist came in through her bedroom window during the night. For several years after the rape she was unable to look at her naked body in the mirror, and when she took a shower she not only locked the bathroom door but also put a chair under the doorknob. At present she continues to be afraid of the dark, and her bedroom must have windows set high in the wall. She still experiences unreasonable guilt with thoughts such as "If I hadn't been standing in front of the shade, he would not have seen me."

Affective Characteristics People suffering from PTSD experience chronic tension. They are often irritable and report feeling edgy, jittery, uptight, and restless. They often experience labile affective responses to the environment. Anxiety is frequent and ranges from moderate anxiety to panic. When environmental cues remind them of the original trauma, the original feelings are experienced in the same intensity.

Guilt is another common affective characteristic of PTSD. When the traumatic event entailed the death of others, the guilt stems from the PTSD sufferer having survived when so many others did not. In addition, war veterans may feel guilty about the acts they were forced to commit to survive the combat experience (Keltner, Doggett, and Johnson, 1983).

Apart from the negative feelings of anxiety, tension, irritability, aggression, and guilt, there is often a psychic numbing of other emotions. It is not unusual for these people to discover they can no longer appreciate previously enjoyed activities. They feel detached from others, and this is accompanied by the inability to experience emotions such as intimacy or tenderness. Obviously, this difficulty in developing emotional closeness with others contributes to many problems with interpersonal relationships.

For approximately two years after returning from Vietnam, Dwight suffered from post-traumatic stress syndrome. He experienced rapid mood swings—he was relaxed one minute and in a furious rage the next, with no known stimulus. During these periods of rage he would shout, throw things, and sometimes brandish weapons in the air. His poor self-image led to his asking permission from others to do things that did not require their permission. When confronted with this behavior, he was able to make decisions for himself.

Cognitive Characteristics A sudden, life-threatening trauma often causes people to reevaluate themselves and their experiences. In the face of imminent death, the myth of personal invulnerability is exploded. This confrontation with severe injury or death results in long-lasting changes in the thinking patterns of the victims.

PTSD sufferers often have difficulty concentrating and may experience some impairment of memory. If the disorder is moderate in intensity, these people will likely have intermittent thoughts about the trauma—thoughts that range from quick flashes to entire recollections of the event. Although this experience is distressing, it may be tolerable if the memories are infrequent. However, for those suffering from severe PTSD, there are frequent recurrent and painful thoughts about the trauma. So intrusive and persistent can these memories be that people become obsessed by them. Recurring nightmares, in which the person reexperiences the event, are also common. Victims may also become preoccupied with thoughts of the trauma recurring. All these cognitive changes contribute to the development of an external locus of control, and the PTSD victims feel themselves at the mercy of the environment.

During the original trauma it is not unusual for victims to experience perceptual changes. Studies of people being held hostage indicate that 25 percent experience auditory or visual hallucinations. These may include a vivid reexperiencing of childhood memories (Lanza, 1986).

Another cognitive characteristic that may accompany PTSD is self-devaluation. For instance, the rape victim may be influenced by cultural myths and begin to believe she was responsible for the act of violence committed against her. Survivors of disasters often feel guilty and may believe they were not worthy to have survived when so many more capable people lost their lives. In returning from Vietnam, many veterans were assailed by society's reproach and indifference. This devaluation became a part of the veteran's self-image. When self-devaluation is compounded by interpersonal and employment difficulties, the self-esteem is further assaulted and the devaluation process continues (Karl, 1989; Keltner, Doggett, and Johnson, 1983; Mullis, 1984).

Dissociative Disorders

Dissociative disorders involve an alteration in conscious awareness, particularly in the area of memory, and an alteration in identity, particularly in the consistency of personality. The alteration in identity may be a loss of identity or the presence of more than one identity. Regardless of the type of dissociative disorder, all who suffer from them at times demonstrate behavior totally different from their usual behavior. As stated earlier, dissociative disorders result from overcontrol in the face of trauma. When traumatic events elicit panic, some people, to maintain and protect the self, dissociate any thoughts and feelings of the events from conscious awareness (Putnam, 1989).

Psychogenic amnesia, amnesia not caused by an organic problem, is usually related to a traumatic event. The most common type of psychogenic amnesia is *localized amnesia,* in which memory loss occurs for a specific time related to the trauma. Psychogenic amnesia may be *selective;* that is, even though it is localized for a specific time, there is a partial remembering of events during that time. The least common types of psychogenic amnesia are *generalized amnesia,* in which there is a complete loss of memory of one's past, and *continuous amnesia,* in which the loss of memory begins at a particular point in time and continues to the present.

> *Salli's firstborn child died of sudden infant death syndrome three months ago. Although she remembers arriving in the emergency department with her baby, she continues to have no memory of finding him in his crib, calling the paramedics, or hearing the physician telling her that her baby was dead.*

Psychogenic fugue is a rare dissociative disorder in which people, by either maintaining their identity or adopting a new identity, wander or take unexpected trips. The disorder is often precipitated by acute stress. The psychogenic fugue may last several hours or several days. During the fugue state, these people may appear "normal" or disoriented and confused; they usually behave in ways inconsistent with their normal personalities and values. The fugue state often ends abruptly, and there is either partial or complete amnesia for that period. Both psychogenic amnesia and fugue are most commonly seen during war and disasters (Putnam, 1989).

Multiple personality is another type of dissociative disorder. This diagnosis is given when at least two personalities are within the same person. Each personality is integrated and complex—that is, each has its own memory, value structure, behavioral pattern, and primary affective expression. The host personality, which is the original personality, has at best only a partial awareness of the other personalities. Thus these people suffer from an alteration in conscious awareness of their total being. Most victims demonstrate anywhere from 8 to 13 personalities, but much higher numbers have also been reported. Usually there is a direct correlation between the severity of the trauma and the age of the victim with the number of personalities. The higher numbers are seen with victims who experienced extreme abuse at a very young age. The more personalities any given person possesses, the greater the likelihood that both genders and a variety of ages will be represented (Kluft, 1987A; Putnam, 1989).

The prevalence of multiple personality disorder is unknown at this time. This is due to the difficulty of making the diagnosis as well as to therapists who have little or no experience in this area and are skeptical of the reality of multiple personality. It has been found that these clients typically spend almost seven years in the mental health system before they are diagnosed with multiple personality disorder. They are most frequently misdiagnosed as schizophrenics, but it is not uncommon to have diagnoses in the categories of affective or personality disorders. As many as 10 percent of all mental health clients may be suffering from multiple personality disorder, with 5,000 cases already diagnosed in North America.

Recent reports agree that the origin of this disorder is severe, sadistic, often sexual, child abuse. This is not to say that all traumatized children will develop multiple personality; rather, it appears to occur in children who symbolize, repress, and dissociate to escape the harsh reality, resolve internal conflicts, and survive the abuse. Other child abuse victims use different defenses in coping with anxiety and thus may develop different disorders (Anderson, 1988; Kluft, 1987B; Putnam, 1989).

Since the model of multiple personality is the most complex dissociative disorder, it is used to illustrate the behavioral, affective, and cognitive characteristics of the dissociative disorder.

Behavioral Characteristics Children are unable to protect themselves adequately from violent abuse by adults. Unpredictable and often cruel, at times these adults protect and nurture, and at times they torment and torture. The victims feel confusion, anxiety, helplessness, and rage. To survive, the host, or original personality, usually behaves passively, trying to placate the abuser. Thoughts and feelings that conflict with passivity are dissociated from the host personality, and new personalities develop around all the dissociated thoughts and feelings.

Each personality has its own behavioral characteristics, sometimes completely opposite from one another. Behavior intolerable in one personality may be expressed when a different personality is in control. One personality may use drugs; one may never use drugs. One may be a prostitute; one may be a faithful spouse. One may be an executive; one may be a parent. One may continually attempt suicide; one may abort the suicide. Physically, one may be blind and one may have no physical sensations. One may have hypochondriasis, one may have bulemia, and one may never be ill. Current research is focusing on the power of the mind to actually change physiology—different personalities demonstrate dramatic differences in brain-wave patterns. Apparently, the brain is able to alter the immune system in that one personality may have extreme allergies while another has no allergies.

Each personality has different preferences in clothing, sexual behavior, vocational skills, and leisure activities. Some may be right-handed while others are left-handed. Each personality may also have a different voice and motor behavior, that is, a different posture, walk, and gesturing pattern. Family members report these people often use and respond to names other than their own.

Some victims are able to switch personalities at will; others cannot control the changes. Personality changes may occur within seconds, or it may take several minutes to make the change. In some cases the switches are so subtle that diagnosis is uncertain. In other cases the differences are abrupt and dramatic. It appears that high stress may contribute to frequent changes in personalities. Even when the alternate personalities are not in complete control, they continue to be able to influence behavior (Bliss, 1986; Kluft, 1987B; Loewenstein, 1987).

Affective Characteristics The host personality, who has either no or limited awareness of the other personalities, experiences bewilderment and fear about "lost" time. When others report what was said and done during the time another personality was dominant, the host personality often feels anxiety and may even suffer from panic. Not infrequently, these clients report feelings that do not seem to be their own. This occurs when an alter personality is trying to influence the personality currently in control (Marmer, 1984).

In 75 percent of the cases, there is at least one personality who does not know any of the others. In 85 percent of the cases, there is at least one personality who knows all the others. All the personalities can be grouped into three categories according to dominant affect and behavior. (Table 8–4 summarizes the personality categories.) Some personalities symbolize the *victim-self* and are pleasant in affect and passive in behavior. Another group is the *aggressive-self,* which tends to dominate during periods of stress. One personality may physically express anger, another may be suicidal, and another may be sexually aggressive. The third group of personalities, the *protective-self* (sometimes called the *inner self-helper*), are rational and calm and have the most awareness of the other personalities; indeed, one of these may have total memory for all the others. The personalities of this group manage new external danger as well as protect against internal helplessness and despair (Anderson, 1988; Fraser and Curtis, 1984; Kluft, 1987B; Putnam, 1989).

Susan is a 33-year-old woman who as a young child was repeatedly raped by her father. In the process of therapy, the following seven personalities emerged. There are two victim-self *personalities, Susan and Little Me. Susan is the host personality who is submissive and childish in her behavior. She dresses very plainly and wears no makeup. She is also the one who is responsible for maintaining the fictions of personality structure, but the host*

Table 8–4 *Categories of Personalities*

Victim-self personalities	
Host	Often unaware of the others; feels powerless
Children	Stay at given ages; contain memories and affect of childhood trauma; may be autistic
Handicapped	May be blind, deaf, paralyzed
Aggressive-self personalities	
Persecutor	Has great deal of energy; may try to harm or kill the others
Promiscuous	Expresses forbidden urges that are often sexual
Substance abusers	Addiction limited to these personalities
Protective-self personalities	
Protector	Counterbalance to persecutor; protects the person from internal and external danger
Inner self-helper	Emotionally stable; can provide information about how the personalities work
Memory tracer	Has most of the memory for the entire life history
Cross-gender	In women, these personalities tend to be protectors; in men, these personalities tend to be "good mother" figures
Administrator	Often this is the personality who earns a living; may be a very competent professional
Special skills	Skills may be related to work, artistic, or athletic activities

personality has no awareness of the other personalities. Little Me is a very small, very young personality who remains at the age of 3, when the original trauma occurred to Susan. There are three aggressive-self *personalities. Barb is the personality who remembers the rape. She is very angry and aggressive in her approach to other people. She dresses in masculine clothing and exhibits much energy in walking and talking. Joyce is the seductive personality who wears excessive makeup, dresses revealingly, and picks up men for casual sexual encounters. Sarah is the personality that is aggressive against the self. She does not believe that life and the struggle is worth continuing. When Sarah is the dominant personality, she attempts to commit suicide. There are also two* protective-self *personalities. Elizabeth is the personality that is the mother to the three children that have been born to Susan. She is able to nurture and discipline the children appropriately. Ruth is the personality who takes Susan away in a trance, either under conditions of high stress or to prevent Sarah from killing all of them. In this way, she functions as an inner self-helper and protector.*

Cognitive Characteristics Periods of amnesia are characteristic of people with multiple personality. Since the host personality has, at best, only partial awareness of the others, the host has no memory of the times when other personalities dominated. In some instances the amnesia is not readily apparent, since the host personality has learned to use confabulation to cope with the "lost" time. Different personalities may learn different skills which may not be transferable between personalities. For example, personality C may be in charge during a class when a particular math procedure is explained. If personality A is in charge when the exam on this procedure is given, personality A is likely to fail since no learning had occurred. Personality A also has no memory for that class.

Not infrequently, the personalities complain about unidentified people trying to influence them or control their minds. A high percentage of people with multiple personality describe hearing voices in their heads. With these two characteristics, it is not surprising that these individuals may be misdiagnosed as schizophrenics (Kluft, 1987B).

One day Susan began to cry and tell her therapist how frightened she becomes at times because she hears voices arguing with each other. One voice (Sarah's) keeps talking about killing Susan and giving very detailed descriptions of how she is going to accomplish this. Another voice (Ruth's) argues back with all the reasons Susan should not be harmed. Susan reports that, at times, the argument becomes very loud and disruptive.

In multiple personality, the defense mechanisms of repression and dissociation are used to manage the anxiety, rage, and helplessness that the child experiences in response to severe abuse. The only way for these people to survive the pain of the trauma is to eliminate it from conscious awareness. Dissociation is accomplished by self-hypnosis, which correlates with the onset of the abuse. This soon becomes the dominant method of managing severe stress, and individuals with multiple personality are able to quickly and spontaneously enter hypnotic trances. What is a life-saving process in childhood becomes a self-destructive tool in adulthood (Bliss, 1986; Marmer, 1984).

Physiologic Characteristics of Anxiety Disorders

A person's expectations of an object, situation, or event influence the interpretation made of physiologic responses. In the same situation, some people expect excitement and fun, whereas others expect misfortune. Although the physiologic responses are identical, they have opposite meanings for the people involved. Thus, what a person thinks and expects determines whether the response is labeled anxiety or excitement.

Two young boys, Joe and Billy, are at the top of a long hill ready to descend on their sleds. Joe is excited because he expects to have a thrilling ride down the hill. Billy is terrified because he anticipates that he will crash his sled and get hurt. Both boys experience the same physiologic response, but Joe interprets it as exhilaration and Billy as terror.

It is expected that a human can, within limits, adapt to anxiety for a time. However, when the cause is unknown, the intensity severe, or the duration chronic, normal physiologic mechanisms no longer function efficiently.

In mild anxiety, people experience an agreeable, perhaps even a pleasant, increase in tension. They may also experience a twitch in the eyelid, trembling lips, occasional shortness of breath, and mild gastric symptoms.

As anxiety increases to the moderate level, the survival response of fight or flight begins. Starting in the cortex of the brain, this response is mediated through the body's nervous system and hormonal system. The sympathetic nervous system and the response of the adrenal glands lead to changes throughout the body. Heart rate increases and blood pressure rises in an effort to force more blood to the muscles. There may be frequent episodes of shortness of breath. The pupils dilate, the person may sweat, and the hands feel cold and clammy. Some body trembling, a fearful facial expression, tense muscles, restlessness, and an exaggerated startle response may all be noticeable. There is an increased blood glucose level due to increased glycogenolysis. The moderately anxious person may verbalize subjective experiences such as a dry mouth, upset stomach, anorexia, tension headache, stiff neck, tiredness, inability to relax, and difficulty falling asleep. There may also be urinary urgency and frequency as well as either diarrhea or constipation. Sexual function complaints may include painful intercourse, erectile failure, orgasmic difficulties, lack of satisfaction, or a decrease in sexual desire.

When anxiety continues to the panic level, the body becomes so stressed it can neither adapt effectively nor organize for fight or flight. At this level of anxiety, the person is helpless to care for or defend the self. As blood returns to the major organs from the muscles, the person may become pale. Hypotension, which causes the person to feel faint, may also occur. Other signs are a quavering voice, agitation, poor motor coordination, involuntary movements, and body trembling. The facial expression is one of terror, with dilated pupils. A person feeling panic may complain of dizziness, lightheadedness, a sense of unreality and, at times, nausea. Some of the most frightening symptoms of the panic level of anxiety are chest pain or pressure, palpitations, shortness of breath, and a choking or smothering sensation (Appenheimer and Noyes, 1987).

Each person tends to experience the physiologic sensations in a pattern that repeats itself with every episode of anxiety. Some people are primarily aware of internal organ reactions, whereas others primarily exhibit symptoms of muscular tension. Still others experience both visceral and muscular responses. (See Table 8–5 for a summary of the physiologic characteristics of anxiety.)

A number of medical conditions may cause secondary anxiety or produce symptoms mimicking panic. These conditions are hypoglycemia, hyperthyroidism, hypoparathyroidism, Cushing's syndrome, pheochromocytoma, pernicious anemia, hypoxia, hyperventilation, audiovestibular system disturbance, paroxysmal atrial tachycardia, caffeinism, and withdrawal from alcohol or benzodiazepine. Individuals with panic disorder, including agoraphobia, have a significantly higher incidence of mitral valve prolapse (MVP) than the general population—57 percent as compared to 5 to 7 percent. The exact relationship between MVP and panic is unclear. The symptoms of MVP—particularly tachycardia, palpitations, and shortness of breath—are similar to the symptoms of severe and panic levels of anxiety. People predisposed to panic attacks often interpret the sensations of MVP as increased anxiety. The interpretation or expectation then evokes panic (Barlow and Cerny, 1988; Matuzas, 1987; Wesner, 1987).

Concomitant Disorders with Anxiety Disorders

There is a high correlation between anxiety disorders and substance abuse. As many as 50 to 60 percent of substance abusers also present with one of the anxiety disorders. Most typically, severe anxi-

Table 8–5 *Physiologic Characteristics According to Levels of Anxiety*

Level of Anxiety	*Physiologic Response*
Absence	Normal respirations Normal heart rate Normal blood pressure Normal gastrointestinal function Relaxed muscle tone
Mild	Occasional shortness of breath Slightly elevated heart rate and blood pressure Mild gastric symptoms such as "butterflies" in the stomach Facial twitches, trembling lips
Moderate	Frequent shortness of breath Increased heart rate; may have premature contractions Elevated blood pressure Dry mouth, upset stomach, anorexia, diarrhea or constipation Body trembling, fearful facial expression, tense muscles, restlessness, exaggerated startle response, inability to relax, difficulty falling asleep
Panic	Shortness of breath, choking or smothering sensation Hypotension, dizziness, chest pain or pressure, palpitations Nausea Agitation, poor motor coordination, involuntary movements, entire body may tremble, facial expression of terror

ety precedes the onset of the abuse, although for some the abuse precedes the anxiety. Believing that alcohol decreases anxiety, these individuals often "self-medicate" in an effort to feel better. In fact, it is now thought that alcohol actually increases anxiety. The combination of increased anxiety, addiction, and continued self-medication contributes to an ever increasing self-destructive cycle (Barlow, 1988).

Not infrequently, depression follows the onset of the anxiety disorders. It is thought that depression and anxiety disorders share a common biologic vulnerability, which may be activated by stress. This hypothesis is based on similar biologic findings in tests such as the nonsuppressive dexamethasone suppression test and in sleep EEG results. (See Chapter 11 for an in-depth discussion of these tests.) A depressive reaction frequently occurs when obsessional or phobic behavior fails to defend against the anxiety of helplessness or powerlessness. The depression, which may range from mild to severe, is actually a response to the failure of the defense mechanisms. When people can no longer maintain perfectionistic standards or control their behavior, the feeling of loss becomes overwhelming and depression ensues. This is usually precipitated by a crisis or unexpected event. In this situation, the depression is secondary to the anxiety disorder (Appenheimer and Noyes, 1987). As with all depressed clients, however, without recognition and intervention, suicide can be a lethal complication of the depressed state (Barlow, 1988).

People with obsessive-compulsive disorders may develop simple phobias, which tend to involve decision making and serve to protect them from internal conflict. There will also be an attempt to hide the phobia from others, since it represents a failure to be in control.

Approximately 30 percent of those suffering from agoraphobia experience a secondary mild-to-moderate depressive disorder. The depression seems to be in response to feelings of hopelessness and helplessness, decreased self-esteem, and severe restrictions on lifestyle. More than 50 percent of agoraphobic persons develop a secondary hypochondriasis, with the majority believing they are suffering from a fatal illness. Alcohol and drug abuse may accompany the agoraphobic disorder. Frequently, these people self-medicate or obtain prescriptions to decrease anxiety and prevent panic. They often continue to increase the amount of medications or alcohol until they are chemically dependent. Additionally, there may be an overlap between agoraphobia and personality disorders. As many as 25 to 50 percent of agoraphobics also have diagnosed personality disorders. These most often are the Cluster C disorders—avoidant, dependent and passive-aggressive (Barlow and Cerny, 1988; Hafner, 1988). (See Chapter 10 for discussion of personality disorders.)

PTSD victims may abuse alcohol or drugs to reduce their anxiety. Often, they begin drinking before sleeping at night in an effort to prevent nightmares. In the Veterans Administration hospital system, 55 percent of all outpatients treated for drug dependence are Vietnam veterans, who also have a high incidence of depression as well as homicidal or suicidal thoughts. There is a 23 percent higher suicide rate among Vietnam veterans than among others in the same age group. With the prolonged physiologic arousal of chronic anxiety, PTSD victims may develop secondary disorders such as migraine headaches, bowel dysfunctions, and hypertension (Atwood, 1987; Keltner, Doggett, and Johnson, 1983).

People with multiple personality also frequently suffer from concomitant disorders. Coons (1984) found that, of 20 people with multiple personality, 55 percent had a secondary diagnosis of somatization disorder. It was also found that 45 percent had a diagnosed substance abuse, 45 percent had a conversion disorder, 25 percent had a secondary affective disorder, and 10 percent had at least one diagnosed antisocial personality.

Sociocultural Characteristics of Anxiety Disorders

People do not live and function in isolation. Dysfunctional behavior affects interpersonal relationships within the family and the community. People who abuse alcohol and drugs are a danger to the community in that they may physically harm others and may turn to crime to support an expensive drug habit. Others, unable to support themselves by employment, may become a burden to their families or their communities. In this regard, everyone is affected by the dynamics of untreated anxiety disorders.

Obsessive-compulsive people erect a protective screen in hopes no one will become aware of their irrational thoughts or behaviors. This secrecy not only keeps family members at an emotional distance, but families also complain that victims appear disinterested and preoccupied. In the middle of conversations, these individuals may be distracted and overwhelmed by obsessive thoughts, and others often accuse them of "not listening." Because obsessive-compulsive behavior takes a great deal of time and energy, there may be little opportunity to develop and maintain intimate relationships. These individuals are two times more likely never to marry than the general population. And if they marry, they are more likely to divorce. Thus, one of the consequences of this disorder is a very lonely lifestyle (Rapoport, 1989).

The impact of agoraphobia on the family system is usually extensive and severe. Those agoraphobics able to leave the home usually depend on family and friends to accompany them. Refusal to remain alone, even in the home, creates an escalation in family stress and tension. The disorder may cause considerable disruption to family patterns of behavior. The family must assume all responsibility for outside activities such as shopping and employment, and this can lead to additional family stress. Unable to attend family gatherings, go out with friends, or attend their children's activities at school or sports events, agoraphobic people, though appearing weak, actually have a great deal of power to control family and friends through their dependence and helplessness.

Advantages from or rewards for being ill are referred to as secondary gains. The secondary gains of agoraphobia are the relinquishing of responsibilities, the indirect satisfaction of dependency needs that cannot be met directly, and the power to control others. In some instances, the phobic behavior is the extreme of the stereotype of female behavior, that is, high dependency and low autonomy. For their phobic behavior, agoraphobics may receive a great deal of attention and positive reinforcement. Often a partner protects the phobic person from overt anxiety and fears. Weakness as a form of control cannot work without another's cooperation. The secondary gains for the partner may be in fulfilling nurturing needs or finding meaning in life by being the main financial and emotional support of the family. In such a case the partner achieves an identity through the role of helper and protector. The family system stabilizes in a pattern that maintains the disorder. The agoraphobic person, fearing abandonment, behaves submissively and believes there is no choice but to remain with the caretaking partner. Also believing there is no choice, the caretaking partner feels compelled to care for the disabled partner. Both may unconsciously fear the relationship will end if there is a change in behavior (Hafner, 1988).

Families of Vietnam veterans with PTSD suffer a great deal of anxiety. One of the veteran's defenses for coping with the trauma of constant brutality is the numbing of emotions, or emotional anesthesia. This process is then extended to the family system. Interpersonal relationships are strained to the limits with the veteran's feelings of detachment, alienation, and doubts about his ability to trust and love. With numbed emotions comes the loss of the ability to communicate feelings, which often leads to marital problems and divorce. The behavior, feeling, and thinking patterns of these veterans are often frightening to female partners. The women may feel overwhelmed by family responsibility in being the primary wage earner, parent, and housekeeper. Some experience guilt over their inability to help the veteran-partner make headway in life. Because of the high incidence of uncontrollable outbursts of anger, physical abuse may occur. Unchecked, the abuse contributes to women's feelings of helplessness and worthlessness (Coughlan and Parkin, 1987; Verbosky and Ryan, 1988).

Causative Theories of Anxiety

No single theory can adequately explain the cause and maintenance of the anxiety disorders. They are best understood as a complex interaction of many theories.

Biologic Theories It appears some component of anxiety runs in families, but the exact vulnerability is unknown at this time. Illustrating this, the rate of panic disorder in families is 20 percent, compared to 4 percent in the general population. Some believe anxious individuals have an overly responsive autonomic nervous system related to a dysfunction of serotonin and norepinephrine neurotransmission. An overly active autonomic nervous system may be responsible for the characteristics of severe and panic levels of anxiety. Research is continuing in the following areas: a deficiency in certain receptors, causing surges of norepinephrine; CNS abnormalities, particularly in the locus ceruleus of the pons, which inhibit the ability to moderate sensory input; and an increased sensitivity to carbon dioxide, leading to rapid breathing and sensations of suffocation. It is believed that some biologic vulnerability is present, which—when combined with certain psychologic, social, and environmental events—leads to the development of anxiety disorders (Barlow and Cerny, 1988; Charney, 1987; Price, 1987).

Research in obsessive-compulsive disorder is now focusing on biologic factors. In this disorder, children experience identical symptoms as adults, whereas, in most of the other mental disorders, children's symptoms are quite different from adults' symptoms. In addition, 50 percent of adults with OCD state their symptoms began when they were children; only 5 percent of adults with other mental disorders report a childhood onset. Of victims of OCD, 20 percent have a first-degree relative with the same problem. Father-son combinations are the most common in these families. It is unlikely the behavior is learned within the family given the high level of secrecy. In addition, children and parents may have very different rituals—for example, the parent may engage in checking rituals whereas the child engages in washing rituals. Tests indicate deficient levels of serotonin in the blood and most probably in the brain of individuals with OCD. The lack of serotonin appears to be involved in the regulation of repetitive behaviors. Additionally, PET scans (positron emission tomography) demonstrate abnormalities in the basal ganglia and portions of the frontal lobes (Rapoport, 1989).

Intrapersonal Theories Intrapersonal theories of anxiety-related behavior state that the person develops defense mechanisms to protect the self from anxiety arising out of internal conflict. The ego experiences conflict between the demands of the id and the reprimands of the superego. The resulting anxiety is pushed out of conscious awareness by the use of repression, projection, displacement, or symbolization. Intrapersonal theories view anxiety disorders as a reaction to anticipated future danger based on past experiences such as separation, loss of love, or guilt. The danger may be internal (disturbing impulses) or external (threats or losses). As stress increases, the defenses become increasingly inefficient, symptoms develop, and the person engages in repeated self-defeating behavior (Atwood, 1987).

People with an internal locus of control view life events as being under their control. Thus, when a stressful life event occurs and anxiety is experienced, they are able to connect the anxiety to the stressor and use the problem-solving approach to manage it. However, persons suffering from anxiety disorders often have an external locus of control. They regard life events as out of their control and occurring by luck, chance, or fate. When stressful events occur, they attribute the feeling of anxiety not to themselves but to external sources, which then can be phobically avoided. This mechanism, displacement, protects people with anxiety disorders from confronting and managing the internal feeling of anxiety. Since an external locus of control forces them to be dependent on others for protection and security, these people are often terrified of being abandoned by their significant others (Emmelkamp, 1982). (Locus of control is considered a social theory as well as an intrapersonal process.)

In dissociative disorders, stressful life events are disowned and kept out of conscious awareness by amnesia. A young girl who is sadistically abused, physically and sexually, remains dependent on her family system. The perpetrator is a trusted parent, and the other parent is incapable of protecting or rescuing her from the situation. The trauma of abuse leaves the child terrified, depressed, angry, and guilty. Dissociating the abuse, displacing it on a new personality, and denying the events allow the child to remain in the family with the least amount of pain (Blake-White and Kline, 1985).

Interpersonal Theories Interpersonal theorists believe persons with anxiety disorders become anxious when disapproval from significant others is sensed or feared. They may feel trapped in unpleasant circumstances but believe they are unable to leave the situation. Since they fear abandonment by others, they are unable to behave assertively during conflict. Thus, the anxiety experienced during interpersonal conflict is displaced onto the immediate surroundings, which allows them to deny interpersonal problems. Obsessive-compulsive or phobic behavior protects the self and the relationship during interactions with significant others (Emmelkamp, 1982).

Cognitive Theory Cognitive theorists believe symptoms develop from individuals' ideas and thoughts. On the basis of limited events, people with anxiety disorders magnify the significance of the past and overgeneralize to the future. They become preoccupied with impending disaster and self-defeating statements. These cognitive expectations then determine reactions to and behavior in various situations (Atwood, 1987; Barlow and Cerny, 1988).

The cognitive theory explains the phobic disorders in a three-part sequence: (1) Phobic people have negative thoughts that increase anxiety and actually precede the feeling of fear in the phobic situation. Phobic people also have irrational thinking and unrealistic expectations about what might occur if the phobic situation is encountered. (2) These anticipatory thoughts and feelings enhance the physiologic arousal level even before the phobic situation is encountered. (3) The physiologic arousal level is misinterpreted. Although thought to be caused by an external object or situation, the arousal is caused by their negative thoughts and irrational expectations. This mislabeling of feelings allows phobic people to displace the feelings onto objects or situations that can be avoided (Emmelkamp, 1982).

Learning Theory Phobias may be learned vicariously from significant others. If a child observes a parent experiencing anxiety in certain situations, the child may learn that anxiety is the appropriate response. For example, if the mother has a phobic avoidance of elevators, the child soon learns to fear entering an elevator. A child can also learn parental fears through information given by the parent. Thus, a father may talk about the dangers of going outside when it is dark, and the child may develop agoraphobia during the nighttime (Emmelkamp, 1982).

Persons who develop dissociative disorders often consider themselves passive and helpless. They are fearful of others' anger and aggressive behavior. Since they are unable to behave assertively or aggressively, they learn to cope by escaping or avoiding the anxiety-producing situations. Thus, they learn to avoid pain through amnesia or the development of multiple personalities.

Behavioral Theory Closely related to learning theory is the behavioral theory of how phobic disorders develop. Behavioral theorists believe phobias are conditioned, learned responses. Classical conditioning occurs when a stimulus results in anxiety or pain. The person then develops a fear of that particular stimulus. An example is a person who becomes phobic of all dogs after being bitten by one dog. The learning component of behavioral theory states that the avoidance of the phobic object or situation is negatively reinforced by a decrease in anxiety. Since the person experiences less anxiety when avoiding the object or situation, avoidance becomes a habitual response.

Sex Role Theory Sex role theory has been used to explain the disproportionate number of women who experience agoraphobia. These theorists believe women have been reinforced to behave dependently, passively, and submissively. This often results in adult women who are unable to assume responsibility for themselves and who view themselves as incompetent and helpless. Often, the symptoms are reinforced by family members who also have been socialized to expect women to be helpless and dependent. Thus, the pattern of withdrawal can continue until the woman is completely homebound (Berlin, 1987; Brehony, 1983).

Medical Interventions

Medications are often used on a short-term basis to assist clients in managing anxiety disorders. Table 8–6 summarizes these medications.

Table 8–6 *Medications Commonly Utilized in Anxiety Disorders*

Generalized anxiety disorder		
Antianxiety agents		Dosage*
buspirone	BuSpar	5–40 mg/day
diazepam	Valium	2–20 mg/day
alprazolam	Xanax	0.75–4.00 mg/day
clorazepate	Tranxene	15–60 mg/day
Tricyclic antidepressant		
imipramine	Tofranil	150–250 mg/day
Panic disorders		
Antianxiety agents		
buspirone	BuSpar	5–40 mg/day
alprazolam	Xanax	0.75–4.00 mg/day
Tricyclic antidepressant		
imipramine	Tofranil	50–150 mg/day
trazodone	Desyrel	50 mg titrated to 300 mg/day
MAOI		
phenelzine	Nardil	15–30 mg/day
Obsessive-compulsive disorder		
Tricyclic antidepressant		
clomipramine	Anafranil	150–250 mg/day
fluoxetine	Prozac	20–80 mg/day
MAOI		
phenelzine	Nardil	15–30 mg/day
Social phobia		
Beta-blockers		
propranolol	Inderal	10 mg before event
atenolol	Tenormin	25 mg before event
Agoraphobia		
Antianxiety agents		
buspirone	BuSpar	5–40 mg/day
Tricyclic antidepressant		
imipramine	Tofranil	50–150 mg/day
MAOI		
phenelzine	Nardil	15–30 mg/day
Posttraumatic stress disorder		
Beta-blockers		
propranolol	Inderal	120–180 mg/day
Adrenergic inhibitors		
clonidine	Catapres	0.2–0.4 mg/day
Antianxiety agents		
buspirone	BuSpar	5–40 mg/day
alprazolam	Xanax	0.75–4.00 mg/day

*Cited dosages are unsuitable for the older client.

In GAD the therapeutic goal in using antianxiety agents is to limit unpleasant symptoms to assist the individual in returning to a high level of functioning. Controversy exists about the effectiveness of the benzodiazepines for people suffering from

GAD. Appenheimer (1987) states the benzodiazepines alleviate symptoms in 70 percent of clients, but Barlow (1988) states they have a very limited therapeutic effect for only several weeks. Additional problems are the addictive and sedative properties of the medications and the withdrawal reactions from them, which result in a higher level of rebound anxiety.

A new nonbenzodiazepine antianxiety agent, buspirone (BuSpar), may prove more effective than benzodiazepines in the management of GAD. Buspirone blocks serotonin receptors and causes minimal sedation. This medication is better than benzodiazepines for the addiction-prone person, since dosage increases result in a general sense of feeling ill. In addition, buspirone reacts only minimally with alcohol, since it interacts very little with other CNS depressants. However, clients should be cautioned not to expect an immediate effect (Dubovsky, 1987).

Since anxiety may be related to a dysregulation of serotonin and norepinephrine, tricyclic antidepressants have been utilized in the medical treatment of GAD. Imipramine (Tofranil) has been found to be the most effective medication in this group (Appenheimer, 1987).

Several types of medications may be utilized in the medical treatment of panic disorders and agoraphobia. As in GAD, buspirone (BuSpar) has been found effective. Alprazolam (Xanax) may significantly reduce panic attacks after six to eight weeks of treatment. However, the addictive properties and strong withdrawal reactions limit the use of this medication. Tricyclic antidepressants, trazodone (Desyrel) and imipramine (Tofranil) and a MAOI, phenelzine (Nardil) seem to prevent panic attacks. Most frequently, clients must take these medications for eight weeks before the therapeutic effect is noticeable. The antianxiety properties of antidepressants reduce anxiety as well as improve the secondary depression resulting from panic disorders and agoraphobia (Barlow, 1988; Mavissakalian, 1987).

Social phobias severe enough to interfere with occupational functioning may be treated with the beta-blockers propranolol (Inderal) or atenolol (Tenormin). They are particularly effective in situations where cardiovascular symptoms of anxiety are disruptive to the individual. Since beta-blockers do not cross the blood-brain barrier, they have no effect on neurotransmission nor do they produce drowsiness or loss of fine motor control (Barlow, 1988; Mavissakalian, 1987).

Of all mental disorders, OCD has generally been considered one of the most resistant to treatment. Based on the theory of serotonin deficiency in OCD, antidepressant medications are being utilized. In clinical studies MAOI seem to be effective only in those individuals who also experience panic attacks. There have been limited case reports of positive response to the tricyclic antidepressant fluoxetine (Prozac). A new tricyclic, clomipramine (Anafranil) shows the greatest promise in the treatment of OCD. This medication has a high potency for preventing serotonin reuptake, thus increasing the available amount of serotonin. Of the many individuals in clinical trials, 70 percent get some relief in that it is easier for them to resist the obsessive-compulsive symptoms. If there is no improvement after eight weeks of medication, Anafranil probably will not be effective (DeVeaugh-Geiss, Landau, and Katz, 1989; Rapoport, 1989).

Medications are used cautiously in clients suffering from PTSD. They are generally reserved for those individuals whose reactions are destructive to general life functioning. To reduce the intensity of somatic symptoms of anxiety, decrease the startle response, and decrease the occurrence of nightmares, propranolol (Inderal) and clonidine (Catapres) have been found effective (Roth, 1988).

Older clients are started on antidepressant medications at lower levels than younger adults. For older clients the maximum levels of imipramine (Tofranil) is 100 mg per day and the maximum of phenelzine (Nardil) is 60 mg per day. Antianxiety agents should begin with a dosage that is no more than half the lowest dosage used for younger adults.

Medications have an important role in medical interventions, but intrapersonal and interpersonal aspects must also be treated. Clients and families need to cope with various aspects of anxiety, learn to take control of their lives, and manage family stress. This is accomplished through individual, family, or group psychotherapy.

Other forms of intervention include

- *Systematic desensitization,* whereby the client is exposed to a graded presentation of the phobic object or situation until the phobic response is no longer elicited and the client is able to maintain a state of relaxation
- *Exposure and response prevention,* whereby the client is gradually exposed to the stimulus for behavior and then restricts the compulsive response such as washing or checking
- *Imaginal flooding,* whereby the client is confronted with the fear in fantasy rather than in reality
- *In vivo flooding,* whereby the client is confronted with the panic-producing object or situation until the fear responses diminish (This is not effective in treating agoraphobia.)

Assessment

Using the knowledge base, the client is assessed. An organized scheme of focused assessment ensures that all areas—that is, behavioral, affective, cognitive, and sociocultural characteristics—are assessed. (See the following focused nursing assessments for examples of the assessment process that use a question format.)

The physiologic assessment must differentiate anxiety response from various organic disorders, such as hypoglycemia, pheochromocytoma, hyperthyroidism, and mitral valve prolapse. Similar symptoms may also occur in withdrawal from barbiturates and in substance intoxications such as caffeine or amphetamines. Anxiety will frequently be seen as another symptom in people who have been diagnosed as schizophrenic, as having a major affective disorder, or as having an eating disorder.

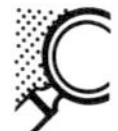

FOCUSED NURSING ASSESSMENT *for the Client with Obsessive-Compulsive Disorder*

Behavioral assessment

What kinds of objects or situations do you feel a need to check or recheck frequently?

How much time during a day do you spend on checking activities?

Describe your daily routine, at home and at work.

Affective assessment

Describe how you experience the feeling of anxiety.

What happens to you when you feel out of control in situations?

Describe your relationships with significant others.

How do these others relate to you?

What are your greatest fears in life?

Cognitive assessment

Describe the qualities you like about yourself.

Describe the qualities you do not like about yourself.

What are your thoughts about your compulsive behavior?

Would you like to decrease the need for your compulsive behavior?

How much time a day do you spend doubting what you have done?

Sociocultural assessment

In what way do habits or thoughts get in the way of work? Social life? Personal life?

Describe situations in which you feel close to and warm with your family members.

In what ways do you feel dependent on your family?

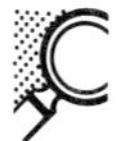

FOCUSED NURSING ASSESSMENT *for the Client with Phobic Disorder*

Behavioral assessment

What situations or objects do you try to avoid in life?

Describe what you do to avoid these situations or objects.

To what degree do these fears interfere with your daily routines?

Are your social or work activities limited to a prescribed geographic area?

How often and in what circumstances are you able to leave home?

Affective assessment

What are your greatest fears in life?

Do you fear others laughing at you? Being humiliated? Being abandoned by others? Being alone in an unfamiliar situation?

What feelings do you experience when you are confronted with the situation or object that you fear?

What else happens to you at this time?

To what degree do you fear having future panic attacks?

Cognitive assessment

Do you dislike being controlled by your fears?

What does the future look like for you?

Describe the qualities you like about yourself.

Describe the qualities you do not like about yourself.

How much support do you need from others to cope with life?

How helpless and dependent on others do you feel?

Sociocultural assessment

Who is able to support you in avoiding your feared situations or objects?

Describe how family living patterns have changed around your fears.

Under what circumstances are you able to socialize with friends?

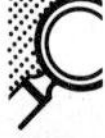

FOCUSED NURSING ASSESSMENT *for the Client with Posttraumatic Stress Disorder*

Behavioral assessment

Under what circumstances do you experience outbursts of aggressive behavior?

In what ways have you been reexperiencing the original trauma?

In what ways do you attempt to avoid situations or activities that may remind you of the original trauma?

How frequently do you participate in social activities?

Have you had any employment difficulties since the original trauma?

Affective assessment

How much time during a day do you feel tense or irritable?

Have you been experiencing panic attacks?

Describe the guilt you have been experiencing in relation to the original trauma.

What types of activities do you enjoy doing?

What are sources of pleasure for you in your life?

Describe relationships in which you feel emotionally close to other people.

Cognitive assessment

Describe difficulties you have had with concentration.

Describe difficulties you have had with your memory.

How often, in a day, do you have recurrent thoughts about the original trauma?

Do you feel you have control over these thoughts?

Describe any nightmares you have.

Describe the qualities you like about yourself.

Describe the qualities you do not like about yourself.

Sociocultural assessment

In what ways do your family and friends tell you that you are distant or cold in your relationships with them?

Describe communication patterns with family and friends.

Describe what happens when you lose control of your anger.

How is violence handled within your family system?

Are you divorced, or have you been threatened with divorce?

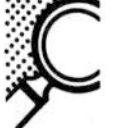

FOCUSED NURSING ASSESSMENT *for the Client with Multiple Personality**

Behavioral assessment

Does the client have widely varying behavior patterns, such as at times being submissive and quiet and at other times loud and outspoken?

Does the client have different styles of dressing that correspond to a change in the client's behavior?

Are vocational or leisure skills inconsistent; that is, are these skills apparent at some times and not at other times?

Does the client's preference in sexual activities and partners change?

Affective assessment

Does the client experience anxiety about "lost" time?

In what ways is the client passive and submissive?

In what ways is the client angry and aggressive?
Has the client been suicidal?

Cognitive assessment
Describe frequency of amnesic periods.
Under what circumstances does this amnesia seem to appear?
Are there times when the client can remember specific events and other times when there is amnesia for the same events?

Sociocultural assessment
Does the family describe the client as having different personalities?
How has the family tried to manage the situation thus far?
Is there a known history of child abuse for the client?
Describe the client's relationship to his or her parents as a child.

*Since the client is unaware of changes in personalities, the assessment data are based on the nurse's observations and family reporting.

Planning and Implementation

The next step in the nursing process is analyzing and synthesizing the client assessment data to form nursing diagnoses. The client's level of anxiety is assessed as well as the behavioral, affective, and cognitive responses to the anxiety. Also assessed by the nurse are the client's self-evaluation, degree of insight, positive coping behavior, defense mechanisms, and family system. Nursing diagnoses are then synthesized to integrate these areas of client assessment. The diagnoses give direction for the development of goals and expected outcomes and help to focus nursing care. The following nursing care plans are written in general terms for clients who are experiencing the anxiety disorders, and so the contributing factors are not individualized. It is expected that the nurse will individualize the process for specific clients.

The goals must be related to the nursing diagnosis and are the connection between the diagnosis and the interventions. The expected outcomes are the basis for evaluation and therefore must be written in behavioral or measurable terminology. Nursing interventions are then planned on the basis of the diagnosis, goals, and expected outcomes and are individualized for each client. (See Table 8–7.)

The client needs to be involved in the planning phase, and expected outcomes should be verified with the client. If the client wants something quite different from what the nurse expects, the nursing care plan will not be appropriate; in fact, it will likely be sabotaged by the client. The overall goal is to help the client improve the response to anxiety and develop more constructive behavior to manage anxiety.

Implementation of the care plan involves the active participation of the client. Implementation is a phase of the nursing process done *with* a client, not *to* a client. If the client does not sense a partnership with the nurse, the implementation phase, too, may be sabotaged by the unconsulted client.

Group therapy is often an effective treatment approach, particularly for clients with phobias and PTSD. Groups of people with similar problems allow each person to establish trust and share with others, and often more significant improvement is seen when compared to individual therapy. Within the group, members are able to identify with others' feelings of anger, fear, guilt, and isolation. This identification increases participation and support for each group member (Hafner, 1988).

Support groups are very helpful to partners of Vietnam veterans. Information that group members receive about the disorder assists the partners in understanding that the veteran is not to blame for the problem. In addition, groups focus on stress management, the problem-solving process, adaptive coping measures, and ways to mobilize other resources (Coughlan and Parkin, 1987).

It is unlikely that beginning practitioners in psychiatric nursing will be assigned to clients with multiple personality disorder, because of the complexity of the diagnosis. Staff may disagree on accepting the diagnosis of multiple personality disorder. Additionally, different personalities may have different relationships with different staff members, leaving each professional with the belief

Table 8–7 Nursing Care Plan for the Client Experiencing Anxiety

Nursing Diagnosis: Anxiety, mild, related to threat to self-concept due to fear of being out of control.
Goal: Client will experience anxiety at a manageable level.

Intervention	*Rationale*	*Expected Outcome*
Access level of anxiety	If anxiety is moderate or severe, client is unable to utilize problem-solving process	
Help client label the feeling as anxiety	Accurate identification is the first step in the problem-solving process	Uses the problem-solving process to decrease anxiety in a single situation and then can extend its use to other situations
Have client identify one anxiety-producing situation	It is more productive to limit diffuse anxiety to a manageable single situation	
Have client identify own thoughts regarding control issues	Control issues need to be acknowledged for them to be addressed	
Help client identify negative anticipatory thoughts	These negative thoughts may be the basis for anxiety	Identifies negative anticipatory thoughts
Help client to analyze fear of losing control and make the connection between the fear and increased anxiety	Connecting client's thinking and feeling processes will help the client remain in control	
Discuss with client the validity of potential loss of control in this situation	Client needs to differentiate between fantasy and reality of the fear	Acknowledges reality of fear
Have client review how anxiety has been handled in the past	Identifying the range and effectiveness of past coping behavior is part of the problem-solving process	Uses variety of coping behaviors when confronted with stressful situations
Teach how mild anxiety can be a drive to change behavior and care for oneself effectively	Client needs to redefine an unpleasant feeling as a positive message for change	
Help client to redefine the sensations of anxiety as sensations of excitement	Client will be less disabled if the expectation is positive rather than negative	Identifies excitement in limited situations
Offer other therapeutic interventions such as a stress management course, relaxation techniques, or biofeedback	These skills will assist client to increase sense of control over life events and anxiety	
Explain that one cannot be relaxed and anxious at the same time, practice relaxation with client	Practice will assist client in gaining mastery over physiologic responses	Utilizes relaxation techniques
Administer antianxiety medications as ordered	These medications decrease anxiety to manageable levels and allow enough energy to use the problem-solving process	Utilizes appropriate level of medication without abuse or addiction

(continued)

Table 8–7 *(continued)*

Nursing Diagnosis: Anxiety experienced at separation from mother.
Goal: Client will feel less anxiety, increased sense of self-worth, and develop coping skills.

Intervention	*Rationale*	*Expected Outcome*
Encourage mother and child to ventilate feelings about separation	Both mother and child must work through feelings associated with separation	Verbalization of feelings by both mother and child
Introduce child to another care giver (eg, have babysitter first visit in home, then have babysitter care for child while mother is in another room); gradually increase the time spent with alternate care giver	Fear that mother will not return increases anxiety	Is able to spend short time with babysitter without increasing anxiety
Have child and mother visit new school and meet the teacher before the start of school. Have the teacher show child around the room, including his or her desk, while mother is in room	Anxiety is intensified in unfamiliar surroundings	
	Builds a trust in the teacher as temporary extension of mother	Is able to attend school for half-day sessions without increased sign of anxiety
	A sense of ownership increases the sense of security	
Repeat visits to school building and playground before the start of school	Reassurance that things are unchanged and familiarity provide a sense of security	
Praise child's accomplishments, identify strengths to build on, and encourage activities child is interested in	Autonomy and sense of accomplishment allows child to separate from mother	Demonstrates pride in work. Is able to make "I" statements that do not include mother
During hospitalization:		
• If possible, allow extended or flexible visiting hours	Illness and unfamiliar surroundings increase anxiety	Minimal amount of anxiety is demonstrated during hospitalization
• Explain procedures slowly and simply, and repeat as needed	Anxiety interferes with the ability to process information	Follows simple instructions with minimal direction
• Give information in intervals; do not overload with information	Consideration for age understanding of child must be made	
• If possible, let child handle equipment, etc	Familiarization decreases fear of the unknown	
• Encourage child to practice procedures (eg, giving injections on a doll)	Role playing helps child work through fears	
• Assign the same nurse to work with child whenever possible; tell child of staff changes in advance	Continuity encourages trust, thus decreasing anxiety (child may fear something terrible has happened to a staff member who does not return to work)	
Explore ways of coping with anxiety when it arises		Discusses ways to cope with anxiety

(Diagnosis continued)

Table 8–7 *(continued)*

Nursing Diagnosis *(continued):* Anxiety experienced at separation from mother.
Goal: Client will feel less anxiety, increased sense of self-worth, and develop coping skills.

Intervention	*Rationale*	*Expected Outcome*
Reinforce coping behaviors, such as: • talking about feelings and fears • deep breathing • relaxation techniques • appropriately removing self from overstimulating situation	Coping behaviors can be learned	Demonstrates use of coping skills on at least two observed occasions

Nursing Diagnosis: Ineffective breathing pattern related to choking or smothering sensations, shortness of breath, and hyperventilation associated with the panic level of anxiety.
Goal: Client will return to a normal respiratory rate.

Intervention	*Rationale*	*Expected Outcome*
Remain with client; maintain calm, direct approach	Client needs support and reassurance that death is not imminent	Verbalizes less fear of choking
Loosen tight clothing	Eases the sensation of choking	Breathing will slow down to normal rate
Assess respiratory status	Ascertains that client is receiving enough oxygen	
Tell client to take slow deep breaths, and breathe with client to demonstrate	Role modeling may be more effective than verbal instructions because of very limited perceptual field	
Have client breathe into a paper bag	Increases CO_2 and prevents acidosis as a result of hyperventilation	

Nursing Diagnosis: Sensory-perceptual alteration related to decreased perceptual field during severe and panic level of anxiety.
Goal: Client will remain safe during episodes of high anxiety.

Intervention	*Rationale*	*Expected Outcome*
Stay with client	Decreases client's fear of being abandoned in a frightening situation	
Give calm reassurance that you will stay and that this attack will go away	Decreases fear of being abandoned and fear that the process will continue indefinitely	
Reassure client of safety	Decreases fear of dying during a panic attack	
Use simple, clear words (eg, "I will stay," "Sit down," "I will help")	The perceptual field is extremely narrowed, and client cannot comprehend complex thoughts and sentences	Responds to brief, clear directions
Speak slowly in a soft voice	Helps set quiet tone and slower tempo	
Decrease environmental stimuli and interaction with other people by asking client to go to a quieter area with the nurse	Decreases anxiety and minimizes the elements of anxiety communicable to and from others in the environment	

(Diagnosis continued)

Table 8–7 *(continued)*

Intervention	*Rationale*	*Expected Outcome*
Direct client to imagine inhaling and exhaling through the soles of the feet	During a panic attack, client does not feel connected to the environment; this imagery will help client feel more connected and therefore safer	Follows directions in breathing imagery
Administer PRN antianxiety agents	To avoid or decrease panic level of anxiety	Verbalizes less anxiety

Nursing Diagnosis: Alteration in thought processes related to difficulty in concentrating and concrete thinking during severe anxiety.
Goal: Client will return to preanxiety level of thought processes.

Intervention	*Rationale*	*Expected Outcome*
Speak to client in simple, concrete language (eg, "Sit down, I will stay")	Perceptual field is so narrowed that client cannot comprehend complex thoughts	Responds appropriately to simple directions
Provide client with simple activities	Attention span is not long enough for complex activities	Participates in simple activities
Stay with client during activities and gently refocus attention	Client will be more successful with activities in presence of nurse	
Instruct client to keep a record of times during the week when anxiety increased	Help client identify the threat or fear and gain understanding of the process of anxiety	Keeps record of anxiety pattern
Explore fear or threat to determine: • if it is in past or present • how the hurt or loss will occur (eg, loss of friendship, threat to self-esteem, etc)	Many "dangers" are in the past and are not realities in the here and now; focusing on the threat of hurt or loss will help find the answers to resolving the anxiety	Identifies fears or threats to self

Nursing Diagnosis: Ineffective individual coping related to inability to ask for help.
Goal: Client will ask for help from others in appropriate situations.

Intervention	*Rationale*	*Expected Outcome*
Have client identify expectations that will occur should help be sought	Client needs to recognize that fear of rejection precludes seeking help	Verbalizes fears of asking for help from others
Use appropriate self-disclosure, which has a therapeutic purpose, regarding situations in which help has been sought	Self-disclosure will help client recognize that asking for help need not result in rejection	
Have client role-play asking for help in a particular situation	Role playing will increase use of unfamiliar skills	Role-plays asking for assistance
Have client evaluate the situation in terms of feelings when help was sought and how others responded	Client needs to appraise change in behavior and assess the reality of fears	Asks for assistance in a given situation

(continued)

Table 8–7 *(continued)*

Nursing Diagnosis: Ineffective individual coping related to checking and rechecking actions or ritualistic behavior.
Goal: Client will gradually decrease ritualistic behavior.

Intervention	*Rationale*	*Expected Outcome*
Do not explain to client that the behavior is pointless and foolish	Client is aware of behavior, so this would only contribute to feelings of inadequacy and failure	
Work with client in modifying the environment and personal schedules so that behavior can be accomplished without interruption of rituals	Support the defense to control anxiety until other coping behaviors can be used	
Implement any necessary safety measures that may be indicated for the behavior (eg, providing dry towels and hand lotion for client who compulsively washes hands)	It is necessary to prevent physical complications resulting from the ritualistic behavior	Physical complications from behavior will not develop
Set limits on destructive ritualistic behavior	Client safety must be maintained	
Provide client with hospital schedule of activities	This will decrease anxiety about the unfamiliar environment	
Follow schedules and fulfill commitments made to client	Demonstrates support for client and fosters development of trust	
Help client identify how the behavior interferes with daily activities	Identification will increase motivation for adopting more effective coping behaviors	Identifies problems that result from compulsive behavior
Use appropriate self-disclosure regarding situations where mistakes have been made (self-disclosure must have a therapeutic purpose)	Assists client in recognizing that mistakes need not result in humiliation	
Explore what purpose the checking or ritualistic behavior serves	Assists client in identifying that the behavior is an effort to control anxiety	
Use problem solving to find other behaviors more effective in managing anxiety	As client learns new ways to manage anxiety, compulsive behavior will decrease	Implements other behaviors to manage anxiety

Nursing Diagnosis: Alteration in family process related to detachment and inability to express feelings.
Goal: Family will verbalize increased feelings of intimacy.

Intervention	*Rationale*	*Expected Outcome*
Help family define and clarify relationships	Increased knowledge of system dynamics will assist family in learning to continuously reassess and redefine nature of relationships	Assesses relationships
Help family members explore how fear of losing self in a close relationship leads to a reaction of distance and alienation	This will increase insight into behavior and assist in differentiation of family members	

(Diagnosis continued)

Table 8–7 *(continued)*

Intervention	*Rationale*	*Expected Outcome*
Help family comprehend the importance of labeling feelings and sharing them with one another	Because the emotional dimension of relationships has a great impact on all other areas of relationships, this needs to be directly confronted	Family labels feelings when they occur
Teach the use of "I" language to express thoughts and feelings (eg, "I think," "I feel")	Each family member needs to assume responsibility for own feelings rather than blaming others (eg, "You make me feel")	Communicates feelings to other family members
Have family members state in behavioral terms what they need from each other to feel cared for and connected emotionally	Intimacy and caring are basic human needs, and the family is a primary source of these	Gives examples of ways in which members can care for one another

Nursing Diagnosis: Alteration in family process related to inability to meet security needs.
Goal: Client will assume more responsibility for meeting own needs.

Intervention	*Rationale*	*Expected Outcome*
Have client examine how excessive helplessness affects relationships with other family members	Increased understanding of family dynamics will assist client in the change process	Identifies the effect of excessive dependent behavior on family system
Have client identify how excessive dependency needs actually increase power and control in family (eg, all must plan schedules and activities around client)	Client needs to identify how his or her helplessness can actually enhance the client's power within the family	
Have family encourage autonomous behavior, and have client seek to meet dependency needs more directly	Fosters the development of healthy interdependence rather than the pattern of a dependent/independent relationship	Implements more autonomous behavior

Nursing Diagnosis: Alteration in family process related to secondary gains of client's partner.
Goal: Partner will decrease behavior that protects phobic client.

Intervention	*Rationale*	*Expected Outcome*
Have partner examine secondary gains that meet own needs (eg, nurturing or control)	To increase insight into behavior and assume responsibility for perpetuating the fears and avoidance	Identifies need to nurture or control
Help family to adjust to changes client is making	Family may feel unneeded, insecure	Manages feelings arising during treatment
Teach the problem-solving process to identify healthier ways of getting needs met	To increase available options and have needs met more directly	Identifies more adaptive methods of meeting needs

(continued)

Table 8–7 *(continued)*

Nursing Diagnosis: Fear related to confrontation with feared object or situation.
Goal: Client will verbalize less phobic fear.

Intervention	*Rationale*	*Expected Outcome*
Have client identify feared object or situations, and make appropriate adaptations in the environment	To limit confrontation with object or situation	Identifies primary source of threat or loss
Allow client to fully express the fears interfering with life	To provide an opportunity to discuss fears without being judged	
Help client search for the source of the original anxiety	Anxiety has been displaced on objects other than self; the original source needs to be confronted and relieved	
Examine each new situation on its own merits	To avoid evaluation of present experiences in terms of the past	
Rehearse various coping behaviors • learn physiologic reactions in sequence • picture event step-by-step • picture self coping effectively • practice relaxation techniques during process or in biofeedback setting	To assist client in reexperiencing those areas of living that have been avoided. Rehearsing how to behave increases sense of control and ability to actually behave in that manner. Visualization helps client move in direction of expectations. Rehearsal reinforces self-image as a person capable of dealing with fear. Relaxation techniques provide client with a means for terminating anxiety when it occurs.	Is able to confront feared object or situation with minimal discomfort
Provide assertiveness training to combat passive style of reacting submissively and fearfully	To increase coping options	Behaves in a more assertive manner
Tricyclic medication or MAOI may be used	To relieve the panic attacks associated with agoraphobia	

Nursing Diagnosis: Powerlessness related to lifestyle of helplessness.
Goal: Client will verbalize more control over lifestyle.

Intervention	*Rationale*	*Expected Outcome*
Don't force client into situations client cannot handle	Support client's defenses as long as they are needed to protect the self	Identifies helpless lifestyle
Don't try to reason away helpless behavior	Client needs behavior to control anxiety	
Give only as much help as is necessary	Gradually help client gain control over life	Assumes more responsibility for fears and behavior
Don't focus attention on phobic behavior. Redirect client to other activity.	It is important to avoid reinforcing maladaptive behavior	
Provide with experiences in which client feels comfortable	Comfort and success will lead to increased self-confidence	

(Diagnosis continued)

Table 8–7 *(continued)*

Intervention	*Rationale*	*Expected Outcome*
Explore beliefs that support a helpless mode of behavior	Cultural beliefs need to be confronted as to their reality and rigidity	
Identify secondary gains such as decreased responsibility and increased dependency	Increased insight into behavior will help client modify behavior appropriately	
Explore alternative methods of meeting these needs	This process will increase self-management	

Nursing Diagnosis: Self-esteem disturbance related to feelings of helplessness, powerlessness, inadequacy and external locus of control.
Goal: Client will verbalize feelings of increased competency.

Intervention	*Rationale*	*Expected Outcome*
Be empathetic, that is, be aware of client's feelings and communicate this awareness to client	Demonstrates understanding and acceptance of client's feelings about self	
Help client focus on relation of self-concept to feelings of anxiety	Client recognizes that anxiety is a warning signal and that resulting behavior is a method of trying to defend self against threats	
Provide experiences in which client can be successful	Success increases self-confidence	
Use the problem-solving process to define and practice behavior that will increase personal adequacy	The problem-solving process gives client an internal locus of control over life and increases feelings of competency	Verbalizes increased confidence in ability to cope
Explore limitations, and help client define realistic goals	Enables client to constructively use energy on things that can be changed in life and not waste energy on things that cannot be changed	Defines realistic goals
Have client identify and participate in pleasurable activities	Provides a sense of control and success	Participates in activities

Nursing Diagnosis: Self-esteem disturbance related to guilt about war acts and survivor's guilt.
Goal: Client will verbalize a decrease in guilt.

Intervention	*Rationale*	*Expected Outcome*
Examine own feelings and beliefs about the war	To prevent an unconscious judgmental process from occurring during the interaction	
Help client identify and label feelings	Enables direct confrontation of feelings	
Help client find ways to directly express feelings	Client may not have had a previous opportunity to discuss guilt	Expresses feelings directly

(Diagnosis continued)

Table 8–7 *(continued)*

Nursing Diagnosis *(continued)*: Self-esteem disturbance related to guilt about war acts and survivor's guilt.
Goal: Client will verbalize a decrease in guilt.

Intervention	*Rationale*	*Expected Outcome*
Refer to clergyperson if appropriate	There is a spiritual dimension to guilt that may be relieved through religious forgiveness	
Refer to a rap group of other combat veterans	This form of group therapy is one of the most effective measures for relieving the guilt of combat veterans	Participates in available rap groups

Nursing Diagnosis: Disturbance in self-concept: self-esteem related to society's devaluation of the Vietnam veteran's worth.
Goal: Client will list worthwhile aspects about self regarding war experience.

Intervention	*Rationale*	*Expected Outcome*
Help client verbalize society's treatment since returning from the war	This may be the first opportunity to discuss individual examples of prejudicial behavior	Verbalizes feelings
Explore sources of internal conflict with client	Client needs to identify anxiety that arises from threat to self-esteem	
Explore ways to increase self-esteem that are not dependent on society's evaluation of the war	Client will benefit from increased insight that much self-validation comes from within	Implements planned methods to increase self-esteem
Refer client to a rap group of other combat veterans	Enables client to receive external validation from others who have been through the same experience	Participates in available rap groups

Nursing Diagnosis: Sleep pattern disturbance related to recurrent nightmares.
Goal: Client will increase hours of restful sleep.

Intervention	*Rationale*	*Expected Outcome*
Keep low light turned on in bedroom at night	A low light will decrease fear and increase orientation when awakening from a nightmare	Verbalizes a decrease in nightmares
Teach relaxation techniques and positive imagery	Help client gain control over nightmares	Reports fewer nightmares
If in the hospital, remain with client after a nightmare	Client needs to be reassured of safety. Remaining with client will increase reality orientation after a nightmare	
Refer to a rap group with others suffering from the same trauma	Talking about nightmares in a supportive and understanding environment will decrease feelings of isolation around this symptom	

(continued)

Table 8–7 *(continued)*

Nursing Diagnosis: Sleep pattern disturbance related to inability to relax enough to fall asleep.
Goal: Client will sleep 6 to 8 hours a night.

Intervention	*Rationale*	*Expected Outcome*
Explore any fears related to falling asleep (eg, loss of control, nightmares, fear of dying)	Identifying the original source of anxiety and confronting the issue directly will increase client's insight into the process	
Teach client to decrease stimuli before bedtime	Helps begin a gradual slowdown of body processes and thought processes	
Explore methods that increase relaxation (eg, warm bath, warm milk, back rub, regular exercise during day)	Client needs to increase the options that will aid falling asleep	Decreases the time needed to fall asleep
Teach progressive relaxation, and have client practice this twice daily and again before sleep	Progressive relaxation will decrease tension and anxiety	Implements relaxation exercises

Nursing Diagnosis: Impaired social interaction related to unsuccessful interpersonal relationships.
Goal: Client will increase amount of time interacting with others.

Intervention	*Rationale*	*Expected Outcome*
Be honest with client and discuss issue of confidentiality	Nurse must prove self as trustworthy	
Allow client to control the amount of self-disclosure that occurs	Until trust is established, client will fear sharing feelings and fears	
Be physically and emotionally accessible to client	Availability is necessary to decrease sense of isolation client is experiencing	
Follow through on commitments made to client	Establishing trust is necessary in satisfying interpersonal relationships	
Gradually increase contact with peers after client feels safe with nurse	Client needs to increase social contact and feelings of competency in interactions	Verbalizes increased comfort when interacting
Explore how isolation increases anxiety	Client needs to be able to relate in an interpersonal world to increase feelings of security and belonging	Identifies the impact of social isolation
Teach that it is acceptable to feel anger and hate toward loved ones as long as feelings are expressed appropriately	Client needs to experience increased comfort with ambivalent feelings rather than using those feelings as an excuse to withdraw from relationships	Verbalizes increased feelings of intimacy with family members
Use appropriate humor and laughter	Sharing laughter increases the feeling of connectedness between two people	
Help client become involved in available therapies (eg, art or dance therapy, cooking, crafts, exercise groups, psychodrama)	One of the goals of these therapies is to increase social interaction among participants	Attends available therapies

(continued)

Table 8–7 *(continued)*

Nursing Diagnosis: Social isolation related to fear of leaving neighborhood or home.
Goal: Client will extend travel distance with minimal discomfort.

Intervention	*Rationale*	*Expected Outcome*
Help client search for the source of the original anxiety	Anxiety has been displaced on situation rather than on self; the original source needs to be confronted and relieved	Identifies primary source of threat or loss
Explore secondary gains with client, such as how a disability can be used to control others	If secondary gains can be identified and understood, these needs can be met more directly	Identifies secondary gains of phobia
Brainstorm many possible ways to handle troublesome situations	This will increase client's available options by changing expectations and increasing client's self-control	Formulates list of alternative behaviors
Refer to a behavior modification program or systematic desensitization therapy	The disorder may need intensive therapy from someone highly trained in the area	Follows through on referral

Nursing Diagnosis: Alteration in thought processes related to egocentricity and grandiose self-beliefs to defend against anxiety.
Goal: Client will exhibit decreased egocentricity and grandiose self-beliefs.

Intervention	*Rationale*	*Expected Outcome*
When exhibition of grandiose behavior occurs, redirect client to other activities or discussion	Redirection will prevent continued focus on problematic behavior	Substitutes other activities for grandiose behavior
Help client find significance in people and situation outside self	This process will decrease egocentricity and increase interpersonal interactions	Interacts appropriately with others
Don't compete with or directly contradict grandiose statements	Such conflict would assault client's defenses and increase anxiety	
Use appropriate self-disclosure to show that being human and fallible need not result in rejection or humiliation	Increased insight enables client to replace defenses with more effective coping behavior	
Help client assess strengths and limitations and verbalize self-doubts	As anxiety decreases, realistic self-appraisal will assist client in giving up egocentricity	Verbalizes decreased anxiety about self-doubts

Nursing Diagnosis: Potential for violence: self-directed or directed at others related to inability to verbalize feelings.
Goal: Client will not harm self or others.

Intervention	*Rationale*	*Expected Outcome*
Identify own feelings of anxiety	Nurse must avoid projection of own anxiety onto client	
Assist client in distinguishing between feelings (eg, anxiety, frustration, guilt, hostility)	Client needs to be able to label feelings to separate the variety of emotions experienced	Labels a variety of feelings accurately
Discuss ways to express feelings appropriately	Client needs to increase options for managing feelings other than destructive behavior	Identifies appropriate methods of expressing feelings

(Diagnosis continued)

Table 8–7 *(continued)*

Intervention	*Rationale*	*Expected Outcome*
Support appropriate expressions of feelings	Client needs to recognize that suppressing any feelings requires energy, which is depleting	
Support direct verbal expression of negative feelings	Client fears potency of negative feelings and fears rejection if these are expressed	Directly expresses negative feelings
Explore relation between high anxiety and destructive behavior against self or others	Anxiety can create hostility, and when anxiety escalates control may be lost; destructive behavior is the overt expression of hostility	
Provide safe physical outlets for negative feelings (eg, exercise, working out in the gym, pounding clay)	Using energy created by unexpressed feelings will prevent escalation of violent behavior	Uses appropriate physical activities to manage energy

Nursing Diagnosis: Potential for violence: self-directed or directed at others related to poor impulse control.
Goal: Client will not harm self or others.

Intervention	*Rationale*	*Expected Outcome*
Identify behavior patterns and clues that indicate increasing anxiety: • verbal—content of remarks, tone of voice • nonverbal—trembling, sweating, pacing, high startle response, pounding fist, angry facial expression	Early identification is necessary to prevent violent behavior associated with loss of control	
Try to find cause of escalating behavior, and remove it if possible	This may prevent an increase in anxiety, frustration, and anger	
Remain calm and available	Anxiety is contagious and may escalate fears; avoidance increases anxiety	
Provide immediate outlets for decreasing tension (eg, hitting pillows, sanding wood, vigorous walking, exercising, using punching bag)	Client needs to use energy of high anxiety in constructive manner	Employs effective behavior to cope with stress and anxiety
Do not personalize aggressive behavior	Loss of objectivity will result in a power struggle, which will increase anxiety	
Assess seriousness of situation, and remove dangerous objects or move client to a safe environment such as a specified quiet room	Nurse must limit possibility of harm to client or others	
Keep staff members with client at all times until client has increased control over self	The presence of staff members will ensure safety until the potential for violence is diminished	
Give limited choices (eg, "You can sit in the chair or lie on the bed as long as you stay in this room")	Allows client to experience some control over situation, which will decrease anxiety	Follows limited choices

(Diagnosis continued)

Table 8–7 *(continued)*

Nursing Diagnosis *(continued)*: Potential for violence: self-directed or directed at others related to poor impulse control.
Goal: Client will not harm self or others.

Intervention	*Rationale*	*Expected Outcome*
When client is calm, explore outlets that can be used to prevent loss of control (eg, sports that offer the opportunity to conquer both physical and emotional tension)	Client needs options other than loss of control to decrease the tension of anxiety	Identifies alternative outlets for energy
Discuss the destructive effects on client when violence is used as a solution to stress	To manage behavior, client needs to increase insight into consequences of behavior and increase responsibility for behavior	Identifies destructive effects of violence

Nursing Diagnosis: Spiritual distress related to a view of the world and people as threatening following a severe traumatic event.
Goal: Client will manage fears.

Intervention	*Rationale*	*Expected Outcome*
Help client search for meaning in the traumatic event	This will assist client in reestablishing a purpose in life	Verbalizes some personal purpose in life
Help client plan interpersonal support systems	To increase feelings of connectedness to others	Seeks out significant others
Encourage sharing feelings of the traumatic event	Allows client to ventilate rather than suppress feelings	Verbalizes feelings
Utilize problem-solving process with client to increase possible self-protection in future	Altering specific behaviors will increase sense of control in some situations	Modifies specific behaviors
If appropriate, refer client to a religious counselor	Processing event may decrease inappropriate guilt or responsibility	Shares feelings with religious advisor

that only he or she understands the client. To prevent manipulation on the part of the client, open communication and frequent team meetings are vital. General interventions involve creating a safe and trusting environment and assisting the client in managing day-to-day living difficulties. It is most helpful if a master chart is made of all the known personalities. The chart should include names, ages, functions, and degrees of influence. This will assist the staff in organizing data and responding appropriately to the various personalities (Anderson, 1988).

These clients can profit from nontherapy group sessions but tend not to benefit from and disrupt group therapy sessions (Putnam, 1989). Other clients may be frightened or confused by the person with multiple personality disorder. Peers may make friends with one personality and then not understand the anger or rejection by another personality.

In all types of anxiety disorders, appropriately implementation includes referrals to support groups or specific treatment programs. Clients and professionals may contact the following groups for further information.

Veteran Outreach Program
Disabled American Veterans
807 Maine Ave., S.W.
Washington, DC 20024

Phobia Society of America
133 Rollins Ave., Suite 4B
Rockville, MD 20852

Obsessive-compulsive Disorder Foundation
Box 60
Vernon, CN 06066

Multiple Personality Clinic
Department of Psychiatry, Rush University
600 S. Paulina
Chicago, IL 60612

Evaluation

The fourth step of the nursing process, evaluation, is the basis for modifying the nursing care plan. It is accomplished by the nurse and client after determining whether the expected outcomes have been met. If they have been met, the nurse determines if the diagnosis is resolved and the client is coping effectively. If the problem is only partially resolved, new outcome criteria need to be developed. When the nurse and client determine that none of the expected outcomes have been met, the problem-solving process is used to determine the cause. It may be that enough time has not elapsed or that outcomes were inappropriate or too long-term. If the outcomes are valid, the interventions are evaluated. Perhaps the interventions were inappropriate or not individualized for the particular client, or perhaps they were not consistently implemented. When the difficulty in the nursing process is identified, modification is made on the basis of the evaluation, to ensure the client's healthier adaptation to anxiety.

SUMMARY

1. Levels of anxiety are described along a four-point scale of absence of anxiety, mild anxiety, moderate anxiety, and panic.

2. Defense mechanisms are unconscious attempts to manage anxiety—attempts that may or may not be successful.

3. Anxiety disorders in childhood are fairly rare, although it is not uncommon for most children to experience fears specific to their developmental stage.

4. Children suffering from separation anxiety disorder present with many somatic complaints as well as morbid fears, phobias, and sleep difficulties.

5. Avoidant disorder is diagnosed in children who are inhibited, shy, tearful, and who suffer great difficulty in speaking or interacting in social situations.

6. Motor restlessness, nail biting, hair pulling, and somatic complaints are indicative of overanxious disorder in the perfectionist, dependent child.

7. An adolescent with identity disorder has impaired social or school functioning and many uncertainties about life goals, friendships, sexual orientation, and value systems.

8. Adolescent adjustment disorder occurs during the transition to adulthood and is characterized by regressive behaviors to decrease the anxiety of assuming a more independent adult role.

Knowledge Base

9. Generalized anxiety disorder (GAD) is the chronic expression of the characteristics of the moderate level of anxiety.

10. Panic attacks may occur unexpectedly and even during sleep. Individuals then develop an intense fear of experiencing another panic attack.

11. People with OCD often display intense and at times bizarre behaviour most typically involving washing, checking, or repeating rituals.

12. OCD is ego-dystonic. Victims recognize the senselessness of their compulsive behaviors and their inability to control their obsessive thoughts.

13. People with phobic disorders suffer from persistent, unreasonable fears that result in avoidance behavior, which often disables the victim. When confronted with the feared object or situation, panic ensues.

14. The major defense mechanisms used in phobias are repression, displacement, symbolization, and avoidance.

15. When severe and unexpected trauma occurs, some people respond with undercontrol and are diagnosed as having PTSD. Other people respond with overcontrol and are diagnosed as having a dissociative disorder.

16. People suffering from PTSD often relive the traumatic event and respond to environmental stimuli with unpredictable irritation and aggression. Related to their need for emotional distance is their difficulty in maintaining intimate relationships.

17. People with a dissociative disorder block thoughts and feelings associated with a severe trauma from conscious awareness. This may take the form of psychogenic amnesia, psychogenic fugue, or multiple personality.

18. The major defense mechanisms used in dissociative disorders are repression and dissociation.

19. It is not unusual for people with anxiety disorders to develop concomitant disorders such as depression or substance abuse.

20. People with anxiety disorders may have a profound effect on their family systems. The family may be expected to assume all responsibilities outside the home or live with detachment and emotional distance.

21. A variety of factors are related to the development of anxiety disorders. These include a biologic vulnerability, external locus of control, fear of disapproval and criticism, expectations of failure, internalization of rigid discipline, learned avoidance responses, and rigid role expectations.

Planning and Implementation

22. A variety of antianxiety agents and antidepressants may be utilized along with individual, family, or group psychotherapy.

23. Planning and implementation of the care plan must be done with the client's active participation. This will avoid sabotage of the plan by an unconsulted client.

24. The majority of nursing diagnoses in this chapter are applicable to many individuals regardless of the specific medical diagnostic category. It is through understanding the issues and problems most significant for each client that plans for care are developed and implemented.

CHAPTER REVIEW

Pam, a client on the adult psychiatric unit, has a history of panic disorder. One day her primary nurse discovers her at the end of the hallway sobbing, talking in a shrill voice about being "frightened to death," and pacing in a small circle. She says she is dizzy and has shortness of breath.

1. Knowing that Pam is experiencing the panic level of anxiety, what would be the most appropriate nursing intervention?
   - (a) Leave her alone so she can get control of herself
   - (b) Stay with her to reassure her of her safety
   - (c) Have her join a group of clients so she will feel better
   - (d) Put her in a waist restraint until she calms down

2. Which one of the following would be the most appropriate PRN medication to give Pam at this time?
   - (a) Imipramine (Tofranil)
   - (b) Phenelzine (Nardil)
   - (c) Benztropine mesylate (Cogentin)
   - (d) Alprazolam (Xanax)

One year after graduation from nursing school, Susan served a one-year tour of duty in Vietnam as an army nurse. She has recently entered counseling for symptoms of PTSD.

3. Which of the following is the most likely factor contributing to Susan's developing PTSD as a result of being in Vietnam?
   - (a) She was very young and impressionable when she went overseas.
   - (b) She has held herself responsible for the death of her patients.
   - (c) She did not have enough nursing experience prior to Vietnam.
   - (d) She thought being in the army would be more glamorous than it actually was.

4. In assessing Susan's affective characteristics, the nurse-therapist is most likely to find that Susan experiences
   - (a) Periods of irritability and emotional detachment from others.
   - (b) Shame about her irrational and sometimes bizarre behavior.
   - (c) Fear and bewilderment about "lost" periods of time.
   - (d) A flat affect and total apathy to changes in her environment.

5. Which one of the following is the most likely nursing diagnosis for Susan?
   - (a) Ineffective individual coping related to need to always "be right."
   - (b) Ineffective individual coping related to checking and rechecking.
   - (c) Self-esteem disturbance related to survivor's guilt.
   - (d) Powerlessness related to lifestyle of helplessness.

REFERENCES

Anderson G: Understanding multiple personality disorder. *J Psychosoc Nurs* 1988; 26(7):26–30.

Appenheimer T, Noyes R: Generalized anxiety disorders. In: *Psychiatric Illnesses, Primary Care.* Yates WR (editor). Saunders, 1987.

Atwood JD, Chester R: *Treatment Techniques for Common Mental Disorders.* Aronson, 1987.

Barlow DH: *Anxiety and Its Disorders.* Guilford Press, 1988.

Barlow DH, Cerny JA: *Psychological Treatment of Panic.* Guilford Press, 1988.

Barrios BA, Hartmann DP: Fears and anxieties. In: *Behavioral Assessment of Childhood Disorders.* Mash EJ, Terdal LG (editors). Guilford Press, 1988.

Berlin S: Women and mental health. In: *The Woman Client.* Burden DS, Gottlieb N (editors). Tavistock, 1987.

Blake-White J, Kline CM: Treating the dissociative process in adult victims of childhood incest. *J Contemp Soc Work* 1985; 65(9):394–402.

Bliss EL: *Multiple Personality, Allied Disorders and Hypnosis.* Oxford University, 1986.

Brehony KA: Women and agoraphobia. In: *The Stereotyping of Women.* Franks U, Rothblum E (editors). Springer, 1983.

Brende JO: Multiple personality: A post-traumatic stress disorder. In: *Dissociative Disorders: 1984. Proceedings of the First International Conference on Multiple Personality Dissociative States.* Braun BG (editor). Chicago: Department of Psychiatry, Rush University, 1984.

Chapman GE: Ritual and rational action in hospitals. *Adv Nurs* 1983; 8(1):13–20.

Charney DS, et al.: Neurobiological mechanisms of panic anxiety. *Am J Psychiatry* 1987; 144(8):1030–1036.

Coons PM: A comprehensive study and followup of 20 multiple personality patients. In: *Dissociative Disorders: 1984. Proceedings of the First International Conference on Multiple Personality Dissociative States.* Braun BG (editor). Chicago: Department of Psychiatry, Rush University, 1984.

Coughlan K, Parkin C: Women partners of Vietnam vets. *J Psychosoc Nurs* 1987; 25(10):25–27.

DeVeaugh-Geiss J, Landau P, Katz R: Treatment of obsessive compulsive disorder with clomipramine. *Psych Annals* 1989; 19(2):97–101.

Dubovsky SL, et al.: Anxiolytics: When? Why? Which one? *Patient Care* 1987; 21(17):60–81.

Emmelkamp P: *Phobic and Obsessive-Compulsive Disorders.* Plenum, 1982.

Fraser GA, Curtis JC: A subpersonality theory of multiple personality. In: *Dissociative Disorders: 1984. Proceedings of the First International Conference on Multiple Personality Dissociative States.* Braun BG (editor). Chicago: Department of Psychiatry, Rush University, 1984.

Goodwin DW: *Phobia: The Facts.* Oxford, 1983.

Guzzetta C, Forsyth G: Nursing diagnostic pilot study: Psychophysiologic stress. *ANS* 1979; 2(1):27–44.

Hafner RJ: Anxiety disorders. In: *Handbook of Behavioral Family Therapy.* Fallon IRH (editor). Guilford Press, 1988.

Hand I: Obsessive-compulsive patients and their families. In: *Handbook of Behavioral Family Therapy.* Fallon IRH (editor). Guilford Press, 1988.

Karl GT: Survival skills for psychic trauma. *J. Psychosoc Nurs* 1989; 27(4):15–19.

Keltner N, Doggett R, Johnson R: For the Viet Nam veteran the war goes on. *Perspect Psychiatr Care* 1983; 21(3): 108–113.

Kluft RP: Making the diagnosis of multiple personality disorder. In: *Diagnostics and Psychopathology.* Flack F (editor). Norton, 1987A.

Kluft RP: First-rank symptoms as a diagnostic clue to multiple personality disorder. In: *Diagnostics and Psychopathology.* Flack F (editor). Norton, 1987B.

Lanza ML: Victims of international terrorism. *Issues Ment Health* 1986; 8(2):95–107.

Liebowitz MR, Klein DF: Agoraphobia: clinical features, pathophysiology and treatment. In: *Agoraphobia: Multiple Perspectives on Theory and Treatment.* Chambless DL, Goldstein AJ (editors). Wiley, 1982.

Loewenstein RJ, et al.: Experiential sampling in the study of multiple personality. *Am J Psychiatry* 1987; 144(1):19–24.

Longo D, Williams R: *Clinical Practice in Psychosocial Nursing.* Appleton-Century-Crofts, 1978.

Marmer SS: The "window of vulnerability" in multiple personality. In: *Dissociative Disorders: 1984. Proceedings of the First International Conference on Multiple Personality Dissociative States.* Braun BG (editor). Chicago: Department of Psychiatry, Rush University, 1984.

Matuzas W, et al.: Mitral valve prolapse and thyroid abnormalities in patients with panic attacks. *Am J Psychiatry* 1987; 144(4):493–496.

Mavissakalian M, et al.: Trazodone in the treatment of panic disorder. *Am J Psychiatry* 1987; 144(6): 785–787.

Maxmen JS: *Essential Psychopathology.* Norton, 1986.

Millon T: *Disorders of Personality: DSM III: Axis II.* Wiley, 1981.

Mullis M: Viet Nam: The human fallout. *J Psychiatr Nurs* 1984; 22(2):27–31.

Ochberg FM: Post-traumatic therapy and victims of violence. In: *Post-Traumatic Therapy and Victims of Violence.* Ochberg FM (editor). Brunner/Mazel, 1988.

Peplau H: A working definition of anxiety. In: *Some Clinical Approaches to Psychiatric Nursing.* Burd S, Marshall M (editors). Macmillan, 1963.

Price L, et al.: Treatment of severe obsessive-compulsive disorder with fluvoxamine. *Am J Psychiatry* 1987; 144(8):1059–1061.

Putnam, FW: *Multiple Personality Disorder.* Guilford Press, 1989.

Rapoport JL: *The Boy Who Couldn't Stop Washing: The Experience and Treatment of Obsessive-Compulsive Disorder.* Dutton, 1989.

Rogers B, Nickolaus J: Vietnam nurses. *J Psychosoc Nurs* 1987. 25(4):10–15.

Roth WT: The role of medication in post-traumatic therapy. In: *Post Traumatic Therapy and Victims of Violence.* Ochberg FM (editor). Brunner/Mazel, 1988.

Salzman L: Obsessions and agoraphobia. In: *Agoraphobia: Multiple Perspectives on Theory and Treatment.* Chambless DL, Goldstein AJ (editors). Wiley, 1982.

Solomon Z, et al.: Reactivation of combat-related post-traumatic stress disorder. *Am J Psychiatry* 1987; 144(1):51–55.

Spitzer C, Franklin J: Hero burnout. *Chicago Tribune.* July 24, 1988; p. 6.

Verbosky SJ, Ryan DA: Female partners of Vietnam veterans. *Issues Ment Health* 1988; 9(1):95–104.

Wesner R: Panic disorder and agoraphobia. In: *Psychiatric Illnesses, Primary Care.* Yates WR (editor). Saunders, 1987.

SUGGESTED READINGS

Barlow DH: New treatment for agoraphobia. *Med Aspects Human Sexuality* 1988; 22(2):98–107.

Hurrelmann K, Engel U: *The Social World of Adolescents.* de Gruyter, 1989.

King JV: A holistic technique to lower anxiety: Relaxation with guided imagery. *J Holistic Nurs* 1988; 6(1):16–20.

Othmer SC, Othmer E: Sexual dysfunction in anxiety disorder. *Med Aspects Human Sexuality* 1989; 23(3): 36–41.

Sachs RG: Recognizing the patient with multiple personality disorder. *Med Aspects Human Sexuality* 1988; 22(12):50–67.

Swanson GL: *Adolescence: The Confusing Years.* Technomic, 1988.

CHAPTER 9

Physiologic Responses to Anxiety

KAREN LEE FONTAINE

How I See my Illness

As I go through each episode I grow but that growth is very costly. The peaks—I sometimes want the euphoria, energy but that lasts only for short moments and then I hit reality and find that it has cost me more than growth, but family and sometimes a friend. The worry I cause others because of this illness may never be repairable. They don't understand that after it gets to a certain point I don't have control. Following comes the depression and I am basically a happy-go-lucky person. It's so hard to smile at times.

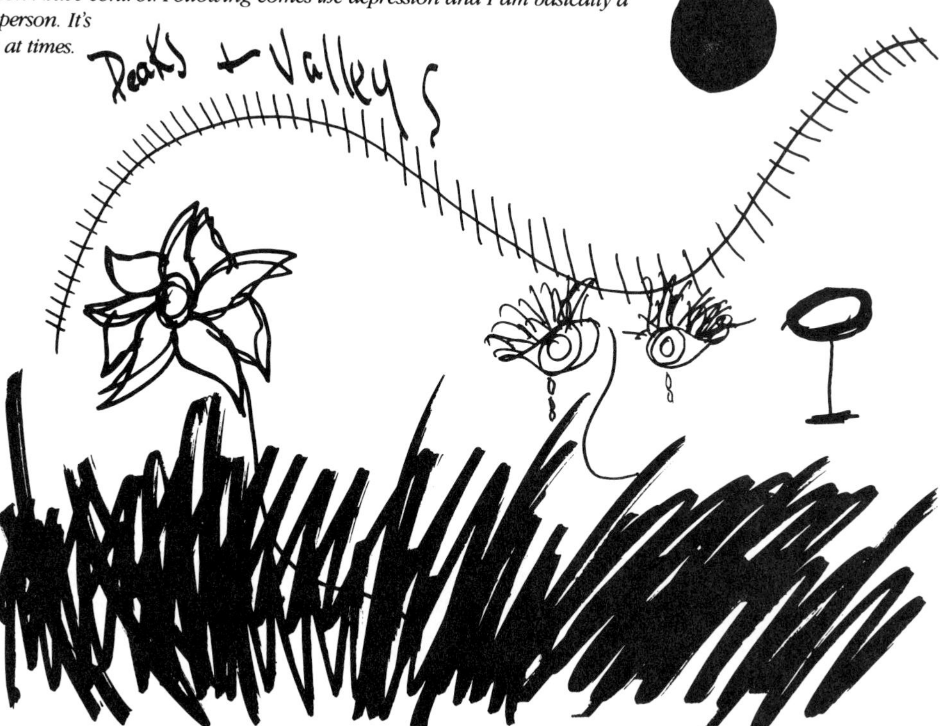

▪ *Objectives*

After reading this chapter the student will be able to

- Distinguish between the characteristics of the somatoform disorders
- Distinguish between anorexia and bulimia
- Analyze sociocultural factors that contribute to the somatoform and eating disorders
- Apply the nursing process when intervening with clients experiencing physiologic responses to anxiety

▪ *Chapter Outline*

Introduction

A number of mental health disorders involve the transformation of anxiety into physical symptoms, which are generally more acceptable in the culture. Some of these resemble organic disorders, but there is no organic basis for the symptoms. Others, such as the eating disorders, develop organic changes as the process continues.

In these disorders, anxiety is repressed, denied, and displaced onto concerns with one's body. This transformation is out of conscious control and provides a protective screen against the direct experience of anxiety. The original source of anxiety often involves acceptance, performance, autonomy, conflict, helplessness, or vulnerability. Initially it is safer for the client to shift the focus onto the body. As the disorders progress, the symptoms often become more of a problem and create greater suffering than the original source of anxiety. In addition, constant use of repression, denial, and displacement takes a great deal of energy; therefore, the client's ability to respond to any other form of stress is decreased.

Secondary gains play a major role in maintaining these disorders. These gains include the right to be nurtured, decreased responsibility, self-punishment for guilt, or punishment of others for a perceived lack of caring. Verbal obsessions about health, food, or weight may serve as an unconscious method of maintaining emotional distance. Others rapidly become bored with this behavior and attempt to avoid the individual.

The disorders presented in this chapter appear in DSM-III-R as the following diagnoses:

300.81 Somatization disorder

300.11 Conversion disorder

307.80 Somatoform pain disorder

300.70 Hypochondriasis

307.10 Anorexia nervosa

307.51 Bulimia nervosa

Somatoform Disorders

The **somatoform disorders**—somatization, conversion, somatoform pain, and hypochondriasis—all involve physical symptoms for which no underlying organic basis exists. People diagnosed with a **somatization disorder** have multiple physical complaints involving a variety of body systems. This is a chronic disorder that usually begins in the teenage years and is seen more often in women then in men. A **conversion disorder**, which involves sensorimotor symptoms, can appear at any age but typically begins and ends abruptly. It is usually precipitated by a severe trauma such as war. Sensory symptoms range from paresthesia and anesthesia to blindness and deafness. Motor symptoms range from tics to seizures to paralysis. The person with a conversion disorder has only one symptom rather than the variety seen in the person with a somatization disorder. Pain that cannot be explained organically is the primary symptom of a **somatoform pain disorder**. Unconscious conflict and anxiety are believed to be the basis for the pain. People with **hypochondriasis** believe they have a serious disease involving one or several body systems, despite all medical evidence to the contrary. Or, they are terrified of contracting certain diseases. These people are extremely sensitive to internal sensations, which they misinterpret as evidence of disease. This disorder usually begins in midlife or late life and affects women and men equally (Black, 1987).

Conversion disorders are rarely seen, but the other disorders are frequently seen in community settings, health care offices, and acute care settings. These three disorders account for a large portion of the medical expenditures in this country. It is estimated that 4 to 18 percent of all physician visits are made by the "worried well." People having these disorders truly suffer, however; they must not be discounted as malingerers or manipulators. For these people, nurses are often able to provide a long-term caring relationship, which may be the most important intervention in preventing needless tests, medications, and surgeries. When these clients feel no one is listening to or caring for them, they often go from one health care professional to another, which results in duplication of previous tests and medical interventions. Knowledgeable, sensitive nurses are able to protect these clients by maintaining them within one health care system (Baur, 1988).

Knowledge Base: Somatoform Disorders

Behavioral Characteristics

Those suffering from somatoform disorders often visit a wide variety of providers of health care. In a desperate attempt to find relief from their disorder, they visit different physicians or chiropractors and receive frequent referrals for specialty consultations, which result in extensive and costly diagnostic exams.

Typically, these clients purchase many over-the-counter medications in an attempt to reduce their symptoms or pain. Inadvertent drug abuse may occur when medications are prescribed for lengthy periods by a variety of physicians. Dependency on pain relievers or antianxiety agents is a common complication of these disorders.

These people frequently discuss their symptoms and disease processes. Many of them adapt their behavior patterns and lifestyles around the disorders. This can range from a minor restriction of activities to the role of a complete invalid.

In the past year Dorothy has been seen by eight health care providers, including her family physician, a cardiologist, an internist, an orthopedist, a chiropractor, a proctologist, a naprapath, and a cancer diagnostician. After extensive and repeated testing, no evidence of organic disease was found. Dorothy continues to complain about the incompetency of these people and is in the process of finding new providers.

Affective Characteristics

The primary gain in somatoform disorders is the reduction of conflict and anxiety. People suffering from them are usually unable to express anger and hostility directly to other people out of fear of abandonment and loss of love. They actively avoid situations where others will become angry with them. As a result, there is an unconscious use of physical symptoms to manage the anxiety experienced with conflicting issues (Baur, 1988).

When relief from the physical symptoms is not obtained, further anxiety is often experienced. This may be manifested by symptoms of anxiety, obsessions about the illness, depression, or phobic avoidance of activities associated with the spread of disease.

Cognitive Characteristics

Somatoform disorder sufferers are obsessively interested in bodily processes, concerns, and diseases. Almost all their attention is focused on the discomfort they are experiencing. So obsessed are they with their bodies, that they are constantly aware of very small physical changes and discomforts that go unnoticed by others. In hypochondriasis, these changes are regarded as concrete evidence of an active disease process.

> *Vera is convinced she has cancer of the bowel in spite of all negative diagnostic tests. She is hyperalert to any bowel noises, twinges, and slight changes in stool. She regards these normal occurrences and sensations as evidence of cancer.*

Denial is a major defense mechanism used by these clients. Initially, there is denial of the source of anxiety and conflict, and the energy is transformed into physical complaints. Along with the physical symptoms is the denial that there could be any psychologic component to the physical symptoms. If confronted with the possibility of a psychologic cause, these clients often change health care providers in an effort to maintain their system of denial. Rarely will they follow through on referrals for psychotherapy.

Some clients with conversion disorders exhibit **la belle indifference**, which is a relative unconcern for their physical symptoms. People showing a sudden onset of symptoms, even severe ones like paralysis or blindness, sometimes seem fairly nonchalant about their condition. This reaction usually occurs in people who do not want to be noticed by others. Other clients with conversion disorders, however, may be very verbal about their distress over the sudden appearance of the symptoms. This reaction is more likely to occur in people with a high need for attention and sympathy.

Physiologic Characteristics

People with a somatization disorder have multiple physical symptoms involving a variety of bodily systems. These symptoms may be vague and undefined, and they do not follow a particular disease pattern. Pain is the primary symptom in somatoform pain disorder. The pain is severe and prolonged and usually does not follow the nerve conduction pathways of the body. Conversion disorder symptoms can occur in any of the sensory or motor systems of the body. The client may become suddenly blind or deaf. Loss of speech may range from persistent laryngitis to total muteness. Body parts may experience tingling or numbness. Motor symptoms range from spasms or tics to paralysis of hands, arms, or legs.

In hypochondriasis, symptoms may be limited to one or several body systems. Most frequent symptoms appear in the head and neck. These symptoms include dizziness, loss of hearing, hearing one's own heartbeat, a lump in the throat, and chronic coughing. Not uncommon are symptoms in the abdomen and chest. These symptoms include indigestion, bowel disorders, palpitations, skipped or rapid heartbeats, and pain in the left side of the chest. Some individuals may also have skin discomfort, insomnia, and sexual problems (Baur, 1988).

> *Six months ago Olivia assumed primary responsibility for the care of her aging parents. She soon began to experience multiple physical complaints and has been seen by a number of physicians. Three months ago, the symp-*

toms became severe, forcing Olivia to quit work. She has a constant stiff neck, is frequently dizzy, and complains of heaviness in her chest when she lies down. She states that her chest feels as though it is cracking into pieces, and she says her esophagus has "fallen," which makes eating very difficult. Olivia is terrified of her symptoms and loss of weight, but she is unwilling to follow through with the recommended psychiatric evaluation.

Sociocultural Characteristics

Within a cultural setting that has little understanding or acceptance of psychologic distress and illness, people may transform emotional distress into physical symptoms. It is often more acceptable to be physically ill than mentally ill. Physical symptoms engender sympathy, support, and care from significant others, whereas emotional symptoms often lead to frustration, anger, and avoidance. Thus, society's values contribute to the incidence of the somatoform disorders.

The media must also be recognized as a contributing factor in these disorders. Magazines, radio, and television bombard us with advertisements for over-the-counter "cures" for every imaginable physical problem. In addition, there has been an emphasis on staying healthy—an emphasis that, at times, seems like a morbid preoccupation with death. A new characteristic of somatoform disorders is an obsessive, unrealistic fear of contracting AIDS. AIDS centers across the country report an increase in calls from low-risk individuals who are terrified they may have AIDS. With such intense media attention, it is hardly surprising that people become obsessed with bodily processes (Baur, 1988).

The somatoform disorders may completely disrupt a person's life. Clients may need to change their vocation to one more adaptable to their physical symptoms. Others may be unable to work in any capacity, either inside or outside the home. The chronic nature of these disorders often places a severe financial and emotional drain on the family. Physician, diagnostic, and hospital expenses may place the family in severe debt. The emotional drain, on both the client and the family, leads to increased stress and interpersonal conflict, especially when there is no physical improvement in the person. This increased level of conflict contributes to the continuation of the disorder, and a vicious cycle is established.

Causative Theories

Intrapersonal theories view anxiety as the major component of the somatoform disorders. The original source of the anxiety is unrecognized, and the discomfort is experienced as physical symptoms or disorders. People with inadequate self-esteem may view their physical symptoms as evidence of their unworthiness. Thus, aches and pains are perceived as a punishment for personal inadequacies. Somatoform disorders may also be the unconscious expression of anger in those unable to communicate feelings of anger and hostility directly. Since physical distress provides an acceptable excuse to avoid certain activities and situations, people with perfectionistic qualities may unconsciously use physical limitations to rationalize their inadequacies and faults. Therefore somatoform disorders are used to excuse the inability to be perfect (Baur, 1988; Black, 1987).

Interpersonal theories focus on the secondary gains for people suffering from somatoform disorders. For those with high dependency needs, the physical symptoms may achieve a great deal of attention and support from significant others. The sympathy and nurturing these people receive may be a major factor in maintaining the disorders. The gain in attention from others may be viewed as a reassurance of care and love or, since sick or weak people are often in a position of great power, as an unconscious attempt to gain power and control.

Since secondary gains are powerful maintainers of the somatoform disorders, the nurse needs to be able to identify secondary gains to assist the clients in meeting their needs in a more adaptive manner.

Behavioral theorists view the somatoform disorders as learned somatic responses. It is thought these individuals are unable to deal directly with stress and habitually respond to stress with physical sensations or symptoms.

Assessment: Somatoform Disorders

The majority of clients suffering from somatoform disorders will be seen in community settings, clinics, physicians' offices, emergency departments, and medical-surgical units. Because these clients often present complicated and detailed medical histories, careful physical assessment is necessary. The nurse needs to remember that, at any time, a client with a somatoform disorder may develop an organic illness. Thus, continual physical assessment is a necessary component of nursing care. As always, assessment questions must be modified to the individual client's cognitive, educational, and language abilities. (See the focused nursing assessment for clients with somatoform disorders, which follows.)

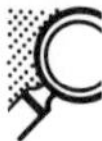

FOCUSED NURSING ASSESSMENT *for the Client with Somatoform Disorders*

Behavioral assessment

What over-the counter medications are you currently taking?
How effective are these medications?
What prescription medications are you currently taking?
How effective are these medications?
What medications have you taken in the past?
What results were obtained with these medications?
Who have you consulted professionally for your illness in the past five years?
What diagnostic procedures have been performed?
What surgeries have you had in your lifetime?
How has your lifestyle been affected by your illness? Work outside the home? Family responsibilities? Social activities? Leisure activities?

Affective assessment

In what situations do you experience feelings of anger?
In what situations do you experience feelings of anxiety?
In what way do you share your feelings with others?
How do you respond when others become angry with you?
How do you respond when you are angry with others?
How do you manage conflict with others?
How sad or depressed are you feeling?

Cognitive assessment

How often, in a day, are you aware of your physical symptoms?
How aware are you of bodily sensations?
Do you believe you have a serious illness?
Has this illness been confirmed by a health care professional?
Has anyone discussed psychologic components of physical illness with you?
Have you ever been referred for counseling?
Describe your level of concern for your physical health.
Describe the positive qualities about yourself.
Do you have a need to do things as perfectly as possible?
What happens to you when you make mistakes?

Sociocultural assessment

How is your family managing with your illness?
Who is supportive to you in this illness?
Who cares for you when you are unable to care for yourself?
Who is frustrated with your lack of physical improvement?
How has your illness affected the family's financial situation?

Diagnosis and Planning: Somatoform Disorders

With the exception of conversion disorders, the somatoform disorders tend to be chronic and lifelong. The most important goal of treatment is to prevent needless diagnostic procedures and surgeries and abuse of medications. The primary intervention is a warm and caring relationship. This enables the client to remain within one health care system, which thus provides continuity of care. Concurrent psychotherapy or family therapy can reduce the unconscious need for the physical symptoms, as can a long-term, empathetic relationship that provides attention and support. If the needs met by the secondary gains can be met in a more adaptive fashion, the client's physical distress will be decreased. (See Table 9–1 for the standard care plan for the client with somatoform disorders.)

Table 9–1 Nursing Care Plan for the Client with Somatoform Disorders

Nursing Diagnosis: Ineffective individual coping related to inability to manage conflict.
Goal: Client will manage conflict directly and reduce physical symptoms.

Intervention	*Rationale*	*Expected Outcome*
Help client identify feelings of resentment and anger	Bringing negative emotions into conscious awareness will decrease the unconscious expression through physical symptoms	Correctly labels feelings of anger and resentment
Role-play methods of direct expression of feelings	Practice of alternative behaviors will increase client's ability to implement new behaviors	Role-plays conflict-resolution techniques
Provide assertiveness training	Assertive behavior may assist client in decreasing use of physical symptoms to avoid conflict	Increases assertive behavior

Nursing Diagnosis: Social isolation related to physical symptoms and disability.
Goal: Client will become more socially active.

Intervention	*Rationale*	*Expected Outcome*
Provide diversional activities (eg, occupational, music, art, and exercise therapy)	To decrease time spent obsessing about physical symptoms	Participates in diversional activities; decreases time spent obsessing about symptoms
Discuss ways to increase social contact within physical limitations	Increasing contact with others will provide additional sources of support and concern	Increases and broadens social contacts
Help client identify groups that may be supportive (eg, self-help groups, volunteer groups)	Becoming involved in a group will decrease isolation	Identifies potential groups

Nursing Diagnosis: Ineffective individual coping related to high need for approval and acceptance.
Goal: Client will be able to meet acceptance needs directly.

Intervention	*Rationale*	*Expected Outcome*
Help client identify positive personal attributes	Ability to give self-approval will decrease excessive dependency needs	Identifies personal strengths
Help client identify ways to increase autonomy and self-confidence	Increasing feelings of competency will decrease excessive need for approval from others	Verbalizes increased self-confidence
Teach client how to assertively ask for attention, support, and nurturing	Asking directly to get needs met will decrease use of physical symptoms to meet emotional needs	Increases assertive behavior

Nursing Diagnosis: Ineffective family coping, compromised, related to struggle for power and control.
Goal: Family system will decrease need for physical symptoms.

Intervention	*Rationale*	*Expected Outcome*
Help family identify how illness maintains family system	The family's perspective will prevent the ill person from being identified as the "sick" family member	Verbalizes understanding of family dynamics
Discuss ways that power can be distributed without using physical symptoms	A more democratic family process will decrease need for illness as an attempt to manipulate others	Verbalizes understanding of relationship between need for power and physical symptoms

Evaluation: Somatoform Disorders

Since these disorders are usually chronic, nurses need to look for small gains in the client's functioning. Through a caring relationship, the client may be able to formulate requests of others more assertively, broaden social contacts, manage conflict more directly, and decrease obsessions with bodily functions. Maintaining the client within one health care system and thus providing continuity of care is a successful outcome of nursing interventions.

Eating Disorders

Anorexia nervosa and **bulimia nervosa** are not single diseases but syndromes with multiple predisposing factors and a variety of characteristics. The most obvious symptom is the eating problem, which is in response to anxiety about self-worth, competency, rejection, and family dynamics. In an effort to limit awareness of the source of the discomfort, anxiety is transformed into an obsession with food and weight.

Restricting anorexics, those with anorexia nervosa, lose weight by a dramatic decrease in food intake, along with a sharp rise in the amount of physical exercise. Some people remain with this pattern throughout the course of the disorder, whereas others move to a bulimarexic pattern. **Bulimarexics**, a descriptive term for those with bulimia nervosa, alternate between periods of excessive and minimal food intake. Those who begin with the bulimarexic pattern most often maintain the pattern. The severity of the disorder is determined by the frequency of the eating binges (Orleans and Barnett, 1984).

The bulimarexic pattern must be distinguished from binge eating in the obese population. The obese tend to follow one of two patterns, neither of which includes purging the body after excessive food intake. The first pattern is overeating in response to losing control over a weight-loss diet. Although these people lose weight in weight-control programs, they regain it after going off the diet. The second pattern is seen in those who overeat because they delight in the taste of food. Because they seldom attempt to diet, there is no sense of loss of control. They are more accepting of their body size and understand it as the result of their enjoyment of food (Gormally, 1984).

To determine the incidence of anorexia nervosa and bulimarexia is difficult because of the variety of definitions that exist. Certainly, the frequency of these disorders has been increasing, but this may be partly due to increased reporting. Estimates are that the eating disorders affect 8 to 20 percent of the population, with 90 to 95 percent of victims being female. The disorders usually develop during adolescence—13 to 17 years of age for restricting anorexics and 17 to 23 years of age for bulimarexics. In the past, these disorders were concentrated in the upper social classes. Today, demographics show a more equal distribution across class lines. It is believed that values relating to body weight, self-control, and achievement in life have become more widespread, contributing to the increased incidence of eating disorders in all social classes. Family size and birth order are not significant factors in the development of eating disorders, nor is the stability of the parent's marriage relationship (Coburn and Ganong, 1989; Dippel and Becknal, 1987).

Nurses encounter clients with eating disorders in a number of clinical settings. In schools, camps, community health settings, pediatric units, medical-surgical units, and intensive care units, nurses need to be alert to the characteristics of the eating disorders so that prompt attention can be given to young people suffering from them. With a mortality rate as high as 22 percent, it is extremely dangerous to overlook eating disorders (Torem, 1986).

Knowledge Base: Obesity

Obesity is the most common form of malnourishment in the United States. It is estimated that one out of five Americans is overweight and that 10 percent of the population is more than 35 percent above the ideal body weight. Since the mental health of obese persons is comparable to that of the general population, obesity is not considered a mental disorder. The only similarity of obesity with the eating disorders of anorexia and bulimia is dissatisfaction with body size and shape (Polivy, 1988). For that reason, a brief overview is presented here, and readers are encouraged to utilize other resources for a more comprehensive description.

Obesity is thought to result from a variety of combinations of physiologic and psychosocial factors. There is no universal cause and therefore no single treatment approach. There are many ways of becoming and staying obese.

A variety of psychosocial factors may contribute to the development and maintenance of obesity. Eating habits are primarily learned patterns of behavior that respond to both hunger (a physiologic sensation) and appetite (social and psychologic cues). Some individuals manage negative feelings —such as anxiety, anger, or loneliness—by overeating. Others may view eating as a reward for themselves. These patterns may have been learned in childhood if parents utilized food as a way to decrease stress or reward good behavior. Because social events are frequently associated with food, some people make a connection between pleasure and eating—a connection that may predispose them to overeating. Not to be underestimated are the social consequences of obesity, for there is a high level of prejudice against obese individuals in America (Balfour, 1988).

Many researchers believe physiologic factors are more significant than psychosocial factors. In 11 percent of the obese population, there appears to be a genetic component, the exact mechanism of which is unknown at this time. It may be a regulatory system malfunction, which causes excessive lipogenesis and an accumulation of adipose tissue. In both obese and nonobese people, the amount of body fat seems to be precisely regulated and maintained. This explains the difficulty most individuals have in changing the amount of their body fat. One explanation of obesity is an elevated weight set point, or the weight that the body tries to maintain. A related theory involves energy balance, with obesity resulting from more energy intake than energy expenditure. There is frequently no clear difference between the amount of food eaten by obese people and that eaten by their nonobese counterparts. Thus the defect seems to be in energy needs and expenditures. There are great individual differences in these areas, and individuals may be predisposed to obesity because of low energy needs or low energy expenditure through metabolic processes (Bennett, 1987; Woods, 1988).

Individuals who are 30 percent or more above ideal body weight are at high risk for developing a number of medical conditions. These include diabetes mellitus, hypertension, cardiovascular disease, hyperlipidemia, gallbladder disease, arthritis, and complications of pregnancy. The effects of mortality are more significant for women than men and more significant for the young than the old (Bennett, 1987).

A wide variety of treatment approaches have been tried. In all the approaches, there is a general tendency of individuals to regain lost weight. At this point prevention of obesity is more effective than treatment programs. Interventions include supervised fasting; dieting; anorectic drugs; weight-reduction groups; exercise groups; jaw wiring; and, for the extremely obese, bowel bypass surgery. Whatever intervention is selected, it is helpful to have family or friends involved in the program, since they may be either allies or adversaries for the individual trying to lose weight.

Knowledge Base: Anorexia and Bulimia

Behavioral Characteristics

Restricting Anorexics For many who become restricting anorexics, an event triggers the syndrome of anorexia. These people tend to be vulnerable to rejection and blame themselves for perceived rejections from male peers. Dieting may begin in an attempt to become more attractive and win boyfriends (Boskind-Lodahl, 1985). Other precipitating events may be separations—such as going away to camp or school, parental divorce, or a death—academic problems, or physical illness (Garfinkel and Garner, 1982).

Anorexic young women have a desperate need to please others, and their feelings of self-worth are dependent on the response from others rather than on their own self-approval. Thus, their behavior is often overcompliant; they always try to meet the expectations of others in an effort to be accepted. They may overachieve in academic and extracurricular activities, but this is usually an attempt to please parents rather than a source of self-satisfaction.

To control themselves and their environment, they develop rigid rules and moralistic guidelines about all aspects of life. The ability to make decisions is hampered by their need to make absolutely correct decisions. Often, this rigidity develops into obsessive rituals, particularly concerning eating and exercise. Cutting all food into a predetermined number or size of pieces, chewing all food a certain number of times, allowing only certain combinations of food in a meal, accomplishing a fixed number of exercise routines, or having an inflexible pattern of exercises are rituals common to restricting anorexics. These rules and rituals help keep anxiety beyond conscious awareness; if the rituals are disrupted, the anxiety becomes intolerable. Paradoxically, all these efforts to stay in control lead to out-of-control behaviors (Landau, 1983; Lilly and Sanders, 1987).

Hopeless, helpless, and ineffective is how anorexics often feel. Because they have been overcompliant and nonassertive with their parents, they believe they have always been controlled by others. Their refusal to eat may be an attempt to assert themselves and gain some power and control in the family system (Burch and Pearson, 1986).

To observe phobias in people with restricting anorexia is not uncommon. Initially the phobia is of weight gain, but this develops into a secondary food phobia. The mechanism of phobic avoidance in anorexics is different from that in nonanorexics. In nonanorexic people, the phobia has an external stimulus, such as an animal or object, a place or situation. Avoidance prevents the escalation of anxiety, but the person receives no pleasure in the process. In anorexic people, the phobia has an internal stimulus, such as a fear of being fat. With these people, avoidance provides a feeling of control and a sense of pleasure when food is avoided and weight is lost (Agras, 1987).

Delilah, 17, is an excellent student, cheerleader, and student council member. In the past six months her weight has dropped from 120 to 95 pounds. Her pattern is to eat only one small meal a day. Her meal consists of food in a series of 10s—eg, 10 peas, 10 kernels of corn, 10 tiny pieces of meat, 10 sips of milk, etc. She has a rigid exercise routine, which she repeats from 5:00 to 7:30 A.M. and from 7:00 to 10:00 P.M. She tries to avoid sitting still, since she believes this will cause weight gain.

Bulimarexics Unlike restricting anorexics, people who begin their eating disorder with a bulimarexic pattern are often overweight before the onset of the disorder. A history of weight-control problems is typical. Becoming involved in athletic activities or being teased about their weight may be the precipitating event. Andersen (1988) found that young men who become bulimarexic often do so to make a specific wrestling weight or to improve other athletic performance. Typically they focus on changing specific body parts, and their usual motive is to remove flab and increase muscle size. Bulimarexics often learn this maladaptive pattern of weight control from peers who have used purging as a method to lose weight. This sort of bulimia may go undetected for years, since frequently there is no significant weight loss. For males and females the behavior rapidly becomes compulsive, and the frequency and severity of the eating disorder tends to increase.

There is a cyclic behavioral pattern in bulimarexia. It begins with skipping meals sporadically and overstrict dieting or fasting. In an effort to refrain from eating, the bulimarexic may use amphetamines, which can lead to extreme hunger, fatigue, and low blood glucose levels. The next part of the cycle is a period of binge eating, where the person ingests huge amounts of food (about 3500 calories) within a short time (about one hour). Some binges have lasted eight hours, with consumption of 12,000 calories. Bingeing usually occurs when the person is alone and at home and is most frequent during the evening. The cycle may occur once or twice a month for some and as often as five or ten times a day for others. The binge part of the cycle may be triggered by the ingestion of certain foods, but this is not consistent for all bulimarexics. Although eating binges may involve any kind of food, they most frequently are limited to junk foods, "fast" foods, and high-caloric foods.

The final part of the cycle involves purging the body of the ingested food. After the excessive eating, these people force themselves to vomit. Often, they abuse laxatives and diuretics in an attempt to purge their bodies from the effects of ingested food. Some bulimarexics have used as many as 50 to 100 laxatives per day. In rare cases, they may resort to syrup of ipecac to induce vomiting. After the purging, the cycle begins all over again, with a return to strict dieting or fasting.

Bulimarexics may engage in sporadic excessive exercise, but they usually do not develop compulsive exercise routines. They are more likely to abuse street drugs to decrease their appetite and alcohol to decrease their anxiety. Since their food binges are often expensive, costing as much as $100 per day, they may resort to stealing food or money to buy the food (Dippel and Becknal, 1987). The bingeing-purging pattern can become so consuming that activities and relationships are disrupted. To keep the secret, the individual often resorts to excuses and lies.

Caroline, 23 years old, is a senior nursing student whose bulimarexia has been carefully hidden from family, friends, and teachers for the past three years. During a typical day after school she stops at the local grocery store to buy two pounds of cookies, which she consumes on the way to the ice cream store. There she buys a gallon of ice cream. She eats that quickly and continues on to a fast-food restaurant, where she has three cheeseburgers, fries, and two milkshakes. Before she goes home, she stops at the drugstore, buys a pack of gum, and steals a box of laxatives so the clerks won't suspect she has an eating disorder. As soon as Caroline arrives home, she forces herself to vomit and then takes the entire package of laxatives. This cycles repeats itself at home during the evening, when she eats any available food.

Affective Characteristics

Restricting Anorexics People with anorexia are often beset by fears. Some fear maturing and assuming responsibilities. Others, because of their need to please others with high achievement levels, fear they are not doing well enough. Almost all have an extreme fear of weight gain and fat. If weight gain (whether real or imagined) occurs, anxiety surfaces to the conscious level and is perceived as a threat to the entire being. Anorexics also fear loss of control. Generally, this is related to loss of control over eating, but it may extend to other physiologic processes such as sleeping, urination, or bowel functioning. The steady loss of weight becomes symbolic of mastery of self and environment. However, if anorexic people lose control and eat more than they believe appropriate, they experience severe guilt (Garfinkel and Garner, 1982).

Bulimarexics Many female bulimarexics exhibit stereotypic gender role characteristics. Their desire to remain dependent on others and to seek approval from friends and family often conflicts with their outstanding professional achievement, which may be viewed as unfeminine behavior. This internal conflict between dependency and independence increases their level of anxiety and may result in an eating disorder. Another possible explanation for the disorder is that women who have succeeded in traditionally male professions greatly feel the strain of their success. In a culture that equates femininity and success with thinness, there may be a great deal of pressure to maintain a low weight level (Orleans and Barnett, 1984).

Because of their need for acceptance and approval, bulimarexics repress feelings of frustration and anger with others. The repression of feelings and avoidance of conflict protect them from their vulnerability to rejection. As the ability to identify feelings decreases, they often confuse negative emotions with sensations of being hungry. Food then becomes a source of comfort and a way to defend against anger and frustration (Loro, 1984).

Like restricting anorexics, bulimarexics experience multiple fears. They fear loss of control, not only over their eating but also over their emotions. They are extremely fearful of weight gain and, with real or perceived changes in their weight, they feel panic. Motivating much of their behavior is fear of rejection (Loro, 1984).

The cycle of the binge-purge syndrome can be understood from the affective perspective as well as the behavioral perspective. Anxiety increases to a high level, whereupon the person engages in binge eating to decrease anxiety. After the period of eating, the person experiences guilt and self-disgust because of the loss of control. The guilt and disgust increase anxiety, and purging, through vomiting and other methods, is then used to decrease this anxiety. Since this is an indirect and ineffective method of anxiety management, the levels rebuild and the cycle starts anew (Dippel and Becknal, 1987).

Cognitive Characteristics

Restricting Anorexics The desire to be thin and the behavioral control over eating are ego-syntonic in the restricting anorexic client. **Ego-syntonic behavior** is behavior in agreement with one's thoughts, desires, and values. Restricting anorexics regard their obsessions with food and eating as conventional behavior. The major defense mechanisms used to define the behavior in an ego-syntonic manner are denial of sensations of hunger, denial of physical exhaustion, and denial of any disorder or illness.

People with restricting anorexia experience distortions in the thinking process that are similar to those experienced by sufferers of other anxiety disorders. These distortions involve food, body image, loss of control, and achievement. One type of distortion is *selective abstraction,* which involves focusing on certain information while ignoring contradictory information. Another distortion is *overgeneralization,* where the person takes information or an impression from one event and attaches it to a wide variety of situations. Restricting anorexics also have a tendency toward *magnification,* where they attribute a high level of importance to unpleasant occurrences. Through *personalization,* or ideas of reference, they believe what occurs in the environment is related to them, even when no obvious relationship exists. There is also a tendency for *superstitious thinking* in people with restricting anorexia. The thinking process is further distorted by *dichotomous thoughts,* an all-or-none type of reasoning that interferes with people's realistic perceptions of themselves. Dichotomous thinking involves opposite and mutually exclusive categories such as eating or not eating, all good or all bad, or sexually celibate or promiscuous. (See Table 9–2 for examples of distortions in the thinking process.)

People suffering from restricting anorexia also experience a severely distorted body image that often reaches delusional proportions. Unable to

Table 9–2 *Examples of Distortions in the Thinking Process*

Selective abstraction
"I'm still too fat—look at how big my hands and feet are."

Overgeneralization
"You don't see fat people on television. Therefore you have to be thin to be successful at anything in life."

Magnification
"If I gain 2 pounds, I know everyone will notice it."

Personalization
"Jim and Bob were talking and laughing together today. I'm sure they were talking about how fat I am."

Superstitious thinking
"If I gain weight, I will never be successful in life."
"If I gain weight, that means I can't control myself and I am a bad person."

Dichotomous thinking
"If I gain even 1 pound, that means I am totally out of control and I might as well gain 50 pounds."
"If I eat one thing, I will just keep eating until I weigh 300 pounds."
"If I'm not thin, I'm fat."

see that their bodies are emaciated, they continue to perceive themselves as fat. Some perceive their total body as obese, whereas others focus on a particular part of the body—such as their hips, stomach, thighs, or face—as being obese. While others see these people as starving and disappearing, they view themselves as strong and in the process of creating a new person. Restricting anorexics believe they are in charge of their lives and in complete control.

They think of food not as a necessity for survival but as something dangerous to survival. Cognitively, fat represents need and loss of control; thinness represents strength and control. Frequently these individuals are secretive about their behavior. The secrecy is not viewed as manipulative but rather protective. From their point of view, anorexia is the solution, not the problem (Orbach, 1985).

Restricting anorexics experience distortion in their perception of internal physical sensations, a distortion referred to as alexithymia. Hunger is not recognized as hunger. When they eat a small amount of food, they often complain of feeling overfull or glutted. There is also a decreased internal perception of fatigue, so these people often push their bodies to physical extremes. Even after long and strenuous exercise, they seem unaware of sensations of fatigue.

Young restricting anorexics are overconcerned with how others view them. Many of them are convinced that other people have more insight into who they are than they themselves do. This self-depreciation and fear of self-definition contribute to fears and beliefs of being controlled by others. Feeling they have no power in their interpersonal relationships, restricting anorexics attempt to please and placate significant others whom they perceive as more powerful (Garfinkel and Garner, 1982).

People with restricting anorexia develop perfectionistic standards for their behavior. They are in such dread of losing control that they impose extremes of discipline on themselves. During the times they are able to maintain control, their perfectionistic behavior and dichotomous thinking lead them to believe they are better than other people. However, these standards of behavior become self-defeating when the anorexic fails consistently to achieve them (Landau, 1983).

> *Mindy, 18, has been diagnosed with restricting anorexia. She does not believe that her 5′ 9″ frame is underweight at 102 pounds. Mindy believes she will look better when she reaches 85 pounds. She says that, when she goes to college, she wants to be active in student government and that fat people are never elected. Her superstitious thinking relates to white clothing, which she feels decreases her hunger.*

Bulimarexics In contrast to restricting anorexics, bulimarexics are troubled by their behavioral characteristics. They experience **ego-dystonic behavior**, that is, behavior that does not conform with the person's thoughts, wishes, and values. Another facet of ego-dystonic symptoms is that one feels the symptoms are beyond personal control. The bulimarexic client feels compelled to binge, purge, and diet; helpless to stop the behavior; and full of self-disgust for continuing the pattern (Andersen, 1987).

Bulimarexic people have usually obtained a significant amount of incorrect nutrition information. Many of them believe that certain foods turn instantly to fat and that other foods contribute nothing to body weight. Some of them believe there is a difference between one calorie and another; that is, they consider 200 calories of ice cream quite different from 200 calories of meat. Many of these people develop excessively rigid guidelines for the dieting phase of the cyclic behavior and have difficulty understanding the need for a balanced diet (Agras, 1987).

Although bulimarexics are not pleased with their body shape and size, they usually do not experience the delusional distortion found in restricting anorexics. There is a direct correlation between the frequency and severity of the disorder and the degree of distortion of body size. Many of them were overweight before the disorder, so there is an obsessional concern about not regaining the lost weight. For them to think of anything other than food, however, is difficult. Since they eat in response to hunger, appetite, and thoughts of food, the obsessions also involve getting rid of the food ingested in an effort to counteract the caloric effects of binge eating (Garfinkel and Garner, 1984).

People with bulimarexia also have a dichotomous thinking process. They have a tendency to relate their problems to weight or overeating. Their fantasy is that if they could only be thin and not overeat, all other problems would be solved. Another example of this all-or-none thinking is the belief that one bite will automatically lead to binge eating. The client may say "As long as I have eaten one cookie, I have failed, so I might as well eat the entire package" (Orleans and Barnett, 1984).

Bulimarexics are also perfectionistic in their personal standards of behavior. Even with their high level of professional achievement, they are extremely self-critical and often feel incompetent and inadequate. They set unrealistic standards of diet control and feel like failures when unable to maintain them. The thought of being a failure is a contributing factor to the binge phase of the cycle. Following the purging phase, they make promises to themselves to be more steadfast and disciplined with their diet. Since these resolutions are unrealistic, they set themselves up for another failure (Loro, 1984; Orleans and Barnett, 1984).

Physiologic Characteristics

There are many physiologic effects of starvation and purging of the body. Vomiting and the abuse of diuretics and laxatives lead to a loss of potassium and hydrochloric acid, which can result in hypokalemic or hypochloremic alkalosis. The kidneys attempt to conserve potassium by increasing sodium loss, which creates a further imbalance. The cardiovascular system demonstrates a decreased blood volume, with a resultant decrease in blood pressure and postural hypotension. The heart rate is slowed, and severe cardiac arrhythmias may develop in response to hypokalemia. Bone marrow hypoplasia results in a mild anemia. Bradypnea is seen in the respiratory system, as is a decrease in oxygen uptake related to anemia. If the person is drinking large amounts of water to decrease hunger, water intoxication may lead to a depletion of sodium. The electrolyte imbalance may cause muscle weakness, convulsions, arrhythmias, and even death (Dippel and Becknal, 1987; Yates and Sieleni, 1987; Zucker, 1989).

People with eating disorders may have elevated blood urea nitrogen. If the protein intake is within normal limits, the elevated blood urea nitrogen is indicative of dehydration with a decreased blood flow to the kidneys, which results in a decreased glomerular filtration rate. This alteration in kidney function makes these individuals prone to edema. In extremely undernourished clients, the presence of ketones in the urine indicates that fat stores are still being mobilized. If there are no ketones in the urine, these clients have exhausted their fat stores and may be approaching death (Garfinkel and Garner, 1982; Spack, 1985).

Gastrointestinal complications may develop as the result of an eating disorder. Constipation is an early sign of a decreased food and fluid intake. The person may abuse laxatives, not only to purge the body but also to relieve the constipation. Laxative abuse can lead to dependency and a cathartic colon. Many of these people complain of feeling bloated much of the time. This is a result of the sharply reduced intake with the decrease in gastric contractibility. Frequent vomiting can lead to esophagitis with scarring and stricture. If perforation or rupture of the esophagus occurs, there is a 20 percent mortality rate even with immediate treatment. Gastric rupture, fortunately a fairly rare occurrence, carries a mortality rate of 85 percent (Spack, 1985; Zucker, 1989).

Amenorrhea is an extremely common occurrence in females with eating disorders. In approximately 6 percent of the cases, the amenorrhea is primary. In about 80 percent of the cases, the amenorrhea precedes the weight loss, and in the remainder the amenorrhea begins shortly after the weight loss begins. Although the exact mechanism is unclear, the amenorrhea is thought to be related to the degree of stress the person is experiencing, the percentage of body fat lost, and the altered hypothalamic function (Spack, 1985).

There is abnormal hypothalamic function in people with eating disorders. At this time, the origin is not known, but three explanations are possible: (1) the state of severe malnutrition itself may alter hypothalamic function, (2) the abnormalities may be a result of emotional stress, or (3) the abnormal hypothalamic function is the primary disorder, with the emotional response being the secondary disorder.

Normal menstrual cycles are correlated with an intact hypothalamic-pituitary-gonadal axis. There is a relationship between the amount of weight lost and the response of the luteinizing hormone (LH) to luteinizing hormone releasing hormone (LHRH). The more severe the weight loss, the more diminished is the LH response to LHRH. The follicle stimulating hormone (FSH) response to LHRH may be slightly reduced. In response to these changes, the level of estrogen is reduced.

The hypothalamus is very sensitive to nutrition status. Elevations in the level of growth hormone and corticotropin are related to starvation and are found whenever there is a marked decrease in food intake. There is a decrease in the serum triiodothyronine (T_3), which is related to the lack of calories as well as a decrease in carbohydrates in the diet. Low T_3 levels are indicative of starvation and evidence of the body's attempt to reduce metabolic rate and thus conserve calories. Vomiting is a strong stimulus to the production of arginine vasopressin (AVP), which is related to one's ability to conserve water. There is a decreased production of antidiuretic hormone (ADH) so that people with eating disorders are unable to concentrate urine to the normal degree. Serum calcium typically remains at normal levels unless the individual is abusing laxatives. As more calcium is drawn from the bones (osteoporosis), fractures occur easily. Neurologically, there is an increased incidence of seizures secondary to hypocalcemia and hyponatremia (Zucker, 1989).

Restricting anorexics usually experience a weight loss of 25 percent, but a loss as high as 50 percent is possible. Bulimarexics do not reach the low levels of weight typical of anorexics and may, in fact, remain at a normal weight level. Since a large food intake speeds up the gastric emptying rate, a significant number of calories are absorbed before the purging begins. If severe weight loss does occur, these people have difficulty regulating body temperature in response to both heat and cold in the environment (Zucker, 1989).

Hair breakage and loss, brittle nails, and the appearance of lanugo on the body are observed in response to the state of malnutrition. Hands and feet may appear cold and blue-tinged. If the person is dehydrated, either from lack of fluid intake or from purging, the skin will be dry and there will be poor skin turgor. If the person is taking in large amounts of water to combat hunger, there may be evidence of edema.

Frequent vomiting affects the person's oral cavity. The acid gastric contents decrease the tooth enamel, which causes an increase in caries and a loss of teeth. There may be a chronic sore throat and, at times, an irritated esophagus from the vomiting. The salivary glands are usually swollen and tender. Some bulimarexics may demonstrate Russell's sign, which is the presence of a callous on the back of the hand. The callous is formed by repeated trauma from the teeth when forcing vomiting (Spack, 1985; Yates and Sieleni, 1987).

The physiologic effects of malnutrition and vomiting are widespread throughout the body's systems. In some cases, death occurs as a result of these disruptions.

Sociocultural Characteristics

In American society, female attractiveness is strongly equated with thinness. Models, actresses, and the media glamorize extreme thinness, which is then equated with success and happiness. In studies of high school students, Garfinkel and Garner (1982) found that between 70 and 80 percent of the girls did not like their bodies and wanted to lose weight, whereas only 20 percent of the high school boys wanted to lose weight. In a survey of 33,000 women it was found that 80 percent believed they had to be thin to be attractive to men. Although only 25 percent were overweight, 41 percent were unhappy with their bodies (Boskind-White, 1985). Additionally, magazines marketed for adolescent women often present diet and weight control as the solution for adolescent crises. Thus the body becomes the central focus of existence, and self-esteem is de-

Table 9–3 *Characteristics of Clients with Eating Disorders*

Characteristic	*Restricting Anorexics*	*Bulimarexics*
Self-evaluation	Are dependent on response from others; are self-deprecatory	Are self-critical; view themselves as incompetent
Decision making	Need to make perfect decisions	Need to make perfect decisions
Rituals	Are obsessive in eating and exercise	Perpetuate cycle of fasting, binging, purging
Sense of control	Create sense of control and achievement by refusing to eat	Set unrealistic standards for own behavior; feel out of control
Phobia	Initially fear weight gain; develop food phobia	None specific
Exercise	Have obsessive routines	Exercise sporadically
Fears	Fear not being perfect, weight gain, fat, loss of control	Fear loss of control, weight gain, rejection
Guilt	Experience guilt when they eat more than they believe appropriate	Experience guilt when they binge and purge
Defense mechanisms	Deny hunger, exhaustion, disease	Do not deny hunger
Insight into illness	Are ego-syntonic—they do not believe they have a disorder; they see anorexia as the solution, not the problem	Are ego-dystonic—they are disgusted with self but helpless to change
Distorted thinking	Practice selective abstraction, overgeneralization, magnification, personalization, dichotomous thinking	Practice dichotomous thinking
Body image	Experience delusional distortion	See themselves as slightly larger
Relationships	Attempt to please and placate others	Experience conflicts between dependency and independence
Social isolation	Tend to isolate themselves to protect against rejection; they tend to be more introverted	Need privacy for binging and purging; they tend to be extroverted
Weight loss	Experience 25–50% weight loss	Maintain normal weight or experience slight weight loss
Death	Results usually from starvation, when body proteins are depleted to one-half normal levels	Often results from hypokalemia (leading cause) and suicide (second most frequent cause)

pendent on the ability to control weight and food intake.

The traditional view of the eating disorders has been that of young women who reject the feminine stereotype and do not wish to mature sexually and thus strive to maintain a preadolescent body shape. A newer perspective suggests these people actually have an exaggerated acceptance of the feminine stereotype, the basis of which is that women define their value and worth in terms of being attractive to and obtaining love from men. Women are encouraged to be dependent on men for confirmation of worth and discouraged from independence and self-reliance. Thus, with a shaky identity and no sense of personal power, some young women are extremely vulnerable to the cultural standards of beauty. The highest priority is then given to controlling one's body shape in an effort to be acceptable and pleasing to others (Boskind-Lodahl, 1985).

Eating disorders may also be an indirect way of achieving power and control in life. The double bind of the subordinate position is that women are expected to be passive and nonassertive while at the same time meeting everyone else's needs. Since no one but the woman can control eating or purging behavior, these disorders help to create an illusion of power (Schwartz and Barrett, 1987).

The exact role of the family system in the development of the eating disorders is not clear at this time. Because the majority of families have not been studied until after the disorder has become serious enough to attract attention and intervention, it is difficult to determine which family factors are predisposing to the disorders and which are a result of a family member's being anorexic. Often, the family struggles with the issues of dependency and hostility, and a variety of systems develop to manage these interpersonal issues (Garfinkel and Garner, 1982).

Some families of restricting anorexics are enmeshed, that is, the boundaries between the members are weak, interactions are intense, dependency on one another is high, and autonomy is minimal. Everybody is involved in each member's concerns; within the family, there is a great deal of togetherness and scant privacy. The enmeshed family system becomes overprotective of the children, which may result in an intense focus on the bodily functions of these children. In contrast, current research indicates that families of bulimarexics are less enmeshed than those of anorexics. Family members tend to be isolated from one another, and eating behavior may be an attempt to decrease feelings of loneliness and boredom (Coburn and Ganong, 1989; Stierlin and Weber, 1989).

Many families of those with eating disorders have difficulty with conflict resolution. An ethical or religious value against disagreements within the family supports the avoidance of conflict. When problems are denied for the sake of family harmony, they cannot be resolved, and growth of the family system is inhibited. The anorexic child often protects and maintains the family unit. In some family systems, the parents avoid conflict with each other by uniting in a common concern for the child's welfare. In other family systems, the issues of marital conflict are converted into disagreements over how the anorexic child should be managed. In both types of systems, the marital problems are camouflaged in an effort to prevent the disruption of the family unit (Schwartz and Barrett, 1987).

Many families of clients with eating disorders are achievement- and performance-oriented, with high ambitions for success of all members. In these families, body shape is related to success, and priorities are established for physical appearance and fitness. The family's focus on professional achievement as well as on food, diets, exercise, and weight control may be obsessional (Root, Fallon, and Friedrich, 1986).

Young women with restricting anorexia usually find that severe dieting does not produce the reward of being sought after by young men. In response to this real or perceived rejection, they feel even more unattractive and undesirable. To protect themselves, they begin to lose interest in social activities and to withdraw from their peers. Dating is minimal or nonexistent, and they purport to have no interest in sexual activities. High scholastic achievement may be an attempt to compensate for the lack of peer relationships (Boskind-Lodahl, 1985).

People with bulimarexia experience shame and guilt about their behavior and may withdraw socially to prevent exposure of their pattern of behavior. They also need privacy for binging and purging, which contributes further to their isolation. The more isolated they become, the more the behavior tends to escalate as food is used to fill in the void and provide a source of comfort. Generally, these people do not become as socially isolated as those with restricting anorexia. Although they are sexually active, they have difficulty enjoying sex because of fears relating to loss of control. They feel inadequate and incompetent and fear the intimacy of a long-term relationship (Boskind-Lodahl, 1985; Garfinkel and Garner, 1984; Loro, 1984).

Causative Theories

The causes of restricting anorexia and bulimarexia are multiple, both within the individual client and in the comparison of a variety of clients. Having a knowledge base about the major theories allows the nurse to understand the individual client from a composite perspective, which is necessary for the individuation of the nursing process.

The *psychodynamic theory* believes the mother is so dominant that the young girl is unable to develop autonomy. This leads to unconscious hostility toward the mother and a rejection of the mother's femininity and sexuality. Maintaining a preadolescent body shape is a passive-aggressive rebellion against the mother's control. Autonomy is sought through control over one's own body. Some theorists believe weight gain is symbolic of pregnancy, and anorexia is a defense against fantasies of maturing sexually and becoming pregnant. Other theorists think that anxiety from any source is transformed into obsessions about food and body. The obsessive-compulsive behavior of an eating disorder is then a defense against the conscious experience of anxiety (Boskind-Lodahl, 1985).

Motivation for losing weight is viewed in terms of how the victim sees herself relating to others. For some the motivation is an attempt to create closeness by gaining attention from parents, siblings, and friends. The motivation for others is to create distance by avoiding identification with a disliked parent. The third possible motivation is a movement against people by using eating behavior as a way to express anger and control parents' behavior (Andersen, 1988).

The *behavioral model* of the eating disorders looks at what the behavior accomplishes rather than at why the behavior occurs. These disorders are considered eating phobias. In this context, anxiety rises with eating and decreases when fasting or purging. Anxiety reduction is the reinforcer for both restricting anorexics and bulimarexics (Minchin, 1978).

The *feminist perspective* views eating disorders as arising out of conflict between female development and traditional developmental theories. Western culture has viewed male development as the norm, with independence being the opposite of dependence. For women, the opposite of dependence is isolation. Conflict arises, then, when women believe they must become autonomous and minimize relationships to be recognized as mature adults. For some, this conflict is acted out in self-destructive eating behavior (Steiner-Adair, 1989).

Cultural stereotypes contribute to women's preoccupation with their bodies. Women are judged as being attractive by how closely they approach the cultural ideal of thinness. Thus identity and self-esteem are dependent on physical appearance. To be disgusted with one's own flesh and fat means having an adversarial relationship with one's own body—a relationship that often results in eating disorders (Worman, 1989).

There are a number of *biologic theories* relating to the eating disorders. Current research is focusing on the relationship between these disorders and the affective disorders. Among the eating-disordered there is a significantly higher rate of depression than in the general population. Studies indicate that anywhere from 20 to 70 percent of those with eating disorders are depressed, with a higher rate in bulimarexics than in restricting anorexics. At this time the exact relationship between the disorders is unclear. There may be some common underlying abnormality; eating disorders may be atypical manifestations of depression, or depression may be secondary to eating disorders. Clients with bulimarexia demonstrate sleep abnormalities similar to those of depressed clients. Both experience a shorter time before REM sleep begins, an increased REM density, and a reduction in slow-wave sleep (Kennedy and Walsh, 1987).

There appears to be similar hypothalamic-pituitary-adrenal axis abnormalities in persons with eating disorders, those with depression, and those with alcoholism. These individuals often demonstrate hypercortisolism as evidenced in a positive dexamethasone suppression test. (See Chapter 11 for an explanation of this test.) Bulimarexic and depressed clients are also more likely to have a positive response in a thyrotropin-releasing hormone stimulation test (Pope, 1986).

There may also be a defect in the feedback control mechanism for certain neurotransmitters such as norepinephrin and serotonin. It is unclear if the neurochemical changes predispose a person to an eating disorder of if self-imposed starvation leads to neurochemical changes. Carbohydrates are involved in the synthesis of serotonin by increasing tryptophan (TRP), which is the precursor to serotonin. Low levels of serotonin may lead to an adaptive need to increase carbohydrate intake; most frequently, bulimarexics binge on high-carbohydrate foods. It is known that serotonin in the hypothalamus acts to suppress eating behavior and therefore that low levels increase the need and desire to eat (Goldbloom, 1987).

The exact role of genetic factors in the development of eating disorders is unknown at this time. There is a 55 percent concordance for monozygotic twins and only a 7 percent concordance for dizygotic twins. Additionally, 43 percent of bulimarexics and 27 percent of restricting anorexics have first-degree relatives (parents, siblings, or children) with alcoholism or an affective disorder (Agras, 1987; Dippel and Becknal, 1987).

Medical Treatment: Anorexia and Bulimia

A number of medications are being tested by clients with eating disorders. So far they seem to be more effective in treating bulimarexia than in treating restricting anorexia. The tricyclic antidepressant imipramine (Tofranil) produces a 70 percent decrease in the frequency of binge eating, a lessening of preoccupation with food, as well as a lessening of anxiety and depressive symptoms. Another tricyclic antidepressant, desipramine (Norpramine), appears to decrease binging in those individuals who do not have current symptoms of depression. Fluoxetine (Prozac) shows promising success in the treatment of eating disorders. Tricyclic antidepressants are started at very low doses (10–25 mg/day) and, over a period of three to four weeks, are increased to a level of 3 mg per kilo of body weight. Typically the medication is continued until six months following the disappearance of symptoms. In some studies lithium has been used alone or in conjunction with tricyclic antidepressants. The results have been positive. Caution must be taken when prescribing lithium for a client who is purging, however. Vomiting will decrease intracellular potassium, and lithium may exacerbate this effect. Similar results have been reported with the use of MAOI, phenelzine (Nardil), and isocarboxazid (Marplan). Medication with MAOI may be dangerous to clients if binging involves foods containing tyramine. The result may be a hypertensive crisis (Herzog and Brotman, 1987; Kennedy and Walsh, 1987; Pope, 1986). (See Chapter 4 for details about medications.)

Assessment: Anorexia and Bulimia

A head-to-toe physical assessment and a focused nursing assessment must be implemented for clients with eating disorders. Table 9–4 provides a guideline for the physical assessment.

Clients with bulimarexia may welcome the opportunity to talk about their disorder with a caring, nonjudgmental nurse. Moreover, discovering the disorder is not unique to them may relieve some of their anxiety and distress. Clients with restricting anorexia, on the other hand, may not be as willing to talk about their disorder. Denial of any problems and illness may interfere with obtaining an accurate nursing assessment. A supportive and caring approach is necessary to establish a rapport. Once a relationship has been established, the client may be more willing to share information, particularly if the client is seeking the approval and acceptance of the nurse.

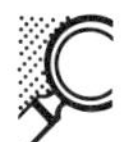

FOCUSED NURSING ASSESSMENT *for the Client with Eating Disorders*

Behavioral assessment

When you were younger, would you describe yourself as an obedient or a rebellious child?

How important is it to you to try and please your parents?

How are your grades in school?

What kinds of extracurricular activities are you involved in?
What kinds of rules do you use to make decisions?
What other kinds of rules do you establish for yourself about how you behave and interact with others?
With whom do you usually eat?
Under what circumstances do you prefer to eat alone?
What type of eating patterns do you have?
Do you have rules for eating? For choosing the place to eat? For the types of foods that can or cannot be combined? For the frequency of eating? Do you cut your food into a certain number of pieces or sizes? Do you chew each bite a certain number of times?
Do you skip meals?
Describe failures you have experienced on diets.
When you break a diet, do you eat a large amount of food?
What time of day do you usually binge?
Where do you usually binge?
How often do you feel compelled to binge?
How long does a binge last?
Are there certain foods that trigger the binge?
Describe your favorite foods to eat on a binge.
How do you obtain the food for a binge?
After a binge, do you vomit to rid your body of the food?
Describe how the use of laxatives and/or diuretics helps rid your body of the food.
How did you discover purging as a method of losing weight?
How much time do you spend exercising in a day?
Do you have a set routine of exercises?
What do you believe will happen if you don't exercise?
How much exercise do you have to do before you feel tired?
How does the use of alcohol help you cope?
How do street drugs help you cope with your problems?

Affective assessment

Tell me about the fears you have.
Do you fear gaining weight?
Being fat?
Not achieving in life?
Rejection by others?
Losing control over eating?
Do you have any other fear about losing control?
What kinds of things make you feel guilty?
What behavior makes you feel ashamed?
What kinds of situations create anxiety for you?
What kinds of situations make you feel frustrated?
What kinds of situations make you feel helpless?
How do you manage anxiety?
What are your feelings when you eat more than your diet allows?
How important is it for you to be liked by others?
In what ways do others approve of you?
How important is it for you to be successful in life?

Cognitive assessment

Do you believe your eating pattern is in any way unusual?
Do you have any desire to alter your eating behavior?
Describe your body to me.
What would you like to change about your body?
Describe what an attractive person looks like.
Describe how thinness is related to success in life.
What would your life be like if you were as thin as you wished?
What will happen if you gain weight?
Describe when you experience feelings of hunger.
Describe what makes you feel bloated.
What do you like most about yourself?
What do others like about you?
What standards of behavior have you set for yourself?
How self-disciplined are you?
What kinds of promises do you make to yourself about eating?
Do you believe these are realistic goals?
What types of food make a person gain weight more quickly?
Tell me what you know about the calories in food.
Describe a balanced diet to me.

Sociocultural assessment

Tell me about the friends you have.
How often do you socialize with friends?
How often do you refuse social activities?
How attractive do others find you?
Are you dating?
How is sexual activity for you?
What do you like most about sex?
What do you like least about sex?
How close-knit is your family?
How much do you depend on one another?
How does one achieve privacy within your family?
How well does your family get along with one another?
What are the rules about disagreements?
How are disagreements managed?
Who fights with whom in the family?
On what topics do family members disagree?

Table 9–4 *Physical Assessment of the Client with Eating Disorders*

Physical assessment data	
Age ______ Height ______	Weight ______
Weight prior to disorder ______	Temperature ______
Blood pressure (lying, sitting, standing) ______	
General physical appearance ______	
Apical pulse ______	Arrhythmias? ______
Evidence of anemia?	Condition of hair?
Respirations?	Condition of fingernails and toenails?
Bloated feelings?	Color of skin? Skin turgor?
Abdominal cramping?	Presence of edema?
Constipation?	Sore throat?
Frequency of bowel movements?	Oral hygiene?
Age at menarche?	Dental caries?
Last menstrual period?	Loss of teeth?
Frequency of menstruation?	Swollen salivary glands?
Muscle weakness or cramping?	Russell's sign?
Laboratory data	
Results of hormonal studies?	Ketones in urine?
Results of electrolyte studies?	Blood glucose?
Blood urea nitrogen?	Dexamethasone suppression test?

What would happen to the family if your eating improved?
How important is it for each family member to be successful?
Describe the family's standards for physical appearance.
Describe the family's standards for physical fitness.
How do other family members control their weight?
Who in the family shares mealtime together?
How do family members view mealtime?
Describe the family's eating patterns.

Diagnosis and Planning: Anorexia and Bulimia

Educating the client and family about eating disorders is a primary concern for nurses. The general public has many misconceptions about these disorders, which interfere with effective treatment. Both the family and client need to become aware of the seriousness of the disorders, as they do the potential complications if the disorders are left untreated. Accurate information will assist the family in problem solving together rather than blaming one another for the onset of the disorder.

Showing firmness, patience, and genuine concern is the most effective approach with these clients, who may view the staff as parental figures and fear the nurses are in an alliance with their parents to force them to gain weight. Clients with restricting anorexia usually deny that they have an eating disorder and are resistant to interventions related to their eating behavior. For other problems—such as social isolation, management of conflict, fear of rejection, and fear of losing control—they may accept help. Interventions designed to assist the client in managing these areas of difficulty will contribute to the overall treatment plan (Deering, 1987).

To help the client create an environment in which the eating disorder is unnecessary is the overall goal of treatment. To this end, nurses should assist clients in identifying the purpose the disorder serves in life. There are many possible purposes, and accurate identification will lead to effective interventions. For some, the purpose is the attainment of the ideal body, with thoughts that this will protect them from all future pain. For others, eating disorders are a way of gaining a sense of control as well as individuating and separating from parents. Eating disorders may develop in response to sibling competition for parental attention; for others it is a respose to depressive feelings. Superimposed on the teenage crisis of identity, eating disorders may represent a regression to a younger and safer time in life. To plan nursing interventions that will help these clients meet their needs in constructive and healthy ways, it is vital that the purpose of the disorder be identified (Andersen, 1988).

Treatment of clients with eating disorders must be planned from a multidisciplinary approach. Medical treatment may include a feeding schedule, tube feeding, IVs, parenteral hyperalimentation, appetite stimulants, potassium supplements, and bedrest. (See Table 9–5 for a list of the nursing diagnoses that apply to these clients.) Psychiatric treatment may include family therapy, cognitive therapy, and systematic desensitization. The majority of centers that treat clients with eating disorders use behavior modification along with individual and family therapy. (See Table 9–6 for a list of organizations that provide information about and treatment of the eating disorders.) Behavioral therapy must be individualized to the particular factors that contribute to and sustain the problematic eating behavior. To achieve maximum effectiveness, the individualized plan should be developed and implemented by the multidisciplinary team (Garfinkel and Garner, 1982; Orleans and Barnett, 1984). (See Table 9–7.)

Table 9–5 *Nursing Diagnoses Related to Physical Condition in the Client with Eating Disorders*

Alteration in bowel elimination: constipation, related to chronic laxative abuse and/or decreased food intake
Alteration in cardiac output: decreased, related to decreased blood volume
Alteration in cardiac output: decreased, related to hypokalemia
Fluid volume alteration: excess, related to increased water intake
Fluid volume deficit, actual, related to diuretic or laxative abuse
Fluid volume deficit, actual, related to inability to concentrate urine
Gas exchange, impaired, related to anemia
Alteration in oral mucous membrane related to frequent vomiting

Table 9–6 *Organizations Established for Information and Treatment of the Eating Disorders*

American Anorexia/Bulimia Association, Inc.
133 Cedar La.
Teaneck, NJ 07666
(201) 836–1800

Anorexia Nervosa and Related Eating Disorders, Inc.
P.O. Box 5102
Eugene, OR 97405
(503) 344–1144

Center for the Study of Anorexia and Bulimia
1 West 91st St.
New York, NY 10024
(212) 595–3449

National Anorexic Aid Society, Inc.
P.O. Box 29461
Columbus, OH 43229
(614) 895–2009

National Association of Anorexia Nervosa and Associated Disorders, Inc.
P.O. Box 7
Highland Park, IL 60035
(312) 831–3438

Bulimic Anorexic Self-Help, Inc.
6125 Clayton Ave., Suite 215
St. Louis, MO 63139
(800) 227–4785; (314) 567–4080

Evaluation: Anorexia and Bulimia

Evaluation of the effectiveness of the nursing care plan is based on the expected outcome. Because changes occur slowly, the nursing staff and the client need a lot of patience. If the client is not actively involved in the planning, implementation, and evaluation process, minimal success will be achieved. When only the client is treated, the rate of cure is between 40 and 60 percent. If the entire family is involved in therapy, the rate of cure is as high as 86 percent (Minchin, Rosman, and Baker, 1978). Unfortunately, these data indicate that be-

Table 9–7 Nursing Care Plan for the Client with Eating Disorders

Nursing Diagnosis: Anxiety related to fears of gaining weight and losing control.
Goal: Client will verbalize fewer fears and show decreased anxiety.

Intervention	*Rationale*	*Expected Outcome*
Discuss fears of weight gain and loss of control	Fears must be openly discussed before they can be managed	Discusses fears
Discuss how obsessions with food and weight are used to protect oneself	Obsessions decrease anxiety and contribute to the avoidance of negative feelings and problems	Identifies purpose of obsessions
Weigh only one or two times a week	Decreasing the frequency of weighing client may decrease the weight obsession	Decreases focus on weight
Discuss how repressing feelings protects client from anticipated rejection	Fears of rejection have been transformed into fears of gaining weight	Discusses fear of rejection
Discuss how feelings are confused with sensations of hunger	The binge eater uses food as a source of comfort and as a way to defend against anxiety	Differentiates emotions from hunger
Help client identify and label feelings	Accurate identification of feelings will decrease distortion of emotions and increase client's trust in own internal experiences	Identifies feelings
Help client identify feelings experienced after losing control over rigid diet	It is important to attach the feelings of shame and guilt to the rigid diet standards rather than to personal inadequacy	Relates guilt and shame to rigid standards
Discuss how weight loss is symbolic of self-control and mastery of self and the environment	Insight into symbolic meaning of the behavior will assist client in establishing more adaptive behavior	Identifies need for self-control
Discuss measures other than weight loss to exert control	Active involvement in the problem-solving process will increase client's use of more adaptive behavior	Implements alternative control measures
Model appropriate ways to share feelings with others	Client may not know how to talk about feelings directly	
Help client share feelings directly	Direct sharing of feelings will decrease the obsession with food to manage unexpressed emotions	Shares feelings directly
Teach client alternative methods to manage fears (eg, relaxation techniques, self-hypnosis, assertiveness training)	Healthful techniques to decrease anxiety will decrease need to use food in an unhealthy manner	Implements alternative measures to manage fears

Nursing Diagnosis: Alteration in nutrition: less than body requirements related to reduced intake.
Goal: Client will increase food intake to meet body requirements.

Intervention	*Rationale*	*Expected Outcome*
With client identify target weight. This is usually set at 90% of average weight for client's age and height	Identifying a reasonable target weight will reassure client that staff will not force her to become overweight	Sets appropriate target weight

(Diagnosis continued)

Table 9–7 *(continued)*

Nursing Diagnosis *(continued)*: Alteration in nutrition: less than body requirements related to reduced intake.
Goal: Client will increase food intake to meet body requirements.

Intervention	*Rationale*	*Expected Outcome*
Choose a weight range of 4 to 6 lb rather than a single target weight	Helps clients learn to accept a certain amount of weight fluctuation	Identifies normalcy of weight variation
Use the term *restore weight*	The term *gain weight* is emotionally laden and increases fears	
Weigh client 3 times a week in morning; weigh with back to scale	To prevent sabotage of plan, client is not told his or her weight until in goal range	Gains 3 pounds a week
When weighing client be alert to techniques of artificially increasing weight such as concealing heavy objects in clothing or drinking large amounts of water	Fear of weight gain may precipitate unusual behavior	Will not artificially increase weight
Be alert for secret disposal of food by client	Client may attempt to get rid of, rather than eat, the food	Eats meals
Implement behavior modification plan for eating behavior	Behavior modification is frequently used to ensure client involvement in the treatment process	Behaves according to established plan
Give social rewards for eating (eg, use of the phone, time in the dayroom); increase rewards as weight is gained	Positive changes reinforced	Reponds to rewards
Begin with a diet low in fats and milk products	Starvation leads to insufficiency of the bowel enzymes necessary for digestion of these foods	
Be supportive but firm in regulating eating behavior	Setting limits will decrease client's self-defeating behavior	Abides by set limits

Nursing Diagnosis: Alteration in nutrition: potential for more than body requirements related to binge eating.
Goal: Client will not engage in binge eating.

Intervention	*Rationale*	*Expected Outcome*
Help client differentiate between emotions and sensations of hunger	Misinterpretation of emotions contributes to binge eating	Differentiates emotions from hunger
Help client identify particular foods that trigger binge eating	Identification of trigger foods will help client gain control of binges	Identifies trigger foods
Help client assess situations that precede binging and problem-solve alternative coping behavior	Insight into high-risk situations will help client gain control of binges	Identifies stressful situations; formulates alternative methods to manage stress
Encourage delay in responding to binge by trying alternative behaviors (eg, talking to staff, calling a friend, relaxation techniques)	Delaying response to urge will interrupt cycle of behavior	Implements plan to avoid binging
During urge to binge, provide sour food (eg, lemon, lime, dill pickle)	Sour taste may decrease craving for sweets	Verbalizes less craving

(Diagnosis continued)

Table 9–7 *(continued)*

Intervention	*Rationale*	*Expected Outcome*
Instruct client to keep a log that records eating behavior, time, situation, emotional state, what was eaten, and purging response	Provides details and structure; links mood changes to disturbed eating	Keeps log and shares it with nurse
Help client solve ways to avoid privacy at usual times of binges	Most binging occurs in isolation; being with others will decrease opportunities to binge	Formulates plan to avoid privacy
Help client identify other positive behaviors (eg, avoiding fast-food restaurants, formulating a list of "safe" foods, shopping for food with a friend)	These activities will inhibit the binging behavior	Implements plan to decrease binge eating
Teach client to eat 3 meals a day and include a carbohydrate at each meal	Interrupts fasting part of cycle; carbohydrate deprivation may lead to binging	Eats 3 meals a day

Nursing Diagnosis: Alteration in nutrition: less than body requirements related to purging.
Goal: Client will not use purging activities to lose weight.

Intervention	*Rationale*	*Expected Outcome*
Discuss with client how purging is used to cope with feelings	Insight into purging behavior as a way to decrease anxiety, guilt, and self-disgust will help client manage the dynamics of the behavior	Associates purging with ineffective management of feelings
If client continues to vomit, restrict bathroom use for one to two hours after meals unless accompanied by a staff member	Staff needs to set limits on purging behavior until client is able to establish own limits	Does not vomit after meals
Encourage client to talk to nursing staff when she feels urge to vomit	Talking about feelings will increase client's ability to control impulsive behavior	Talks to staff to decrease urge to vomit
Check belongings for laxatives, diuretics, diet pills on admission and when returning from pass	Compulsive need to purge may result in secretive behavior	Does not use medication to purge

Nursing Diagnosis: Alteration in thought process related to dichotomous thinking, overgeneralization, personalization, obsessions, and superstitious thinking.
Goal: Client will verbalize a logical and realistic thinking process.

Intervention	*Rationale*	*Expected Outcome*
Help client identify that weight loss is symbolic of other problems, which must be identified and solved	Client uses overgeneralization in the belief that all life's problems will be solved if enough weight is lost	Identifies problems that need to be solved
Help client avoid defining the "perfect" body as the solution to all problems	Client believes all problems in life relate to the body	Separates interpersonal problems from physical problems
Discuss topics other than food and weight	Client needs to be redirected from obsessional thought content	Decreases obsessional talk about food

(Diagnosis continued)

Table 9–7 *(continued)*

Nursing Diagnosis *(continued)*: Alteration in thought process related to dichotomous thinking, overgeneralization, personalization, obsessions, and superstitious thinking.
Goal: Client will verbalize a logical and realistic thinking process.

Intervention	*Rationale*	*Expected Outcome*
Confront all-or-none thinking patterns	Decreasing dichotomous thinking will increase realistic perceptions	Verbalizes less dichotomous thinking
Discuss how perfectionism influences client's perception of reality	Client needs to understand relationship between need for perfectionism and cognitive distortion	Identifies perfectionistic thinking
Discuss unrealistic goals and promises to self	Rigid goals and promises contribute to client's superstitious thinking	Identifies rigidity of goals and superstitious thinking
Help client formulate realistic goals	Realistic goals will help client remain in control and decrease feelings of helplessness	Establishes reasonable goals

Nursing Diagnosis: Knowledge deficit about nutrition value of foods.
Goal: Client will implement accurate nutrition knowledge.

Intervention	*Rationale*	*Expected Outcome*
Teach about nutrition, calories, food values, and balanced diets	Accurate information will dispel magical beliefs about food	Verbalizes accurate knowledge of nutrition
Teach about foods that contribute to normal bowel function	Client may be abusing laxatives to stimulate bowel function	Uses food rather than laxatives for laxative effect
Teach about healthful patterns of eating	Preventing the excessive dieting and fasting may control urge to binge	Identifies need for at least 3 meals a day
Have client plan meals	Active involvement with meal planning will increase client's feeling of control	Plans balanced meals

Nursing Diagnosis: Body image disturbance related to delusional perception of body.
Goal: Client will verbalize a realistic perception of the body.

Intervention	*Rationale*	*Expected Outcome*
Discuss with client the client's perception of his or her body	Nurse needs to understand the particular distortions of the client	Verbalizes perceptual distortions
Do not argue with client's perceptions	Arguments will increase client's need to defend the delusions	
Point out your perceptions and objective data about client's body	Introduction of reality may assist client in focusing on a more realistic body image and decrease self-criticism	Listens to nurse's perceptions
Discuss cultural stereotypes of thinness and attractiveness	Ability to recognize unrealistic cultural standards will assist client in establishing more realistic goals	Identifies cultural stereotypes that have influenced perceptions

(Diagnosis continued)

Table 9–7 *(continued)*

Intervention	*Rationale*	*Expected Outcome*
Discuss client's perceptions of other people's bodies	Ability to accurately perceive others' bodies will assist client in becoming more realistic about his or her own body	Verbalizes realistic perception of others' bodies
Minimize comments about actual weight gain	Comments may increase phobia of weight gain	

Nursing Diagnosis: Self-esteem disturbance related to striving to please others to obtain acceptance.
Goal: Client will verbalize a more adequate self-esteem.

Intervention	*Rationale*	*Expected Outcome*
Help client identify own interests (eg, pleasurable activities, ways to spend leisure time, vocational interests)	Identifying own interests will increase client's ability to define and control self and decrease feelings of powerlessness	Makes list of interests; formulates plan of action around interests
Have client identify positive attributes about himself or herself	Increased self-acceptance and approval will decrease overdependency on others	Verbalizes positive qualities about self
Help client identify from whom he or she wants acceptance and healthy ways to seek acceptance	Focusing on significant others will decrease the wishful thinking of needing acceptance from all people	Identifies important persons in his or her life; implements plan to seek acceptance in ways that are not self-depreciating

Nursing Diagnosis: Impaired social interaction related to withdrawal from peer group and fears of rejection.
Goal: Client will increase the amount of socialization time.

Intervention	*Rationale*	*Expected Outcome*
Teach interpersonal communication and socialization skills through information and role playing	Social isolation may have occurred from fears of inadequacy in interpersonal relationships	Verbalizes feelings of competency in social settings
Help client problem-solve how to increase socialization and with whom	Focusing on particular people and situations will prevent client from feeling overwhelmed when attempting to change behavior	Implements plan to increase socialization
Help client problem-solve ways to spend leisure time without the need to be productive	Client needs to be able to relax without the rigid self-demand for productivity and achievement	Spends leisure time relaxing; verbalizes enjoyment of leisure time
Refer client to local self-help groups	Decreases social isolation and increases sense of belonging	Attends groups

Nursing Diagnosis: Potential for injury related to excessive exercise.
Goal: Client will not harm himself or herself.

Intervention	*Rationale*	*Expected Outcome*
Discuss physiologic result of excessive exercise	Client may have inaccurate information about physiology and effects of exercise	Verbalizes understanding of information

(Diagnosis continued)

Table 9–7 *(continued)*

Nursing Diagnosis *(continued)*: Potential for injury related to excessive exercise.
Goal: Client will not harm himself or herself.

Intervention	*Rationale*	*Expected Outcome*
Set limits on excessive exercise; check on client when alone in room	Client must be protected until client can protect himself or herself	Does not exercise to extremes
Help client problem-solve an appropriate exercise pattern	Realistic goals and patterns will decrease the potential for injury	Implements a safe, realistic exercise routine
Help client identify alternative activities when feeling the need to exercise	These activities may limit time and urge for excessive exercise	Utilizes other activities

Nursing Diagnosis: Altered family processes related to enmeshed family system.
Goal: Family will assist client toward autonomy.

Intervention	*Rationale*	*Expected Outcome*
Discuss inappropriate dependency on family	Extreme dependency inhibits normal separation and autonomy of adolescents and young adults	Identifies examples of inappropriate dependency
Problem-solve ways to increase independence appropriate to client's age	Increasing autonomy will decrease use of food as a method of passive-aggressive rebellion	Implements plan to increase independence from family unit
Problem-solve ways to obtain appropriate privacy within the family	Decreasing family's overinvolvement in client's life will increase feelings of self-control	Implements plan to increase privacy within family unit
Explore family patterns that support client's behavior	Family may have inadvertently supported the eating disorder	Identifies maladaptive family patterns
Explore secondary gains of all family members when client maintains disordered eating patterns	To help family identify other ways to meet their needs	Formulates alternative plans to meet needs

Nursing Diagnosis: Ineffective family coping, compromised, related to inability to manage conflict.
Goal: Family will manage conflict constructively.

Intervention	*Rationale*	*Expected Outcome*
Help family identify that disagreements are inevitable and normal within the family system	Normalizing feelings of anger will prevent the denial of negative emotions	Verbalizes feelings of anger with one another
Teach interpersonal communication skills to family	Improvement in communication pattern will decrease need to deny problems	Communicates directly and openly with one another
Provide assertiveness training to family members	Direct communication of thoughts, feelings, and needs will increase the adaptability of the family system	Increases assertive behavior
Teach constructive methods to manage anger and frustration	Managing feelings directly decreases the denial of family conflict	Implements plan to manage conflict within family

(continued)

Table 9–7 *(continued)*

Nursing Diagnosis: Powerlessness related to having no control over bulimarexic behavior pattern.
Goal: Client will verbalize internal locus of control.

Intervention	*Rationale*	*Expected Outcome*
Point out to client that binging and purging began as a method of control that is now out of control	Insight into the paradox of the behavior will assist client in finding alternative methods of control	Formulates alternative plan to gain control
Acknowledge the client's strengths	Client often feels no sense of strength when focused on symptoms	Identifies positive qualities of self
Practice effective social skills with client (eg, assertiveness, effective communication)	Client often feels lack of control in relationships	Has more successful interactions with others

Nursing Diagnosis: Ineffective denial related to not perceiving danger of disorder and resistance to intervention.
Goal: Client will participate in treatment plan.

Intervention	*Rationale*	*Expected Outcome*
Allow client to express anger at being coerced into treatment	Acknowledges and validates feelings	Expresses anger appropriately
Set limits	Establishes consistency, decreases manipulation, fosters trust	Abides by established limits
Avoid authoritarian approach	Client may view nurse as an enemy in alliance with parents	
Focus on problems client identifies as priority issues	May accept help for problems not directly related to eating	Participates in problem-solving process

tween 14 and 60 percent of the young people suffering from these disorders are not helped by the current therapeutic models. Professionals need to continue striving to find effective interventions for clients with eating disorders.

SUMMARY

Somatoform Disorders

1. The somatoform disorders all involve physical symptoms for which no organic basis exists.

2. People with a somatoform disorder spend a great deal of money on physician visits and over-the-counter medications, which are related to their obsession with bodily processes and diseases. Denial is used to transform anxiety into physical symptoms.

3. The physical symptoms may be interpreted as a punishment for perceived inadequacies, an excuse to avoid unwanted activities, or a way to achieve secondary gains such as nurturing or power and control.

4. The most important nursing goals for these clients are to maintain the clients in one health care system, to prevent needless diagnostic procedures and abuse of medications, and to assist clients to meet secondary gains in a more adaptive fashion.

Eating Disorders

5. Obesity is the most common form of malnourishment in the United States and results from a combination of physiologic and psychosocial factors.

6. The eating disorders are a person's response to anxiety about self-worth, competency, rejection, and family dynamics.

7. Behaviors associated with the eating disorders are compulsions and rituals about food and exercise, pho-

bias, eating binges, purging, and abuse of laxatives and diuretics.

8. Affective characteristics include multiple fears, dependency, and a high need for acceptance and approval from others.

9. Cognitive characteristics include selective abstraction, magnification, personalization, dichotomous thinking, distorted body image, self-depreciation, and perfectionistic standards of behavior.

10. The eating disorders affect the cardiovascular system, alter fluid and electrolyte balance, cause gastrointestinal complications, lead to amenorrhea, and result in a weight loss of 25 to 50 percent.

11. The family system of a person with an eating disorder may be enmeshed, have difficulty with conflict resolution, and have high ambitions for achievement and performance.

12. There are a variety of theories about the cause of eating disorders. The disorder may result from the person's trying to achieve autonomy, to reduce anxiety, to maintain family unity, or it may be related to chemical changes in the brain.

13. Treatment of clients with eating disorders must be planned from a multidisciplinary approach that involves medical interventions for the organic complications, family therapy, and individual behavior modification.

14. The most effective nursing approach with these clients is a combination of firmness, patience, and genuine concern.

15. Nursing goals should include assisting clients with social isolation; management of conflict, multiple fears, and distorted thinking processes; and maintaining adequate nutrition.

CHAPTER REVIEW

In the past year Dorothy has been seen by eight different health care providers. Results of all diagnostic tests have been normal. In spite of this, Dorothy continues to have multiple physical complaints involving a variety of body systems. The symptoms are vague and undefined and do not follow a particular disease pattern.

1. Dorothy has a number of prescriptions for pain relievers and antianxiety agents. The danger to her is that
   (a) The medications may mask her symptoms
   (b) The medications are likely to interfere with her work performance
   (c) She is at risk for developing drug dependency
   (d) She is likely to use the medications to commit suicide

2. A priority goal is to develop a warm, caring relationship with Dorothy to help her remain within one health care system. The best rationale for this is
   (a) To convince her of the need for psychiatric care
   (b) To provide continuity of care to prevent needless diagnostic tests
   (c) To take the burden of meeting her emotional needs off her family
   (d) To make certain her insurance company will continue payments

Caroline, 23 years old, has been bulimarexic for the past three years and has successfully hidden her disorder from her family and friends.

3. Caroline takes 50 laxatives a day. Physically she is in danger of developing
   (a) Primary amenorrhea
   (b) Bone marrow hypoplasia
   (c) Hypochloremic acidosis
   (d) Hypokalemic alkalosis

4. Caroline has been admitted to an eating disorders unit. In assessing her behavior pattern the nurse is most likely to find that Caroline
   (a) Has a cycle of fasting, binging, and purging
   (b) Refuses to eat in an attempt to assert herself
   (c) Has a rigid and excessive exercise routine
   (d) Isolates herself to protect against rejection

5. When Caroline returns to the unit from a day pass, the nurse will implement all the following interventions. Which one is most important in terms of safety?
   (a) Asking Caroline how she managed urges to purge
   (b) Discussing Caroline's feelings about the pass
   (c) Checking Caroline and her belongings for laxatives
   (d) Checking Caroline's eating log to see if she binged

REFERENCES

Agras WS: *Eating Disorders.* Pergamon Press, 1987.

Andersen AE: Anorexia nervosa, bulimia, and depression. In: *Diagnostics and Psychopathology.* Flack F (editor). Norton, 1987. 131–139.

Andersen AE: Anorexia nervosa and bulimia nervosa in males. In: *Diagnostic Issues in Anorexia Nervosa and Bulimia Nervosa.* Garner DM, Garfinkel PE (editors). Brunner/Mazel, 1988. 166–207.

Balfour JD, et al.: Behavioral and cognitive-behavioral assessment. In: *Assessment of Addictive Behaviors.* Donovan DM, Marlatt GA (editors). Guilford Press, 1988. 239–273.

Baur S: *Hypochondria.* University of Calif Press, 1988.

Bennett GA: Behavior therapy in the treatment of obesity. In: *Eating Habits.* Boakes RA, Popplewell DA, Burton MJ (editors). Wiley, 1987. 45–74.

Black DW: Somatoform disorders. In: *Psychiatric Illness, Primary Care.* Yates WR (editor). Saunders, 1987. 711–723.

Boskind-Lodahl M: Cinderella's stepsisters, a feminist perspective on anorexia and bulimia. In: *Psychology of Women: Selected Readings,* 2nd ed. Williams J (editor). Norton, 1985.

Boskind-White M: Bulimarexia: A sociocultural perspective. In: *Theory and Treatment of Anorexia Nervosa and Bulimia.* Emmett SW (editor). Brunner/Mazel, 1985. 113–126.

Burch GW, Pearson PH: Anorexia, bulimia and obesity in adolescence. In: *Eating Disorders: Effective Care and Treatment.* Larocca FEF (editor). Euro American, 1986. 183–195.

Coburn J, Ganong L: Bulimic and non-bulimic college females' perceptions of family adaptability and family cohesion. *J Adv Nurs* 1989; 14:27–33.

Deering CG: Developing a therapeutic alliance with the anorexia nervosa client. *J Psychosoc Nur* 1987; 25(3): 10–17.

Dippel NM, Becknal B: Bulimia. *J Psychosoc Nurs* 1987; 25(9):12–17.

Garfinkel PE, Garner DM: *Anorexia Nervosa: A Multidimensional Perspective.* Brunner/Mazel, 1982.

Garfinkel PE, Garner DM: Bulimia in anorexia nervosa. In: *The Binge-Purge Syndrome.* Hawkins RC et al. (editors). Springer, 1984.

Goldbloom DS: Serotonin in eating disorders. In: *The Role of Drug Treatment for Eating Disorders.* Garfinkel PE, Garner DM (editors). Brunner/Mazel, 1987. 124–149.

Gormally J: The obese binge eater. In: *The Binge-Purge Syndrome.* Hawkins RC et al. (editors). Springer, 1984.

Herzog DB, Brotman AW: Use of tricyclic antidepressants in anorexia nervosa and bulimia nervosa. In: *The Role of Drug Treatment for Eating Disorders.* Garfinkel PE, Garner DM (editors). Brunner/Mazel, 1987. 36–58.

Kennedy S, Walsh BT: Drug therapies for eating disorders. In: *The Role of Drug Treatment for Eating Disorders.* Garfinkel PE, Garner DM (editors). Brunner/Mazel, 1987. 3–35.

Landau E: *Why Are They Starving Themselves?* Julian Messner, 1983.

Lilly GE, Sanders JB: Nursing management of anorexic adolescents. *J Psychosoc Nurs* 1987; 25(11):30–33.

Loro AJ: Binge eating: A cognitive-behavioral treatment approach. In: *The Binge-Purge Syndrome.* Hawkins RC et al. (editors). Springer, 1984.

Minchin S, Rosman B, Baker L: *Psychosomatic Families: Anorexia Nervosa in Context.* Harvard, 1978.

Miner DC: The physiology of eating and starvation. *Holistic Nurs Pract* 1988; 3(1):67–74.

Orbach S: Visbility/invisibility. In: *Theory and Treatment of Anorexia Nervosa and Bulimia Nervosa.* Emmett SW (editor). Brunner/Mazel, 1985. 127–138.

Orleans CT, Barnett LR: Bulimarexia: Guidelines for behavioral assessment and treatment. In: *The Binge-Purge Syndrome.* Hawkins RC et al. (editors). Springer, 1984.

Polivy J, et al.: Cognitive assessment. In: *Assessment of Addictive Behaviors.* Donovan DM, Marlatt GA (editors). Guilford Press, 1988. 274–295.

Pope HG, et al.: Treatment of bulimia with thymoleptic medications. In: *Eating Disorders: Effective Care and Treatment.* Larocca FEF (editor). Euro American, 1986. 151–172.

Powers PS, et al.: Perceptual and cognitive abnormalities in bulimia. *Am J Psychiatry* 1987; 144(11):1456–1460.

Rau JH, Green RS: Neurological factors affecting binge eating: Body over mind. In: *The Binge-Purge Syndrome.* Hawkins RC et al. (editors). Springer, 1984.

Root M, Fallon P, Friedrich WN: *Bulimia: A Systems Approach to Treatment.* Norton, 1986.

Schwartz RC, Barrett MJ: Women and eating disorders. In: *Women, Feminism and Family Therapy.* Braverman L (editor). *J Psychother and Family* 1987; 3(4):131–144.

Spack NP: Medical complications of anorexia nervosa. In: *Theory and Treatment of Anorexia Nervosa and Bulimia.* Emmett SW (editor). Brunner/Mazel, 1985. 5–19.

Steiner-Adair C: Developing the voice of the wise woman. In: *The Bulimic College Student.* Whitaker L, Davis WN (editors). Haworth Press, 1989. 151–165.

Stierlin H, Weber G: *Unlocking the Family Door.* Brunner/Mazel, 1989.

Torem MS: Eating disorders and dissociative states. In: *Eating Disorders: Effective Care and Treatment.* Larocca FEF (editor). Euro American, 1986. 11141–50.

Woods SC, Brief DJ: Physiological factors. In: *Assessment of Addictive Behaviors.* Donovan DM, Marlatt GA (editors). Guilford Press, 1988. 296–322.

Worman V: A feminist interpretation of college student bulimia. In: *The Bulimic College Student.* Whitaker L, Davis WN (editors). Haworth Press, 1989. 167–180.

Yates WR, Sieleni B: Anorexia and bulimia. In: *Psychiatric Illness, Primary Care.* Yates WR (editor). Saunders, 1987. 737–744.

Zucker P: Medical complications of bulimia. In: *The Bulimic College Student.* Whitaker L, Davis WN (editors). Haworth Press, 1989. 27–40.

SUGGESTED READINGS

Brumberg JJ: *Fasting Girls.* Harvard University Press, 1988.

Geary MC: A review of treatment models for eating disorders. *Holistic Nurs Pract* 1988; 3(1):39–45.

Kopeski LM: Diabetes and bulima: A deadly duo. *Am J Nurs* 1989; 89(4):483–485.

Leininger MM: Transcultural eating patterns and nutrition. *Holistic Nurs Pract* 1988; 3(1)16–25.

McBride AB: Fat: A women's issue in search of a holistic approach to treatment. *Holistic Nurs Pract* 1988; 3(1):9–15.

Rossi LR: Feminine beauty: The impact of culture and nutritional trends on emerging images. *Holistic Nurs Pract* 1988; 3(1):1–8.

CHAPTER 10

Personality Disorders

J. SUE COOK and KAREN LEE FONTAINE

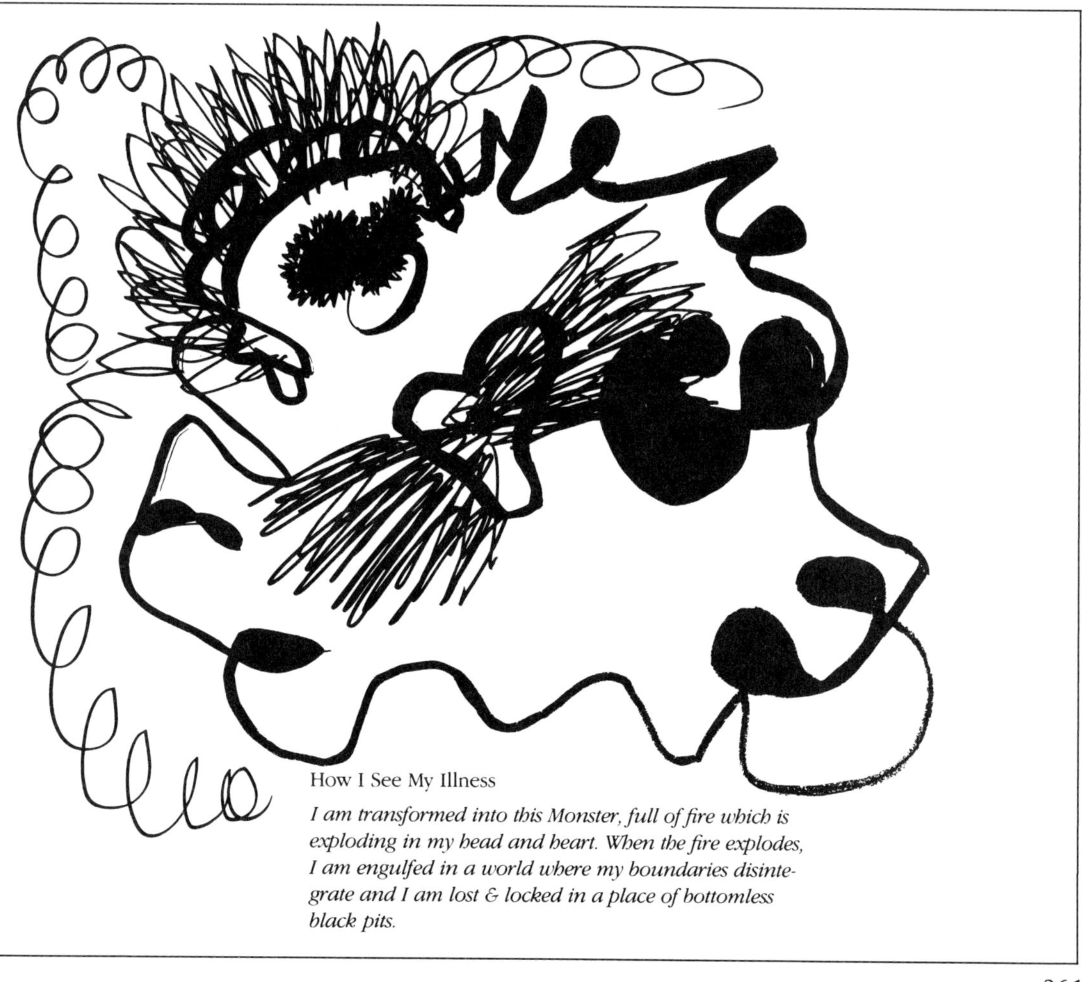

How I See My Illness

I am transformed into this Monster, full of fire which is exploding in my head and heart. When the fire explodes, I am engulfed in a world where my boundaries disintegrate and I am lost & locked in a place of bottomless black pits.

▪ *Objectives*

After reading this chapter the student will be able to

- Define the concept of personality disorder
- Describe the behavioral, affective, cognitive, and sociocultural characteristics of clients with a personality disorder
- Discuss causative theories underlying personality disorders
- Identify the subtypes of personality disorders
- Apply a focused nursing assessment to assess clients with a personality disorder
- Identify nursing diagnoses appropriate to clients with various personality disorders
- Prepare nursing care plans for clients with the various subtypes of personality disorders
- Discuss the evaluation of nursing care for clients with the various subtypes of personality disorders

▪ *Chapter Outline*

Introduction

Psychiatric disabilities lying within the category of personality disorders are among the most difficult of any form of mental illness to treat. Most people with personality disorders will never enter a psychiatric hospital, seek or receive outpatient treatment, or even undergo a diagnostic evaluation. With those who do come into the mental health system, mental health professionals find the limits of their expertise tested. Clients with personality disorders constitute many of the treatment failures; they frequently drop out of clinics, and often accumulate numerous referrals to other agencies.

To understand the nature of this pathology, it is helpful to review the concept of personality. Most people refer to a certain quality or set of qualities that a person has when trying to describe that person's personality. These qualities are often called *personality traits.* The traits or behaviors are enduring patterns of how one perceives, relates to, and thinks about the environment. It is only when a personality trait is maladaptive, rigid, causes subjective distress, or impairs social or occupational functioning that it constitutes a *disorder.* There is a high degree of overlap among the personality disorders, and many individuals exhibit traits of several disorders. Typically, personality disorders become apparent before or during adolescence and persist throughout life. In some cases the symptoms become less obvious by middle or old age (Gunderson, 1988).

Incidence of Personality Disorders

It is extremely difficult to estimate the incidence of personality disorders. Many people with personality disorders never come to the attention of the mental health system. The best estimate is that 15 percent of the general population suffer from some disruption serious enough to be diagnosed as a personality disorder (Gunderson, 1988).

Because of their refusal to seek treatment, the incidence is unknown for those experiencing paranoid, schizotypal, histrionic, narcissistic, avoidant, dependent, and passive-aggressive personality disorders. Within the general population about 2 percent are diagnosed with schizoid personality disorder, 3 percent with antisocial personality disorder, 2 percent to 4 percent with borderline disorder, and 2 percent with obsessive-compulsive personality disorder. Males are more likely to be diagnosed with paranoid, schizoid, and antisocial personality disorders. Females are more likely to be diagnosed with borderline and histrionic personality disorders (Gunderson, 1988; Reid, 1989).

Significance of Personality Disorders to Mental Health Nursing

Although it is unlikely there will be an accompanying psychiatric diagnosis, the nurse will frequently encounter people who manifest the problems of inflexible and maladaptive personality traits. Any person, in the presence of sufficient stress, might retreat to more primitive and rigid defense mechanisms in coping with anxiety. Since the nurse's contact with clients is usually brief, it is rarely possible to know if or to what extent these problems have been significant over time. Without this knowledge, no diagnosis of personality disorder can be made. However, it is never the diagnosis that creates the condition, so the nurse needs to consider the possibility that the client's manner of perceiving and relating are typical for him or her.

Personality disorders rarely result in psychiatric hospitalization for the client, but the nurse will likely encounter persons with these problems in every other health care setting. When psychiatric hospitalization is necessary, it usually occurs for persons having a diagnosis of borderline, antisocial, or schizotypal personality disorder.

Knowledge Base

Behavioral Characteristics

It is important to remember that the problems associated with this diagnostic group are not only of long duration but also thoroughly interwoven within the personality. Invariably, a *pattern* of acting and responding signals the presence of a personality disorder. It follows that no single behavior, either in isolation or as a transitory response, distinguishes this diagnostic group. Table 10–1 summarizes the major behavioral characteristics for each personality disorder by cluster.

The first, and most prevalent, set of behavioral characteristics for the entire category of personality disorders encompasses the various manifestations of **narcissism**. Whether the behavior-disordered person assumes a posture of self-centeredness, vanity, grandiosity, or entitlement, the pervasive stance is narcissistic. People who regularly speak and act as if their own concerns were of supreme importance, while hardly recognizing others', fit this description.

A second characteristic shared by people with personality disorders is that these clients' behaviors are particularly annoying and abrasive. They have a unique capacity to "get under the skin" of others. In fact, many therapists find these clients so trying that they will not accept them for private therapy. When therapists do work with these clients, the therapists frequently experience intense countertransference reactions. Typically, these clients appear untroubled by their own behaviors while the therapist and others are in turmoil (Vaillant and Perry, 1985).

A third behavioral characteristic for the person with a personality disorder is a pattern of inflexible and maladaptive responses to most interpersonal situations. These responses are not only repetitive but also typically undermine the person's effectiveness in all interpersonal relationships.

Affective Characteristics

For years, it was believed that clients with personality disorders feel no subjective discomfort, that they experience no anxiety. This belief arose be-

Table 10–1 *Behavioral Characteristics in Personality Disorders*

	Dominant Traits	*Behavioral Control*	*Occupational Functioning*	*Deficits*
Disorders in Cluster A				
Paranoid	Craves solitude	Hypervigilant, unable to relax	Needs rigid routines	Argumentative
Schizoid	Craves solitude	Constricted	Has some interference with function	Anxious in social situations
Schizotypal	Craves solitude	Eccentric	Has some interference with function	Odd speech content
Disorders in Cluster B				
Antisocial	Craves excitement, immediate gratification	Impulsive, irresponsible	Typified by frequent job changes	Poor internal control of behavior, pathologic lying, impersonal sex life, transient lifestyle
Borderline	Alternates between isolation and high sociability; often bored	Impulsive	Uncertain of career, low achievement in work/school	Self-mutilation, frequent suicide gestures, impulsive sexual behavior
Histrionic	Craves excitement, immediate gratification	Is overly reactive	Has some interference with function	May be seductive
Narcissistic	Often bored	Emphasizes self-importance	Strives for power and success	Exploitative
Disorders in Cluster C				
Avoidant	Avoids activities with others, needs rigid routine	Is rigid	Usually in careers with minimal contact with others	Easily hurt by criticism
Dependent	Has difficulty doing things alone	Needs much advice and reassurance	Usually in careers with minimal independence	Unable to make decisions
Obsessive-Compulsive	Leaves tasks incomplete, is task-oriented	Needs to be in control	Incapacitated in careers requiring decisionmaking and deadline meeting	Inflexible, perfectionistic
Passive-Aggressive	Is dependent on others to perform activities	Exhibits resistant behaviors	Shows ineffective functioning	Stubborn

cause the disorders are considered **ego-syntonic**, which means these clients are not disturbed by their own behaviors. It is now understood that many people who have a personality disorder do feel anxiety.

If there is one common affective feature that can be said to exist across the group, it is one more significant for its absence than its presence. Many clients with a diagnosis of personality disorder are unable to see or feel the world from another person's vantage point, that is, they have an inability to feel empathy.

Table 10–2 summarizes affective characteristics in each personality disorder by cluster. Again, it is essential to remember there are wide variations in the affective characteristics of clients within this

Table 10–2 *Affective Characteristics in Personality Disorders*

	Expression of Affect	*Stability of Affect*	*Emotional Reactions*
Disorders in Cluster A			
Paranoid	Minimal	Stable	Quick anger, avoids blame and guilt, fears losing power
Schizoid	Minimal; flat or blunted	Stable	Indifference to criticism, fears intimacy, suspicious of others
Schizotypal	Constricted or inappropriate	Restricted range of lability	Social anxiety
Disorders in Cluster B			
Antisocial	Quick but shallow	Intolerance of frustration	Quick anger, no sense of guilt
Borderline	Intense	Labile eruptions of rage; intolerant of frustration	Frequent lack of control of anger, suspicious of others, often anxious and depressed
Histrionic	Changing and excessive	Stable	Fairly good control of anger
Narcissistic	Changing	Can exhibit lability	Rages against criticism, avoids blame and guilt, fears helplessness and humiliation, often depressed, may experience panic
Disorders in Cluster C			
Avoidant	Avoids expression	Stable	Anger at self, fears embarrassment and disapproval, may develop depression, often anxious
Dependent	Passive	Stable	Fears abandonment and rejection, depression common, anxiety common when others disapprove
Obsessive-Compulsive	Restricted	Stable	Controls anger, depressed mood common, fears disapproval and criticism, fears losing control
Passive-Aggressive	Passive	Stable	Fears conflict and anger, often depressed, often anxious

general category. Specific affective characteristics are directly related to the particular personality disorder. Clients with paranoid personality disorder, for example, are likely to be cold, hypersensitive, and humorless. On the other hand, clients diagnosed as histrionic may express feelings of helplessness and insecurity. Clearly, broad generalizations are not possible.

Cognitive Characteristics

Several distinctive cognitive characteristics do apply across all personality disorders. These are directly related to the pattern of inflexible responses so typical for clients with these diagnoses.

Since the demands of everyday living require adaptability and flexibility to achieve creative solu-

Table 10–3 *Cognitive Characteristics in Personality Disorders*

	Identity/ Self-Image	*Self-Confidence*	*Decision Making*	*Deficits*
Disorders in Cluster A				
Paranoid	Guarded	Avoids intimacy	Is secretive	Transient ideas of reference
Schizoid	Self-consumed	Prefers to be left alone	Is indecisive, has vague plans for future	Absent-minded
Schizotypal	Guarded	Anxious in social settings	Makes poor decisions	Ideas of reference, magical thinking, unusual perceptual experiences, illusions
Disorders in Cluster B				
Antisocial	Grandiose	Egocentric, extremely confident	Has no long-range plans	Egosyntonic, lack of remorse
Borderline	Identity diffusion, unstable changing body image	Egocentric	Has no long-range plans	Dichotomous thinking, splitting
Histrionic	Self-centered	Egocentric	Needs approval of others	Overly concerned with other's perceptions
Narcissistic	Grandiose view of self	Superficially confident, egocentric	Lacks empathy	Dichotomous thinking, perfectionistic, inability to accept failure
Disorders in Cluster C				
Avoidant	Timid	Avoids social contacts	Follows set routine	Overly sensitive to opinions of others
Dependent	Belittles self	Needs constant approval	Allows others to make most decisions	Passive, dependent
Obsessive-Compulsive	Controlled	Seeks to control all contacts with others	Delays decisions because of fear of mistakes	Overly conscientious, moralistic, perfectionistic
Passive-Aggressive	Stubborn	Lacks self-confidence	Procrastinator	Argumentative, resentful of authority

tions for the problems everyone faces, it is easy to see that rigid patterns of perceiving situations and responding to them would severely limit the ability to function effectively. These clients frequently interpret situations from their own rigid vantage point and are unable to consider alternative perspectives. As a result, they tend to have difficulty in both reality testing and problem solving.

Although these clients may have normal or even very high IQs, their limited capacity to see or accept creative solutions frequently impedes their success on the job. Often they are seen as rigid and unyielding, unable to understand the "big picture." This inflexibility often leads to mistakes in judgment, making them prone to job problems and other difficulties in functioning. Table 10–3 summarizes major cognitive characteristics in each personality disorder by cluster.

Sociocultural Characteristics

Rather than considering that a problem may rest within themselves, clients with personality disorders tend to believe the rest of the world is out of step. As a result, all interpersonal relationships with others are difficult at best, including those within the family. However, since the behavior patterns are of long duration and typical for the client, family members frequently perceive the client as simply "being that way."

Families that are accepting and nonjudgmental will tolerate a member who displays these pathologic personality patterns of thinking and acting. Some families, on the other hand, will exclude or isolate a member whose behavior they find persistently annoying. Often, these clients have a long history of strained or broken relationships with siblings or even parents. Further, marriage or other longterm interpersonal commitments are not easily formed or maintained. Table 10–4 summarizes sociocultural characteristics of personality disorders by cluster.

Clusters of Personality Disorder Subtypes

There are twelve different personality disorders. DSM-III-R has grouped eleven of them into three clusters:

Cluster A

Paranoid
Schizoid
Schizotypal

Cluster B

Antisocial
Borderline
Histrionic
Narcissistic

Cluster C

Avoidant
Dependent
Obsessive-compulsive
Passive-aggressive

The label "personality disorder not otherwise specified" is used for mixed conditions.

People with diagnoses from **Cluster A** usually appear eccentric. People with diagnoses from **Cluster B** appear dramatic, emotional, or erratic. People with diagnoses from **Cluster C** are those who appear anxious or fearful (American Psychiatric Association, 1987).

Cluster A The common characteristics of the personality disorders under Cluster A are odd, eccentric behavior, suspicious ideation, and social isolation.

Paranoid Personality Disorder. Behaviorally, these individuals are very secretive about their entire existence. Confiding in other people is perceived as dangerous and is not likely to occur, even within family relationships. Paranoid people are hyperalert to danger, search for evidence of attack, and become argumentative as a way of creating a safe distance between themselves and others. They rarely seek help for their personality problems and they seldom require hospitalization.

Affectively, paranoid people typically avoid sharing their feelings except for a very quick expression of anger. They may never forgive perceived slights and bear grudges for long periods of time. There is a prevalent fear of losing power or control to others. These individuals experience a chronic state of tension and are rarely able to relax.

Cognitively, paranoid people are very guarded about themselves and secretive about their decisions. They expect to be used or harrassed by others. When confronted with new situations, they look for hidden, demeaning, or threatening meanings to rather benign remarks or events and respond with criticism of others. For example, if there is an error in a bank statement, the paranoid person may say the bank did it to ruin his or her credit rating.

Socioculturally, paranoid people have great difficulty with intimate relationships. They interact in a cold and aloof manner, thus avoiding the per-

Table 10–4 *Sociocultural Characteristics in Personality Disorders*

	Characteristics of Relationships	*View of Others*	*Needs from Others*
Disorders in Cluster A			
Paranoid	Pathologically jealous, minimally intimate	Views others as threatening, expects to be used or harmed by others, critical of others, suspicious	Does not need others
Schizoid	Not desirous of relationships or intimacy	Is suspicious of others	Is indifferent to praise or criticism
Schizotypal	Impaired relationships, minimal intimacy	Suspicious of others	Wants no interpersonal relatedness
Disorders in Cluster B			
Antisocial	Successfully manipulative, detached and distant, often abusive	Disregards rights and feelings of others	Uses others for self-gratification
Borderline	Intense stormy relationships, manipulative	Is suspicious of others, idealizes and then devalues others	Alternates between dependency and self-assertion
Histrionic	Manipulative	Is concerned about others' perceptions of self	Needs attention, reassurance, praise
Narcissistic	Manipulative	Objectifies others, idealizes and then devalues others	Expects others to meet all needs and be available; needs attention and praise
Disorders in Cluster C			
Avoidant	Avoids but yearns for social contact	Is sensitive to reactions of others	Needs constant unconditional love
Dependent	Dependence on others	Is sensitive to reactions of others	Needs constant companionship, wants others to like them
Obsessive-Compulsive	Formal quality to relationships	Controls others by using rules, procedures	Needs others to maintain standards
Passive-Aggressive	Passive resistance to demands from others	Practices covert aggression, resents authority figures	Places no specific demands on relationships

ceived dangers in intimacy. Because they expect to be harmed by others, they question the loyalty or trustworthiness of family and friends. Pathologic jealousy of the spouse or sexual partner frequently occurs. (American Psychiatric Association, 1987; Gunderson, 1988).

Harold, a 40-year-old single man, met Katherine when he went to her home to repair her television set. Katherine asked him if he would like some coffee, and Harold concluded that she was "coming on to him." As Harold was leaving, he decided to ask Katherine out to dinner. When Katherine told Harold she was married, he became irate and accused her of trying to "play games" with him. Later in the day Harold called Katherine, told her he didn't believe she was married, and asked why she wouldn't go out with him. Katherine hung up, and Harold called her back. Katherine had to threaten to call the police before Harold would stop calling.

Schizoid Personality Disorder. *Behaviorally,* people with schizoid personality disorder are loners who prefer solitary activities, since social situations and interactions increase their level of anxiety. They may be occupationally impaired if the job requires interpersonal skills. However, if work may be performed under conditions of social isolation, eg, being a night guard in a closed facility, they may be capable of satisfactory occupational achievement.

Schizoid people have a stable but restricted range of emotional experience and expression and their *affect* is described as blunted or flat. They rarely experience strong emotions such as anger or joy. Because they are suspicious of others they are fearful of intimate relationships.

Socioculturally, they interact with others in a cold and aloof manner, have no close friends, and prefer not to be in any relationships. They are indifferent to attitudes and feelings of others, and thus are not influenced by praise or criticism. Males with this disorder have great difficulty dating and rarely marry. Females may passively accept being courted and subsequently marry (American Psychiatric Association, 1987; Gunderson, 1988).

Juan, a 34-year-old dishwasher, has been employed by the same restaurant for the past 18 years. Juan started this job when he left high school at 16. Juan prefers to work alone and, when he does, he can do the work of three men. Juan works the late afternoon and early evening shift. Juan does not socialize with his coworkers. Juan's boss is the only one who knows that Juan is single and lives in a residential hotel. Juan eats his meals at the restaurant, in the back of the kitchen, alone.

Schizotypal Personality Disorder. People with schizotypal personality disorder have a considerable disability, with peculiarities of ideation, appearance, and behavior that are not severe enough to meet the criteria for schizophrenia. Under periods of extreme stress and anxiety they may experience transient psychotic symptoms that are not of sufficient duration to make an additional diagnosis.

Behaviorally, they exhibit odd speech and their appearance may be rather eccentric. They prefer solitary activities and often experience occupational difficulties.

Their *affect* is typically constricted, and may be inappropriate to the situation at times. Social situations create anxiety for those with schizotypal personality disorder,

Cognitively, schizotypal disturbances may include paranoid ideation, suspiciousness, ideas of reference, odd beliefs, and magical thinking. They may have impoverished speech that is digressive, vague, and inappropriately abstract. It is difficult for them to make decisions.

Socioculturally, they fear intimacy and desire no relationships with family or friends. Thus they are very isolative and are usually avoided by others (American Psychiatric Association, 1987; Gunderson, 1988).

Carol, a 24-year-old unemployed single female, lives in a roominghouse. She keeps to herself, and most of the other boarders in the roominghouse find her to be eccentric. Carol is preoccupied with the idea that her dead father was a movie star who left her a fortune with which her guardian absconded. Carol has a habit of saying odd things like, "So go the days of our lives." Most of the roominghouse boarders avoid Carol because of her strange behaviors.

Cluster B The common characteristics of the personality disorders under Cluster B are impulsive and dramatic behavior, intolerance of frustration, and exploitive interpersonal relationships. The three unstable types, borderline, narcissistic, and histrionic, can barely be distinguished from one another. More so than with other disorders, the diagnosis may be influenced by personal bias and cultural preferences on the part of the professional (Kroll, 1988).

Antisocial Personality Disorder. A diagnosis of antisocial personality disorder requires that the characteristics appear before the age of 15. In boys, the behavior typically emerges during childhood, while for girls it is more likely to occur around puberty. *Behaviorally,* predominant childhood manifestations are lying, stealing, truancy, vandalism, fighting, and running away from home. In adulthood the pattern changes to failure to honor financial obligations, inability to function as a responsible parent, a tendency to lie pathologically, and an inability to sustain consistent work behavior. People with antisocial personalities conform to rules only when it is useful to them and often commit antisocial acts for which they may be arrested.

There is a high correlation between substance abuse and antisocial personality disorder. In several studies it has been found that the rate of antisocial personality disorder is as high as 50 percent among male opiate addicts and alcoholics. At times it is difficult to separate these disorders, as substance abuse is itself an antisocial behavior that causes problems similar to those of the personality disorder. Thus substance abusers may be divided into two groups: *primary antisocial addicts,* whose antisocial behavior is independent of the need to obtain drugs, and *secondary antisocial addicts,* whose antisocial behavior is directly related to drug use (Gerstley, 1990).

Affectively, antisocial people express themselves quickly and easily, but with very little personal involvement. Thus, they can profess undying love one minute and terminate the relationship the next minute. In addition, they are very irritable and aggressive. They have no concern for others and experience no guilt when they violate society's rules.

Cognitively, antisocial people are egocentric and grandiose. They are extremely confident that everything will always work out in their favor because they believe they are more clever than everyone else. The disorder is ego-syntonic and they have no desire to change in any way. They make no long-range plans for the future.

Socioculturally, these individuals are generally unable to sustain lasting, close, warm, and responsible relationships. Their sex life is impersonal and impulsive. They disregard the feelings and rights of others. With their quick anger, poor tolerance of frustration, and lack of guilt they are often emotionally, physically, and sexually abusive to others (American Psychiatric Association, 1987; Gunderson, 1988).

Stephen, a divorced 20-year-old, works as a busperson at a pizza parlor, but he has a new job every other month. Stephen has an arrest record going back to high school. There he was often truant and was picked up many times by the police for using marijuana and receiving stolen goods. Stephen often took money from his mother's purse, and once fenced the family silver for drug money. Stephen married when he was 18, but the marriage lasted only six months—Stephen liked having women on the side, and his wife wasn't very understanding. When she nagged him about going out, Stephen beat her up. Stephen is working as a busperson to get enough money together to start a marijuana crop. As soon as he has enough money to buy some starter plants, Stephen plans to go into business for himself.

Borderline Personality Disorder. The clinical features of this disorder are not limited to borderline personality disorder; they are extremely varied and even contradictory. The dramatic symptoms and chaotic lifestyle may resemble other mental disorders, which complicates diagnosis and treatment. There is a great overlap between the symptoms of borderline personality disorder and posttraumatic stress disorder (see Chapter 8). Borderline symptoms can appear and disappear rapidly and they may fluctuate from mild to severe. Even though the majority of research on personality disorders has focused on borderline, it is probably the least understood of the personality disorders (Kroll, 1988).

The predominant *behavioral* characteristic is widespread impulsivity, especially of a physically self-destructive type. Borderline people often drive recklessly, abuse substances, binge eat, shoplift, engage in assaultive behavior, self-mutilate, or attempt suicide. It is thought that this behavior is an attempt to escape from intolerably intense feelings. This is the only personality disorder in which people are deliberately self-destructive. They may manipulate others to act against them in a negative or aggressive way. At other times they appear helpless and incompetent. They alternate between periods of isolation and frantic efforts to avoid real or imagined abandonment.

Most noticeable in these individuals is their intense and labile *affect*. They experience much anxiety and depression, are intolerant of frustration, and express these feelings intensely and dramatically. They lack control over their anger and unexpectedly fly into rages. At times they are able to express their sense of loneliness and inner emptiness.

There are noticeable *cognitive* difficulties, many of which may be related to past traumatic experiences. These individuals often suffer from partial amnesias, changing identities and body images, and changing sexual orientations, all of which may be indications of transient dissociative states. This may be a form of multiple personality disorder with the same antecedent of childhood sexual abuse (see Chapter 8). Another cognitive characteristic is that of dichotomous thinking, that is, things are either all good or all bad. For example, borderline people are unable to see both positive and negative qualities in the same person at the same time.

Socioculturally, borderline individuals have a history of intense, unstable, and manipulative relationships. They shift rapidly from extremes of dependency to extremes of independency. It is not uncommon for them to escalate the relationship to extreme closeness and then abruptly abandon the partner or perceive themselves to be abandoned. The process of being idealized and then devalued provokes strong feelings and responses in friends and family (Everett, 1989; Zanarini, 1990).

Julie, a 25-year-old parttime college student, frequently tells her friends how inconsiderate her parents are because they don't take care of her the way they "should" and, conversely, how awful it is because she can't become independent and live on her own. At times she tries to manipulate her friends into doing things for her and at other times she barely acknowledges that they exist. After dating Greg for two weeks she has told everyone he is absolutely perfect and they are "madly in love." One afternoon Greg tells Julie he can't see her that evening because he must study for an exam. Julie flies into a rage, jumps into her car and goes to a local bar, where she impulsively picks up a stranger and has sex with him in the parking lot. Returning home, she scratches her wrists with a broken bottle and calls Greg to tell him it is all his fault that she slashed her wrists and is going to die.

Histrionic Personality Disorder. The most prominent *behavioral* characteristic of people with histrionic personality disorder is that of seeking stimulation and excitement in life. Their behavior and appearance focus attention of themselves in an attempt to evoke and maintain the interest of others. They are seen as colorful, extroverted, and seductive individuals who seem always to be the center of attention.

The best description of histrionic people's *affect* is overly dramatic. Even minor stimuli causes emotional excitability and exaggerated expression of feelings. They often seem to be on a roller coaster of joy and despair.

Cognitively, they are very self-centered. They become overly concerned with how others perceive them because of a high need for approval. Histrionic people have a vague and fanciful way of thinking that is reflected in their style of speech, which is expressionistic but lacking in detail.

Socioculturally, they constantly seek assurances, approval, or praise from family and friends. There is often exaggeration in their interpersonal relationships, with an emphasis on their acting out the role of victim or princess. Histrionic people commonly have flights of romantic fantasy, though the actual quality of their sexual relationships is variable. They may be overly trusting and respond very positively to strong authority figures, who they think will magically solve their problems (American Psychiatric Association, 1987; Gunderson, 1988).

Leticia, a 25-year-old hairdresser, is popular with her clients. Leticia is very attractive, with long black hair and elegantly sculptured nails. She always wears the latest fashions and lots of jewelry. Leticia enjoys entertaining her customers with tales of exploits with the many men in her life. Recently Leticia told of meeting a handsome cowboy in a bar and deciding to go to Las Vegas with him for the weekend. Leticia claimed he treated her like a queen, hiring a chauffeured limo, dining by candlelight, and dancing until dawn. However, Leticia doesn't plan to see the young man again because she lives by the motto "So many men, so little time!"

Narcissistic Personality Disorder. The *behavioral* pattern for those with narcissistic personality disorder is one of striving for power and success. Failure is intolerable because of perfectionistic standards. Occupational functioning can be impaired by unreasonable goals or enhanced by an unquenchable thirst for success.

Affectively, narcissists are often labile. If criticized they may fly into a rage. At other times they may experience anxiety and panic and short periods of depression. They try to avoid feelings of blame and guilt because of intense fear of humiliation. When their needs are not met they may react with rage or shame, but mask these feelings with an aura of cool indifference. Their obsession with personal success contributes to chronic envy of others who appear more successful.

The primary *cognitive* style of those with narcissistic personality disorder is arrogant and egotistical. They are even more grandiose than histrionic people. They have a tendency to exaggerate their accomplishments and talents. They expect to be noticed and treated as special whether or not they have achieved anything. Their feelings of specialness may alternate with feelings of special unworthiness. They are preoccupied with fantasies of unlimited success, power, brilliance, beauty, and ideal love. Underneath this confident manner is a very fragile self-esteem.

Socioculturally, narcissistic people have disturbed relationships. They have unreasonable expectations of favorable treatment and exploit others to achieve personal goals. Friendships are made on the basis of how the other person can profit them. Romantic partners are used as objects to bolster the narcissistic person's self-esteem. They are unable to develop a relationship based on mutuality (American Psychiatric Association, 1987; Gunderson, 1988).

Michael, a 28-year-old real-estate broker, has never been married. He lives in an expensive apartment and drives a foreign sports car. Michael thrives on letting others know how successful his business is and about all the luxuries it affords him. Michael may be seen frequently with attractive women, but he loses interest when they get serious. Michael likes to throw large parties and enjoys watching people rave over his apartment. Michael claims, "Everybody loves me." At a recent party a colleague enraged Michael by failing to recognize the aesthetic value of Michael's newest piece of French sculpture. Instead of acting out his rage, Michael cooly said, "It is obvious you have no eye for the elegance of French sculpture." Then he turned to another guest and continued bragging about his find.

Cluster C The common characteristics of the personality disorders under Cluster C are high levels of anxiety and fearfulness.

Avoidant Personality Disorder. Social discomfort is the primary *behavioral* characteristic of persons with avoidant personality disorder. Any social or occupational activities that involve significant interpersonal contact are avoided. Rigid routines of behavior are employed to avoid the possibility of failure or rejection.

Affectively, these individuals are fearful and shy. Avoidant people are easily hurt by criticism and devastated by the slightest hint of disapproval. They are distressed by their lack of ability to relate to others and often experience depression, anxiety, and anger for failing to develop social relationships.

Cognitively, avoidant people are overly sensitive to the opinions of others. They suffer from exaggerated needs for acceptance. Rigid routines decrease the risk of failure with the accompanying disapproval from others.

In the *sociocultural* area, avoidant people are reluctant to enter into relationships without a guarantee of uncritical acceptance. Since unconditional approval is not guaranteed, they have few close friends or confidants. In social situations avoidant people are afraid of saying something inappropriate or foolish or of being unable to answer a question. They are terrified of being embarrassed by blushing, crying, or showing signs of anxiety before other people (Reid, 1989).

> *Eric, a 22-year-old college senior, is considered shy by other students. Eric stays in his room studying and generally avoids attending parties. He has no real friends at college and spends his time watching television when he has no homework. Eric has a hard time in some of his classes, especially those that require him to speak in front of the group. He frets for hours over being embarrassed by something he might say that will make him look foolish. In class Eric never sits next to the same person twice because this helps him avoid having to socialize. He has been admiring a girl named Jennie in his philosophy class, but he has never attempted to speak to her. Eric has been trying to find a way to ask Jennie out. However, everything he plans to say seems foolish. He is afraid Jennie will say no.*

Dependent Personality Disorder. Dependent and submissive *behavior* are the major features of dependent personality disorder. Dependent people have difficulty doing things by themselves and in getting things done on their own. They go to great lengths not to be alone and always agree with others for fear of rejection. With a strong need to be liked, dependent people volunteer to do unpleasant or demeaning things to increase their chances of acceptance. They avoid occupations in which they must perform independent functions.

Affective characteristics center around fears of rejection and abandonment. They feel totally helpless when they are alone. Dependent people are easily hurt by criticism and disapproval and are devastated when close relationships end. These fears contribute to a chronic sense of anxiety and they may develop depression.

Cognitively, dependent people have a severe lack of self-confidence and belittle their abilities and assets. They are unable to make everyday decisions without an excessive amount of advice and reassurance from others and often allow others to make important decisions for them.

Socioculturally, those with dependent personality disorder desire constant companionship because they feel so helpless when they are alone. Since they passively resist making decisions, they often force their spouses or partners into making decisions such as where to live, where to work, with whom to socialize and in what activities to participate (Gunderson, 1988).

> *Alice, a 39-year-old homemaker, calls her mother daily. Alice's mother lives less than a mile from her, and they sometimes spend the day together watching television. Alice never makes any decisions, leaving everything to her husband Gene. She will not go anywhere unless Gene or her mother go with her. Alice relies on her mother to help her pick out clothing for the children and for herself. Alice feels she has no taste and is too stupid to know what the children would like.*

Obsessive-Compulsive Personality Disorder. Perfectionism and inflexibility are essential *behavioral* features of obsessive-compulsive personality disorder. The need to check and recheck objects and situations demands much of these people's time and energy. They are industrious workers, but because of their need for routine they are usually not creative and may fail to complete projects because of unattainable standards. No accomplishment ever seems good enough.

Obsessive-compulsive people are polite and formal in social situations, which allows them to maintain emotional distance from others. They are very protective of their status and material possessions, so they have difficulty freely sharing with other people.

The primary *affective* characteristic is one of inability to express emotions. To alleviate the anxiety of helplessness and powerlessness, obsessive-compulsive people need to feel in control. Total control means that emotions, both tender and hostile, must be held in check or denied, which decreases their emotional experiences. Life and interpersonal relationships are intellectualized. The blocking of feelings and emotional distance are attempts to avoid losing control over themselves and their environment.

Because defenses are rarely adequate to manage anxiety, these people develop a number of fears. They fear disapproval and condemnation from others, and for that reason avoid taking risks. They dread making mistakes and when mistakes occur they experience a high level of guilt and self-recrimination, thus becoming their own tormentors. Obviously, losing control is also feared. Rules and regulations are an attempt to remain in control at all times. Still fearful that things could go wrong, obsessive-compulsive people invent rituals in an attempt to ensure constancy and increase their feelings of security. As they try to control fear with a narrow focus on details and routines, the need for order and routine escalates.

Cognitively, obsessive-compulsive people have difficulty making decisions. Procrastination and indecision are common, because they would rather avoid commitments than experience failure. Before making a decision, they accumulate many facts and try to figure out all the potential outcomes of any particular decision. When a decision finally is made, doubts and fears that an alternative decision would have been better plague the obsessive-compulsive person. Since there is a constant striving to be perfect in all things, doing nothing is often considered better than doing something imperfectly.

Questioned as to how they view themselves, obsessive-compulsive people say they are conscientious, loyal, dependable, and responsible—descriptions that are in conflict with an underlying low self-esteem and beliefs of inadequacy.

In the *sociocultural* area, obsessive-compulsive people's need for control extends into interpersonal relationships. Regarding themselves as omnipotent (all-powerful) and omniscient (all-knowing), they expect their opinions and plans to be acceptable to everyone else; compromise is hardly considered. Frequent demands on their families to cooperate with their rigid rules and detailed routines undermine feelings of intimacy within the family system. For obsessive-compulsive people to see that other family members have their own, perhaps completely different, needs and styles of coping is difficult. Since they view dependency as being out of control and under the domination of the partner, they may abuse or oppress their partners so that an illusion of power and control can be maintained.

When interacting, obsessive-compulsive people have an overintellectual, meticulous, detailed manner of speaking that is designed to increase feelings of security. They unconsciously use language to confuse the listener. By bringing in side issues and focusing on nonessentials, they distort the content of the subject, which is a source of great frustration to the listener (Reid, 1989).

Jim, a 42-year-old midlevel executive for a food processing plant, is always in trouble with the plant manager because he fails to get reports in on time. Jim blames his secretary for the problem, saying "I can't get anything done right unless I do it myself." However, Jim's secretary promptly types exactly what he gives her. Jim then adds new details and reorganizes the report, and she has to type a new version. Jim keeps all the drafts of the report and documents the time it takes for the secretary to type them. This he stores in a file that only he is allowed to use. Jim lost his "to do" list one morning and had his secretary help him try to find it for over half an hour. Jim yelled at the secretary when she suggested that he try to remember what was on the list.

Passive-Aggressive Personality Disorder. The primary *behavioral* characteristic of passive-aggressive disorder is passive resistance to requests and demands from others. It is very manipulative interpersonal behavior. These individuals assume a role of chronic submissiveness and compliance but beneath this facade is a great deal of anger and a refusal to comply with requests.

There are many varieties of passive aggression. One form is forgetting. Chronic forgetters are unable to assert themselves openly by saying no. Instead they passively agree to everything and then forget to do it. Forgetfulness is selective to situations that are unimportant to them but important to others. Another form of passive aggression is chronic misunderstanding, which is expressed with a pretense of sincerity. They say, "Oh my, I thought you meant . . ." as the other person experiences acute frustration. Procrastination is a very common form of passive aggression. Chronic procrastinators either refuse to set a fixed date or time or passively refuse to accomplish what was agreed to. Additionally, they attempt to make others feel guilty about their requests by saying, "Slow down. You're too hyper. You'll never live long at this rate." People who are chronically late are indirectly expressing their hostility toward those kept waiting. The message to others is, "I am more important than you, you will just have to wait." Typically, these latecomers are very creative with excuses for their behavior. Some passive aggressors express their hostility by never learning from previous experiences. They force others to request the same thing over and over. They may know that the garbage has to go out every day but passively force the partner to verbalize the request every single time. The frustration is increased when they add, "Calm down. If you want me to do it, just ask me."

In all forms of passive-aggressive behavior, there is a verbal expression of compliance or agreement. Passive aggressors achieve an inner sense of satisfaction when they do not comply and their victims are left irritated and frustrated.

Affectively, passive-aggressive people appear concerned, interested, and sympathetic. However, there is an underlying tone of hostility that contradicts the superficial message. The passive behavior is the only way they know to express hostility. They fear overt expression of anger and conflict, believing that will lead to rejection and isolation.

Cognitively, passive aggressors lack self-confidence. They have little insight into their behavior and usually believe they are doing a better job than others seem to think. There is little recognition that their behavior is responsible for their interpersonal difficulties.

Socioculturally, passive aggressors are very manipulative in presenting themselves as innocent and well intentioned. Their victims end up feeling guilty and hesitant to confront them for fear of being accused of bullying behavior. Family and friends of passive aggressors need to set limits on, and consequences for, this irritating behavior (Reid, 1989).

> *Marilyn, a 45-year-old community college instructor, irritates her colleagues by procrastinating in everything she does. Each semester the bookstore manager has to call Marilyn several times to get her book order. Marilyn brings her exams to be typed the afternoon she plans to give them. She forgets faculty meetings. Marilyn didn't speak to her department chair for several weeks after finding out she had to teach a class she didn't want to teach. She told one of her colleagues, "I'm one of the best teachers here and that old dingbat makes me teach a section I hate!" Marilyn goes on to say, "I'll show the old goat. I'll show up to class only when I feel like it. Let him find a substitute!"*

Personality Disorder Not Otherwise Specified The category "**personality disorder not otherwise specified**" is used when a person does not meet the full criteria for any one personality disorder, yet there is significant impairment in social or occupational functioning or in subjective distress (American Psychiatric Association, 1987).

Causative Theories

As with other psychiatric disorders, a number of theories have been offered to identify the causes of personality disorders. With continuing refinement of diagnostic criteria for each category of personality disorder, it will become possible to conduct useful research on specific populations that have been accurately diagnosed. In the past wide differences in the application of specific diagnostic labels precluded the gathering of reliable data. Since there was so little agreement about whether a person should be included in the category at the outset, it is easy to understand why the search for any common factors—in genetics, early experiences, family patterns, or any other variables—failed to yield results from which general conclusions could be drawn.

Remaining obstacles are the refusal to seek treatment on the part of the client and the relatively infrequent need for psychiatric hospitalization. This has greatly limited research to those persons seeking therapy (most often borderline personality disorder) or those being referred through the criminal system (most often antisocial personality disorder).

Genetic Theory The perspective that aberrant behavior is biologically or genetically determined has been investigated in relation to the whole category of personality disorders. The most convincing study (Vaillant and Perry, 1985) has been done in the United States. The researchers divided 15,000 pairs of twins into two groups, identical and fraternal. Each set of siblings was reared in their own home, so that each member of the pair was exposed to the same environment, parenting style, and so forth. By controlling the variables of environment and parenting, the variable of heredity could be more accurately examined. In the group of identical twins, the incidence of a personality disorder existing in both twins was considerably greater than in the group of fraternal twins. This incidence is known as a *concordance rate,* and it points to the possibility of a genetic link in the transmission of personality disorders. Although this research does suggest that heredity plays a part in personality disorders, more research is needed.

Studies of adoptive twins indicate there may be a genetic predisposition to antisocial personality disorder. Biologic relatives demonstrate a higher rate of incidence than that of the general population for both antisocial behavior and alcohol abuse. There is also a higher incidence of antisocial personality disorder in children of convicted felons than in control children in adoptee studies. At this time it is difficult to sort out genetic from family and environmental factors (Gerstley, 1990; Gunderson, 1988; Reid, 1986).

Psychodynamic Theory Those persons experiencing Cluster A personality disorders (paranoid, schizoid, schizotypal) have been studied minimally, since they seldom request or are forced into treatment. Psychodynamic theory suggests that the primary defense mechanism is one of projection, that is, they project their own hostility on others and respond to them in a fearful and distrustful manner. Additionally, it is thought that they defensively withdraw from others for fear they will be hurt (Gunderson, 1988).

With the Cluster B disorders (narcissistic, histrionic), psychodynamic theory focuses on the parent-child relationship. Johnson (1987, p. 52) describes the parental message to the child: "Don't be who you are, be who I need you to be. Who you are disappoints me, threatens me, angers me, overstimulates me. Be what I want and I will love you." Johnson goes on to say that the child is forced to reject the real self and develop a false self. Individuation is prevented when the child is forced to become the idealized person the parents desire. As adults, these individuals become grandiose in an attempt to live up to exaggerated parental expectations. In an attempt to prove the false self to others and compensate for the rejected real self, these people focus on having the right clothes, home, car and career. Perfectionist standards become the defense against unrealistic expectations.

Psychodynamic theory explains antisocial personality disorder as a developmental delay or failure. It is believed that these individuals have an underdeveloped superego, in that authority and cultural morals have not been internalized. With an inadequate superego, conformity to cultural expectations is situational and superficial, and there is an inability to experience guilt when rules are violated (Kegan, 1986).

Borderline personality disorder is viewed as a failure in ego development occurring during the early childhood stage of separation-individuation. During the symbiotic period of age 2 to 6 months, infants experience parents as part of themselves. From 6 to 36 months infants begin to individuate, that is, to develop boundaries between parents and themselves. They begin to see parents as both gratifying and frustrating and learn to live with these conflicting emotions. Inconsistent parenting that alternates between clinging to and withdrawing from the infant is believed to contribute to borderline personality disorder. As adults, these individuals struggle with the fear of losing themselves in an intimate relationship, while desiring nurturance at the same time. To decrease anxiety and shame, feelings of uselessness, lack of worth, and hostility are projected onto others (Everett, 1989; Fine, 1989).

Environmental Theory Cluster B personality disorders (antisocial, borderline, histrionic, and narcissistic) may be a response to society's increasing complexity. Some believe that industrialization, for example, has contributed to a changing value system. Thus, we recognize values such as: personal needs are more important than group needs; expediency is more important than morality; and appearance is more important than inner worth. With additional upheavals such as political and religious scandals and the threat of nuclear holocaust or chemical warfare, some people learn to distrust authority figures and focus on personal survival. Those with Cluster B personality disorders believe that survival depends solely on themselves and they develop a value system of "Every person for herself or himself" and "Take care of number 1 first" (Gunderson, 1988; Reid, 1986).

Recent research is focusing on emotional, physical, and sexual abuse during childhood as a primary cause of borderline personality disorder. Initial data suggests that the rate of abuse among people diagnosed with borderline personality disorder is much higher than the general population. Since more women were childhood victims of abuse than men, this theory accounts for the disproportionate number of women given this diagnosis. In fact, the symptom picture is very similar to adult survivors of child sexual abuse (Chapter 16) and for victims of posttraumatic stress disorder (Chapter 8). Continued research is necessary to identify the components of abuse that contribute to the development of or protection from borderline traits. Some of these components may be: age at time of abuse, duration of abuse, number of abusers, relationship with abuser, peer relationships, family interaction, and community support systems. Failure to recognize that these individuals are adult survivors of sexual abuse will result in ineffective treatment approaches (Kroll, 1988; Shearer, 1990).

Family Theory Those individuals with antisocial personality disorder are thought to come from families with inconsistent parenting that resulted in emotional deprivation of the children. Because of their own personality or substance abuse problems, parents may be unable to supervise and discipline their children, or may even model antisocial behavior for the children (Gunderson, 1988; Reid, 1986).

Passive-aggressive personality disorder seems to be related to parental issues with anger and conflict. Normal growth and development includes children's ability to express anger and manage conflict appropriately. In a family where any overt expression of anger is unacceptable to parents and is not tolerated, children learn to express their hostility with subtle rebellious behavior.

Family theorists view borderline personality disorder as a dysfunction of the entire family system across several generations, with similar dynamics of blurred generational boundaries of the incestuous family (See Chapter 16). The borderline personality disorder usually occurs in a family system in which members are immersed in and absorbed by one another. With a high family value on children's loyalty to parents, adult children cling to their parents even after marriage. As a result, the marital couple is unable to attach and bond with one another. When children are born to this couple, the children are encouraged to cling, and normal separation behavior is discouraged. Often the children end up in a caretaking role with parents and must assume a high level of family responsibility. During late adolescence these children are unable to separate from their parents because of an incorporated family theme that separation and loss are intolerable. It is within the third or fourth generation of enmeshed families that borderline traits develop into the personality disorder. Male children with borderline personality disorder tend not to marry and remain connected with their families of origin. Female children with borderline personality disorder often marry, but tend to pick passive and distant partners who are enmeshed with their own families (Everett, 1989).

Medical Treatment

Not uncommonly, those with personality disorders may suffer with another concurrent mental disorder such as depression, an anxiety disorder, or substance abuse problems. Treatment for these disorders is described throughout this text.

At present there is no appropriate medication therapy for those suffering from the personality disorders. Common treatments used today are psychotherapy, family therapy, marital therapy, behavior therapy, and self-help groups. Few of these clients are able to make significant and lasting changes.

Assessment

As with other psychiatric disorders, data collection serves as the starting point for the nursing process for the client with a personality disorder.

The Nursing History

When the nurse suspects a personality disorder, the general history becomes an important part of the knowledge base. For any of the personality disorders, the focused nursing assessment must be based firmly on the nurse's knowledge that there has been a persistence of the identified patterns of behavior over time. By understanding these patterns, the nurse will be able to arrive at the appropriate nursing diagnoses and subsequent plan of care. A focused nursing assessment of the client suspected of a personality disorder follows.

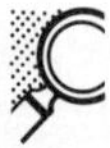

FOCUSED NURSING ASSESSMENT ***for the Client with Personality Disorder***

Social and behavioral history

What is your usual pattern of daily activities?
Describe any anxiety in conjunction with completing these activities.
Describe how you are responsible for your own behavior.
Has anyone ever told you your behavior was a problem? If so, what did they tell you?
How do you usually relate to others?
When do you prefer to be alone?
When do you prefer to be with others?
What causes you to become upset with others?
How do you resolve conflicts with others?
Describe any problematic behavior you displayed as a teenager.
Describe any unsuccessful attempts you have had in trying to modify your behavior patterns.

Emotional history

Do others ever describe you as detached, cold, or aloof? If so, what do they say?
Describe the differences in your business and social relationships.
Describe your sensitivity to others: Are you affectionate, empathetic, etc.?
How do you react to criticism?
How many close relationships with others do you have? Describe the relationships.
How often are you rejected or feel you are rejected by others?
Describe your feelings when in a group. Are you anxious?
Describe your usual mood.
How often do you feel people make fun of you?
Would you describe yourself as dependent or independent?

Cognitive and perceptual history

Have you ever been told that your ideas are illogical by your friends or others? If so, describe their comments.
Have you ever heard voices? If so, describe the voices.
Have you ever been concerned about being harmed by others? If so, describe the incident(s).
Describe how you view yourself. Are you better than, the same, or not as good as the next person?
How often do you worry about making mistakes?
How important are details when you are completing an assignment for work or school?
Are you more efficient, less efficient, or as efficient as other people?
When people do you favors, how important is it to you to return the favor?

Physical and motor history

What physical symptoms worry you?
What do you do for headaches?
What do you do for muscle pains?
What do you do for (other symptoms listed by the client)?
What medications do you take regularly? How do these medications help you?

When do you usually eat? How many meals? Snacks? How much and what kind of fluid?
How much do you sleep in 24 hours? When do you sleep? Do you take naps? How do you feel after sleeping?
How much physical activity do you do during a week? What kinds of activities do you enjoy most? Least?
How often do you engage in sexual activity?
Have you ever been diagnosed as epileptic? If so, what type?
Describe your general health.

The Nurse's Emotional Response to the Client

The next area to consider is the nurse's emotional response to the client. Since it is uncommon for clients to identify their personality as troublesome, the first clue the nurse may have is his or her emotional reaction to the client. On careful examination of the feelings that surface during and after contacts with the client, the nurse may consider the possibility that similar responses are evoked in others as well. However, it is essential that nurses understand themselves well enough not to misinterpret the origin of the difficulty. It could be that the nurse's own anger, frustration, or irritation existed before the encounter with the client and that the client is merely the vehicle for its emergence.

The Client's Subjective Perceptions

The next area to assess includes the client's perceptions, feelings, and behaviors. The main obstacle to the nurse in conducting this component of the assessment is the probability that the client will not perceive that a problem exists. In exploring the client's perceptions of relationships with others, the nurse can determine first whether any close relationships exist and, if so, the duration and quality of these relationships. This information will help indicate the degree to which the client is capable of establishing significant, mature, and enduring relationships with others.

To maintain an alliance with the client, the nurse needs to be sensitive in the interview so that the client does not become guarded or defensive. The nurse should consider relationships from all areas of a client's present life and past experience to discover themes around issues such as trust, dependence, isolation, impulsivity, exploitation, control, and so forth. The client's sphere of activity will indicate which persons to consider: family members, spouse or other long-term relationships, friends, or coworkers.

The two main themes to identify and understand about all the client's relationships are (1) what the client wants from them and why and (2) what the client gets from them and how. Of course, these questions cannot be posed directly, so the nurse must listen carefully as the client presents perceptions and descriptions to discern the answers.

Elsie, a 23-year-old woman hospitalized following a ruptured ectopic pregnancy, has steadily accelerated her demands on the nursing staff since admission. It is now the third postoperative day, and she has insisted on one nurse's undivided attention for most of the morning. The client seems quite theatrical in describing her recent experience to other clients and friends who telephone or visit. Her story seems to grow more dramatic with each telling. The nurse is initially alerted to the situation by two occurrences: her excessive demands on the nursing staff for time and attention and the drama surrounding descriptions of her experience.

After examining his or her own feelings, the nurse concludes that the client's behaviors are atypical and warrant further investigation. The nurse spends 30 minutes in conversation with the client to assess relationships with her spouse, mother, several friends who have been mentioned, children, and neighbors. The nurse accomplishes this by open-ended comments such as, "You seem to have a number of friends," which encourages the client to focus and elaborate. The nurse elicits further detail by encouraging the client to describe how she feels about the friendships—for example, how concerned others are, how aware they are of her needs, and whether these relationships are satisfying to her. It is essential to discover the client's view of what the client gives to these friendships.

The nurse's analysis leads to the conclusion that the client feels the need for constant reassurance from her friends, seems to place heavy demands on others for attention, consistently places herself in the center of attention, and appears quite inconsiderate of others' needs. Although these data are limited, they do lend considerable support to the nurse's hypotheses that the client's behaviors represent a longstanding pattern of problematic relating.

Interpersonal Relations with the Client

The fourth area of assessment includes the perception and experience of others who have some degree of intimacy with the client. They may be as close as a spouse or parent or someone slightly more removed, such as a casual friend or employer. The availability of these people for a systematic assessment varies widely, and often the nurse has no direct control over being able to interview any of them. However, in certain clinical situations it may be possible for the nurse to arrange interviews with one or two people closely associated with the client. More typically, the nurse will make use of a serendipitous opportunity to speak with a family member or friend who visits the client. It is imperative that the nurse exercise professional judgment in seeking information from others about their relationships with the client. Although the objective is to obtain a description of the client's functioning within various family and social contexts, the nurse must be certain that the client's rights are protected. By remaining alert to the potential for a breach of confidentiality, the nurse can ensure that neither the legal nor the ethical limits of the professional domain are exceeded. Such questions as, "In your view, how does your wife seem to be handling this?" will open the door to permit further exploration. To gain a broader perspective of the client's pattern of adaptation, the nurse may ask a relative or friend of the client for a comparison between the spouse's view and the client's usual style of coping in everyday situations.

Physical Assessment

As part of the assessment of clients with personality disorders, the nurse needs to be aware of the potential for drug or alcohol abuse. This is particularly true for persons suffering from antisocial, histrionic, or passive-aggressive personality disorders and is thought to be associated with the style of coping that has developed over time.

Persons with passive-aggressive or histrionic personality disorder frequently experience alcohol dependency or abuse as a complication of their emotional illness. Many times, problems associated with the use of alcohol bring the client to the attention of the health care system, and the personality disorder is diagnosed secondarily.

Persons with a diagnosis of antisocial personality disorder constitute a large segment of prison populations and are frequently seen in the courts. Often mental health agencies and personnel become involved by direction of the court rather than in response to a request for services from the client. Nearly 70 percent of those in this diagnostic group have a history of excessive use of alcohol (Kaplan, 1986). Alcohol or drug use may have also played a part in related arrests for assault or violent behavior, vandalism, or driving while intoxicated. A history of polydrug use is also common.

The nurse should include an assessment of the history of drug or alcohol use for any of these clients. (See Chapters 12 and 13 for assessment tools.) When signs of acute intoxication or influence are present, it may be necessary to seek information from the family, friends, or in case of prior legal intervention, the police. If alcohol intoxication was suspected during an arrest, a test to determine blood alcohol content may have been performed. The results of this test will provide the nurse with an estimate of the amount of alcohol consumed before the arrest.

Other obvious signs of recent substance use include changes in the client's neurologic functioning reflected in difficulties in speech, coordination, perception, and cognition. The presence of unidentified capsules, powders, pills, or drug paraphernalia indicate the need for a thorough investigation of the amounts and patterns of use.

To ascertain a client's pattern of drug or alcohol use when there are no manifest signs is more difficult. The nurse is faced with the problem of introducing the topic to the client in a way that does not create defensiveness or evoke denial. One strategy that may prove helpful is to ask the length of time the person has been drinking (or using drugs if this is indicated) rather than to ask if the person uses either of these substances. It is considerably easier for the client to respond negatively to a question like, "Do you drink regularly?" than to a question like, "How long have you been drinking?" (See Chapters 12 and 13 for further information on assessment strategies for alcohol and drug use.)

In addition to considering possible alcohol and substance abuse, the physical assessment must also include a review of the client's history with regard to the presence of temporal lobe epilepsy, since it is associated with the general diagnostic category of personality disorders and seems to influence the severity of behavioral and affective problems.

Nursing Diagnosis and Planning

Nursing diagnoses identify both the probable and potential problems for each category of personality disorders. The nurse needs to remember that no client fits neatly into any theoretically determined diagnostic category and that no standardized list or table can provide a comprehensive description of the problems specific to an individual client. The diagnoses that follow in Table 10–5 can serve as a framework for nursing care, but they cannot replace a comprehensive, individualized assessment of the client.

Clients falling into the general diagnostic category of personality disorders experience many different behavioral and affective problems, so no one standard plan of care can address the entire array of potential problems. Therefore, the nursing diagnoses listed in Table 10–6 review some of the diagnoses common to the client with personality disorder. Although no client is likely to manifest this particular cluster of problems, the care plan will assist the student in applying the nursing process to actual clients.

Nurses should approach persons experiencing Cluster A personality disorders (paranoid, schizoid, schizotypal) in a gentle, interested, and nonintrusive manner that is respectful of the client's need for distance and privacy. Task-oriented groups and sheltered work programs may be helpful for these clients in learning social skills and building relationships.

Clients with Cluster B personality disorders (antisocial, borderline, histrionic, and narcissistic) require much more patience and structure on the part of nurses. The milieu must be one of consistency. Roles of clients and staff, as well as rules concerning appropriate behavior and consequences, must be clearly defined. The desired outcome of this type of milieu is that clients gain ability to delay impulsive actions and thus are able to enhance day-to-day functioning. Clients are encouraged to talk about feelings rather than acting them out impulsively. Peer interactions should be assessed so that nurses can help clients understand how their behavior affects others and modify their maladaptive interpersonal patterns. Clients are encouraged to explore new behaviors to meet their needs in more adaptive ways. Structured, task-oriented groups are useful. Often these groups focus on the practical issues of life, such as nutrition, living arrangements, budgets, employment, and relationships, to increase clients' adaptation outside the hospital environment.

A variety of approaches are appropriate for clients experiencing Cluster C personality disorders (avoidant, dependent, obsessive-compulsive, passive-aggressive). Group therapy helps these clients learn to express feelings and opinions openly. Through the group process they have increased interactions and an opportunity to learn empathy and to give support to others. In individual therapy, gentle confrontation about their avoidance issues is helpful. This helps them identify what they gain

Table 10–5 *Nursing Diagnoses by Personality Disorder Subtype*

Cluster A

Paranoid personality disorder
- Ineffective individual coping related to inability to trust
- Fear related to perceived threats from others or environment
- Potential for noncompliance related to denial of problem

Schizoid personality disorder
- Ineffective individual coping related to self-absorption
- Social isolation related to inability to form relationships
- Fear related to "people phobia"

Schizotypal personality disorder
- Ineffective individual coping related to unusual perceptions and communication
- Social isolation related to lack of empathy
- Impaired thought processes related to peculiar interpretations of stimuli
- Impaired social interaction

Cluster B

Antisocial personality disorder
- Ineffective individual coping related to deviance from social norms and/or manipulation of others
- Potential for violence directed at others related to impulse control deficit
- Potential alteration in parenting related to unmet developmental needs

Borderline personality disorder
- Ineffective individual coping related to unstable mood
- Disturbance in self-concept with personal identity confusion related to splitting
- Potential for violence directed at self related to faulty reality testing

Histrionic personality disorder
- Ineffective individual coping related to extreme emotional reactions
- Powerlessness related to feelings of helplessness
- Potential for sexual dysfunction related to stereotypic gender behaviors

Narcissistic personality disorder
- Ineffective individual coping related to extreme self-centeredness
- Social isolation related to lack of empathy
- Potential for noncompliance related to denial of problem

Cluster C

Avoidant personality disorder
- Ineffective individual coping related to extreme interpersonal sensitivity
- Disturbance in self-concept with reduction in self-esteem related to devaluation of self-achievements
- Impaired social interaction
- Social isolation related to need for approval

Dependent personality disorder
- Ineffective individual coping related to inability to function independently
- Disturbance in self-concept with reduction in self-esteem related to lack of self-confidence
- Fear related to feelings of abandonment

Obsessive-compulsive personality disorder
- Ineffective individual coping related to rigidity
- Disturbance in self-concept with reduction in self-esteem related to fear of making a mistake
- Potential for traumatic injury related to reactive depression

Passive-aggressive personality disorder
- Ineffective individual coping related to inadequate role performance
- Potential for traumatic injury related to reactive depression
- Potential for noncompliance related to resistance

from avoiding anxiety, anger, or open conflict. Additional nursing interventions include teaching socialization skills, problem-solving skills, and assertiveness training.

Evaluation

Expected outcomes serve to forecast results of nursing intervention. Before evaluation, it is important for the nurse to determine the length of time necessary to pursue the proposed intervention before evaluating its effectiveness. Since problems associated with personality disorders have been in place for a long time, they are unlikely to yield readily to intervention strategies. The nurse may need to define incremental steps to forecast eventual improvement. The nurse should not abandon a valid intervention before there has been sufficient opportunity for it to effect change.

When no improvement occurs, the nurse needs to decide whether it is the intervention that is

(continues page 393)

Table 10–6 Nursing Care Plan for the Client with Personality Disorder

Nursing Diagnosis: Ineffective individual coping related to inability to function independently.
Goal: During the course of treatment client will operationally define independent functions.

Intervention	*Rationale*	*Expected Outcome*
Acknowledge client's feelings of helplessness	Recognition of feelings promotes a working relationship with client and conveys empathy	Identifies wishes and preferences
Set limits by defining amount of time you will give to client	Client will understand that nurse will be available in consistent and predictable times in a structured relationship	
Work with client to identify his or her preferences in two situations	Independent decision making is a skill client does not possess and needs to develop	Expresses opinions in appropriate settings
Role-play assertive behaviors in one situation	Practice in nonthreatening situation increases self-confidence and the likelihood of testing new behavior	Demonstrates effective way of functioning
Plan time to test new behaviors	Conveys collaboration and makes exercises real	
Remain with client during and after implementation of new techniques	Withdrawing support from client would lead to false conclusion that independent actions result in abandonment	
Help client improve skills based on performance in practice: • set daily expectations • work with client to determine what tasks client wishes to perform daily • elicit feedback from client on work completed	Increased effectiveness will help client gain pleasure from knowing what he or she wants and getting it; fostering independence will assist client in changing behavior	Engages in appropriate assertive behaviors to satisfy needs

Nursing Diagnosis: Ineffective individual coping related to deviance from social norms and/or manipulation of others.
Goal: During the course of treatment client will attempt to conform to accepted social standards of the agency.

Intervention	*Rationale*	*Expected Outcome*
Initiate a one-to-one relationship with client	Will assist client in learning to relate to others	Attempts to participate in treatment
Clearly communicate by: • matter-of-factly stating unit routines and expectations • keeping focus on client behaviors • setting limits on behaviors • confronting client with his or her behaviors • validating reality for client • direct client to discuss problems he or she believes he has with a staff member, with that staff member	Will assist client in keeping behavior within acceptable limits	Does not play one staff member against another

(Diagnosis continued)

Table 10–6 *(continued)*

Nursing Diagnosis *(continued):* Ineffective individual coping related to deviance from social norms and/or manipulation of others.
Goal: During the course of treatment client will attempt to conform to accepted social standards of the agency.

Intervention	*Rationale*	*Expected Outcome*
Set limits on manipulative behavior: • clearly state behavioral expectations • prevent client from harming others • tell client you will not stretch rules • be firm and consistent • avoid arguing with client • validate information if client tells you another staff member gave permission • refer client to the staff member who has jurisdiction over situation	Setting limits reduces the manipulation of staff by client	Attempts to follow unit rules

Nursing Diagnosis: Impaired social interaction related to poor impulse control.
Goal: During the course of treatment the client will reduce aggression and manipulation of others.

Intervention	*Rationale*	*Expected Outcome*
Assess aggressive and manipulative behaviors	Assists in identifying behaviors in need of change	Identifies aggressive and manipulative acts
Confront aggressive and manipulative behavior	Assists client in recognizing inappropriate behaviors	States consequences of aggressive and manipulative behavior
Identify consequences of continued aggressive and manipulative behavior	Makes client aware of effects of behavior on self and others	Attempts to use constructive behaviors
Explore constructive ways of coping with social situations when aggressive or manipulative behavior is used	Client learns new coping skills with which to replace maladaptive behaviors	
Evaluate and give feedback to client when he or she attempts to use more constructive social behaviors	Reinforces socially acceptable behaviors and assists client in identifying effective behaviors	

Nursing Diagnosis: Impaired social interaction related to disorganized thinking.
Goal: During the course of treatment the client will identify feelings that lead to poor social interaction.

Intervention	*Rationale*	*Expected Outcome*
Establish a one-to-one relationship with the client	Learning to interact with a nurse will assist client in learning to interact with a person in a new situation	Verbalizes any discomfort in interacting with nurse and other staff
Assist client in participating in social interactions	Removes the opportunity for the client to isolate self from others	Attempts to verbalize with nurse and other staff
Explore effects of client behaviors on social interactions	Assists client in understanding how others perceive him or her	Identifies behaviors that interfere with social interactions
Develop a schedule for client's participation in specific social interactions	A regular schedule assists in reducing client anxiety about social interactions	Willingly attends and participates in group activities

(continued)

Table 10–6 *(continued)*

Nursing Diagnosis: Impaired social interaction related to lack of self-esteem.
Goal: During the course of treatment the client will make changes in social behaviors and improve interpersonal relationships.

Intervention	*Rationale*	*Expected Outcome*
Assess client's social interaction patterns	Understanding usual coping patterns assists in developing new patterns	Verbalizes patterns of social interactions
Assist client in identifying patterns that cause discomfort	Assists in identifying patterns in need of change	Verbalizes feelings related to social interaction patterns
Use role playing to assist in the development of new interaction patterns	Practicing new behaviors makes client more comfortable in their use	Participates in activities to learn new interaction patterns
Identify negative factors in self-concept	Assists client in identifying areas of change needed in self-concept	Identifies positive areas of self-concept

Nursing Diagnosis: Social isolation related to inability to form relationships.
Goal: During the course of treatment client will begin at least one new relationship.

Intervention	*Rationale*	*Expected Outcome*
Assess client's pattern of social interactions	Assists the nurse in remembering that longstanding problems are slow to change	Verbalizes enjoyment from interactions
Offer self as a person with whom client can begin a relationship	Nurse can be objective, trustworthy, and undemanding	Seeks company of another person on own accord
Set aside time each day to spend with client	Building trust allows freedom for client to risk contact	Plans to develop new relationships
Begin where client is; do not demand a level of interaction for which client is not ready	Forcing complex interactions beyond level of client's social skills defeats purpose of interactions	
When client is ready, invite one other person to join in a nonthreatening, noncompetitive activity (eg, looking at a magazine, watching TV)	Nurse's support allows expansion of social group	

Nursing Diagnosis: Potential for violence: directed at others related to impulse control deficit.
Goal: During the course of treatment client will maintain behavior within defined limits of environment.

Intervention	*Rationale*	*Expected Outcome*
Define rules of conduct, consequences for violation, and means of negotiation to change rules (eg, weekly staff meetings only)	Potential for violence is reduced when structure is imposed on environment	Verbalizes knowledge of rules of conduct
Ensure that all staff members know and agree on rules, consequences, and procedures to modify	Staff's consistency prevents client from creating confusion	States that he or she is in a secure, consistent environment
Provide information to client about rules; use a written contract	Prevents possibility of client not knowing rules and consequences	Behavior remains within appropriate limits

(Diagnosis continued)

Table 10–6 *(continued)*

Nursing Diagnosis *(continued)*: Potential for violence: directed at others related to impulse control deficit.
Goal: During the course of treatment client will maintain behavior within defined limits of environment.

Intervention	*Rationale*	*Expected Outcome*
Firmly, kindly, and consistently enforce limits according to predetermined criteria	Consistency provides safety and structure and allows client to experience consequences of actions	
If behavior becomes violent: • use more than one nurse if the situation warrants • remove client to a quiet area • talk to client about feelings • let client know you will provide control • stay with client, remain calm	Imposing structure and control aids in reducing violence	

Nursing Diagnosis: Disturbance in self-concept: self-esteem related to lack of self-confidence.
Goal: During the course of treatment client will work on developing a realistic sense of self-worth.

Intervention	*Rationale*	*Expected Outcome*
Recognize that "difficult" behaviors often result from low self-esteem	Nurse may avoid "difficult" client or feel annoyed by behaviors if the underlying cause is not recognized	Demonstrates more socially acceptable behavior
Spend brief amounts of time with client in addition to times client requests attention	Conveys your belief in the client's intrinsic worth; prevents client from feeling ignored and devalued	States that he or she feels valued
Anticipate client's needs and meet these before a request is made	Builds client's self-esteem by recognizing client's worth	States acceptance of self
Convey respect for client by listening, encouraging, and supporting		
Plan activities in which client can succeed and demonstrate ability (eg, going for a walk)	Provides an opportunity for client to succeed	Demonstrates improved self-esteem
Offer realistic praise and recognition for accomplishments	Genuine praise for real success can translate to real-life situations	

Nursing Diagnosis: Ineffective individual coping related to inability to trust.
Goal: While in the hospital environment client will state feelings of safety and comfort.

Intervention	*Rationale*	*Expected Outcome*
Provide information about normal hospital routines (eg, visiting, meals, etc)	Creates a climate of openness, which will increase client's feeling of security	Decreased level of suspicion
Identify personnel to client by title, name, and role	Diminishes opportunity for doubt in client	
Be punctual and reliable in keeping commitments made to client	Provides stable relationship with nurse and promotes trust	States feelings of security

(Diagnosis continued)

Table 10–6 *(continued)*

Intervention	*Rationale*	*Expected Outcome*
Keep communication clear, unambiguous, direct, and open	Reduces the potential for misinterpretation	
Avoid behaviors that could be interpreted as secretive or deceptive: • make matter-of-fact statements • give honest responses • be consistent • don't make promises that cannot be kept	Will reduce any anxiety underlying suspicions	
Honor client's requests whenever possible; if necessary to refuse, be honest	Conveys nurse's respect for client	

Nursing Diagnosis: Ineffective individual coping related to inadequate role performance.
Goal: Throughout the course of treatment client will function according to defined expectations.

Intervention	*Rationale*	*Expected Outcome*
Develop a warm, trusting relationship with client	Client's behaviors are irritating and can create frustration and anger in staff if no relationship is developed	Reduced resistance to expectations
Recognize resistance to recommended actions as sign of illness, not stubbornness	Growth toward a more mature way of behavior can occur only in response to a positive relationship	States satisfaction in role performance
Define expectations in specific terms (eg, attend OT 3× a week for 1 hr)	Setting clear limits provides structure	
Build system of rewards to recognize compliance with defined expectations	Client must gain more from meeting expectations than from resisting them	
Be objective and neutral in stating and enforcing limits	Limits should not be punitive; punitiveness leads to further resistance	

Nursing Diagnosis: Ineffective individual coping related to inability to ask for help.
Goal: Client will ask for help from others in appropriate situations.

Intervention	*Rationale*	*Expected Outcome*
Have client identify expectations that will occur should help be sought	Client needs to recognize that fear of rejection precludes seeking help	Verbalizes fears of asking for help from others
Use appropriate self-disclosure regarding situations in which help has been sought	Self-disclosure will help client recognize that asking for help need not result in rejection	
Have client role-play how to ask for help in a particular situation	Role playing will increase use of unfamiliar skills	Role-plays asking for assistance
Have client evaluate the situation in terms of feelings when help was sought and how others responded	Client needs to appraise change in behavior and assess the reality of fears	Asks for assistance in a given situation

(continued)

Table 10–6 *(continued)*

Nursing Diagnosis: Ineffective individual coping related to need to always "be right," which keeps others at a distance.
Goal: Client will exhibit less perfectionistic behavior.

Intervention	*Rationale*	*Expected Outcome*
Initiate the learning and change process, without getting caught in an obsessional struggle for control with client	A struggle for control in being right will reinforce client's maladaptive behavior	Appropriately admits to errors in a given situation
Help client accept responsibility for behavior and explore how this affects other people and how others respond	When client sees self more realistically in relation to others, client may be able to behave in a more socially effective manner	Identifies how behavior affects others
Use relevant humor and laughter regarding perfectionism as a relief from tension and anxiety	Humor allows client to risk speaking about need to be right in a socially accepted way without fear of ridicule	Expresses a sense of humor about minor mistakes
Teach that humor used appropriately is a highly valued attribute in this culture	Humor allows pleasure for the self and others and decreases emotional distance	

Nursing Diagnosis: Ineffective individual coping related to verbal manipulation: superficiality, defocusing, getting off the subject.
Goal: Client will stay focused on topic and goals during one-to-one session.

Intervention	*Rationale*	*Expected Outcome*
Move slowly from nonthreatening topics to anxiety-producing topics	If move is made too quickly, client will feel threatened and escalate verbal manipulation	
Note immediately where client introduces extraneous content; point out this behavior, and link the behavior to anxiety	Client needs to clearly identify the verbal responses to increased anxiety	Identifies how superficiality and defocusing are responses to anxiety
Bring client back to the point under discussion, and do not allow digression unless anxiety becomes too intense	Confronting the anxious feelings directly rather than through verbal manipulation will help client manage anxiety more effectively	Increases length of time spent in focusing on goals

Nursing Diagnosis: Ineffective individual coping related to checking and rechecking actions or ritualistic behavior.
Goal: Client will gradually decrease ritualistic behavior.

Intervention	*Rationale*	*Expected Outcome*
Do not explain to client that the behavior is pointless and foolish	Client is aware of behavior, so this would only contribute to feelings of inadequacy and failure	
Modify the environment and schedules so that behavior can be accomplished without interruption of rituals	Support the defense to control anxiety until other coping behaviors can be used	
Implement any necessary safety measures that may be indicated for the behavior (eg, providing dry towels and hand lotion for client who compulsively washes hands)	It is necessary to prevent physical complications resulting from the ritualistic behavior	Physical complications from behavior will not develop

(Diagnosis continued)

Table 10–6 *(continued)*

Intervention	*Rationale*	*Expected Outcome*
Set limits on destructive ritualistic behavior	Client safety must be maintained	
Provide with hospital schedule of activities	Decreases anxiety about the unfamiliar environment	
Follow schedules and fulfill commitments made to client	Demonstrates support for client and fosters development of trust	
Help client identify how the behavior interferes with daily activities	Identification increases motivation for adopting more effective coping behaviors	Identifies problems that result from compulsive behavior
Use appropriate self-disclosure regarding situations where mistakes have been made	Assists client in recognizing that mistakes need not result in humiliation	
Explore what purpose the checking or ritualistic behavior serves	Assists client in identifying that the behavior is an effort to control anxiety	
Problem-solve other behaviors more effective in managing anxiety	As client learns new ways to manage anxiety, compulsive behavior will decrease	Implements other behaviors to manage anxiety

Nursing Diagnosis: Ineffective individual coping related to need to use rules and routines to maintain a steady environment.
Goal: Client will verbalize increased comfort with ambiguity in the environment.

Intervention	*Rationale*	*Expected Outcome*
Accept client's self-concept, and respect personal rights	Instills confidence and feelings of worth and helps client develop adequate self-concepts	
Keep the environment and routines consistent	Prevents anxiety from increasing to unmanageable levels	
Protect client from the need to make decisions until there is increased comfort with the process	Decision making increases anxiety, and the defenses protect client from this anxiety	Makes minor decisions on the basis of logical thought process
Introduce changes slowly and help client through new experiences	Defenses are formed to avoid anxiety and change	Tolerates minor changes without evidence of increased anxiety
Reassure client that the rules and routines will be abandoned when the need for control of self is decreased and self-esteem increased	Client fears rejection by others if rules are broken; disobedience to rules increases guilt and anxiety	
Evaluate new experiences in the here and now rather than on the basis of past experiences	Past experiences may so dominate thinking that new behavior may be evaluated from the past rather than the present	
Develop plans for trying out new solutions to decrease anxiety	If nurse does not guarantee success with new solutions the nurse does not assume responsibility for client's behavior	

(continued)

Table 10–6 *(continued)*

Nursing Diagnosis: Powerlessness related to perfectionistic behavior to guard against inferior feelings.
Goal: Client will exhibit less perfectionistic behavior.

Intervention	*Rationale*	*Expected Outcome*
Link perfectionistic behavior to feelings of anxiety and helplessness	Client will benefit from increased insight into need for this behavior	Verbalizes feelings of anxiety
Explore the fear of being judged inferior by others	Helps client evaluate if this is a realistic appraisal of others' response	
Explore factors in childhood that led to feelings of inadequacy	Helps client understand the relation between childhood experiences and present behavior	
Help client assess self realistically and set appropriate goals	Helps client gain insight into true abilities and limitations	Realistically appraises self
Use appropriate self-disclosure in admitting to deficiencies	Assists client in recognizing that this need not result in humiliation	
Assign client to make three purposeful mistakes a day and to record feelings in response to the mistakes (eg, setting the table incorrectly, giving wrong directions, putting postage stamps on upside down)	Increases client's sense of control over errors and helps client recognize that many mistakes are not serious	Practices mistakes in a controlled setting
Provide feedback for changes client makes	Reinforces behavior and increases client's ability to accurately appraise self	
Help client to acknowledge that an anxiety-free life is impossible	Client needs to give up striving for perfection	

Nursing Diagnosis: Powerlessness related to overuse of intellectualization and denial of emotions to support sense of control.
Goal: Client will decrease frequency of intellectualization.

Intervention	*Rationale*	*Expected Outcome*
Move slowly from content to feeling level	Confronting feelings creates anxiety; client needs to feel safe before giving up denial system	
Focus on the here and now	Allows for the least distortion, and present is more available for emotional reactions	Expresses feelings when they occur
Help client to identify and label feelings as they occur	This process will assist client in abandoning denial system	Verbalizes decreased anxiety when confronting feelings
Help client connect feelings with intellectual description of events	Decreases use of intellectualization as an ineffective defense	
Role-play expression of feelings	Helps client change defensive behavior patterns in a safe situation	
Explore the issue of emotional consideration in the decision-making process	Helps client understand that many decisions are based on taste or preference rather than on factual data	Considers emotions in the decision-making process

(Diagnosis continued)

Table 10–6 *(continued)*

Intervention	*Rationale*	*Expected Outcome*
Use appropriate humor and laughter	Humor will increase client's ability to be spontaneous and will increase pleasure	
When client talks as if emotions are understood but continues to deny feelings, point out this process	Provides immediate feedback to enable client to learn to modify behavior	

Nursing Diagnosis: Disturbance in self-concept: self-esteem related to fear of being exposed as worthless resulting in perfectionistic standards.
Goal: Client will verbalize feelings of competency and increased self-esteem.

Intervention	*Rationale*	*Expected Outcome*
Adapt environment to avoid situations in which client could be humiliated	Client's defenses need to be protected until able to employ more adaptive coping behavior	
Let client set pace for self-disclosure	If the connection between fear of worthlessness and perfect standards is made too early in the process, client will attempt to prove nurse wrong	Verbalizes fear of being inadequate
Find familiar activities at which client can be successful	Decreases the frustration of not being perfect with unfamiliar activities	
Provide realistic feedback about talents and positive qualities	As self-esteem improves, client will be better able to withstand attacks against defenses	
Explore the value of human qualities apart from degree of perfection	Helps client decrease the use of perfection as means of validating self and thereby decreases anxiety	Realistically appraises self
Explore how perfectionism is uncomfortable and what client fears is the worst thing that will occur with failure	Helps client put failure in a realistic perspective and thereby decreases anxiety	Identifies fears of failure
Assign client to make three purposeful mistakes a day and to record feelings in response to the mistakes (eg, cooking steaks rare instead of medium, purchasing something not needed at the grocery store)	Helps client take risks, face the possibility of failure, and recognize there is no demand to be perfect all the time	Tolerates mistakes without high anxiety

Nursing Diagnosis: Alteration in thought processes related to egocentricity and grandiose self-beliefs to defend against anxiety.
Goal: Client will exhibit decreased egocentricity and grandiose self-beliefs.

Intervention	*Rationale*	*Expected Outcome*
When exhibition of grandiose behavior occurs, redirect client to other activities or discussion	Redirection will prevent continued focus on problematic behavior	Substitutes other activities for grandiose behavior

(Diagnosis continued)

Table 10–6 *(continued)*

Nursing Diagnosis *(continued)*: Alteration in thought processes related to egocentricity and grandiose self-beliefs to defend against anxiety.
Goal: Client will exhibit decreased egocentricity and grandiose self-beliefs.

Intervention	*Rationale*	*Expected Outcome*
Help client find significance in people and situation outside self	This process will decrease egocentricity and increase interpersonal interactions	Interacts appropriately with others
Don't compete with or directly contradict grandiose statements	Such conflict would assault client's defenses and increase anxiety	
Use appropriate self-disclosure in that being human and fallible need not result in rejection or humiliation	Increased insight enables client to replace defenses with more effective coping behavior	
Help client assess strengths and limitations and verbalize self-doubts	As anxiety decreases, realistic self-appraisal will assist client in giving up egocentricity	Verbalizes decreased anxiety about self-doubts

Nursing Diagnosis: Alteration in thought processes related to indecision and doubting decisions to avoid the anxiety of failure.
Goal: Client will verbalize increased ease in making decisions.

Intervention	*Rationale*	*Expected Outcome*
Do not make unnecessary decisions for client	If done, this will reinforce client's view of self as inadequate and a failure	
Point out destructive effects of indecision	Helps client understand that an imperfect decision may be less harmful than no decision	Identifies negative effect of indecision
Help client recognize that absolute guarantees of the future are unrealistic	Client's need for absolute guarantees interferes with the decision-making process	Verbalizes that future is not guaranteed
Explore how many decisions in life can be remade	Client believes that decisions are always final and therefore fears failure if the "perfect" decision is not made	
Teach the problem-solving process	Increases skills in decision making and helps client see there are a variety of choices that can be made, tested, and evaluated	
Model decision-making behavior	Modeling enables client to see the active process	
Encourage and support client in making decisions	Client needs to test new behavior in a supportive environment	Uses the problem-solving process to make decisions
Give feedback for decisions that client makes	Client needs reinforcement of positive changes in behavior	

(continued)

Table 10–6 *(continued)*

Nursing Diagnosis: Alteration in thought processes related to omniscience of thought.
Goal: Client will verbalize a decrease in omniscience of thought.

Intervention	*Rationale*	*Expected Outcome*
Help client identify anxiety related to omniscience of thought	In the past, client has not connected feelings with beliefs. This connection increases client's insight	Distinguishes between thoughts and actions
Explain that others cannot know client's thoughts unless they are verbalized	Client's underlying fear of being exposed as a failure contributes to fear that people know what client is thinking and are threatening to uncover inadequacies	
Discuss how unverbalized thoughts cannot influence other people or events	Client is fearful of doing harm to someone else through thoughts	Identifies that thoughts cannot harm others
Explore how client's ritualistic acts serve to decrease anxiety when believing self all-powerful	This will increase client's insight into the internal conflict between belief of being powerful and fear of being inadequate	Decreases ritualistic acts of undoing

Nursing Diagnosis: Alteration in family process related to rigidity in functions and roles.
Goal: Family will demonstrate increased flexibility in role functions.

Intervention	*Rationale*	*Expected Outcome*
Have family members share fears and anxieties that the rigid rules serve to protect	Identification of perceptions and belief systems precedes change of rules	Shares fears and anxieties
Help family explore the effect of rigidity on relationships	Rigidity and lack of spontaneity lead to remaining dependent on narrowly defined role structures	Verbalizes how rigid rules affect the family system
Identify family members' roles and functions	Specific identification precedes modification of roles and functions	
Involve family members in planning the changes in roles and functions	Family will function more effectively with increased available options and through use of the process of renegotiation of relationship contracts	Plans reasonable changes in functions and roles

inappropriate or the original nursing diagnosis. A meeting with other colleagues involved in the client's care is a valuable tool in reaching this decision and exploring alternatives.

Behaviorally defined outcomes stated in measurable terms are an additional aid in evaluation. In some cases, this is a simple task. For example, an outcome criterion for the diagnosis of social isolation states, "Client will seek company of a third person on his own." This is a behaviorally defined outcome that could be made even more specific by stating a date for its accomplishment, a specific length of time for the client to spend with this "third person," and so forth. Unfortunately, client goals cannot always be reduced to strict behavioral terms; still, the nurse should try to be as specific as possible.

When a change in the client's affective response is the goal, measurement techniques are much less precise. To obtain data, the nurse can observe cues in nonverbal behavior, such as facial expression or posture. The client's verbalizations about mood state are another source of information. However, the nurse must always consider the potential difficulties inherent in asking a client who has not been sensitive to internal feeling states to verbalize a change in this area. For example, it would be unrealistic to assess the attempt to improve a client's self-esteem by simply asking the client. In spite of the difficulties in evaluating outcomes for affective change, nurses must not abandon efforts to provide corrective emotional experiences for clients. (See Table 10–7 for an example of an evaluation of the care of a client with a personality disorder.)

The case example that follows involves a client with a borderline personality disorder. The nurse and client are in a general hospital setting.

CASE EXAMPLE

A Client with a Borderline Personality Disorder

Cindi Duncan, a 35-year-old divorced woman, was admitted to the hospital for a drug overdose. Cindi had attempted suicide before. During each hospitalization Cindi was very demanding of the staff. Cindi constantly seemed angry. If her breakfast was on time it was "too much food" or the "stupid kitchen workers" got her order mixed up. Cindi seemed to need a nurse in constant attendance.

Nursing History

Location: Medical floor, General Hospital
Client's name: Cindi Duncan Age: 35
Admitting diagnosis: Drug overdose secondary to borderline personality disorder
T=99.5, P=100, R=18, BP=140/80

Health history
Height: 5′3″
Weight: 103 lbs but six months earlier weighed 175 lbs
Allergies: None
Medications: None

Clinical data
Not applicable at this time

Nursing observations
Cindi has been married three times and divorced three times. One child was born from each of these relationships. The youngest son, age 9, is mentally retarded and suffers from seizures. It was the ingestion of this boy's phenobarbital that precipitated this admission. During a diagnostic evaluation, Cindi demonstrated identity confusion problems in several ways. First, she reported a history of dramatic weight changes. When questioned about this extreme weight loss, Cindi reported she frequently went on diets because, "I don't know if I like myself skinny or fat." A second example of identity problems centered on the recent death of her stepfather. Cindi stated that at the time of his death, she wasn't sure whether it had been he or she who had actually died. At the time of his death, Cindi had been thinking of suicide and took a combination of pills in the house. After the funeral, she felt "mixed up about who died." This confusion occasionally recurred. Cindi's behavior on the unit was volatile and unpredictable. She was extremely critical of the staff and responded with intense anger whenever her wishes were not met. At the same time, she reported feelings of loneliness, isolation, and depression. Multiple self-inflicted cigarette burns were noted on Cindi's arms and legs.

Analysis/Synthesis of Data

Concerns	*Nursing Diagnoses*
Impulsiveness	Impaired verbal communication
Unpredictability	Ineffective individual coping
Self-damaging behavior	Disturbance in self-concept: personal identity
Unstable relationships	Social isolation
Lack of control of anger	Ineffective family coping: disabling
Identity confusion	Dysfunctional grieving
Mood swings	Potential for injury: trauma
Loneliness	
Boredom	

Suggested Care Planning Activities

1. Determine the priorities for Cindi's care.
2. Determine the themes related to Cindi's personality disorder.
3. Determine whether Cindi has any support system.
4. Determine the developmental aspects to be considered in Cindi's case.
5. Identify nursing goals for Cindi.
6. Identify the special needs in relation to rehabilitation in Cindi's situation.
7. Suggest some therapeutic communication techniques that may be helpful in dealing with Cindi.
8. List and provide a rationale for nursing interventions in Cindi's care.

Table 10–7 *Example of Evaluation of Nursing Care of a Client with a Personality Disorder*

Plan	*Evaluation*
1. The nurse will acknowledge the client's feelings of helplessness.	On 12/23, the nurse assisted Carmen in wrapping her Christmas packages after Carmen verbalized her frustration at being so stupid that she couldn't even wrap them.
2. The nurse will assist the client by role-playing assertive behaviors in a situation.	On 12/24, the nurse assisted Carmen in verbalizing her wishes about whether to go out on leave for Christmas Eve dinner with her family.
3. The nurse will set limits on the amount of time to be spent with the client.	On 12/25, the nurse told Carmen she would have to wait until everyone had their packages before any assistance could be given for opening Carmen's packages. Carmen calmly waited her turn.

SUMMARY

1. Long-standing problems of behavior, mood, and perception closely woven into the personality constitute a simple description of personality disorder.

2. Nurses are likely to encounter clients with personality disorder in every health care setting.

Knowledge Base

3. The chief behavioral characteristic for the entire category of personality disorders is various manifestations of narcissism.

4. Clients with a personality disorder have a unique ability to "get under the skin" of others.

5. Clients with personality disorders have a pattern of inflexible and maladaptive responses to most interpersonal situations.

6. Clients with personality disorders are ego-syntonic, not disturbed by their own behaviors, and are unable to feel empathy.

7. Cognitively, clients with personality disorders are inflexible and rigid in their responses. It has been said that they are unable to see "the big picture."

8. The causes of personality disorders are unknown. The possibility of genetic origins has been studied inconclusively. Psychodynamic theory focuses on parent-child relationships resulting in altered development of the ego or superego. Childhood sexual abuse appears to be a key factor in borderline disorder as well as intergenerational family system pathology.

9. Common treatments for personality disorders are psychotherapy, family therapy, behavior therapy, and self-help groups.

Subtypes of Personality Disorder

10. The subtypes of personality disorders are divided into three clusters: Cluster A includes paranoid, schizoid, and schizotypal; Cluster B includes antisocial, borderline, histrionic, and narcissistic; and Cluster C includes avoidant, dependent, obsessive-compulsive, and passive-aggressive.

11. The term *paranoid personality disorder* refers to the client who is suspicious and secretive with pathologic jealousy.

12. *Schizoid personality disorder* refers to the client who has a tendency to be emotionally cold and aloof and has very few friends.

13. *Schizotypal personality disorder* refers to the client with oddities of thought, perception, speech, and behavior.

14. *Antisocial personality disorder* refers to the client with antisocial behavior manifested by consistent violation of the rights of others as well as the rights of society.

15. *Borderline personality disorder* refers to the client with a pattern of instability in self-image, interpersonal relationships, and mood.

16. *Histrionic personality disorder* refers to the client who is overdramatic, reactive, and intensely expressive.

17. *Narcissistic personality disorder* refers to the client with an exaggerated sense of achievement and talent who focuses on what the client sees as the unique nature of personal problems.

18. *Avoidant personality disorder* refers to the client who is shy, introverted, lacking in self-confidence, and extremely sensitive to rejection.

19. *Dependent personality disorder* refers to the client who defers to the judgment, desires, and decisions of others.

20. *Compulsive personality disorder* refers to the client who is seen by others as cold, methodic, stubborn, and controlling.

21. *Passive-aggressive personality disorder* refers to the client who procrastinates, finds fault, indirectly expresses resistance, and performs inadequately.

22. *Personality disorder not otherwise specified* refers to the client who fits the general criteria for the category of personality disorder but does not meet the specific criteria of any of the subtypes.

Assessment

23. The focused nursing assessment must be based firmly on the nurse's knowledge that there has been a persistence of the identified patterns of behavior over time.

24. It is not uncommon for the nurse to have an emotional reaction to the client because people with personality disorders are difficult to deal with.

25. Clients typically do not perceive that a problem exists within themselves.

26. The nurse must maintain a sensitivity in the interview process so that the client does not become guarded or defensive.

27. It is important to assess the perception and experience of others who have some degree of intimacy with the client. Care must be taken not to violate the rights of the client in obtaining this information.

28. There is a potential for alcohol and drug abuse in clients with a personality disorder, especially clients with antisocial, histrionic, and passive-aggressive subtypes.

29. Ineffective individual coping is the nursing diagnosis common to all subtypes of personality disorder.

30. In evaluating the care of the client with a personality disorder, it is important to remember that the disorder has been in place for a long time and is unlikely to yield readily to intervention strategies. The nurse should give the client sufficient opportunity to change.

CHAPTER REVIEW

1. A behavioral characteristic common to persons with personality disorders from Cluster A is
   - (a) Social isolation
   - (b) Manipulation by the use of narcissism
   - (c) High sociability
   - (d) Impulsive antisocial acts

2. An affective characteristic common to persons with personality disorders from Cluster B is
   - (a) Flat or blunted affect
   - (b) Intense and changing expression
   - (c) Passive affect
   - (d) Minimal expression

3. A cognitive characteristic common to persons with personality disorders from Cluster C is
   - (a) Indecision or poor decisions
   - (b) Lack of long-range plans
   - (c) Procrastination in making decisions
   - (d) Secretiveness in making decisions

4. A person with which of the following personality disorders has a tendency to interpret the actions of others as deliberately demeaning or threatening?
   - (a) Antisocial
   - (b) Dependent
   - (c) Obsessive-compulsive
   - (d) Paranoid

5. The person with which of the following disorders has persistent identity disturbances about major life issues such as self-image, sexual orientation, long-term goals, career choice, types of friends or lovers, and values?
   - (a) Schizoid
   - (b) Avoidant
   - (c) Borderline
   - (d) Passive-aggressive

6. Which one of the following nursing diagnoses is applicable to the client with a borderline personality disorder?
   - (a) Fear related to perceived threats from others or environment
   - (b) Social isolation related to lack of empathy
   - (c) Potential for noncompliance related to denial of problems
   - (d) Ineffective coping related to unstable mood

REFERENCES

American Psychiatric Association: *Diagnostic and Statistical Manual of Mental Disorders,* 3rd ed., revised. American Psychiatric Association, 1987.

Everett C et al.: *Treating the Borderline Family.* Harcourt Brace Jovanovich, 1989.

Fine, R: *Current and Historical Perspectives on the Borderline Patient.* Brunner/Mazel, 1989.

Gerstley LJ et al.: Antisocial personality disorder in patients with substance abuse disorders. *Am J Psychiatry,* 1990. 147(2):173–77.

Gunderson JG: *New Harvard Guide to Psychiatry.* Harvard University Press, 1988.

Johnson SM: *Humanizing the Narcissistic Style.* WW Norton, 1987.

Kaplan CA: The challenge of working with patients diagnosed as having a borderline personality disorder. *Nurs Clin North Am,* 1986. 21(8):429–38.

Kegan RG: The child behind the mask: Sociopathy. In: *Unmasking the Psychopath: Antisocial Personality and Related Syndromes.* Reid WH et al. (editors). WW Norton, 1986. 45–77.

Kroll J: *The Challenge of the Borderline Patient.* WW Norton, 1988.

Reid WH et al.: *Unmasking the Psychopath: Antisocial Personality and Related Syndromes.* WW Norton, 1986.

Reid WH: *The Treatment of Psychiatric Disorders.* Brunner/Mazel, 1989.

Shearer SL et al.: Frequency and correlates of childhood sexual and physical abuse histories in adult female borderline inpatients. *Am J Psychiatry,* 1990. 147(2): 214–16.

Vaillant GE, Perry, JC: Personality disorders. In: *Comprehensive Textbook of Psychiatry,* 7th ed. Vol 1. Kaplan HI, Sadock BJ (editors). Williams & Wilkins, 1985.

Zanarini MC, et al.: Discriminating borderline personality disorder from other anix II disorders. *Am J Psychiatry,* 1990. 147(2):161–67.

SUGGESTED READINGS

Freeman SK: Inpatient management of a patient with borderline personality disorder. *Arch Psychiatr Nurs,* 1988. 2(6):360–65.

Gallop R et al.: How nursing staff respond to the label "borderline personality disorder." *H & CP,* 1989. 40(8): 815–19.

Gorton G, Akhtar S: The literature on personality disorders. *H & CP,* 1990. 41(1):39–51.

Johnson M et al.: Conflicts in the inpatient treatment of the borderline patient. *Arch Psychiatr Nurs,* 1988. 2(5):312–18.

Vaccani JM: Borderline personality and alcohol abuse. *Arch Psychiatr Nurs,* 1989. 3(2):113–19.

Wester CM: Managing the borderline personality. *Nurs Manage,* 1989. 20(2):49–51.

Zanarini MC, et al.: Cognitive features of borderline personality disorder. *Am J Psychiatry,* 1990. 147(1):57–63.

CHAPTER 11

Affective Disorders

KAREN LEE FONTAINE

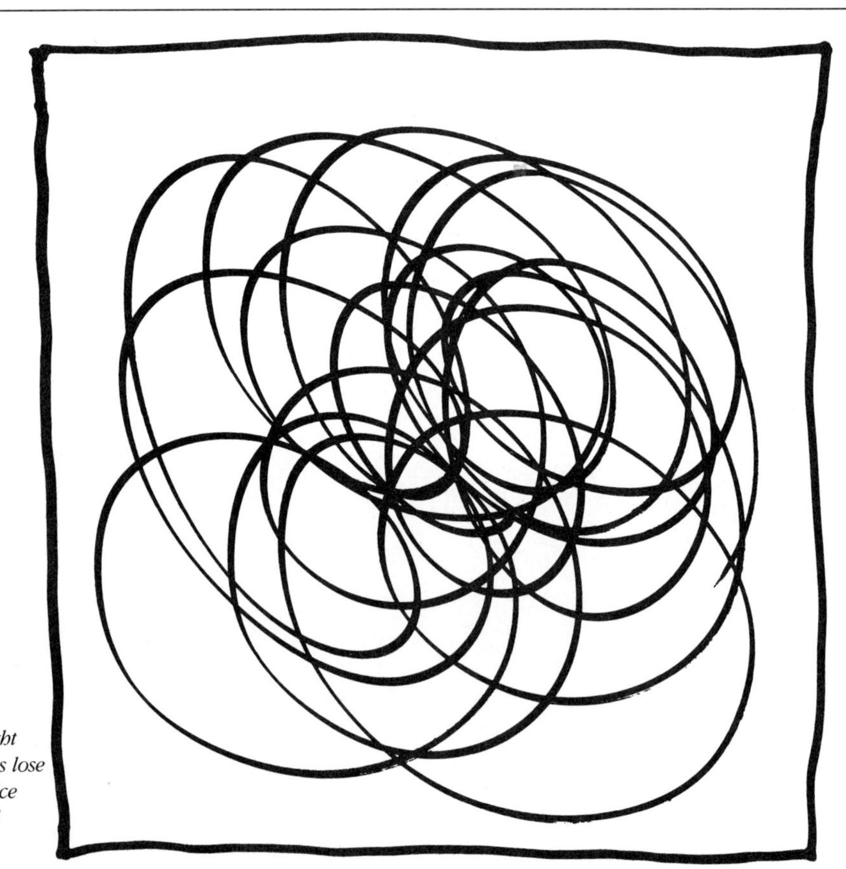

Molecule in an ice cube

When I'm depressed every thought moves so slowly that I sometimes lose it. It's like being encased in an ice cube. No way out of a cold and dark place.

■ *Objectives*

After reading this chapter the student will be able to

- Distinguish among affective disorders across the lifespan
- Compare and contrast a person having unipolar disorders with a person having bipolar disorders
- Analyze sociocultural factors that contribute to the incidence of depression
- Discuss the impact of affective disorders on the family and the family's response
- Explain altered neurotransmission in persons with affective disorders
- Describe alterations in biologic rhythms during affective disorders
- Discuss how the amount of sunlight may contribute to depression
- Discuss how losses and anger are related to depression
- Discuss how negative thinking contributes to depression
- Apply the nursing process to clients experiencing affective disorders

■ *Chapter Outline*

Introduction

Affect is the term used to describe the emotional tone of a person. It is the verbal and nonverbal communication of the person's internal feelings. Verbal cues are words used to describe feelings such as elation, happiness, pleasure, frustration, anger, or hostility. Nonverbal cues to feelings include facial expressions, such as beaming, smiling, frowning, and looking downcast or blank. Another nonverbal cue to feelings is motor activity, such as sitting comfortably and calmly, wringing one's hands, or constantly swinging one's foot. Still another nonverbal cue is physiologic responses, such as profuse sweating, rapid heart rate, and increased respirations. A person may choose not to communicate feelings verbally but to prevent its nonverbal expression is almost impossible.

Descriptors of Affect

A variety of descriptors of affect are used to facilitate communication among health care professionals. **Appropriate affect** indicates the emotional tone is in agreement with the current situation. If a client has an **inappropriate affect**, the emotional tone is not related to the person's immediate circumstances. A **stable affect** is one resistant to sudden changes when there is no provocation in the environment. A **labile affect** denotes sudden shifts in a person's emotional tone that cannot be understood in the context of the situation. An **elevated**

Table 11–1 *Behavioral Examples of Affective Descriptors*

Affect	*Behavior*
Appropriate	Juan cries when learning of the death of his father.
Inappropriate	When learning that her daughter has made the honor roll, Sue begins to scream and curse.
Stable	During a bridge party, Dan smiles and laughs at the appropriate social interchanges.
Labile	During a friendly checker game, Dorothy, who has been laughing, suddenly knocks the board off the table in anger. She then begins to laugh and wants to continue the game.
Elevated	Sean bounces around the dayroom, laughing and singing and telling the other clients how wonderful everything is.
Depressed	Leo sits slumped in a chair with a sad facial expression, teary eyes, and minimal body movement.
Overreactive	Karen screams and curses when her child spills a glass of milk on the kitchen floor.
Blunted	When Tom learns of his full tuition scholarship, he responds with only a small smile.
Flat	When Juanita is told about her best friend's death, she says "Oh" and does not give any indication of an emotional response.

affect refers to a feeling of euphoria, whereas a **depressed affect** indicates feelings of despondency or sadness. An **overreactive affect** is appropriate to the situation but out of proportion to the stimulus in the environment. A **blunted affect** accompanies a dulled emotional response to a situation, and a **flat affect** gives no visible cues to the person's feelings. (See Table 11–1.)

Affect can also be pictured along a continuum that ranges from depression, through normal, to manic. The normal range of affect is stable and appropriate to the situation. People diagnosed with one of the following affective disorders from DSM-III-R (1987) experience disrupting mood disturbances at varying points along the continuum.

296.2 Major depression, single episode

296.3 Major depression, recurrent

296.6 Bipolar disorder, mixed

296.4 Bipolar disorder, manic

296.5 Bipolar disorder, depressed

301.13 Cyclothymic disorder

300.40 Dysthymic disorder

The medical diagnosis of **major depression** (also called unipolar depression) is given when, along with a loss of interest in life, a person experiences an unresponsive mood that moves from mild to moderate with the severe level lasting at least two weeks. A **dysthymic disorder** is similar but remains in the mild to moderate range and is not as long lasting as a major depression. A medical diagnosis of **bipolar disorder** is given when a person's mood runs the entire gamut over a period of time. The bipolar disorder is further clarified as

- *Mixed:* The person alternates between depressed and manic every few days
- *Manic:* The person is presently in the manic phase
- *Depressed:* The person is in the depressive phase but has a history of manic episodes

In the bipolar disorder the manic phase begins suddenly and the depressive phase is shorter than that experienced in a major depression. These people often experience times of normal affect between the pathologic phases. **Cyclothymic disorder** is a chronic problem with an affective range from moderate depression to hypomanic, which may or may not include times of normal mood. See Figure 11–1.

Incidence of Disorders

Major, or unipolar, depression is 10 times more common than bipolar disorder. At any given time there are approximately 30 to 40 million people in the United States who are suffering from depression. It is thought that 8 to 12 percent of men and 18 to 25 percent of women will suffer a major de-

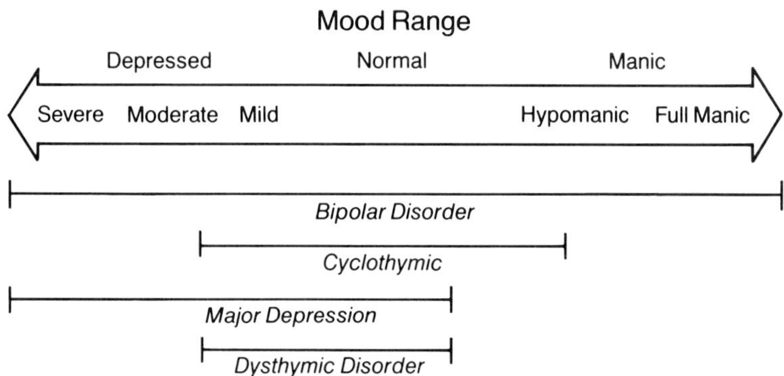

Figure 11–1 *Affective disorders and mood ranges.*

pression in their lifetime. It is not uncommon for women to experience multiple episodes of depression. Estimates are that only 25 to 50 percent of these individuals receive treatment. An untreated major depression lasts six months to a year. Full recovery occurs 80 percent of the time; the remaining 20 percent of the victims suffer from chronic depression (Haas and Clarkin, 1988; McBride, 1988; Yapko, 1988).

The incidence of depression in children of depressed parents ranges from 14 percent to almost 50 percent. In the prepubertal years, depressive symptoms are twice as common in boys; after puberty, symptoms are seen twice as often in girls. Additionally, the rate of depression from preadolescence to adolescence doubles. In adolescents between the ages of 14 and 16 Kashani (1987) found a prevalence rate of 4.7 percent for major depression and 3.3 percent for dysthymic disorder, for a total rate of 8.0 percent. The rate of depression in people over the age of 65 is estimated at 10 to 15 percent for major depression and 30 percent for mild depression. Many of these individuals may be misdiagnosed, since depression in the elderly often simulates dementia. Depression, viewed as pseudodementia, increases the older person's chances of being institutionalized due to an inability to accomplish ADLs (Ronsman, 1987; Rutter, 1986; Trad, 1987).

In the total population there is a risk factor of 7 percent for depression. When a first-degree relative (parent, child, or sibling) experiences a depression, the risk factor rises to 20 percent. If both parents are depressed, the risk leaps to a high of 74 percent (Cytryn, 1986).

Another risk factor is marital status. At highest risk are women who are separated, divorced, or widowed. The second-highest risk is among men who have never been married or who are divorced or widowed. At a lower risk are married women. Women who have never been married and married men are at the lowest risk for developing a depression. Considering marriage alone, married men are less depressed than single men, whereas married women are more depressed than women who have never married (Gove, 1987).

In the bipolar affective disorder, the female-male ratio is fairly even, with both sexes being equally at risk. Usually, the bipolar disorder is diagnosed when the client is in his or her early thirties. Bipolar disorder affects about 1.2 percent of the adult population. The manic phase rarely occurs before puberty. Untreated, the depressive phase may last six to nine months and the manic phase two to six weeks. It is difficult to predict the course of the disorder—some individuals may have only one episode every 10 years but others may have three or more episodes a year. About 15 percent of individuals with bipolar disorder suffer from a rapid cycle, that is, they experience frequent and almost continuous disruptions in well-being. For unknown reasons these individuals are more likely to be women. The majority of people with bipolar disorder have a lifetime average of 11 episodes. The genetic factor ranges from 20 to 50 percent risk among first-degree relatives (Cytryn, 1986; Davenport and Adland, 1988; Haas and Clarkin, 1988; Wehr, 1988).

The high rate of the affective disorders makes them a major concern for nurses. Preventive measures can be instituted for those individuals and families who are at higher risk because of either family history or situational stress. Since the majority of depressed people do not initiate requests for professional help, nurses, as community members, need to be alert to the need for referrals for family, friends, and neighbors. Depressed clients are found in all types of clinical settings and are not restricted to the psychiatric unit. It is vital that nurses be alert to cues, since a lethal complication of untreated depression is suicide. As many as 15 percent of people with affective disorders go on to commit suicide (Haas and Clarkin, 1988).

Knowledge Base

The signs and symptoms people develop when experiencing an affective disorder vary from person to person.

Depression in Children and Adolescents

DSM-III-R does not clearly distinguish childhood and adolescent depressions from adult depression, indicating there are more similarities between the two than differences. Other sources disagree and discuss different characteristics for varying ages and developmental levels. Depressive features increase in complexity as developmental levels progress. Depression in infants may be recognized in a sad face, immobility, decreased appetite, and an inability to be consoled. Depressed preschoolers may be irritable when in the presence of others but quiet and less demanding when left alone. Additional symptoms include decreased appetite, sleep changes, and somatic complaints. School-age children exhibit nonspecific changes indicating depression or some other problem. These changes may include problems with peers, poor school performance and low achievement, misbehavior, and temper tantrums. The important cue is the change in behavior along with a sad or depressed affect (Emde, 1986; Kashani and Carlson, 1987; Kazdin, 1988).

Adolescents experiencing depression also exhibit age-specific characteristics such as antisocial behavior, aggression, labile moods, difficulties in school, withdrawal from peer and family activities, fatigue, and hypersomnia. They are extremely sensitive to rejection in their romantic relationships. Adolescents are less likely than adults to experience hallucinations, delusions of guilt, and feelings of persecution. However, they frequently complain of not being understood. In the 1987 study by Kashani 75 percent of depressed teens also suffered from an anxiety disorder, 25 percent abused alcohol, and 25 percent abused drugs. The chemical abuse is often an attempt to dull the pain of depression and feel better. It is not uncommon for adolescent depression to be masked by substance abuse, school phobia, eating disorders, or conduct disorders. (These disorders are discussed in detail in Chapters 6, 8, 9, 12, and 13.) The first manic episode of bipolar disorder may occur during adolescence and is characterized by marked instability of behavior and intense adolescent turmoil (Kashani, 1987; Petti and Larson, 1987).

Although the signs and symptoms of an affective disorder vary from person to person, they tend to be fairly constant for any given person. Thus, clients can learn to recognize the warning signs of an impending disruption and seek professional attention. Though specific changes vary in people, all areas of life are affected when the disorder is severe. The depressed or manic client exhibits behavioral, affective, cognitive, physiologic, and sociocultural changes. To ascertain the specific difficulties the client is experiencing, the nurse must complete a thorough assessment in all areas.

Behavioral Characteristics

One of the changes seen in affective disorders is in the *will or desire to participate in activities.* In a mild depression, people avoid complex tasks because of difficulty in completing them. There is a decreased desire to participate in activities that do not bring immediate gratification. As the depression deepens, there is a further decrease in participation. One study (Rothblum, 1983) found that unemployed depressed women had a higher level of impaired performance than employed depressed women. The housewives had no interest in housework and needed assistance in fulfilling normal responsibilities, whereas the employed women continued to fulfill their outside work responsibilities. As the level and quality of activity decrease, people regard themselves as incompetent and inadequate. This further contributes to feelings of discouragement and, in severe depression, results in a complete paralysis of the will. There is no desire to do even the simple ADLs. To suggestions the client often responds, "It's pointless to even try because I can't do it."

In the early stages of an elevated mood, people with a bipolar disorder increase their work productivity. This leads to positive feedback from employers and family members, which contributes to increased self-esteem around the issues of competency and power. When these people reach the manic end of the continuum, however, their productivity decreases because of a short attention span. Manic clients are interested in every available activity and are supremely confident of being able to accomplish them all perfectly.

Interaction with other people is altered when people experience an affective disorder. In the beginning of a depressive episode, people may avoid social activities that are not highly interesting and stimulating. As the depression deepens, the tendency is to withdraw from most social interactions because they are too demanding and require too much effort. There may be concurrent fantasies of living in an isolated spot where there would be no need to interact with others. Depressed people say they feel lonely but also say they feel helpless to halt the process of withdrawal and isolation. Family and friends, frustrated with the withdrawal and separation, often respond with criticism and anger. This intensifies the depressed person's self-dissatisfaction, which contributes to further isolation (Yapko, 1988). In depression, people may experience more friction, tension, and conflict than usual when interacting with family and friends. Difficulty communicating often leads to disputes and hostility within the family. So painful can interactions become that some clients become silent as a way to decrease unpleasant interactions.

> *Ellen described her interactions with her son in this way: "I have a 3-year-old son, and I want to be able to take care of him. I've been so short with him lately. I don't seem to have any patience with him, and I just don't have any energy. This isn't fair to him."*

People experiencing a manic episode are unusually talkative and gregarious. Their interactions are effusive, and they are unable to control the impulse to interact with everyone in the environment. They spend a great deal of time on the telephone and write letters to many people. These people are oblivious of the social convention of not interrupting a private discussion. And, while interacting with others, they may share intimate details of their lives with anyone who will listen. When their mood returns to its normal range, they are often embarrassed about what they have said to others.

A change in *affiliation needs* also occurs in the affective disorders. People unable to love and care for themselves believe themselves inherently unlovable and thus attempt to earn love. Their only security with family and friends is based on their attempts to meet all the needs of significant others. Since they have difficulty defining themselves as individuals, they need the presence of others to maintain self-worth. Depending on the depth of the depression, normally self-sufficient people also experience an increase in dependency. This begins with a desire to have others participate in activities with them. As the depression progresses, they seek advice and assistance in work responsibilities and leisure activities. Affiliation needs are frequently expressed as demands or through whining complaints. If these demands, unrealistic though they are, are rejected by others, depressed people view this as validation of their being unlovable and unwanted by family and friends. If, on the other hand, intense assistance is given to depressed people, their dependency needs are reinforced, which contributes to a lack of self-confidence. In severe depression, people tenaciously cling to significant others. They no longer want advice only—they want total care and attention. If others leave them for even a short time, they may become maudlin about the significance and length of the separation. At this level, as the need to cling to others becomes incessant and extreme, agoraphobia may develop (Yapko, 1988).

Those experiencing a shift in affect toward elation show a decreased need for affiliation. They neither seek nor heed advice. They view themselves as independent and completely self-sufficient. They have confidence in their ability to be self-sustaining while believing themselves beneficial to others.

Affective Characteristics

The *mood* in depression begins with an intermittent sense of sadness or low spirits. Statements are made such as "I feel down in the dumps" or "I feel blue today." Stimulation from family and friends or other pleasurable experiences can sometimes elevate a person's mood. As depression deepens, however, people become more gloomy, melancholic, and dejected, and responding to pleasurable stimuli becomes more difficult. One hears "There is no joy in my life anymore" or "I really feel unhappy." In severe levels of depression, there is a sense of desolation. These people despair over the past, present, and future; the misery is uninterrupted. Cues to the depth of the feeling are "I'll always feel this wretched" or "I feel awful all the time."

On the manic end of the continuum, there is an unstable mood state. Beginning with cheerfulness, it escalates toward euphoria. People in this state are exuberant, energetic, and excitable. One hears statements such as "Everything is just wonderful" or "I feel so high and great." The instability of mood is observed when, with minimal environmental stimulus, the person suddenly becomes irritable, argumentative, and openly hostile. Arrogance contributes to an intolerance of criticism, under which the person rapidly becomes combative. As the stimulus is withdrawn, however, the person's mood returns to one of euphoria.

Guilt is another common affective experience on which depressed people focus. For some the source of guilt is vague; for others, specific. Perfectionistic people have difficulty admitting to themselves and others that they need attention and support. When the need is recognized, they feel guilt. When there are no concrete problems yet there is deep depression, guilt may be experienced. A cue to this is a comment such as "I have a loving husband and good children, a nice house, and no money problems. But I'm so unhappy. I shouldn't be feeling this way. It's terrible for me to be so miserable." Guilt sometimes occurs in people who blame themselves for all the difficulties in their life. Evidence of this is heard in "It's my fault I'm so depressed. If I had been a better wife, my husband would not have beaten me." Depressed people ruminate over incidents they feel guilty about, and it is difficult to change their focus of attention.

> *Mark is a 27-year-old client who has had multiple hospital admissions over the past nine years. He has just been readmitted for a suicide attempt. Three years ago his father had coronary artery bypass surgery and is doing very well. Mark's mother died two years ago from cancer. He talks about guilt in relation to both of his parents. About his father he says: "Dad is very sick. I feel guilty about leaving him alone while I'm here in the hospital." About his mother he says: "I yelled at my mom the night before she died. Now I can't say I'm sorry. If I killed myself, I would be able to tell her I'm sorry." These two themes are continually repeated throughout the day.*

During a manic episode, people are unable to experience any sense of guilt. Confronted with behavior that has hurt another person, they respond with indifference, laughter, or anger. It is as if a temporary shutdown of the conscience occurs during the elevated mood state. The ability to experience guilt returns when the affect returns to a normal level.

Crying spells may be evidenced during a depressive state. In mild and moderate depressions, people have an increased tendency to cry in situations that would not normally provoke tears. Where the cultural norm dictates that men ought not to shed tears, depressed men who cry may feel a sense of shame. In a severe depression, there is often an absence of crying, although there may be a desire to cry; it is as if there is not even enough energy to shed tears. The depth of despair is indicated by a comment such as "Why can't I cry? I want to, but the tears just won't come." During the manic phase, sudden and unpredictable crying spells may occur. These may last only 20 to 30 seconds, and the stimulus is probably unknown to others. The individual often returns rapidly to a euphoric mood.

Peoples' feelings of *gratification* are altered in affective disorders. In a mild depression, there is a narrowing of interest in pleasurable activities, and there may be a shift from active to passive participation. As the depression increases, the person may resort to activities that result in immediate gratification such as excessive eating, drinking, or drug taking. At this point, there is a decrease in formerly pleasurable activities. This is exhibited by remarks such as "I don't enjoy playing the piano anymore. It doesn't do anything for me. I just sit and watch TV all day" and "I can't seem to get interested in my stamp collection any more. I used to enjoy spending an hour a day working on it." In severe depression, people become *anhedonic,* that is, they are incapable of experiencing pleasure (Yapko, 1988). Cues to this level are comments such as "I don't remember anything that was ever any fun" and "I don't deserve to enjoy anything."

Manic people, on the other hand, try to participate in every available pleasurable activity. Skillfulness is not a concern; they enjoy the activity regardless of the outcome. There is a constant need for fun, excitement, and stimulation.

Accompanying a depressive state is a loss of *emotional attachments.* It begins with decreased affection for family members and friends, along with a dissatisfaction with these relationships. In a moderate depression, people often become indifferent to others, and remarks are made such as "I don't even think about home or my wife or children. I just don't care anymore." As the depression intensifies, a severe disengagement from family members and a repudiation of all significant relationships may occur. Statements are heard such as "I don't have a family anymore. We hate each other" and "I hate teenagers. I hope I never see my kids again."

People in a manic state form intense emotional attachments very rapidly. During their euphoric moods, they feel affectionate toward everyone in the environment. They "fall in love" in a matter of minutes and with a number of people, and they become preoccupied with sex. The person in a manic state does not think it inappropriate to have simultaneous intimate relationships. Values and ethics held in a normal mood do not appear to influence behavior during a manic episode.

The alterations in the affective experience of depressed and manic people are both broad and deep. In depression, there is a sense of hopelessness that the future will bring any changes in mood, pleasure, or loving relationships. In a manic state, there is little recognition that they have not always felt this euphoric and wonderful.

Carla describes her changes in this way: "I worry about what's going to happen to me. I mean, I didn't have this numbness a month ago. I could be lying here dying and not even know it. I just don't have any feeling anymore."

Dale describes himself in this way: "I feel so good since I stopped taking my lithium. I'm not sick and I never needed it anyway. You know Susan who was just admitted yesterday? Well, we really hit it off and are thinking about getting married as soon as we get out of the hospital."

Cognitive Characteristics

A person's thoughts about personal worth and value contribute to the overall sense of self-esteem. In the affective disorders, there is an alteration in *self-evaluation.* In mild depression, people overreact to mistakes they may make; for even minor errors, they reproach themselves. Their self-evaluation is flexible at this level because they are still able to recognize some positive attributes in themselves. As the depression worsens, however, people focus much of their attention on past and present failures.

A good deal of their thinking is self-deprecatory and self-accusatory. They blame themselves for feeling depressed and attribute the depression to a personal defect or inadequacy. This magnification of failures is called **catastrophizing.** These negative thoughts then make them feel more depressed, which causes more self-depreciation. They believe the depression proves they are weak and inferior to others. Severely depressed people have a global negative view of themselves. One hears statements such as "I am completely incompetent" or "I am a total failure at everything." Severely depressed people withdraw from family and friends, because they believe they are a burden to them. Incorrectly, they assume responsibility for negative events; if it is possible to blame themselves for some unpleasantness, they will do so, however scant the justification. This type of distorted thinking process is referred to as **personalization** (Dreyfus, 1988).

> *Peter, age 29, was admitted following a suicide attempt with an overdose of Xanax. He stated: "I know my wife doesn't love me anymore. Even my kids don't care what happens to me. I tried to commit suicide because I had a fight with my mother. I'm a failure as a father, husband, and son."*

People on the manic end of the continuum have an exaggerated evaluation of themselves. They have grandiose beliefs about their physical and intellectual talents. In any undertaking, there is a supreme sense of self-confidence. During these episodes, they do not regard their behavior as inappropriate, nor do they realize their need for professional assistance.

> *Claire, who is exhibiting manic behavior, says the following: "I write poetry and songs, which I am going to have published. I am also going to be an aerobics instructor. That's how I really express myself. I'm not crazy. I am well enough to go home and start my own psychotherapy business using my special religious insights."*

People's *expectations* of themselves, others, and the future are altered during the affective disorders. Persistent negative expectations reinforce depressive behaviors. In the beginning of a depression, people have a pessimistic view of outcomes, particularly in ambiguous situations. Often, they ignore positive experiences or misinterpret them as negative ones. This **overgeneralization** is a distortion in the thinking process. As the depression continues, the view of the here-and-now and the future becomes more gloomy still. Persistent negative expectations reinforce depressive behaviors. **Dichotomous thinking** suggests that experiences will be either all good or, more likely, all bad. Statements are made such as "I can't do it," "I'll fail anyway," or "It won't do any good." In severe depression, the present and future are viewed as completely hopeless. Even simple goals are unachievable because of people's self-perceived inadequacies. Past events are used to prove that there is no hope for the future and that things will never change. They see no reason to make an effort, since life is not worth living and they might as well be dead. The inability to cope is evidence of an external locus of control.

> *Wendy is a severely depressed young woman. She verbalizes her negative expectations in the following way: "Dr. Lee isn't doing anything. The antidepressants aren't working. I'm getting worse, and I won't get better this time. There is nothing anyone can do to help me. I wish I would just die."*

In contrast, manic persons have inordinate expectations of themselves, others, and the future. They become involved in activities without considering any possible negative outcomes. For instance, because of their certainty that every investment will be a wonderful success, they are open to abuse in business ventures. And they often go on buying sprees without concern for the consequences of incurring great debt.

> *Jorge and Ava have been married for 12 years and are experiencing severe marital problems centering on financial issues. Jorge has had multiple episodes of bipolar disorder. Eighteen months ago they took a $10,000 home equity loan to pay off all the bills Jorge had run*

up during a manic phase. At that time they agreed that their credit cards would be used only for an emergency. Two weeks ago Ava needed to use the credit card to pay for some medication and found that the card was up to its limit of $5000. During a confrontation with Jorge, Ava found out that he had received two new credit cards and had taken a cash advance of $5000 on each card. He could not explain what he had done with the $15,000.

Self-criticism is another cognitive facet of an affective disorder. Often, it begins with perfectionistic standards impossible to meet. People respond to failure with feelings of inadequacy, guilt, and shame rather than question their excessively high standards. As the depression deepens, the criticism becomes more harsh. The depressed person pays close attention to actions or statements of others that might be construed as disapproval or indifference. These are interpreted as rejection and translated into an angry rejection of themselves (Dreyfus, 1988).

In bipolar manic episodes, people lose their ability to be critical of their own behavior. Past and present accomplishments as well as future goals are exaggerated. Their elated self-esteem allows them to approve of all of their behavior. Concurrently, they are very sensitive to criticism from others and become irate if they sense disapproval from others.

People's *decision-making ability* deteriorates during the process of affective disorders. In mild depressions, people show an obsessiveness about making decisions. They need to look at every possible choice and potential result before deciding on a course of action. There is a high priority on doing "the right thing." They often seek advice and affirmation from others before making the decision. As the depression extends, so does the difficulty in decision making. There is a decreased ability to concentrate on a subject long enough to formulate a decision. A person might stand in front of the closet for 20 minutes, trying to decide what clothes to wear to work. To plan meals, do shopping, or concentrate on homework may also be difficult. In severe depressions, people are incapable of making decisions. Because they cannot concentrate, they cannot recall information from the past to help them. Lack of concentration also interferes with their ability to compare alternatives and potential outcomes in the problem-solving process (Yapko, 1988).

In manic episodes, people also have difficulty making decisions. So easily are they distracted by stimuli in the environment, they cannot concentrate long enough to go through the problem-solving process. Their short attention span causes them to respond impulsively to stimuli. Since there is an inability to think through the consequences of behavior before impulsively engaging in it, manic clients often have poor judgment and self-control.

Mario and his wife Tanya have been fighting more as Mario's manic phase progresses. At the end of one day Tanya refuses to take Mario over to the service station to pick up his car, which had been repaired. She says, "You have treated me badly all day. I won't take you to get your car. You can take the bus or ask a neighbor to take you." Thirty minutes later a stretch limousine with a chauffeur arrives in front of the house, and Mario gets in it. Tanya becomes very angry at Mario's lack of judgment and impulsive behavior—they simply cannot afford this extra expense.

Flow of thought is disrupted during the affective disorders. Along the continuum of depression, there is a gradual retardation in the rate and number of thoughts. This may be evidenced by slowed speech, an inability to think of specific words, or not completing sentences. Frustrated, others may react by completing the depressed person's thoughts. In a severe depression, it may take the person several minutes to respond to a question; mutism may even be present.

In manic episodes, flight of ideas is often present. The flow of thought is fragmented by any external stimuli. Thoughts come so quickly that there is not enough time to completely express one idea before another idea is stimulated. These thoughts may be connected by a theme or by alliteration, rhymes, or puns. The following is an example of flight of ideas.

> *"I didn't kill anyone. I won't do any harm. I am upset. I am worried about these people taking drugs, people ruining others' lives. I have heart problems because I was born with a hole in my heart. I saw people dying after heart surgeries, and I wanted to help them but I couldn't. I have smoked grass since I was 19. Grass does the same thing as my Lanoxin and lithium, so I don't take my medication. I trust in God to help me. I am a religious person. I like to see pictures of God. I am afraid of being hurt by evil spirits. Evil spirits can kill people and even make them have heart problems."*

Thoughts about *body image* are also distorted during the affective disorders. In mild or moderate depression, distortion begins as an obsessional concern over physical appearance, with a focus on the disliked body parts. As depression worsens, people believe that there is an actual change in the body and that they are more unattractive. In severe depression, there may be an erroneous perception of the body as being disfigured or deformed.

People in a manic state also have an incorrect perception of their body image. Exaggerated self-esteem contributes to their believing they look like well-known people or famous beauties. If others challenge this perception, they often respond with a great deal of anger.

> *Vera is 5 feet tall and weighs 150 pounds. She has long frizzy hair that is several shades of blonde and brown. She approaches the nurse and says, "Don't I look like Marilyn Monroe? Look at my hair, I just washed it. Isn't it a pretty shade of blonde? And look at me, I look just like her. I think I will go into the movies. Maybe I can make it as a Marilyn Monroe look-alike."*

Faulty perceptions of body image may extend into *delusions* in the affective disorders. In depression, there may be somatic delusions during which people believe themselves to be hopelessly ill. At times, there are delusions that part of the body is deformed or that the body has been infected or contaminated by outside agents. Manic clients may experience delusions of grandeur that center on beliefs of being famous or having a personal relationship with prominent, well-known people. Not uncommonly, delusions include paranoid content.

> *Recent violent episodes at home forced Melina's husband to bring her to the hospital. Melina tells the nurse, "I am stressed out and misunderstood. My husband is doing things to upset me, and he is trying to set me up. He has the phone tapped. I know he has been unfaithful. I have trouble with my thinking. My husband is controlling my thoughts."*

Hallucinations occur in 15 to 25 percent of people with both unipolar and bipolar affective disorders and may be the result of sleep deprivation. These are usually auditory hallucinations with the voices condemning them or telling them what to do. As Brenners, Harris and Weston (1987) discuss, those with affective disorders who hallucinate often believe they are talking with God or well-known people.

> *Sherry describes her hallucinations this way: "I'm hearing voices telling me to kill myself. I hear them all the time. I feel like I'm going crazy. The voices are getting clearer. They tell me to kill myself and I'll be at peace. Kill yourself and your problems will be solved." The next day Sherry says: "I'm getting worse. Now I'm seeing the person as well as hearing the voice. It's a man, and it started last night."*

Loss of faith is a common experience during depressive episodes. People lose faith in their ability to do things, in their ability to ever experience joy again, in the possibility of their negative thoughts ever improving, as well as in God or a Supreme Being. This loss of faith contributes to an overwhelming sense of spiritual distress.

Physiologic Characteristics

Vague physical complaints and somatic preoccupation may be the only symptoms of depression in the elderly. Other depressed older persons commonly exhibit changes in appetite, sleeping, and elimination, as well as a loss of energy (Ronsman, 1987).

Clients who are not elderly often experience many physiologic symptoms of depression and other affective disorders. A change in *appetite* accompanies the affective disorders. In a mild or moderate depression, there may be a diminishing of appetite and complaints that food is not as tasty. Depressed people may omit meals without feeling hungry. Severely depressed people may abhor food and have to force themselves to eat. Others discover their appetites increase when they become depressed, and their eating patterns cause them to gain weight throughout the disorder. This pattern of weight gain is more common in women than in men. Another pattern is for people to overeat and gain weight when mildly depressed and to lose their appetite and weight when severely depressed. Statements are heard such as "I don't even want to eat anymore," "Nothing tastes good to me," and "I can't eat, I feel like there is a big knot in my throat." Manic clients may not obtain sufficient food and fluid. This is related both to their inability to remain still long enough to eat a meal and to their attention span, which is so short that they forget to finish meals. The consequences of a change in appetite depend on the severity of the reduction or increase in food and fluid intake. The change may become life-threatening (Frank, 1988).

Sleep patterns are disrupted during unipolar and bipolar affective disorders. In a mild depression, people may sleep more than usual or they may awaken earlier in the morning. As the depression deepens, some people sleep 12 hours a day, whereas others awaken one or two hours earlier in the morning. In a severe depression, people usually have difficulty falling aleep; sleep is sporadic and awakenings are frequent. The person often awakens in the early morning and is unable to return to sleep. Moreover, these people obsess about their lack of sleep and believe they need much more sleep than they actually do (Beck, 1979). Remarks are made such as "I've had insomnia, so I haven't been able to sleep. I need sleep so badly. I'm tired all the time, but I just can't sleep." Their difficulty sleeping is demonstrated with changes in the REM cycle of sleep. Nondepressed people have more REM activity toward the end of the sleep period, whereas depressed people have more REM activity in the beginning of the sleep period. Additionally, depressed people experience less slow-wave sleep throughout the night. These sleep changes may or may not be evident in depressed children, but they are apparent by adolescence (Emslie, 1987; Kazdin, 1988).

People experiencing the depressed phase of a bipolar disorder tend to sleep more than eight hours and report their sleep is restful. When in the manic phase of the disorder, they have a dramatic decrease in the amount of sleep. Although they may sleep only one or two hours a night, they are refreshed and full of energy in the morning. They have great difficulty taking naps or relaxing during the day to compensate for their lack of sleep.

In the affective disorders, there is a change in the level of *sexual desire*. In depression, this begins with a mild loss of interest in sexual activity, both autoerotic and with a partner. The depressed person often decreases initiation of sexual activity but continues to give and receive pleasure in the usual pattern. With deepening depression, further change in sexual activity is common. Some people, needing comfort, seek out the partner more frequently. Others may change their patterns by increasing sexual behavior that takes less energy such as cuddling or oral sex. Without clear and direct communication, the nondepressed partner may interpret these changes as an increase in sexual desire rather than as a need to be comforted or a lack of energy. In severe depressions, most people experience a complete loss of sexual desire and fulfillment. The partner needs to understand that this inhibited sexual desire is a symptom of the depression, not necessarily a reflection of the relationship.

In manic states, there is an exaggerated sexual desire, which is often acted out with a variety of partners. People's ethical and moral restraints on sexual activity do not function during the elevated mood state. Seductive behavior, frequency of activity, and number of sexual partners all increase. Families are often angry and hurt, and this may be the particular behavior that forces a hospitalization. At the height of manic episodes, a paradoxic decrease in sexual behavior may occur. Because clients may be constantly trying to seduce everyone in the environment, there is no time for consummating any of the relationships. When mood levels return to normal, these people often feel embarrassed and guilty about their behavior.

Another change during the affective disorders is in *activity level.* It begins with people's tiring more easily and extends to their becoming fatigued with all activities. At the depth of depression, people say they are too tired to do anything, even basic ADLs. Some depressed people experience a retardation in their motor activity. They walk slowly with a trudging gait. When speaking, they use a minimum of gestures to illustrate their thoughts. The pitch of the voice is lowered, and there is little speech inflection. Immobility becomes so severe in some people that they appear catatonic. Others experience increased motor activity during a depressive state. This is observed as constant and nonpurposeful activity such as wringing of the hands, picking at the skin, or agitated pacing (Yapko, 1988).

In manic states, people experience hyperactivity without being aware of fatigue. They move constantly and have great difficulty remaining seated for more than a few minutes. When they are seated, constant swinging of the legs is typical. The voice is pitched higher and is much louder than normal. And dramatic arm and facial gestures accompany their speaking. Because they are unaware of fatigue, they are in danger of total physical exhaustion.

Bowel activity may be a problem in both unipolar and bipolar disorders. In depression, constipation may be caused by markedly decreased food and fluid intake and by a slowing of the body processes in response to decreased physical activity. Constipation in manic episodes is related to distractibility and therefore the ignoring of bodily signals or to the refusal to take the time to have a bowel movement.

More easily than others, depressed people develop *secondary physical illness* related to an impairment of the immune system. The immune system, in current thinking, is one way psychologic signals are transformed into physical effects. The neurotransmitters epinephrine, norepinephrine, and serotonin suppress lymphocyte function; acetylcholine and vasopressin enhance it. Endorphins function as either suppressors or enhancers, depending on a variety of factors. It is unclear if the immune response changes are a direct result of depression or arise from associated behaviors, such as decreased nutrition, sleeplessness, heavy smoking, and heavy drinking (Levy and Krueger, 1988).

People's *physical appearance* often is indicative of an altered mood state. Depressed people tend to wear colorless clothing that may not fit well because of either lost or gained weight. They may wear the same clothes for days without laundering them. Personal hygiene may be poor because they do not have the desire or energy to brush their teeth, shower, or wash their hair. There may be no energy to shave or apply cosmetics. In a manic state, people often wear gaudy, brightly colored clothes. Separates, such as skirts, pants, and tops, may clash and seem to be chosen for their brightness rather than for their coordination. Some manic people change clothes as often as every hour. Personal hygiene may become a problem if restlessness and distractibility interfere with normal ADLs. Women who wear makeup and jewelry have extravagant tastes in an elevated mood state. Their cosmetics are very bright and may be carelessly applied. And to see five or six rings and pins or several necklaces and earrings worn at once is not unusual. (See Table 11–2 for a summary of these characteristics.)

Pam has been diagnosed as having a bipolar disorder, manic phase. Since admission 4 days ago, she has been averaging 2 hours of sleep a night. The rest of the nighttime hours are spent pacing hallways and talking to staff. She is in constant motion and brags about how energetic she is. Her clothing consists of startlingly bright miniskirts, low-cut sweaters, and high heels. Every few hours she reapplies her makeup to match each change of clothing.

Sociocultural Characteristics

A variety of sociocultural conditions may contribute to a person's depressive feelings of powerlessness, hopelessness, and loss of self-esteem. *Racism, sex-*

Table 11–2 *Characteristics of Clients with Affective Disorders*

Characteristic	*Depressed Client*	*Manic Client*
Desire to participate in activities	Decreased to absent	Interested in all activities
Interaction with other people	Limited; client withdraws	Talkative, gregarious
Affiliation needs	Increased dependency	Independent, self-sufficient
Mood	Despair, desolation	Unstable: euphoric and irritable
Guilt	High level	Unable to experience guilt
Crying spells	Frequent crying to inability to cry	May have brief episodes
Gratification	Loss of interest in pleasurable activities	Constantly seeking fun and excitement
Emotional attachments	Indifference to others	Forms intense attachments rapidly
Self-evaluation	Focuses on failures; sees self as incompetent; exercises catastrophizing and personalization	Grandiose beliefs about self
Expectations	Believes present and future hopeless; overgeneralizes one experience or fact	Inordinate positive expectations; unable to see potential negative outcomes
Self-criticism	Harshly critical of self; is a perfectionist; anticipates disapproval from others	Approves of own behavior; irate if criticized by others
Decision-making ability	Decreased ability or inability to make decisions	Difficulty due to distractibility and impulsiveness
Flow of thought	Decrease in rate and number of thoughts	Flight of ideas
Body image	Believes self unattractive or ugly	Believes self unusually beautiful
Delusions	Somatic delusions	Delusions of grandeur
Hallucinations	15–25%	15–25%
Appetite	Increased or decreased in mild and moderate depression, decreased in severe depression	Difficulty eating due to inability to sit still
Sleep pattern	Increased or decreased in mild and moderate depression, decreased in severe depression	Sleeps only one or two hours a night
Sexual desire	Loss of desire	Increase in activity and partners
Activity level	Motor activity retarded	Hyperactivity
Bowel activity	Constipation	Constipation
Physical appearance	Unkempt, poor hygiene	Bright clothing, frequently changes clothing

ism, and *ageism* are three of the most predominant sociocultural characteristics of today. However minority groups are defined, they experience discrimination psychologically, educationally, vocationally, and economically. When one is the object of cultural stereotypes in comments or jokes, it is difficult not to feel inadequate and shameful. When education has been substandard, one cannot expect to be as successful without remedial work. To feel hopeful about advancing in one's career when promotions are based on race, gender, and age is difficult, as is combating the helplessness felt when one's pay is clearly below what the position calls for.

There is a much higher rate of depression among women than among men. One of the factors contributing to this may be the stress of being a single parent. With the high divorce rate, there is an increasing number of single parents, 85 percent of them women. These women must deal with financial worries, parenting problems, loneliness, and lack of a supportive adult relationship. A major predisposing factor for depression in women is having three or more children under the age of 14 living at home. When the children grow up and leave home, the rate of depression decreases. This is contrary to the theory that depression results from the empty nest syndrome. It appears that being responsible for children is a source of stress that contributes to depression (McBride, 1988; Rothblum, 1983).

> *June is 49 years old, married, and the mother of six children between the ages of 17 and 27. She says she is very close to all her children and continues to feel responsible for them. She describes her situation in this way: "I don't know what it feels like to be happy. I know a lot of my stress is from my kids. They always come to me for help, money, or when they're in trouble. I just can't say no, I feel too guilty. I don't have any fight left—I'm so tired of being a parent."*

Some women feel a great deal of pressure from society to fulfill the roles of "superwives" and "supermothers." Much of their time and energy is devoted to meeting the needs of their families and communities. When this is done to the exclusion of their own needs and desires, they may be more susceptible to a depressive episode. Women who do not work outside the home experience more profound and longer-lasting depressions than women who do. It is believed that employment is a positive factor because it improves the financial situation, increases social contacts, decreases boredom, and strengthens the sense of achievement and self-esteem (McBride, 1988).

Another sociocultural factor that may contribute to depression is the occurrence of *significant life events.* (See Chapter 6 for discussion of crisis situations.) Some events involve expansion of the family system through marriage, births, adoptions, or other people moving into the home. Other events involve a reduction of the family system through children leaving, marital separations, divorce, or death. Some life events involve a threat, such as job problems, difficulties with the police, or illness. Others are emotionally exhausting, such as holidays, changing residences, or arguing with family and friends. One study (Hume, 1988) found that the number and frequency of life events experienced by people with affective disorders was greater than the number and frequency experienced by the general population. There was also a peaking of these events one month before the onset of the disorder. Among depressed women, marital difficulty was the event most frequently reported. Compared to non-depressed women, there was a higher incidence of *communication problems* and lack of intimacy. It is believed that the physiologic responses to these types of stress may predispose people to depression.

A number of factors influence the degree of stress that accompanies significant life events. (See Figure 11–2.) The presence of a *social support network* can decrease the impact an event may have on a person. Those who lack network support are more susceptible to developing a depressive reaction. People who have developed adaptive coping patterns—such as problem solving, direct communication, and use of resources—are more likely to maintain their normal affective range. Those who feel out of control, are unable to problem-solve, and ignore available resources are more apt to feel depressed. Thus an individual's perception and in-

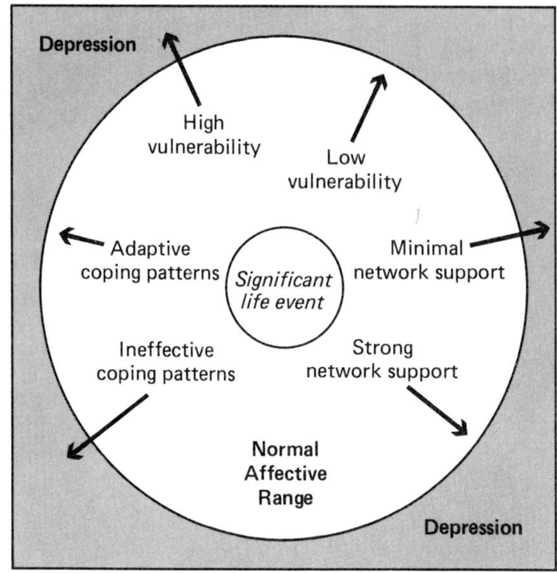

Figure 10-2 Relationship between life events and depression.

terpretation of significant events may contribute to depression.

People's vulnerability to specific illnesses, including depression, varies. The system through which stress is expressed depends on genetic makeup, enzyme defects, hormonal deficiencies, and health patterns. Some people develop ulcers, some experience cardiac problems, and some become depressed in response to significant life events (Hume, 1988).

Michelle, who is moderately depressed, has been divorced for 6 months and is struggling to raise her three children with minimal financial or emotional support from her former husband. She has had to return to work as a hair stylist after having been a full-time homemaker for 10 years. Much of her leisure time is spent in her children's sport and cultural activities. As a result she has little time to socialize and has become isolated from her support network.

The impact of affective disorders on the family must not be underestimated. Not surprising is the family's frustration, confusion, and anger in response to the multiple changes these disorders cause. Initially, family members may respond with support and concern. In some families, when the depression does not improve, the support changes to frustration and anger. A vicious cycle may be established. Increased conflict causes increased symptoms, further rejection, and deepening depression. Other families may become overly solicitous and assume total care of the depressed person. Total care may contribute to increased symptoms because the individual feels helpless and indebted to the family.

During manic episodes the family may be subjected to bizarre, hostile, and even destructive behavior. It is not uncommon for the family to call the police to protect themselves and their property. Untreated bipolar disorder often leads to a downward spiral in interpersonal, economic, and occupational functioning.

Marital problems may lead to separation and divorce. In one study of recently divorced couples (Garvey, 1985), 40 percent of the women and 34 percent of the men suffered from a major depression. In 40 percent of these cases, depression was identified as a factor contributing to the divorce rather than depression as a result of the divorce. Another study (Henker, 1985) found that the divorce rate was 57 percent for couples in which one person suffered from bipolar disorder. The risk for divorce increased with each successive occurrence of the manic state.

Causative Theories

Multiple theories have been developed to explain the cause of the affective disorders. It is now thought that these disorders are largely a clinical syndrome with common features caused by a variety of factors. In understanding the individual client from these theoretic perspectives, the student needs to look at how these different factors interacted within the person's past and how they interact in present circumstances. A person may have a genetic predisposition to changes in neurotransmission. The actual changes may occur only if certain psychologic mechanisms are present, and these mechanisms may occur only if particular social interactions occur. Many factors in individuals and environments increase or decrease the risk for affective disorders. It is by applying the biologic, intrapersonal, learning, cognitive, and social status theories that the nurse approaches the client from a holistic perspective.

Biologic Theories Some evidence suggests that people who experience affective disorders may have a *genetic predisposition* to the syndrome. There is a higher incidence of the syndrome in first-degree relatives of people diagnosed with either unipolar or bipolar disorders than in the general population. The risk to first-degree relatives is 10 to 20 times higher. Relatives of victims of bipolar disorder may develop either bipolar or unipolar disorder, whereas relatives of victims of unipolar disorder primarily develop unipolar disorder. Studies of the incidence of unipolar and bipolar disorder in twins documented that, in 75 percent of monozygotic twins, both twins developed a disorder. Only 20 percent of dizygotic twins developed a disorder. Although the specific genetic marker is unknown at this time, recent studies of the Amish population have indicated a link between bipolar disorder and an abnormality on chromosome 11 (Targum, 1988; Yates, 1987). The genetic mechanism remains unclear, however.

One thought is that the amount of monoamine oxidase secreted in the brain may be under genetic control. Another hypothesis is that there is a genetic predisposition to a lower threshold for stress. Thus those with a low threshold are more susceptible to the chemical changes that occur with stressful events.

The *amine hypothesis* is specifically concerned with the levels of norepinephrine, serotonin, and dopamine in the CNS. As the electric impulse travels to the nerve endings, stored amines are released at the synaptic juncture. These amines react with the neuronal receptors, which allow the impulse to be conducted through the next nerve cell. It is believed that there is a functional deficiency of these amines during a depressive episode and a functional excess during a manic episode. (See Figure 11–3.)

One way this imbalance may occur is through the action of the enzyme monoamine oxidase (MAO), which is responsible for inactivating the amines after they have been released for impulse conduction. If there is an excess of MAO, it will result in a low amine level, which will decrease transmission of impulses. If, however, the level of MAO is not sufficient to inactivate the amines, these amines will accumulate at the synapse and increase transmission of impulses (Janowsky, 1987).

This theory may be one explanation for the higher incidence of depression in women and older persons. Throughout life, women have consistently higher levels of MAO than do men. The result of this may be a functional decrease in the necessary neurotransmitters. As people age, the MAO level increases, which may explain the higher risk factor for depression in the aged population.

Another part of the amine hypothesis does not concern an actual deficit or excess of amines but rather the sensitivity of the neuronal receptor to them. During depression, it is thought that the receptor is subsensitive, so that fewer impulses are transmitted. In the manic phase, there may be a supersensitivity of the receptors to the amines. If so, the result is that there is an increase in the transmission of impulses. The sensitivity of the receptor is influenced by the hormone triiodothyronine (T_3). Thus people with hypothyroidism are at a higher risk for a depressive episode, and those with hyperthyroidism are at a higher risk for a manic episode (Green, 1988).

Some depressed people have hyperactivity of the hypothalamic-pituitary-adrenal axis (HPA), which is thought to be related to hypersecretion of corticotropin releasing hormone (CRH) from neurons in various areas of the central nervous system.

An endogenous amphetamine, phenylethylamine (PEA), contributes to mood state and the ability to concentrate. In some unipolar disorders, there is a decrease in the amount of PEA produced; in bipolar disorder, there is an increase in PEA production (Gold, 1987; Fawcett and Kravitz, 1985).

The brain amines have an important role in the

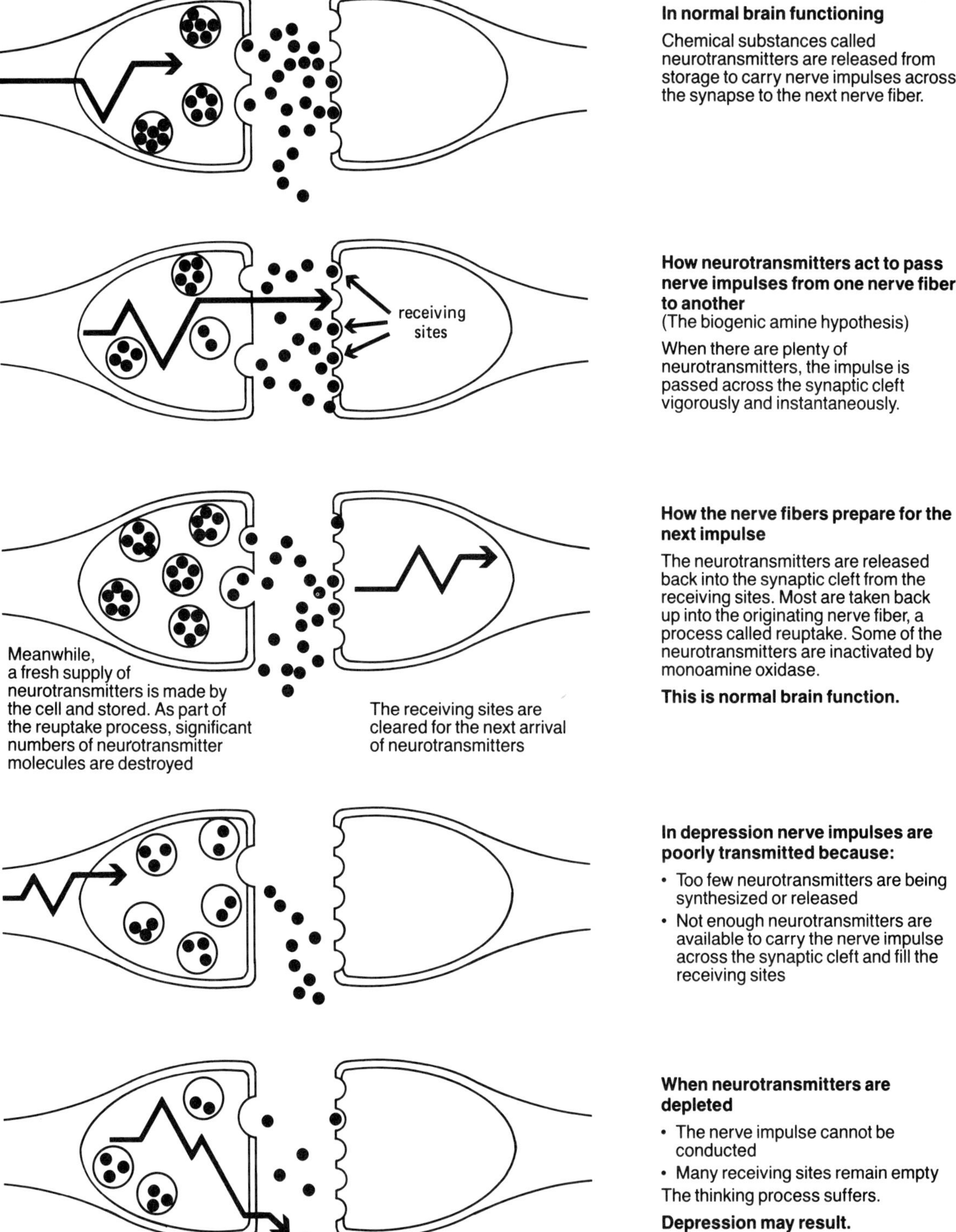

Figure 11–3 *Amine hypothesis of depression.* Source: The Chemical Origin of Depression. *Merrell Dow Pharmaceuticals. Adapted with permission.*

regulation of motor behavior, sleep, appetite, will, enjoyment, emotions, and sex drive. A deficiency or excess of amines alters the person's ability to respond to stimuli, both internally and externally. Continuing research into the relationship between stress and the affective disorders indicates that the limbic system of the brain is the major site of stress adaptation. With stress, the production of the amines in the limbic system increases. When the stress becomes chronic or recurrent, the body can no longer adapt as efficiently, and a shortage of brain amines occurs. In manic episodes, there appears to be a defective feedback mechanism in the limbic system. After the stressful event has been resolved, the limbic system continues to produce excessive amines; the increased transmission of impulses continues. Different areas of the limbic system play a major role in the regulation of emotions such as fear, rage, excitement, and euphora. The signs and symptoms of limbic dysfunction correlate to the characteristics seen in the affective disorders, that is, alterations in the pleasure mechanisms, mood, and activity levels (Risch, 1987).

Another hypothesis concerns *biologic rhythms.* **Circadian rhythms** are regular fluctuations of a variety of physiologic measures over 24 hours. The biologic "clock" is located in the hypothalamus and may be desynchronized by external or internal factors. An example of external desynchronization is jet lag, where rapid time zone changes result in decreased energy level, concentration ability and mood variations. In some individuals, internal desynchronization may result in depression.

One measure of desynchronization is change in adrenal rhythm. The adrenal cortex produces cortisol, which affects diurnal activity. If a client is in a depressive phase, the level of cortisol does not drop as low as it should in late evening and in the early part of sleep. The change in biologic rhythms can also be measured by temperature patterns and sleep patterns. In the depressed person the feeling of tiredness appears four to six hours earlier than the change in body temperature, and REM sleep is greatest during the early part of the sleep cycle rather than toward the end of the cycle. In the manic phase, the temperature and activity patterns do not correlate. The temperature pattern remains on a 24-hour cycle, whereas the activity pattern changes to a 50-hour cycle. In depression there is no early morning peak of the thyroid stimulating hormone, and the total production of it is decreased. In both bipolar and unipolar disorders, there is an increased production of growth hormone during periods of being awake. It is unclear if changes in circadian rhythms cause mood disturbances or if changes in mood alter circadian rhythms (Beck-Frils and Wetterberg, 1987; Groos, 1988; Mendelwicz, 1987; Monk, 1988).

Some forms of depression are related to the time of year and the amount of available *sunlight.* These are referred to as **seasonal affective disorders (SAD)** in which depression occurs annually between October and March and normal mood or hypomania occurs in spring and summer. The depression appears directly related to the amount of light, since symptoms disappear if the person is exposed either to more sunlight or to special lights that simulate the sun. SADs have been studied primarily in adults, but as many as one third of adult victims report that the onset began in childhood or adolescence. The majority of victims are female who have a family history of affective disorders. Unlike unipolar depression, in which the symptoms for children and adults differ, children and adults with SADs exhibit similar symptoms: fatigue, decreased activity, irritability, sadness, crying, worrying, and decreased concentration. However, adults tend to sleep more and children tend to sleep less during the winter depressive phase. In 70 to 85 percent of SAD cases, sufferers have an increased appetite, carbohydrate craving, and weight gain. In unipolar or bipolar depression, these symptoms are seen in only 15 to 30 percent of the cases. During the summer adults and children with SAD experience high levels of energy and talkativeness (Jacobsen and Rosenthal, 1988; Sonis, 1989; Thase, 1989; Trad, 1987; Wehr, 1987).

One hypothesis for this seasonal disorder is related to the pineal gland, which is located in the middle of the brain. Light signals travel along the optic nerve and affect the gland's secretion of the hormone melatonin. During periods of darkness, the pineal gland secretes more melatonin, with the normal peak of production between 1:00 and 3:00 A.M. Light has an inhibiting effect on melatonin production. The least secretion occurs about 2:00 P.M. This response to light has been documented in studies of blind people, who do not demonstrate this typical circadian rhythm. High levels of melatonin affect one's mood, sensations of tiredness, and sleepiness. It is thought that people with SAD are very sensitive to increased levels of melatonin. So, during the short photoperiods of winter, they respond with a depressive reaction (Wehr, 1987).

Another hypothesis about the effect of diminished sunlight is related to calcium and vitamin D. The body's calcium level is also on a circadian, or 24-hour, cycle. In some people, a lower calcium level increases tension and mood swings, which may contribute to depression. Vitamin D is necessary for the absorption of calcium in the diet and is produced by exposure to sunlight. During winter photoperiods, many people rely on supplements of synthetic vitamin D. Although helpful, this synthetic form is not as effective for calcium absorption as natural vitamin D. Elderly people may be especially prone to depression because of their hesitation or inability to be outside in the sunlight during northern winter months.

Affective disorders are heterogeneous. A variety of neurologic and endocrinologic factors as well as a variety of psychosocial factors may lead to the disruption of well-being.

Intrapersonal Theory Intrapersonal theory centers on the theme of loss, either real or symbolic. The loss may be of another person, a relationship, an object, self-esteem, or security. The process of grief is time-limited. After grief the person who sustained the loss maintains the self-concept with minimal self-criticism. When grief is unrecognized or unresolved, depression may result. A normal feeling that accompanies all losses is anger. People who have been taught that anger is an inappropriate feeling to experience and express learn to repress it. The result is that anger is turned inward and against the self. Some theorists believe this repressed anger and aggression against the self is the cause of the depressive episode. Along with the internalized anger, depressed people have very critical superegos, as evidenced by their high levels of guilt and extreme self-criticism. What is more, these people have many narcissistic needs arising out of the id component of the personality. They become involved with themselves to the exclusion of others. Other theorists , however, believe that anger is not the primary cause of depression. They believe the cause is the inability to achieve desired goals, the loss of these goals, and a feeling of lack of control in life (Yapko, 1988).

Intrapersonal theory relates the tendency for affective disorders to occur in families to impaired parenting. When one or both parents are depressed, the disorder causes them to relate in an unresponsive, detached, and helpless manner with their children. As a result, the children have difficulty attaining a sense of mastery and competence. They may be at risk for future depression (Trad, 1987).

Intrapersonal theory is also applicable in explaining the high incidence of depression in women and older people. Traditionally, women have been taught to depend on others' opinions and approval to form and maintain their own identities and self-esteem. When the source of self-worth is external rather than internal, people have scant self-control, which leads to feelings of helplessness; therefore, they are more vulnerable to loss. Losses become more incapacitating when they are considered a threat to identity and self-esteem. Older people, too, are at a higher risk for depression because of the multiple losses they have experienced. These may include the loss of a job, friends, loved ones, roles, economic security, and even the home. With the accumulation of losses, coping patterns are stretched to their limits, and depression results (Gove, 1987).

Learning Theory Learning theory states that people learn to be depressed in response to an external locus of control as they perceive lack of control over life experiences. Throughout life, depressed people have experienced little success in achieving gratification and positive reinforcement for their attempts to cope with negative incidents. These repeated failures teach them that what they do has no effect on the final outcome. The more stressful life events that occur, the more their sense of helplessness is reinforced. When people reach the point of believing they have no control, they no longer have the will or energy to cope with life and a depressive state ensues. Learned helplessness is viewed as a failure to adapt to others and their environment (Yapko, 1988).

The stereotypical socialization process for women has encouraged them to be passive, nonaggressive, and noncompetitive. Adaptive coping skills are often not taught to females on the assumption that they will move from dependency on parents to dependency on the husband. This expectation of dependency reinforces beliefs of helplessness. When men are viewed as the head of the family, women often feel powerless and fearful of asserting themselves and are thereby more susceptible to depression (McBride, 1988). Older people may experience an increase in stressful life events at a time when they have decreased resources to manage these. As a result, more failures may occur, and these contribute to a feeling of loss of control and an increase in depressive reactions.

Cognitive Theory Beck (1979) has developed a cognitive model of depression in which life events activate negative thinking. There are three interdependent components to the cognitive model. The first component, the cognitive triad, relates to views of the self, the present, and the future. Depressed people have learned to view themselves as incompetent, unworthy, and unlikeable. Present experiences are seen as negative events, and for the future there is no hope. The second component concerns cognitive patterns, or ways of interpreting information. Depressed people focus on the negative messages in the environment and ignore positive experiences. These negative patterns contribute to the third component, cognitive errors. Depressed people have a tendency to make global judgments and personalize negative incidents. They think dichotomously; that is, situations are either good or bad, things are either clean or filthy, life is either a success or a failure. There is no middle category in viewing the world, and they consistently put themselves on the negative side. This distorted thinking creates the affective characteristics of depression.

Social Status Theory The social status theory relates to the intrapersonal, learning, and cognitive theories with an added emphasis on society and culture. The theory is holistic in that it considers psychologic, sociologic, and economic components of depression. Although it is primarily applied to women and older people, its principles can sometimes be applied to depressed men and adolescents.

In the definition of mental health there has, in the past, been a double standard for women and men. A healthy woman has been described as acquiescent, subdued, dependent, and emotionally expressive. A healthy man, on the other hand, has been described as logical, rational, independent, aggressive, and nonemotional. These stereotypes have had unfortunate consequences for both women and men. However, there is movement toward an androgynous definition of mental health. This perspective stresses positive human qualities such as assertiveness, self-reliance, sensitivity to others, intimacy, and open communication—qualities that legitimately belong in the repertoire of both women and men.

Socialization in Western culture has taught women traditional feminine values. The ideal woman should not express anger or behave assertively. She should be compliant, helpless, and passive when interacting with other adults. Women who internalize these cultural expectations develop few coping skills to deal with stress and are more vulnerable to depressive episodes. When the Prince Charming myth dissolves in the reality of life, many women experience hurt, guilt, frustration, anger, and perhaps depression.

Rigid expectations about gender role continue to linger and contribute to higher rates of depression among women. Women who are full-time homemakers may develop no identity outside that of wife and mother. The tremendous duties of managing a household are often indiscernible and certainly not prestigious. Positive feedback or positive reinforcement such as compliments or a paycheck hardly exist. What is more, the position is continuous, 24 hours a day. Since one lives in the workplace, there is no stimulation from a change in the environment. Indeed, being a full-time homemaker is one of the most isolating professions in our present-day society.

Women who are employed outside the home may or may not fare better than women who remain home. For some women, this means assuming the responsibility for two full-time jobs with minimal or no support from other family members. Other families adapt by redefining home management as the responsibility of all members. Even still, conflict between traditional and nontraditional roles for married women may contribute to their developing depression. Data demonstrate that married women are more depressed than married men, and unmarried women are less depressed than unmarried men (Gove, 1987).

In addition to role conflict, employed women often must accept lower pay, inferior jobs, and fewer opportunities for career advancement. The legal system has been slow to redress employment discrimination, which increases women's frustration, anger, and distress. In this situation, some women begin to view themselves as incompetent and as failures. Thoughts of the future center on the hopelessness of their situations and contribute to depression.

Social status theory can also be applied to the situation in which some older people find themselves. In a society that places a premium on youth, older people feel useless, unimportant, incapable, and at times even repulsive. Role changes and losses may threaten their self-esteem. With aging, physiologic changes may lead to their perceiving themselves unfit, which then extends to further thoughts of being ineffectual and inferior. All these changes may contribute to a despair about one's entire life and a sense of hopelessness about the limited future. Considering these effects, it is scarcely surprising to find a higher rate of depression among older people. (See Table 11–3 for a summary of the theories of depression that have been discussed in this chapter.)

Medical Treatment

The initial phase of medical intervention for the client with an affective disorder begins with an in-depth assessment. The physician needs to determine if any drugs are contributing to or causing the client's depression. Most commonly, these drugs are alcohol, barbiturates, tranquilizers, and certain antihypertensive agents. At the same time, the physician treats any medical conditions, since poor physical health may increase the severity of a clinical depression (Akiskal, 1985).

Antidepressant and antimanic medications are often prescribed for clients with affective disorders. Most frequently, antidepressant medications are given in divided doses for one to two weeks at which point the total dose can be given at bedtime. Maintenance continues until clients are free of symptoms for four months to one year. Then the drugs are slowly discontinued. Approximately 30 percent of clients do not respond to antidepressants used alone, but they often respond when 600 mg per day of lithium or 25 μg per day of triiodothyronine (T_3) are added. An acute manic state is a medical emergency, since exertion may exceed safe limits. Acutely manic clients are given antipsychotic medications for rapid calming since lithium does not achieve its clinical effect for about ten days. In some cases, rapid cycling bipolar disorder may be initiated by antidepressant medications. If this occurs, the medications are discontinued and lithium is the only medication prescribed (Dreyfus, 1988; Garbutt, 1988; Reid, 1989; Wehr, 1988).

One of the difficulties with clients continuing on these medications at home may be secondary sexual dysfunctions. It is not uncommon for men to experience ejaculatory problems and for women to become nonorgasmic. Given these dysfunctions, some people personally elect to stop taking their medication (Nurnberg and Levine, 1987).

Therapeutic response to tricyclic antidepressants is better determined by blood plasma levels than dosages. Nortriptyline (Pamelor) has the most

Table 11–3 *Theories of Depression in Women and the Elderly*

Theory	*Main Points*	*Relevance to Women and Older People*
Genetic	Increased sensitivity to chemical changes related to stress	
Amine	Impaired neurotransmission; limbic dysfunction	Higher levels of monoamine oxidase in CNS in women and older people
Biologic rhythms	Internal desynchronization of circadian rhythms	
Sunlight	Decreased exposure to sunlight increases production of melatonin and decreases vitamin D production	Older people do not go outside as much during the winter months thus making less vitamin D and absorbing less calcium, which contributes to mood swings
Intrapersonal	Loss of person, object, self-esteem; hostility turned against the self; goals unachieved	Women are more dependent on others for self-esteem; older people suffer multiple losses
Learning	Lack of control over experiences; learned helplessness; failure of adaptation	Expectations of women's dependency reinforces helplessness; older people have increased stress with decreased resources, which contributes to loss of control
Cognitive	Negative view of self, the present, and the future; focus on negative messages; cognitive errors	
Social status	Internalization of cultural norms of behavior; rigid gender-role and age expectations	Women's identity may be limited to homemaker role. Employment positions less prestigious. May hold two full-time jobs. Older people suffer from the cultural value on youth; many role changes and losses.

specific therapeutic range of 50–150 ng/mL. Levels above or below this range are associated with a lack of response. Amitriptyline (Elavil) is most effective at a plasma level near 300 ng/mL; exceeding this level causes toxicity. The plasma level for desipramine (Norpramin) is 100–250 ng/mL, and the level for imipramine (Tofranil) is 100–300 ng/mL in adults and 100–225 ng/mL in children. Clients taking fluoxetine (Prozac) do not need blood levels drawn as this medication is frequently effective at a dose of 20–40 mg per day. (Harris, 1988; Trad, 1987). (See Chapter 4 for an in-depth discussion of these medications.)

When prescribing tricyclic antidepressants for older clients, particular care must be taken for several reasons. The older person metabolizes tricyclic medications at a slower rate because of a decrease in hepatic enzyme activity. As people age, they develop more body fat in comparison to their total body mass. This results in a longer duration of action of the tricyclic medications, since they are stored in body fat. In addition, the CNS of an elderly person is more sensitive to psychoactive medications.

The physician must determine if the benefits of tricyclic therapy outweigh the risks for the elderly client. The anticholinergic properties of these medications may lead to short-term memory problems, disorientation, and impaired cognition. These side effects may then be mistaken for organic brain disease (pseudodementia) in the elderly client. The physician is able to determine if the client's confusion is due to the tricyclic therapy by administering physostigmine, 1–2 mg IM. This medication increases the acetylcholine at the sites of cholinergic transmission, and the symptoms are temporarily reversed if they are related to the side effects of the medication.

There are additional problems with the anticholinergic properties of these medications. If the client has dentures, an extremely dry mouth can lead to gingival erosion. If the older male client has prostatic enlargement, the anticholinergic effect of urinary retention can cause very serious problems. Anticholinergic properties can also intensify an unsuspected glaucoma, resulting in an increase in intraocular pressure. Many older people experience orthostatic hypotension as part of the aging process. Tricyclic medications may cause orthostatic hypotension with the result that the older client is at higher risk for dizzy spells and falls.

Compared to younger adult clients, older clients are started on tricyclic medications at lower levels, which are gradually increased to lower maximum levels. Imipramine (Tofranil, SK-pramine) and amitriptyline (Amitid, Elavil, Endep) have a maximum level of 100 mg per day for the older client. Desipramine (Pertofrane, Norpramin) has a maximum daily dosage level of 150–200 mg.

Amitriptyline (Amitid, Elavil, Endep) has the most potent anticholinergic properties of the tricyclic group. Desipramine (Pertofrane, Norpramin) and maprotiline (Ludiomil) are the least anticholinergic, the least sedating, and the least likely to cause orthostatic hypotension. Therefore these medications are the drugs of choice for elderly clients. Another choice is trazadone (Desyrel). Although trazadone has no anticholinergic properties and minor hypotensive effects, it does have sedating effects that may be undesired. Fluoxetine (Prozac) may be the antidepressant of choice for the elderly as there are few anticholinergic side effects with this medication.

Since the production of monoamine oxidase increases with age, the monoamine oxidase inhibitors (MAOI) may be a possibility for the elderly client. The maximum dosage for phenelzine (Nardil) is 60 mg daily, and for tranyleypromine (Parnate) and isocarboxazid (Marplan) the dosage is 30 mg daily. The disadvantage of this group of antidepressant medications is the potential for toxicity and strict dietary limitations. Many older clients' nutritional options are limited because their finances are; thus, they may find it difficult to follow the severely restricted diet.

Lithium toxicity may occur with conditions causing fluid loss, such as vomiting or diarrhea, or with decreased glomerular filtration rate, which is most often seen in the elderly or pregnant client. In the normal aging process there is a decreased glomerular filtration rate in the kidneys. When an older client is on lithium therapy for bipolar affective disorder, there is delayed excretion of the lithium and therefore an increased risk of lithium toxicity. If the older client is concurrently on a sodium depleting diuretic, the risk for toxicity increases rapidly. The therapeutic range of blood lithium levels for the younger adult is 0.8–1.2 Eq/L. In the older adult, the therapeutic range lowers to 0.5–1.0 Eq/L (Reid, 1989).

Electroconvulsive therapy (ECT) may be used for those clients who do not respond to or who cannot tolerate the use of antidepressant medications. ECT has been found to be effective in those clients who experience rapid cycling bipolar disorder. ECT may be a safer alternative for older clients at high risk from the side effects of antidepressant medications. ECT appears to have a noticeable clinical effect more quickly than medications, a fact that may be significant when faster results are important. Lithium must be discontinued before ECT is used because the combination will decrease the therapeutic effects of lithium and increase the neuropsychologic side effects (Friedman, 1985).

A new medical treatment for depression is *sleep deprivation*. This may be total, for 36 hours, or partial, with the individual being awakened after 1:30 A.M. and kept awake until the next evening. During this time clients may be alone, in a group, or participating in activities. Some individuals improve steadily after only one night of sleep deprivation. Others respond better if the deprivation is conducted once a week for several weeks. Younger clients respond better than older clients.

It is thought the treatment normalizes the disturbance in the circadian rhythm and increases the amount of slow-wave sleep (Pflug, 1988).

Phototherapy is often the treatment of choice for SAD. Clients are exposed to very bright full-spectrum fluorescent lamps for two to six hours a day. Clinical improvement is typically seen within three to five days. Phototherapy may be used prophylactically with clients susceptible to SAD. It is thought the bright light suppresses the production of daytime melatonin and normalizes the disturbance in the circadian rhythm (Jacobsen and Rosenthal, 1988; Rosenthal, 1989).

Assessment

In assessing a client with an affective disorder, nurses organize interviews and observations around the knowledge base.

Nursing History

To increase the client's comfort, privacy should be provided for compiling the general nursing history and conducting a focused nursing assessment. Since a depressed client tires easily and a manic client is unable to remain seated for long periods, the interviewing will likely have to be completed over two or three sessions. The following focused nursing assessment is set up in a question-and-answer format. However, the interview will be more successful if the nurse uses his or her own words to guide discussions. The purpose of the focused nursing assessment is to establish a pattern for and a picture of the client.

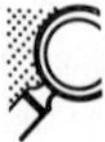

FOCUSED NURSING ASSESSMENT
for Clients with Affective Disorders

Behavioral assessment

Desire for activity
- Has there been a change in your activity level?
- How are you managing work/household responsibilities?
- What are your leisure activities?
- What kinds of activity demands are there on you?
- Are you having any difficulty doing basic activities of daily living?

Interaction with others
- Do you enjoy doing things with other people?
- Under what conditions do you like to be alone?
- Under what conditions do you like to be with others?
- Do you feel isolated from others?
- What are the sources of friction or conflict with others?
- How are disagreements handled?
- Would you define yourself as passive, aggressive, or assertive?

Dependency
- Do you need others around you to feel secure?
- In what way do you see yourself needing others?
- What kind of attention do you want from family and friends?
- Do you see yourself as an equal in adult relationships?

Affective assessment

Mood
- How would you describe your overall mood?
- Do you have mood swings?
- Under what conditions do you experience anger?
- Under what conditions do you experience anxiety?
- What kinds of things cause you frustration?

Guilt
- What kinds of things make you feel guilty?
- How much time a day do you spend thinking about failures or guilt?

Crying
- Under what conditions do you find yourself crying?
- How often do you cry?
- Have other people commented on your crying?

Gratification
- What activities in the past have given you pleasure?
- What activities give you pleasure at the present time?
- How would you describe your sense of humor?
- Tell me one of your favorite jokes.
- How have you used food, alcohol, or drugs to increase your pleasure?

Emotional attachments
- Who lives in your household?
- Do you make friends easily?
- How many friends do you have at present?
- To whom do you feel close?
- Who feels close to you?

Cognitive assessment

Self-evaluation
- What qualities do you like about yourself?
- How would you describe your level of self-confidence?

Give me an example of past successes in your life.
Do others like you?
How much do you need approval from others?
Give me an example of past failures in your life.
What would you like to change about yourself?
Do you feel in control of your life?
Are you feeling helpless?

Expectations
What do you expect will be the outcome of this illness/hospitalization?
What are your hopes for the future?
What goals do you have for the future?
How much effort will it take for you to change your situation?
Do you feel hopeless?
In what ways have you been investing/spending money recently?

Self-criticism
Overall, how would you evaluate your past life?
Do you have a need to do things perfectly?
How would you describe your standards for your own behavior?
How do others value you?
Do others criticize you a great deal?
How often do you feel rejected by others?
What does criticism and rejection by others mean to you?
To what degree do you evaluate situations as either all good or all bad?

Decision making
Do you feel a need to make a perfect decision?
Do you make decisions easily?
Do you think through the consequences before making a decision?
Has anyone commented on your difficulty or ease in making decisions?
Are you having difficulty concentrating?

Flow of thought
Does it seem as though your thoughts come slowly or quickly?
Do you have difficulty remembering what you were saying or going to say?

Body image
What do you like best about your body? Least?
Has your body changed in any way?
How much time a day do you spend thinking about your body?
How would you describe your overall appearance?

Delusions
Are you presently ill?
What makes you an important person?

Hallucinations
Are you hearing voices? What do they say?
Do you see things that others say they don't see?
What kinds of feelings do you have when you hear or see these things?

Physiologic assessment

Appetite
How has your appetite changed?
Do you skip a meal without even realizing it?
How much food do you eat a day? Can you recall your diet for the last 24 hours?
How much fluid do you drink a day?
How much weight have you gained or lost? In what length of time?
What are your favorite foods?

Sleep patterns
Describe your normal patterns of sleep before illness.
Are you having difficulty sleeping?
Do you awaken during the night?
Tell me about the dreams you have.
When you wake up do you feel tired? Energetic?
Do you nap during the day?
How much sleep do you believe you need?

Sexual desire
Before your illness how often did you engage in sexual activity?
Was this a source of enjoyment and satisfaction for you?
Tell me how your desire for sexual activity has changed.
Has your partner commented on a change in your level of desire?

Activity level
Do you tire easily?
What kinds of activities tire you?
Do you have a high level of energy?
Do you have difficulty sitting still?

Bowel activity
What is your normal pattern for bowel movements?
How has this changed?
What measures do you use at home when you are constipated?

Sociocultural assessment

Communication
With whom do you communicate most easily?
What areas of your life do you have difficulty sharing with others?
How clearly are you able to communicate during a crisis?

Network
Who can you depend on in a crisis?

Who can depend on you in a crisis?
Roles
What roles and responsibilities do you assume in your family?
What type of feedback do you receive about these roles?
To what degree are roles flexible in your family?
Significant life events
What kinds of losses have you sustained during the past year?
Relationships? Separations? Divorce? Deaths? Jobs? Roles? Self-esteem?
Describe the significance of these losses.
How have you managed these losses?

Goal assessment
Where do you hope to be in one month? Six months? One year?
Give me a word picture of what you will be like when you achieve your goals (use measurable data).
What do you need to do to achieve your goals?
How do you envision the nursing staff helping you meet your goals?

Physical Assessment

It is important for the nurse to complete a head-to-toe physical assessment of clients with affective disorders. Since some medical disorders have a high incidence of associated depression, these clients may be admitted to the medical service rather than the psychiatric service. In that case, it is important to consider the possibility of a concurrent depression. Clients who suffer from eczema or psoriasis may find that their skin disorder worsens with a depressive episode. Other disorders associated with depression are AIDS, carcinoid syndrome, CNS tumors, strokes, Cushing's syndrome, adrenal insufficiency, hypoglycemia, Parkinson's disease, thyroid disorders, parathyroid disorders, metal poisonings, Huntington's chorea, mononucleosis, hepatitis, multiple sclerosis, pancreatic carcinoma, and systemic lupus erythematosus (Gold and Herridge, 1988). Table 11–4 presents guidelines for conducting a physical assessment of the client with an affective disorder. Treatment of the primary medical disorder needs to be accompanied by psychiatric intervention for depressed clients.

Table 11–4 *Physical Assessment for Clients with Affective Disorders*

Medical history
Past illnesses/surgery:
Past hospitalizations:
Current illnesses:
Current medications:
Presenting complaints:
Family history of psychiatric problems:
Personal history of psychiatric problems:

Appearance
Hygiene:
Clothing:
Eye contact:
Posture:

Motor activity
Gait:
Hand gestures:
Responsiveness to environment:

Verbal
Rate of speech:
Amount of speech:
Tone and volume of voice:

Laboratory results
CBC:
T_3:
Serum electrolytes:
DST:
Sleep EEG:
TRH stimulation test:
ITT (children):

Some clients experience a depressive episode related to the medications they are receiving for medical disorders. When this occurs, it is referred to as an **iatrogenic depression.** In this instance, the medication is often discontinued, and a different medication is substituted. The following drugs have been associated with depression: opiates, antineoplastics, phenothiazines, digitalis, guanethidine, hydralazine, methyldopa, propranolol, reserpine, levodopa, sedatives, and steroids (Cohen, 1988; Ronsman, 1987; Yates, 1987).

It is important to note the serum electrolytes in clients with affective disorders. Some clients have an inappropriate secretion of antidiuretic hormone, which can lead to hyponatremia. Clients with low levels of sodium may present symptoms that mimic either depression or a manic psychosis. Restoring the sodium level removes the manifestations of the affective disorder (Santy and Schwartz, 1983).

If the physician has ordered the dexamethasone suppression test (DST), the nurse should note the results. Dexamethasone (0.5 mg) is administered orally at midnight. This is the critical time for ACTH release within the 24-hour biologic rhythm, and it is when the hypothalamic-pituitary-adrenal axis can be most accurately measured. Plasma cortisol levels are measured the next day in the late morning and late afternoon. The oral steroid blocks ACTH release for 28 hours in a nondepressed person. This blockage is demonstrated by low cortisol levels (5 mcg/100 mL or below) at both times of measurement. Depressed clients have suppressed cortisol levels in the morning, but these return to normal by the afternoon. The more severe the depression, the earlier the plasma cortisol levels return to normal. The more severe the depression, the more likely that the client will be a nonsuppressor. The accuracy of DST is 40 to 50 percent in clients with major depression, 67 percent in clients whose depression includes psychotic features, and 78 percent in clients who are seriously suicidal. This test is accurate for depression in both unipolar and bipolar disorders, but it is not indicative during the manic phase of the bipolar disorder. This test is not accurate for clients suffering from SAD. Clients who experience several bouts of depression a year have been found to return to nonsuppression one to two weeks prior to clinical relapse (Reid, 1989; Rose, 1987).

Several factors may influence the DST results, and they must be taken into consideration. The DST may not be accurate below the age of 18 or above the age of 60. Weight loss may contribute to nonsuppression, and so can severe or acute medical illness. Concurrent use of alcohol, sedatives, or anticonvulsants may increase nonsuppression (Arana and Baldessarini, 1987).

Another predictive test measures serum thyroid stimulating hormone (TSH) after administration of thyrotropin releasing hormone (TRH). After an overnight fast, the client is placed in a recumbent position and 0.5 mg of TRH is administered IV. For 2 minutes clients may experience discomfort such as nausea, urinary urgency, flushing, or general sensations of warmth. Blood samples are collected at 0, 15, 30, and 45 minutes to measure the level of TSH. Depression causes a blunted response in 25 to 70 percent of clients who have otherwise normal thyroid functioning. False positive results may be related to old age, starvation, chronic renal failure, or medications (glucocorticoids, thyroid hormones, opiates, or salicylates). False negative results may occur in clients with SAD or those receiving lithium, dopamine blockers, iodine dyes, theophylline, or spironolactone. Because of the short rise in blood pressure, the TRH test is not usually done for persons with hypertension or heart disease. The test is not performed for people with seizure disorders, because the test may precipitate a seizure (Looser, 1988).

For depressed children, an insulin tolerance test (ITT) may be ordered. Normally when there is an insulin-induced hypoglycemia, the body responds with an increased production of growth hormone. Children who are depressed demonstrate a hyposecretion of growth hormone in response to an ITT (Puig-Antich, 1986).

Nursing Diagnosis and Planning

The general nursing history and focused nursing assessment provide the data from which the nurse develops the plan of care. To guide the planning process, the nurse needs to ask the following:

1. In what areas does the client have the most difficulty functioning?
2. Which problems does the client define as priority problems?
3. What are the priority nursing diagnoses?
4. What are reasonable goals?
5. Are these in agreement with the client's goals?
6. What will be the most effective interventions?
7. What expected outcomes will appropriately measure the effectiveness of the plan of care?
8. Has the client been included during this planning process?

See Table 11–5 for the nursing care plan for the client with affective disorders. The care plans have

(continued page 437)

Table 11–5 Nursing Care Plan for the Client with Affective Disorders

Nursing Diagnosis: Constipation related to decreased activity, decreased intake, ignoring bodily signals, or side effects of antidepressant medications.
Goal: Client will have normal bowel function.

Intervention	*Rationale*	*Expected Outcome*
Keep a record to assess any problems with elimination; review client's normal pattern of bowel movements	To establish baseline data	
Have client set a regular time for elimination	Establishment of routine will increase perception of body signals	Bowel movements become regularized
Encourage physical activity	Exercise increases bowel motility	
Increase raw or bulk foods in diet	Foods with a natural laxative effect will stimulate bowel motility	Selects foods that aid in elimination
Increase fluid intake	Fluid maintains stool softness and aids in elimination	Increases fluid intake
Encourage not to delay urge to defecate	Failure to defecate when defecation reflexes are excited causes reflexes to become progressively less strong over time	
Offer warm fluids in early morning	Stimulation of morning gastrocolic and duodenocolic reflexes causes mass movement in large intestine	

Nursing Diagnosis: Impaired verbal communication related to retardation in flow of thought.
Goal: Client will experience an increase in flow of thought.

Intervention	*Rationale*	*Expected Outcome*
Stand or sit in a position that is in client's direct line of vision	Client may be unaware of your presence or interest if you are not easily visible	Indicates awareness of your presence
Introduce only one topic or question at a time	To decrease fragmentation of thought process	
Give client time to verbally respond	Time is needed to organize thought processes	Responds to topics or questions
Avoid answering for client	Responding for client as if he or she were incapable decreases self-esteem	
Assure client you will remain even if he or she chooses not to talk	Conveying to client that your acceptance is not dependent on his or her ability to communicate will increase feelings of worth	Indicates client does not feel pressured to communicate
If verbalization is difficult, suggest activities (eg, a 10-minute walk, looking at a magazine together, a simple OT project)	Helps client feel connected to others and decreases sense of isolation	Participates in nonverbal activities

(continued)

Table 11–5 *(continued)*

Nursing Diagnosis: Impaired verbal communication related to flight of ideas.
Goal: Client will experience a decrease in flow of thought.

Intervention	*Rationale*	*Expected Outcome*
If you can't follow what client is saying, say you are having difficulty (eg, "Your thoughts are coming too quickly for me to follow what you are trying to say")	Client may be unaware of not communicating clearly	Identifies that others cannot follow client's thought process
Ask client to try and slow down the communication (eg, "Let's talk about one thought at a time" or "Let's stay with this idea for a minute")	Helping client organize thoughts will improve communication	Talks about one topic for a short time
Try and identify theme or content thread of client's flight of ideas	To increase comprehension of what client is attempting to communicate	
Validate theme with client (eg, "You seem to be mentioning lithium often. Are you concerned about your medication?")	Client must have the opportunity to validate or correct your perception of communication	Responds to questions that seek clarification
Keep conversational topics on a concrete level	Abstraction will overstimulate client	Talks coherently about concrete topics
Decrease environmental stimuli (eg, "I think it's noisy here. Let's go to another area")	Flight of ideas are partially in response to multiple stimuli in the environment	

Nursing Diagnosis: Decisional conflict related to inability to concetrate; need to make perfect decisions.
Goal: Client will be able to make logical decisions with minimal difficulty.

Intervention	*Rationale*	*Expected Outcome*
Assess degree of impairment	Establish degree of difficulty before planning interventions	
Give limited choices when client is having difficulty making decisions (eg, "Would you like to take your shower before or after breakfast?")	Activity is directed while giving client limited control until decision-making ability is improved	Makes decisions within limited context
Allow as much control in situations as client is able to manage effectively	Increases self-confidence and self-esteem	Assumes control when possible
When client talks about being overwhelmed by all the decisions that have to be made, have him or her identify only one to work toward	Narrowing the focus to one decision at a time decreases feelings of helplessness	Focuses on one decision at a time
Use the problem-solving process	Old rigid patterns of problem solving decrease creativity in formulating alternatives	Uses new skills in the problem-solving process
Help client describe thoughts and feelings after the process	Client may believe that adequacy is related to perfect decisions	Verbalizes feelings related to decision making
Encourage client to delay making major decisions until the affective disorder has improved	Major decisions require optimal functioning of client	Delays major decisions until feeling better

(continued)

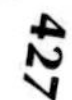

ntinued)

iosis: Altered role performance related to high affiliation needs.
Goal: ll verbalize a balance between dependence and independence.

Intervention	*Rationale*	*Expected Outcome*
Help client identify dependency needs (eg, who client feels dependent on and under what conditions)	Identification of situations that increase dependency will aid client's insight into problems	Identifies situations that increase dependency needs
Have client discuss impact of this dependency on others and provide feedback	Increased perception of effect on others will enable client to modify behavior	Verbalizes effect of client's behavior on others
Discuss how others also have rights and needs of their own	Assists client in seeing self as separate from others	Identifies rights and needs of others
Help client identify internal strengths that will decrease clinging dependency	Developing feelings of control will decrease the learned helplessness that contributes to depression	Verbalizes increased feelings of control and independence
Discuss responsibility for meeting own needs	Increases internal locus of control	Lists several needs that can be met without help
Encourage appropriate independent action	Increases active responsibility	Implements identified plan
Help client identify a variety of support systems	Having a variety of support systems will increase client's options under stress	Describes a network of support systems

Nursing Diagnosis: Hopelessness related to negative expectations of self and future; anger toward self.
Goal: Client will verbalize increased hope and less anger toward self.

Intervention	*Rationale*	*Expected Outcome*
Assist client in expressing feelings	Feelings need to be expressed before they can be managed	Verbalizes feelings
Explore with client sources of anger or guilt	Understanding that anger and guilt are responses to hurts or threats increases insight into the emotions	Identifies situations that cause anger or guilt
Help client plan appropriate ways to express anger, verbally and physically	Anger not expressed but turned inward is experienced as guilt	Expresses anger outwardly in an appropriate manner
Consult RT and OT for activities to vent anger	Physical discharge of the energy of anger will prevent escalation of anger	Uses available activities
Help client decide if hopeless feelings are validated by reality	Assisting client to see that these feelings are not substantiated by reality may lessen the hopelessness	Reports understanding that reality is not as hopeless as client may perceive
Remind client that feelings of hopelessness are part of disorder	The hopeless feelings will decrease as the depression lifts	
Avoid promising or giving false reassurance about recovery	Client will interpret this as lack of understanding and appreciation of his or her depth of despair	
If client is religious, use spiritual resources to focus on hope for future	Religious beliefs that encourage hope and faith may counteract feelings of sadness and hopelessness	Uses religious resources

(continued)

Table 11–5 *(continued)*

Nursing Diagnosis: Deficit in diversional activity related to decrease in gratification.
Goal: Client will verbalize pleasure in a variety of activities.

Intervention	*Rationale*	*Expected Outcome*
Be direct in encouraging participation in unit activities if client says there is no purpose in attending them	A severely depressed client may not have the energy or desire to initiate activity	Participates in one unit activity each day
Select activities that provide immediate gratification and that ensure success	This will help motivate client to continue with activity schedule and will temporarily decrease feelings of incompetence	Verbalizes feelings of gratification
Select activities that client has enjoyed and been successful with in the past	It is difficult to learn new skills during a severe level of the affective disorders	Uses familiar skills in activities
Reinforce verbal and nonverbal expressions of enjoyment	To reinforce and enhance feelings of gratification incongruous with depression	Acknowledges positive reinforcement
Have client gradually assume responsibility for activities and structure daily routine	Reinforcement of client's ability to rely on self	Schedules and participates in a variety of activities

Nursing Diagnosis: Fatigue related to lack of energy and tiring easily.
Goal: Client will increase amount of motor activity.

Intervention	*Rationale*	*Expected Outcome*
Explain the purpose of exercise to client, that is, that it has an antidepressant effect by decreasing sadness and tension	Explaining the rationale of the treatment plan will increase client's collaboration with the plan	Verbalizes the antidepressant effect of exercise
Ask client what particular physical activity would be the most enjoyable	Planning with client demonstrates respect for client's ability to collaborate and control life	Identifies acceptable exercises
Schedule frequent, short walks and activities throughout the day and evening	Having a schedule will emphasize the importance of exercise and reinforce the necessity to avoid immobility	Plans an exercise routine
Be firm in helping client to participate in the schedule	There may not be enough energy or desire to maintain the schedule	Carries through with planned exercises
Provide client with materials to keep a record of activities	Provides an objective measurement of activity performance	Keeps record of exercises
After activities, ask client to evaluate feelings and note any changes	Provides a subjective measurement of the effects of exercise	Verbalizes subjective effects of exercise

(continued)

Table 11–5 *(continued)*

Nursing Diagnosis: Fatigue related to hyperactivity and decreased awareness of physical exhaustion.
Goal: Client will not reach total physical exhaustion.

Intervention	*Rationale*	*Expected Outcome*
Assess level of activity during 24 hours	Establish baseline data	
Ask client to sit with you for 5 minutes every half hour	Provide frequent periods of rest	Sits for set periods of time
Be direct and supportive when client rests for short periods every 2 hours	Client is unable to monitor activity to prevent physical exhaustion	Rests in room every 2 hours
Decrease environmental stimuli	Hyperactivity is partially in response to stimuli in environment	Decreases activity in quieter surroundings

Nursing Diagnosis: Alteration in nutrition: less than body requirements related to anorexia or hyperactivity.
Goal: Client will maintain or attain normal nutritional intake.

Intervention	*Rationale*	*Expected Outcome*
Keep accurate records of food intake	To establish baseline data	
Find out food likes and dislikes	Providing preferred foods will increase intake	Eats preferred foods
Provide small, frequent feedings	Frequent feedings increase gastric motility; small feedings decrease sensations of bloating	Eats enough food to maintain normal 24-hour intake
Sit and interact with client while he or she eats	Social interaction increases the perception of eating as a pleasurable experience; client may increase intake under pleasant conditions	Verbalizes that mealtime is a pleasurable experience
Encourage physical activity	Physical activity stimulates appetite	Verbalizes an increase in appetite
Provide a quiet mealtime environment for hyperactive client	Client may eat more if there is less distraction during mealtime	
Provide hyperactive client with high-calorie foods that can be eaten while walking (eg, sandwich, milkshake)	Intake must be sufficient to provide energy for high activity level	Eats high-calorie, high-nutrient foods
Weigh client every other day	Any losses or gains in weight must be measured, which provides feedback to client and staff	Weight will be maintained or gained

Nursing Diagnosis: Powerlessness related to passivity, dependency, or external locus of control.
Goal: Client will verbalize increased feelings of control and power.

Intervention	*Rationale*	*Expected Outcome*
Help client identify sources of values relating to the maintenance of passivity (eg, "Who do you think taught you to be dependent and passive in relationships?")	The ability to identify sources of values is the first step in the process of clarifying values	Verbalizes how value of passivity was developed

(Diagnosis continued)

Table 11–5 *(continued)*

Intervention	*Rationale*	*Expected Outcome*
Help client identify secondary gains in remaining passive and dependent (eg, "How does your dependency protect you?" or "What is your reward for remaining passive?")	Bringing unconscious secondary gains to conscious awareness will assist client in formulating alternative ways to meet these needs	Identifies secondary gains that maintain passivity
Help client set realistic, daily goals specific to assuming more control of self and environment	To increase feelings of mastery and decrease learned helplessness by planned actions and objective measurement	Accomplishes daily goals
Provide assertiveness training	New options in relating to others will increase an internal locus of control	Responds assertively rather than passively in familiar situations

Nursing Diagnosis: Bathing/hygiene self-care deficit related to low energy level and decreased desire to care for self or to distractibility in completing ADLs.
Goal: Client will maintain ADLs.

Intervention	*Rationale*	*Expected Outcome*
If client is unable to do basic hygiene, provide these measures	Providing hygiene for client will prevent social embarrassment and improve body image	Is clean and neatly dressed each day
Assist client in gathering hygienic articles and clean clothing	Client's inability to make decisions may interfere with ADLs	
Encourage client to assume responsibility for own hygiene	Self-directive behavior will increase self-esteem	Initiates self-care measures
Provide positive feedback for assuming responsibility	Positive feedback reinforces behavioral changes	Maintains positive changes in behavior

Nursing Diagnosis: Deficit in diversional activity related to short attention span and high energy level.
Goal: Client will participate in diversional activities.

Intervention	*Rationale*	*Expected Outcome*
Keep activities simple and short (eg, painting, clay projects, wood-sanding projects)	To ensure success, which will increase self-esteem	Verbalizes feelings of success
Avoid activities that need intense concentration such as complicated games or puzzles	Attention span is insufficient for client to be successful at these activities	Completes projects
Provide activities that make constructive use of high energy levels	To expend energy in a creative manner that will increase self-worth	Discharges energy appropriately
Provide nonstimulating activities such as individual projects or quiet games	To avoid escalating hyperactive behavior by competition	
As client improves, provide activities with increasing complexity	To further develop client's feelings of mastery	Completes more complex activities

(continued)

Table 11–5 *(continued)*

Nursing Diagnosis: Nursing Diagnosis: Altered thought processes related to overgeneralization, dichotomous thinking, catastrophizing or personalization.
Goal: Client will verbalize a logical and realistic thinking process.

Intervention	*Rationale*	*Expected Outcome*
Assess client for distorted thinking	Establish baseline before planning interventions	
Help client understand that depression is not related to a personal defect or a sign of inferiority	Decreasing catastrophizing will increase self-esteem	Verbalizes improved self-esteem
Confront all-or-none thinking	Decreasing dichotomous thinking will increase realistic perceptions	Verbalizes less dichotomous thinking
Help client identify positive attributes and experiences	Decreasing overgeneralization will increase logical thinking processes	Identifies positive qualities and successes
Confront client with tendency to blame self for all unpleasantness	Decreasing personalization will increase realistic perceptions	Verbalizes less negative responsibility

Nursing Diagnosis: Family coping: potential for growth related to knowledge of affective disorders.
Goal: Client and family will verbalize adequate understanding of disorders.

Intervention	*Rationale*	*Expected Outcome*
Assess client and family's knowledge	Begin teaching at the appropriate level	
Teach the symptoms and typical course of the disorder	Prevents client and family from being overwhelmed by disorder	Lists signs and symptoms
Explain basic neurotransmission as it relates to disorder and medications	Helps client give up responsibility for causation; does not mean client gives up responsibility of working towards recovery	Verbalizes understanding of neurotransmission
Explain medical treatments and medications	Knowledge will decrease anxiety and increase cooperation with treatment plan	Verbalizes basic action of medications and purpose of treatment
Provide written materials	Reinforces verbal instruction	Refers to written materials
Encourage questions from client and family	Clarifies issues; increases active participation in learning	Asks questions
Teach symptoms of relapse	Ensures earlier treatment if relapse occurs	Lists symptoms
Discharge planning (eg, activity schedules, stress management, communication, problem solving, when to contact physician)	Assists family in not abandoning client out of frustration	Plans for discharge

(continued)

Table 11–5 *(continued)*

Nursing Diagnosis: Altered family processes related to rigidity in functions and roles.
Goal: Client and family will demonstrate increased flexibility in functions and roles.

Intervention	*Rationale*	*Expected Outcome*
Help client identify sources of gender role expectations, ie, family of origin, nuclear family, extended family, friends, cultural myths	Identifying sources of past and present expectations will assist the client in validating these expectations	Validates gender role expectations with current reality
Have client list all the roles by which he or she defines self	The fewer defining roles there are for a person, the higher the risk for depression	Lists roles
Have client describe any role changes or losses that have occurred	The more changes and losses of roles, the higher the risk of depression	Describes recent changes
Help client describe sources of positive reinforcement for each role	Lack of positive reinforcement and approval contribute to depression	Verbalizes need for positive reinforcement
Help client identify secondary gains for each family member related to rigidity of functions and roles	Bringing secondary gains to conscious awareness will assist client in formulating alternative ways to meet these needs	Describes secondary gains that maintain rigid roles
Ask client to predict what might occur if roles became less rigid	The predictive process allows the client to articulate vague fears and concerns	Verbalizes specific fears regarding change
Help client formulate ways to give self approval for functions and roles	Learning to give self-approval will increase self-esteem and decrease depressive feelings	Describes methods of self-approval
Involve nuclear family members in the problem-solving process related to home management functions and roles	Every family member contributes to maintenance of rigid roles and must be involved in any planned changes	Evaluation by all family members of roles and functions
Provide assertiveness training for client and family	Assertiveness skills are necessary if relationships are to be restructured	Uses assertive techniques when interacting
Help client identify possible new or additional functions and roles in life	Increasing sources of gratification and positive reinforcement will lessen depressive feelings	Lists new roles/functions

Nursing Diagnosis: Potential fluid volume deficit related to decreased intake.
Goal: Client will maintain normal fluid intake.

Intervention	*Rationale*	*Expected Outcome*
Keep accurate records of fluid intake	To establish baseline data	
Find out fluid likes and dislikes	Providing preferred fluids will increase intake	Identifies preferred fluids
Offer preferred fluids at frequent intervals in small amounts	Large amounts of fluid will increase sensations of bloating	Drinks enough fluids to maintain normal 24-hour intake (1200–1500 cc)
If client has a high activity level, provide containers of fluid that can "travel"	Adaptations for fluid intake must be considered in light of client's activity level	

(continued)

Table 11–5 *(continued)*

Nursing Diagnosis: Self-esteem disturbance related to guilt, criticism, and negative self-evaluation.
Goal: Client will verbalize positive self-concept.

Intervention	*Rationale*	*Expected Outcome*
Assess negative thought patterns for logic and validity; ask client if these are realistic evaluations	Global statements about guilt and inadequacy contribute to a negative self-esteem; cognitive errors increase feelings of depression	Verbalizes fewer feelings of inadequacy and guilt
Confront perfectionism in the client	Identification of unrealistic demands will decrease the associated guilt	Verbalizes decreased need for perfectionism
Help client formulate realistic standards for self	Realistic standards will be achievable and thereby increase self-esteem	Identifies realistic self-evaluation criteria
Set limits on the amount of time client spends discussing past failures	Rumination will intensify the guilt and negative self-esteem	Decreases the time spent focusing on failures
Review past achievements and present successes	To remotivate and encourage positive cognitions	Identifies successes in life
Help client write out list of positive attributes	Increases client's ability to see alternatives to negative self-view	Develops list
Give verbal recognition of positive thought patterns	To reinforce client's attempt to view self in a different way	Acknowledges positive reinforcement

Nursing Diagnosis: Self-esteem disturbance related to delusions and grandiosity.
Goal: Client will verbalize a realistic body image.

Intervention	*Rationale*	*Expected Outcome*
Do not argue about the client's delusions	An argument will place the client in the position of having to defend the delusions	
Set limits on the amount of time the client can discuss body image, eg, "We will talk about your body for 5 minutes and then we will talk about something else for 15 minutes."	Excessive preoccupation will increase negative self-concept in the depressed client and increase grandiose perceptions in the manic client	Decreases the amount of time spent focusing on body image
Provide accurate feedback as to how you perceive the client's body	To assist client in identifying that his or her body image is distorted and to provide reality testing	Verbalizes a changing body image that is more congruent with reality

Nursing Diagnosis: Sexual dysfunction related to lack of desire.
Goal: Client will report a return of sexual desire.

Intervention	*Rationale*	*Expected Outcome*
Introduce topic of sexuality with client and partner	To enable client and partner to share concerns they may have	Discusses sexual concerns/problems
Ascertain what, if any, problems existed prior to the depression	Preexisting sexual problems may be unrelated to the affective disorder	Identifies preexisting sexual problems
Explain to the client and partner that sexual desire usually returns as the depression improves	The knowledge that lack of sexual desire is a symptom of depression will decrease feelings of hurt, inadequacy, or guilt	Identifies lack of desire as a symptom of the disorder

(Diagnosis continued)

Table 11–5 *(continued)*

Intervention	*Rationale*	*Expected Outcome*
Stress the importance of physical affection such as hugging and holding each other	Touch is a very comforting and reassuring form of communication	Receives and gives touch with partner
Refer for sex therapy if the dysfunction continues after the depression has lifted	The dysfunction may be related to other difficulties that need specialized intervention	Follows up on referral to therapist

Nursing Diagnosis: Altered sexuality patterns related to impulsive increase in activity.
Goal: Client will report a return to previous level of sexual behavior.

Intervention	*Rationale*	*Expected Outcome*
Introduce topic of sexuality with client and partner	To enable client and partner to share concerns they may have	Discusses sexual concerns/problems
Ascertain what, if any, problems existed prior to the manic episode	Preexisting sexual problems may be unrelated to the affective disorder	Identifies preexisting sexual problems
Explain to the client and partner that the impulsive sexual behavior is not an indication of a change in ethics and values	The knowledge that impulsive sexual behavior is a symptom of the manic state during which the behavior is out of the client's control will decrease feelings of embarrassment, anger, and rejection	Identifies change in sexual behavior as a symptom of the disorder
Reassure client and partner that sexual behavior patterns usually return to normal as the manic episode improves	To help client and partner recognize that there is not a permanent change in ethics and values	
Protect the client from sexual acting out	To assume control over inappropriate behavior until the client is able to assume own control	Does not engage in inappropriate sexual behavior

Nursing Diagnosis: Sleep pattern disturbance related to insomnia and frequent awakenings.
Goal: Client will attain normal sleep pattern.

Intervention	*Rationale*	*Expected Outcome*
Ask client about past and present patterns; keep record of present pattern	To establish baseline data	
Ask what measures to improve sleeping have been successful in the past	Past measures may be adaptable to present setting	Suggests measures to improve sleep
Discuss alternative methods to facilitate sleep • Increase physical activity • Avoid exercise right before bedtime • Relaxation techniques • Avoid caffeine • Avoid emotional upsets prior to bedtime • Warm bath • Warm drink • Decrease amount of daytime napping	Natural sedative measures may improve the client's sleeping pattern	Initiates and evaluates measures that improve sleep; reports that sleep is more restful

(Diagnosis continued)

Table 11–5 *(continued)*

Nursing Diagnosis *(continued)*: Sleep pattern disturbance related to insomnia and frequent awakenings.
Goal: Client will attain normal sleep pattern.

Intervention	*Rationale*	*Expected Outcome*
Encourage client to read, watch television, or talk to someone when unable to sleep	Nighttime may increase feelings of hopelessness and sleepless periods are often spent ruminating over problems; redirection decreases excessive focus on problems	Initiates positive activities when unable to sleep

Nursing Diagnosis: Sleep pattern disturbance related to high energy level.
Goal: Client will attain normal sleep pattern.

Intervention	*Rationale*	*Expected Outcome*
Ask client about past and present sleep patterns; keep record of present pattern	To establish baseline data	
Provide a quiet environment at periodic times during the day	A quiet environment will decrease stimulation and hyperactivity	Decreases activity level in response to quiet environment
Be direct and supportive when client rests for short periods every 2 hours	Client is unable to monitor activity to prevent physical exhaustion	Rests in room every 2 hours
Have client participate in quiet activities prior to bedtime	Decreased stimulation may increase ability to sleep	Decreases activity level prior to bedtime
Encourage client to remain in bed for at least 3 hours during night	Client is unaware of need for relaxation and sleep	Remains in bed for 3 hours each night

Nursing Diagnosis: Social isolation related to withdrawal and decreased desire to interact with others.
Goal: Client will interact with staff and peers.

Intervention	*Rationale*	*Expected Outcome*
Do not overwhelm with scheduled activities when client is severely depressed	If client feels overwhelmed, he or she will further withdraw to protect self	
Participate in solitary activities with the client	Participation will stimulate client's interest in the activity	Interacts during activities on a one-to-one basis
Give positive feedback when client expresses interest in interactions	Positive changes in behavior must be supported and reinforced	Acknowledges positive reinforcement
Encourage participation in groups on unit	Attending and verbalizing will decrease sense of isolation	Participates in available groups
Remain with client while gradually adding peers to the interactions	Providing security will enable client to increase interactions with others	Interacts with peers
Help client identify benefits of social interaction	Positive gains will reinforce change in behavior	Identifies personal benefits of interaction with others

(continued)

Table 11–5 *(continued)*

Nursing Diagnosis: Impaired social interaction related to decreased perception of appropriate social behavior.
Goal: Client will interact with others according to social standards.

Intervention	*Rationale*	*Expected Outcome*
Encourage client to verbalize feelings rather than acting them out	Appropriate communication of feelings will decrease antisocial behavior	Verbalizes feelings
Set limits on behavior that interferes with peers and visitors	Inappropriate behavior will alienate client from peers and may result in angry outbursts	Does not interfere with interactions of others
Redirect client to activities that have minimal social interaction	Environmental stimulation escalates manic behavior	Demonstrates control over behavior
Set limits on behavior that is amusing and funny to the other clients	Client may suffer later embarrassment about behavior during manic episode	
Do not allow the client to give money to or buy gifts for other clients	The client in a manic state is easily manipulated by others; protect client until he or she can protect self	Does not spend money inappropriately

Nursing Diagnosis: Spiritual distress related to no purpose or joy in life; lack of connectedness to others; misperceived guilt.
Goal: Client will verbalize less spiritual distress.

Intervention	*Rationale*	*Expected Outcome*
Review with client past joys and successes in life	To identify past sources of spiritual comfort	Recalls past
Help client identify "small" purposes of current life (eg, contributions to family, value to friends, goals for next month)	Client is often overwhelmed with long-range goals; helps client move toward integrity rather than despair	Identifies appropriate purposes
Help client identify possible new functions/purposes in life	Positive reinforcement will help counteract depressive feelings	Lists new purposes
Help client evaluate if guilt feelings are validated by reality	Assisting client to see guilt is not substantiated by reality may lessen spiritual distress	Identifies reality of guilt
Help client identify a variety of available supportive people	Having a variety of people will increase sense of connectedness to others	Contacts support systems
If client is religious, use spiritual resources to decrease distress	Religious beliefs encouraging purpose, joy, and connectedness to others may counteract feelings of distress	Uses religious resources

been developed with a variety of clients in mind and need to be individualized to the specific client for whom one is caring. Standard care plans should not be used without adaptation. Individual clients are not expected to adapt to the care plan, the care plan must adapt to the individual client. (See Chapter 16 for care plans for suicidal clients.)

Evaluation

The evaluation step of the nursing process is accomplished by determining the client's progress toward achieving the expected outcomes. If progress is not being made, the nurse must ascertain if the interventions or diagnoses need to be modified. It is through evaluation that the nursing process is validated. Use of all steps of the nursing process is ongoing and will ultimately assist the client to achieve a higher level of wellness.

SUMMARY

1. Affect is the verbal and nonverbal communication of one's internal feelings.

2. In their lifetimes 8 to 12 percent of men and 18 to 25 percent of women will suffer a major depression. More male children are depressed then female children.

3. Many depressed elderly are misdiagnosed as having dementia and are at risk for being institutionalized.

Knowledge Base

4. Untreated depressions may last 6 to 9 months and untreated manic phases may last 2 to 6 weeks.

5. Depressive features are related to developmental levels from infancy to old age, and they exhibit age-specific characteristics.

6. Depressed people withdraw from activities and other people; experience feelings of despair, guilt, loss of gratification, loss of emotional attachments; and suffer from self-depreciation, negative expectations, distorted thinking processes, and self-criticism. They also have difficulty making decisions and experience a retarded flow of thought.

7. Manic people engage in any available activity and are effusive in interactions with others. They experience feelings of euphoria and form intense emotional attachments quickly. Thoughts center on grandiose expectations for themselves, exaggerated accomplishments, and a positively distorted body image. Distractibility and flight of ideas interfere with decision making.

8. Physiologically, depressed people experience anorexia, insomnia, inhibited sexual desire, decreased mobility, constipation, and an impaired immune system.

9. Manic people experience hyperinsomnia, exaggerated sexual desire, hyperactivity, and constipation.

10. Families may be oversolicitous or may become frustrated when the client is unable to change affect, behavior, or cognition. Abandonment and divorce is not uncommon.

11. Racism, sexism, and ageism contribute to depression by increasing feelings of powerlessness, hopelessness, and loss of self-esteem.

12. People experiencing multiple significant life events along with minimal support networks and maladaptive coping patterns are at higher risk of developing a depressive disorder.

13. There appears to be a genetic predisposition to affective disorders. The specific genetic marker is unknown at this time.

14. In the affective disorders, there may be a change in the amount of brain amines or a change in the sensitivity of the receptors to the amines, thus disrupting the transmission of electrical impulses.

15. The affective disorders may involve a desynchronization of circadian rhythm in some individuals.

16. A seasonal affective disorder (SAD) is cyclic and may be a variation of the more common affective disorders.

17. Repressed hostility, losses, unachieved goals, learned helplessness, external locus of control, negative thinking, and general role conflict all contribute to depression.

18. Tricyclic antidepressants, monoamine oxidase inhibitors, lithium, ECT, sleep deprivation, and phototherapy may be used in the treatment of the affective disorders. Blood plasma levels are important in determining the dosage of some medications.

Nursing Assessment

19. Clients with affective disorders must be assessed behaviorally, affectively, cognitively, physically, and socioculturally.

20. Clients must be assessed for a variety of medical disorders that can cause secondary depression.

21. The nurse must assess results of medical tests. Relevant tests may include the DST, sleep EEG, TRH, and ITT.

Diagnosis and Planning

22. Nursing diagnoses are formulated on the basis of the data collection.

23. Nursing interventions are individualized and expected outcomes are developed and dated.

Evaluation

24. Based on evaluation, nursing care plans are modified and continued until all expected outcomes have been met.

CHAPTER REVIEW

Claire, age 23, is admitted voluntarily to the psychiatric unit. Her family states she has had little sleep for three days, has been too busy to eat, and has been calling friends and neighbors "to talk" during the middle of the night. Her family has attempted to take her credit cards from her, since she has gone on spending sprees in the past. These attempts were met with Claire screaming and running out of the house. Her family reports that Claire stopped taking her lithium about six weeks ago. During the first several days of hospitalization, she talks about how famous she is and how she writes poetry and songs that will be published soon. She states further that she will start her own psychotherapy practice when she is discharged, since she has the gift of special religious insights.

1. Claire states, "I stopped my lithium. Now I feel like myself. I'm not going to take the lithium anymore. I feel better than I've ever felt. I'm great!" Your best response would be
   (a) "Stop talking so fast. I can't understand a word you are saying."
   (b) "It's good to see you feeling so positive about yourself."
   (c) "You should not stop any medication without consulting your doctor."
   (d) "I hear you expressing several ideas. Can we focus on your stopping your lithium?"

2. You encourage Claire to participate in diversional activities. The most appropriate activity is
   (a) An exercise group
   (b) A Ping-Pong tournament
   (c) A chess match
   (d) A monopoly game

3. You overhear Claire talking about her sex life to other clients. You interrupt the conversation and remove Claire from the situation. Your rationale for this intervention is to
   (a) Protect the other clients from embarrassment
   (b) Protect Claire from future embarrassment
   (c) Improve the moral aspect of the milieu
   (d) Improve Claire's moral behavior

Several weeks have gone by, and Claire has moved into the depressive phase of her bipolar disorder.

4. Claire talks about her relationship with her parents and siblings. She states, "Before I came into the hospital I was so impatient with them. I snapped at the least little thing, and often I screamed at them when they were just trying to help me. I feel so guilty. I'm such a bad person." Your best response is
   (a) "Guilty? I don't understand. I'm sure you're a good daughter and sister."
   (b) "Your family will understand that you've been under stress."
   (c) "You shouldn't feel guilty. Everyone gets impatient at times."
   (d) "I can see you feel a lot of pain when you act that way."

5. Claire isolates herself in her room. She comes to the dining room for meals, sits by herself, and does not interact with her peers. How can you best intervene in this problem?
   (a) Let her continue this behavior until the antidepressants work.
   (b) Sit with Claire at mealtime and have a cup of coffee.
   (c) Force Claire to sit with a group of clients at mealtime.
   (d) Ask Claire's physician to ask her to stay out of her room.

REFERENCES

Akiskal HS: The challenge of chronic depression. In: *Depression in Multidisciplinary Perspective.* Dean A (editor). Brunner/Mazel, 1985.

American Psychiatric Association: *Diagnostic and Statistical Manual of Mental Disorders,* 3rd ed, revised. Washington, DC: American Psychiatric Association, 1987.

Arana GW, Baldessarini RJ: Developmental and clinical application of DST in psychiatry. In: *Hormones and Depression.* Halbreich U (editor). Raven Press, 1987. 111–133.

Beck AT et al.: *Cognitive Therapy of Depression.* Guilford Press, 1979.

Beck-Frils J, Wetterberg L: Melatonin and the pineal gland in depressive disorders. In: *Hormones and Depression.* Halbreich U (editor). Raven Press, 1987. 195–206.

Brenners DK, Harris B, Weston PS: Managing manic behavior. *Am J Nurs* 1987; 87(5):620–623.

Cohen GD: *The Brain in Human Aging.* Springer, 1988.

Cytryn L, et al.: Developmental issues in risk research. In: *Depression in Young People.* Rutter M, Izard CE, Read PB (editors). Guilford Press, 1986. 163–188.

Davenport YB, Adland ML: Management of manic episodes. In: *Affective Disorders and the Family.* Clarkin JF, Haas GL (editors). Guilford Press, 1988. 173–195.

Dreyfus JK: The treatment of depression in an ambulatory care setting. *Nurs Pract* 1988; 13(7):14–33.

Emde R, et al.: Depressive feelings in children. In: *Depression in Young People.* Rutter M, Izard CE, Read PB (editors). Guilford Press, 1986. 135–160.

Emslie GJ, et al.: Sleep EEG findings in depressed children and adolescents. *Am J Psychiatry* 1987; 144(5): 668–670.

Fawcett J, Kravitz HM: Current research in affective illness. In: *Nursing Interventions in Depression.* Rogers CA, Ulsafer-VanLanen J (editors). Grune & Stratton, 1985. 13–38.

Frank E, et al.: Sex differences in recurrent depression. *Am J Psychiatry* 1988; 145(1):41–45.

Friedman MJ: Diagnosis and treatment of depression in the elderly. In: *Depression in Multidisciplinary Perspective.* Dean A (editor). Brunner/Mazel, 1985.

Garbutt JC: L-triiodothyronine and lithium in treatment of tricyclic antidepressant nonresponders. In: *Psychobiology and Psychopharmacology,* no. 2. Flach F (editor). Norton, 1988. 109–120.

Garvey MJ: Decreased libido in depression. *Med Aspects Human Sexuality* 1985; 19(2):30–34.

Gold M, Herridge P: The risk of misdiagnosing physical illness as depression. In: *Affective Disorders,* no. 3. Flach F (editor). Norton, 1988. 64–76.

Gold PW, et al.: Corticotropin releasing hormones. In: *Hormones and Depression.* Halbreich U (editor). Raven Press, 1987. 161–169.

Gove WR: Mental illness and psychiatric treatment among women. In: *The Psychology of Women.* Walsh MR (editor). Yale University Press, 1987. 102–126.

Green AI, et al.: The biochemistry of affective disorders. In: *The New Harvard Guide to Psychiatry.* AM, Jr (editor). Harvard University Press, 1988. 129–138.

Groos, GA: Physiological basis of circadian rhythmicity. In: *Biological Rhythms and Mental Disorders.* Kupfer DJ, Monk TH, Barchas JD (editors). Guilford Press, 1988. 121–141.

Haas GL, Clarkin JF: Affective disorders and the family context. In: *Affective Disorders and the Family.* Clarkin JF, Haas GL (editors). Guilford Press, 1988. 3–28.

Harris E: The antidepressants. *Am J Nurs* 1988; 88(11): 1512–1518.

Henker FO: Coping with a manic depressant spouse. *Med Aspects Human Sexuality* 1985; 19(4):29–32.

Hume AJA, et al.: Manic depressive psychosis. *J Adv Nurs* 1988; 13(1):93–98.

Jacobsen FM, Rosenthal NE: Seasonal affective disorder and the use of light as an antidepressant. In: *Affective Disorders,* no. 3. Flach F (editor). Norton, 1988. 215–229.

Janowsky DS, et al.: Psychopharmacologic-neurotransmitter-neuroendocrine interactions in the study of the affective disorders. In: *Hormones and Depression.* Halbreich U (editor). Raven Press, 1987. 151–160.

Kashani JH: Depression, depressive symptoms and depressed mood among a community sample of adolescents. *Am J Psychiatry* 1987; 144(7):931–933.

Kashani JH, Carlson GA: Seriously depressed preschoolers. *Am J Psychiatry* 1987; 144(3):348–350.

Kazdin AE: Childhood depression. In: *Behavioral Assessment of Childhood Disorders,* 2nd ed. Mash EJ, Terdal LG (editors). Guilford Press, 1988. 65–78.

Levy EM, Krueger R: Depression and the immune system. In: *Affective Disorders,* no. 3. Flach F (editor). Norton, 1988. 186–198.

Looser P: The TRH test in psychiatric disorders. In: *Affective Disorders,* no. 3. Flach F (editor). Norton, 1988. 52–63.

McBride AB: Mental health effects of women's multiple roles. *Image,* 1988; 20(1):41–47.

Mendelwicz J: Chronobiology, sleep and hormones in depressive disorders. In: *Hormones and Depression.* Halbreich U (editor). Raven Press, 1987. 229–238.

Monk TH: Circadian rhythms in human performance. In: *Affective Disorders,* no. 3. Flach F (editor). Norton, 1988. 199–214.

Nurnberg HG, Levine PE: Spontaneous remission of MAOI-induced anorgasmia. *Am J Psychiatry* 1987; 144(6):805–807.

Petti TA, Larson CN: Depression and suicide. In: *Handbook of Adolescent Psychology.* VanHasselt VB, Hersen M (editors). Pergamon Press, 1987. 288–312.

Pflug B: Sleep deprivation in the treatment of depression. In: *Affective Disorders,* no. 3. Flach F (editor). Norton, 1988. 175–185.

Puig-Antich J: Psychobiological markers. In: *Depression in Young People.* Rutter M, Izard CE, Read PB (editors). Guilford Press, 1986. 341–381.

Reid WH: *The Treatment of Psychiatric Disorders:* Brunner/Mazel, 1989.

Risch SC, et al.: Muscarinic mechanisms in neuroendocrine regulation and depression. In: *Hormones and Depression.* Halbreich U (editor). Raven Press, 1987. 207–228.

Ronsman K: Therapy for depression. *J Gerontol Nurs* 1987; 13(12):18–25.

Rose RM: Endocrine abnormalities in depression and stress. In: *Hormones and Depression.* Halbreich U (editor). Raven Press, 1987. 31–47.

Rosenthal ME et al.: Seasonal affective disorder. *Arch Gen Psychiatr* 1984; 40:72.

Rosenthal NE, et al.: Phototherapy for seasonal affective disorder. In: *Seasonal Affective Disorders and Phototherapy.* Rosenthal NE, Blehar MC (editors). Guilford Press, 1989. 273–294.

Rothblum ED: Sex-role stereotypes and depression in

women. In: *The Stereotyping of Women,* Franks V, Rothblum ED (editors). Springer, 1983.

Rutter M: The developmental psychopathology of depression. In: *Depression in Young People.* Rutter M, Izard CE, Read PB (editors). Guilford Press, 1986. 3–30.

Santy P, Schwartz M: Hyponatremia disguised as an acute manic disorder. *Hosp Community Psychiatry* 1983; 34(12):1156.

Sonis, WA: Seasonal affective disorder of childhood and adolescence. In: *Seasonal Affective Disorder and Phototherapy.* Rosenthal NE, Blehar, MC (editors). Guilford Press. 46–54.

Targum SD: Genetic issues in treatment. In: *Affective Disorders and the Family.* Clarkin JF, Haas GL (editors). Guilford Press, 1988. 196–212.

Thase ME: Comparison between seasonal affective disorder and other forms of recurrent depression. In: *Seasonal Affective Disorders and Phototherapy.* Rosenthal NE, Blehar MC (editors). Guilford Press, 1989. 64–78.

Trad PV: *Infant and Childhood Depression.* Wiley, 1987.

Wehr TA, et al.: Eye versus skin phototherapy of seasonal affective disorder. *Am J Psychiatry* 1987; 144(6): 753–757.

Wehr TA: Rapid cycling affective disorder. *Am J Psychiatry* 1988; 145(2):179–184.

Yapko MD: *When Living Hurts.* Brunner/Mazel, 1988.

Yates WR: Depression. In: *Psychiatric Illness, Primary Care.* Yates WR (editor). Saunders, 1987. 14(4): 657–668.

SUGGESTED READINGS

Kerr NJ: Signs and symptoms of depression and principles of nursing intervention. *Perspect Psychiatr Care* 1987/88; 24(2):48–63.

Oakley LD: Marital status, gender role attitude and black women's report of depression. *J Natl Black Nurses Assoc* 1986; 1(1):41.

Rosenbaum JN: Depression: Viewed from a transcultural nursing theoretical perspective. *J Adv Nurs* 1989; 14:7–12.

Weiner RD, Coffey CE: When ECT is recommended for your patient. *Med Aspects Human Sexuality* 1988; 22(6):20–24.

CHAPTER 12

Alcohol Abuse

J. SUE COOK

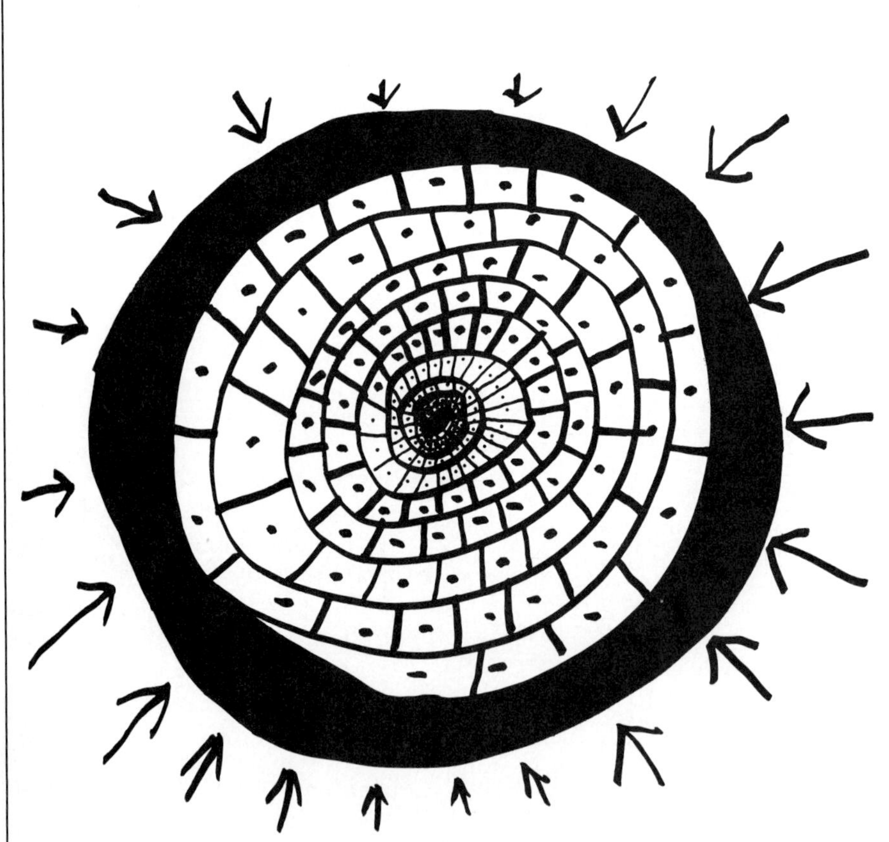

How I See My Illness

Engulfed in Darkness
Spiraling inward, weaving
a web that is ultimately
devastated by a darkness
whose victim I
always have been but
always hope to never be.

■ *Objectives*

After reading this chapter the student will be able to

- Discuss the significance of alcohol abuse to mental health nursing
- Describe the reasons underlying the development of alcohol abuse
- Explain the DSM-III-R diagnostic criteria for alcohol abuse and alcohol dependence
- Apply a focused nursing assessment to clients significantly affected by alcohol
- Relate abnormal findings in the assessment of an alcoholic client
- Identify nursing diagnoses for clients with acute alcohol intoxication, alcohol withdrawal, and chronic alcoholism
- Prepare nursing care plans for clients with acute alcohol intoxication, alcohol withdrawal, and chronic alcoholism
- Discuss the evaluation of nursing care of the client with acute alcohol intoxication, alcohol withdrawal, and chronic alcoholism
- Apply the five steps of the nursing process to clinical situations involving clients with alcoholism

■ *Chapter Outline*

Introduction

As many as one third of the clients admitted to general hospitals have alcohol-related problems, but seldom is the admitting diagnosis alcoholism. Rather, the diagnoses are indirectly associated with or directly the result of alcohol abuse (Tweed, 1989). For example, a client may be admitted for upper gastrointestinal bleeding, but only after nursing assessment is it realized that the client's condition is a result of alcoholism. The following case illustrates this point.

Manuel, a 30-year-old farm laborer, was admitted to the medical floor with upper gastrointestinal bleeding. During the nursing history interview Manuel told the nurse that he was not a heavy drinker. When asked how much he drank, Manuel admitted to drinking at least a six-pack of beer a day. Manuel asked the nurse why his drinking behavior was so important. Manuel said he did not consider his drinking to be heavy, nor did he think his drinking behavior had any connection to his gastrointestinal bleeding.

Because alcoholism is frequently not stated as part of the client's admitting diagnosis, nurses need to become familiar with background information about the problem of alcoholism.

Incidence of Alcoholism in the United States

Alcoholism is a major public health problem in the United States. Of the estimated 100–110 million alcohol users in the United States, 18 million are problem drinkers. Each of those drinkers affects one to four people, largely spouses and children, or an additional 40 million people. (See Figure 12–1.)

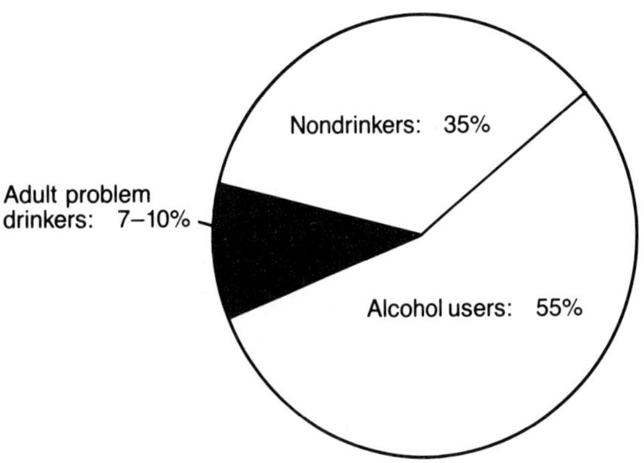

Figure 12–1 *Alcohol use in the United States*

Fetal alcohol syndrome is the third leading cause of birth defects in the United States. Studies indicate that 50 percent of all deaths from falling accidents as well as 50 percent of all fires are related to alcoholism. Alcohol is a frequent contributing factor in auto accidents, assaults, rapes, homicides, and suicides. Alcoholism is the most expensive addiction for business and industry; 40 percent of industrial deaths and 47 percent of industrial injuries are caused by the use of alcohol (Amaro, 1990; Campbell and Graham, 1988). (See Figure 12–2.)

Abuse of alcohol among culture groups in the United States varies a great deal. The rate among Native North Americans may be as high as 50 percent. Following in decreasing order are the Irish, French, Scandinavians, English, and Germans. Italians have very low rates. Extremely low rates of alcoholism are found among the Semitic races, the Africans, and the Asians (Campbell and Graham, 1988).

In the 1987 Report to Congress, the National Institute on Alcohol Abuse and Alcoholism estimated the cost of alcohol abuse in the United States to be $117 billion for 1983. Of this $117 billion, loss of employment and reduced productivity accounted

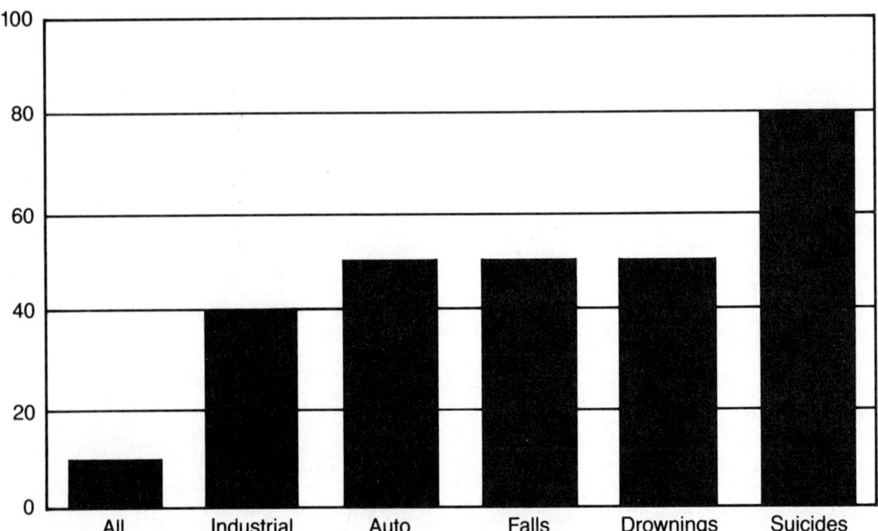

Figure 12–2 *Alcohol and fatal accident-related problems*

Sources: Campbell and Graham, 1988; *Chicago Tribune,* 1990; Schenk, 1989.

for $71 billion and health care costs accounted for $15 billion. The estimated per capita consumption of alcohol in the United States is 2.65 gallons of alcohol per year. This figure represents a decrease in consumption since 1977. Consumption reached a peak in 1980 and 1981 and then began a gradual decline.

Half of the alcohol consumed in this country is consumed by 10 percent of the drinking population. Generally women drink less heavily than men. However, the level of drinking for women ages 35 to 64 has increased. Ninety-two percent of high school students and 90 percent of college students report using alcohol at least one time. Thirty percent report drinking regularly. This rate has remained fairly stable for the past 15 years. How much and how often a person drinks is determined by a complex set of interactions including demographics, social variables, economics, and biologic factors (U.S. Department of Health and Human Services, 1987; World Almanac, 1990).

Significance of Alcoholism to Mental Health Nursing

Because the use and abuse of alcohol is a prevalent problem that causes a good many personal and social consequences, it is a major concern to the nursing profession. Nurses are likely to come into contact with people significantly affected by alcohol in a variety of settings. But regardless of the setting, nurses need to be prepared to complete assessments and intervene effectively to assist the client toward recovery.

Nurses also need to realize that alcoholism cuts across all ages, cultures, genders, and occupations. Recently, attention has been given to the severity of the problem among health professionals, including nurses. Many state nurses' associations, supported by the national nursing organizations, have established peer support systems to assist impaired nurses in recovering from alcoholism. These programs often depend on volunteers to help the impaired nurse toward recovery. Unimpaired nurses have a responsibility to their professional colleagues to help them find ways of coping with the stress in health care settings.

Finally, nurses need to examine their own values, attitudes, and behaviors in relation to alcohol abuse. Effective client interventions will be difficult unless nurses are able to identify their feelings about the use and abuse of alcohol. Alcoholic clients are acutely aware of the emotional overtones present in interactions, and those overtones can affect whether the client decides to stay in treatment or continue using alcohol. To judge and reject clients because of their use of alcohol is not professionally ethical.

Knowledge Base

There is no precise definition of alcoholism. At best, alcoholism can be described as a biologic, psychologic, and sociocultural disorder. The American Medical Association (AMA) and the World Health Organization (WHO) (Tweed, 1989) regard alcoholism as a specific disease entity. The AMA defines alcoholism as

> an illness characterized by significant impairment that is directly associated with persistent and excessive use of alcohol. Impairment may involve physiological, psychological, or social dysfunction.

The WHO defines alcoholics as

> those excessive drinkers whose dependence on alcohol has attained such a degree it shows a noticeable mental disturbance or an interference with their bodily and mental health, their interpersonal relations and their smooth social and economic functioning, or who show the prodromal signs of such developments.

Because there are many different patterns of alcohol abuse, it is impossible to use quantity and frequency of drinking as criteria in the definition of alcoholism. Treating it as a chronic, progressive, and potentially fatal disease has led to better acceptance of treatment by many alcoholics. Since there are many definitions of alcoholism, this text utilizes Bigby, Clark, and May's (1990, p. 147), working definition of **alcoholism** as "anyone who repetitively has multiple problems because of drinking over a period of time."

DSM-III-R divides criteria related to alcohol use into two categories: Alcohol Dependence and Alcohol Abuse. The diagnostic criteria are patterns of use, associated features, course, prevalence, and familial pattern. Each criterion consists of typical patterns of behavior that profile the client who uses alcohol.

Patterns of use:

1. Regular daily intake of large amounts of alcohol
2. Regular heavy drinking limited to weekends
3. Long periods of sobriety interspersed with binges of daily heavy drinking lasting for weeks or months

Associated features:

1. Often associated with the abuse of other psychoactive drugs such as cannabis, cocaine, heroin, amphetamines, sedatives, and hypnotics. Most commonly seen in people under 30.
2. Nicotine dependence very common.
3. Often associated with depression. However, the depression appears to be a consequence, rather than the cause, of the drinking.

Course:

1. Natural course varies for males and females.
2. Male onset is usually in late teens or early twenties, with an insidious course. He may not be aware of dependence on alcohol until his thirties. The first hospitalization usually occurs in the man's late thirties or early forties. Symptoms rarely appear for the first time after age 45.
3. Female onset often occurs later in life than onset for males. Females with alcohol dependence have been studied less extensively than males.
4. Tolerance develops as people drink more over days, months, and years. That is, the person must drink more to get the desired effect.
5. Tolerance may also be inborn, because people vary in the amount of alcohol they can tolerate. After drinking very small amounts of alcohol, some people develop a headache, upset stomach, or dizziness; others drink large amounts with hardly any ill effects.

Prevalence:

1. It is predicted that by 1995 there will be 18.4 million people over the age of 17 who are problem drinkers. This represents a 4 percent increase since 1985 (Finley, 1989).

Familial pattern:

1. There is a tendency for alcohol dependence to cluster in families.
2. Adoption studies indicate that alcohol dependence from one generation to another does not require environmental exposure to family members with alcohol problems. This suggests a genetic influence in the disorder (American Psychiatric Association, 1987).

Behavioral Characteristics

Many attempts have been made to organize information on the behavioral and developmental patterns of problem drinking. E. M. Jellinek was a pioneer in this area, and his work has withstood the test of time in that it is referred to in almost all major sources. Jellinek identified four phases of alcohol addiction. (See Table 12–1.)

The course of alcoholic behavior is one of highs and lows sometimes referred to as remissions and exacerbations. Lack of control of drinking is the central behavioral characteristic. This lack of control is both insidious in origin and inconsistent, especially in the early and middle stages. At times the alcoholic can drink with control and at other times cannot control the drinking behavior (Bigby, Clark, and May, 1990).

Table 12–1 *Jellinek's Four Phases of Alcohol Addiction*

Phase	*Behavior*
1—The prealcoholic symptomatic phase	Drinking is used to relieve tension Tolerance for tension decreases steadily for a period of six months to two years Drinking takes place on practically a daily basis Larger and larger amounts of alcohol are required to reach the desired stage of sedation
2—The prodromal phase	Onset of blackouts—that is, after a relatively moderate amount of alcohol, the drinker will not show signs of intoxication and is able to carry on a conversation and participate in elaborate activities with little recollection the next day Surreptitious drinking Preoccupation with alcohol Heavy consumption of alcohol
3—The crucial phase	Loss of control Any intake of alcohol begins a chain reaction that is felt as a physical demand for alcohol Drinks until is too intoxicated or too ill to ingest more alcohol Rationalizes behavior by producing "alibis" Grandiose behavior to compensate for drinking Marked aggressive behavior generating guilt and remorse Alcohol-centered lifestyle Neglect of nutrition Decreased sexual drive Increased social pressures from parents, spouse, employers, and friends warning the drinker of behavior
4—The chronic phase	Prolonged periods of intoxication Ethical deterioration Marked impairment of thinking Loss of tolerance, half of the previously required amount of alcohol is enough to bring about a sedated state Experiencing of indefinable fears Tremors Signs of physical deterioration

Source: Adapted from E. M. Jellinek, Phases of alcohol addiction. In: D. J. Pittman, C. R. Snyder (editors). Society, Culture & Drinking Patterns (Wiley, 1962), pp. 356–368. Reprinted with permission.

As the course of alcoholism continues, there may be behaviors such as starting the day off with a drink, sneaking drinks through the day, gulping alcoholic drinks, shifting from one alcoholic beverage to another, and hiding bottles at work and at home. Some alcoholics skip meals in order to drink. Often they give up hobbies and other interests in order to have more time to drink. It is not unusual for alcoholics to engage in what is called telephonitis, which is making telephone calls to family and friends at inappropriate times, such as the middle of the night. As alcohol becomes more central to the person's thinking, there is a tendency to make more verbal references to drinking (Tweed, 1989).

Since alcohol decreases inhibitions, many alcoholics become hostile, argumentative, loud, boisterous, and even assaultive when they are drinking. There may be multiple arrests for assaults and fights. Other alcoholics become withdrawn, tearful, depressed, and socially isolated when they drink.

Behavioral characteristics are also noted in terms of employment. Many alcoholics have frequent absences from work, especially on Mondays and Fridays. If they are drinking at noon, their work productivity decreases in the afternoon. They often suffer from interpersonal problems at work that are related to their alcoholic behavior. Frequently they experience loss of a promotion, loss of a job, and/or frequent job changes (Tweed, 1989). See Table 12–2 for an overview of behavioral characteristics of alcoholics.

Their drinking behavior often gets alcoholics into legal difficulties. Statistics show that 75 percent of people arrested for the first time for driving while intoxicated (DWI) are alcoholics. People who cannot stop drinking and driving after the first arrest certainly have an alcohol problem. This is sup-

Table 12–2 *Behavioral Characteristics of Alcoholism*

Lack of control of drinking
Starting the day off with a drink
Sneaking drinks
Gulping drinks
Shifting from one alcoholic beverage to another
Hiding bottles at home or work
Skipping meals in order to drink
Giving up hobbies or other interests in order to drink
Telephonitis
Making verbal references to drinking
Hostile, argumentative, assaultive
Arrests for fights or DWI
Withdrawn, tearful, socially isolated
Employment difficulties

ported by the data that 95 percent of second-time DWI arrests and 99.9 percent of third-time DWI arrests are alcoholics (Bigby, Clark, and May, 1990; Tweed, 1989).

Behavioral characteristics are also related to blood alcohol levels (BAL). One ounce of hard liquor, one glass of wine, or one can of beer raises the blood alcohol level by about 0.025. Metabolism of alcohol in the liver takes place at about 0.66 to 1.0 ounces of hard liquor per hour and 8 to 12 ounces of beer per hour. There is also an individual response to BAL, in that chronic drinkers can function at much higher levels of alcohol because of acquired tolerance. Inexperienced drinkers may become comatose at relatively low levels of alcohol consumption. See Table 12–3 for an overview of BAL and behavior (Lerner et al., 1988).

Mary McCormick, a 35-year-old homemaker, was recently released from the Recovery Resources program for alcoholics. Mary was trying to stay away from alcohol but had a few relapses and drunken episodes. Mary's oldest son came home from school and found his mother sneaking a glass of whiskey from a bottle hidden in the garage. Mary's son was trying to take the glass from Mary to check it when Mary slapped him across the face. Realizing what she had done, Mary tried to apologize to her son. However, he screamed "I hate you!" and ran from the garage. Mary broke the top off the whiskey bottle and slashed her wrists.

Table 12–3 *Blood Alcohol Level and Behavior*

*Blood Alcohol Level**	*Behavior*
0.05	Changes in mood Changes in normal behavior Judgment and restraint are loosened Person feels carefree
0.08–0.10	Voluntary motor action clumsy Legal level of intoxication
0.20	Brain motor area depression causes staggering Easily angered Shouting Weeping
0.30	Confusion Stupor
0.40	Coma
0.50	Death (usually due to medullar respiratory blocking effects)

*Percentage of alcohol in blood

Affective Characteristics

Many alcoholics experience guilt for their behavior. At times they are able to acknowledge responsibility for their actions and experience the painful feeling of regret that is called guilt. Shame is probably the most typical and deeply experienced emotion for alcoholics. Shame is a more difficult emotion to manage than guilt, since shame is a painful feeling about oneself as a person. Shame is a matter of personal identity, and shameful people believe they have no choices and no power. They experience themselves as failures and feel tormented, isolated, and lonely. Shame is reflected in statements such as: "I'm hopeless. I'm no good. Nothing about me is good." Alcoholics often drink in an attempt to decrease their feelings of shame, but in the end their shame is increased because of their drinking behavior and its life-damaging consequences (Bradshaw, 1988; Potter-Efron, 1989).

Many alcoholics find themselves in a state of depression and despair. These feelings arise out of behaving in ways that do not match their value system, hurting people they love and care about, and not living up to their potential (Bigby, Clark and May, 1990).

One of the affective characteristics of advanced alcoholism, which may be related to brain damage, is alcoholic jealousy. This is seen when the alcoholic person becomes convinced that his or her partner is seeking relationships with others or having an affair. The alcoholic is certain this is an effort by the partner to humiliate or abandon him or her (Potter-Efron, 1989). (See Table 12–4 for an overview of affective characteristics.)

Table 12–4 *Affective Characteristics of Alcoholism*

Guilt
Shame
Torment
Feeling like a failure
Depression
Despair
Alcoholic jealousy

Theron Sanders, a 40-year-old autoworker, was feeling a little depressed over the Christmas holidays because he had been laid off until after the first of the year. Theron resented having to go to visit his wife's parents—he knew they didn't respect him very much. Theron had never provided enough for "their little girl," and when he was around them he felt as though he didn't measure up. Theron started drinking in the mornings to keep from feeling nervous. When his wife begged him not to drink, Theron screamed at her, "Woman leave me alone. I know when to stop." When Theron's wife began to cry, he stormed out of the house and jumped into the car. He drove around randomly, not really knowing where he was headed.

Cognitive Characteristics

Because of behavioral and affective characteristics, most alcoholics have inadequate self-esteem and an internal sense of being flawed as a person. Grandiose thoughts may be an attempt to compensate for these beliefs.

Denial is the major defense mechanism maintaining dependence on alcohol. Denial is the process of self-deception and an unconscious attempt to maintain self-esteem in the face of out-of-control behavior. Denial also functions to underestimate the amount of alcohol consumed and to avoid recognizing the impact of alcoholic behavior on others. Supporting the denial is the use of projection, minimizing, and rationalization. Projection, seeing others as being responsible for one's drinking, is heard in: "My three teenagers are driving me crazy. It's their fault I drink." Minimizing, not acknowledging the significance of one's behavior, is heard in: "Don't believe everything my wife tells you. I wasn't so drunk I couldn't drive." Rationalization, giving reasons for their behavior, is heard in: "I only drink because I'm so unhappy in my marriage" (Bigby, Clark, and May, 1990; Tweed, 1989).

These defense mechanisms are considered consequences, not causes, of alcoholism. They serve to protect self-esteem and perpetuate the problem. Denial can be a major obstacle to treatment, for no treatment will be effective until the alcoholic acknowledges that the drinking is out of control.

Blackouts are a fairly early sign of alcoholism. They are a form of amnesia for events that occurred during the drinking period. The alcoholic may carry out conversations and elaborate activities with no loss of consciousness, but have total amnesia for those activities the next day (Tweed, 1989).

A more advanced cognitive characteristic of alcoholism is Wernicke's encephalopathy. This is characterized by abnormal patterns of thinking and receptive aphasia. Without treatment the client may progress to the irreversible condition of Korsakoff's psychosis. At this stage the person is unable to retrieve longterm memory events and is also unable to retain new information. Confabulation, making up information to fill memory blanks, develops in an attempt to protect self-esteem when confronted with loss of memory. Wernicke's encephalopathy and Korsakoff's psychosis are caused by severe thiamine deficiency and the direct neuro-toxic effect of alcohol (Lerner et al., 1988). (See Table 12–5 for an overview of cognitive characteristics.)

Table 12–5 *Cognitive Characteristics of Alcoholism*

Inadequate self-esteem
Gradiose thoughts
Denial
Projection
Minimizing
Rationalization
Blackouts

Juanita Wilson, a 55-year-old homemaker, had been a closet drinker for about ten years. She kept her drinking a secret from her husband and friends by using breath mints and strong perfume to cover the alcohol odor. Juanita's family had noticed that she was getting forgetful and had a hard time getting a simple meal on the table. When the children would come over for Sunday dinner, Juanita couldn't get everything on the table at the same time, and she burned or undercooked everything she served. Juanita's husband noticed that she had some bruises and was falling frequently. When he confronted Juanita, she passed it off by saying, "Well, dear, that's what happens when you get old!" Juanita's husband became very concerned when he came home to find her sleeping on the sofa while the iron smoldered on one of his dress shirts.

Physiologic Characteristics

Alcohol is a CNS depressant. Every cell in the body is adversely affected by the chronic use of alcohol. Several organ systems become so impaired that the effect is clinically obvious; these are the respiratory, cardiac, gastrointestinal, hematopoietic, immune, and nervous systems. Organ system damage results primarily from malnutrition. Indeed, alcohol may be an important cause of malnutrition in the United States. Consuming large amounts of alcohol decreases the appetite and causes inadequate food intake. Alcohol provides 200 calories per ounce; thus, an intake of one pint of 86-proof whiskey contains 1300 calories. This is one half a person's daily energy requirement. These two factors, decreasing appetite and substituting alcohol for nutrients, cause alcoholics to lose weight. Malabsorption, disturbed nutrient metabolism, and increased nutrient requirements are frequent problems of alcoholics.

Two nutrition disorders are related to alcoholism: Wernicke's encephalopathy and Korsakoff's psychosis. In DSM-III-R these disorders, which are due to thiamine deficiency, are classified as alcohol amnesic disorders.

In Wernicke's encephalopathy, neuronal and capillary lesions are found in the gray matter of the brain stem. The encephalopathy is characterized by delirium; memory loss; confabulation; apathy; apprehension; ataxia; clouding of consciousness; and, sometimes, coma. If Wernicke's encephalopathy is not treated early with large doses of thiamine, Korsakoff's psychosis may develop.

Korsakoff's psychosis is primarily the result of thiamine deficiency, but niacin deficiency also plays a role in its development. The result is degeneration of the cerebrum and peripheral nerves. Korsakoff's psychosis is characterized by amnesia, confabulation, disorientation, and peripheral neuropathy.

Wernicke's encephalopathy and Korsakoff's psychosis are treated by withdrawal from alcohol and vitamin supplements. Improvement can occur in Wernicke's encephalopathy, but most clients retain a certain degree of cognitive and emotional impairment. In Korsakoff's psychosis, impairment of memory is a residual effect even when slight improvement occurs (Cohen, 1982; Donald, 1985). See Chapter 15 for discussion of dementia.

Cecil McDonald, a 60-year-old electronics assembly-line worker, had been using alcohol to cope with job and home stress for the last 20 years. Cecil noticed that he had developed tremors to the point that he could barely lift his coffee cup and hold it still. He found that he had to make up data to put on his assembly inspection reports because he couldn't remember what he had done during the day. Cecil's coworkers found his memory lapses very amusing. In his latest episode, Cecil panicked because he couldn't find his car in the parking lot. A coworker reminded him that he had come to work on the bus that morning.

Sociocultural Characteristics

Alcoholism is a family problem. The most devastating impact on the family is when the alcoholic is the parent. Alcoholism leads to the deterioration of the couple system and power struggles occur between the alcoholic and nonalcoholic partner. Family relationships begin to deteriorate, and the family is trapped in the alcoholic cycle of shame, anger, confusion, and guilt.

The inability to discuss the alcohol problem openly contributes to family denial. To avoid embarrassment, family members make excuses to outsiders for the alcoholic's behavior. The nonalcoholic partner may remain in the relationship because of emotional dependency, money, family cohesion, religious compliance, or outward respectability. Other nonalcoholic partners may threaten to or actually leave the alcoholic. At this point the alcoholic promises never to drink again, the family is reunited, the promise is usually broken, and the family becomes locked into dysfunctional relationships.

Co-dependence is the term used to describe the nonalcoholic partner who remains in the relationship. Co-dependents operate out of fear, resentment, helplessness, hopelessness, and the desire to control the alcoholic's behavior. The co-dependent tries obsessively to solve the problems created by the alcoholic. Not effective, the co-dependent becomes exhausted and depressed but unable to stop the "helping" behavior. Co-dependents often suffer from low self-esteem and fear of abandonment. Co-dependents are caretakers, and this caretaking activity may be a compensation for feelings of inadequacy. Women may be more vulnerable to co-dependent behavior because they have been socialized to be responsible for the family and often feel they are expected to be loyal to their partner at all costs (Sullivan, Bissell, and Williams, 1988).

Co-dependents tend to experience one of four response patterns. The *alienated* ignore the alcohol problem as well as their own feelings of pain and hope it will all go away. *Bullies* manage their own pain by lashing out and constantly criticizing the alcoholic, hoping that will stop the drinking. *Managers* take care of everything and shield the alcoholic from distress and problems. *Martyrs* passively endure their pain, hoping their partners will feel guilty enough to change their alcoholic behavior (Earle and Crow, 1989).

It is estimated that there are 28 to 30 million adults in the United States who grew up in alcoholic homes. Children who grow up in homes where one or both parents are alcoholics often suffer the effects their entire lives. Dysfunctional family rules develop around the impact of alcoholism. Very early in life, children of alcoholics learn not to talk about the alcohol problem, even within the family. They are taught not to talk about their own feelings, needs, and wants. These children are also taught not to feel. Eventually they learn to repress all feelings and become numb to both pain and joy. Children of alcoholics are expected always to be in control of their behavior and their feelings. They are expected to be perfect and never make mistakes. However, within the family system, no child can ever be perfect enough. Consistency is necessary for building trust, and alcoholic parents are very unpredictable. Children of alcoholic parents do not expect reliability in relationships. They learn very early that if you don't trust another person you will not be disappointed (Scavnicky-Mylant, 1990).

Children of alcoholics tend to develop one of four patterns of behavior. The *hero,* often the oldest child, becomes the competent caretaker and works on making the family function. The *scapegoat* acts out at home, in school, and in the community. This child takes the focus off the alcoholic parent by getting into trouble and becoming the focus of conflict in the family. The *lost child* tries to avoid conflict and pain by withdrawing physically and emotionally. The *mascot,* often the youngest child, tries to ease family tension with comic relief that is used to mask his or her own sadness (Earle and Crow, 1989; Treadway, 1989).

In dysfunctional families, roles are necessitated by the need of the family system to keep the family in balance. Each role is a way to handle the distress and shame of having an alcoholic parent. Each role gives the family member a sense of some control, even though the roles do not change the family systems' dysfunction (Bradshaw, 1988).

Adult children of alcoholics often feel a need to change others or to control and fix the environment for the good of others. It is typical of these adult children to deny powerlessness and try to solve all problems alone. Adult children blame themselves for not being able to achieve what no one can achieve. Obsessions are a common form of defense and may take a variety of forms such as constant worrying about situations, preoccupations with work or other activities that bring about good feelings, and compulsive achievement. This obsessive pattern covers the feelings of helplessness and blocks the feelings of anxiety, inadequacy, and fear of abandonment (Bradshaw, 1988; Scavnicky-Mylant, 1990).

The majority of Americans take a moralistic attitude toward alcoholism. It is viewed as a sin or as the result of a weak will. Alcoholics are seen as totally responsible for their situation and are expected to use will power to control themselves and become respectable members of society once again. Women are especially stigmatized by this perspective. Women are expected to be "lady-like" at all times and when they drink too much are quickly labeled "loose women" or "drunks" (Bigby, Clark, and May, 1990; Hughes, 1989).

A group even more stigmatized by American society is that of lesbian alcoholics. They suffer as women in a male-dominated culture, as well as carrying the stigmata of being lesbian and being alcoholic. Lesbian women have a higher rate of alcohol consumption than heterosexual women. They also attempt suicide 7 times more often and have higher rates of suicide completion than heterosexual, nonalcoholic women. Lesbian women suffer from being labeled self-centered, ridiculous, immature, promiscuous, immoral, and emotionally disturbed. In an anti-gay culture such as the United States, coming to terms with one's homosexuality and accepting a gay identity are very painful. It is thought that depression, alcohol use, and suicide among lesbians may be related to the effects of stigmatization (Hall, 1990).

Women who have been abused physically and sexually are at greater risk for becoming alcoholics than nonabused women. Increased use typically follows the first incident of abuse. It is believed that this may be an attempt to self-medicate while coping with the physical and emotional consequences of abuse (Amaro, et al, 1990). (See chapter 16.)

Sonja Walker, a 14-year-old high school student, had been an excellent student when suddenly her grades dropped dramatically. She tearfully confessed to her high school counselor that personal problems were affecting her grades. Sonja explained that her father had had a "drinking problem" but had been going to AA for several years. Three months ago, Sonja's father lost his job and was unable to get another. A month ago, he started a pattern of binge drinking. Sonja was reluctant to talk because she knew her mother would be furious if she knew Sonja had revealed the family secret. Sonja's mother was working overtime to keep the family going. When Sonja's mother was home she fought constantly with her husband about his drinking. Her father tried to get Sonja to buy alcohol for him after his wife poured his supply down the drain. When Sonja tried to explain that she was too young to purchase alcohol, her father screamed at her "Get out of my sight, you're useless!" When her father was sober he tried to be Sonja's best friend. Sonja stopped bringing friends home because she didn't know what to expect. She was too nervous to do homework, always worrying about what her father might do. Sonja told the counselor "I don't want him to be my friend. I don't even want him for a father anymore!"

Causative Theories

Years of research in intrapersonal theories of alcoholism have now yielded to models that combine biologic, psychologic, and sociocultural components of alcoholism. Most likely there are a number of subtypes of alcoholism with different combinations of these predisposing components. At this time it is unclear how genes and environment interact and contribute to the development of alcoholism (Gordis et al., 1990).

Biologic Theories Beginning around 1970, research has focused on family studies in an attempt to determine if a predisposition to alcoholism is inherited. Twin studies have demonstrated that monozygotic (identical) twins have 2 times the rate of alcoholism of dizygotic (fraternal) twins of the same sex. Adoption studies indicate that children of a biologic alcoholic parent who were adopted by nonalcoholic families are 3 times more likely to become alcoholic than adopted children of biologic *non*alcoholic parents. It is unknown at this time if the genetic defect is in alcohol metabolism, mood regulation, nutritional absorption, neurologic function, hormonal regulation, or personality patterns.

In 1990 the first study was published indicating there is a strong link between alcoholism and a dopamine gene on chromosome 11. Further research is indicated as to the role of dopamine, serotonin, and norepinephrine in the brain's reward system. Initial findings indicated that 69 percent of the alcoholics studied had the specific dopamine gene, while the gene was not present in 80 percent of the nonalcoholics studied. The fact that the gene did not show up in all alcoholics and was not absent in all nonalcoholics indicates that other genes may be involved and that alcoholism may not be a purely genetic disorder (Blum et al., 1990; Hughes, 1989).

Continuing research in the genetics of alcoholism will provide a greater understanding of the physiology of alcoholism. In combination with additional psychosocial research, the results can be expected to lead to new methods of prevention and treatment.

Intrapersonal Theories For many years intrapersonal theories were the only explanations for alcoholism and they contributed to the development of the moral perspective of alcoholism. These theories describe alcoholism as being determined by personality traits and developmental failures. More recent research has made these theories much less popular (Hughes, 1989).

In the psychoanalytic category, Freud was the first to explain alcoholism as the result of fixations at the oral, anal, or Oedipal stages of childhood. He also felt alcohol provided the mechanism for regression and a release from anxiety-ridden reality. The earlier the stage of fixation and regression, Freud felt, the poorer the prognosis for recovery from alcoholism. Menninger advanced the "self-destructive drive" as the major component of alcoholism. Adler attributed the cause to powerful feelings of inferiority and a desire to escape responsibility. Believing that childhood overindulgence and excessive coddling led to an inability to face adulthood frustrations, Adler said people used alcohol to counter adulthood demands.

Personality theories, the second group of psychologic theories, may be correlated with psychoanalytic theories. Allport, whose studies focused on traits of the individual, gave attention also to traits specific to the alcoholic. Sullivan claimed that personality, including the personality of an alcoholic, was a pattern of interpersonal situations characterizing the person's life. Lewin's research focused on the social aspects of the alcoholic's personality. For Lewin, the alcoholic operated in "life space," which existed for the person at that moment. Alcohol was seen as the intangible to which the self had some type of relationship within the life space.

Behavioral/Learning Theories Behavioral theories look at the antecedents of drinking behavior, prior experiences with drinking, and the beliefs and expectations surrounding drinking behavior. This perspective looks at which reinforcement principles operate in alcoholism. Consequences for continuing to drink or deciding not to drink, such as increasing pleasure or decreasing discomfort, are studied. These theorists also look at activities associated with drinking, social pressure, rewards, and punishments for drinking.

Learning theories state that alcoholics have learned maladaptive ways of coping. It is thought that drinking is a learned, maladaptive means of decreasing anxiety. Drinking behavior is viewed on a continuum from no use, to moderate use, through excessive to dependent use. All of these behaviors are learned responses. These theorists look at childhood exposure to drinking role models, quantity of alcohol considered appropriate and safe, customs surrounding the use of alcohol, and the symbolic meaning of alcohol (Hughes, 1989).

Sociocultural Theory Sociocultural theorists look at how the cultural values and attitudes influence people's drinking behavior. Those cultures whose religious or moral values prohibit or extremely limit the use of alcohol have lower incidences of alcoholism.

This theory is based on the idea that values, perceptions, norms, and beliefs are passed on from one generation to another. Alcohol is part of everyday life in some families, while in other families there is infrequent use or abstinence from alcohol. Exposure to the use or abuse of alcohol may influence the development of alcoholism. For example, a child growing up in a neighborhood where people are drinking on the streets is more likely to become alcoholic than a child in a more abstinent environment. Likewise, a child reared by one or two alcoholic parents is more likely to become alcoholic than a child with nondrinking parents (Campbell and Graham, 1988).

Recovery Movement People involved in the recovery movement do not consider alcohol addiction as a symptom of some other problem but rather view addiction as an illness in itself. The responsibility for recovery is on the client and any attempt to shift responsibility to others, such as the family or staff, is confronted directly. Recovery is considered a life long, day-to-day process and is accomplished with the support from peers with the same addiction. Recovery programs typically are 12-step programs first introduced by Alcoholics Anonymous in which honesty is a very high value. These programs are deeply spiritual and recovery is thought to be dependent in part on a faith in a "higher power" (Nowinski, 1990).

Medical Treatment

Alcoholism treatment modalities can be grouped into three areas: biologic, psychologic, and social. Studies indicate that internists and general practitioners have been the most successful of all primary therapists in the treatment of alcoholism. They are followed next by social workers and last by psychiatrists. Other literature indicates that Alcoholics Anonymous (AA) has the highest success rate in the treatment of alcoholism (Sugerman, 1982). However, before reaching conclusions about the success of any particular kind of treatment, one must consider the type of treatment given. Often, the general practitioner and internist place the alcoholic client on antianxiety drugs. This treatment shifts the client from one addiction to another, so one must ask if this is a successful treatment for alcoholism. The psychiatric nurse needs to take all forms of treatment into consideration in planning the care of the alcoholic client.

Biologic Treatments This treatment model includes emergency medical care for (1) acute intoxication and injuries related to intoxication, (2) detoxification or withdrawal, (3) inpatient hospitalization, and (4) medication therapy.

Acute intoxication. The major management problem in acute intoxication is determining if a medical emergency exists. Many alcoholics are confused or in a coma when they are brought into the emergency department. The nurse should attempt to learn from friends, family, and witnesses what and how much the client drank and over what period of time. The BAL is a general guide for management of the client who is acutely intoxicated. The client ABCs—airway patency, breathing, and circulation—are assessed to determine if ventilatory support is necessary. The most common cause of death in acute intoxication is respiratory failure.

Blood pressure must be determined. Hypotension may be related to occult bleeding from trauma or esophageal varices. Vomitus and stool are tested for occult blood. Temperature is assessed, since the client may be hypothermic from exposure. An ECG is often ordered to look for alcohol-induced arrhythmias. Head to toe assessment is necessary, since the client may be suffering traumatic injuries from falls, fights, or accidents. The nurse should look for signs of infection since intoxication and chronic alcoholism predispose the client to aspiration and pneumonia. A drug screen is ordered when symptoms indicate that additional toxic substances may have been ingested (Lerner et al., 1988).

Alcohol withdrawal. The process described by the terms detoxification, withdrawal, and "drying out" can include a broad range of symptoms of differing severity. Alcohol withdrawal syndrome can be progressive, with minor symptoms of agitation, anorexia, and nausea. It can also include major symptoms such as seizures and delirium tremens.

Withdrawal symptoms typically begin about 6 to 8 hours after the last ingestion of alcohol. Early symptoms include irritability, anxiety, insomnia, tremors, and a mild tachycardia. Withdrawal *seizures* typically occur 6 to 96 hours after the last ingestion of alcohol with 90 percent of the seizures occurring between 7 and 48 hours. Seizures are usually grand mal and may last for a few minutes or less. Status epilepticus occurs in 3 percent of withdrawal clients. During withdrawal, *hallucinations* may occur 6 to 96 hours after the last ingestion of alcohol with the peak at 48 to 72 hours and typically lasting for 3 days. Hallucinations range from "bad dreams" to visual, auditory, olfactory, or tactile hallucinations. *Delirium tremens* (DTs) usually occur on days 4 and 5 but may appear as late as 14 days after the last drink. During DTs clients experience confusion, disorientation, hallucinations, tachycardia, hyper- or hypotension, extreme tremors, agitation, diaphoresis, and fever. DTs usually last about 5 days and still carry a 15 percent mortality rate, usually from cardiovascular failure. (See Table 12–6 for an overview of withdrawal symptoms.)

Table 12–6 *Physiologic Responses to Alcohol*

Related medical conditions

- Acute pancreatitis
- Alcohol-induced hypoglycemia
- Alcoholic ketoacidosis
- Alcoholic myopathy
- Gastrointestinal bleeding, especially from varices
- Hepatic precoma and encephalopathy
- Hypothermia
- Infections

Withdrawal responses

Response	*Time range*	*Peak time*
Seizures	6–96 hours	7–48 hours
Hallucinations	6–96 hours	48–72 hours
Delirium tremens	3–14 days	4–5 days

The nurse should assess vital signs frequently. Increasing heart rate and blood pressure may indicate the onset of DTs. Rapid respirations may lead to respiratory alkalosis. Additional assessment includes the area of concomitant disorders. (See Table 12–6 for these related disorders.)

Medical management utilizes a keep-open IV line. This can be used to administer necessary medications. If the client is out of control and a danger to self or others, haloperidol (Haldol) may be given IV. If the client is exhibiting signs of Wernicke's encephalopathy, thiamin HCl is given IV. Since magnesium is necessary for thiamine to be effective, low serum magnesium levels indicate a need for replacement therapy. With signs of hypoglycemia, glucose may be administered IV. A variety of medications may be used to treat early withdrawal and prevent seizures and DTs. These medications are started at fairly high doses and tapered off over a period of 5 days (Lerner et al., 1988; Powell and Minick, 1988). (See Table 12–7 for these medications.)

The environment should allow the client to relax as much as possible and feel comfortable. Helping the client maintain contact with reality is extremely important. This is done by keeping enough light in the environment to avoid casting shadows, orienting the client, having a clock close by, and having staff present or within a short distance. Experts disagree on whether radios, television sets, and telephones should be present in the room. Some contend these objects add to the client's confusion, but others say they help the client maintain contact with reality. Nursing judgment should be used, taking the client's condition and response to the environment into consideration. Of utmost concern is client safety. Although an alcoholic in the midst of withdrawal can be difficult to manage, restraints are a therapeutic measure that should be used judiciously and avoided if at all possible.

The client's activity level will be determined by his or her orientation to reality, physical condition, and amount of medication. For initial periods of confusion and sedation, bedrest may be indicated. As physical difficulties and confusion subside, the client should be encouraged to walk and complete

Table 12–7 *Medications used during alcohol withdrawal*

Medication	*Route*	*Dose*
Chlordiazepoxide (Librium)	po; IV	25–50 mg; q 4–6 hours
Diazepam (Valium)	po; IV	5–10 mg; qid
Lorazepam (Ativan)	po; IM; IV	2 mg; prn
Clorazepate dipotassium (Tranzene)	po	15 mg; qid
Oxazepam (Serax)	po	15–30 mg; qid
Thiamine HCl	po; IM; IV	100 mg per day
Haloperidol (Haldol)	IM	5 mg; q 30–60 minutes
Magnesium sulfate	IV	As necessary

ADLs (Burkhalter, 1975; Estes, Smith-DiJulio, and Heinemann, 1980; Powell and Minick, 1988).

Complete recovery from withdrawal may take as long as two or three weeks. An important component to successful treatment is consistent contact and development of a relationship with another person such as a nurse or nurse-therapist. For any treatment to be successful, family members or significant others should be included. Furthermore, as part of discharge planning, it is wise to introduce alcohol counselors, social workers, or therapists. Representatives of Alcoholics Anonymous can be very helpful in laying the groundwork for long-term treatment (Hough, 1989; Powell and Minick, 1988).

Inpatient hospitalization. Recently, alcohol treatment programs have been added to general hospital services. These programs have been newly offered for several reasons: (1) public awareness of the problem of alcoholism has increased, (2) hospitals have been responding more to community needs, (3) insurance coverage for alcoholism treatment has increased, and (4) more medical schools have been preparing physicians to diagnose and treat alcoholism. The most successful hospital treatment programs have been affiliated with Alcoholics Anonymous. The average length of stay for alcoholism clients ranges from two to four weeks, depending on the treatment program (Weisberg and Hawes, 1989). As a result of this trend, many psychiatric hospitals do not admit alcoholic clients until detoxification is complete.

Medication therapy. Disulfiram (Antabuse) is an enzyme inhibitor which some alcoholics choose to utilize as a medical treatment. Disulfiram inhibits aldehyde dehydrogenase (AldDH) and leads to accumulation of acetaldehyde if alcohol is consumed, causing a chemical reaction called a disulfiram-alcohol reaction. This reaction can occur within 5 to 10 minutes of ingestion of alcohol and may last from 30 minutes to several hours. Symptoms include flushing, nausea and copious vomiting, thirst, diaphoresis, dyspnea, hyperventilation, throbbing headache, palpitations, hypotension, chest pain, syncope, anxiety, blurred vision, weakness, and confusion. In severe reactions, arrhythmias accompanied by myocardial infarction, cardiovascular collapse, respiratory depression, coma, convulsions, and death can occur. Nursing interventions for clients experiencing a disulfiram-alcohol reaction include monitoring vital signs, maintaining an adequate airway, fluid replacement, and the administration of oxygen (Townsend, 1990).

An initial dose of 500 mg is administered each morning for two weeks. Following this, the client is maintained on a range of 125 mg to 500 mg daily; the average dose is 250 mg. Disulfiram is continued until permanent self-control is obtained, which may be from a few months to several years.

Disulfiram should be used only under careful medical and nursing supervision. It is essential that the client understand the consequences of the therapy. The client must understand, for example, that disulfiram takes 14 days to be removed from the system following discontinuation of the medication. Consumption of alcohol during this two-week time period will result in a disulfiram-alcohol reaction. The client should be warned about all sources of alcohol: mouthwash, cough syrups, the external application of liniments and shaving lotion, and so forth. These preparations are dangerous, since they

Table 12–8 *Items to Avoid While Taking Disulfiram (Antabuse)*

Substances	*Foods*
Antianxiety agents	Flavorings, especially vanilla extract
Anticoagulants	Food prepared with wine
Liquid cough-cold medications	Salad dressings
Liquid analgesics	Sauces
Mouthwashes	Caffeine
Rubbing alcohol	
Alcohol swabs	
Back-rub preparations	
Shaving lotion	
Colognes	
Nail polish remover	

can be absorbed through the skin and produce a disulfiram-alcohol reaction. (See Table 12–8 for foods and substances to be avoided while taking disulfiram.) Other client teaching should include an appraisal of disulfiram-induced side effects. The client should know that drowsiness, fatigue, headache, peripheral neuritis, erectile problems, and metallic or garliclike tastes should subside after approximately two weeks of therapy. The longer disulfiram is taken, the more sensitive the client will become to alcohol. The client should be encouraged to purchase a Medic-Alert identification bracelet or carry a card that identifies his or her use of disulfiram. Some agencies require clients to sign an informed consent before disulfiram medication begins. It is recommended that supportive psychotherapy be a part of disulfiram therapy (Townsend, 1990).

Psychologic Treatments The psychologic treatments for alcoholism are extremely varied. The most common and current trend in treating the alcoholic is using the combined efforts of the hospital and a mental health alcoholism treatment unit. Following crisis intervention and detoxification, alcoholics are referred to an inpatient mental health alcoholism treatment unit. The treatment unit uses a variety of methods, including referral for outpatient treatment, individual psychotherapy, group psychotherapy, family therapy, and milieu therapy. The major goals of these modalities are to assist clients in (1) recognizing they have a drinking problem, (2) accepting their drinking problem, (3) developing adaptive coping mechanisms, (4) reducing or eliminating problem drinking, and (5) improving their self-concept (Estes, Smith-DiJulio, and Heinemann, 1980; Levin, 1987; Sugerman, 1982).

Group therapy provides a setting in which alcoholics can face their excessive drinking problems and learn new coping mechanisms for facing the stresses in their lives. Group therapy may be expanded to include family members, or it may be focused on family therapy in an effort to identify the communication patterns within the family structure that encourage alcoholic behavior.

Other treatment options are outpatient treatment, after-school or work programs, partial hospitalization, short-term residential care, long-term care, and halfway houses. A newer experience being utilized in some adolescent and young adult programs is the Therapeutic Adventure. This experience, which is several days long, is modeled after the Outward Bound programs. This experiential learning exercise works on individual and group issues around such concepts as trust, cooperation, help-seeking, autonomy, and communication. Clients work as a group on a survival course with the goal of increased self-esteem and group identity and cohesiveness (Nowinski, 1990).

Sociologic Treatments The best known of the sociologic treatments is Alcoholics Anonymous (AA), a nonprofessional 12-step counseling program focusing on person-to-person and group relationships. For clients to profit from AA, they must acknowledge their drinking problems. AA clients are not allowed to drink and are encouraged to look at alcoholism as a problem bigger than they are. See Table 12–9 for the 12 Steps of AA.

In 1990, there were more than 76,000 AA groups worldwide. AA is open to teenagers and adults with drinking problems and is a self-help group. Only first names are used to protect the identity of the alcoholic. AA provides the support structure to socialize the client into a new way of life. Testimonials from recovering alcoholics assist new members with their drinking problems.

Table 12–9 *The 12 Steps of Alcoholics Anonymous*

We
1.—Admitted we were powerless over alcohol, that our lives had become unmanageable
2.—Came to believe that a Power greater than ourselves could restore us to sanity
3.—Made a decision to turn our will and our lives over to the care of God as we understood Him
4.—Made a searching and fearless moral inventory of ourselves
5.—Admitted to God, to ourselves, and to another human being the exact nature of our wrongs
6.—Were entirely ready to have God remove all these defects of character
7.—Humbly asked Him to remove our shortcomings
8.—Made a list of all persons we had harmed and became willing to make amends to them all
9.—Made direct amends to such people wherever possible, except when to do so would injure them or others
10.—Continued to take personal inventory and when we were wrong promptly admitted it
11.—Sought through prayer and meditation to improve our conscious contact with God as we understood Him, praying only for knowledge of His will for us and the power to carry that out
12.—Having had a spiritual awakening as the result of these steps, we tried to carry this message to alcoholics and to practice these principles in all our affairs

Source: Alcoholics Anonymous World Services. *A.A.: 44 Questions.* Alcoholics Anonymous World Services, 1952. Reprinted with permission.

Other groups affiliated with AA serve as support groups for families of alcoholics. Al-Anon is designed to help family members share common experiences and to gain an understanding of alcoholism. Alateen is designed to be a support group for teens whose parent(s) are alcoholic, and Alatots is a similar group for children.

Another community agency that provides occupational retraining and employment for recovering alcoholics is the Salvation Army, best known for its work with the homeless alcoholic population.

The final major sociologic treatment group is the clergy. The role of the clergy has become somewhat like that of a catalyst, that is, the clergy stimulates and challenges society to examine the moral and spiritual aspects of critical issues such as alcoholism. The religious community serves as a resource for people trying to find meaning in life. Clergy are trained and skilled in counseling. Those clergy trained to avoid using guilt and remorse are helpful in assisting the alcoholic through recovery (Hancock, 1982).

Despite the availability of the numerous treatment programs for alcoholics, many problem drinkers are not receiving treatment. It is estimated that 65–70% of alcoholics do not seek treatment (Fingarette, 1988). Successful treatment is linked to early detection of the drinking problem, the person's recognizing the need for treatment and availability of adequate treatment facilities.

Assessment

The foundation of the nursing process in alcoholic clients is data collection. Primary data sources are the client, the client's family or significant others, medical records, social records, diagnostic test results, and nursing records. A thorough nursing history and physical assessment are essential to identify problems in the alcoholic client's health status and to identify nursing diagnoses related to these problems. In interviewing alcoholic clients, the nurse needs to realize that clients may downplay the amount of drinking they actually do. So it is important to be direct in questioning; ask "How much do you drink?" rather than "Do you drink?" The nurse should be nonjudgmental and matter-of-fact in posing questions to the client.

Nursing History

Since use of alcoholic beverages is so common in our society, it is important to include questions about alcoholic consumption when compiling a general nursing history. After completing an initial history and discovering frequent intake of alcoholic beverages, the nurse needs to appraise the situation further by obtaining data related to drinking behavior. These data can be critical in recognizing the potential for impending alcoholic withdrawal and other potential emergency conditions. Table 12–10 presents a quick appraisal tool helpful for gathering data.

Table 12–10 *Quick Appraisal Tool for Impending Withdrawal and Emergencies**

Assessments Related to Withdrawal

When was your last drink?
When did you start this drinking episode?
When was your last drinking episode before this episode?
What have you been drinking? In what quantities?
How much alcohol did you consume each day during this drinking episode?
How much alcohol do you usually consume during a drinking episode?
What kinds of reactions do you experience when you stop drinking?

_____ Tremors _____ DTs
_____ Hearing things _____ Convulsions
_____ Seeing things _____ Other

Have you ever taken medications for any of the above reactions?

_____ Valium _____ Dilantin
_____ Librium _____ Thorazine
_____ Paraldehyde _____ Vistaril
_____ Chloral hydrate _____ Other

Are you taking any medications now?

_____ Prescription Kind:
_____ Over-the-counter Kind:
_____ Street drugs Kind:

Do you have any drug allergies? Which drugs?

Assessments Related to Emergency Conditions

Have you had any recent accidents or injuries?

_____ Falls
_____ Fistfights
_____ Auto accidents
_____ Other accidents

Have you experienced any of the following symptoms recently?

_____ Pain _____ Difficulty balancing
_____ Bleeding Where: _____ Blurred or double vision
_____ Breathing problems _____ Confusion
_____ Vomiting _____ Loss of memory
_____ Diarrhea _____ Other

Do you have any of the following chronic health problems?

_____ Diabetes _____ Stomach
_____ Lung (COPD, bronchitis) _____ Liver
_____ Heart _____ Skin
  _____ Other

*This guide is particularly useful for emergency department nurses and nurses working in psychiatric outpatient settings such as mental health centers.

Once a diagnosis of alcoholism is confirmed, the nurse should complete a focused nursing assessment of the alcoholic client. The assessment, which follows, is divided into five areas: behavioral, affective, cognitive, physiologic, and sociocultural. The assessment may be made in a single sitting or in several separate sittings.

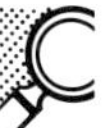

FOCUSED NURSING ASSESSMENT
for the Alcoholic Client

Behavioral assessment

What made you come to this agency?
What type of help do you want most at this time?
How old were you when you had your first drink? When you started drinking regularly?
When did you begin to have problems with alcohol?
How often do you now drink alcoholic beverages? What kind of alcoholic beverages do you consume?
How much alcohol do you consume in one day? Do you drink that much every day?
What quantity of each type of alcoholic beverage do you drink?
When was your last drink?
When did you begin your present drinking episode?
How frequent are your drinking episodes?
What were you drinking before you came to this agency?
Are you taking any medications? Are these medications prescription, over-the-counter, or street drugs? What is the name of the drug?
Are you taking any other medications that you haven't mentioned?
What is the name of the drug?
How do you take your drugs? As directed? More than directed? Less than directed?

Affective assessment

What is your usual mood?
What in your life makes you feel guilty?
Describe to me what areas of your life make you feel like a failure.
How does your drinking make you feel out of control of your life?
What feelings make you want to drink?
Have you had mental or emotional problems? Depression? Anxiety (nervousness)? Loneliness? Attempted suicide? Other?

Cognitive assessment

What do you plan to do about your drinking after you leave this agency?

What kinds of things do you have difficulty remembering?

Have you ever invented stories to make up for forgetting? What kinds of stories?

What kinds of voices do you hear?

Have you ever seen things that others didn't? What were the things?

Physiologic assessment

What physical problems do you have?

(The following questions are related to specific systems that may be mentioned by the client.)

Gastrointestinal system

What have you been eating during your drinking episodes?

How do you usually eat? When you are in a drinking episode? When you are not drinking?

Have there been recent changes in your appetite?

Have you had a recent change in your weight? How much lost? How much gained?

Are you eating a special diet?

What liquids do you drink besides alcohol? How much? How often?

Have you had irritation in your mouth and throat recently?

Do you have pain in your stomach? What is it like?

Are you bothered by heartburn or gas? Do you belch frequently?

Have you been nauseated recently? How long before you came to this agency?

Have you been vomiting or had dry heaves? Have you vomited blood?

Do you have ulcers or other stomach problems?

Are you bothered by diarrhea or constipation?

Do you have hemorrhoids?

Do you have esophageal varices?

Have you ever bled from the bowels?

What color are your bowel movements?

Has your skin ever turned yellow? The whites of your eyes?

Have you ever been told you have liver problems? Problems with your pancreas? Diabetes?

Do you take medicine for diabetes? What kind?

Cardiovascular and respiratory systems

Have you ever been told you have heart trouble? What kind?

Do you have difficulty with shortness of breath?

Do your hands and feet swell?

Have you had chest pain?

Do you take any medicine for heart problems? What kind?

Have you ever had pneumonia?

Do you smoke? How much?

Do you have any lung problems? Cough? Spitting up blood?

Neurologic system

Have you ever had a blackout or a period in which you don't remember what you did while you were drinking?

Do you have tingling, pain, or numbness in your hands or feet?

Do you have muscle pain in your legs and arms?

Have you changed the amount of alcohol you drink to get the effect you desire? Does it take more? Does it take less?

What reactions do you have when you stop drinking? Tremors? DTs? Seizures? Hear things? See things?

Do you take any medications for convulsions? If so, what?

Have you had any problems with your vision?

How well do you sleep? How many hours when drinking? How many hours when sober? Does drinking affect how well you sleep?

Sociocultural assessment

What is your marital status?

With whom do you live?

How many children do you have? How are you involved with them? How much time do you spend with them each day?

Does the person with whom you live drink with you?

Have you had major losses in the past six months?

Has the amount of stress you have been under in the last six months changed? How?

Are you currently employed? How many hours do you work a week? Will this treatment affect your employment?

What are your hobbies?

Describe a typical day you spend at home.

Do you participate in a religious group?

Do you have close friends, neighbors, or others with whom you drink?

Do you attend AA? A counseling program? Have you in the past? If so, when?

Physical Assessment

Physical assessment is a critical and overwhelming task with the alcoholic client. A physical examination or assessment should accompany the interview of the alcoholic client. The complete physical assessment is necessary because alcohol affects so many major body systems. The physical assessment is begun by reviewing the client's responses to the general nursing history. The nurse looks first at the client's general appearance, takes vital signs, and examines the client in cephalocaudal (head-to-toe) order.

Skin and Scalp Depending on the stage of alcoholism, the type of trauma the client may have been exposed to, poor hygiene, and malnutrition, the nurse needs to examine for changes in the integrity of the skin and scalp. Ecchymoses, lacerations, color, evidence of healed injuries, bumps, scars, and diaphoresis may be present. Bruises, lacerations, and numerous scars are evidence of frequent trauma from bumps, falls, and fights. Decreased prothrombin production in advanced liver disease causes easy bruising. Dermatitis, seborrhea, and skin sensitivity to light results from vitamin B deficiencies (Tweed, 1989). Poor hygiene results in unkempt skin and nails and increases the probability of impetigo, scabies, and lice. Spider angiomas are found on the face and sometimes on the chest of many advanced alcoholics. Diaphoresis may be a sign of impending alcohol withdrawal. Dependent edema may indicate liver involvement. Statis dermatitis indicates the edema has been present for some time.

Head The nurse observes the client's facial expression for shape and symmetry of facial structures. Orbital ridges and bony areas around the eyes should be palpated for evidence of fractures. Advanced alcoholism frequently causes facial edema, or a puffy face with flushed cheeks and nose.

The eyes need to be inspected thoroughly. Icterus may be present in the sclera from hepatitis or cirrhosis. The lids may have infected glans. Extraocular movements are assessed to look for nystagmus and palsies of the lateral and conjugate gaze. When these signs are positive, Wernicke's syndrome is suspected. Pupil shape, equality, and reactivity to light evaluate normal nerve function. Pupil sluggishness indicates nerve damage (Schenk, 1989).

The ear canals need to be examined. Increased redness is an indication of infection. Since trauma is often seen in alcoholics, the ear canal is inspected for the presence of foreign objects, exudate, blood, and lesions.

The nasal mucosa is inspected for the presence of infection, which would be indicated by redness. Alcoholics frequently have nasal fractures and sometimes a perforated septum due to trauma. Rhinophyma, acne roseacea or "brandy nose," and nasal spider veins may be observed as late signs of alcoholism.

The lips are observed for signs of trauma and cheilosis. Lip peeling and corner fissures are early signs related to vitamin B deficiencies. Since alcoholics often have poor oral hygiene habits and teeth in poor repair, the teeth need to be inspected for caries, cracks, missing teeth, shape, state of repair, and tenderness. The gums are observed for color, inflammation, consistency, bleeding, and retraction.

The tongue is inspected for color, edema, ulceration, coating, variation in size, and variation in position. White caking, increased papilla on the tip of the tongue called "strawberry tongue," and fissures are a result of niacin deficiency. A smooth red tongue might be seen in pyridoxine deficiencies. In advanced disease, when the hypoglossal nerve is degenerating, fasciculations are found. In chronic alcoholism, a tongue with a verticle furrow and purplish vessels with cyanosed discoloration indicates a chronically congested liver.

Malodorous breath is an obvious sign. When noted, the nurse needs to include the questions related to drinking habits in the focused nursing assessment for the alcoholic client. Since denial is common, it may take more than one encounter to obtain adequate data. Alcohol breath odor is particularly helpful in alerting the nurse to young problem drinkers and others who do not match the alcoholic stereotypes.

The neck is observed for color, skin texture, scars, masses, symmetry, range of motion, and visible pulsations. Chronic alcoholics may have cardiomyopathy with CHF, causing increased venous pressure and distended jugular veins. Esophageal varices may cause swallowing difficulties.

Chest Since debilitated alcoholics are at risk for pneumonia and tuberculosis, the rate and character of respirations need to be noted. Auscultation can reveal altered breath sounds with lung consolidation. The presence and character of the sputum should be observed and cultured for AFB if physical findings support the possibility of tuberculosis.

Palpation may reveal tenderness from rib fractures. Gynecomastia is common with cirrhosis or chronic liver disease. The heart rate, peripheral and apical pulses, major neck vessels, and blood pressure need to be assessed. Tachycardia and transient hypertension may occur in withdrawal.

Abdomen Gross nutrition status can be observed by surveying the client's weight distribution. Difficulty in losing weight may be the presenting problem. Dieting without success may be due to the excessive calories from drinking. Observation of abdominal contour may reveal obesity with normal distribution of excess fat, bulging flanks indicative of abdominal fluid retention, and tense glistening skin resulting from ascites. Portal hypertension may be indicated if the nurse finds dilated veins at the umbilicus, esophageal varices, gastrointestinal bleeding, and hemorrhoids.

Gastrointestinal problems, such as esophagitis, gastritis, pancreatitis, and alcoholic hepatitis are a frequent complication of alcoholism. Alcohol has a toxic effect on the intestinal mucosa, which inhibits normal nutrient absorption. With decreased absorption, there is an increased need for nutrients. Alcohol also decreases storage and increases excretion of valuable nutrients. The metabolism of alcohol depends on vitamin B, so that there is an increased need for the B complex vitamins (Schenk, 1989).

Bowel sounds may be increased because of gastrointestinal irritability or gastrointestinal bleeding. To identify bleeding, the nurse checks for hematemesis, black or tarry stools, or frank rectal bleeding. Stool samples need to be hematested (guaiaced). The abdomen is percussed to identify organomegaly, fluid retention, gaseous distention, and masses. An enlarged liver, percussed at greater than 12 centimeters from the midclavicular line, can indicate alcoholic hepatitis or cirrhosis. Complaints of anorexia, nausea, vomiting, fever, and presence of liver tenderness are all early signs of hepatitis. Later signs of hepatitis are pale stools, dark urine, and jaundice. Jaundice may be more readily identified on the abdomen because of its being less exposed to the sun. However, in a dark-skinned person it may be necessary to use the sclera of the eyes to identify jaundice.

Musculoskeletal System The review of the musculoskeletal system should include observation of body parts for size, symmetry, deformities, contour, edema, and discoloration. The chief presenting complaint in early alcoholics may be fractures. In chronic alcoholism, bone structure becomes impaired because calcium is absorbed poorly and excreted readily, and muscle wasting is common because of inadequate protein intake (Weisberg and Hawes, 1989).

Genitourinary System Urine should be observed for specific gravity, color, clarity, and odor. Fluid balance, dehydration, and possible infection may be indicated from these findings. Alcoholics may exhibit polyuria, dehydration or overhydration, and urinary tract infections.

In chronic alcoholic men, testicular atrophy and sexual dysfunction may be present. In chronic alcoholic women, there is an increased incidence of amenorrhea and gynecological problems.

Neurologic System The major areas observed in assessing the neurologic status of the alcoholic are consciousness, mentation, and motor function. Neurologic disorders associated with chronic alcoholism are primarily related to nutrition deficiencies (Luckman and Sorensen, 1987). A change in behavior with confusion may be the result of a shortage of glucose to the brain. Adequate glucose may be present, but no energy is produced when the body's supply of niacin and thiamine is depleted as a result of the alcohol metabolism (Tweed, 1989).

Consciousness may be assessed as the client converses with the nurse. Deviations may be observed in relation to the client's arousability, responses to commands, and response to painful stimuli. There are alterations of consciousness when the client is in an alcoholic stuporous state. Because the alcoholic may be disoriented, the nurse needs to note the client's orientation to time, place, and person. Mood swings are also characteristic of alcoholics.

Motor function is assessed by observing the client's nerve function, eating behavior, facial expression, speech, and movement. Tremors at rest and intention tremors are seen in advanced alcoholism. Flapping tremor (asterixis) is seen in the prehepatic coma state (Luckman and Sorensen, 1987). Ataxia and a wide stance are frequently seen with intoxication. Hyperreflexia is present during alcohol withdrawal. Changing the temperature, applying a pinprick or cotton-tipped applicator, and placing a tuning fork along long bones are methods of evaluating sensory function. In alcoholic neuropathy, the vibratory sense is the first sense to disappear as peripheral neuropathies develop.

After completing the history and physical assessments and appraising the knowledge base, the nurse is ready to analyze and synthesize the information. To do this, the nurse compares the information about the client with the information from the knowledge base on alcoholism. From this comparison, the client's strengths and health concerns can be identified. The phase culminates by identifying the nursing diagnoses related to the client (Griffith and Christensen, 1986).

Diagnosis and Planning

Several nursing diagnoses related to health concerns of the alcoholic can be affected by nursing intervention. These diagnoses are designed to provide a common language for nurses dealing with alcoholic clients. They are grouped into diagnoses related to (1) acute intoxication, (2) alcohol withdrawal, and (3) chronic alcoholism. (See Table 12–11 for the common nursing diagnoses related to these three areas.) It should be remembered that nursing diagnoses are made after data collection and are tentative because they depend on individual client response. Often, further assessment, validation, and adaptation of diagnoses is required.

After identifying nursing diagnoses specific to

Table 12–11 *Nursing Diagnoses of the Alcoholic Client*

Acute intoxication
- Impaired swallowing, potential
- Injury, potential for: trauma
- Gas exchange, impaired: potential
- Nutrition, alteration in: less than body requirements
- Sleep pattern disturbance
- Fear
- Self-care deficit: feeding, bathing/hygiene, dressing/grooming, toileting

Alcohol Withdrawal
- Sleep pattern disturbance
- Impaired swallowing
- Injury, potential for: trauma
- Fluid volume deficit, potential
- Activity intolerance, potential
- Nutrition, alteration in: less than body requirements
- Sensory-perceptual alteration: visual, auditory, kinesthetic, gustatory, tactile, olfactory
- Skin integrity, impairment of: potential
- Thought processes, alteration in
- Fear
- Anxiety
- Urinary elimination, alteration in pattern

Chronic alcoholism
- Impaired adjustment
- Coping, ineffective individual
- Family process, alteration in
- Health maintenance, alteration in
- Infection, potential for
- Injury, potential for: trauma
- Knowledge deficit
- Nutrition, alteration in: less than body requirements
- Self-care deficit: feeding, bathing/hygiene, dressing/grooming, toileting
- Sexual dysfunction
- Social interaction impaired
- Social isolation
- Spiritual distress
- Violence, potential for: self-directed or directed at others

the client, planning the care of the alcoholic client is the next phase of the nursing process. From the list of diagnoses, the nurse needs to determine the priority for meeting the needs of the individual client. The nurse will use a variety of concepts, principles, models, and theories in setting priorities. Generally, diagnoses related to life-threatening concerns take priority over potential concerns. Developmental concerns also need to be considered. The teenager, housewife, retiree, and corporate manager all have varying developmental needs. Maslow's model has often been used to establish priorities for the alcoholic client. Usually several diagnoses are dealt with concurrently, as the nursing care plans later in this chapter will indicate.

Once priorities have been decided on, goals must be set for the alcoholic client. Ideally, the client and the nurse will have similar goals. However, since the nurse's knowledge base is greater than the client's, it is the nurse's responsibility to assist the client in understanding the concerns and diagnoses related to alcoholism. (See Table 12–12 for goals related to nursing diagnoses of alcoholic clients.)

After the nurse has identified the alcoholic client's goals, nursing actions or interventions are selected to assist the client in meeting these goals. Tables 12–13, 12–14, and 12–15 offer examples of nursing interventions along with the rationale for the interventions (Carpenito, 1989).

Table 12–12 *Alcoholic Client Goals for Some Specific Nursing Diagnoses*

Nursing Diagnosis: Potential impaired gas exchange.
Goal: For an 8-hour shift client will have a patent airway.

Nursing Diagnosis: Alteration in nutrition; less than body requirements.
Goal: In a 24-hour period client will take a minimum of 1500 calories.

Nursing Diagnosis: Sensory-perceptual alteration: visual, auditory, kinesthetic, gustatory, tactile, olfactory
Goal: Client will state his/her name, where he/she is, the date, and the time.

Nursing Diagnosis: Sleep pattern disturbance.
Goal: Client will sleep or rest for 4- to 6-hour intervals.

Nursing Diagnosis: Alteration in family process.
Goal: Client's family will help client abstain from drinking one day at a time.

Nursing Diagnosis: Social isolation.
Goal: Client will attend AA meetings daily for 90 days.

Table 12–13 Nursing Care Plan for the Client with Acute Alcohol Intoxication

Nursing Diagnosis: Impaired gas exchange potential related to depressant effect of alcohol.
Goal: Client will maintain a patent airway for at least 24 hours.

Intervention	*Rationale*	*Expected Outcome*
Monitor, record, and report alterations in vital signs	Increased and/or decreased pulse and respirations are due to changes in the respiratory center in the brain stem	Stabilized vital signs
Observe changes in skin color and nail beds	Cyanosis is associated with depression in hemoglobin-oxygen saturation	Adequate O_2 intake to maintain body functions
Monitor arterial blood gases (ABG's)	Mechanical ventilatory support is indicated if pCO_2 is elevated	
Assess gag reflex	Cranial nerve function may be depressed from alcohol and interfere with respirations	
Encourage coughing and deep breathing	Will assist in maintaining an open airway	
Place in semi-Fowler's position	Ascites in advanced alcoholism can place pressure on the diaphragm	
Monitor blood alcohol level (BAL)	To determine the level of client intoxication	Decreased BAL

(continued)

Table 12–13 *(continued)*

Nursing Diagnosis: Alteration in fluid volume excess related to excessive alcohol intake.
Goal: Client will maintain fluid and electrolytes within normal limits within 24 hours.

Intervention	*Rationale*	*Expected Outcome*
Monitor intake and output (I & O)	Dehydration can occur with excess alcohol use, because alcohol initially exerts an antidiuretic effect	Fluid and electolytes come within normal limits
Monitor lab reports on electrolytes	Assists in asessing fluid and electrolyte imbalance	Body hydration comes within normal limits

Nursing Diagnosis: Alteration in nutrition: less than body requirements related to use of alcohol instead of food.
Goal: Client will increase tolerance for food within 24 hours.

Intervention	*Rationale*	*Expected Outcome*
Monitor dietary intake by noting amount and frequency of meals	Will ensure nutritional intake for basic metabolism and cell maintenance	Takes nutrition within caloric limit prescribed
Offer diet as tolerated, usually bland foods	Dental status and nausea may alter the type of diet client can eat	
Give medications as needed for GI distress	GI irritation is common; relief of irritation will aid in retaining food and fluids and prevent further irritation of gastric mucosa with possible perforation	Retention of nutrients taken in

Nursing Diagnosis: Disturbance in sleep pattern related to excessive alcohol intake interrupting sleep.
Goal: Client's environment will be established to be conducive to sleep.

Intervention	*Rationale*	*Expected Outcome*
Monitor client activity	Assists in determining client's sleep difficulties	Sleeps at least 6 hours
Provide a quiet, temperate room with altered lighting	Will maximize client's ability to sleep	
If tolerated, give a warm beverage (eg, milk)	Will prevent disturbance from hunger or GI irritation	
Give sleeping medications, if indicated	Sleeping medications (eg, Benadryl) are effective for a short-term sleeping disturbance	

Nursing Diagnosis: Potential impaired swallowing related to altered level of consciousness resulting from excess alcohol intake.
Goal: During the course of treatment the client will experience no episodes of aspiration.

Intervention	*Rationale*	*Expected Outcome*
Loosen clothing around neck	Prevents pooling of secretions	No pooling of secretions
Place in lateral or semiprone position	Assists in drainage of secretions	No episodes of aspiration
Suction trachea	Removes excess secretions	

(continued)

Table 12–13 *(continued)*

Nursing Diagnosis: Potential for injury: trauma related to potential for seizures or alcohol withdrawal and altered sensorium.
Goal: During treatment and/or hospitalization client will sustain no further injuries.

Intervention	*Rationale*	*Expected Outcome*
Monitor client activity	Will assist in assessment of client safety	Appropriate measures to protect client from injury
Bed in low position	Will protect client from falls	
Place Side rails up		
Place call light within reach		
Use restraints if necessary	Protects client from potential injury	

Nursing Diagnosis: Fear related to loss of control from excessive alcohol intake.
Goal: Client will demonstrate decreased anxiety within 72 hours.

Intervention	*Rationale*	*Expected Outcome*
Orient client to time, place, and person	Will reduce the confusion related to fear responses	Responds appropriately to environment
Explain procedures		Maintains orientation to time, place, and person
Maintain a nonjudgmental attitude	Client is sensitive to the caretaker's attitude	Does not attempt self-injury
Use comfort measures (eg, warm bath, restful environment)	Will reduce client anxiety by assisting client to regain control	
Remain calm and use a firm voice	Will assist in developing a constructive relationship	
Use listening skills	Will encourage client to vent feelings	

Nursing Diagnosis: Deficit in self-care: feeding, bathing/hygiene, dressing/grooming, toileting related to impaired ability as a result of excessive alcohol intake.
Goal: During the course of treatment the client will express feelings of self-worth and dignity.

Intervention	*Rationale*	*Expected Outcome*
Determine need for personal hygiene	Intoxicated persons may neglect grooming needs	Maintains self-care activities insofar as is capable
Assess client capabilities	Will aid in determining what client is able to do and what assistance is required	
Discuss routines and explain procedures	Including client in decisions enhances self-esteem	
Consult with client before making treatment choices		
Provide supplies, grooming tools, and assistance as needed	Will encourage client to maintain responsibility for self	Maintains behavioral control
Assist with toileting by providing needed equipment	Prompt response to client's requests will avoid embarrassment	

Table 12–14 Nursing Care Plan for the Client Experiencing Alcohol Withdrawal

Nursing Diagnosis: Deficit in fluid volume potential related to extensive diaphoresis, excessive vomiting, and/or gastrointestinal bleeding.
Goal: During the period of withdrawal client will maintain an optimal level of fluid and electrolyte balance.

Intervention	*Rationale*	*Expected Outcome*
Monitor vital signs	Hypotension, increased pulse rate, and increased body temperature are defining characteristics of fluid volume deficit	Vital signs come within normal limits
Maintain balanced oral or IV fluid intake	To prevent excessive fluid loss from profuse perspiration, agitation, and vomiting	Retains fluids
Monitor I & O	Assists in assessing fluid and electrolyte balance	Output correlates with intake
Monitor electrolyte values and hematocrit	Electrolytes are lost with excessive vomiting; hematocrit increases with excess perspiration and decreases with hemorrhage	Lab values come within normal limits
Test urine specific gravity	Decreased urinary output concentrates the urine	
Observe for signs and symptoms of fluid volume deficits (eg, skin turgor, dry mucous membranes)	Decreased skin turgor and dry mucous membranes are present in hypovolemia	Skin and mucous membranes return to normal
Daily weight	Weight loss is an indicator of hypovolemia	
Hematest (guaiac) stools and emesis	Screening for occult blood assists in assessing bleeding	

Nursing Diagnosis: Alteration in nutrition: less than body requirements related to anorexia, nausea, and/or vomiting caused by withdrawal from alcohol.
Goal: During the period of withdrawal client will maintain optimal nutritional intake.

Intervention	*Rationale*	*Expected Outcome*
Assess ability to chew and swallow	Shaking, tremors and/or seizure activity may alter client's ability to chew and swallow food	Takes in adequate nutrients to maintain body function
Give antiemetic medications before meals	Nausea and vomiting often accompany withdrawal	Retains food
Provide food in a form appropriate to client's condition	Will increase probability of client's ability to take in nutrients	No complaints of GI distress
Give vitamins as ordered	Assists in replacing nutrition deficits	
Assist client as necessary; it may be necessary to feed client	Tremors prevent client from helping self	
Give small, frequent feedings of bland foods	Nausea and gastric distress are reduced by nonirritating foods; small amounts of foods are more readily retained	

(continued)

Table 12–14 *(continued)*

Nursing Diagnosis: Intolerance for activity potential related to alcoholic tremors or delirium tremens.
Goal: Client will demonstrate acceptance of activity limitations.

Intervention	*Rationale*	*Expected Outcome*
Monitor vital signs	Psychomotor hyperactivity causes instability of vital signs	Stabilized vital signs Decreased tremors
Maintain activity as tolerated	Bedrest may be indicated for client with agitation and tremors	Verbalizes understanding of activity restrictions No client injuries

Nursing Diagnosis: Potential for injury: trauma related to musculoskeletal, visual, auditory, or sensory disturbances related to alcohol abuse.
Goal: Client will be free from injury until capable of returning to normal activities.

Intervention	*Rationale*	*Expected Outcome*
Assess client's ability to protect self from injury	Mental impairment and/or decision-making ability may be reduced because of hallucinations	No client injuries
Orient client to time, place, and person	Will assist in evaluating cognitive ability and determine whether client is confused	Maintains orientation to time, place, and person
Use strategies to protect client from injury (eg, side rails, bed in low position, call light in reach, restraints)	Confused clients may attempt to climb out of bed or wander, increasing likelihood of injury	Client stays in bed
Supervise client while he or she smokes	Uncontrolled tremors increase potential for injuries	
Take seizure precautions (eg, use oral airway or bite stick, padded side rails, suction equipment, etc)	Convulsions may occur in severe withdrawal reactions	No seizures
Suicide precautions (eg, remove harmful objects from environment, closely observe client—one-to-one day and night or q 15 minutes at intermittent, irregular intervals as necessary—know client's whereabouts, etc)	Alcohol withdrawal can cause depression and increase potential for self-harm	
Remain with client while he or she takes medications	Reduces the potential for aspiration and prevents hoarding of medications	

Nursing Diagnosis: Impairment of skin integrity potential related to altered nutrition status, altered sensation, alterations in skin turgor, and/or use of restraints.
Goal: For the duration of treatment client will maintain hygiene and promote integrity of the skin.

Intervention	*Rationale*	*Expected Outcome*
Daily assessment of skin integrity	Will assist in early detection of skin breakdown	Skin is protected
Correct nutrition deficits	Proper nutrients will aid in tissue repair and prevent skin breakdown	Proper diet maintained

(Diagnosis continued)

Table 12–14 *(continued)*

Intervention	*Rationale*	*Expected Outcome*
Protect skin (eg, blot dry rather than rub, use lotion or oil)	Will prevent further skin breakdown	Adequate circulation maintained
Provide appropriate treatments for wounds, cuts, and lesions	Will promote client comfort and restore skin integrity	
Release restraints q 1 hour and massage extremity gently	Will assist in maintaining circulation to the skin of the area affected by the restraint	

Nursing Diagnosis: Disturbance in sleep pattern related to disorientation, restlessness, and physical discomfort from alcohol withdrawal.
Goal: Throughout course of treatment client will sleep at regular intervals of at least 4 hours.

Intervention	*Rationale*	*Expected Outcome*
Provide a quiet and comfortable environment	Overstimulation increases tremors and agitation	Sleeps at least 4 hours at intervals throughout a 24-hour period
Restrict visitors to significant others Use dim light in room	Decreases agitation and has a calming effect on client; also assists client in maintaining orientation	
Administer benzodiazepines as ordered (eg, tapered and discontinued after 7 to 10 days)	Will prevent DTs and seizures	

Nursing Diagnosis: Alteration in sensory perception: visual, auditory, kinesthetic, gustatory, tactile, olfactory potential related to the long-term effects of alcohol on the brain.
Goal: During the withdrawal period client will be in contact with reality and will respond appropriately to environmental stimuli.

Intervention	*Rationale*	*Expected Outcome*
Assess stimuli present in the environment that may alter sensory-perceptual function	Decreasing or eliminating stimuli that intensifies sensory-perceptual alteration will assist in restoring function	Elimination of distracting environmental stimuli
Orient client to reality by • calling client by name • stating correct time • identifying self • stating information about surroundings • maintaining eye contact with client • reinforcing behaviors that are reality-oriented	Will assist client in maintaining contact with reality	Client maintains contact with reality No evidence of hallucinations, delusions, or illusions
Make environment meaningful: • have a clock • have a calendar • wear a name tag • explain all procedures • clarify client's misperceptions	Will assist in decreasing extraneous environmental stimuli	
Use safety precautions (eg, bedrails up, bed in low position, call light in reach, sharp objects out of client's reach)	Will decrease and prevent self-injury	

(Diagnosis continued)

Table 12–14 *(continued)*

Nursing Diagnosis *(continued):* Alteration in sensory perception: visual, auditory, kinesthetic, gustatory, tactile, olfactory potential related to the long-term effects of alcohol on the brain.
Goal: During the withdrawal period client will be in contact with reality and will respond appropriately to environmental stimuli.

Intervention	*Rationale*	*Expected Outcome*
Maintain a pleasant physical environment (eg, control noise; reduce unnecessary traffic and personnel; explain sights, sounds, and smells in the environment)	Will assist in promoting client comfort	

Nursing Diagnosis: Alteration in thought process related to a change in problem-solving ability resulting from long-term alcohol use.
Goal: By the end of the withdrawal period client will demonstrate a constructive interpretation of reality.

Intervention	*Rationale*	*Expected Outcome*
Listen to client's communication	Analysis of behavior assists in representing reality to client	Client verbalizes realistic interpretations of reality
Observe client's nonverbal communication		
Use therapeutic communication techniques: • clarifying • open-ended statements • challenge distortions • validation of thoughts and feelings	Will assist client in clarifying reality	
Involve client as much as possible in the daily routine	Will enhance client's responsibility for self-care	

Nursing Diagnosis: Fear related to emotional responses to changes in sensory perception.
Goal: During the course of withdrawal client will verbalize reduced fear or no fear.

Intervention	*Rationale*	*Expected Outcome*
Assist client in identifying the source of fear	Client's recognition of dangers causing fear will assist in reducing fear	Reduction of fear
Observe client for fearful reactions: • pupil dilation • panic • increased agitation • increased pulse and respirations • diaphoresis	Early recognition of signs of fear will minimize the effects of the reaction	Absence of fear
Remain with client during hallucinations	Often hallucinations will dissipate by the mere presence of nurse	
Use a calm, matter-of-fact voice	Maintains client's comfort and promotes reassurance	

(continued)

Table 12–14 *(continued)*

Nursing Diagnosis: Anxiety related to distress created by physical symptoms of alcohol withdrawal.
Goal: During the withdrawal period client will be able to cope with increased anxiety.

Intervention	*Rationale*	*Expected Outcome*
Assess level of anxiety: • mild • moderate • severe • panic	Will assist in determining the interventions necessary to reduce anxiety	Reduced anxiety Demonstration of coping strategies Verbalizes insight into causes for anxiety
Extreme anxiety: Provide comfort measures (eg, warm bath, back rub, calm environment)	Will have a calming effect on client, thereby reducing anxiety	
Use short and simple phrases with a calm, firm voice	Reciprocal anxiety will increase client's anxious reaction	
Mild to moderate anxiety: Encourage client to state the presence of anxiety	Client's early recognition of anxiety will prevent its escalation to the panic level	
Encourage client to express and explore apprehensions	Client's involvement in problem solving will assist in the development of new coping strategies	
Involve client in diversional activity (eg, simple concrete tasks, walking)	Teaching new coping strategies will increase client's ability to reduce anxiety	
Maintain confidentiality; inform client of his or her right to confidentiality	Client's knowledge of legal rights will decrease anxiety and guilt related to diagnosis of alcoholism	

Nursing Diagnosis: Alteration in pattern of urinary elimination related to alcoholic neuropathy.
Goal: During the course of withdrawal client will overcome incontinence.

Intervention	*Rationale*	*Expected Outcome*
Assess normal urinary patterns	Assists in planning care	Reduction in number of incontinent episodes
Take to the toilet or offer urinal or bedpan at regular intervals	Assists in maintaining a regular elimination pattern	
Observe for cues indicating an incontinent episode (eg, restlessness, picking at clothes, holding self)	Assists in identifying need to urinate	
Change bed immediately after each incontinent episode	Prevents skin breakdown and avoid embarrassment	Client's self-esteem is maintained
Avoid belittling client when an incontinent episode occurs	Assists client in maintaining self-esteem	
Record frequency of incontinent episodes	Assists in planning care	

Table 12–15 Nursing Care Plan for the Client with Chronic Alcoholism

Nursing Diagnosis: Alteration in nutrition: less than body requirements related to use of alcohol instead of food.
Goal: Client will alter nutrition patterns weekly.

Intervention	*Rationale*	*Expected Outcome*
Determination of client's nutrition patterns	Will assist client in recognizing nutrition deficits	Reduces and/or discontinues use of alcohol
Counsel client to reduce and/or discontinue the use of alcohol	Persistent use of alcohol causes loss of appetite, malabsorption, and disturbed nutrient metabolism	Eats regular balanced meals Takes vitamin supplements
Teach client about essential nutrients and vitamins	Greater client awareness and knowledge will assist in altering nutrition patterns	Verbalizes understanding of nutrition Weight gain

Nursing Diagnosis: Alteration in health maintenance related to unhealthy lifestyle.
Goal: Client will assume responsibility for health maintenance after one month in a rehabilitation program.

Intervention	*Rationale*	*Expected Outcome*
Provide health maintenance information	Increased knowledge will assist client in altering poor health practices	Attempts to maintain health Controls alcoholic behavior
Assist client in identifying health maintenance goals	Involving client in health maintenance planning will increase compliance	Uses health maintenance resources
Referral to health care and community agencies	Use of support systems for health maintenance will assist in restructuring client health practices	

Nursing Diagnosis: Deficit in self-care: feeding, bathing/hygiene, dressing/grooming, toileting related to alcohol-impaired self-care abilities.
Goal: As soon as possible after entering rehabilitation program, client will develop self-care capabilities.

Intervention	*Rationale*	*Expected Outcome*
Provide client with a list of ADL requirements	Will assist client in developing more readily accomplished short-term goals and increase client's experience with success	States self-care capabilities Gains control over ADLs Makes choices concerning self-care
Give client positive feedback on accomplishment of self-care activities	Will increase client's self-esteem and reinforce the behavior	Verbalizes positive self-esteem
Refer to job counseling if employable	Will provide economic security	Seeks employment
Refer to social services if unemployed	Will provide adequate support while attempting to overcome difficulties	If employed, maintains regular work hours

Nursing Diagnosis: Sexual dysfunction related to excessive alcohol use.
Goal: Following a counseling session client will recognize the relationship of sexual dysfunction and alcohol intake.

Intervention	*Rationale*	*Expected Outcome*
Explain why loss of libido occurs to client	Client understanding will decrease anxiety about sexuality and may motivate client to curtail drinking	Verbalizes understanding of alcohol's effect on sexual functioning

(Diagnosis continued)

Table 12–15 *(continued)*

Intervention	*Rationale*	*Expected Outcome*
Counsel client to discontinue and/or curtail the use of alcohol	Alcohol blocks the synthesis of testosterone in the gonads and decreases libido	Return of sexual function

Nursing Diagnosis: Potential for injury: trauma related to high blood alcohol level.
Goal: Client will attempt to abstain from drinking one day at a time.

Intervention	*Rationale*	*Expected Outcome*
Provide instruction on the effects and consequences of alcohol consumption	Will decrease the denial of alcohol-related injuries	Discontinues the use of alcohol No alcohol-related injuries
Assess level of motivation to prevent trauma	Will assist in identifying client's needs in regard to protection from injury	Follows treatment program

Nursing Diagnosis: Potential for violence: self-directed or directed at others related to a dysfunctional family pattern disrupted by chronic alcoholism.
Goal: During the rehabilitation period client will identify patterns of family violence and plan interventions with other family members.

Intervention	*Rationale*	*Expected Outcome*
Encourage client to verbalize rather than act out violent feelings	Will reduce potential harm from violent behavior	Reduction in violent behavior
Remove potentially dangerous items from environment (eg, items that could be used as weapons)		
Explain consequences of violent behavior: • calling security • use of additional staff • use of tranquilizing medications	Client's understanding of behavioral consequences reduces violent actions	Identifies alternatives for dealing with aggression
Use of seclusion if indicated	Removal from environment contributing to aggression will assist in regaining self-control	
Assist client and family members to identify situations that provoke violence	Will assist client and family members to explore alternatives for dealing with violent feelings	
Observe client for signs of depression	As a means of dealing with anger, alcoholics are often depressed	Identifies alternatives for dealing with depression
Institute suicide precautions if necessary	Will protect client from self-inflicted harm	Client verbalizes that he or she will not commit self-harm
Assist client in identifying situations that trigger depression	Will assist client in gaining control over drinking behaviors	No suicide attempts
Teach client measures to counteract depression	Learning physical releases for frustration will reduce factors precipitating depression	

(continued)

Table 12–15 *(continued)*

Nursing Diagnosis: Ineffective individual coping related to inappropriate coping mechanisms for meeting life's demands.
Goal: During the rehabilitation period client will develop healthier coping responses to stress.

Intervention	*Rationale*	*Expected Outcome*
Establish a therapeutic relationship	Consistency in relationships increases client's potential for recovery	Identifies constructive coping mechanisms
Assist client in identifying stress-producing situations	Knowledge of factors producing stress will reduce stress	Attends AA meetings as needed Accurately assesses stress level
Teach methods for coping with stress: • problem solving • relaxation techniques • physical exercise	Will assist client in developing new coping skills	
Help client learn to socialize without using alcohol	Simulating social situations can assist client in learning to say no safely	
Encourage client to discuss the consequences of drinking behaviors	Recognition of effects of drinking on self, family, work, and social situations will assist client in finding alternative behaviors	

Nursing Diagnosis: Social isolation related to inappropriate behavior patterns (ie, chronic use of alcohol).
Goal: During the course of treatment the client will learn to participate in social and/or leisure activities.

Intervention	*Rationale*	*Expected Outcome*
Assess social history	Will assist in identification of potential support system	Elimination of social isolation
Develop a trusting therapeutic relationship	Developing a one-to-one relationship assists client in learning communication skills	Participation in social activities that do not involve drinking
Encourage client to discuss feelings of loneliness	Will assist client in identifying intimacy needs	
Explore alternative ways of reaching out to others without the use of alcohol (eg, role playing)	Will improve client's coping skills when confronted with difficult situations and assist in meeting nondrinking peers	

Nursing Diagnosis: Deficit in knowledge related to effects of alcohol on the brain.
Goal: Throughout the treatment program client will participate in rehabilitation planning.

Intervention	*Rationale*	*Expected Outcome*
Assess knowledge deficit	Understanding of deficits will assist in setting realistic goals	Uses knowledge from treatment program to make health care decisions
Use information, terms, and strategies appropriate to client's level of understanding	Will assist in increasing client's understanding	Carries out health care activities that increase well-being
Give clear, explicit directions	Will assist client in comprehending what needs to be learned	

(continued)

Table 12–15 *(continued)*

Nursing Diagnosis: Alteration in family process related to a family system unable to meet members' emotional needs.
Goal: During the rehabilitation period client will communicate with family members to resolve alterations in family process.

Intervention	*Rationale*	*Expected Outcome*
Assess family role relationships	Will assist in identifying family structure	Demonstration of mutual support within family
Assist client and family members to identify each other's role expectations	Will assist family members to assess willingness to meet role expectations	Verbalization of mutual respect
Assist client and family members to negotiate differences	Will increase family member's ability to respond to each other	Plans alternative living arrangements as necessary
Refer to Al-Anon for spouse and Alateen for children if counseling indicated	Will provide resources for dealing with client's alcoholism	

Nursing Diagnosis: Spiritual distress related to moral implications of therapeutic intervention.
Goal: Client will be able to reduce feelings of guilt by verbalizing spiritual concerns as needed.

Intervention	*Rationale*	*Expected Outcome*
Assess client's spiritual concerns	Will assist in clarifying client's spiritual beliefs and values	Expresses feelings of guilt and remorse
Be an advocate for client's spiritual needs: • refer client to a spiritual advisor • prepare client for spiritual rituals • provide spiritual atmosphere	Will assist in alleviating feelings of alienation from spiritual ties	Decrease in a sense of alienation with a spiritual being or God Finds comfort in moral decisions Verbalizes feelings of help and assistance from a spiritual being
Be accepting of cultural differences related to spiritual beliefs	Will decrease client's sense of loneliness and separation from others	

Nursing Diagnosis: Impaired adjustment related to impaired cognition resulting from alcohol used to solve personal problems.
Goal: Client will develop a greater sense of autonomy in current life situation.

Intervention	*Rationale*	*Expected Outcome*
Promote the development of trust in the nurse-client relationship	Promotes mutual acceptance and increases communication	Seeks out situations to discuss problems
Assess coping skills that have been previously effective	Helps client look at other coping mechanisms besides using alcohol	Identifies techniques for coping with stress
Encourage client to become involved in activities and/or identify potential job skills	Working on short-term attainable goals increases client's self-esteem	Verbalizes sense of positive self-esteem
Encourage client to develop a relationship with another adult(s) (eg, attend AA meetings)	Reinforces the new coping strategies learned	Attends AA meetings

(continued)

Table 12–15 *(continued)*

Nursing Diagnosis: Potential for infection related to the pathologic changes resulting from alcoholism.
Goal: Client will be afebrile and there will be no evidence of active infectious process during the course of treatment.

Intervention	*Rationale*	*Expected Outcome*
Assess vital signs, especially temperature	Elevated or low-grade fever may be the first indicator of infection	Client will be afebrile
Determine the types of infections to which the client is prone	Assists in planning care	Client appears well
Assess any complaints of pain, tenderness, or redness	Assists in identifying potential infections quickly	No complaints of pain, tenderness, or redness
Complete a physical assessment on a regular basis	Assists in identifying changes in physical status	
Assess environment to which client will be returning, including health status of family members	Assists in planning for prevention of potential infections	

Nursing Diagnosis: Impaired social interaction related to disorganization in cognition resulting from alcohol use.
Goal: Client will identify factors leading to poor social interactions.

Intervention	*Rationale*	*Expected Outcome*
Develop a therapeutic relationship with client to allow client to test new behaviors	Assists client in learning to interact appropriately with others	Seeks out nurse for interactions
Encourage client to participate in group interactions	Will provide a social environment to assist client in learning to effectively interact with others	Attends group sessions and participates in discussions
Assist client in identifying behaviors that interfere with development of satisfactory relationships	Recognizing actions affecting relationships may improve ability to interact with others	Verbalizes factors interfering with the development of relationships

Standard Care for the Client with Acute Alcohol Intoxication

Acute alcohol intoxication is a medical emergency. The client may appear drunk but deny alcohol intake. Blood alcohol levels are generally obtained to document the level of intoxication. (See Table 12–3 for the criteria for behaviors related to blood alcohol levels.) The nurse needs to be alert in observing for the problem of mixed addiction. Depending on the level of alcohol in the bloodstream, the neurologic status, and the presence of other injuries, it may be necessary either to hospitalize the client or admit the client to a detoxification unit. (See Table 12–16 for a list of the four classes of intoxication found in the emergency room.)

Clients generally need to sleep off their alcoholic intoxication. While the client sleeps, the nurse needs to observe the client closely. The client should be monitored for signs of CNS depression. If the client is noisy and belligerent, sedative medications may be necessary. Before administering intravenous infusions, medications, or completing treatments that affect neurologic status, the client needs to be assessed for head injuries and other trauma.

General considerations for nursing care during acute alcohol intoxication include

Table 12–16 *Classes of Intoxication in the Emergency Room*

Class I	Awake, but clinically drunk (supported by BAL): slurred speech, ataxic gait, slowed mental activity, uncooperative and belligerent
Class II	Semicomatose: in a deep sleep but responsive to painful stimuli, most reflexes present
Class III	Comatose: not responsive to painful stimuli, some reflexes still present
Class IV	Deep coma: not responsive to painful stimuli, no reflexes but no respiratory or circulatory impairment

- Providing a quiet environment to avoid excessive stimulation that could increase the client's agitation
- Protecting the client from injury by, for instance, using the side rails
- Monitoring the client's vital signs to allow for the necessary physical assessment data on which to make nursing care decisions on appropriate interventions
- Attending to the self-care activities that the client may be unable to carry out

(See Table 12–13 for a nursing care plan for the client with acute alcohol intoxication.)

Standard Care for Alcohol Withdrawal

Alcoholic withdrawal constitutes a serious medical problem. The primary concern in alcohol withdrawal is the development of an acute toxic state called delirium tremens (DTs). This is a serious life-threatening occurrence in the alcoholic client. Adequate medical and nursing care are essential for client recovery.

The primary treatment goal of clients in withdrawal from alcohol with delirium tremens pending is to give proper amounts of sedation and support to enable the client to rest and recover without injury. Sedative medication is necessary to temporarily duplicate the depressant action of alcohol in the CNS. To assist in titrating the proper level of sedative medication, it is important to monitor the client's vital signs, especially the pulse and blood pressure. Elevations in these vital signs indicate the need for increased sedation.

The client should be placed in an environment that will decrease the potential for agitation. Generally, this means a private or semiprivate room. Lighting in the room should be maintained, especially at night, to decrease the possibility of misinterpretation of stimuli and shadows. If the client is in a private room without someone in constant attendance, it may be necessary to restrain the client for safety and protection from injury.

Because the client suffering from alcohol withdrawal is agitated and perspires profusely, adequate fluid replacement is needed. If the client is unable to maintain oral intake, intravenous fluids may be necessary. Hypoglycemia may accompany alcoholic withdrawal; therefore, it is important to give orange juice and other carbohydrates to stabilize the blood sugar and decrease tremors. Decaffeinated coffee is recommended because caffeine increases tremors. For the client unable to retain fluids, parenteral dextrose may be indicated. Since clients experiencing alcohol withdrawal usually have nutrition deficits, a high-protein, high-carbohydrate diet supplemented with vitamins is indicated as soon as the client is able to retain solids.

Because convulsions may occur, the client should be placed on seizure precautions, including an oral airway or bite stick (depending on agency protocol), suction equipment, padded side rails, and close observation. Once the client has overcome the critical phase of withdrawal, it is important to refer the client for rehabilitative or follow-up treatment. (See Table 12–14 for a nursing care plan for the client experiencing alcohol withdrawal.)

General considerations for nursing care during alcohol withdrawal include

- Providing the proper amount of sedation and support to enable the client to rest and recover without injury
- Monitoring the client's vital signs to assist in titrating the proper level of sedation
- Providing an environment free from excessive stimuli to decrease potential agitation

- Giving adequate fluids to the client to replace fluids lost by perspiration
- Giving a diet high in protein and carbohydrates as soon as client is able to retain solids
- Placing client on seizure precautions in case of convulsions

Standard Care for Chronic Alcoholism

The primary focus of continuing treatment for alcoholic clients is assisting them to accept that they cannot drink. The client should be made aware that relapses may occur as attempts are made to abstain from the use of alcohol.

Planning for leisure activities and diversions is an important part of the convalescent period; not only does it assist in alleviating anxiety and loneliness, but it provides a learning base of activities not related to drinking. It is important to require the client to follow through and complete projects.

The client should be encouraged to make decisions. The client should also be made responsible for keeping appointments, maintaining personal appearance, and eating regular meals. Any manipulative behavior should be confronted. The client should continue to be observed frequently, especially for symptoms of depression. Regular routines of rest, work, and socialization should be planned. Help the client build ego strength by exploring alternatives to destructive behaviors.

It is important to introduce outpatient services while the client is still hospitalized. Referral to Alcoholics Anonymous and attendance at meetings while hospitalized is also recommended. Teaching the client about alternative ways of handling stress and medical problems aggravated by alcohol should be included in the client's plan of care. Goals are directed toward assisting the client to accept a new way of life without alcohol. (See Table 12–15 for a nursing care plan for the client with chronic alcoholism. See Table 12–17 for referral resources.)

General considerations for nursing care during chronic alcoholism include

- Assisting client to accept that he or she cannot drink alcohol

Table 12–17 *Resources for Client Referral*

Alcoholics Anonymous
World Services Office
PO Box 459, Grand Central Station
New York, NY 10163
212-686-1100

Al-Anon Family Group Headquarters, Inc.
(For Al-Anon, Alateen, Alatots, ACOA)
PO Box 862 Midtown Station
New York, NY 10018-0862
1-800-356-9996
Canada: 613-722-1830

Adult Children of Alcoholics (ACOA)
Central Service Board
PO Box 3216
2522 W. Sepulveda Blvd, Suite 200
Torrance, CA 90505
213-534-1815

National Council on Alcoholism, Inc.
12 W 21st Street
New York, NY 10010
212-206-6770

- Planning leisure activities to alleviate anxiety and loneliness
- Encouraging client to make responsible decision for maintaining a normal lifestyle
- Assisting the client to plan regular outings for work, rest, and socialization
- Referring client to AA as a follow-up support service (Eells, 1986; Throwe, 1986)

Evaluation

The nurse evaluates care of the alcoholic client by comparing the client's health status to the previously identified goals. As nursing care is implemented, the nurse appraises the alcoholic client's response to nursing interventions and determines whether the client is progressing toward the identified goals. Based on the client's response, the nurse may modify the care plan.

The nurse determines whether appropriate scientific theory has been applied as the basis for decisions regarding the care of the alcoholic client. The client data are reviewed for accuracy and comprehensiveness, and the need for additional information is ascertained. The nurse reviews the nursing diagnoses identified for the client and determines the appropriateness of the diagnoses for the client. The nurse reviews the plan of care to determine if the interventions are eliciting a therapeutic client response. Finally, the nurse modifies the plan to incorporate the findings obtained by reviewing the outcomes.

The focus on outcomes is useful because changes in the client's behavior and health status can be observed. Outcomes are written in measurable terms, and documentation of the outcomes can be found in the client's record. (See Table 12–18 for an example of an evaluation of the care of a client with acute alcohol intoxication, Table 12–19 for an example of the evaluation of the care of a client in alcohol withdrawal, and Table 12–20 for an example of the evaluation of the care of a client with chronic alcoholism.)

Using the expected outcomes as a base, the nurse can expect to observe the following:

- Client demonstrates uncomplicated recovery from withdrawal symptoms.
- Client states knowledge of adverse effects of alcohol.
- Client practices alternative behaviors for coping with stress.
- Client participates in support groups like Alcoholics Anonymous.

Table 12–18 *Example of Evaluation of Nursing Care of a Client with Acute Alcohol Intoxication*

Plan	*Evaluation*
1. The nurse will record intake and output every 8 hours and total every 24 hours.	On 10/21, the 24-hour oral and intravenous intake was 2300 cc, and the 24-hour output was 2100 cc.
2. The client will sleep or rest for a 4- to 6-hour interval.	On 10/21, the client slept 5 hours during the night shift.
3. The client will have no injuries during a 24-hour period.	On 10/21, the client hit head on headboard during a convulsion, causing a bruise on the forehead.

Table 12–19 *Example of Evaluation of Nursing Care of a Client with Alcohol Withdrawal*

Plan	*Evaluation*
1. The nurse will orient client to time, place, and person at least q 2 hours.	On 10/23, Manuel was unable to verbalize his name, the date, or the time without prompting from the nurse.
2. The nurse will validate any misperceptions noted in the client's communication.	On 10/23, Manuel was informed by the nurse that spiders were not on his body.
3. The nurse will explain all procedures and treatments to the client.	On 10/23, Manuel was informed by the nurse that restraints were in place for his protection.

Table 12–20 *Example of Evaluation of Nursing Care of a Client with Chronic Alcoholism*

Plan	*Evaluation*
1. The nurse will monitor caloric intake for a 24-hour period.	On 12/15, Esther ate 1200 calories in a 24-hour period.
2. The nurse will encourage the client to complete ADLs.	Before her group session on 12/15, Esther dressed and put on make-up without prompting from staff.
3. The nurse will encourage the client to abstain from drinking one day at a time.	On 12/16 and 12/17, Esther went home on a pass. The family and the client reported no alcohol intake during the entire time the client was home.

- Client obtains support from family in changing alcoholic behavior.

CASE EXAMPLE

A Client Withdrawing from Alcohol

Donald Spier, a 35-year-old sales manager for a computer store, was admitted to an orthopedic unit following an automobile accident in which he received multiple injuries including a fractured right hip. Twenty-four hours following his admission, Mr.

Spier became noticeably restless and irritable. His hands were tremulous, and he was confused about where he was. On entering the room, the nurse found Mr. Spier extremely agitated. He yelled, "Get these ants off of me! They are eating me alive!"

Nursing History

Location: General Hospital, Orthopedic Unit
Client's name: Donald Spier Age: 35
Admitting diagnosis: MVA with multiple trauma and fracture of the right hip
T=99.2, P=60, R=18, BP=130/70

Health history
Height: 5′10″
Weight: 130 lb
Eats: 1–2 meals a day
Sleeps: 3–5 hours at night
Smokes: 2 packs of cigarettes a day
Drinks: 3–4 cocktails daily and at least 6 beers nightly for the past 4 years

Social history
Marital status: separated from wife for one month
Employment status: fired from job on the date of the accident
Living arrangements: local hotel room

Clinical data
Laboratory findings:
BAL (on admission to ER): 0.15%

CBC:		Urinalysis:
WBC:	8.0	Color: Amber
RBC:	4.2	Clarity: Cloudy
Hgb:	12.8	Sp gr: 1.080
Hct:	38.4	Protein: neg
MCV:	88	Glucose: neg
MCH:	30	Acetone: neg
MCHC:	32.4	WBC: none
		RBC: none

Nursing observations
Mr. Spier remained agitated and was unable to sleep during the first 24 hours of hospitalization. He was very talkative and told the nurses he had been fired from his job on the day of his accident. He became upset by the loss of his job and went to a tavern near the computer store where he had been employed. Mr. Spier had 4–5 whiskeys; he could not remember the exact number. Mr. Spier ran a red light and hit another car on his way to another tavern. Mr. Spier argued with the nurses and became belligerent when his demands were not immediately met. The morning following his admission, Mr. Spier's temperature went up to 99.2, his pulse rose to 80, his respirations rose to 28, and his blood pressure rose to 150/80. He was tremulous and perspiring profusely. By the afternoon, Mr. Spier continued to have diaphoresis, his vital signs were T=101, P=100, R=32, and BP=180/100. Mr. Spier was trying to crawl out of bed and was screaming at the nurses to get the ants that were crawling on him.

Analysis/Synthesis of Data

Concerns	*Nursing diagnosis*
Decreased weight	Alteration in nutrition: less than body requirements
Inadequate sleep	Disturbance in sleep patterns
Decreased respiratory capability due to smoking	Potential for impaired gas exchange
Hallucinations	Alteration in visual sensory perception
Fractured hip	Activity intolerance
Ambulating with a fractured hip	Potential for injury: trauma

Suggested Care Planning Activities

1. Determine the priorities for Mr. Spier's care.
2. Determine the developmental aspects to be considered in the care of Mr. Spier.
3. Identify the support systems available to Mr. Spier.
4. Describe the client teaching necessary to assist Mr. Spier toward recovery.
5. Describe the significance of the laboratory findings.
6. Describe the significance of the change in vital signs.
7. Identify nursing goals for Mr. Spier.
8. List and provide a rationale for nursing interventions in the care of Mr. Spier.

SUMMARY

Significance of Alcoholism

1. Alcohol abuse is a major public health problem in the United States. It spans all ages, cultures, genders, and occupations.

2. Nurses are likely to care for clients with alcohol abuse problems in a variety of settings, including the acute care hospital, emergency rooms, detoxification units, substance abuse treatment centers, inpatient psychiatric units, and outpatient units.

Knowledge Base

3. A working definition of an alcoholic is anyone who repetitively has multiple problems because of drinking over a period of time.

4. Behavioral characteristics of alcoholism include lack of control over drinking, skipping meals to drink, giving up other interests to drink, telephonitis, hostility, withdrawal, employment problems, and arrests for fights or DWI.

5. Affective characteristics of alcoholism include guilt, shame, torment, despair, depression, alcoholic jealousy, and feeling like a failure.

6. Cognitive characteristics of alcoholism include inadequate self-esteem, grandiose thoughts, denial, projection, minimization, rationalization, blackouts, Wernicke's encephalopathy, and Korsakoff's psychosis.

7. Alcohol affects all body systems, causing a number of medical complications.

8. Alcoholism is a family problem. Co-dependents are the caretakers in the family systems and may respond in certain patterns such as alienated, bullies, managers, and martyrs.

9. Children of alcoholics tend to become heros, scapegoats, lost children, or mascots.

10. Family roles develop as a way to handle the distress and shame of having an alcoholic member and in an attempt to keep the family in balance.

11. Alcoholic women are more severely stigmatized than alcoholic men and certain groups of women are at higher risk for alcoholism, i.e., abused women and lesbians.

12. There is a recognized genetic component to the development of alcoholism. Biologic research indicates that a dopamine gene on chromosome 11 may be predisposing to alcoholism.

13. Intrapersonal theories such as psychoanalytic and personality theories have not been supported by recent research.

14. Learning theories center around reinforcement principles and maladaptive ways of coping.

15. Sociocultural theories look at the interaction of cultural values and attitudes with drinking behavior.

16. The recovery movement focuses on the alcoholic's responsibility for recovery and the values of honesty and spirituality.

Assessment

17. Nurses must assess the acutely intoxicated client for airway, breathing, circulation, blood pressure, trauma, and infection.

18. The client in alcohol withdrawal may experience the following symptoms after the last drink: irritability, anxiety, insomnia, and tremors (6–8 hours); seizures (6–96 hours); hallucinations (6–96 hours); and DTs (3–14 days). A variety of medications may be utilized to manage alcohol withdrawal.

Diagnosis and Planning

19. Disulfiram (Antabuse) is used with some clients to help them remain abstinent. Careful client teaching must accompany the use of disulfiram.

20. AA, Al-Anon, Alateen, Alatots, and ACOA are 12-step programs where alcoholics and their families are able to share common experiences and receive emotional support as part of recovery and healing.

21. Although most nursing diagnoses may be applied to alcoholic clients, those related to mental and emotional well-being are of primary consideration in mental health nursing.

22. General nursing interventions during acute alcohol intoxication include monitoring vital signs, protecting the client from injury, and providing a quiet environment.

23. General nursing interventions for clients in alcohol withdrawal include monitoring vital signs, fluid replacement, preventing seizures and DTs, and providing a quiet environment.

24. General nursing interventions for clients with chronic alcoholism include assisting clients to recognize the need for abstinence, encouraging responsible decision making, stress management, and referral to support groups.

Evaluation

25. Nurses evaluate the effectiveness of the nursing care plan on the basis of the client's achievement or nonachievement of the outcome criteria.

26. Based on evaluation, the client and nurse modify the plan of care.

CHAPTER REVIEW

1. Which of the following statements indicates why nurses should have a knowledge base about persons affected by alcohol?

(a) Alcoholism may not be stated as part of the client's admitting diagnosis, but his or her condition may be a direct result of alcohol abuse.

(b) Since there is no precise definition of alcoholism, the nurse must use physical assessment to identify the long-term use of alcohol.

(c) Having a knowledge base prevents nurses becoming involved in the abuse of alcohol.

(d) The nurse is able to plan care and make interventions more effectively by identifying his or her feelings of disapproval of the client's use of alcohol.

2. Women may be more vulnerable to co-dependent behavior because:
   (a) They are less able than men to manage their emotions and behavior.
   (b) They have been socialized to be responsible for everyone in the family system.
   (c) There are many more alcoholic husbands than there are alcoholic wives.
   (d) They wish to protect their children from future physical and sexual abuse.

3. Nursing assessment includes checking for blackouts in alcoholic clients. Which of the following statements by a client best indicates a blackout?
   (a) "I know you just told me where I am but I can't remember what you just said."
   (b) "I only drink because of job stress. If I had a different boss I wouldn't drink."
   (c) "My wife told me I was the life of the party last night but I don't remember anything."
   (d) "You know, I think I have several different personalities. I never can control who is in charge."

4. Which one of the following has been one of the most effective treatment methods for the alcohol-dependent client?
   (a) Inpatient detoxification units
   (b) Group therapy
   (c) Medication therapy
   (d) Alcoholics Anonymous

5. In securing a nursing history of a client you suspect abuses alcohol, it is important to remember that the client may downplay the amount of drinking he or she actually does. Which one of the following would be the best question to ask to avoid this interview problem?
   (a) "Do you drink regularly?"
   (b) "When was your last drink?"
   (c) "Do you drink every day?"
   (d) "When do you drink?"

6. The nurse observes that an alcoholic client has teeth in poor repair, gum lesions, fissures around the mouth, and poor personal hygiene in general. Which one of the following nursing diagnoses is most appropriate to these findings?
   (a) Activity intolerance, potential
   (b) Fluid volume deficit, actual
   (c) Infection, potential for
   (d) Thought processes, alteration in

REFERENCES

Alcoholics Anonymous World Services: *A.A.: 44 Questions.* Alcoholics Anonymous World Services, 1983.

Amaro H, et al.: Violence during pregnancy and substance use. *Am J Public Health* 1990; 80(5):575–579.

American Psychiatric Association: *Diagnostic and Statistical Manual of Mental Disorders,* 3rd ed, revised. Washington DC: American Psychiatric Association, 1987.

Bigby J, Clark WD, May H: Diagnosing early treatable alcoholism. *Patient Care* (Feb 15) 1990; 24(3):135–156.

Blum et al.: Allelic association of human dopamine D_2 receptor gene in alcoholism. *JAMA* (April 18) 1990; 263(15):2055–2060.

Bradshaw J: *Healing the Shame That Binds You.* Health Communications, Inc., 1988.

Burkhalter PK: *Nursing Care of the Alcoholic and Drug Abuser.* McGraw-Hill, 1975.

Carpenito LJ: *Handbook of Nursing Diagnosis 1989–90.* Lippincott, 1989.

Campbell D, Graham M: *Drugs and Alcohol in the Workplace.* Facts on File Pub., 1988.

Cohen S: Alcohol and malnutrition. *Drug Abuse and Alcoholism Newsletter* (Oct) 1982; 11:1–4.

Donald W: Alcoholism and alcoholic psychoses. In: *Comprehensive Textbook of Psychiatry,* 4th ed. Vol. I. Daplan HI, Sadock BJ (editors). Williams and Wilkins, 1985.

Earle R, Crow G: *Lonely All the Time.* Pocket Books, 1989.

Estes NJ, Smith-DiJulio D, Heinemann ME: *Nursing Diagnosis of the Alcoholic Person.* Mosby, 1980.

Fingarette H: *Heavy Drinking: The Myth of Alcoholism as a Disease.* University of California Press, 1988.

Finley B: The role of the psychiatric nurse in a community substance abuse prevention program. *Nurs Clin N Am* 1989; 24(1):121–136.

Gordis E, et al.: Finding the gene(s) for alcoholism. *JAMA* (Apr 18) 1990; 263(15):2094–2095.

Griffith JW, Christensen PJ: *Nursing Process.* Mosby, 1986.

Hall JM: Alcoholism in lesbians: developmental, symbolic, interactionist, and critical perspectives. *Health Care for Women International* 1990; 11(1):89–107.

Hancock DC: Alcohol and the church. In: *Alcohol, Science & Society Revisited.* Gomberg EL, White HR, Carpenter JA (editors). University of Michigan Press, 1982.

Hough ES: Alcoholism: Prevention and treatment. *J Psychosoc Nurs* 1989; 27(1):15–19.

Hughes TL: Models and perspectives of addiction: Implications for treatment. *Nurs Clin N Am* 1989; 24(1):1–12.

Jellinek EM: Phases of alcohol addiction. In: *Society, Cul-*

ture & Drinking Patterns. Pittman DJ, Snyder CR (editors). Wiley, 1962.

Lerner WD, et al.: Alcoholic emergencies. *Patient Care* (May 30) 1988; 22(10):112–136.

Levin JD: *Treatment of Alcoholism and Other Addictions.* Aronson, 1987.

Luckman J, Sorensen RC: *Medical-Surgical Nursing: A Psychophysiologic Approach,* 4th ed. Saunders, 1987.

Nowinski J: *Substance Abuse in Adolescents and Young Adults.* Norton, 1990.

Potter-Efron RT: *Shame, Guilt and Alcoholism: Treatment Issues in Clinical Practice.* Haworth Press, 1989.

Powell AH, Minick MP: Alcohol withdrawal syndrome. *Am J Nurs* 1988; 88(3):312–315.

Scavnicky-Mylant M: The process of coping among young adult children of alcoholics. *Issues Men Health Nurs* 1990; 11(2):125–139.

Schenk E: Substance abuse. In: *Medical-Surgical Nursing,* 2nd ed. Long BC, Phipps WJ (editors). 1989. pp. 263–289.

Sugermann AA: Alcoholism: An overview of treatment models and methods. In: *Alcohol, Science & Society Revisited.* Gomberg EL, White HR, Carpenter JA (editors). University of Michigan Press, 1982.

Sullivan E, Bissell L, Williams E: *Chemical Dependency in Nursing.* Addison-Wesley, 1988.

Townsend MC: *Drug Guide for Psychiatric Nursing.* Davis, 1990.

Treadway DC: *Before It's Too Late: Working with Substance Abuse in the Family.* Norton, 1989.

Tweed SH: Identifying the alcoholic client. *Nurs Clin N Am* 1989; 24(1):13–32.

U.S. Department of Health and Human Services: *Sixth Special Report to the U.S. Congress on Alcohol and Health.* DHHS publication no. (ADM)87:1519. U.S. Department of Health and Human Services. 1987.

Weisberg J, Hawes G: *Rx for Recovery.* Franklin Watts, 1989.

World Almanac and Book of Facts. World Almanac, 1990.

SUGGESTED READINGS

Alcoholics Anonymous World Services: *A Message to Teenagers . . . How to Tell When Drinking Is Becoming a Problem.* Alcoholics Anonymous World Services, 1988.

Castiglia PT: Influences on children's attitudes toward alcohol consumption. *Pediatric Nurs* 1989; 15(3):263–266.

Doenges ME, Townsend MC, Moorhous MF: *Psychiatric Care Plans.* Davis, 1989.

George VD: Alcoholism: A major Black health problem. *J Natl Black Nurs Ass.* (1988 Fall–1989 Winter). 3(1): 8–11.

George VD: Nurses' attitudes toward alcohol abuse and alcoholism. *J Natl Black Nurs Ass.* (1988 Fall–1989 Winter). 3(1):12–22.

Goldberg J, et al.: A twin study of the effects of the Vietnam conflict on alcohol drinking patterns. *Am J Public Health* 1990; 80(5):570–574.

Marcus RN, Katz JL: Inpatient care of the substance-abusing patient with a concomitant eating disorder. *Hosp & Comm Psychiatry* 1990; 41(1):59–63.

Rynerson BC: Cops and counselors: Counseling issues with prison inmate substance abusers. *J Psychosoc Nurs* 1989; 27(2):12–17.

Vaccani JM: Borderline personality and alcohol abuse. *Arch Psychiatr Nurs* 1989; 3(2):113–119.

CHAPTER 13

Drug Abuse

J. SUE COOK

Being in the Hospital

In a secure place being deflated of power, fear, unreal feelings and/or depression.

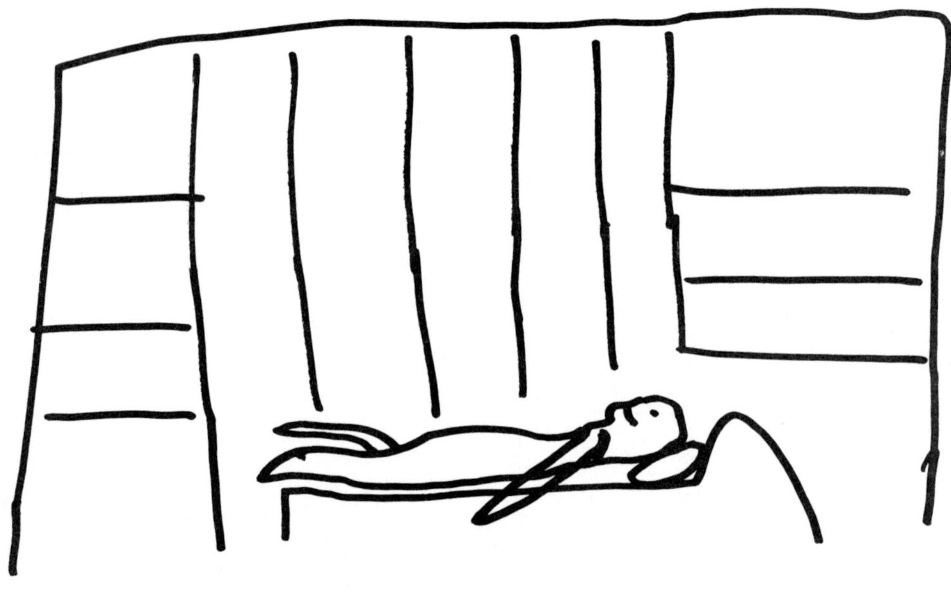

Objectives

After reading this chapter the student will be able to

- Distinguish between drug abuse and drug dependence
- Explain the criteria for choosing a diagnosis of drug abuse versus drug dependence
- Discuss the significance of drug abuse to the mental health nurse
- Describe the theoretic knowledge base underlying the development of drug abuse
- List commonly abused categories of drugs, along with the names of the drugs, street names for the drugs, the actions of the drugs, and the signs and symptoms of abuse
- Discuss the abuse of caffeine and tobacco
- Make a focused nursing assessment of a client with drug abuse
- Relate abnormal physical findings in the assessment of the drug-abusing client
- Identify nursing diagnoses for clients with drug intoxication/withdrawal and drug overdose
- Prepare nursing care plans for clients with drug intoxication/withdrawal and drug overdose
- Discuss the evaluation of nursing care of the client with drug intoxication/withdrawal and drug overdose

Chapter Outline

Introduction

The abuse of drugs is classified as a mental disorder. In our society, many people use drugs recreationally to modify mood or behavior; however, wide sociocultural variations in the acceptability of drug use exist. For example, peyote is used by the Southwestern Plains Indians to induce a hallucinogenic religious experience (Hahn, Barkin, and Klarmen Oestreich, 1982). In the broader American culture, the use of almost all drugs for recreational purposes is illegal. Alcohol, caffeine, and tobacco are considered the socially acceptable forms of drug use for recreational purposes. Aside from alcohol, the most commonly abused drugs in our society are narcotics, sedatives, stimulants, antianxiety drugs, and hallucinogens.

DSM-III-R classifies the pathologic use of drugs as psychoactive substance use disorders. Historically, the term **addiction** has been used to describe the habitual ingestion of narcotic drugs in increasing proportions to the point of physical dependence. Thus the term *addiction* has a primary physiologic focus. Currently the term **chemical** (or substance) **dependence** is used to reflect the biopsychosocial model of substance use disorders. Chemical dependence is viewed as a continuum that ranges from mild to moderate to severe dependence.

Some people distinguish between substance abuse and substance dependence. **Abuse** is defined as the purposeful use of a drug which results in adverse effects to oneself or others.* *Dependence* occurs when the use of the drug is no longer under personal control and continues despite adverse effects. Table 13–1 lists the diagnostic criteria for dependence and Table 13–2 lists the diagnostic criteria for abuse. Other people are attempting to eliminate the distinction between abuse and dependence because they view it as arbitrary. Chemical dependence is a physical and emotional disorder in which individuals are dependent on the use of substances to alter and control mood states, have a compulsion to use these substances, and experience some form of distress if they are deprived access to the substances (Donovan, 1988; Sullivan, Bissell, and Williams, 1988; Treadway, 1989).

Tolerance means that the user must take increased amounts of the psychoactive substance to achieve the desired effect. **Withdrawal** refers to the psychoactive substance–specific syndrome that occurs after cessation or reduction in intake of the psychoactive substance.

*(See Chapter 12 for discussion of alcohol abuse)

There are nine classes of psychoactive substances associated with chemical dependence:

- Alcohol
- Amphetamines and similarly acting sympathomimetics
- Cannabis
- Cocaine
- Hallucinogens
- Inhalants
- Opioids
- Phencyclidine (PCP) and similarly acting arylcycloalkylamines
- Sedatives, hypnotics, and anxiolytics

Diagnostic Criteria for Classes of Psychoactive Substances

Amphetamines and Similarly Acting Sympathomimetics The drugs associated with this classification are the substances known as "speed." The group includes amphetamines, dextroamphetamine, and methamphetamine. Some ap-

Table 13–1 *The Diagnostic Criteria for Substance Dependence*

The diagnostic criteria for psychoactive substance dependence are
1. At least three of the following:
   (a) Larger amounts of the drug taken over a longer period of time than the person intended.
   (b) Persistent desire to cut down or control drug use or one or more unsuccessful efforts to cut down or control drug use.
   (c) A great deal of time spent in activities necessary to obtain, take, or recover from the effects of the drug.
   (d) Intoxication or withdrawal symptoms when expected to fulfill major role obligations at work, school, or home.
   (e) Important social, occupational, or recreational activities reduced or given up because of drug use.
   (f) Continued drug use despite knowledge of having social, psychological, or physical problems caused by the use of the drug.
   (g) Evidence of tolerance or need for increase amounts of the drug to achieve intoxication or desired effect. (This criteria may not apply to cannabis, hallucinogens, or phencyclidine.)
   (h) Withdrawal symptoms.
   (i) Taking drug to relieve or avoid withdrawal symptoms.
2. The disturbance has persisted for at least one month or has occurred repeatedly over a longer period of time.

Source: Adapted from American Psychiatric Association, *Diagnostic and Statistical Manual of Mental Disorders,* 3rd ed., revised (Washington, DC: American Psychiatric Association, 1987). Reprinted with permission.

Table 13–2 *The Diagnostic Criteria for Substance Abuse*

The diagnostic criteria for psychoactive substance abuse are as follows:
1. A maladaptive pattern of drug use according to one of the following:
   (a) Continued use despite knowing that social, occupational, psychologic, or physical problems are caused or exacerbated by use of the drug.
   (b) Recurrent use in situations in which use is physically dangerous.
2. Symptoms of disturbance have persisted for at least one month or have occurred repeatedly over a longer period of time.
3. Drug use never met the criteria for psychoactive substance dependence for the drug.

Source: Adapted from American Psychiatric Association, *Diagnostic and Statistical Manual of Mental Disorders,* 3rd ed., revised (Washington, DC: American Psychiatric Association, 1987). Reprinted with permission.

petite suppressants also fit into this category. These drugs are taken orally, intravenously, and sometimes by nasal inhallation. A new form of these substances is the methamphetamine known as "ice" on the streets. Ice is ingested by smoking it and its effect is described as similar to crack cocaine. The difference is that the effect of ice lasts as long as 14 hours. Abuse and dependence criteria for amphetamines may be summarized as follows.

- *Pattern of use:* Episodic, almost daily, or daily use. Binging on weekends is a common form of episodic use. There is a general increase in the dose over time.
- *Associated features:* Users are often also dependent on alcohol or sedatives, hypnotics, or anxiolytics to alleviate the unpleasant aftereffects of amphetamine intoxication. Psychologic and behavioral changes include depression, irritability, anhedonia, anergia, social isolation, sexual dysfunction, paranoid ideation, attentional disturbances, and memory problems.
- *Course:* Intravenous administration tends to cause dependence within a few weeks or months. Intranasal administration may take months or years after initial use to create dependence. Continuing use appears to be a result of persistent craving for the drug rather than attempts to avoid withdrawal symptoms.
- *Prevalence:* Of the adult population, 2 percent have used amphetamines at some time during their lives.

Nancy, a 30-year-old secretary, decided to get some diet pills to lose weight. When she went to her doctor to get the pills, she found he would not give her a prescription for amphetamines. Nancy knew of a drug dealer, so she decided to take matters into her own hands. Nancy liked the effects of the pills she got; they gave her extra energy on the job. On weekends she would double her dose because she liked the feeling of "flying high" and found she didn't eat all weekend. Nancy's coworkers began to notice that Nancy had lost a lot of weight suddenly. They attributed her memory problems and irritability on the job to her loss of weight.

Cannabis This classification includes marijuana and hashish. These drugs are most often smoked and occasionally taken orally, mixed with food. Delta-9-tetrahydrocannabinol (THC) is the psychoactive ingredient in marijuana and hashish. The content of THC ranges from 1 to 5 percent in marijuana, while hashish can contain up to 15 percent THC (Youcha and Seixas, 1989). The following is a summary of the criteria for abuse and dependence of cannabis.

- *Patterns of use:* Cannabis is thought to have low abuse potential, and many people start using the drug because of this factor. They do not realize the capacity of the drug for causing dependence. Dependence is most often seen with daily or almost daily use. Abuse is seen in maladaptive behavior such as driving while cannabis-intoxicated. There is less social, occupational, and physical impairment with cannabis dependence than with other drugs.

- *Associated features:* Cannabis is often used in combination with other substances, especially alcohol and cocaine. The psychologic symptoms associated with cannabis include lethargy, anhedonia, attention problems, and memory problems.
- *Course:* Dependence usually develops with repeated use over a long period of time. Tolerance may develop and cause increased consumption and frequency of use.
- *Prevalence:* Cannabis is the mostly widely used illicit drug in the United States. Sixty million people in the United States have tried cannabis and some 20 million continue to use it regularly (McCormick, 1989).

Juan, a 15-year-old high school student, began smoking pot when he was in sixth grade. Juan used to hang around the middle school with some older guys who introduced him to the drug. At first the guys were real good to Juan—they let him take drags off their reefers. Once Juan got into the middle school, the guys changed. They expected Juan to buy the reefers. Juan didn't have his own money, so he started taking money from his mother's purse. By the time he was in ninth grade, Juan smoked every day. Juan sold his bicycle so he could buy a stash of weed. He told his mother the bike had been stolen. Juan had always done fairly well in school, but his grades slipped to barely passing. Juan spent most of his free time smoking with his friends.

Cocaine There are several types of cocaine preparations, all of which are made from the coca leaf. The preparations can be chewed, smoked, inhaled, or injected. The most commonly used form of cocaine in the United States is cocaine hydrochloride powder, which is generally inhaled through the nostrils.

Since 1984 the prevalence of smoking cocaine has greatly increased, and "crack," or "rock" cocaine, has been readily available for this purpose.

Crack is cocaine hydrochloride mixed with baking soda and water, heated, allowed to harden, and broken into small pieces. These pieces are smoked in cigarettes or glass waterpipes (Gianelli, 1986; Levy, 1987). The deadliest aspect of crack is that it is relatively cheap. It costs from $5 to $50 on the street, making it easily available to many teenagers.

The high received from crack is rapid and intensely euphoric. This euphoria is followed by a crash that is called coming down. Within a few seconds to a few minutes after coming down, users feel the need to smoke more crack. It is not until they can no longer support their habit that many users seek help. The crack user has the following symptoms: irritability, paranoia, depression, wheezing, coughing blood and black phlegm, increased heart rate and blood pressure, weight loss, and parched throat and lips. Cardiac arrhythmias and seizures are common and may cause death (Gianelli, 1986; Levy, 1987).

The following summarizes the criteria for cocaine dependence and abuse.

- *Patterns of use:* The major patterns of use vary from episodic to daily. Binging is the most common form of episodic use and is most often associated with smoking or intravenous use. Chronic use is often associated with increases in doses over time.
- *Associated features:* The user often abuses alcohol, sedatives, hypnotics, or anxiolytics to alleviate the aftereffects of cocaine intoxication. The psychologic and behavioral changes associated with cocaine use include depression, irritability, anhedonia, anergia, social isolation, sexual dysfunction, paranoid ideation, attentional disturbances, and memory problems.
- *Course:* Smoking and intravenous administration tend to produce abuse or dependence within a few weeks or months. Intranasal administration produces a more gradual abuse or dependence over a period

of months or years. Tolerance is common and usually there is an increase in dose to produce desired effects. Continued use of the substance is driven by cravings for the drug rather than by attempts to avoid withdrawal symptoms.

- *Prevalence:* Approximately 0.2 percent of the adult population have abused cocaine at some time during their lives.

Larry, a 25-year-old insurance salesperson, had been a partier since high school. Larry usually drank beer and sometimes hard liquor, but recently one of his clients had introduced him to cocaine. Larry had never experienced the high with alcohol that he did with cocaine. Larry thought he had everything under control because he used cocaine only on weekends. Larry noticed that he wanted to use cocaine during the week to unwind—his evening beer wasn't doing the job. Soon he was using cocaine nightly.

Hallucinogens Drugs in this classification are taken orally and include those that involve 5-hydroxytryptamine neuronal pathways, such as LSD, MDA, MDMA, TMA, DOM and DMT; and phenylethylamines, such as mescaline and psilocybin. The following summarizes the criteria for abuse and dependence of hallucinogens.

- *Patterns of use:* Most people begin using hallucinogens by experimenting. Use is almost always episodic because the effects of the drugs impair normal cognitive function to the point that daily activities must be interrupted. Abuse is more common than dependence.
- *Associated features:* Hallucinogens are frequently contaminated with other drugs such as phencylidine (PCP) and amphetamines. Hallucinogen users frequently smoke cannabis and abuse alcohol.
- *Course:* The course is unpredictable and is most likely related to the underlying pathology that precipitated the onset of use. Most people resume their former lifestyle after a brief period of abuse.
- *Prevalence:* People seeking help for dependence on hallucinogens are extremely rare. Approximately 0.3% of the adult population have abused hallucinogens at some point in their lives.

Anna, a 20-year-old college student, liked to keep to herself and study. She had always needed extra time to learn and tried to avoid a lot of people when she was studying. Anna was considered a recluse by her college classmates, but they continued to encourage her to join them for parties. One evening after finals, for which she'd studied extra hard, Anna felt she wanted to escape. She had a few alcoholic drinks and decided to go to a party with her roommate. Some people there were smoking mescaline, and Anna decided she would like to try it. After smoking it, Anna thought she was floating on a cloud. The music sounded wonderful. The colors were bright and vivid, and Anna was the life of the party with the descriptions of her visions.

Inhalants This classification of drugs includes aliphatic and aromatic hydrocarbons found in substances such as gasoline, glue, paint, paint thinner, and spray paint. Other types of inhalants are amyl nitrite, butyl nitrite, and nitrous oxide. The nitrites cause vasodilatation which results in a sudden drop in blood pressure and an increased heart rate within 15 to 30 seconds after inhalation. The user experiences an intense euphoric high which lasts about 3 minutes. It is said to increase sexual stimulation and intensify orgasm. Nitrous oxide is a general anesthesia used in dentistry and is abused for its euphoric effects and mild hallucinations. The drugs are either inhaled through the mouth or the nose. The following summarizes the criteria for abuse and dependence of inhalants.

- *Patterns of use:* Generally, inhalant users come from dysfunctional families and have school or work adjustment problems. There is a high incidence of inhalant use among minority youths living in economically depressed areas. Use of inhalants may begin as young as age 9. Use gradually increases through adolescence and young adulthood.

- *Associated features:* Nearly all inhalant users use other drugs as well. There may be significant physical and mental problems.
- *Course:* Inhalants may be used several times a week, on weekends, or after school. The pattern may persist for many years.
- *Prevalence:* No information is available.

Ricky, an 11-year-old student, lives in the inner city with his family. Ricky is the third of five children. He and his brothers and sisters live in a two-bedroom apartment. Ricky hangs out after school with a group of friends at the park. They steal glue from the five-and-dime in the neighborhood and take it to the park bathroom to sniff.

Opioids This classification of drugs includes heroin, morphine, codeine, and synthetic drugs that act like morphine—hydromorphine, meperidine, methadone, oxycodone, and so on. These drugs can be taken orally, intravenously, by nasal inhalation, or by smoking. The following is a summary of the criteria for abuse and dependence on opioids.

- *Patterns of use:* There are two major patterns of use. The first is the less frequent and involves the person originally obtaining the opioid by prescription for the treatment of pain. The person may go to several physicians to obtain sufficient supplies of the drug. The second pattern involves young people who obtain the opioid from illegal sources to obtain a high.
- *Course:* Once the pattern of opioid abuse or dependence is established, the person's life is dominated by the procurement and use of the drug. There is a high death rate for those dependent on opioids from physical complications and for many, a violent lifestyle.
- *Associated features:* Most people who use opioids also use alcohol, amphetamines, cannabis, hallucinogens, nicotine, sedatives, hypnotics, anxiolytics, and nonprescription cough syrups.
- *Prevalence:* Approximately 0.7 percent of the adult population have abused opioids at some time during their lives.

Diana, a 19-year-old hairdresser, lives at home with her parents and seven brothers and sisters. Her brother, Ramon, belongs to a gang and Diana recently started dating José, one of the gang members. José taught Diana how to shoot herself up with heroin. Diana uses most of her earnings to buy heroin from José.

Phencyclidine (PCP) and Similarly Acting Arylcycloalkylamines This group of drugs includes phencyclidine (PCP) and ketamine. The criteria for abuse and dependence of this classification of drugs are as follows.

- *Patterns of use:* PCP is usually taken episodically in binges or runs that last several days. There are a few people who use PCP on a daily basis. It is not clear whether tolerance or withdrawal symptoms develop with this drug.
- *Associated features:* Heavy users of PCP also use alcohol and cannabis.
- *Course:* Abuse or dependence develops after a short period of occasional use. The motivation for continued use is the euphoric effect of the drug.
- *Prevalence:* The use of PCP by people seeking help for dependence is relatively rare.

Nineteen-year-old Jean-Paul was found by his friends in a confused and stuperous state after ingesting a mixture of PCP and alcohol. He was unable to speak coherently or walk or sit without assistance. After admission to the emergency department, he was transferred to an inpatient chemical-dependence unit, because of his history of polysubstance abuse.

Sedatives, Hypnotics, and Anxiolytics This classification of drugs includes sleeping pills and drugs used to treat anxiety. Commonly abused drugs in this category are: ethchlorvynol, glutethimide, chloral hydrate, methaqualone, and the barbiturates. Drugs in this category are usually taken orally. The following are the criteria for the abuse and dependence on sedatives, hypnotics, and anxiolytics.

- *Patterns of use:* There are two major patterns of use. In the first clients obtain the drug by prescription for anxiety or insomnia and gradually increase the dose and frequency on their own. In the second, young people obtain the drugs from illegal sources.
- *Course:* The most common course is heavy daily use resulting in dependence.
- *Associated features:* Some people use these drugs to enhance the euphoria of opioids or to counteract the stimulant effects of cocaine or amphetamines.
- Approximately 1.1 percent of the adult population have abused or have been dependent on sedatives during their lives.

Jane, a 65-year-old widow, received a prescription for barbiturates for insomnia when her husband died. Jane continued to take the "sleeping capsules" because she had a hard time sleeping. Jane often doubled up on the capsules in order to sleep through the night. When her doctor wouldn't give her another prescription, Jane went to a different doctor because the only way she could get any rest was with her sleeping capsules.

Incidence of Drug Abuse

Statistics on the number of drug abusers are difficult to provide. The illicit nature of drug use makes it nearly impossible to retrieve accurate information. Young people have been the major indicators of use because they are often the leaders of social change.

In the 1960s, psychedelics, hallucinogens, and amphetamines were the major drugs. In the 1970s, heroin, marijuana, and sedative hypnotic drugs were the most popular drugs. The decade of the 1980s was the era of cocaine. In the United States the average age at which marijuana and alcohol are tried is 13. Teenage use of illicit drugs other than cocaine has declined in recent years but still continues to be a significant problem. The Institute for Social Research at the University of Michigan has conducted a drug use survey of U.S. high school seniors each year since 1975. Table 13–3 presents the Institute's findings for the high school graduating classes of 1979 and 1986 (Johnston et al. 1987; Piercy and Nelson, 1989).

It is estimated that 7 percent of adults, and 19 percent of teens age 14 to 17, suffer from chemical dependence. As many as 33 percent of all Americans, 12 years and older, have used an illegal drug during their lives. Men are more likely to be dependent on cocaine, marijuana, and opioids; women are more likely to abuse sedatives, antianxiety agents, and amphetamines (Bluhm, 1987; Sullivan, Bissell, and Williams, 1988).

Significance of Drug Abuse to Mental Health Nursing

Because we live in a pill-oriented society, nurses must be familiar with attitudes, practices, and illnesses that are related to chemical dependence. Drugs for all types of maladies are advertised and used daily. Caffeine in coffee helps keep many people awake, and nicotine in cigarettes helps relieve many people's tension. Doctors readily prescribe sedatives and antianxiety agents for anxiety, stress, and insomnia.

Recently, attention has been given to the severity of the problem of chemical dependence among professionals—nurses and physicians who work in high-stress situations and have easy access to narcotics are especially prone to dependence. Because women who abuse substances are judged more harshly than are men, female nurses are more

Table 13–3 *Comparison of the Prevalence and Recency of Drug Use by High School Seniors in the Class of 1979 and Class of 1986*

	Percent Ever Used		*Percent Used Last Month*		*Percent Used Last Year*	
Type of Drug	*1979*	*1986*	*1979*	*1986*	*1979*	*1986*
Alcohol	93.0	91.3	71.0	65.3	16.3	19.2
Amphetamines	24.2	23.4	9.9	5.5	8.4	7.9
Barbiturates	14.6	8.4	4.4	1.8	5.5	2.4
Cigarettes	74.0	67.6	34.0	29.6	39.6	38.0
Cocaine	15.4	16.9	5.7	6.2	6.3	6.5
Heroin	1.1	1.1	0.2	0.2	0.3	0.3
LSD	18.6	7.2	5.5	1.7	7.3	2.8
Marijuana	60.4	50.9	36.5	23.4	14.3	15.4
PCP	12.8	4.8	2.4	1.3	4.6	1.1

Adapted from Johnston, 1987.

likely than male physicians to suffer job termination, arrest, prosecution, and loss of license. Many state nurses' associations have established peer-support systems, and health care systems are beginning to establish employee assistance programs to help nurses overcome their drug dependence (Hughes and Sullivan, 1989; Sullivan, Bissell, and Williams, 1988).

Since drug abuse is a major public health problem in the United States, nurses are likely to have clients that are being treated for complications associated with the abuse of specific drugs. Nurses need a clear understanding of the nature of these drug abuse disorders to intervene effectively with clients and their significant others.

The nurse's values, attitudes, and behaviors toward the drug addict should be examined. The drug user is very sensitive to the attitudes of care givers. Condemning or condoning drug use can hamper the client's attempts at recovery. The client is responsible for trying to change drug-seeking and drug-using behavior, and the nurse is responsible for supporting those efforts without making judgments about them.

Knowledge Base

Behavioral Characteristics

As with alcoholism, there is no definitive set of indicators for drug abuse. The nurse appraises the information given by the client and compares those appraisals with his or her understanding of the complexities of drug abuse behaviors. It is the consequences of the drug abuse behaviors—the grave social and personal problems arising as a result of drug use—that bring the drug abuser to the attention of the nurse. One behavior common to drug abusers is a strong desire or need to use the drug continually. Other primary behaviors associated with drug abuse are uncooperative and belligerent behavior (Schnoll, 1983).

The behaviors associated with drug abuse also characterize other disorders, so the nurse needs to be attuned to look for other behavioral indicators when these primary behaviors are observed. Of course, the simplest way of recognizing the drug abuser is by the client's admission of a drug problem. But because drug abusers rarely seek help in overcoming drug problems, the nurse needs to look for other behaviors to confirm suspicions of drug abuse. The client may seek new prescriptions frequently or may seek prescriptions from more than one physician. This can be confirmed by calling the pharmacies where the client's prescriptions are being filled. Sudden behavior changes can be another indicator of drug abuse. For example, an ordinarily docile person may become aggressive, or someone who is fastidiously neat, may become sloppy and poorly groomed. Frequent job changes or loss of job with no explanation may also point to drug abuse problems.

The client's lifestyle may be drastically affected by the use of drugs. Clients who obtain their drugs through legal prescriptions may be able to live normally without arousing suspicion, but those who use illegal drugs may have to alter their lifestyles. This latter group often become involved in a drug subculture in which self-protection, prostitution, theft, and burglary prevail. As a result of this kind of lifestyle, clients often find themselves in legal difficulties.

Affective Characteristics

Psychoactive substances are used by some people as stimulants to overcome feelings of boredom and depression. Others use these substances as depressants to manage their anxiety and stress. Their overall intention is to decrease negative feelings and increase positive feelings. The affective manifestations of specific drugs range from anxiety and fear to drastic mood swings and paranoia. When chemically dependent people try to control their use of drugs and fail in this attempt, they experience feelings of guilt and shame. When the problem becomes public knowledge, they are likely to feel embarrassed and humiliated (Donovan, 1988).

Many chemically dependent people suffer from depression, which may have preceded or may have resulted from the substance abuse. Research is currently focusing on the incidence of anxiety disorders and panic attacks in chemically dependent individuals. Cocaine, PCP, marijuana, organic solvents, and caffeine can all induce panic attacks. It is believed that as many as 64 percent of regular cocaine users develop an acquired form of panic disorder related to the effect of cocaine on CNS excitability. Once the panic attacks are established, the disorder persists even after the use of cocaine is stopped (Louie et al. 1989).

Cognitive Characteristics

Research on personality traits of the drug abuser is inconclusive. There are some common characteristics, since to maintain drug dependence the person must be capable of deception, dishonesty, and camouflage. For example, the person may have to invent new ailments or change doctors to continue receiving prescriptions, or may have to resort to criminal activity to obtain illegal drugs.

Chemically dependent people often experience disturbances of concentration, attention span, or the ability to follow directions. The ability to make rational decisions is impaired. *Denial* is the major defense mechanism maintaining the dependence. Denial of a problem is a person's unconscious attempt to maintain self-esteem in the face of out-of-control behavior. Supporting the denial is the use of *rationalization,* heard in such comments as: "I use drugs because I was an abused child," or "I use drugs because I have to escape from the stress of my job."

Gaming, rounding, and imaging are other defenses exhibited by many chemically dependent persons. *Gaming* is the skill of swindling or practicing deception to achieve an end. *Rounding* is the verbal avoidance of unpleasant or unproductive subjects. *Imaging* is the projection of a personality that is considered desirable and acceptable to those trying to help the client.

Physiologic Characteristics

Abused drugs have either a stimulant or depressant effect on the CNS. The physical and psychologic dependence on these drugs is frequently associated with debilitated physical states. Malnutrition with associated hypovitaminosis and dehydration is common. Respiratory problems such as pneumonia, pulmonary emboli, abscesses, and respiratory depression may occur. Skin problems, sepsis, and hepatitis often result from contaminated drug paraphernalia. Death can occur because of accidental overdose (Hahn, Barkin, and Klarmen Oestreich, 1982). Medical sequelae are common in drug abusers and may be related to the method the client uses to administer the drug. Clients who smoke their drugs may have chronic bronchitis and throat irritations. Clients who snort (take by insufflation) may have nasal lesions and irritation, chronic nasal stuffiness, and postnasal drip. Intravenous drug abusers commonly have infections such as hepatitis, cellulitis, and endocarditis. Intravenous drug abusers often have "tracks," or needle marks over veins, from repeated injections. Contaminated needles are a leading cause of AIDS. Among IV drug users, it is estimated that 50 to 60 percent are HIV positive. This group and their sexual partners are the fastest growing segment of AIDS cases (Schleifer et al. 1990). See Table 13–4 for a summary of the physiologic effects of various abused drugs.

Sociocultural Characteristics

Chemical dependence not only affects the individual, it affects families, peers, health systems, and society as a whole. In some instances family members and old friends will be abandoned for new relationships within the subculture of drug abuse. In other cases, chemically dependent people simply become more isolated as drugs become the main focus of their lives. Yet others are successful in keeping their drug use hidden from their colleagues and most of their significant others.

Chemical dependence is a family problem. The most devastating impact on the family is when the abuser is the parent. Substance abuse leads to the deterioration of the couple system. Power struggles occur between using and nonusing partners. The inability to discuss the drug problem openly contributes to family denial. To avoid embarrassment, family members make excuses to outsiders for the user's behavior. Family roles and responsibilities shift according to the crisis of the day. In spite of all this chaos, the nonabusing partner may remain in the relationship because of emotional dependency, money, family cohesion, religious compliance, or outward respectability.

Co-dependence is the term used to describe the nonabusing partner who remains in the relationship. Co-dependents operate out of fear, resentment, helplessness, hopelessness, and desire to control the user's behavior. Women may be more vulnerable to co-dependent behavior, because they have been socialized to be devoted to and responsible for the family and are expected to be loyal to their partners at all costs. Co-dependents often suffer from low self-esteem and often fear abandonment. The intensity of chaos and crisis is mistaken for intimacy. Obsession with the user's behavior is mistaken for love. Co-dependents tend to experience one of four response patterns. The *alienated* co-dependents ignore the drug problem, as well as their own feelings of pain, and hope that it will all go away. *Bullies* manage their own pain by lashing out and by constantly criticizing the user with hopes that this will stop the drug abuse behavior. *Managers* take care of everything and shield the user from distress or problems. *Martyrs* passively endure their pain in hopes that their partners will feel guilty enough to change (Earle and Crow, 1989).

Children who grow up in homes where one or both parents are chemically dependent often suffer effects their entire lives. Very early in life they learn not to talk about the drug problem—not even within the family. Children learn by fear of verbal or physical assault that they should keep all feelings to themselves. Often it is difficult for them to trust others, because consistency is necessary for building trust, and chemically dependent parents are very unpredictable. Children tend to develop one of four patterns of behavior. The *hero,* often the oldest child, becomes the competent caretaker and works on making the family function. This child may grow up and become a caretaker of a dysfunctional partner or may become a workaholic. The *scapegoat* acts out at home, in school, and in the community. This child takes the focus off the parental user by getting into trouble to become the focus of conflict in the family. This child may grow up to become another substance abuser. The *lost child* tries to avoid conflict and pain by withdrawing physically and emotionally. As an adult, this person has difficulty forming close relationships and may turn to chemicals to decrease the feeling of isolation. The *mascot,* often the youngest child, tries to ease family tension with comic relief, which is used to mask his or her own sadness (Earle and Crow, 1989; Treadway, 1989).

A sociocultural characteristic primarily limited to cocaine abuse is that of sexual acting-out behavior. Cocaine is a CNS stimulant which relaxes inhibitions, increases sexual fantasies, and increases sexual desire. Some people begin experimenting with cocaine specifically for this sexual high. High doses of cocaine can produce compulsive masturbation, multipartner marathons, group sex, partner swapping, and even sexual abuse of children. It is not uncommon for cocaine abusers to go on marathon binges of cocaine and sex (Cocores and Gold, 1989).

Causative Theories

Theories of causation of chemical dependence parallel those of alcoholism. Some believe that those vulnerable to chemical dependence have a genetic deficiency of endorphins. Psychoactive substances are then used to achieve the effects of the missing endorphins. The biopsychosocial view states that there is no single cause of chemical dependence. Social learning, physiologic effects, and meaning of the experience all combine in some way to produce chemical dependence (Bluhm, 1987; Donovan, 1988). Polydrug-use situations are common. Individuals choose to use a variety of drugs to

- enhance the effects of another drug
- counteract the effects of another drug
- substitute for preferred but unavailable drugs
- conform to patterns of use in peer group.

Burkhalter (1975) identified two broad categories of proposed causes of drug abuse: (1) factors related to the initiation of drug abuse and (2) factors related to the continuation of drug dependence.

Factors Related to the Initiation of Drug Abuse Several aspects constitute this category. One hypothesis is that the person's basic nature is to search for altered states of consciousness. The result of this unconscious search is substance dependence. Another hypothesis is related to the person's desire to seek out and discover new experiences. Because of the affluence of American society and readily available illicit drugs, this makes adolescents and young adults particularly vulnerable.

A third explanation for initiating drug abuse is societal and parental example. The United States is a drug-oriented society. Advertisements offer medicinal cures not only for minor aches and pains but also for major health problems. Adolescents and young adults see their parents use various substances such as alcohol, caffeine, tranquilizers, nicotine, and sedatives. With sanction from television advertising and parental example, these young people see nothing wrong with trying various drugs.

Another explanation for initiating drug abuse is escape. The economic and emotional deprivation seen in inner-city ghettos have been posed as reasons for drug use, which the user sees as a means of temporary release from dismal surroundings. One young man illustrated this explanation in an interview by defensively stating, "How would you know what it's like to always want and have nothing? My drugs are my dream house and Caribbean cruise!"

Rebellion has also been hypothesized as an explanation for initiating drug abuse. Unlawful or undesirable behavior is one of the most effective means of expressing contempt or defiance of authority. Peer group pressure can be associated with rebellion. Being a member of a peer group is an important need to many adolescents and some young adults. So, if the peer group is experimenting with illicit drugs, other members of the group are likely to follow suit.

Factors Related to the Continuation of Drug Dependence The first and most potent reason to continue using a drug is physical depen-

Table 13–4 *Manifestations of Drug Abuse*

Name of Drug (Street Name)	*Action*	*Mode of Administration*	*Tolerance*	*Dependence*	*Cognitive Manifestations*
Cannabis Cannabis and hashish (Mary Jane, J, hay, joints, reefer, pot, grass, hash, stuff, dope, tea, hemp, love, weed, reach, Acapulco gold, hash oil, baby, Aunt Mary, bhang, blonde, bule saze, bobo, bo, burnie, bash cannabix, Chicago green, Colombian, dagga, ding, doobies, fu, rick sticks, roach rope, TJ, wheat, yerba)	CNS depressant	Smoked, swallowed	No, reverse tolerance sometimes occurs	Psychologic	Slowed sense of time Short-term memory impairment Colors are brighter
Stimulants Cocaine (snow, dust, coke, happy dust, C, stardust, majo, bernies, flake, gold dust, crack) Amphetamines (uppers, pep pills, wake-ups) Benzedrine (bennies, greenies, footballs, cartwheels, hearts, peaches, roses) Methedrine (ice, speed, crystal, meth) Dexedrine (dexies, Christmas trees, hearts, oranges)	CNS stimulant	Oral, subQ injection, IV injection Cocaine: insufflation	Yes	Psychologic	Delirium can occur Variable LOC Loss of cognitive abilities Disoriented Severe short-term memory loss Unable to perform simple mental tasks May have paranoid delusions Denial and rationalization
Hallucinogens and Phencyclidine (PCP) LSD (acid, blue acid, the hawk, royal blue, sugar cubes, pearly gates, heavenly blue, 25, instant Zen, trip) Mescaline (mesc, Big Chief, cactus, the buttontops, half moon, a moon, P, tops, mescal beans, the mescal button, the bad seed) PCP (peace pill, angel dust, hog, synthetic marijuana)	Unknown	Oral, some are injected or inhaled	Potential	Potential psychologic	Preoccupied by perceptual changes Illusions Disorientation Inability to perform simple tasks Poor fundamental knowledge of performance

Affective Manifestations	*Signs and Symptoms of Abuse*	*Withdrawal and Symptoms*	*Physical Complications*	*Death*
Sense of pleasure may progress to euphoria Apathy Feeling of being removed from one's surroundings May experience anxiety progressing to panic At times may be suspicious or paranoid	Nervous system: auditory, personality, and visual disturbances: personality alteration Respiratory system: cough	None	Bronchitis, conjunctivitis	No
Feeling of extreme self-confidence Exaggerated sense of competence and self-worth Euphoria May be hypervigilant, grandiose, elated, and agitated	Nervous system: seizures, muscle spasms, anesthesia, paresthesia, hallucinations, headaches; auditory, personality, and visual disturbances: hearing impairment, personality alteration, mydriasis Cardiovascuar system: circulatory collapse or shock, tachycardia, hypertension, vasoconstriction Respiratory system: rapid or deep breathing, slow or labored breathing Digestive system: anorexia, dysphagia, salivation, dry oral mucosae, nausea and vomiting, diarrhea, abdominal pain Skin and mucous membranes: dermatitis inflammation, needle marks Urine and breath: polyuria, urobilinogenuria	None	Malnutrition Amphetamines: needle contamination Cocaine: nasal septum perforation	Amphetamines: seizures, coma, cerebral hemorrhage Cocaine: seizures, respiratory failure
Euphoria Anxiety Emotional lability Grandiosity Belligerence Impulsivity Unpredictability	Nervous system: coma, ataxia, tetanic rigidity, seizures, muscle weakness or paralysis, anesthesia, paresthesia, hallucinations; auditory, personality, and visual disturbances: personality alteration, blurred vision, color distortions, blank stare, mydriasis Cardiovascular system: tachycardia, hypertension, hypotension Respiratory system: rapid or deep breathing, respiratory paralysis Digestive system: nausea and vomiting Skin and mucous membranes: rash, urticaria	None	Rare	Potential

(continued)

Table 13–4 *(continued)*

Name of Drug (Street Name)	*Action*	*Mode of Administration*	*Tolerance*	*Dependence*	*Cognitive Manifestations*
DOM (STP)					Sensation of slowed time
TMA					
DMT (businessman's LSD)					
MDA (the love drug)					
MDMA (ecstasy)					
Opioids	CNS depressant, analgesic	Oral, smoked, insufflation, "skin popped" (injected under skin), IM injection, IV injection	Yes	Psychologic, physiologic	Reduced LOC
Morphine (Miss Emma, morf, morphie, monkey, M, dreamer, white stuff, hokus, unkie)					Slurred speech Loss of coordination
Heroin (H, junk, shit, stuff, horse, dope, boy, hard stuff, joy, powder, skag, smack, Lady Jane, Mexican mud)					Orientation not impaired Manifestations of withdrawal
Codeine (junk, schoolboy)					Denial of problem drug use
Dilaudid (lords, D)					
Meperidine (Demerol)					
Methadone (dollies, dolls, 10-8-20, dolophine, amidone, adanon)					
Sedatives, hypnotics, or anxiolytics (downers, barbs, sleepers, candy, cap)	CNS depressant	Oral, IM injection, IV injection	Yes	Psychologic, physiologic	Similar to alcohol in regard to intoxication and withdrawal
Amytal (blue heaven, blue devils, blue angels, blue birds)					Reduced LOC
Nembutal (yellow jackets, dolls, goof balls, nimbie)					Loss of cognitive abilities
Seconal (seggy, red devils, red birds, seccy, reds)					Changes in perception of the environment
Placidyl					
Methaqualone (sopors, luding, quaalude, soapers, the love drug, heroin for lovers, mandrakes)					May insist drugs are necessary for the treatment of a legitimate illness
Valium Librium Equanil Miltown					

Affective Manifestations	*Signs and Symptoms of Abuse*	*Withdrawal and Symptoms*	*Physical Complications*	*Death*
		None	Rare	Potential
Altered moods Demanding Manipulative Angry	Nervous system: coma, tetanic rigidity, seizures, muscle weakness or paresthesia, hallucinations, headaches; auditory, personality, and visual disturbances: tinnitus, personality alteration, blurred vision, miosis Respiratory system: slow or labored breathing, respiratory paralysis Digestive system: anorexia, thirst, nausea and vomiting, colic, bloody stools, constipation, abdominal pain Skin and mucous membranes: pruritis, dryness, flush, pallor, dermatitis inflammation, alopecia, needle marks Urine and breath: glycosuria, proteinuria Hematologic disorders: anemia	Yes: tremors, spasms, abdominal pain, nausea, and vomiting; tearing; goose bumps, sweating, and chills; hypertension, increased respirations, tachycardia; anxiety; irritability; drug craving; depression	Infections, hepatitis, endocarditis, vascular disorders, pulmonary embolism	Yes: coma, respiratory failure, shock
A feeling that drug use is rising above everyday life Romanticized view of drug use	Nervous system: coma, ataxia, seizures, anesthesia, paresthesia, hallucinations, headaches; auditory, personality, and visual disturbances: personality alteration, blurred vision, miosis Cardiovascular system: circulatory collapse, bradycardia or tachycardia, hypotension, hemorrhage, petechiae, purpura Respiratory system: rapid or deep breathing, slow or labored breathing, respiratory paralysis Digestive system: constipation Skin and mucous membranes: rash, urticaria, pallor, cyanosis, bullae, dermatitis inflammation, hirsutism, needle marks	Yes: nausea, vomiting, diarrhea; bleeding; tremors; diaphoresis; hypertension and hypotension; sleep disturbance; irritability, hostility, restlessness, agitation; acute brain syndrome; impaired cognitive function; seizures	Overdose	Yes: coma, respiratory failure, shock

dence. Many abused substances cause tolerance and a physical craving for the drug. (See Table 13–4.) Another explanation is the positive reinforcement resulting from taking the drug. The rush, or high, that creates mental or physical ecstacy is a major reward. Other sensations associated with drug use are feelings of calmness, avoidance of conflict, and a perception of philosophic insight.

Avoiding withdrawal is another explanation given to the continuation of drug use. This has been termed negative reinforcement; that is, the drug user continues to take the drug to avoid the adverse affects of withdrawal symptoms.

Personality characteristics have been proposed as a potential explanation for continued drug abuse. Psychoanalytic theory proposes that drug abusers suffer from affective dysregulation (tension and depression alleviated by drug use) or a disorder in impulse control that is dominated by a search for pleasure. Opioid dependence has been linked with narcissistic character disorders. Epidemiologic studies of personality have found the following in drug abusers: placement of high value on independence and low value on academic achievement, more tolerance for deviance, and signs of delinquency before first experimentation with drugs (Jaffe, 1985).

Still another explanation proposed for continued drug use is lifestyle. The living patterns and rituals associated with obtaining and administering drugs contribute to continued drug use. A drug-oriented peer group reinforces drug dependence as a way of maintaining acceptance in the group. The abuser has a sense of belonging and security as a result of the lifestyle.

Medical Treatment

Because the drugs and problems are varied, no one treatment can deal with drug abuse problems. The complexity of treatment is compounded by complications such as malnutrition, infections, hepatitis, pancreatitis, family disruption, and social problems (Brunner and Suddarth, 1988). The major modalities for drug abuse treatment are detoxification programs, inpatient programs, outpatient programs, residential programs, day care programs, therapeutic communities, and psychotherapy. Since there are a variety of drug abuse and treatment modalities, treatment for specific drugs is presented.

Treatment for Users of Amphetamines or Similar Sympathomimetics Frequently amphetamines are withdrawn abruptly from chronic abusers. However, gradual tapering of dosage over several days appears to be more effective. There may be a potential for amphetamine psychosis in chronic abusers. Treatment requires supportive measures. It is important to approach both the psychotic and the intoxicated amphetamine user in a subdued manner. That is, do not speak in a loud voice, do not move too quickly, do not touch the client unless you are fairly sure it is safe, and do not approach the client from behind (Schnoll, 1983; Sullivan, Bissell, and Williams, 1988).

Elimination of amphetamines is facilitated by using ammonium chloride to acidify the urine. Because of the tendency to be combative and assaultive, amphetamine psychotics frequently must be kept in a hospital. After residual amphetamine is out of the user's system, antipsychotics such as the phenothiazines or haloperidol may be prescribed. Usually these antipsychotics are prescribed only for a few days for severe psychotic reactions.

Depression occurs frequently following amphetamine withdrawal, and tricyclic antidepressants may be indicated for a month or longer. Because of the client's tendency to return to drug use, it is important to establish antidepressant therapy during the initial withdrawal period (Grinspoon and Bakalara, 1985; Luckman and Sorensen, 1987; Schnoll, 1983).

Treatment for Cannabis Users Usually clients using cannabis, or marijuana, are not admitted to acute care units for treatment. Because this substance is not physically addicting, it requires no detoxification treatment. The primary treatment for the chronic marijuana user is emotional support (Gary and Trenznewsky, 1983). Since so many marijuana users are young people, health education covering marijuana's effect on decreasing testosterone levels and sperm production is also important.

Cannabis is often used simultaneously with other drugs, and personality alterations often occur with chronic polydrug use. Therefore, use of this drug needs to be assessed in acute and follow-up settings.

Treatment for Cocaine Users Chronic cocaine abuse is becoming an increasingly common problem in the United States. One reason it is difficult to treat is that anxiety and depression occur when the drug is stopped. (See Chapters 8, 9, and 11 for a discussion of treatment for anxiety and depression.) For the client who has become cocaine dependent, psychotherapy may fail to relieve anxiety and solve personal problems. Generally, diazepam (Valium) is used for chronic abusers in a state of anxiety.

Cocaine overdose is an acute emergency. Oxygen should be administered with the client's head in Trendelenburg's position. Seizures may occur and diazepam (Valium) is given intravenously to reduce the seizures. An anxiety reaction may be accompanied by tachycardia and hypertension. This reaction is treated with intramuscular or intravenous diazepam (Valium). Propranolol (Inderal) may be indicated in severe cocaine overdose, because it is a specific antagonist to the sympathomimetic effects of cocaine (Brunner and Suddarth, 1988; Luckman and Sorensen, 1987).

Treatment for Hallucinogen Users LSD is not as popular today as it was in the 1960s. Long-term use of hallucinogens like LSD is uncommon. Adverse reactions to LSD are responsible for prolonged treatment. Persons with schizoid and prepsychotic personalities are most likely to be hospitalized for mental instability produced by taking LSD. Therapy has included psychotherapy, antianxiety agents, antipsychotics, or antidepressants.

Treatment for Users of Inhalants Tolerance for inhalants does not seem to occur; craving for the substance is more common. Some people experience a withdrawal syndrome when they stop inhalant use. These clients are treated symptomatically for restlessness, anxiety, and irritability. The client who has taken large doses of inhalants should rest, because heart failure may occur. Inhalation psychosis may develop and should be treated the same as other psychoses in which hallucinations and paranoid delusions are common. (See Chapter 14 for discussion of psychoses.) Stimuli should be kept to a minimum, and the environment should be supportive and protective (Luckman and Sorensen, 1987).

Treatment for Users of Opioids The bulk of the literature on drug abuse treatment focuses on narcotic, or opioid, addiction. Treatment for opioids may be divided into overdose treatment measures, detoxification, and rehabilitation. In addition, there are treatments for the medical-surgical problems that occur as a result of opioid use.

The client's willingness to accept treatment means the client must make major lifestyle changes in attitude, family dynamics, and maybe geographic location. From the outset, the client must be aware that he or she is responsible for making the changes (Jaffe, 1985).

For the client presenting signs and symptoms of narcotic overdose, the treatment of choice is intravenous naloxone (Narcan). The client should be hospitalized for at least 24 hours and monitored for vital signs and level of consciousness. Initially, the client should be monitored every 15 minutes. Once the condition has stabilized, monitoring should occur once every hour. Consultation with a mental health agency is highly recommended before discharging the client from the hospital.

Detoxification or withdrawal is difficult for the narcotic abuser; relapses occur frequently. Detoxification can be done on an outpatient or an inpatient basis. Methadone is most often used to complete withdrawal, because it is the only opioid permitted by federal regulation. Clients will have to expect some discomfort: the purpose of using methadone is not to suppress withdrawal but to make withdrawal tolerable. It is not uncommon for the client to use manipulative behavior during the withdrawal period. The initial dose of methadone is 10–20 mg by mouth, which can be repeated in two hours if signs of withdrawal continue. Usually the stabilizing dose does not require more than 40 mg of methadone in 24 hours. Withdrawal may take three to six weeks (Greenbaum, 1983; Judson, Carbary, and Carbary, 1981; Quinones et al., 1979).

Following detoxification, the addict may be maintained on methadone or may participate in a therapeutic community. These two forms of treatment, which came about in the 1960s, currently are the primary methods of rehabilitating the narcotic abuser (Schnoll, 1983). The theory underlying methadone maintenance is to eliminate the drug-seeking behavior preoccupying the client, thereby allowing the client more energy for rehabilitation and useful productivity. Government regulations specify 21 days as the time allowed for maintenance on methadone, but programs vary in respect to long-term goals and dosages for clients.

Residential drug-free programs are available for those who need intensive intervention. Clients enter these programs for anywhere from 6 to 24 months. The therapeutic milieu is family-like, and each person assumes the responsibility for his or her personal behavior as well as the responsibility for the entire family group.

Treatment for Users of PCP or Similar Drugs PCP is a dangerous drug since overdose of PCP can be life threatening. Treatment goals include life-support measures, isolation, and detoxification. Respiratory depression is the most severe effect of PCP overdose. The airway must remain patent, and suctioning may be needed to prevent aspiration. Respiratory assistance may be required to maintain adequate ventilation. Seizures may occur and are treated with intravenous diazepam.

Isolation of the PCP client is necessary to reduce sensory stimulation. Ideally, one person should stay with the client in a quiet room with dim lighting. If the client is too agitated and there is a possibility of violence, it may be necessary to place secure restraints on the client to avoid injury to the client. To keep the client manageable, tranquilizing agents such as haloperidol may be used.

Detoxification is accomplished by gastric lavage. Urine is acidified by ammonium chloride. Acidification of the urine continues for 10 to 14 days to eliminate any remaining PCP. Occasionally, ascorbic acid and cranberry juice are given to accomplish this acidification of urine.

Psychosis can result from withdrawal of PCP. This may occur from a few days to a few weeks after abstinence. Depression, suicidal impulses, and violence to others are common. Psychiatric inpatient care is generally indicated (Greenbaum, 1983). (See Chapter 14 for a discussion of the treatment for psychosis.)

Treatment for Users of Sedatives, Hypnotics, or Anxiolytics Hypnotics produce tolerance necessitating detoxification or withdrawal as the primary modality.

Sources (Grinspoon and Bakalara, 1985; Schnoll, 1983) emphasize that the barbiturate abuser needs to go through withdrawal in the hospital to prevent death by accidental overdose. Pentobarbital is the drug of choice for completing barbiturate withdrawal. Since barbiturate users often are unreliable about giving an accurate account of the amount of drug used daily, an intoxicating dose must be determined. To do this, 200 mg of pentobarbital is given by mouth on an empty stomach. An additional 100 mg is given every hour until the client is intoxicated. Some users require up to 2.5 gms in a 24-hour period. Users taking 800 mg or more of the barbiturate daily are candidates for a psychosis resembling alcoholic delerium tremens. Symptoms of psychosis generally begin between the third and eighth day after abstinence and may last as long as two weeks.

Once the intoxicating dose is established, withdrawal is started. The client should be stabilized on the intoxicating dose for one to two days; then the dosage is gradually reduced by 10 percent each day. This treatment is somewhat like substituting methadone for heroin. After detoxification is complete

(10 days to 2 weeks), follow-up treatment is necessary. Common modalities are outpatient therapy and other community resources.

The other major treatment modality associated with barbiturates is treatment for overdose. Six percent of all suicides are a result of barbiturate overdose. The goals of treatment for barbiturate overdose are to support vital organ function, to prevent further absorption of the drug, and to promote drug elimination (Gary and Trenznewsky, 1983).

Withdrawal from these CNS depressants necessitates detoxification in the acute care setting. The withdrawal from these drugs is more serious and life threatening than the withdrawal from heroin. Because of the long half-life of these medications, withdrawal symptoms may not occur until 7 to 10 days after the last dose. The goal of treatment is to prevent seizures and minimize discomfort. Withdrawal is accomplished either by gradually decreasing doses of the drug or a substitute for it. Most typically, pentobarbital or Valium are the drugs of choice. Withdrawal from CNS depressants causes a rebound CNS hyperexcitability resulting in anxiety, elevated vital signs, psychosis, and a decreased seizure threshold. Since these drugs affect the hypothalamus, withdrawal may cause the body's temperature control mechanism to become dysfunctional. A temperature rise to 102°F is considered a medical emergency; an uncontrolled high fever can result in death (Bluhm, 1987; Sullivan, Bissell, and Williams, 1988).

The other major treatment modality associated with CNS depressants is treatment for overdose. Valium overdose is the second leading cause of drug-related emergency department admissions in the United States. It is especially life-threatening when combined with other CNS depressants. The goals of treatment for overdose are the support of vital organ function, the prevention of further absorption of the drug, and the promotion of drug elimination (Bluhm, 1987).

To meet the treatment goals, priority goes to maintaining an adequate airway and ventilation, and supporting the cardiovascular system. Once this has been done, gastric lavage is performed to empty the stomach. Oral activated charcoal may also be administered to absorb the drug. Drug elimination may be accomplished by hemoperfusion and dialysis. Nursing care should be provided in the intensive care unit until the client is out of danger. Referral to mental health services should be initiated while the client is hospitalized.

Other Clinical Phenomena Associated with Drug Use

Caffeine and Tobacco Use

Caffeine and tobacco are considered nondrugs by the general population but are included in DSM-III-R. The major conditions related to the use of caffeine and tobacco are caffeine intoxication, tobacco withdrawal, and tobacco dependence. These conditions will be briefly discussed because so many mental health clients exhibit one or more of these patterns along with their primary disorders.

Caffeine intoxication is considered commonplace. Caffeine acts as a CNS stimulant. Although the exact incidence of caffeine intoxication is unknown, it is estimated that more than 60 percent of all Americans over 10 years of age have used caffeine in some form. The average amount of caffeine in a cup of brewed coffee is 100 to 150 mg. Roughly one third of all Americans consume more than 500 mg of caffeine a day, but daily doses of 250 mg are considered large. In hospitalized psychiatric patients, more than 20 percent report consuming in excess of 750 mg of caffeine a day from various sources (Doyle, Quinones, and Lauria, 1982).

Clinical manifestations of caffeine intoxication include diuresis, restlessness, tremulousness, hyperactivity, irritability, dry mouth, sensory disturbances, hyperesthesia, ringing in the ears, ocular dyskinesias, flashes of light, headache, tachycardia, diarrhea, lethargy, epigastric pain, and insomnia. Other reported manifestations include accentuation of stress, exacerbation of psychosis, interactions with drugs like lithium, interference with laboratory tests, and interactions with psychotropic drugs.

Withdrawal symptoms may occur after three hours in high-caffeine consumers. Abstinence can produce anxiety and muscle tension, but headache is the most common symptom in withdrawal. Other reported withdrawal symptoms are drowsiness, lethargy, rhinorrhea, irritability, nervousness, a vague feeling of depression, and nausea.

Treatment of caffeinism consists primarily of discontinuing the use of caffeine. Client compliance is a problem because most clients view their symptoms skeptically. No long-term data are available on the effects of abstinence on behavior.

Tobacco use is widespread in the United States; approximately 50 million Americans smoke. Although the number of adult smokers continues to decrease, more than 29 percent of American men and nearly 28 percent of American women smoke.

Tobacco use has been considered a psychosocial coping mechanism. The nicotine in tobacco has multiple pharmacologic effects, but primarily acts as a ganglionic stimulant.

Tobacco dependence is characterized by mild anxiety; subtle guilt or shame; possible development of a secretive pattern of tobacco use; or an angry, defensive style supporting continued use of the substance.

The symptoms of tobacco withdrawal include irritability, restlessness, dullness, sleep disruptions, gastrointestinal disturbances, headache, impaired concentration and memory, anxiety, and increased appetite.

Recently, clinics have been developed to aid smokers in breaking their habit. Clinics vary in their approach. Some use contracts, some use behavior modification, and some use relaxation techniques (Doyle, Quinones, and Lauria, 1982; Hahn, Barkin, and Klarmen Oestreich, 1982).

Intravenous Drug Use and AIDS

In the United States in 1988, 30 percent of those with Acquired Immune Deficiency Syndrome (AIDS) were intravenous drug abusers. Estimates place the number of intravenous drug users in the United States at over one million people. In some major cities it is estimated that between 50 and 80 percent of the heroin users are seropositive for HIV. This creates a special problem for the mental health nurse working with these clients. Unless the clients present themselves for treatment, they are likely to become statistics. Once the client comes in for treatment, the nurse must teach him or her about changing sexual and needle-sharing practices (Bateson and Goldsby, 1988; Schleifer et al. 1990; Morbidity and Mortality Weekly Report. June 2, 1989). Chapter 17 discusses the care of clients with AIDS.

Assessment

The foundation of the nursing process with the drug abuse client, as with the alcoholic client, is data collection. Although the client remains the primary source of data, it may be necessary to validate the client's reports because the client is likely to understate the type, amount, and number of drugs used. Other data sources include the client's family or significant others, medical records, social records, diagnostic test results, nursing records, and legal records. When the general nursing history reveals drug use, a focused nursing assessment and physical assessment should be completed. These will identify the drug abuser's health status and nursing diagnoses related to these alterations.

Nursing History

The general nursing history should contain simple questions such as "What medications do you take on a regular basis?" The nurse needs to use sensitivity in pursuing questions related to drug use. Less intrusive questions such as "Do you smoke cigarettes?" or "Do you use other forms of tobacco?" should precede questions on other drugs. Questions related to the use of prescription drugs should follow. The nurse needs also to ask questions about the client's use of alcoholic beverages. Then the nurse can proceed to ask questions about past and present use of illicit drugs. Because marijuana use is considered socially acceptable, asking about its use is likely to lead to more honest responses about other drugs. Positive responses to these initial questions indicate the nurse may need to do a more in-depth history on specific patterns of drug use.

As with other history-taking interviews, the nurse needs to plan a sufficient amount of time to complete an extensive drug use history. The focused nursing assessment that follows may be used in a single sitting or on separate occasions. The assessment begins with substance use history. These questions provide essential data for determining whether a withdrawal reaction can be expected. The assessment continues with questions related to the extent of drug use, treatment history, and expectations for future use. The assessment ends with questions about the psychosocial ramifications of drug use.

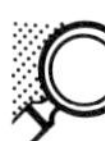

FOCUSED NURSING ASSESSMENT *for Substance Abuse Clients*

Behavioral assessment

Describe any physical conditions requiring physician-prescribed medications.
What is the name(s) of the condition(s)?
What medications are prescribed?
How long have you taken these medications?
Do the medications help your medical problem?
Do you take other drugs not prescribed by your physician?
If so, which of the following drugs have you taken (circle yes or no)?

- Marijuana yes no
- Tranquilizers (specific drug) yes no
- Barbiturates (specific drug) yes no
- Other sedatives/hypnotics (specific drug) yes no
- Cocaine yes no
- Amphetamines (specific drug) yes no
- Hallucinogens (specific drug) yes no
- Syrups with codeine yes no
- Heroin yes no
- Morphine yes no
- Other opiates/synthetics (specific drug) yes no
- Nonprescription methadone yes no
- Other over-the-counter drugs (eg, cough syrup) (specific drug) yes no

How frequently do you use these drugs? What is your usual dose? How do you administer these drugs?

Drug	Frequency	Dose	Method of use
Marijuana			oral smoking inhalation
Tranquilizers specific drug:			oral IM IV
Barbiturates specific drug:			oral IM IV
Other sedatives/ hypnotics specific drug:			oral IM IV
Cocaine			oral IM IV inhalation
Amphetamines			oral subQ IV
Hallucinogens specific drug:			oral IV inhalation
Opiates specific drug:			oral smoked "skin popped" inhalation IM IV

When was the last time you took any of these drugs?
How old were you when you started taking these drugs?
How do these drugs help you?
What happens to you when you stop taking these non-prescription drugs?
Do these drugs have any effects you do not want while under their influence?
Have you ever attempted to harm yourself while under the influence of these drugs? Following the use of these drugs?

Have you ever been injured because of taking drugs?
Have you ever overdosed on any of these drugs?
Have you ever missed work because of drug use?
How do you procure your drugs:
From different physicians? yes no
From street sources? yes no
Have you ever received treatment for using drugs? If so, what kind?
Have you had any periods during the time you have taken drugs that you have been drug-free? How long do the drug-free periods last?
Are you currently receiving treatment for using drugs?
If so, do you feel treatment is helpful? yes no
If no, describe how the treatment could be improved.
Do you plan to continue using drugs?
When do you envision you will stop taking drugs?
Do you want to stop taking drugs? What goals do you have to accomplish this?
What would your life be like without drugs?

Affective assessment
At what times do you feel most anxious?
In what way does your drug use decrease your anxiety?
When do you feel most bored or depressed?
In what way does your drug use decrease your boredom or depression?
What kinds of comments have others made to you about your rapid mood swings?
Under what circumstances do you experience guilt and shame?
What drug-abusing behavior has led you to feel embarrassed and humiliated?
Under what circumstances do you feel suspicious of others?
How often have you experienced panic attacks?

Cognitive assessment
Do you believe you have a chemical dependence that is out of your control?
What reasons do you give others for explaining your use of drugs?
Have you ever had blackouts following use of drugs?
Poor memory: yes no
Short attention span: yes no
Lack of concentration: yes no
Problems following directions: yes no
Difficulty making decisions: yes no
Suicidal thoughts: yes no
Hallucinations: yes no

Sociocultural assessment
Who do you consider the most significant person in your life?
Can you confide in this person?
Does anyone in your family have a drug problem?
Who knows about your drug use? Wife/husband? Significant other? Family members? Friends?
Do you try to conceal your drug-taking activities from your family?
How has your sexual behavior changed with your drug use?

Physical Assessment

Physical assessment for the drug abuse client is aimed at identifying impending drug withdrawal, the extent of CNS depression, adverse drug reactions, and physical complications. Data gathered from the focused nursing assessment guide the nurse in assessing the physical health of the drug abuser.

Vital signs should be taken. Common in withdrawal from heroin are elevation in pulse, respiration, temperature, and blood pressure. Bradycardia is common with use of codeine, narcotics, and sedatives/hypnotics. Tachycardia may be present in use of amphetamines, caffeine, cocaine, methaqualone, and PCP. Hypertension may occur with the use of amphetamines, PCP, and caffeine, whereas hypotension may be a result of using barbiturates, methaqualone, chloral hydrate, LSD, meprobamate, and narcotics.

The head and scalp should be inspected and palpated for evidence of traumatic injury. Accidental falls while intoxicated may leave the drug abuser with facial and scalp lacerations or fractures. Pupil shape, equality, and reactivity to light should be evaluated. Miosis (pinpoint pupils) is present with the use of barbiturates, caffeine, chloral hydrate, codeine, heroin, and morphine. Mydriasis (enlarged pupils) is present with amphetamines, cocaine, and hallucinogens.

The nasal mucosa should be inspected for irritation. A perforated septum is common in cocaine abusers who snort the drug. Runny nose may be indicative of cocaine use or opiate withdrawal, and dry mucous membranes are most common with heroin and morphine use. Malnutrition and poor oral hygiene may contribute to inflammation, color change, and bleeding in the mouth and around the teeth.

The chest should be examined next. This is a good time to thoroughly inspect the skin, which should be observed for color, texture, moisture, turgor, and edema. Sweating may be an indicator of impending drug withdrawal. Skin is sometimes flushed with the use of amphetamines, codeine, and morphine. Pallor is often noted in abusers of barbiturates, cocaine, and heroin. Cyanosis is sometimes noted following the use of barbiturates, especially in barbiturate overdose. Jaundice is often present when chloral hydrate is abused. Bullae are sometimes present in barbiturate abusers. Cocaine abusers may have skin burns, irritation, and corrosive ulcers. Dermatitis may be present in abusers of amphetamines, chloral hydrate, cocaine, and morphine. Hirsutism is occasionally noted in abusers of barbiturates. The most common skin abnormality noted in intravenous drug abusers is tracks or needle marks.

Respiratory status is reviewed when examining the chest. Depressed respirations are often indicative of drug overdose. Rapid respirations frequently accompany drug withdrawal. Respiratory paralysis can occur in overdoses of barbiturates, opiates, and PCP.

The abdomen should be examined for presence and nature of bowel sounds. Distribution of body weight should be noted. Anorexia and weight loss often accompany the abuse of amphetamines, cocaine, and morphine. Dysphagia is common in abusers of cocaine. Thirst is an indicator of chloral hydrate and morphine abuse. Salivation occurs with cocaine and morphine abuse. Nausea and vomiting accompany the abuse of caffeine, cocaine, codeine, LSD, marijuana, and opiates. Diarrhea occurs with abuse of chloral hydrate and cocaine. Morphine abuse can lead to bloody stools. Constipation accompanies the abuse of barbiturates, codeine, and morphine. Gastroenteritis can occur with the abuse of chloral hydrate, codeine, and sedative/hypnotics.

The assessment of the CNS of the drug user is comprehensive, since virtually all abused substances exert their effects on this system. Headaches accompany the abuse of barbiturates, caffeine, cocaine, and morphine. Muscle weakness or paralysis may occur in abuse of hallucinogens, morphine, and PCP. Muscle spasms may occur with the abuse of cocaine, and methaqualone. Ataxia and incoordination occur in abusers of barbiturates, cocaine, hallucinogens, opiates, and PCP.

Abuse of barbiturates, cocaine, and PCP can cause anesthesis. Paresthesia occurs in the abuse of barbiturates, hallucinogens, and morphine. Hallucinations are common in the abuse of amphetamines, barbiturates, caffeine, cocaine, LSD, morphine, and PCP.

More severe CNS problems such as seizures can result from the abuse of amphetamines, barbiturates, caffeine, cocaine, meprobamate, methaqualone, opiates, and PCP. Tetanic rigidity may result from abuse of caffeine, methaqualone, morphine, and PCP. The most severe CNS problem—coma—can occur with abuse of amphetamines, barbiturates, chloral hydrate, diazepam, meprobamate, methaqualone, narcotics, PCP, and sedatives/hypnotics (Burkhalter, 1975; Hahn, Barkin, and Klarmen Oestreich, 1982; Schultz and Dark, 1982).

Once the nurse has completed the client's history and physical assessment, the information is appraised and ready for synthesis and analysis. To accomplish this, the nurse compares the knowledge gathered about the client with the general knowledge base about drug abuse. Any gaps in the data base and patterns are identified. Then standards related to drug abuse are compared to the information gathered about the client to identify the client's strengths and health concerns.

Table 13–5 is a guideline for completing the physical assessments.

Nursing Diagnosis and Planning

Almost all the nursing diagnoses on the accepted list of nursing diagnoses can be related to the health concerns of the drug abuser. In turn, these nursing diagnoses guide the nurse in planning interven-

Table 13–5 *Physical Assessment Tool for Substance Abuse Clients*

What physical symptoms do you experience when you stop taking the drug (circle yes or no):

- Restlessness yes no
- Runny nose yes no
- Tearing yes no
- Sweating yes no
- General anxiety yes no
- Muscle weakness yes no
- Anorexia yes no
- Nausea and vomiting yes no
- Psychomotor hyperactivity yes no
- Disorientation yes no
- Confusion yes no
- Tremors yes no
- Seizures yes no

Do you have skin problems related to drug use?
Do you have frequent respiratory problems? Pneumonia?
Do you have frequent irritation in your throat and mouth?
Do you experience any tingling, pain, or numbness in your extremities?
Have you had problems sleeping?
Are you allergic to any drugs? If so, which drugs?

tions for the care of drug abuse clients. Since drug abuse is so complex and dependent on individual client responses, nursing diagnoses for drug abuse clients have been grouped into those related to intoxication/withdrawal and those related to overdose. (See Table 13–6 for a list of nursing diagnoses for the substance abuse client.)

As soon as nursing diagnoses for the specific client have been identified, the nurse begins to plan the care for the client. From the list of diagnoses generated, the nurse needs to determine the priority of the client's needs; Maslow's hierarchy of needs is often applied to the drug abuse client.

The nurse, in cooperation with the client, will establish goals related to the client's identified nursing diagnoses. This is an extremely important aspect of the plan because the drug abuser is prone to relapses of drug use and has difficulty remaining in treatment.

Once mutually acceptable nurse-client goals have been established, the nurse is able to select interventions that will assist the client in meeting those goals.

Care for Acute Drug Intoxication/Withdrawal

Drug intoxication may or may not require medical attention; that is, since the drug abuser is using a drug to create intoxication, the pleasure derived from intoxication is a primary motivator for drug-taking behavior. When behavior gets out of control and personal difficulties arise from a drug-induced intoxication, the nurse is most likely to see the client in a health care setting. Nurses must plan care for drug abusers in a variety of settings: the emergency room, detoxification unit, and general nursing units.

Drug intoxication affects individual clients differently. If the drug taken is not known to the treatment team, it is necessary to complete a blood and urine screen to identify the drug. Once the drug has been identified, the nurse needs to be concerned about the type of withdrawal reaction the client may experience. Finally, the nurse determines whether the intoxication is so severe that overdose is a possibility.

General considerations for nursing care during acute drug intoxication/withdrawal include

- Determination of the substance causing intoxication
- Identifying the type of withdrawal reaction the client may experience
- Determining whether an overdose from the drug may occur
- Maintaining a nonjudgmental attitude toward the client
- Screening visitors from the client's peer group to prevent smuggling in of more drugs

The nurse needs to maintain a nonjudgmental attitude because clients are sensitive to the attitudes and biases of those caring for them. Visitors should be limited, especially if they are from the abuser's drug-using peer group, because they may try to give

Table 13–6 *Nursing Diagnoses for the Client Who Abuses Drugs*

Intoxication/Withdrawal	*Overdose*
Anxiety, potential for	Airway clearance, ineffective
Communication, impaired: verbal	Bowel elimination, alteration in: incontinence
Coping, ineffective family: compromised	Breathing pattern, ineffective
Coping, ineffective individual	Gas exchange, impaired
Family process, alteration in	Impaired swallowing, potential for
Fear, potential for	Injury, potential for: trauma
Health maintenance, alteration in	Self-care deficit: feeding, bathing/hygiene, dressing/grooming, toileting
Infection, potential for	Skin integrity, impairment of: potential
Injury, potential for poisoning	Sleep pattern disturbance
Nutrition, alteration in: less than body requirements	Urinary elimination, alteration in patterns of
Powerlessness	
Self-concept, disturbance in: body image, self-esteem, role performance, personal identity	
Sensory-perceptual alteration: visual, auditory, kinesthetic, gustatory, tactile, olfactory	
Sexual dysfunction, potential for	
Impaired social interaction	
Thought processes, alteration in	
Violence, potential for: self-directed or directed at others	

the client drugs. (See Table 13–7 for the nursing care plan for the client with acute drug intoxication/withdrawal.)

Care for Drug Overdose

Drug overdose is an acute medical emergency. If not treated promptly, death can result. The primary concern in drug overdose is maintaining a patent airway because respiratory depression is frequent. It is also important to assess the client's level of consciousness. (See Table 13–8 for a list of levels of consciousness.)

General considerations for nursing care during drug overdose follow.

- Recognize that drug overdose is a life-threatening emergency.
- Maintain a patent airway because respiratory depression is common.
- Assess the client's level of consciousness.
- Maintain a quiet, calm environment with constant attendance by the nurse.
- Monitor the client's vital signs at least every 15 minutes.
- Maintain the client's hydration and monitor fluid intake and output.
- Once the critical period is overcome, recommend detoxification and rehabilitation.

Table 13–7 Nursing Care Plan for the Client with Acute Drug Intoxication/Withdrawal

Nursing Diagnosis: Potential for anxiety related to distress caused by physical symptoms of withdrawal.
Goal: During the withdrawal period client will recognize that anxiety may be increased. During the withdrawal period client will be able to cope with increased anxiety.

Intervention	*Rationale*	*Expected Outcome*
Assess level of anxiety: • mild • moderate • severe • panic	Will assist in determining the interventions necessary to reduce anxiety	Reduced anxiety Decreased psychomotor agitation Demonstration of coping strategies Verbalizes insight into causes for anxiety
Extreme anxiety: • provide comfort measures (eg, warm bath, calm environment) • use short, simple phrases with a firm, calm voice	Will reduce anxiety by providing a calming effect Reciprocal anxiety increases client's anxious feelings	
Mild to moderate anxiety: • encourage client to state when anxiety is present • encourage client to verbalize and explore apprehensions • involve client in diversional or leisure activity as tolerated (eg, simple concrete tasks, walks)	Client's early recognition will prevent anxiety escalation Client's involvement in problem solving assists in developing new coping strategies Teaching new coping strategies will assist client in learning to cope with anxiety	

Nursing Diagnosis: Impaired verbal communication related to physical condition resulting from drug intoxication.
Goal: During the withdrawal period client will demonstrate increased verbal communication.

Intervention	*Rationale*	*Expected Outcome*
Complete treatments necessary to reduce drug intoxication	Will decrease physical limitations and restore client's ability to verbally communicate	Client relates messages in an understandable manner
Reduce environmental stimuli and maintain a calm, accepting atmosphere	Distractions impair client's attempts to communicate	Congruence in verbal and nonverbal communication
Assist client in modifying verbal skills (eg, use of gestures)	Will increase understanding of client's concerns	Expresses feelings in an appropriate manner
Encourage client to verbalize perceptions	Will assist in increasing client's awareness and ability to communicate with others	
Use clear, concise statements	Client's cognitive abilities may be impaired	Client gives appropriate responses
Use therapeutic techniques of communication: • reflection • focusing • validation • clarification • open-ended questions • stating observations • exploring • confrontation • summarizing	Will assist in clarifying client responses	

(Diagnosis continued)

Table 13–7 *(continued)*

Intervention	*Rationale*	*Expected Outcome*
Use active listening skills	Will assist in identifying appropriate therapeutic communication strategies	Client attempts to communicate needs to nurse
Avoid use of street-drug jargon	Avoids reinforcement of ties to the drug culture	Client uses appropriate terminology

Nursing Diagnosis: Ineffective family coping: compromised related to drug-oriented lifestyle.
Goal: Client will recognize and state the effects of drug use on family relationships.

Intervention	*Rationale*	*Expected Outcome*
Initiate a one-to-one relationship with client	Will serve as a foundation in assisting client to build appropriate relationships	Client relates effectively with family members
Encourage client to explore the family's value orientation	Identifying value discrepancies will assist client toward understanding family relationships	Client seeks help from family members to decrease drug use
Encourage client to discuss role relations and expectations within family		
Encourage client to develop a family support system	Will assist in developing effective family communication	

Nursing Diagnosis: Ineffective individual coping related to maladaptive drug-oriented lifestyle.
Goal: Client will state plans for new coping strategies to replace the use of drugs before discharge.

Intervention	*Rationale*	*Expected Outcome*
Initiate a one-to-one relationship with client	Will provide a foundation for developing new coping strategies	Client abstains from drug use one day at a time
Client teaching on effects of drug(s) abused	Client knowledge and understanding assists in abstaining from further use of drugs	Demonstration of new coping strategies
Client teaching on: • problem-solving skills • decision-making skills • communication skills • relaxation skills	Will assist client in identifying new coping strategies	
Assist client in identifying behaviors in need of change and potential coping behaviors necessary to complete change		
Confront denial and other defense mechanisms	Will assist client in recognizing emotional reactions	
Restrict visitors if necessary	Assists client in avoiding the temptation of using drugs that may be smuggled in	

(continued)

Table 13–7 *(continued)*

Nursing Diagnosis: Alteration in family process related to social deviance of drug-using member.
Goal: Before discharge client will explore ways of reducing alterations in family process.

Intervention	*Rationale*	*Expected Outcome*
Assess family structure	Understanding family role relationships will assist in identifying reasons for client's drug abuse	Roles are adapted to meet all family members' needs
Encourage client to verbalize perceptions of family functions	Will assist in assessing the interdependence of family members	Demonstration of mutual support within family structure
Teach client about: • coping skills • communication techniques	Will assist client to relate more effectively within family unit	Discussions and negotiations about new role relationships
Encourage client to identify stressors within the family		

Nursing Diagnosis: Potential fear related to disruptions in perception caused by drug intoxication.
Goal: During the course of drug withdrawal client will verbalize reduced or no fear.

Intervention	*Rationale*	*Expected Outcome*
Observe client for signs of fear: • pupil dilation • panic • increased agitation • increased pulse, respirations, blood pressure • diaphoresis	Early recognition of a fear reaction will assist in reducing the reaction	Absence of fear Reduction of fear
Assist client in identifying the source of fear	Will promote client comfort	Client will verbalize fear/source of fear
Maintain a quiet, calm environment and use a calm, firm voice		
Explain all procedures	Client understanding of situation will reduce fear	

Nursing Diagnosis: Alteration in health maintenance related to maladaptive lifestyle.
Goal: Client will assume responsibility for health maintenance on discharge from treatment for withdrawal.

Intervention	*Rationale*	*Expected Outcome*
Assess health maintenance skills	Will guide in planning for health teaching	Attempts to maintain health
Teach client about health maintenance	Client's knowledge and understanding will assist in altering poor health practices	Controls drug use behavior
Assist client in identifying health maintenance goals	Client involvement in goal setting will increase compliance	Uses health maintenance resources
Make referrals to health care and community agencies as necessary	Use of support systems will assist in restructuring client health practices	

(continued)

Table 13–7 *(continued)*

Nursing Diagnosis: Potential for infection related to use of contaminated drug paraphernalia.
Goal: Client will alter lifestyle to reduce risk factors.

Intervention	*Rationale*	*Expected Outcome*
Assess risk factors (eg, IV drug use techniques, malnutrition, drug impurities)	Knowledge of risk factors assists in planning care	Verbalizes risk factors connected to current lifestyle
Provide information about risk factors	Client's understanding of risk factors can promote behavior change	
Provide positive reinforcement when client attempts to change behavior	Increases the potential of the client continuing the new behavior	Attempts to make changes in current lifestyle
Review laboratory studies (eg, UA, CBC, chem panel, VDRL, HIV)	Assists in identifying possible causative agents related to infection	Normal laboratory results
Monitor vital signs	Elevated temperature is often first indicator of infection	Vital signs within normal limits

Nursing Diagnosis: Potential for injury: poisoning related to unknown substances in street drugs.
Goal: During the course of treatment client will state toxic effects of drugs prepared by unknown sources.

Intervention	*Rationale*	*Expected Outcome*
Provide health teaching materials on specific drugs used by client	Knowledge will increase client's understanding of problem	Verbalizes lethal doses of abused drugs

Nursing Diagnosis: Alteration in nutrition: less than body requirements related to side effects of abused drugs.
Goal: Client will plan a balanced diet for use after discharge.

Intervention	*Rationale*	*Expected Outcome*
Assess client's nutrition patterns	Will assist in identifying nutrition deficits	Controls drug intake
Frequently give foods high in calories, protein, and vitamins; teach client to choose these foods; make snacks readily available	Small meals may be more attractive than large meals and encourage client to eat proper nutrients	Eats regular, balanced meals Verbalizes understanding of essential nutrients
Counsel client to discontinue using drugs	Will increase intake of nutrients Persistent use of drugs decreases client's interest in food and decreases appetite	Gains weight

Nursing Diagnosis: Powerlessness related to dependence on drugs and resulting in lack of self-control.
Goal: Client will admit powerlessness over control of drug habit.

Intervention	*Rationale*	*Expected Outcome*
Assist client in recognizing the drug problem	Assists client in avoiding the common problem of denial	Verbalizes dependency on drugs
Assist the client in identifying ways drug problem is interfering with life	Enables client to confront drug dependency's effect on ADLs and goals	Verbalizes how drugs control life

(Diagnosis continued)

Table 13–7 *(continued)*

Nursing Diagnosis *(continued)*: Powerlessness related to dependence on drugs and resulting in lack of self-control.
Goal: Client will admit powerlessness over control of drug habit.

Intervention	*Rationale*	*Expected Outcome*
Teach alternate coping mechanisms, (eg, adequate diet, rest, exercise, biofeedback)	Will assist in returning feelings of power and self-control to the client	Engages in new coping behaviors
Encourage client to participate in treatment	Participation in treatment is necessary to overcome the use of drugs	

Nursing Diagnosis: Disturbance in self-concept: body image, self-esteem, role performance, personal identity related to lack of direction in life and disrupted lifestyle caused by drug use.
Goal: Before discharge client will state the role of drugs in personal identity.

Intervention	*Rationale*	*Expected Outcome*
Initiate a one-to-one relationship with client	Will assist client in relating concerns to a caring person	Client states realistic body image
Teach client about: • methods of improving body image • new roles without drugs • problem solving • normal developmental crises	Knowledge and understanding will assist client in developing a more positive self-concept	Maintains a constructive level of self-esteem Develops new roles free of drug use
Assist client in improving personal appearance	Will increase client's self-esteem	Expresses satisfaction with identity
Encourage client to verbalize concerns and anxieties related to personal identity	Will assist client in subjectively defining personality manifestations	
Encourage client participation in daily activities	Will increase client's feelings of acceptance and self-worth	
Assist client in defining new roles: • role clarification • role playing • role rehearsal	Will assist in client acceptance of new roles	

Nursing Diagnosis: Potential alteration in senses and perception: visual, auditory, kinesthetic, gustatory, tactile, olfactory related to decreased problem-solving abilities induced by drug intake.
Goal: By the end of the withdrawal period client will be in contact with reality and will respond appropriately to environmental stimuli.

Intervention	*Rationale*	*Expected Outcome*
Assess stimuli in environment that may alter sensory-perceptual function	Excessive stimuli intensify sensory-perceptual alterations	Reduction and/or elimination of distracting environmental stimuli
Orient client to reality by: • calling client by name • giving client correct time • giving information about surroundings • maintaining eye contact with client • identifying self • reinforcing reality-oriented behaviors	Assists client in maintaining contact with reality	No loss of contact with reality No hallucinations, delusions, and/or illusions

(Diagnosis continued)

Table 13–7 *(continued)*

Intervention	*Rationale*	*Expected Outcome*
Make environment meaningful for client: • provide a clock • provide a calendar • wear a name tag • explain all procedures • clarify client misperceptions	Assists client in maintaining contact with reality	
Use safety precautions: • bed rails up • bed in low position • call light in client's reach • sharp objects out of client's reach	Will prevent accidental injury when client is confused	
Maintain a pleasant environment: • control noise • reduce unnecessary personnel and traffic • explain sights, sounds, and smells in the environment	Will promote client comfort	

Nursing Diagnosis: Potential sexual dysfunction related to disruption of sexual response from excessive drug use.
Goal: Following a counseling session client will recognize the relationship of sexual dysfunction and drug use.

Intervention	*Rationale*	*Expected Outcome*
Explain the relationship of libido and drug use	Client knowledge and understanding will decrease anxiety about sexuality and may motivate client to stop taking drugs	Discontinues drug use Verbalizes understanding of effect of drug use on sexual function
Counsel client to discontinue and/or curtail the use of drugs	Hypothalamic nerve pathways that control the secretions of gonadotropins are inhibited by drugs acting on the CNS	

Nursing Diagnosis: Impaired social interaction related to unsuccessful social interaction behaviors while under the influence of psychoactive drugs.
Goal: Client recognizes that drug use alters social interaction behaviors.

Intervention	*Rationale*	*Expected Outcome*
Assess client's perception of social isolation	Provides nurse with information on which to base care	Client verbalizes feelings of social isolation
Spend time with the client	Indicates nurse's positive regard for the client	Client seeks interaction with nurse
Assist client in learning new social skills by role playing	Client learns new skills with less anxiety	Client participates in role playing with nurse
Encourage client to become involved in new social situations that do not involve drugs or drug-using friends	Assists the client in developing positive social behaviors	Attempts to involve self with others

(continued)

Table 13–7 *(continued)*

Nursing Diagnosis: Alteration in thought processes related to drug impairment of abstract thinking, problem solving, and decision making.
Goal: By the end of the withdrawal period client will demonstrate a constructive interpretation of reality.

Intervention	*Rationale*	*Expected Outcome*
Use active listening when client communicates	Analysis of behavior assists in representing reality to client	
Observe client's verbal and nonverbal communication		Client verbalizes realistic interpretations of reality
Maintain a nonjudgmental attitude toward client	Addicts are very sensitive to the attitudes of care givers	Constructively relates with others
Orient client to reality, if necessary: • have client state name • have client state date and time • have client state location • maintain eye contact with client • identify self	Assists in maintaining contact with reality	
Use therapeutic communication techniques: • open-ended statements • clarifying • validation • confrontation • restatement	Will assist client in clarifying reality	
Provide opportunities for client to contribute to own treatment plan	Will enhance the reality of necessary self-care	
Assist client in examining the effect of behavior on others	Will increase client's ability to relate realistically with others	
Involve client as much as possible in self-care activities	Will assist in motivating client toward self-care and increase contact with reality	

Nursing Diagnosis: Potential for violence: self-directed or directed at others related to a dysfunctional family pattern disrupted by drug abuse.
Goal: Before the end of the withdrawal period, client will identify patterns of family violence. Client will reduce attempts at self-directed violence during the course of withdrawal.

Intervention	*Rationale*	*Expected Outcome*
Encourage client to verbalize rather than act out violent feelings	Will reduce potential harm from violent behavior	Reduction in violent behavior
Use of seclusion, if necessary	Will assist client in regaining self-control	Identifies alternatives for dealing with aggression
Explain consequences of violent behavior: • calling security • use of additional staff • use of restraints	Understanding will reduce client's violent actions	Demonstrates new coping strategies for dealing with aggression

(Diagnosis continued)

Table 13–7 *(continued)*

Intervention	*Rationale*	*Expected Outcome*
Assist client and family members to identify and discuss situations that provoke violence	Will assist family to explore alternatives for dealing with violent feelings	
Refer to family counseling		
Observe and assess client for signs of self-inflicted harm	Drug-altered thoughts may cause client to attempt self-harm	No injuries observed No suicide attempts

Table 13–8 *Levels of Consciousness*

Level of Consciousness	*Client Responses*	*Assessment Strategies*
Alert	"Normal" responses. Aware of self and environment.	Ask client's name, date, time, and location in a normal voice.
Lethargic	Falls asleep when not stimulated. Carries out simple commands. May move as if intoxicated.	Ask client's name in a louder voice. Firmly ask client to perform a simple task.
Obtunded	Must be shaken or given a painful stimulus to produce a response. May make purposeful attempt to remove painful stimuli, but attempts are very slow.	Pinch skin, shake client, prick with pin.
Stuporous	No verbal response even to painful stimuli. Movement occurs as a patterned response that is not meaningful in relation to stimuli.	Pinch skin, shake client, prick with pin.
Coma	No output when maximally stimulated. No response to deep pain, reflexes (corneal, pupillary, pharyngeal, swallowing, and cough) absent. Incontinence of urine and feces.	Apply pressure to Achilles tendon, supraorbital notch, sternum, or calf muscles in legs. Check corneal, pupillary, and pharyngeal reflexes.

Because of the acute nature of the problems associated with drug overdose, the client will probably need care in ICU following emergency treatment. The client's privacy should be maintained. It is recommended that the environment be kept as calm as possible and that a nurse be in constant attendance.

The client's vital signs should be monitored at least every 15 minutes. In severe cases, it may be necessary to monitor vital signs electronically to detect any sudden changes. Because no food or fluids can be given by mouth, an IV will be necessary to maintain the client's hydration. A nasogastric tube is frequently placed for gastric lavage, and a Foley catheter will be necessary to maintain accurate urine output.

Once the client has overcome the critical period of overdose, it is important to recommend detoxification and rehabilitation. (See Table 13–9 for the nursing care plan for the client with drug overdose; and Table 13–10 for community referral resources.)

Evaluation

The nurse evaluates the care of the drug-abusing client by comparing the client's health status to the mutual goals previously agreed on. As the nursing care plan is implemented, the nurse appraises the drug abuser's response to nursing interventions.

Table 13–9 Nursing Care Plan for the Client with Drug Overdose

Nursing Diagnosis: Ineffective airway clearance related to drug-induced respiratory depression.
Goal: Client will maintain a patent airway for the course of treatment.

Intervention	*Rationale*	*Expected Outcome*
Auscultate lungs	Will assist in assessing breath sounds	Airway remains patent
Tilt head back	Will prevent tongue from obstructing airway	Adequate ventilation
Suction secretions as necessary	Excess mucus and secretions block air passageway	Evidence of physical and psychologic comfort
Have setup prepared for possibility of endotrachial tube insertion	Endotrachial tubes maintain an open airway	
Provide mechanical breathing assistance if indicated	Mechanical assistance is required when respirations are severely depressed	
Administer oxygen if ordered	Will assist in maintaining adequate ventilation	
Provide oral care as needed	Will keep client comfortable	

Nursing Diagnosis: Alteration in bowel elimination: incontinence related to involuntary passage of stool.
Goal: Client will regain bowel function after the critical period subsides.

Intervention	*Rationale*	*Expected Outcome*
Pad linen on bed	Will aid in removing fecal matter without agitating client	No skin breakdown
Provide adult diapers, if indicated	Will promote client comfort	Return of normal bowel function
Clean area after each incontinent episode	Will prevent breakdown of skin and promote client self-esteem	

Nursing Diagnosis: Ineffective breathing pattern related to drug-induced respiratory depth changes.
Goal: Client will have adequate lung expansion and ventilation.

Intervention	*Rationale*	*Expected Outcome*
Auscultate lungs	Will assist in assessing breathing patterns	Full expansion of lungs
Monitor vital signs at least every 15 minutes—noting the character of the respirations	Frequent monitoring will provide significant data regarding client's condition	Adequate ventilation indicated by no use of accessory muscles, respiratory rate within normal limits, and symmetrical chest on inspiration and expiration
Administer oxygen as needed	Will assist in maintaining adequate ventilation	
Elevate head of bed unless contraindicated (eg, spinal cord injury)	Will assist in achieving full lung expansion	
Turn frequently, at least every 2 hours		

(Diagnosis continued)

Table 13–9 *(continued)*

Intervention	*Rationale*	*Expected Outcome*
Assist with any procedures necessary to maintain adequate ventilation (eg, tracheostomy, chest tube insertion, endotrachial tube insertion)	Essures adequate intake of air	

Nursing Diagnosis: Impaired gas exchange related to drug interference with respiratory center activity.
Goal: Client will maintain adequate ventilation and physical comfort.

Intervention	*Rationale*	*Expected Outcome*
Auscultate lungs	Will assist in assessing changes in breath sounds	ABGs within normal limits: pH: 7.35–7.45 Po_2: 80–95 mm Hg Pco_2: 35–45 mm Hg O_2 saturation: 95–99% Breathing without difficulty (eg, no use of accessory muscles, even, unlabored) Respiratory rate within normal limits Other vital signs within normal limits
Monitor: • vital signs • ABGs	Adequate oxygenation is required for brain function and early indicators of hypoxia assist in maintaining adequate function	

Nursing Diagnosis: Potential for impaired swallowing related to altered level of consciousness resulting from intake of drugs.
Goal: Client will experience no episodes of aspiration.

Intervention	*Rationale*	*Expected Outcome*
Assess the client for symptoms of aspiration	Indicates whether further treatment is necessary	No evidence of aspiration
Place client on side or in prone position unless contraindicated	Prevents aspiration of stomach contents	

Nursing Diagnosis: Impaired gas exchange related to drug interference with respiratory center activity.
Goal: Client will maintain adequate ventilation and physical comfort.

Intervention	*Rationale*	*Expected Outcome*
Elevate head of bed, unless contraindicated	Will assist client in fully expanding lungs	
Turn frequently, at least every 2 hours		
Administer oxygen as necessary	Assists in maintaining adequate ventilation	
Explain care being given and what is planned	Will decrease client's anxiety level and increase psychologic comfort	

(continued)

Table 13–9 *(continued)*

Nursing Diagnosis: Potential for injury: trauma related to altered level of consciousness.
Goal: Client will survive drug overdose episode.

Intervention	*Rationale*	*Expected Outcome*
Prepare appropriate medications to combat effects of drugs (eg, Narcan)	Some medications reverse the effects of drugs and combat circulatory collapse	Stabilized condition within 24 hours following drug ingestion
Insert nasogastric tube (if lavage is indicated for specific drug ingested)	Gastric lavage aids in removing some types of ingested drugs from the system	No injuries
Assess client's level of consciousness (eg, pupil reactions, presence of reflexes, hand grips)	Will assist in identifying variables leading to increased susceptibility	
Maintain NPO status	Food and/or fluid may cause aspiration in semiconscious clients	
Administer IV fluids as ordered	Will assist in flushing drugs from circulatory system	

Nursing Diagnosis: Deficit in self-care: feeding, bathing/hygiene, dressing/grooming, toileting related to altered state of consciousness.
Goal: Client will maintain a sense of dignity and self-worth in the presence of self-care deficits.

Intervention	*Rationale*	*Expected Outcome*
Assess client's self-care capabilities	Will assist in planning nursing interventions for presenting deficits	Adequate intake and output
Provide parenteral, nasogastric, or spoon feeding as necessary	Body cells need adequate nutrition to function and to maintain normal activity	Skin intact
Provide comfort and hygiene measures	Will promote client's sense of well-being	
Tend to toileting needs	Adequate elimination is needed to maintain normal function	
Turn at least every 2 hours	Promotes adequate ventilating and prevents skin breakdown	
Administer artificial tears (or normal saline) at least every 4 hours	Prevents drying of cornea when client is unable to blink	Adequately moistened cornea

Nursing Diagnosis: Potential for impairment of skin integrity related to altered metabolic state.
Goal: During the course of treatment client will have no skin breakdown.

Intervention	*Rationale*	*Expected Outcome*
Assess skin daily	Will assist in identifying abnormalities (eg, reddened areas)	Skin warm, dry, and has adequate turgor
Change client's position at least every 2 hours, ideally every hour	Will assist in maintaining adequate circulation to the skin	Adequate circulation
Use lotion if indicated	Dry skin is more likely to break down	Skin protected
Place on air or water mattress, if available; eggcrate mattress will suffice	Will relieve pressure over bony prominences	

(continued)

Table 13–9 *(continued)*

Nursing Diagnosis: Disturbance in sleep pattern related to drug-induced lethargy.
Goal: Client's environment will be established to be conducive to sleep.

Intervention	*Rationale*	*Expected Outcome*
Monitor client's activity and level of consciousness	Assists in assessing disruptions in sleep patterns	Sleeps between procedures
Reduce environmental stimuli • reduce noise • provide a temperate climate • complete procedures at regular intervals	Noise, bright lights, and extraneous stimuli in ICU can induce a psychoticlike reaction	Sleeps uninterrupted for at least 4 hours

Nursing Diagnosis: Alteration in urinary elimination patterns related to involuntary passage of urine.
Goal: Client will return to normal urinary patterns following critical period.

Intervention	*Rationale*	*Expected Outcome*
Reduce contributing physiologic factors: • complete procedures to remove drugs • place Foley catheter as ordered	Will assist in reducing incontinence	Patterns of voiding return to normal No incontinence No skin breakdown
Monitor Foley catheter (eg, patency)	Prevents urinary retention and promotes excretion of ingested drugs	No urine odor
Monitor I & O	Assists in assessing hydration	
Change bedding and clean skin around catheter	Prevents skin breakdown	
When client indicates ability to control urine flow, clamp catheter at regular intervals	Will assist in reestablishing a normal pattern for emptying the bladder	

Table 13–10 *Referral Resources for Chemical Dependency*

Cocaine Anonymous
PO Box 1367
Culver City, CA 90232
213-559-5833

Impaired Nurse Network
Pat Green, Chairperson
1020 Sunset Drive
Lawrence, KS 66044
913-842-3893

Naranon Family Groups
PO Box 2562
Palos Verdes, CA 92704
213-547-5800

Narcotics Anonymous
PO Box 9999
Van Nuys, CA 92409
818-780-3951

National Clearinghouse for Drug Abuse Information
10A-43 Parklawn Building
5600 Fishers Lane
Rockville, MD 20857

National Nurses Society on Addictions
2506 Gross Point Road
Evanston, IL 60201
708-475-7300

Progress toward goals and discrepancies are then identified. The care plan may need to be modified.

Client progress is measured by reviewing outcomes. From nursing observations, the client's observations, and the documents in the client's record, the nurse determines whether the client's behavior or health status has changed. Client outcomes have been included in Tables 13–6 and 13–9. It should be noted that the outcomes presented in these tables are measurable and relate to specific interventions for each of the conditions. (See Table 13–11 for an example of evaluation of a client with acute drug intoxication/withdrawal, and Table 13–12 for an example of evaluation of a client with drug overdose.)

Case examples illustrating a variety of drug abusers follow.

Table 13–11 *Example of Evaluation of Nursing Care of a Client with Acute Drug Intoxication/Withdrawal*

Plan	Evaluation
1. The nurse will initiate a one-to-one relationship with the client.	On 8/16, the client requested that nurse stay with him for a few minutes.
2. Restrain client if violent behavior is demonstrated.	On 8/15, the client attempted to strike several nurses. Restraints were placed with good results. The client fell asleep.
3. The client will rest and sleep for at least 6 hours during a 24-hour period.	On 8/17, the client slept for 4 hours without interruption.

Table 13–12 *Example of Evaluation of Nursing Care of a Client with Drug Overdose*

Plan	Evaluation
1. The client will maintain a patent airway for at least 24 hours.	On 9/2, an oral airway was placed following an episode of respiratory distress.
2. The client will have no injuries for a 24-hour period.	On 9/3, client attempted to get out of bed without assistance and fell. No injuries were apparent.
3. The nurse will complete self-care requirements for the client during the period of acute illness.	On 9/3, the client received a bedbath, oral care, skin care, and Foley catheter care.

CASE EXAMPLE

A Client with Cannabis Abuse

Jason Thomas, a 15-year-old high school student, was referred to his high school counselor for failing grades. Jason told the counselor he wasn't into school and had been using marijuana daily for the past 2 years.

Nursing History

Location: Family Counseling Center
Client's name: Jason Thomas Age: 15
Admitting diagnosis: Cannabis dependence
Vital signs: Not applicable to this setting

Health history
Height: 5′7″
Weight: 140 lbs
Eats three meals a day plus snacks
Sleeps 8–12 hours a night
Smokes one pack of regular cigarettes a day and four to six marijuana cigarettes daily
Drinks beer with friends on weekends

Social history
Lives at home with a mother and stepfather
Has three other siblings at home
Has been ditching school to party with friends
Plans to drop out of school

Clinical data
Not applicable to this setting

Nursing observations
During the initial interview, Jason was indifferent to the concerns of the high school counselor who had referred him for counseling. Jason stated that he had been using marijuana daily since he was 13. Jason had kept his use of marijuana from his family and stated that "the shit hit the fan" at home when his stepfather found out he had been ditching school and smoking grass. Jason said he had no goals for treatment; in fact, he had no interest in quitting his marijuana consumption. Jason told the nurse-counselor he was coming to therapy only because his parents made him after they talked to his school counselor.

Analysis/Synthesis of Data

Concerns	*Nursing diagnoses*
Disruption in growth and development	Impaired verbal communication
Disturbance in coping mechanisms	Ineffective individual coping
Communication problems	Alteration in family process
Disturbance in thought and cognitive processes	Disturbance in self-concept: self-esteem and role performance
	Alteration in thought processes

Suggested Care Planning Activities

1. Determine the developmental aspects to be considered in the care of Jason.
2. Identify the support systems available to Jason.
3. Identify potential stumbling blocks to Jason's progress in rehabilitation.
4. Describe the client teaching necessary to assist Jason toward recovery.
5. Identify nursing goals for Jason.
6. Determine the priorities for Jason's rehabilitation.
7. List and provide a rationale for nursing interventions in the care of Jason.

CASE EXAMPLE

A Client with Cocaine Abuse

Kevin Hale, a 32-year-old executive for an engineering firm, was found unconscious in a motel room. Kevin was raced to the emergency room. When Kevin reached the ER, he was barely breathing and went into respiratory arrest shortly after arrival. Kevin was resuscitated, moved to ICU, and placed on a respirator. Lab reports showed high levels of cocaine and heroin.

Nursing History

Location: Emergency Room
Client's name: Kevin Hale Age: 32
Admitting diagnosis: Drug overdose (probably heroin and cocaine)
T=102.4(R), P=120, R=10, BP=140/80

Health history
Height: 6′0″
Weight: 190 lbs

(Note: The remainder of the history was incomplete because client was comatose.)

Clinical data
Urine screen indicated a high level of cocaine, a trace of heroin, and other unidentified substances
BS: 26

Nursing observations
Kevin was intubated and placed on a respirator. He was listed as a John Doe until he could be identified. Kevin remained unconscious on a respirator for the first 48 hours of his hospitalization, at which time he was identified and relatives were notified of his condition. Kevin's mother was able to give additional history. Kevin was recently divorced because of his problems with the use of cocaine. Kevin had been using cocaine for the past 3 years. Kevin is employed as an executive with a major engineering firm, and his mother learned of his drug use only when Kevin's wife filed for divorce. Kevin had moved home after his wife asked him to leave and filed for the divorce. Kevin's mother stated that Kevin had gone to the motel on the evening he was found with $10,000 in cash to purchase a large amount of cocaine from a dealer. Kevin's mother became concerned when he did not return home after two days and notified authorities of his disappearance. It was at this time that Mrs. Hale learned her son was possibly in the hospital. Kevin's mother was able to positively identify him in ICU and was obviously distraught during the interview with the nurse. Kevin remained in a coma on a respirator for 14 days. From interviews with other family members and the authorities, it was determined that Kevin had been a victim of foul play. He had been given an injection with a large dose of cocaine mixed with heroin, and it was suspected the dose had been cut with insulin. Kevin progressed enough on his 16th hospital day to be moved to a private room on a medical floor.

Analysis/Synthesis of Data

Concerns	*Nursing diagnoses*
Continued bowel and bladder incontinence	Alteration in urinary elimination patterns
Change in mental status	Alteration in bowel: incontinence
Unable to feed self	Deficit in self-care: feeding, bathing/hygiene, dressing/grooming, toileting
Perceptual disturbances	Potential for injury: trauma
Emotional regression	Impaired verbal communication
	Disturbance in self-concept: body image, self-esteem, role performance, personal identity
	Alteration in thought processes

Suggested Care Planning Activities

1. Determine the priorities for Mr. Hale's care.
2. Determine the developmental aspects to be considered in the care of Mr. Hale.
3. Identify the support systems available to Mr. Hale.
4. Describe the client teaching necessary to assist Mr. Hale toward recovery.
5. Describe the significance of the laboratory findings.
6. Describe the methods for obtaining data when the client is unable to give information.
7. Identify nursing goals for Mr. Hale.
8. List and provide a rationale for nursing interventions in the care of Mr. Hale.

CASE EXAMPLE

A Client with Opioid Dependence

Teresa Jones, a 21-year-old prostitute, was admitted to a medical unit for recurrent pelvic inflammatory disease (PID). Teresa readily admitted she was a prostitute and stated that prostitution was how she supported her $200-a-day heroin habit. Teresa agreed to talk to drug counselors and decided to enter the methadone treatment program on her release from the hospital.

Nursing History

Location: Methadone Treatment Program
Client's name: Teresa Jones Age: 21
Admitting diagnosis: Opioid Dependence
T=99, P=80, R=16, BP=120/60

Health history
Height: 5′8″
Weight: 120 lbs
Eats one meal and snacks each day
Sleeps 4–6 hours during the day
Smokes one or two packs cigarettes per day
Drinks one or two cocktails a day

Social history
Divorced from spouse 5 years
Lives with a pimp and three other prostitutes addicted to heroin
Seven-year-old daughter lives with client's mother, but spends several days a month with Teresa
Has been a prostitute for the past 5 years, since her divorce, to support her heroin habit

Clinical data
Positive Pap smear for gonorrhea
Positive VDRL

Nursing observations
Teresa was interviewed by a drug treatment nurse-counselor while she was hospitalized on a medical unit for treatment of PID. In the interview, Teresa told the nurse-counselor she was worried about the effects of her lifestyle on her daughter. Teresa's daughter, now 7, was beginning to pressure Teresa to live with her. Teresa is afraid her daughter will learn of her drug problem and occupation. Teresa says she understands how difficult it will be for her to kick her drug habit because she will have to completely change her life. Teresa tells the nurse-counselor she is ready to "clean up her act."

Analysis/Synthesis of Data

Concerns	*Nursing diagnoses*
Physical symptoms related to withdrawal	Anxiety
Lifestyle pattern incompatible with stated goals	Ineffective family coping: compromised
Anxiety	Ineffective individual coping
Disturbed family dynamics	Alteration in family process
	Alteration in health maintenance

Suggested Care Planning Activities

1. Determine the developmental aspects to be considered in the care of Ms. Jones.
2. Identify the support systems available to Ms. Jones.
3. Describe the client teaching necessary to assist Ms. Jones toward drug-free living.
4. Identify the priorities for Ms. Jones for the course of her rehabilitation.
5. Describe the lifestyle changes necessary for Ms. Jones to be rehabilitated.
6. Determine the priorities for Ms. Jones's rehabilitation period.
7. Identify nursing goals for Ms. Jones.
8. List and provide a rationale for nursing interventions in the care of Ms. Jones.

CASE EXAMPLE

A Client Using Phencyclidine

Kimberly Adams, a 16-year-old high school student, was admitted to a psychiatric inpatient unit. She stared lethargically into space and, at times, was unresponsive. She was also irritable and refused to eat. Kim's mother was not very cooperative with the staff. When Kim's lab results revealed PCP, Kim's mother admitted that Kim had been known to smoke marijuana cigarettes laced with PCP.

Nursing History

Location: Psychiatric Inpatient Unit
Client's name: Kimberly Adams Age: 16
Admitting diagnosis: PCP intoxication
T=101, P=130, R=30, BP=110/80

Health history (given by mother)
Height: 5′4″
Weight: 110 lbs
Eats several small snacks a day
Sleeps 8–10 hours at night

Social history (given by mother)
Lives with her mother and stepfather
Biologic father is unknown
Mother lives on public assistance
Mother has used drugs in the past

Clinical data
Urine screen positive for PCP

Nursing observations
Kim was unresponsive to the staff and her mother. She lay in her bed, lethargically staring into space. Kim became irritable when attempts were made to feed her. Kim's mother admitted to the nurse that Kim may have smoked a marijuana cigarette laced with PCP. Kim's mother was concerned that authorities would take Kim from her care because of her own drug history.

Analysis/Synthesis of Data

Concerns	*Nursing diagnoses*
Ineffective parenting	Ineffective family coping: compromised
Disturbance in normal growth and development	Alteration in family process
Possible hallucinations	Potential for injury: poisoning
Decreased nutrition	Alteration in nutrition: less than body requirements
Potential for drug overdose	Alteration in senses and per ception: visual

Suggested Care Planning Activities

1. Determine the developmental aspects to be considered in the care of Kim.
2. Identify the support systems available to Kim.
3. Describe the legal implications related to Kim's case.
4. Describe the significance of Kim's urine screen.
5. Determine the priorities for Kim's care.
6. Describe the client teaching necessary for Kim's family to assist Kim toward recovery.
7. Identify nursing goals for Kim.
8. List and provide a rationale for nursing interventions in the care of Kim.

CASE EXAMPLE

A Client with Sedative Dependence

Chris Lambert, a 40-year-old homemaker, found it more and more difficult to get through the day without her Valium. Chris's husband became alarmed when he came home and found Chris semiconscious on the livingroom sofa. Chris, it was discovered, had accidentally taken an overdose of Valium.

Nursing History

Location: Emergency Room
Client's name: Chris Lambert Age: 40
Admitting diagnosis: Drug overdose, Valium
T=97.6, P=56, R=8, BP=90/60

Health history
Height: 5′4″
Weight: 140 lbs
(Note: The remainder of the history was incomplete because Chris was comatose.)

Social history (given by husband)
A homemaker with two teenage children living at home
Has been married 20 years
Has been depressed and anxious since the death of her mother, so family physician prescribed Valium for "nerves"

Clinical data
Urine screen indicated presence of Valium

Nursing observations
Chris was intubated and had an NG tube placed. Chris received gastric lavage and was sent to ICU after care in the emergency room. Physicians referred Chris to mental health clinic before

her discharge from the hospital. Chris told the nurse-counselor she had found it more and more difficult to get through the day without the Valium her doctor had prescribed for "nerves." Chris said she didn't mean to take so many pills, but she often forgot what time she had taken her last pill. Chris said she did not think she was "hooked" on Valium.

Analysis/Synthesis of Data

Concerns	*Nursing diagnoses*
Pathologic depression	Impaired verbal communication
Potential suicide	Ineffective family coping: compromised
Disturbance in coping mechanisms	Ineffective individual coping
Disturbed family relationships	Alteration in family process
	Disturbance in self-concept: role performance
	Potential for violence: self-directed

Suggested Care Planning Activities

1. Determine the priorities for Mrs. Lambert's care.
2. Identify the support systems available to Mrs. Lambert.
3. Describe the significance of the urine screen findings.
4. Describe the significance of the admitting vital signs for Mrs. Lambert.
5. Determine the developmental aspects to be considered in the care of Mrs. Lambert.
6. Describe the client teaching necessary to assist Mrs. Lambert toward recovery.
7. Identify nursing goals for Mrs. Lambert.
8. List and provide a rationale for nursing interventions in the care of Mrs. Lambert.

SUMMARY

1. Because of the illegal and illicit nature of drug abuse, it is difficult to retrieve information on the amount of drug abuse in the United States.

2. Recreational drug use is widespread among adolescents, young adults, and others.

3. Some forms of drug use such as caffeine and tobacco are socially acceptable.

4. Accurately assessing the drug-taking habits of clients is a major responsibility of the mental health nurse.

5. Drug use is divided into two categories: psychoactive substance abuse and psychoactive substance dependence. Psychoactive substance abuse involves the use of a drug that results in adverse effects to oneself and others and psychoactive substance dependence when use of the drug is no longer under personal control and when use continues despite adverse effects.

6. Classes of drugs linked to dependence are amphetamines or similarly acting sympathomimetics; cannabis; cocaine; hallucinogens; inhalants; opioids; phencyclidine (PCP) or similarly acting arylcycloalkylamines; and sedatives, hypnotics, and anxiolytics.

Knowledge Base

7. There are biologic, physiologic, psychologic, and sociocultural considerations underlying the initiation of drug abuse and factors related to the continuation of drug dependence.

8. The treatment modality for drug abuse varies with the specific drug abused. The major treatment modalities are detoxification programs, inpatient programs, outpatient programs, residential programs, day care programs, therapeutic communities, and individual psychotherapy.

Assessment

9. Nursing assessment of the drug abuse client is developed around behavioral, affective, cognitive, physiologic, and sociocultural aspects of the knowledge base.

Nursing Diagnosis and Planning

10. Many of the accepted nursing diagnoses may be applied to the drug abuse client; however, the mental health nurse focuses on those diagnoses related to the emotional health of the client.

Evaluation

11. There are many digressions and progress often seems slow as the client attempts to change drug-seeking behaviors. The nurse develops patience and persistence when dealing with drug-abusing clients.

CHAPTER REVIEW

1. Jim has been chemically dependent on marijuana for 15 years. His wife, Mary, has never used drugs. During a family assessment the nurse has determined that Mary is a co-dependent of the *alienated* type. Which of Mary's behaviors contributes to this assessment conclusion?

(a) She has ignored Jim's drug problem, thinking it will change.

(b) She has been shielding Jim from problems related to his marijuana.

(c) She endures her pain, hoping that Jim will feel guilty and change his behavior.

(d) She constantly criticizes Jim for his use of marijuana.

2. A slang term for amphetamines is
(a) Coke
(b) Speed
(c) Angel dust
(d) Mary Jane

3. The psychoactive ingredient in cannabis that causes euphoria is
(a) Hashish
(b) Marijuana
(c) Delta-9-tetrahydrocannabinol
(d) 5-hydroxytryptamine

4. Which one of the following is an opioid?
(a) Methaqualone
(b) Phencyclidine
(c) LSD
(d) Heroin

5. The nurse caring for the client experiencing drug overdose should
(a) Place the client in Trendelenberg's position
(b) Continually assess the client's level of consciousness
(c) Restrain the client
(d) Recognize that drug overdose is a common medical problem

6. The nursing history of a cocaine abuser indicates that the client has been smoking crack daily or nearly daily over the past 6 months. The client's mother is an alcoholic, and there is a drug-abusing stepfather. Although the mother knew the client had been smoking crack, she did nothing to stop the behavior. Which of the following nursing diagnoses would be consistent with these findings?
(a) Growth and development, alteration in
(b) Communication, impaired: verbal
(c) Family process, alteration in
(d) Social isolation

REFERENCES

American Psychiatric Association: *Diagnostic and Statistical Manual of Mental Disorders.* 3d ed. Revised. Washington DC: American Psychiatric Association, 1987.

Bateson MC, Goldsby R: *Thinking AIDS.* Addison-Wesley, 1988.

Bluhm J: *When You Face the Chemically Dependent Patient: A Practical Guide for Nurses.* Ishiyaku Euro-America, 1987.

Brunner LS, Suddarth DS: *The Lippincott Manual of Nursing Practice.* 4th ed. Lippincott, 1988.

Burkhalter PK: *Nursing Care of the Alcoholic and Drug Abuser.* McGraw-Hill, 1975.

Cocores JA, Gold MS: Substance abuse and sexual dysfunction. *Med Aspects Human Sexuality* (2) 1989:23:22–31.

Donovan DM: Assessment of addictive behaviors. In: *Assessment of Addictive Behaviors,* Donovan DM, Marlatt GA (editors). Guilford Press, 1988. 3–48.

Doyle KM, Quinones MA, Lauria DB: Treating the drug abuser. *Public Health Rev* (Jan/Mar) 1982:77–98.

Earle R, Crow G: *Lonely All the Time.* Pocket Books, 1989.

Gianelli D: Very addictive, appealing to youth, crack poses major health worries. *Am Med News* (Sept) 1986:12.

Greenbaum DM: Clinical aspects of drug intoxication: The St. Vincent's Hospital symposium—Part 1. *Heart Lung* (3) 1983:12:109–21.

Grinspoon L, Bakalara JB: Drug dependence: Nonnarcotic agents. In: *Comprehensive Texbook of Psychiatry,* 4th ed. Vol. 1. Kaplan HI, Sadock BJ (editors). Baltimore: Williams and Wilkins, 1985. 1010–11.

Hahn AB, Barkin RL, Klarmen Oestreich SJ: *Pharmacology in Nursing.* 15th ed. St. Louis: Mosby, 1982.

Hughes TL, Sullivan EJ: Attitudes toward chemically dependent nurses: Care or curse? In: *Addiction in the Nursing Profession.* Haack MR, Hughes TL (editors). Springer. 1989. 20–34.

Jaffe JH: Opioid dependence. In: *Comprehensive Textbook of Psychiatry,* 4th ed. Vol. 1. Kaplan HI, Sadock BJ (editors). Baltimore: Williams and Wilkins, 1985. 992.

Johnston LD, et al: *National Trends in Drug Use and Related Factors among American High Students and Young Adults, 1975–1986.* National Institute on Drug Abuse. 1987.

Judson I, Carbary C, Carbary N: Angle dust. *J Nurs Care* (Nov) 1981:17–18.

Levy DB: Providing crack care. *Emerg Med* (8) 1987:19:16–17.

Louie AK, et al: Treatment of cocaine-induced panic disorder. *Am J Psychiatry* (1) 1989. 146:40–44.

Luckman J, Sorensen KC: *Medical Surgical Nursing: A Psychophysiologic Approach,* 3d ed. Philadelphia: W. B. Saunders, 1987. 1851.

McCormick M: *Designer-Drug Abuse.* Franklin Watts. 1989.

Piercy FP, Nelson TS: Adolescent substance abuse. In: *Treating Stress in Families.* Figley CR (editor). Brunner/Mazel. 1989. 209–30.

Quinones MA, et al: Evaluation of drug abuse rehabilitation efforts: A review. *Am J Public Health* (11) 1979: 69:1164–69.

Schleifer SJ, et al: HIV seropositivity in inner-city alcoholics. *Hosp Community Psychiatry* (23) 1990:41: 248–49.

Schnoll SH: Aiding the drug abuser. *Hosp Med* (Aug) 1983:116–17.

Schultz JM, Dark SL: *Manual of Psychiatric Nursing Care Plans.* Boston: Little, Brown, 1982.

Sullivan E, Bissell L, Williams E: *Chemical Dependency in Nursing.* Addison-Wesley. 1988.

Treadway DC: *Before It's Too Late: Working with Substance Abuse in the Family.* WW Norton, 1989.

Youcha G, Seixas JS: *Drugs, Alcohol, and Your Children.* Crown. 1989.

SUGGESTED READINGS

Alper J: Tranquilizers: A user's guide. *Health* (11) 1988: 20:35–39, 86–87.

Eller RA, et al: Responding to the chemically dependent nursing student. *J Nurs Educ* (2) 1989:28:87–88.

Kirmer DA: Caffeine use and abuse in psychiatric clients. *J Psychosoc Nurs* (11) 1988:26:20–24.

Rynerson BC: Cops & counselors: Counseling issues with prison inmate substance abusers. *J Psychosoc Nurs* (2) 1989:27:12–17.

CHAPTER 14

Schizophrenic Disorders

J. SUE COOK

Asking for Help

Inside myself is the person who yells out for help. Outside is the person with no mouth to ask for help. Also I'm asleep so anyone who sees me won't ask me, the sleeping person, if I need help. I want HELP.

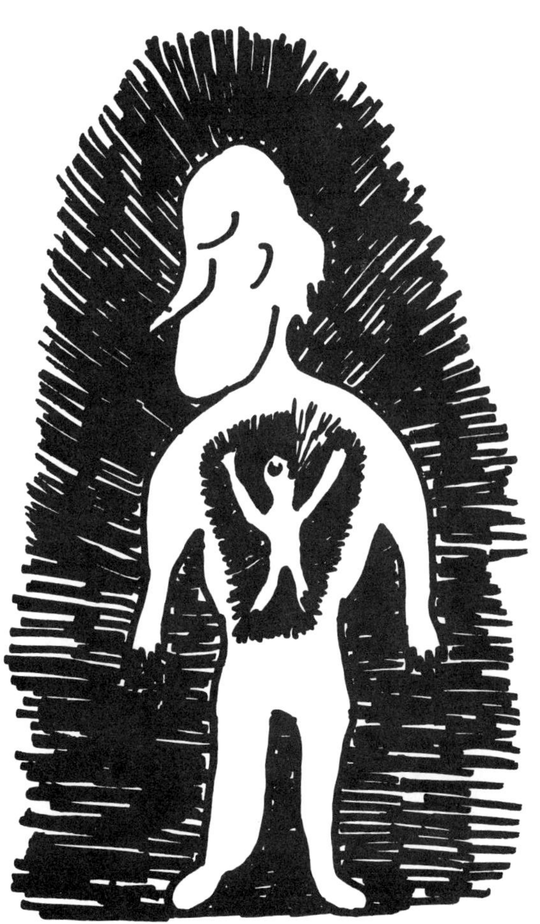

■ *Objectives*

After reading this chapter the student will be able to

- Define terms commonly used in diagnosing schizophrenia
- Describe the characteristics of the five subtypes of schizophrenia
- Discuss the current theories of causation related to the diagnosis of schizophrenia
- Make a focused nursing assessment of clients with schizophrenia
- Relate considerations relative to interviewing the schizophrenic client
- Identify nursing diagnoses appropriate to the five subtypes of schizophrenia
- Prepare nursing care plans for clients with the subtypes of schizophrenia
- Discuss the evaluation of nursing care of the client with schizophrenia

■ *Chapter Outline*

Introduction

A popular belief about schizophrenia is that those who suffer from it have a "split" personality; this, however, does not accurately describe the complexity of the disorder. The split, as it were, is between the body and the mind, not within the personality. That is, the schizophrenic experience involves a disharmony of the thinking, feeling, and acting components of behavior. Moreover, the split is with reality and does not refer to two personalities. There are four essential indicators of **schizophrenic disorder**:

- Certain psychotic features during the active phase of the illness
- Deterioration from a previous level of functioning
- Onset before 45 years of age
- At least a six-month duration

Many classification systems have been presented in the literature over the years. Bleuler (1911) developed what has been called the 4-A classification: ambivalence, avoidance, autism, and associative looseness. This system focuses on underlying disturbances in these four psychologic processes. **Ambivalence** refers to opposing emotions, **avoidance** to moving away from strong emotion, **autism** to preoccupation with self, and **associative looseness** to illogical thinking.

The weakness of Bleuler's system is that the 4-A symptomology can be seen in other psychiatric disorders. DSM-III-R recognizes schizophrenia as a group of disorders involving characteristic symptoms from multiple psychologic processes. The following are the DSM-III-R diagnostic criteria for a schizophrenic disorder:

A. Presence of active psychotic symptoms from categories 1, 2, or 3 for at least one week.
   1. Two of the following:
      (a) Delusions
      (b) Hallucinations
      (c) Incoherence or marked loosening of associations
      (d) Catatonic behavior
      (e) Inappropriate or flat affect
   2. Bizarre delusions, e.g., being controlled by a dead person, thoughts being broadcast, etc.
   3. Prominent hallucinations, e.g., two or more voices conversing with one another, a voice keeping a running commentary on the person's behavior, etc.
B. Functioning in work, social relations, and self-care is markedly below the highest level achieved before the onset of symptoms. In the case of onset in childhood or adolescence, failure to achieve the expected level of social development.
C. Other diagnoses, such as schizoaffective disorder, have been ruled out because of the total duration of the active and residual phase of the disturbance.
D. At least six months of continuous signs of disturbance.
E. Inability to establish that an organic factor initiated and maintained the disturbance.
F. A history of autistic disorder.

Schizophrenia is complex and presents a clinically variable picture. It is difficult to apply a single set of criteria for diagnosis of the disorder. Because of this complexity, DSM-III-R also contains criteria for five subtypes of schizophrenia:

- Disorganized
- Catatonic
- Paranoid
- Undifferentiated
- Residual

Incidence of Schizophrenia in the United States

More than 2 million Americans have been affected at some time during their lives by schizophrenia. Historically, at least in the last 100 years, schizophrenia has been diagnosed in 1 to 2 percent of the population. According to the U.S. Department of Health and Human Services, 40 percent of the beds in mental hospitals are occupied by schizophrenics. The annual cost of schizophrenia in the United States is between $10 and $20 billion, the bulk of which is due to the lack of productive employment by the schizophrenic (American Psychiatric Association, 1987; Baker, 1989; Tsuang and Faraone, 1988).

Significance of Schizophrenia to Mental Health Nursing

Nurses are likely to care for schizophrenic clients in many institutional settings. The nurse should not personalize the client's distant and seemingly unfeeling response to interpersonal approaches. Often the nurse is left feeling inadequate because little progress is observed. The nurse needs to realize that change in the schizophrenic is very slow. To feel successful in dealing with the schizophrenic client, it is extremely important to set small, achievable, short-term goals. Moreover, the nurse needs a great deal of energy because progress is so slow and the schizophrenic client's sense of hopelessness so draining. Sharing goals with a treatment team and using the team as a support system are helpful.

Subtypes of Schizophrenia

Catatonic Type The catatonic type is the least common form of schizophrenia. Medical care is often needed because of the problems created by nonmovement, malnutrition, exhaustion, hyperpyrexia, or self-inflicted injury (American Psychiatric Association, 1987).

Yolanda, a 35-year-old with a history of severe episodes of schizophrenia, participates in a sheltered workshop in her city. Yolanda usually takes the bus to the workshop, where she uses hand tools to assemble the parts of small appliances. Yolanda's supervisor became alarmed when Yolanda did not come to the workshop for three days in a row; she notified the Mental Health Department. A Mental Health Department community worker went to Yolanda's boardinghouse and found her sitting in a rocking chair, staring out into space. The owner of the boardinghouse said that Yolanda had not answered his knocks on the door, so he assumed Yolanda had gone to work.

Disorganized Type The disorganized type, formerly called hebephrenic, is primarily identified by incoherence and altered affect. The disorganized schizophrenic has no systematized delusions or hallucinations; delusions or hallucinations, if present, are fragmented, without a coherent theme. Features common to the disorganized schizophrenic are odd behaviors; extreme social withdrawal; mannerisms; hypochondriac complaints; and blunted, inappropriate, or silly affect. Odd behaviors typical of disorganized schizophrenics are strange grimaces, sniffing, blowing out the cheeks, wrinkling the forehead, and ritualistic activities.

Tyrone, a 23-year-old private school janitor, had been treated for two episodes of schizophrenia within the past three years. Tyrone lived at home with his mother, grandmother, and two siblings. The school principal noticed that Tyrone was giggly and silly while he was supposed to be cleaning the school lavatory. On the way in to the lavatory to check on Tyrone, the principal could see that Tyrone had not shaved. Tyrone's clothes were mismatched and looked as if they had been slept in, and he had obvious body odor. The giggling got louder, and the principal saw Tyrone dump mop water over his head.

Paranoid Type The paranoid type of schizophrenia is identified by preoccupation with one or more systematized delusions. Also, there can be frequent auditory hallucinations related to a specific single theme. The primary features associated with the paranoid type are unfocused anxiety, anger, argumentativeness, and violence. Interpersonal interactions are often stilted, formal, and extremely intense. Functional impairment may be minimal unless the delusional material is acted upon. Those with the paranoid type of schizophrenia usually have symptoms later in life and have a better prognosis than those with the other types—in terms of occupational functioning and independent living.

Max was a 32-year-old bank teller. Max was well liked at the bank because he rarely made errors and was meticulous at his job. During his first episode of schizophrenia he locked himself in the bank over a weekend and was not discovered until Monday morning. Max told the bank manager that he had discovered a plot by the Mafia to take over the bank. Max had worked nonstop all weekend, trying to identify the Mafia accounts that were taking over the accounts of the good customers.

Undifferentiated Type The undifferentiated type is identified and primarily marked by prominent psychotic symptoms outside the categories previously described. Mixed schizophrenic symptoms, such as inappropriate affect like the disorganized type and delusions like the paranoid type, characterize the disorder. This is the most commonly listed diagnosis for clients in residential institutional settings.

Sandy, a 24-year-old schizophrenic, lived with her mother in a small downtown apartment. Sandy had never worked outside the home. She often looked unkempt and would not go outside for days at a time. Sandy heard voices coming from the television set when it wasn't on. When it was on, Sandy thought the television controlled her mind. One day Sandy tried to strangle her mother because she thought her mother was involved in a cult that spoke in a code over the television set. Sandy thought the cult had told her mother to poison Sandy. Sandy is now institutionalized and has been in and out of three different treatment facilities in the past two years.

Residual Type The residual type is a category used when there has been at least one episode of schizophrenia. This type is called **chronic**, and common features are emotional blunting, social withdrawal, eccentric behavior, illogical thinking, and loose associations.

George, a 47-year-old streetperson, is well known to the local general hospital staff and mental health authorities. George is often seen pushing a grocery cart and mumbling to himself as he finds garbage cans to rummage through. One day, on a downtown boulevard, George was cursing a motorist and was attempting to hurl a bottle at the motorist's car. George lost his balance, fell into the street, and was hit by an oncoming car.

Knowledge Base

The behavioral, affective, and cognitive characteristics of schizophrenia can be divided into two groups of symptoms. **Positive symptoms** include behaviors that are different from the usual patterns of most people; these are most typically seen during the acute phase of schizophrenic disorders. **Negative symptoms** are described as the absence of usual and important behaviors of most people; these tend to be chronic problems. See Table 14–1 for an overview of positive and negative symptoms.

Behavioral Characteristics

The bizarre behavior of the schizophrenic was described in earlier times by labels like "madness," "lunacy," and "insanity." The abnormal speech patterns and unusual motor behaviors that result from acting out disordered thoughts make the schizophrenic's behavior appear bizarre indeed.

Table 14–1 *Positive and Negative Characteristics of Schizophrenia*

Positive Characteristics	*Negative Characteristics*
Behavioral	*Behavioral*
Catatonic excitement	Catatonic stupor
Stereotypes	Posturing
Echopraxia	Minimal self-care
Echolalia	Social withdrawal
Verbigeration	Stilted language
	Poverty of speech
Affective	*Affective*
Inappropriate affect	Blunted affect
Overreactive affect	Flat affect
	Anhedonia
Cognitive	*Cognitive*
Delusions	Concrete thinking
Hallucinations	Symbolism
Loose associations	Blocking
Neologisms	

Positive behavioral characteristics include catatonic excitement, stereotypies, echopraxia, echolalia, and verbigeration. The term *catatonic excitement* is used to describe the hyperactive behavior that may occur during the acute phase. The excitement may become so great that it threatens the safety of the schizophrenic or those around him or her. *Stereotypies* are repetitive meaningless movements or gestures; ticlike grimacing, particularly in the perioral area, is often observed. Some clients exhibit *echopraxia,* the imitation of an observed person's movements and gestures; *echolalia,* the repetition of an interviewer's question in answer to the question; or *verbigeration,* a senseless repetition of the same word or phrase that may continue for days.

Negative behavioral characteristics are catatonic stupor, posturing, minimal self-care, social withdrawal, stilted language, and poverty of speech. The term *catatonic stupor* is used to describe a reduction of energy, initiative, and spontaneity. There is a loss of natural gracefulness in body movements that results in poor coordination; activities may be carried out in a robotlike fashion. The client is *posturing* when he or she holds unusual or uncomfortable positions for a long time. Another characteristic typical of schizophrenic clients is a deterioration in appearance and manners. *Self-care* may become minimal; clients may need to be reminded to bathe, shave, brush their teeth, and change their clothes. Because of confusion and distraction, schizophrenics may not conform to social norms of dress and behavior. *Social withdrawal* is noticed when greetings are not returned or when conversations are ignored. They may resist involvement in social activities, and may also show a lack of consideration for the presence or feelings of others. *Stilted language* refers to the use of formal and quaint language in social situations. Clients are described as having *poverty of speech* when they say very little on their own initiative or in response to questions from others; they may be mute for several hours to several days (Lehmann and Cancor, 1985; Tsuang and Faraone, 1988). (See Table 14–2 for examples of verbal behavior characteristics of schizophrenics.)

Affective Characteristics

Positive affective characteristics include inappropriate affect and overreactive affect. *Inappropriate affect* occurs when the person's emotional tone is not related to the immediate circumstances. An *overreactive affect* is appropriate to the situation, but out of proportion to it. (See Chapter 11 for examples.)

Negative affective characteristics include blunted affect, flat affect, and anhedonia. A *blunted affect* describes a dulled emotional response to a situation, and a *flat affect* describes the absence of visible cues to the person's feelings. *Anhedonia,* the inability to experience pleasure, causes many schizophrenics to feel emotionally barren; some eventually commit suicide (Tsuang and Faraone, 1988).

Cognitive Characteristics

A word frequently used to describe thought patterns of the schizophrenic is *autistic,* which refers to a preoccupation with one's own experiences. Autistic thinking is intelligible only to the individual autistic person. Schizophrenics think and express their thoughts according to private, complicated rules of logic. This type of thinking interferes with the schizophrenic's speech, and effective communication with others becomes difficult.

Positive cognitive characteristics of schizophrenia are delusions, hallucinations, loose associations, and neologisms.

Delusions are the client's fixed false idiosyncratic ideas that cannot be corrected by reasoning. There are two phases in the development of delusions: (1) *trema*—Clients become aware that some-

Table 14–2 *Examples of Verbal Behavior Characteristics of Schizophrenics*

Behavior	*Example*
Mutism	Nurse: Good morning, Juanita. Client: (no verbal response; client sits stoically and stares ahead) Nurse: Juanita, can you hear me? Client: (still no response)
Echolalia	Nurse: Are you hearing voices? Client: Are you hearing voices? Nurse: What are the voices like? Client: What are the voices like?
Verbigeration	Nurse: What brought you in for treatment? Client: Why did I come to the clinic? Why did I come to the clinic? Because I'm crazy. I'm crazy. Why did I come to the clinic?
Stilted language	Nurse: Hi, my name is Brenda. I am your nurse today. Client: I must say Miss Brenda, I am very pleased to make your acquaintance. Your services are certainly to be admired.

thing threatening is happening to them. They feel harassed and powerless, and then become anxious, irritable, and depressed; and (2) *apophany*—Clients then experience sudden revelations and become absolutely sure of new facts.

Delusions meet the schizophrenic's internal emotional needs and "help" the schizophrenic deal with life's problems and stresses. When there is an extensively developed central delusional theme from which conclusions are logically deducted, the delusions are termed *systematized.* There are a number of delusional types: grandiose, persecution, sin and guilt, control, somatic, religious, ideas of reference, thought broadcasting, thought withdrawal, and thought insertion (Tsuang and Faraone, 1988).

Delusions of grandeur develop as a result of the client's feelings of inadequacy, insecurity, and inferiority. By becoming some well-known figure of importance, the client is able to escape from the emotional insecurity. *Delusions of persecution* develop as a result of dissatisfaction with the self projected toward others. Clients often believe someone is trying to harm them, and therefore any failures in life are the fault of these harmful others. *Delusions of sin and guilt* develop as a result of rationalizing remorse; guilt feelings are then allayed by self-punishment. *Delusions of control* develop when the schizophrenic attempts to shift the responsibility for failure to others since others are seen as controlling all aspects of life. *Somatic delusions* occur when clients believe something abnormal and dangerous is happening to their bodies. *Religious delusions* involve false beliefs with religious or spiritual themes. *Ideas of reference* are remarks or actions by another person that in no way refer to the client, but are interpreted by the client as relating to him or her. *Thought broadcasting* delusions are occurring when the client believes that his or her thoughts can be heard by others. *Thought withdrawal* is the belief that others are able to remove thoughts from the client's mind; *thought insertion* is the belief that others are able to put thoughts into the client's mind. (See Table 14–3 for examples of delusions.)

The primary perceptual disorder in the schizophrenic client is the *hallucination,* a sensory experience without external stimuli—that is, a hallucination is part of the client's mental life. Usually triggered by anxiety, the hallucination is a projection of needs, of enhancement of self-esteem, of self-criticism, of a sense of guilt, of self-punishment, or of repressed impulses onto reality (Williams, 1989). Dreams during sleep in the normal person may resemble the hallucinations during wakeful hours in the schizophrenic client. The most common hallucination is the *auditory hallucination,* or the hearing of voices. The voice is often that of God, of the devil, of neighbors, or of relatives; the voice may say either good or bad things. The next most common type are *visual hallucinations.* These are usually in proximity, are clearly defined, and are moving. Visual hallucinations almost never occur alone; they are usually accompanied by hallucinations of the other senses. *Tactile, olfactory,* and *gustatory hallucinations* are uncommon and are more likely to occur in clients undergoing substance withdrawal than in schizophrenics.

Hallucinations may considerably control the behavior of the schizophrenic, who may be preoccupied with the voices and oblivious to the environment. It is not unusual for the client to carry on a conversation with one of these voices. After a period of time in the mental health system, many clients realize that if they admit that they hear voices, they will be labelled "sick." To avoid treatment they may be very evasive about their hallucinations (Williams, 1989).

The remaining two positive cognitive characteristics of schizophrenia are loose associations and neologisms. The client is described as having *loose association* when there is no apparent relationship between thoughts. For example:

> PATIENT: I got to get out of here. I had steak last night for dinner. Do you work for the government? I got to get out of here. It's sunny outside. Do you fish?

Neologism is the creation of new words to express concepts for which ordinary words may or may not exist. An example of this is:

Table 14–3 *Examples of Types of Delusions*

Type of delusion	*Example*
Grandiose	"I've been on the President's Cabinet since the Kennedy years. No president can do without me. If it weren't for me, we would probably be in World War IV by now."
Persecution	"The CIA and the FBI are both out to get me. I am constantly being followed. I'm certain that one of these other patients in here is really a CIA agent and is here to spy on me."
Sin or guilt	"I know I often hurt my parent's feelings when I was growing up. That's why I can't ever keep a job. When I get a job and start doing good, I have to quit it to make up for my bad behavior."
Control	"I have this wire in my head and my family controls me with it. They make me wake up and make me go to sleep. They control everything I say. I can't do anything on my own."
Somatic	"My esophagus is being torn apart. I have this rat in my stomach and sometimes he comes all the way up to my throat. He's eating away at my esophagus. Look in my throat now—you can probably see the rat."
Religious	"As long as I wear these 10 religious medals and keep all these pictures of Jesus pinned to my clothes, nothing bad can happen to me. No one can hurt me as long as I do all of this."
Idea of reference	"People on TV last night told me I was in charge of saving the environment. That's why I'm telling everyone to stop using their cars. It's my job because that's what they told me last night."
Thought broadcasting	"I'm afraid to think anything. I know you can read my mind and know exactly what I'm thinking."
Thought withdrawal	"I can't tell you what I'm thinking. Somebody just stole my thoughts."
Thought insertion	"You think what I'm telling you is what I'm thinking, but it isn't. My father keeps putting all these thoughts in my head. They are not my thoughts."

NURSE: What are you eating?

CLIENT: (holding out a banana) What you have here is a *falana-in-lania.*

The negative cognitive characteristics of schizophrenia are concrete thinking, symbolism, and blocking. *Concrete thinking* is characterized by a focus on facts and details, and an inability to generalize or think abstractly. An example is:

NURSE: What brought you to the hospital?

CLIENT A car.

Symbolism is the preoccupation with witchcraft, religion, philosophy, and invisible forces. An example is:

NURSE: What is your name?

CLIENT: Jesus. He is a spirit. God made me a spirit. Therefore I must be Jesus.

The term *blocking* describes what occurs when the client's thoughts suddenly stop and do not continue for a period of time. The client seems frozen for this time. When thoughts return they may not be related to the topic that preceded the blocking. An example of this is:

> NURSE: What should we make for our cookout tomorrow?
>
> CLIENT: I would like to cook . . . (period of silence for 2 minutes) What time does group therapy start today?

Physiologic Characteristics

Recent research on the neurochemical basis of schizophrenia has focused on neurotransmitters, serum creatine phosphokinase, CNS structures, cerebral blood flow, and CNS electroactivity.

Since 1976 many studies have been conducted to review the role of the neurotransmitters dopamine and norepinephrine in schizophrenia. Overactivity of dopaminergic synapses is thought to be related to the symptoms of delusions, hallucinations, and sterotyped behavior. Insufficiency of synaptic norepinephrine is thought to be related to blunted or flat affect, anhedonia, and withdrawal experienced by schizophrenics (Kety and Matthysse, 1988).

Elevated serum creatine phosphokinase (CPK) levels have been found in half of newly diagnosed schizophrenics. This elevation is related to skeletal muscle abnormalities, and is also thought to be related to CNS neurotransmitter abnormalities, such as increased dopaminergic activity (Weiner, 1985).

Computed tomography (CT) scans demonstrate enlarged ventricles in schizophrenics. Cerebral blood flow studies have demonstrated several abnormalities. Some schizophrenics have a decreased blood flow to the entire brain, some have a decreased blood flow to the frontal lobes, and some have an increased blood flow to the left hemisphere. Brain electroactivity mapping (BEAM) demonstrates lower than normal electrical activity in the temporal and frontal lobes. Positron emission tomography (PET) scans of untreated schizophrenics demonstrate decreased glucose metabolism in the frontal cortex and temporal lobes, and increased glucose metabolism in the basal ganglia. When these clients are managed with antipsychotic medications, glucose metabolism returns to normal, except in the frontal cortex. Further research is needed to understand the specific role of brain abnormalities in schizophrenia (Mathew and Wilson, 1990; Buchanan et al. 1990; Tsuang and Faraone, 1988).

Drug-induced psychoses have also been studied. Hallucinogens and amphetamines can trigger schizophrenialike illnesses in some persons. Acute phencyclidine intoxication is precipitating psychotic reactions with increasing frequency.

Sociocultural Characteristics

The family, especially the mother, has long been blamed for and studied as the potential cause of the schizophrenic's behavior. Mental health professionals have not questioned the studies suggesting that disruptions in family relationships are the primary cause of schizophrenic behavior. However, in recent decades there has been a family self-help trend to ensure that schizophrenics get adequate treatment and that the blame is removed from the family (Lamb et al. 1986).

The parents of schizophrenics are no more perfect or imperfect than any other parents. Some research indicates that highly enmeshed families may have dysfunctional members with any number of disorders. It has been noted that families with high expressed emotion—that is, families that are highly critical, hostile, and overinvolved—and who also have schizophrenic members may contribute to the schizophrenic's relapse (Fallon et al. 1984). If there is a pattern of "schizophrenic motherhood," it may be that mothers of schizophrenics are more overprotective of their suffering children and overempathetic with their children's emotions. The least that can be said of having a schizophrenic in the household 24 hours a day is that stress levels are extremely high (Walsh, 1985).

Families with schizophrenics experience severe and chronic stress. Primary sources of stress are demands on family resources, loss, stigma, guilt, and realignment of family structure. These stresses can burden the family unit intensely (Baker, 1989).

Walsh (1985) developed the concept of no-fault schizophrenia, a perception of schizophrenia that did not blame mothers, fathers, doctors, society, or the client for the illness. Walsh believed that professionals should focus their energies on finding the cause and cure for the disease, thereby substituting positive action instead of blame.

Over their lives, 50 to 60 percent of schizophrenics recover completely or are able to live fairly independent lives. Currently researchers are examining the differences between those whose outcome is positive and those who suffer from prolonged mental illness. World studies indicate that schizophrenics have a better illness outcome in developing countries. The following factors may be related to this improved prognosis (Lefley, 1990):

- The cause of mental illness is viewed as being imposed from the outside.
- The affected person and the family are not blamed for the illness.
- There is less social rejection of mentally ill persons.
- Extended social and family relationships are a source of strength for the mentally ill person and the family.
- Families are viewed as treatment allies instead of being blamed for the illness.

Understanding these differences may lead to modification of treatment approaches in industrialized countries. Instead of assuming family pathology, professionals should stress that family strengths be supported; families should have a collaborative role in treatment. Support through extended social and family systems and the use of community resources should be encouraged.

Causative Theories

The causes of schizophrenia are complex. No single theory accounts for all variabilities. Schizophrenia is a multitiered problem influenced by genetic factors, sociology, family and environmental actions, and culture. Theories of causation in schizophrenia are categorized as biologic, family relationship, sociocultural, and psychoanalytic. Many of these theories are not empirically based and are speculative.

Biologic Theories Genetic studies have centered on family studies, twin studies, and adoption studies. In the general population, the risk for developing schizophrenia is 0.6 percent. Family studies indicate that the risk of schizophrenia for children with one schizophrenic parent ranges from 8 to 18 percent; if both parents are schizophrenic, the risk jumps to between 15 and 55 percent. Because social as well as genetic factors could be involved in transmission, researchers sought to gain further evidence on the relationship of genetics and schizophrenia by studying twins. Most twin studies demonstrate a 40 to 50 percent rate of schizophrenia in a second twin (where one has been diagnosed schizophrenic) in identical (monozygotic) twins and a 9 to 10 percent rate in fraternal (dizygotic) twins. In adoption studies, the prevalence of schizophrenia was approximately what one could have expected from other family studies. These genetic factors are significant but not uniform. They are clustered in some families and absent in others. This finding may indicate a variety in the causes of schizophrenia (Kety and Matthysse, 1988).

Recently, in Great Britain, scientists found a link between schizophrenia and an abnormally functioning gene on chromosome 5. The gene or gene cluster is still unidentified, but the discovery of its approximate location will assist in looking at abnormalities. This research is important because it provides solid evidence of the biologic cause of schizophrenia and may help in further identifying subtypes of schizophrenia. New studies of the genetic cause of schizophrenia are expected to narrow research to a single gene or gene cluster (Press release, 1988).

Family Relationship Theories Across the United States, investigators have observed similar deviances in families of schizophrenics. Bateson et al. (1956), in his paper "Toward a Theory of Schizophrenia," coined the term **double bind** to describe situations where options seem to be offered but where, in reality, no choice is available. In a double-bind interaction the primary message is followed by a secondary message that contradicts the first. For example, the first message to the recipient may be "If you take this action, you will suffer consequences." This is followed by the second message: "If you don't take this action, you will suffer consequences." This creates the proverbial "damned if you do, damned if you don't" situation. For double-bind communication to contribute to schizophrenia, the recipient must be exposed to these messages repeatedly and not be able to escape the situation (Bateson et al., 1956). The following is an example of a double-bind situation.

John's family was one of turmoil. His father constantly enlisted him as an ally to battle his mother. John's mother was at best ineffectual and was usually distant and aloof. Any evening could turn into a fiasco.

FATHER: (addressing John) Come here and chat with me. You know how much I love to chat with you.

JOHN: (sitting next to his father on the sofa) I had a very interesting day today . . .

(John's mother reads the newspaper and ignores the circumstances around her.)

FATHER: Don't be so noisy boy; can't you see your mother is trying to read the newspaper? You need to start respecting your parents more!

Although double-bind theory was presented in the 1950s, it was several decades before researchers began to test it. In tests of Bateson's theory, there was difficulty in identifying double-bind situations and some difficulty in telling the difference between the communications of parents with a normal child and the communications of parents with a schizophrenic child. There have been no studies to support the double-bind theory. Yet, the theory still persists in professional literature (Walsh, 1985).

The primary commonality in family studies of schizophrenia regards vulnerability. Studies show that the less one is able to learn to think clearly and to relate to unambivalent messages in the home, the more vulnerable one is to fragmented thinking. The implication is that a premorbid person is vulnerable to human relationships. Research seems to indicate that clients with a successful premorbid history of peer relationships and intimacy have a greater tendency to recover from schizophrenia. The most recent trend in family studies has been to avoid placing blame on the family and to focus efforts on family self-help (Lamb et al. 1986; Tsuang and Faraone, 1988).

Sociocultural Theories Sociocultural theories have been difficult to substantiate empirically; at best, only some facts are known. It is apparent that those with lower socioeconomic status have a greater chance of developing schizophrenia than those with higher socioeconomic status. One theory, called *downward drift,* refers to a phenomenon that occurs over several generations when marginal members of society pass on the weakest aspects of the gene pool. Adaptive abilities are affected; a gradual increase of disease frequency in the lower classes of society results. A factor that contributes to downward drift is the inability of lower-class families to care for schizophrenic members. The family of an upper-class schizophrenic can afford to provide care at home or in a private facility. The economically disadvantaged schizophrenic, on the other hand, must continue to fend for himself or herself. The continuing pressure aggravates the disease and results in lessened cognitive and social abilities, which in turn weaken earning power, and the schizophrenic drifts downward on the socioeconomic ladder.

The *stress theory* is also related to the sociologic view of schizophrenia. Children born into poverty are exposed to excessive stressors such as poor nutrition, inadequate housing, inadequate clothing, crime, and street violence. Inadequate medical care, poor prenatal care, increased obstetric complications, and inadequate early childhood medical care are additional stressors. Schizophrenia may be a consequence for the deprivation and distress associated with poverty existence (Tsuang and Faraone, 1988; Weiner, 1985).

Psychoanalytic Theories These theories are descriptive, but do not offer reasons why some people do develop schizophrenia and others do not. Freud postulated the original psychoanalytic concepts that pertain to schizophrenia; these concepts continue to undergo modification. More recently psychoanalytic theories have centered on the intense ambivalence, anxiety, and infantile ego mechanisms that schizophrenics use in their relationships with objects (Meissner, 1985).

As can be seen, the search for the cause of schizophrenia has been extensive, but no conclusive answers have been found. The search has not been without value, because these theories have given rise to a number of treatment modalities.

Medical Treatment

Eclectic approach is the best term to describe treatment for schizophrenia. No treatment "cures" schizophrenia, but evidence suggests that various strategies are helpful at different phases of the illness.

Since the introduction of phenothiazine drugs in the 1950s, the majority of schizophrenics have been treated as outpatients. The schizophrenic being treated for the first episode has an 80 to 90 percent chance of being discharged in a few weeks to a few months following the acute episode. However, 45 percent of those admitted for the first episode are readmitted during the first year after the initial treatment. Approximately one third of those treated for schizophrenia remain symptom-free for five years, and approximately 10 percent have permanent disability. Schizophrenics who have a history of multidrug use also have a poor record of recovery. The remaining people show some personality impoverishment and episodic psychotic behavior. They are the group on which prevention efforts should focus. As previously stated, research data suggest that clients with a good premorbid history of peer relationships and intimacy have a greater tendency to recover (Coleman, Butcher, and Carson, 1984; Sulliger, 1988; and Weiner, 1985).

The major step in management is to be certain of the diagnosis. In the initial evaluation, careful consideration needs to be given to where treatment should take place. With modern community mental health laws, it may be difficult to keep clients in the hospital for the length of time sufficient for adequate treatment. The primary psychosocial treatment approaches have been individual, group, family, and community support (Liberman, 1985; Schultz, 1985).

Antipsychotic Agents No empirical evidence indicates the superiority of one antipsychotic drug over another, although some persons respond better to one drug than another. (See Table 14–4 for a list of commonly used antipsychotic drugs.)

Many factors must be taken into account when using antipsychotic drugs with the schizophrenic client: family history of drug responsiveness; potential side effects; initial sedation, which may be advantageous for the young, agitated client but unacceptable for the elderly or infirm; and long-acting substances, which may be more appropriate for the chronic client than for the client with an acute episode. The primary mode of action of antipsychotic agents is the blocking of postsynaptic dopamine receptors in the brain. This action leads to a compensatory increase in dopamine synthesis and increase in dopamine destruction. These actions are thought to be responsible for the extrapyramidal side effects of the phenothiazine drugs (Townsend, 1990).

Antipsychotics are used for their behavioral effects. Symptoms of excessive psychomotor activity, panic, fear, and hostility respond well to phenothiazines. The relief of these symptoms lessens the client's response to delusions and hallucinations.

Some adverse behavioral effects of antipsychotics are feelings of lassitude, fatigability, and depression. There is also an increased risk of suicide for psychotic clients receiving antipsychotic medications. (See Chapter 16 for nursing care of suicidal clients.) Other clients may experience feelings of excitement and restlessness. The wide range of side effects in antipsychotic drugs may be due to the secondary action of the drug on the central nervous system or autonomic nervous system, or to idiosyncratic reactions or allergic reactions. The most common side effects of antipsychotic drugs are extrapyramidal symptoms, which include acute dystonic reactions, akathisia, and parkinsonism. *Acute*

Table 14–4 *Commonly Used Antipsychotic Drugs*

Generic Name	*Trade Name*	*Dosage for Acute Episodes (mg)*	*Maintenance Dose (mg)*	*Side Effects*
Chlorpromazine	Thorazine	25–800	100–300	Sedation or sleep, ataxia, dry mouth, constipation, dermatitis, extrapyramidal symptoms, orthostatic hypotension, blood dyscrasia such as agranulocytosis, jaundice, antiemetic, blurred vision, hypothermia, tachycardia, nasal congestion, photosensitivity, tardive dyskinesia, pigmented retinopathy
Chlorprothixene	Taractan	75–600	25–50	Sedation or sleep, ataxia, dry mouth, constipation, orthostatic hypotension
Triflupromazine	Vesprin	100–150	150	Sedation or sleep, ataxia, dry mouth, constipation, dermatitis, extrapyramidal symptoms, orthostatic hypotension, blood dyscrasia, jaundice, convulsions, antiemetic, blurred vision
Thioridazine hydrochloride	Mellaril	300–800	100–300	Sedation or sleep, ataxia, dry mouth, extrapyramidal symptoms, orthostatic hypotension, blurred vision, hypothermia, nausea and vomiting, edema, impotence
Loxapine	Loxitane	60–100	30–50	Sedation or sleep, extrapyramidal effects
Mesoridazine besylate	Serentil	100–400	25–200	Sedation or sleep, ataxia, dry mouth, constipation, dermatitis, extrapyramidal symptoms, orthostatic hypotension, hypothermia, impotence, bradycardia
Molindone hydrochloride	Moban	40–225	10–75	Sedation or sleep, ataxia, dry mouth, constipation, orthostatic hypotension, extrapyramidal effects
Piperacetazine	Quide	1–160	40–160	Sedation or sleep, extrapyramidal symptoms, orthostatic hypotension, convulsions, antiemetic, impotence, increased appetite, photosensitivity
Fluphenazine hydrochloride	Prolixin, Permitil	5–20	1–15	Sedation or sleep, ataxia, dry mouth, constipation, dermatitis, extrapyramidal symptoms, orthostatic hypotension, blood dyscrasia, jaundice, antiemetic, blurred vision, nasal congestion, edema
Perphenazine	Trilafon	16–64	8–16	Sedation or sleep, ataxia, dry mouth, constipation, dermatitis, extrapyramidal symptoms, orthostatic hypotension, blood dyscrasia, jaundice, antiemetic, blurred vision
Trifluoperazine hydrochloride	Stelazine	10–60	4–30	Sedation or sleep, ataxia, constipation, dermatitis, extrapyramidal symptoms, orthostatic hypotension, blood dyscrasia, jaundice, antiemetic, blurred vision, nasal congestion, edema
Thiothixene hydrochloride	Navane	6–100	4–30	Sedation or sleep, dry mouth, dermatitis, extrapyramidal symptoms, orthostatic hypotension, convulsions, blurred vision, hypothermia, tachycardia, edema, photosensitivity
Haloperidol	Haldol	1–100	1–15	Blood dyscrasia, extrapyramidal symptoms, blurred vision, dry mouth, urinary retention, menstrual irregularities, gynecomastia, rash

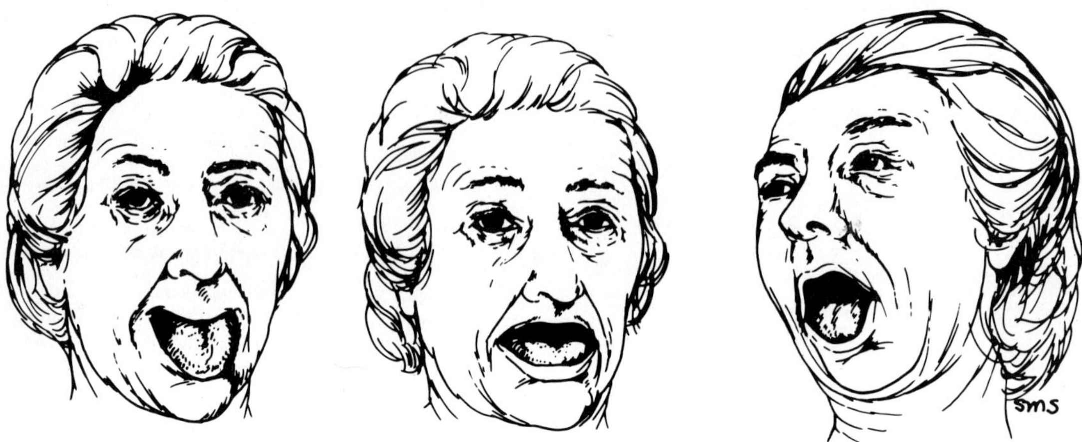

Figure 14–1 *Tardive dyskinesia—abnormal movements of the mouth, tongue, and jaw*

dystonic reactions have an abrupt onset, with frightening muscular spasms in the head and neck. These reactions usually occur within the first two days of therapy or when dosage of the medication is significantly increased and are most likely caused by higher doses. *Akathisia* is the inability to sit or stand still. The client has a subjective feeling of anxiety, for which antiparkinson agents are given. *Parkinsonism* produced by antipsychotics is distinguished from classic parkinsonism by the initial effects on the muscles of the face and neck, which then spreads to the shoulders and trunk. To combat this side effect, antiparkinson agents such as Cogentin or Artane are given (Townsend, 1990).

Tardive dyskinesia is an unpleasant side effect of antipsychotic drugs that occurs in up to 20 percent of clients receiving them. Symptoms of tardive dyskinesia include movements of the tongue, mouth, face, and jaw; mouth puckering; chewing movements; and involuntary movement of the extremities. (See Figure 14–1.) There is no known treatment to counteract this side effect. Some cases of tardive dyskinesia are not reversible. The greatest incidence of tardive dyskinesia appears in elderly females and clients with organic brain syndrome on high-dose therapy. An anticonvulsant, the benzodiazepine derivative clonazepam (Klonopin, Rivotull) has shown promise in treating tardive dyskinesia. It is thought that a reduction in gamma aminobutyric acid (GABA) transmission in the CNS plays a role in the development of tardive dyskinesia. Clonazepam potentiates the action of GABA and thus reduces the symptoms of tardive dyskinesia. Studies have demonstrated that 50 to 83 percent of clients showed improvement in their symptoms of tardive dyskinesia on 2 to 10 mg daily doses. Other research has looked at the role of vitamin E in the treatment of tardive dyskinesia. It is thought that vitamin E neutralizes the byproducts of dopamine metabolism in the CNS. Studies have shown a 30 percent improvement in symptoms (Elkashef et al. 1990; Thaker et al. 1990).

Autonomic effects of antipsychotics include anticholinergic effects, antiadrenergic effects, and convulsant effect. *Anticholinergic effects* include dry mouth, constipation, urinary retention, and failure of accommodation for near vision. *Antiadrenergic effects* include vasodilation and orthostatic hypotension. Convulsions occur with extremely high doses—epileptics are more susceptible to this side effect.

Antipsychotics can cause changes in the heart rate. This effect can increase the client's vulnerability to arrhythmias. Common electrocardiograph changes are depressed S-T segments, flattened T-waves and U-waves, and prolonged Q-T intervals. A particularly hazardous side effect of Mellaril is the activation of the ventricular ectopic pacemaker which can lead to ventricular fibrillation and death.

An allergic response to an antipsychotic usually

causes a skin reaction. Rashes and photosensitivity are the most common reactions. Rarely do other allergic responses—such as agranulocytosis, thrombocytopenic purpura, hemolytic anemia, and pancytopenia—occur.

Endocrine and metabolic effects of antipsychotics include sexual disturbances, some of which are also due to autonomic nervous system effects. Sexual disturbances are decreased libido, with difficulty in achieving and maintaining erection. The client may be unable to reach orgasm, and retrograde ejaculation can occur. Mellaril is the drug most likely to cause sexual dysfunction. Other side effects are amenorrhea, lactation, hirsutism, and gynecomastia. Weight gain can also occur. The endocrine mechanism involved is unclear (Townsend, 1990).

Psychosocial Intervention Psychosocial intervention is the major component of treatment for schizophrenics. It may be argued that the use of antipsychotic drugs is the major treatment for schizophrenia, but coping skills for a greater quality of life are not a result of drug intervention. Rather, these skills are learned through psychosocial interventions in which schizophrenics learn social and personal survival skills.

There is considerable overlap among treatment modalities for schizophrenia. Specific interventions vary from individual therapy, to family or group therapy, to therapeutic communities. The location of treatment may be the hospital, private office, clinic, mental health center, board and care facility, or home. Treatment approaches range from behaviorally oriented ego-supportive token-economy strategies to psychodynamic approaches.

Milieu Therapy Milieu therapy is the purposeful use of people, resources, and events in the client's immediate environment to promote positive client behavior, including improved interpersonal relationship skills and skills to allow optimal functioning outside an institution. Milieu therapy has been used in inpatient units, day care, rehabilitation clubs, board and care homes, and sheltered workshops. Treatment modalities vary from behavior therapy to humanistic approaches. Most milieu therapy programs

- Emphasize group or social interaction
- Have rules or expectations mediated by peers to maintain adaptation
- View clients as responsible human beings rather than having a "dependent patient" role
- Emphasize client's rights
- Emphasize client's involvement in goal setting, freedom of movement, and informal relationships with staff
- Strive for clear interdisciplinary and goal-oriented communication

The body of literature on milieu therapy is large, but data indicate certain structural elements associated with favorable outcomes.

- Milieu groups should be small in relation to size and census.
- There should be high staff-to-client ratios and staff stability.
- The client group should be heterogeneous, optimally having a mix of two thirds higher-functioning acutely ill clients and one third lower-functioning chronic clients.
- There should be clarity and consistency in the staffing roles and status.
- The average hospital episode should be no longer than three months.

The focus of treatment in a therapeutic milieu is on the practical, adaptive aspects of everyday behavior. Clearly defined and time-limited goals are set for clients. There is a schedule of prosocial activities. Although there is a variety of psychosocial treatments, one frequently used model is the social learning–token economy. This treatment model has been successful in remediating bizarre behaviors, social deficits, and self-care deficits. Client behavior is assessed, and the psychosocial strategy of choice is the focus of therapy (Liberman, 1985; Mosher and Keith, 1981).

Group Therapy Group therapy for schizophrenics has theoretic, operational, and procedural qualities. For example, one group may be organized around a specific theoretic approach such as behaviorism. The same group has operational procedures for conducting itself, and the procedures for group members are clear. Some groups are highly structured, whereas others are spontaneous and insight-oriented. Therapy groups for schizophrenics have been used in hospitals, clinics, and private offices. Groups focus on peer support, with emphasis on the development of insight and skill, and on behavior change. Groups have also been used for social support and maintenance. As with other types of groups, the leader of a group for schizophrenics uses the interactional dynamics of the group to improve outcomes. The factor in group therapy that seems to have the most favorable impact on outcomes is cohesion (Plante, 1989).

Family Therapy The focus of family therapy, a specialized type of group therapy, is to change the emotional climate of the family to reduce relapse of the schizophrenic client. Family therapy studies have indicated that overinvolved attitudes and feelings of relatives are among the most powerful predictors of relapse in the schizophrenic client. Family therapy takes place in a variety of settings, such as the hospital, the clinic, the private office, and the home. The common element in most approaches to family therapy is an emphasis on educating the client and family members about schizophrenia and its treatment. Time is spent on helping the family understand the symptoms and prognosis of the disorder. The importance of antipsychotic drugs is also emphasized so that family members realize they must help the client comply with the pharmacotherapeutic regimen.

Family therapy ranges from systems methods to supportive methods. Many therapists use a therapeutic relationship to move the family to change its rules and reactions. Supportive family therapies employing educational and skill-building methods have proved among the most successful (Liberman, 1985; Plante, 1989).

Individual Therapy In individual therapy for the schizophrenic client, the setting is extremely important because the schizophrenic is highly sensitive to the environment. To ensure the safety of the therapist and client, the environment should allow for physical distance between the client and therapist. In individual therapy, respect for the client is essential. A regular schedule of appointments should be maintained. If the therapist will be late, the client should be notified.

The most successful therapists in some way convey an emotional involvement with the client. The therapist's expecting that the client will improve assists the client to participate more actively in therapy. Mutual goal setting with consensus about goals also fosters effective individual therapy. Listening is essential as a technical intervention in forming a therapeutic relationship with the schizophrenic client.

Rehabilitation Regardless of the treatment modality, the ultimate aim is rehabilitation. To plan for the schizophrenic's rehabilitation, first it is necessary to assess the client's support system. Has the client held a job? Does the client's family accept and want this person? Is the client capable of acting in his or her own behalf? See Chapter 4 for a review of the general principles related to psychiatric rehabilitation.

To assist the schizophrenic in adapting is a major goal of rehabilitation. How clients view their illness is a primary factor in rehabilitation. Some clients want to deny they are ill and do not take prescribed medications or participate in other treatments. If this is the case, the nurse needs to help the client accept the responsibility for getting better by modifying the nursing care plan.

Problems after discharge from acute care can be anticipated. Clients may need to change their type of work, especially if they have been in jobs where they are under stress and time pressures. The client may need to take a job with fewer responsibilities. These changes may mean the client will be paid less. The client may then have difficulty remaining in treatment and meeting living expenses, thus creating additional stress on an already vulnerable client. Many schizophrenic clients have a need for ongoing supportive care, perhaps for a lifetime. A major goal in rehabilitation is to identify individual potential, ways to maintain potential, and ways to increase quality of life.

Because social isolation can be a problem for schizophrenic clients, rehabilitation needs to emphasize behavioral skills to assist the client in adaptation. Simple skills like making eye contact during a conversation are important to emphasize. What to wear and how to dress needs to be taught, as does the importance of keeping appointments and completing forms correctly (Plante, 1989).

Special Problems Related to Schizophrenia

Childhood Schizophrenia

Care of children with schizophrenia is a specialized area in pschiatric nursing. There is a stigma associated with its diagnosis, and the prognosis tends to be poor no matter what the age of onset through adolescence. Although the cause is unknown, childhood schizophrenia may be related to a dysfunctional cholinergic system (Cantor, 1988).

Preschizophrenic Symptoms Most of these children appear normal at birth and during the first year of life. During the second and third years of life, preschizophrenic symptoms may become obvious. *Behaviorial characteristics* include the inability to engage in fantasy play with toys and a tendency toward repetitive sensorimotor play such as stacking blocks up for long periods of time. They may also exhibit deviant social behavior such as ignoring peers, moving away from peers, or interacting with only one peer at a time. By the age of three, many of these children exhibit some form of unusual behavior such as rocking constantly, head banging, or touching everything in sight. *Affective characteristics* are primarily fear and anger in response to loud noises. *Cognitive characteristics* are preoccupation; others find it difficult to attract and maintain the child's attention. *Physical characteristics* include deficits in fine and gross motor function, which limits the child's ability to explore the environment. These children appear to have a hyperaroused sensory system and often try to avoid sensory stimulation.

Schizophrenic Symptoms The diagnosis of childhood schizophrenia usually cannot be made before the child is 5 or 6 years old, at which point he or she can communicate disruptions in thought process and content. The schizophrenic symptoms are as follows: *Behavioral characteristics* include speaking in a monotone voice, exhibiting poverty of speech, and echolalia. Frequently the child engages in perseveration behavior which is defined as repetitive actions or words. *Affective characteristics* include constricted and inappropriate affect. The child suffers from chronic anxiety and morbid fears and is easily frightened by unfamiliar objects or situations. *Cognitive characteristics* include concentration difficulties, fragmented thought processes, and loose association. There may be evidence of a paranoid ideation. If delusions are present they typically involve personal identity. These children may believe they are animals or cartoon characters. Hallucinations are rare before puberty. *Physical characteristics* include hypotonic muscles and decreased muscle power. Many of these children exhibit poor posture and abnormal gaits. They may exhibit a worried facial expression much of the time. Very often their skin remains soft and velvety (as in infancy) up through adolescence (Cantor, 1988).

The goal of treatment is to help schizophrenic children and their families learn to live and compensate for the behavioral, affective, cognitive, and physical deficits. The ideal treatment setting is within the public-school setting. A classroom of schizophrenic children should not contain more than six to eight children. The staff should consist of a special education teacher, a child psychiatric nurse, an occupational therapist, and a family therapist (Cantor, 1988).

Homelessness

Between 1955 and 1980 the state hospital populations were reduced from 559,000 to 132,000 (Riesdorph-Ostrow, 1989). With the deinstitutionalization of those with chronic mental illness such as schizophrenia, homelessness has become a problem. Poor systems of aftercare and community support add to the problem.

The homeless mentally ill are difficult to serve. They are usually unwilling or unlikely to seek out community mental health service. They are unlikely to seek outpatient service. The fact that they have no home makes them difficult to reach. Mental health services should be available to the homeless and perhaps should be a part of the community plan for shelter, food, and health care (Ryan, 1989). Chapter 17 discusses the problem of homelessness in detail.

Assessment

Nursing History

Data collection is the starting point of the nursing process for the schizophrenic client. Because of the client's deficits, it is sometimes difficult to use the client as the primary source of data. This is especially so for the delusional and hallucinating client. Family members and nursing observations may become primary data sources in assessing the schizophrenic client. Table 14–5 presents a guideline for recording observations related to disordered thoughts in the schizophrenic client.

Table 14–5 *Behavioral Observation Tool for Schizophrenic Clients*

Behaviors exhibited	*Yes*	*No*	*Frequency*
Delusions	☐	☐	
Auditory hallucinations	☐	☐	
Other hallucinations	☐	☐	
Loose associations	☐	☐	
Illogical thinking	☐	☐	
Incoherence	☐	☐	
Flat affect	☐	☐	
Other inappropriate affect	☐	☐	
Neglect in self-care	☐	☐	
Odd mannerisms	☐	☐	
Ideas of reference	☐	☐	
Bizarre thinking	☐	☐	
Autistic thoughts	☐	☐	
Suspiciousness	☐	☐	
Excitement	☐	☐	
Stupor	☐	☐	
Waxy flexibility	☐	☐	
Negativism	☐	☐	
Echolalia	☐	☐	
Stereotyped motor activity	☐	☐	
Voice tone	☐	☐	
Potential for violence	☐	☐	

A general nursing history (such as the history in Chapter 2) should be obtained as soon as the client is able to respond to questions. The information obtained from the general nursing history assists in planning initial nursing interventions.

Since schizophrenia is a multidimensional disorder and antipsychotic drugs affect several body systems, it is essential for the nurse to complete a focused nursing assessment specific to the schizophrenic client. The interview may take several sessions and will be based on a combination of observations and client answers. The focused nursing assessment for clients with schizophrenia follows.

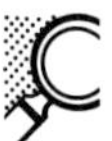

FOCUSED NURSING ASSESSMENT
for the Client with Schizophrenia

Behavioral Assessment

What is your usual pattern for activities of daily living?
- Is this a change from your previous level of functioning?
- How are you able to balance your work/household and leisure activities?

What do you do for leisure activities?

How do you relate to other people?
- When do you prefer to be alone?
- When do you prefer to be with others?
- What causes you to become upset with others?
- How do you resolve conflicts with others?

Affective Assessment

How do you emotionally react to stressful situations?
- When you are under stress, do you experience conflicting emotions? Describe them.
- What kinds of situations cause you to be angry?
- What kinds of situations cause you to be anxious?

Who are the people most significant to you?
- How many close friends do you have now? Have you had?
- When do you turn to friends?

Describe your usual mood.

What causes you to feel guilty?

Cognitive Assessment

Do you describe yourself as intellectual?
- When do you find decision making difficult?

When do you make decisions quickly? Slowly?
What decisions are easiest for you to make?
Have you ever heard voices?
Are you hearing voices now?
What do the voices say to you?
How do you feel when you hear these voices?
Have you ever seen things other people don't see?
What things do you see?
How do you feel when you see these things?
Have you ever felt anyone is deliberately trying to harm you?
Why do you think people try to harm you?
Have you been injured by others?
Have you ever thought about harming yourself?
Have you ever thought you were someone else?
Who were you?
What would you do if you found a wallet in the street?
What do the following statements mean: "A rolling stone gathers no moss" and "People in glass houses should not throw stones."

Physical Assessment
What physical symptoms worry you?
What do you do for headaches?
What do you do for muscle pains?
What do you do for indigestion?
What do you do for [other symptoms listed by client]?
Are you taking any medications?
What are these medications?
How do these medications help you?
What are your eating patterns?
How many meals do you eat a day? Snacks?
How much and what kind of fluid do you take each day?
Have you recently gained or lost weight? How much?
Is your mouth unusually dry? What do you do for this?
What is your usual sleeping pattern?
What disturbs your sleep?
How do you feel after sleeping?
How do you feel after activity?
What activities do you enjoy most? Least?
How often do you engage in sexual activities?
Have you experienced dizzy spells when you first get up?
Have you noticed any changes in your gait?
Have you experienced tremors in your hands? Other parts of the body?
How is your general health?
Have you experienced blurred vision?
What are your usual vital signs?
Have you had problems with constipation? What do you do for this?
Have you noticed any edema (swelling) of your hands or feet?
What mannerisms do you find annoying?
How is your perspiration compared to others?
Do you have trouble keeping your balance?
What kind of skin problems do you have?
Do you sunburn easily?
Have you noticed a yellow tint to your skin?
What kinds of rashes or irritations do you have?
Has your hair become dry?

Physical Assessment

General observations relative to the physical assessment of the schizophrenic begin when the vital signs are taken. The nurse should look for evidence of orthostatic hypotension and abnormal changes in the heart rate and blood pressure as possible indications of medication side effects. The client's general appearance is often unkempt. The client may exhibit strange motor activity, such as grimacing and erratic movements.

During acute episodes, the nurse needs to be alert for dilated pupils, elevated heart rate and blood pressure, excess perspiration, and general sympathetic excitement. Other physical findings in schizophrenia include disturbances in gait such as ataxia, disturbances in balance, hyperreflexia, sensory abnormalities, and parkinsonlike movements. In some schizophrenic women, hirsutism and amenorrhea occur. A diminished sex drive is a side effect of antipsychotic medication experienced by some clients of both sexes. In males, retarded ejaculation is most common; however, they may also report episodes of retrograde ejaculation or erectile problems (Hagerty, 1984; Townsend, 1990).

Considerations in Interviewing Schizophrenic Clients

Specific suggestions for interventions are found in nursing care plans later in this chapter. In general, however, nurses who interview schizophrenic clients should keep several considerations in mind.

Nurses should remember that since schizophrenic clients have disturbances in several areas of psychologic functioning, it is not uncommon to see two diagnosed schizophrenics with totally different symptoms. Being prepared for this variation assists the nurse in more thorough assessment.

Certain conflicts may appear as themes in the interview with a schizophrenic. One theme is the problem with personal identity. On the one hand, the client wishes to have a personal identity, but the fear of isolation or abandonment may block the client's reaching it. The client may view the nurse as an extension of an earlier relationship with a mother figure, which may arouse fears of a symbiotic merger. The resulting conflict within the client may leave the nurse feeling that whatever is said or done in the interview is wrong. Distortions in body image further complicate the theme of personal identity. It is not uncommon for the schizophrenic client to borrow an identity from someone else. The client may use the borrowed identity when conversing with the nurse, thereby complicating the interview process further.

A second theme common to the interview with a schizophrenic client is dependency. The schizophrenic client lacks adaptive coping skills and is often dependent on the assistance of others to gratify needs. The schizophrenic client may regress to a conflict between trust and mistrust. A lack of self-confidence further complicates the dependency theme. The fantasized, as well as the actual, helplessness perceived by the client leads to regressive behavior. Passivity and submissiveness may dominate an interview. This dependency makes it difficult for the client to establish any interpersonal contacts. The security and self-esteem derived from being independent eludes the schizophrenic client. The result may be ambivalence that can interfere with the client's participation in an interview.

The final theme is the struggle for power and control over the interview. The schizophrenic client maintains hostile feelings over the issues described in this section. The fear of expressing this hostility is suppressed, and expressed by apathy. To compensate for the feelings of inadequacy brought on by the suppressed rage, the client may attempt to control the interview. Also, the severe anxiety related to suppressed or repressed conflicts may cause the schizophrenic client to avoid any discussion of content that may tap the anxiety. Avoiding references to such content is another way the client can control the interview.

These conflicts make it difficult to establish rapport with the schizophrenic client. The nurse needs to be patient. Since the client's thinking is disorganized, effective communication in an interview becomes a task. It is important to consciously follow the conversation with the schizophrenic client. If the nurse becomes confused or angry with the client, it should not be ignored, for communication will further deteriorate, and the client will become anxious. Instead, the nurse needs to clarify any lack of understanding by saying something like, "I'm not following you." A crucial consideration in interviewing the schizophrenic client is to allow for secrecy and privacy, because the client has a great need for them. If this need, which is related to the client's problem with personal identity, is not met, the client may withdraw from the interview. (Coleman, Butcher, and Carson, 1984; Liberman, 1985; Sarason and Sarason, 1984; Schultz, 1985).

There is no specific set of rules and techniques that can be universally applied to interviewing schizophrenic clients. However, if the client is viewed as a troubled human being rather than a psychiatric problem, the outcome for both the nurse and the client is more positive. When the nurse tries to understand the world the client is experiencing, the client is more likely to feel that the nurse is helpful. The nurse should recognize that progress will be slow but can be gratified when a relationship based on trust and understanding has been developed.

The Importance of Developing a Trusting Relationship

A trusting relationship is important in dealing with clients experiencing psychiatric disorders. The trusting relationship is paramount with the schizophrenic, and establishing it is one of the nurse's primary interventions. From the nurse's first introduction to the client, it is essential to clarify and explain the roles within the therapeutic milieu of both the nurse and the client. For additional information on developing a therapeutic milieu, refer to Chapter 4.

The nurse must make the expectations for the relationship clear to the client. That means honesty becomes a priority. Glossing over or ignoring a client's bizarre behaviors is not part of that honesty.

The nurse should set specified periods to be spent with the client. Then consistency is necessary to maintain client security. Setting limits on unacceptable client behavior may be necessary as well. The nurse may find it useful to offer alternatives to the client when behavior is bizarre or unacceptable.

The nurse has a responsibility to help the client identify the problems that led to treatment or hospitalization. That responsibility includes assisting the client to vent feelings and learn more effective coping mechanisms.

Finally, the nurse should help the client plan for a support system, a follow-up treatment, or a rehabilitation program as needed to overcome maladaptive behaviors. The nurse's caring and efforts toward building a trusting relationship improve the client's progress toward recovery.

Table 14–6 *Nursing Diagnoses in the Acute Schizophrenic Client*

Anxiety
Communication, impaired verbal
Coping, ineffective individual
Diversional activity deficit
Family process, alteration in
Fear
Health maintenance, alteration in
Home maintenance management, impaired
Nutrition, alteration in: less than body requirements
Self-care deficit: feeding, bathing/hygiene, dressing/grooming, toileting
Self-concept, disturbance in: body image, self-esteem, role performance, personal identity
Sensory-perceptual alteration: visual, auditory, kinesthetic, gustatory, tactile, olfactory
Sleep pattern disturbance
Social interaction, impaired
Social isolation
Thought processes, alteration in
Violence, potential for

Nursing Diagnosis and Planning

The primary nursing diagnoses in this text are related to the psychiatric symptoms of schizophrenia. Those symptoms relate to the disrupted thoughts and perceptions of the client. (See Table 14–6 for a list of the nursing diagnoses in the acute schizophrenic client, Table 14–7 for a list of the diagnoses specific to each subtype of schizophrenia, and Table 14–8 for a list of diagnoses related to antipsychotic drugs.)

The nursing care plan for schizophrenic clients is based on nursing diagnoses identified for the specific client. Since establishing mutual goals for a client who may be out of contact with reality is a potential problem in planning care for the schizophrenic, it is necessary to review common nursing concerns. Initially, the nursing goal may be simply to ensure adequate rest for schizophrenic clients. Often, because clients may think they are on a mission of great importance, there is a high energy level at the beginning of an acute episode. The client, unable to filter external stimuli, assigns a personal meaning to everything in the environment. The nurse has to assume responsibility for meeting the client's physical needs until the client is able to assume self-care. Another common concern for the nurse of a schizophrenic is reducing anxiety, which may be profound in the client experiencing a psychotic episode for the first time. The nurse should focus on interventions to reduce anxiety.

Clients will need assistance at first in establishing control over their behavior. Assisting the client in maintaining control consists of setting firm limits, encouraging and rewarding self-control, and maintaining safety. Establishing a therapeutic rela-

Table 14–7 *Nursing Diagnoses for Specific Subtypes of Schizophrenia*

Disorganized
Communication, impaired verbal
Diversional activity, deficit
Injury, potential for: trauma
Nutrition, alteration in: less than body requirements
Social interaction, impaired
Thought processes, alteration in

Catatonic
Activity intolerance
Bowel elimination, alteration in: constipation
Communication, impaired verbal
Fluid volume deficit, potential
Injury, potential for: trauma
Mobility, impaired physical
Nutrition, alteration in: less than body requirements
Skin integrity impairment, potential for
Social interaction, impaired
Urinary elimination, alteration in patterns

Paranoid
Coping, ineffective individual
Knowledge deficit
Noncompliance
Nutrition, alteration in: less than body requirements
Sensory-perceptual alteration: visual, auditory, kinesthetic, gustatory, tactile, olfactory
Social isolation
Thought processes, alteration in
Violence, potential for: self-directed or directed at others

Undifferentiated
Communication, impaired verbal
Self-care deficit: feeding, bathing/hygiene, dressing/grooming, toileting
Self-concept, disturbance in: body image, self-esteem, role performance, personal identity
Social interaction, impaired

Residual
Coping, ineffective individual
Diversional activity deficit
Health maintenance, alteration in
Home maintenance management, impaired
Knowledge deficit
Noncompliance
Powerlessness
Social isolation

tionship is essential in planning the care of the schizophrenic client. To understand the client's conversation, the nurse needs to listen for themes in the client's communication. Because it may be difficult to understand the schizophrenic client, the nurse will need to use techniques for validating nurse-client communication.

Table 14–8 *Nursing Diagnoses Related to Antipsychotic Drugs*

Activity intolerance, potential for
Anxiety, potential
Bowel elimination, alteration in: constipation
Fluid volume deficit, potential for
Injury, potential for poisoning
Noncompliance due to fear of drug
Oral mucous membrane, alteration in
Sexual dysfunction
Skin integrity impairment, potential for
Sleep pattern disturbance
Urinary elimination, alteration in patterns

Medication compliance is a major factor in determining the client's ability to be in the community. Maintaining a medication schedule will assist the client in dealing with cognitive and perceptual distortions. The nurse must also teach social skills to assist the client in overcoming problems related to socialization (Plante, 1989).

Standard Care for the Client with Acute Schizophrenia

The care of the client having an acute schizophrenic episode might best be handled in an inpatient setting. For a client out of contact with reality, this is probably the safest environment. General nursing considerations for the client suffering from acute schizophrenia include

- Ensuring the client's safety
- Meeting the client's physical needs
- Instituting a therapeutic nurse-client relationship to assist the client in developing more constructive behaviors
- Reducing the client's anxiety
- Assisting the client in behavioral control by setting limits

(See Table 14–9 for the nursing care plan for the client with acute schizophrenia.)

Table 14–9 Nursing Care Plan for the Client with Acute Schizophrenia

Nursing Diagnosis: Anxiety related to feelings of diffuseness caused by reduced contact with reality.
Goal: During the course of treatment client will be able to reduce anxiety.

Intervention	*Rationale*	*Expected Outcome*
Assess level of anxiety	Will assist in identifying appropriate nursing interventions	Reduced anxiety
Extreme anxiety: • maintain a calm milieu • remove threats (eg, orient the client to time, place, and person) • remove client from environment if necessary • use short, simple sentences • administer antipsychotic drugs as ordered • remain calm and avoid reciprocal anxiety • use firm tone of voice • stay with client	Will assist in reducing anxiety and promoting contact with reality	Uses adaptive coping strategies to reduce anxiety Verbalizes no anxiety States name, date, and place correctly
Moderate anxiety: • assist client in recognizing presence of anxiety • have client identify thoughts before becoming anxious • teach client about problem solving, large muscle relaxation • do simple concrete tasks (eg, folding clothes) • go for a walk • encourage client in noncompetitive sports (eg, jogging)	Will assist client in developing insight into anxiety and develop adaptive coping skills	

Nursing Diagnosis: Impaired verbal communication related to multiple psychotic symptoms such as disorientation, reluctance to speak, inability to organize words, use of unfamiliar words, message inappropriate to context, false perceptions, inappropriate emotional expression, and imaginary perceptions.
Goal: During the course of treatment client will be able to reduce communication impairment.

Intervention	*Rationale*	*Expected Outcome*
Initiate a one-to-one relationship with client	Will assist client in obtaining appropriate input	Gives appropriate input (eg, client is oriented to time, place, and person)
Encourage client interactions: • increase language skills • modify language skills • correct faulty perceptions • client's expression of emotions	Will assist client in appropriately focusing communication	Communicates accurate perceptions Uses words appropriately (eg, no clang associations, embololalia, echolalia, etc.)
Use concrete, short, simple statements	Will reduce the stimuli to which client must respond and encourage appropriate responses	Presents appropriate affect

(Diagnosis continued)

Table 14–9 *(continued)*

Nursing Diagnosis *(continued)*: Impaired verbal communication related to multiple psychotic symptoms such as disorientation, reluctance to speak, inability to organize words, use of unfamiliar words, message inappropriate to context, false perceptions, inappropriate emotional expression, and imaginary perceptions.
Goal: During the course of treatment client will be able to reduce communication impairment.

Intervention	*Rationale*	*Expected Outcome*
Use therapeutic communication techniques: • reflection • validation • summarizing • clarification • stating observations • confrontation • providing feedback	Will assist in clarifying incongruent thoughts, preventing inaccurate assumptions, refocusing thinking, establishing understanding, correcting misperceptions	
Use active listening skills	Will assist in identifying misperceptions	
Be consistent in verbal and nonverbal behavior	Will assist client in learning more effective communication	

Nursing Diagnosis: Ineffective individual coping related to incorrect interpretation of environment and impaired communication skills.
Goal: During the course of treatment client will be able to develop new responses to emotional reactions.

Intervention	*Rationale*	*Expected Outcome*
Initiate a one-to-one relationship with client	Will assist client toward developing accurate appraisals of events	Interprets events accurately
Encourage client to describe daily events	Will assist in assessing client's perceptions	Sets clear, realistic goals
Encourage client to describe fears, angers, etc	Will assist client in developing an awareness of emotional reactions	Decreases regressive behavior
Set daily goals and expectations with client	Will assist client in coping with regressive behaviors	Communicates well enough to identify needs
Use directive approach with client	Too many choices increases client's anxiety	

Nursing Diagnosis: Deficit in diversional activity related to regressive behavior and social isolation.
Goal: During the course of treatment client will increase participation in diversional activities.

Intervention	*Rationale*	*Expected Outcome*
Assess client's ability to participate in activities	Will assist in identifying client's limitations	Client takes responsibility for diversional activity selection
Use one-to-one activities at first, gradually introduce group activities	Clients have difficulty with abstract concepts, competition, and maintaining attention	Observed doing activity
Encourage clients to choose a diversional activity based on ability level (eg, finger painting, modeling clay)	Will assist client in engaging in diversional activity	

(continued)

Table 14–9 *(continued)*

Nursing Diagnosis: Alteration in family process related to multiple disruptions such as system unable to meet emotional needs of members, inability to express feelings, members use distance to maintain homeostasis, use of member for scapegoating, failure to send and receive clear messages, and impaired communication.
Goal: During the course of treatment client will begin to alter communication when relating to family members.

Intervention	*Rationale*	*Expected Outcome*
Assess family structure and role relationships	Will assist in identifying peculiarities in family communication patterns	Mutual respect demonstrated between client and family members during visits
Assess: • family stressors • overt and covert rules • degree of interdependence • types of conflicts • discipline techniques	Will assist client in resolving alterations in family process	Client negotiates with family members Uses problem solving to identify family needs
Teach client about: • problem-solving skills • communication techniques • positive reinforcement for constructive family behaviors • medication compliance	Will assist client in changing communication patterns within family structure Will assist client in dealing with cognitive and perceptual distortions	Plans for follow-up treatment
Refer client and family for follow-up treatment	Will assist in resolving alterations in family structure	

Nursing Diagnosis: Fear related to reduced contact with reality.
Goal: During the course of treatment client will be able to reduce or prevent fear.

Intervention	*Rationale*	*Expected Outcome*
Assist client in identifying perceived dangers by: • indirect questioning • open-ended questions • verbalizing feelings • stressing ability to cope with danger	Will assist in reducing fear	Demonstrates no hallucinations States fears
Assist client in coping with fear(s): • stay with client • avoid overstimulation • engage in conversation • avoid acknowledging faulty perceptions (eg, hallucinations) • validate what is real and what is unreal • avoid arguing with client	Client will learn to rely on nurse for a sense of security	
Avoid situations that increase fear (eg, hallucinations)	Hallucinations are indicators that client is upset; however, nurse should only acknowledge client's being upset and clarify that he or she can't hear or see what client hears or sees	

(continued)

Table 14–9 *(continued)*

Nursing Diagnosis: Alteration in health maintenance related to inability to assume responsibility for meeting basic health practices.
Goal: During the course of treatment client will begin to assume responsibility for health maintenance.

Intervention	*Rationale*	*Expected Outcome*
Assess client's health maintenance knowledge and capabilities	Will assist in planning for the cognitive restructuring necessary for change in behavior	Identifies personal health goals
Use behavior modification techniques: • self-monitoring (recording behavior) • guided practice • cuing • tailoring • positive reinforcement • contracting	Will assist client in gaining control over inappropriate health practices	Controls thoughts related to maladaptive behaviors Identifies potential community resources
Provide information on community resources	Will assist client in developing a support system	Uses community resources

Nursing Diagnosis: Impaired home maintenance management related to reduced contact with reality.
Goal: During the course of treatment client will begin to adapt lifestyle to promote safety within home environment.

Intervention	*Rationale*	*Expected Outcome*
Assess client's home management skills	Will assist in identifying risk factors making it difficult for client to maintain the home	Identifies home maintenance as a problem
Assist client in planning for home maintenance: • teach roles • determine needed equipment • practice home maintenance skills • present available resources	Will assist client toward realistically performing daily home maintenance	Plans lifestyle adaptations Demonstrates home maintenance skills
Encourage client to participate in maintaining own area/room while under care	Will increase client awareness and ability in home maintenance skills	

Nursing Diagnosis: Alteration in nutrition: less than body requirements related to multiple factors such as unaware of hunger or thirst, apathy toward food, or fear of eating.
Goal: During the course of treatment client will identify factors interfering with nutritional intake.

Intervention	*Rationale*	*Expected Outcome*
Assess client's perceptions of food and nutrition	Will assist in identifying factors interfering with desire to eat	Adequate nutrition: • erect body posture • good skin turgor • clear skin • clear eyes • firm muscles • regular elimination • normal body weight • mental alertness • energy to perform tasks
When client is actively hallucinating: • get client's attention • offer client foods • give client directions on eating • give favorite foods • spoon-feed if necessary	Hallucinating client may not be able to complete simple skills like eating and may need directional support	

(Diagnosis continued)

Table 14–9 *(continued)*

Intervention	*Rationale*	*Expected Outcome*
Offer assistance to client in selecting foods: • high in calories • from each food group • with nutritional content (eg, don't offer dessert; offer fruit or gelatin)	Will aid client in maintaining an adequate calorie intake	Selects basic foods: • meats • milk • fruits • vegetables • breads
Offer foods in a manner appealing to client: • small meals • frequent meals • fluids and snacks between meals	Clients may not be able to tolerate stress of sitting in a group or taking a long time for meals	
Teach client about nutrition, when client is able to understand and process information	Knowledge of proper nutrition will assist client in overcoming nutrition deficits	

Nursing Diagnosis: Deficit in self-care: feeding, bathing/hygiene, dressing/grooming, toileting related to perceptual impairment and loss of contact with reality.

Goal: Before discharge client will assume control over self-care activities.

Intervention	*Rationale*	*Expected Outcome*
Assess client's self-care capabilities for feeding, bathing/hygiene, dressing/grooming, toileting	Will assist in planning physical care of client	Initiates eating and requires no assistance Initiates and completes own bath
Assist client with feeding, bathing, grooming, and personal hygiene as needed	Will assist client in learning appropriate skills and teach client to be more socially acceptable	Clean body, hair, nails, teeth Initiates and completes own grooming and dressing Wears appropriate attire, combs hair, etc
If deficits in any area, give client directions for completing care (eg, "Brush your teeth," "Wash your face," etc)	Will reduce psychotic symptoms and move client to a reality orientation	Uses toilet and cleans self No urine or fecal odor
Encourage client to initiate self-care activities	Client's self-esteem will be enhanced	
Acknowledge client's attempts to complete self-care activities	Positive feedback is important for maintaining client's participation in self-care activities	

Nursing Diagnosis: Disturbance in self-concept: body image, self-esteem, role performance, personal identity related to multiple factors such as feelings of depersonalization and derealization, self-depreciation, role ambivalence, and confusion about personal identity.

Goal: During the course of treatment client will regain ego boundaries.

Intervention	*Rationale*	*Expected Outcome*
Assess client's perceptions of self-concept	Will assist in identifying the defining characteristics of client's reduced self-concept	Decrease in subjective manifestations Improved mental functioning

(Diagnosis continued)

Table 14–9 *(continued)*

Nursing Diagnosis *(continued)*: Disturbance in self-concept: body image, self-esteem, role performance, personal identity related to multiple factors such as feelings of depersonalization and derealization, self-depreciation, role ambivalence, and confusion about personal identity.
Goal: During the course of treatment client will regain ego boundaries.

Intervention	*Rationale*	*Expected Outcome*
Initiate a one-to-one relationship built on trust and caring	Sincere interest will assist client in building self-esteem	Oriented to reality Participation in therapy
Provide a structured environment that is quiet and nonstimulating	A structured setting increases client's chances for success	
Assist client in discriminating between the real and unreal in the environment	Will assist client in reintegrating ego functions within reality	
Encourage client to participate in all treatment modalities (eg, medication therapy, group therapy, etc)		
Encourage client contact with others: • one-to-one contact first, then • small groups, then • community groups		
Demonstrate respect for client	Will increase client's feelings of self-worth and build self-confidence	
Acknowledge achievements (eg, wearing new clothes)	Will assist client in maintaining a positive self-image	

Nursing Diagnosis: Alteration in senses and perception: visual, auditory, kinesthetic, gustatory, tactile, olfactory related to inaccurate interpretation of stimuli.
Goal: During the course of treatment client will be able to decrease or eliminate hallucinations.

Intervention	*Rationale*	*Expected Outcome*
Assess environmental stimuli for: • intensity • quantity • movement • change • clarity • ambiguity • incongruity	Will assist in removing any stimuli fostering client's disordered thought processes	Increased orientation to reality Knows person, time, and place No hallucinations Stable emotional tone
Recognize and reduce environmental stimuli that may be misinterpreted; remove client from room if necessary	Television, stereos, etc may increase hallucinations	Appropriate verbal feedback and behavior in relation to perceptions of stimuli
Use direct, concrete terms with client	Use of abstract ideas may add to client confusion	No bizarre behavior
Maintain verbal contact, eye contact, touch; with paranoid client, avoid touch	Will assist client in maintaining contact with reality	
Structure routines	Will assist in eliminating extraneous stimuli from environment	

(Diagnosis continued)

Table 14–9 *(continued)*

Intervention	*Rationale*	*Expected Outcome*
Orient to reality: • address client by name • repeat self-introduction as needed • state time regularly • have clock in plain view • regularly state location • state date • have calendar in plain view • explain routines and policies • interpret sights, sounds, and smells in the environment		

Nursing Diagnosis: Impaired social interaction related to inability to establish supportive relationships as a result of schizophrenic symptoms.
Goal: Attempts to initial interactions with others.

Intervention	*Rationale*	*Expected Outcome*
Limit the number of care givers assigned to the client	Will assist the client in developing trust	Responds positively to care giver by eye contact during conversation.
Encourage client to participate in interactions with others	Will establish a reality-based environment	Attempts to talk to others
Be available as a support person when client attempts to interact with others	Will provide a feeling of security as the client attempts a new venture	Can interact for short periods

Nursing Diagnosis: Social isolation related to multiple factors such as hallucinations, depersonalization, unacceptable social behavior, and mistrust.
Goal: During the course of treatment client will be able to reduce or eliminate social isolation.

Intervention	*Rationale*	*Expected Outcome*
Establish a trusting one-to-one relationship with client: • convey trust in client • encourage client regarding improvement • recognize client's fears of interpersonal closeness • maintain appropriate distance from client • make visits brief (10 minutes), gradually increase amount of time spent together • speak slowly • let client know when you are leaving and when you are returning • use silence as a therapeutic technique • do not push client to talk	Will assist client in maintaining contact with others and prevent further withdrawal	Identifies feelings of isolation Verbalizes fears about relating with others No hallucinations Participates in conversations with nurse Participates in conversations with others Attends occupational therapy
Assess social history	Will assist in planning nursing interventions	

(Diagnosis continued)

Table 14–9 *(continued)*

Nursing Diagnosis *(continued)*: Social isolation related to multiple factors such as hallucinations, depersonalization, unacceptable social behavior, and mistrust.
Goal: During the course of treatment client will be able to reduce or eliminate social isolation.

Intervention	*Rationale*	*Expected Outcome*
Observe for hallucinations. When hallucinations occur: • sit with client • engage client in some type of activity to distract from hallucination • make comments at intervals to gain client's attention • medicate as ordered • listen to hallucinatory content and focus client on content related to actual events	Reducing and/or eliminating hallucinations prevents client from withdrawing from social contact	
Client teaching for social skills: • how to make conversation • how to make requests from others • participation in occupational therapy as ordered	Will encourage client to build a new set of social behaviors and decrease isolation from others	

Nursing Diagnosis: Alteration in thought processes related to inaccurate interpretations of stimuli.
Goal: During the course of treatment client will develop accurate interpretations of reality.

Intervention	*Rationale*	*Expected Outcome*
Assess client's perceptions of reality	Will assist in identifying hallucinations, ideas of reference, delusions, and other disrupted thought patterns	Clear conversations Reduced generalizations
Use active listening: • listen to verbal and nonverbal communication • analyze communication patterns (eg, loose associations, echolalia, etc) • identify themes • identify feeling tone • identify reality-oriented ideas		No hallucinations No delusions No ideas of reference Expression of thoughts and feelings in group settings
Use communication techniques to clarify reality: • clarify generalizations • explore deletions • challenge distortions • assist client in elaborating on reality-oriented ideas • correct misconceptions • avoid reinforcing ideas of reference or delusions • use clear, direct terms • avoid generalizations • avoid whispered comments • focus on real things and real people	Will assist client in realistically and constructively interpreting reality	Increased contact and conversations with others

(Diagnosis continued)

Table 14–9 *(continued)*

Intervention	*Rationale*	*Expected Outcome*
• do not let client think you understand delusions; let client know you are trying to understand • comment on understandable conversation		
Administer medications as ordered	Antipsychotic drugs reduce psychotic symptoms, making client more amenable to other therapy	
Assist client in developing positive relationships with others: • provide group experiences (when client is ready) • encourage client to express wants and needs • help client examine effect of behavior on others	Will assist client in experiencing reality in a controlled setting	

Nursing Diagnosis: Disturbance in sleep pattern related to anxiety and fear resulting from loss of contact with reality.
Goal: Client will sleep for 4–6 hours.

Intervention	*Rationale*	*Expected Outcome*
Assess factors related to client's sleep pattern disturbance: • fears about going to sleep • misperceptions of environment (eg, shadows on the wall) • daytime naps • amount and type of antipsychotic drugs (give at bedtime unless contraindicated)	Loss of contact with reality increases client's anxiety and fear at night Divided doses will interfere with sleep and alertness; H.S. dose will assist client in sleeping	Able to fall asleep without using sleeping medications Expresses no fear of going to sleep Sleeps for 4–6 hours without disruption
Assist client to relax: • offer warm beverage (eg, warm milk) • encourage slow, deep breathing • turn on soft, soothing music • decrease lighting to reduce shadows • maintain temperate climate	Will create a setting conducive to sleep	No symptoms of inefficient sleep (eg, yawning, tired appearance) States satisfaction with sleep

Nursing Diagnosis: Potential for violence: self-directed or directed at others related to misperceived messages from others.
Goal: During the course of treatment client will be able to reduce or eliminate violent behavior.

Intervention	*Rationale*	*Expected Outcome*
Assess client's potential for violence, both self-directed and directed at others	Will assist in planning for client safety	Self-control Builds trusting relationship
Establish a trusting relationship with client: • be honest • be clear, concise • maintain a stable environment • establish short-term goals with client • follow through	Will convey empathy and concern to client	Verbalizes fears, frustration, anger, etc No episodes of dangerous behavior Uses thought expressions rather than physical expressions

(Diagnosis continued)

Table 14–9 *(continued)*

Nursing Diagnosis *(continued)*: Potential for violence: self-directed or directed at others related to misperceived messages from others.
Goal: During the course of treatment client will be able to reduce or eliminate violent behavior.

Intervention	*Rationale*	*Expected Outcome*
For self-directed harm establish precautions: • remove harmful objects from the environment • closely observe client • know client's whereabouts	Will maintain client safety	Participates in therapy
For harm directed at others: • encourage client to talk instead of act out physically • be a role model (eg, be calm, verbalize feelings) • remove items that can be used as weapons • set limits on aggressive behavior and episodes • use seclusion if necessary	Will assist in eliminating potential for violent behavior	
Use methods to decrease agitation: • replace aggression with physical activity • administer medications as ordered • maintain one-to-one interaction • avoid touching client unless you explain rationale • remain calm • allow client to maintain personal space	Will assist in reducing factors precipitating violent behavior	

Antipsychotic drugs are so commonly given that the nurse needs to be aware of specific nursing actions that will enhance the client's compliance to treatment. (See Table 14–10 for the nursing care plan for the client taking antipsychotic drugs.)

Tables 14–11 through 14–15 offer nursing diagnoses and care specifically related to each subtype of schizophrenia.

Evaluation

The nurse evaluates care of the schizophrenic client by comparing the client's progress to established goals. When discrepancies are noted, the nurse looks at the outcomes for clues to alter the plan. It may be necessary to alter strategies and interventions to meet client needs better.

In caring for schizophrenic clients, small setbacks are not uncommon. The nurse continually refocuses on assisting the client in developing a better self-image. The process of dealing with schizophrenics is long-term, so the nurse needs to show patience in evaluating the effectiveness of interventions. It is wise to keep expectations simple and develop short-term objectives.

It may be necessary to contact other staff members when evaluating the care of the schizophrenic client. Evaluation conferences add data on which to plan care more effectively. Retrospective analysis may be necessary to locate evidence in client's records of behavior changes. The client's physiologic responses are readily apparent by observation and documentation. Using these data, the nurse is able to determine the client's appropriate response to stimuli.

Consideration should be given to specifically stating goals in behavioral terms. The concreteness will reduce stress for the client while encouraging the nursing staff when progress is noted. (See Table 14–16 for an evaluation of the care of a client with schizophrenia.)

Table 14–10 Nursing Care Plan for the Client Taking Antipsychotic Drugs

Nursing Diagnosis: Potential activity intolerance related to side effects of medication such as orthostatic hypotension or sedation.
Goal: Client will be able to develop a regular routine for activity while taking antipsychotic drugs.

Intervention	*Rationale*	*Expected Outcome*
Assess effects and side effects of antipsychotic medications taken by client	Will provide data for planning appropriate interventions	No sedation No dizziness on arising
Teach client about the effects and side effects of antipsychotic drugs	Client's knowledge of drugs will assist in identifying activities to avoid (eg, operating equipment)	Active participation in daily routine
Encourage client to report side effects of antipsychotic drugs	Will assist in planning for an optimal level of functioning	
Teach client about behaviors to reduce side effects of antipsychotic drugs: • gradual increase in activity • rising slowly from prone or sitting position • dangle feet while sitting	Assists in avoiding dizziness due to orthostatic hypotension	
Establish a daily routine within client's physical limitations	Will assist in overcoming the side effects of antipsychotic drugs	
Monitor client for signs of orthostatic hypotension: • dizziness or fainting when arising from prone or sitting position • tachycardia when arising from prone or sitting position • drop in BP with change in position		

Nursing Diagnosis: Potential anxiety related to the development of extrapyramidal side effects of antipsychotic drugs.
Goal: During the course of treatment client will be able to reduce anxiety by identifying extrapyramidal effects of antipsychotic drugs.

Intervention	*Rationale*	*Expected Outcome*
Assess client for signs of extrapyramidal effects: • tremor • masklike facial expression • rigidity • drooling • restlessness	Early recognition of extrapyramidal side effects can reduce or eliminate anxiety related to frightening nature of symptoms	Reduced anxiety No extrapyramidal effects Reduced extrapyramidal effects

(Diagnosis continued)

Table 14–10 *(continued)*

Nursing Diagnosis *(continued)*: Potential anxiety related to the development of extrapyramidal side effects of antipsychotic drugs.
Goal: During the course of treatment client will be able to reduce anxiety by identifying extrapyramidal effects of antipsychotic drugs.

Intervention	*Rationale*	*Expected Outcome*
• fatigue • abnormal posturing • perioral spasms with tongue protrusion • mandibular movements • weakness in arms and legs • continually moving hands, mouth, and body • opisthotonos		
Reassure client that extrapyramidal effects are reversible	Will assist in reducing the anxiety created by frightening symptoms	
Teach client about extrapyramidal effects of antipsychotic drugs: • pseudoparkinsonism • dystonias • akathisia • dyskinesia		
Administer medications as ordered to reverse extrapyramidal reaction	Antiparkinson agents (eg, Cogentin) may produce a reversal of symptoms	

Nursing Diagnosis: Alteration in bowel elimination: constipation related to side effects of antipsychotic drugs.
Goal: Client will develop a regular pattern of bowel elimination while taking antipsychotic drugs.

Intervention	*Rationale*	*Expected Outcome*
Monitor client's patterns of elimination: • record stools • maintain I & O record • observe for abdominal distention	Will assist in recognition of potential problem with constipation	Eats bulk foods Drinks eight to ten glasses of water a day
Prevent constipation by encouraging: • bulk in diet • adequate fluid intake • regular exercise appropriate for client's physiologic state • use of laxatives when other measures are ineffective	Diet, fluids, and exercise assist in developing regular bowel patterns	Maintains a daily exercise regimen Bowel movements at least every 3 days No habitual use of laxatives

Nursing Diagnosis: Deficit in fluid volume related to side effects of antipsychotic drugs such as dry mouth, nausea, vomiting, diaphoresis, etc.
Goal: Client will be able to achieve fluid replacement while on antipsychotic drugs.

Intervention	*Rationale*	*Expected Outcome*
Monitor: • vital signs • client weight • skin turgor • I & O • electrolyte values	Will assist in identifying need for fluid replacement	Vital signs in normal limits Good skin turgor Moist mucous membranes No thirst

(Diagnosis continued)

Table 14–10 *(continued)*

Intervention	*Rationale*	*Expected Outcome*
Teach client about: • actions to prevent fluid deficits • what foods and fluids to take (eg, oranges, orange juice, bananas) • what food and fluids to avoid (eg, coffee, caffeinated drinks)	Will be able to prevent development of actual fluid deficit by involving client in self-monitoring	Balanced intake and output Electrolyte values within normal limits Can explain actions to prevent fluid loss

Nursing Diagnosis: Potential for injury: poisoning related to overuse of antipsychotic drugs.
Goal: Client will state correct dose and time for taking antipsychotic drugs while under treatment.

Intervention	*Rationale*	*Expected Outcome*
Assess client's cognitive ability and decision-making ability	If client is unable to understand, nurse should seek out a family member to be responsible for giving client antipsychotic medications	States dosage, times for administration, and side effects of antipsychotic drugs prescribed
Provide information on all antipsychotic medications ordered for the client: • dosage • administration • side effects	Client understanding will decrease the possibility of incorrect dosage	No over- or underuse of antipsychotic drugs

Nursing Diagnosis: Deficit in knowledge related to preventing undesirable side effects of antipsychotic drugs.
Goal: Client will demonstrate increased understanding of antipsychotic drugs while undergoing drug therapy.

Intervention	*Rationale*	*Expected Outcome*
Include information on antipsychotic drugs as part of discharge planning: • explain importance of regular blood work • explain importance of eye examinations • cite signs and symptoms of side effects to report	Laboratory tests on blood will assist in identifying agranulocytosis, etc Eye tests will assist in identifying pigmented retinopathy	States signs and symptoms of side effects of antipsychotic drugs Has regular laboratory blood tests Has regular eye examinations

Nursing Diagnosis: Noncompliance related to fear of drug actions.
Goal: Client's fear of antipsychotic drugs will be reduced after explanation of purpose for medication.

Intervention	*Rationale*	*Expected Outcome*
Assess client's understanding of purpose for antipsychotic drugs	Will assist in identifying alterations in client's perceptions regarding antipsychotic medications	Client will take antipsychotic drugs as ordered
Encourage client to monitor behavior and misconceptions about drugs	Will assist in alleviating fears related to use of antipsychotic drugs	Accurate perceptions and conceptions about drugs

(Diagnosis continued)

Table 14–10 *(continued)*

Nursing Diagnosis: *(continued)*: Noncompliance related to fear of drug actions.
Goal: Client's fear of antipsychotic drugs will be reduced after explanation of purpose for medication.

Intervention	*Rationale*	*Expected Outcome*
Correct client's misperceptions and misconceptions about drugs	Expresses feelings and beliefs about antipsychotic medications	
Provide information on antipsychotic drugs (eg, specific drug and what it will do)		

Nursing Diagnosis: Alteration in oral mucous membrane related to side effects of antipsychotic drugs such as tardive dyskinesia.
Goal: Client will maintain adequate hydration while taking antipsychotic drugs.

Intervention	*Rationale*	*Expected Outcome*
Assess oral mucosa	Will assist in determining presence of dry mucous membranes	Good oral color
Monitor I&O		Moist mucous membranes
Check urine specific gravity		Takes 8–10 glasses of water daily
Encourage adequate fluid intake, 8–10 glasses of water a day	Will assist client in achieving adequate hydration	Intake congruent with output
		Urine specific gravity within normal limits: 1.001–1.040
Explain side effects of antipsychotic drugs	Will reinforce importance of adequate fluid intake	
Provide hard sugarless candy or gum	Will increase salivation and moisture in oral cavity	
	Sugarless candy and gum will prevent cavities and prevent weight gain	
Lubricate lips	Will prevent skin breakdown of lips	
Encourage oral hygiene	Will maintain normal function of mucous membranes	
Observe for signs and symptoms of water intoxication	Some clients overhydrate when taking antipsychotic drugs	

Nursing Diagnosis: Sexual dysfunction related to side effects of antipsychotic drugs.
Goal: Client will be able to relate sexual dysfunction to side effects of antipsychotic drugs.

Intervention	*Rationale*	*Expected Outcome*
Assess client's understanding of sexual functions	Client may not know normal sexual functions	Reports no concern over sexual function
Provide information on specific effects of antipsychotic drugs on sexual function	Will assist in reducing stress related to concerns about sexual functioning	States specific side effects of antipsychotic drugs related to sexual function
Suggest client inform physician about problems with sexual function	Changes in medications can often relieve symptoms of sexual dysfunction	

(continued)

Table 14–10 *(continued)*

Nursing Diagnosis: Potential impairment of skin integrity related to side effects of antipsychotic drugs.
Goal: Client will protect skin when planning to be in the sun while taking antipsychotic drugs.

Intervention	*Rationale*	*Expected Outcome*
Assess client's skin: • color • texture • irritation • abrasions, etc	Will assist in identifying disruptions in skin integrity	Verbalizes understanding of photosensitivity Uses protective measures for skin against sun
Explain potential for photosensitivity	Antipsychotic drugs increase sensitivity to sunburn	No sunburns No loss of skin integrity
Encourage client to use: • broad-brimmed hats • umbrellas • long sleeves • sun block		

Nursing Diagnosis: Disturbance in sleep pattern related to antipsychotic drugs interrupting sleep.
Goal: Client will sleep 6–8 hours at night.

Intervention	*Rationale*	*Expected Outcome*
Establish a regular bedtime routine: • establish regular rising and retiring time • go to bed only when sleepy • if unable to fall asleep within 30 minutes, get out of bed and complete some type of activity	Will assist in establishing a regular sleep pattern supportive of client's circadian rhythms	Reports sleeping 6–8 hours No naps States satisfaction with sleep
Establish a daily routine conducive to satisfactory sleep: • no naps • eliminate caffeine from diet • avoid alcohol • exercise regularly • eat regular meals • avoid spicy foods	Diet, exercise, and medications affect normal sleep patterns	

Nursing Diagnosis: Alteration in urinary elimination pattern related to urinary retention caused by side effects of antipsychotic drugs.
Goal: Client will be able to monitor voiding pattern while taking antipsychotic drugs.

Intervention	*Rationale*	*Expected Outcome*
Teach client to: • monitor hydration • monitor voiding pattern • establish voiding schedule • methods to promote micturition (eg, adequate fluid intake)	Client understanding of normal functions will assist in maintaining a regular pattern of voiding and prevent urinary retention	No urinary retention Intake congruent with output

Table 14–11 Nursing Care Plan for the Client with Disorganized Schizophrenia

Nursing Diagnosis: Impaired verbal communication related to blunted, inappropriate, or silly affect and incoherent, disorganized behavior.
Goal: During the course of treatment client will demonstrate improved communication patterns.

Intervention	*Rationale*	*Expected Outcome*
Assess affect and communication patterns, both verbal and nonverbal	Will assist in identifying appropriate therapeutic communication techniques	Affect congruent with situation
Clarify client's disturbances in communication (eg, symbolic words, actions, etc)	Clarification will assist in deciphering client's meaning and give clues to thoughts and feelings	Use of appropriate communication Behavior congruent with situation
Avoid reinforcing inappropriate affect: • no smiling or laughing at odd behavior • avoid nodding • avoid anger at client's mannerisms	Amusement or disgust at client's bizarre behavior and communication creates a nonsupportive and nontherapeutic environment	Responds to relevant stimuli

Nursing Diagnosis: Deficit in diversional activity related to disorganized behavior.
Goal: During the course of treatment client will engage in appropriate level of diversional activity.

Intervention	*Rationale*	*Expected Outcome*
Assess activity pattern: • observe for excessive activity • observe for social withdrawal • odd behaviors (eg, tics) • grimaces	Will assist in identifying client's ability to participate in diversional activity	Reduction in odd behaviors such as grimaces, mannerisms, etc Completion of tasks Reduced random activity and disorganized behavior Completes daily routines
Structure daily routine: • limit client's environment • set limits on client's behavior • remove excess stimuli	Will provide for client safety and enhance client's sense of security	
Choose a diversional activity that is: • meaningful to client • simple enough not to frustrate client • within the client's capabilities	Focusing client on meaningful and realistic activities will reduce psychotic symptoms	
Give positive feedback on client's accomplishments	Will encourage client to engage in appropriate diversional activity	

Nursing Diagnosis: Potential for injury: trauma related to bizarre behavior.
Goal: During the course of treatment client will experience no injuries.

Intervention	*Rationale*	*Expected Outcome*
Identify hazards in environment: • stairs • windows • harmful objects	Removing physical risks reduces the potential for injury	No injuries Recognizes factors that increase risk for injury

(Diagnosis continued)

Table 14–11 *(continued)*

Intervention	*Rationale*	*Expected Outcome*
Supervise client's activity	Will ensure client does not become agitated	
Monitor: • mood • temperament • stress level	Will reduce risk of injury	
Provide protective measures if necessary (eg, seclusion)	Will protect client from injury	

Nursing Diagnosis: Alteration in nutrition: less than body requirements related to excessive activity increasing the body's demand for nutrients.
Goal: During the course of treatment client will modify activity level to obtain enough nutrients to maintain body function.

Intervention	*Rationale*	*Expected Outcome*
Weigh weekly	Will assist in monitoring weight loss	Normal weight level for body build
Provide foods in appropriate form for client: • small, frequent feedings • finger foods • favorite foods • high-protein, high-calorie foods • foods easy to swallow and easy to chew • liquid supplements (eg, Ensure)	Will provide adequate intake of nutrients	Good skin turgor Clear skin Firm muscles Mental alertness Energy level adequate to perform ADLs

Nursing Diagnosis: Alteration in thought processes related to nonthematic hallucinations and fragmentary delusions.
Goal: During the course of treatment client will develop constructive interpretations of reality.

Intervention	*Rationale*	*Expected Outcome*
Assess potential for aggressive behavior	When clients are out of contact with reality, they may act out as a means of self-defense	Verbalizations clear
Assess client's representations of reality: • observe for fragmentation • presence of themes • loose associations	Will assist in understanding client's bizarre thoughts and behaviors	Oriented to reality, to time, place, and person No hallucinations No delusions
Avoid accepting distortions of reality: • confront distortions • clarify misperceptions • focus on real things and real people	Will assist in refocusing client's thoughts	Able to problem solve
Encourage client to relate positively with others: • validate thoughts • validate feelings • expression of feelings	Will assist client in gaining control over distorted thoughts	

Table 14–12 Nursing Care Plan for the Client with Catatonic Schizophrenia

Nursing Diagnosis: Activity intolerance related to emotional status affecting psychomotor function.
Goal: During the course of treatment client will develop activity pattern.

Intervention	*Rationale*	*Expected Outcome*
Assess disruption in psychomotor function: • stupor • negativism • rigidity • excitement • posturing	Will assist in planning nursing interventions to alter activity level	Appropriate posture Attempts to participate in self-care No cyanosis in body or extremities No waxy flexibility
Assess for: • patchy cyanosis in body or extremities • waxy flexibility of extremities • hypostatic edema	Client remaining in one position for long periods affects physiologic function	
Administer antipsychotic medications as ordered	Will make client more amenable to "talk" therapy	
Passive exercise if necessary	Will assist in maintaining adequate mobility	
Suggest modifications for disruption in activity: • sit with client • attempt to involve client in self-care activities • make client get out of bed		

Nursing Diagnosis: Alteration in bowel elimination: constipation related to decreased activity level and immobility.
Goal: During the course of treatment client will alter behavior to prevent constipation.

Intervention	*Rationale*	*Expected Outcome*
Assess: • abdominal distention • bowel sounds • frequency of stools • volume of stools • straining to pass stool • swollen rectal veins	Will assist in identifying presence of constipation	Eats bulk in diet Takes 8–10 glasses of water a day Participates in at least a 15-minute walk daily
Monitor I & O		Verbalizes urge to defecate
Encourage: • bulk in diet • daily fluid intake • no posturing, rigidity	Will prevent constipation	Bowel movement at least every 3 days
Give laxatives and enemas as ordered	Will assist in repatterning the bowel	

(continued)

Table 14–12 *(continued)*

Nursing Diagnosis: Impaired verbal communication related to reliance on nonverbal communication and mutism.
Goal: During the course of treatment client will be able to resolve impaired communication.

Intervention	*Rationale*	*Expected Outcome*
Initiate a one-to-one relationship	Demonstrating genuine care and concern for client encourages attempts to verbalize	Attempts to communicate with others No mutism
Assess communication patterns: • echolalia • echopraxia • muteness	Will assist in determining type of catatonic reaction, withdrawn or excited	No inappropriate patterns (eg, echolalia, echopraxia) Understandable messages
Use therapeutic techniques of communication: • focusing • validation • silence • clarification • stating observations • providing feedback	Will assist in encouraging client to communicate appropriately	
Attempt to engage client in conversations: • sit with client • encourage client's self expression • point out odd nonverbal behaviors • point out misinterpreted verbal attempts		

Nursing Diagnosis: Potential deficit in fluid volume related to altered fluid intake.
Goal: During the course of treatment client will increase fluid intake.

Intervention	*Rationale*	*Expected Outcome*
Monitor: • vital signs • weight • skin turgor • I & O • electrolyte values • urine specific gravity	Will assist in assessing adequate fluid intake	Normal vital signs Good skin turgor Mucous membranes moist
Offer fluids frequently: • offer juices preferred by client • offer fluids each time with client • administer IV fluids as ordered, if necessary	Will maintain fluid replacement	Congruent intake and output Major electrolytes within normal limits: Na: 135–145 mEq/L K: 3.5–5.0 mEq/L Cl: 100–106 mEq/L HCO_3: 20–30 mEq/L Urine specific gravity: 1.001–1.035

(continued)

Table 14–12 *(continued)*

Nursing Diagnosis: Potential for injury: trauma related to developmental level being inappropriate for environment.
Goal: During the course of treatment client will have no injuries.

Intervention	*Rationale*	*Expected Outcome*
Assess environment for potential dangers (eg, heating vents, stairs, etc)	Will assist in reducing the risks for injury	Demonstrates new methods for coping with emotions
Assess client's behavior: • negativistic • passive cooperation • automatic obedience • posturing • rigidity • enraged • destructive	Will assist in identifying psychomotor factors increasing the risk of injury	No posturing No rigidity No excitable episodes No injuries
Teach client skills for avoiding injury	Will assist in preventing injury	
Use protective measures: • restraints if necessary • seclusion (for excited client) • side rails up • bed in low position		

Nursing Diagnosis: Impaired physical mobility related to refusal to attempt to move.
Goal: Client will return to normal musculoskeletal function before discharge.

Intervention	*Rationale*	*Expected Outcome*
Assess: • posturing • rigidity • presence of edema • vital signs • lung sounds	Will assist in identifying alterations in musculoskeletal functions, cardiovascular functions, etc	Normal ROM for all joints Demonstration of muscle strength Participates in self-care activities Normal vital signs
ROM two to three times a day Work through movements with client Attempt to change client's position at least every 2 hours	Will assist in maintaining normal musculoskeletal function during acute psychotic period	Clear lungs No pedal edema Normal venous return No posturing
Suggest movements to client	Clients may automatically respond to requests	No rigidity

Nursing Diagnosis: Alteration in nutrition: less than body requirements related to lack of interest in food.
Goal: Client will take in adequate nutrients to maintain body function.

Intervention	*Rationale*	*Expected Outcome*
Assess: • ability to chew and swallow • willingness to ingest food	Will assist in planning strategies for feeding client	Intake of at least 1200–1500 calories daily Good skin turgor

(Diagnosis continued)

Table 14–12 *(continued)*

Intervention	*Rationale*	*Expected Outcome*
Provide foods in form appropriate for client: • soft • finger foods • high-protein liquids	Foods easily ingested are more likely to be taken by client	Clear skin Clear eyes Firm muscles No weight loss
Feed client if necessary	Will ensure adequate nutrients to maintain body function	
Monitor weight, at least weekly; daily, if necessary		
Insert NG tube as ordered if necessary	May be necessary when client exhibits negativism and refuses attempts at feeding	

Nursing Diagnosis: Potential impairment of skin integrity related to physical immobility.
Goal: During the course of treatment client will have no skin breakdowns.

Intervention	*Rationale*	*Expected Outcome*
Assess skin daily for: • turgor • reddened areas • broken areas • bruised areas • blisters • edema	Will assist in identifying impairments in skin integrity	Skin warm and dry to touch Good color Adequate turgor Adequate moisture
Maintain adequate circulation: • change client's position at least every 2 hours • ROM • massage feet and hands (avoid massaging legs) • place support stockings if necessary		
Protect skin: • keep clean and dry • lubricate skin with oil or lotion	Clean and adequately lubricated skin is less likely to break down	

Nursing Diagnosis: Alteration in urinary elimination pattern related to retention and refusal to urinate.
Goal: Client will return to normal pattern of urinary elimination by the time of discharge.

Intervention	*Rationale*	*Expected Outcome*
Assess and monitor: • hydration • I & O • voiding pattern	Will assist in maintaining as normal a pattern as possible	Voids at least 1000–1500 cc daily Intake congruent with output
Establish voiding schedule	Will remind client of need to urinate	
Catheterize as ordered if necessary	Will prevent urinary retention	

Table 14–13 Nursing Care Plan for the Client with Paranoid Schizophrenia

Nursing Diagnosis: Ineffective individual coping related to inaccurate appraisal of threats.
Goal: During the course of treatment client will be able to develop alternative responses to suspicious behaviors.

Intervention	*Rationale*	*Expected Outcome*
Initiate a one-to-one relationship with client Encourage client to explore perceptions of events	Will give nurse an opportunity to refocus incorrect interpretations of events	Accurate appraisal of events No delusions No hallucinations Appropriate expression of feelings No violent behavior Use of problem solving, decision making, and other new coping skills
Give feedback on behaviors observed and feelings expressed by client	Will assist client in developing an awareness of emotional responses	
Assist client in identifying the needed behavioral changes	Will assist client in developing new coping responses to stress	
Teach client: • problem solving • decision making • goal setting • evaluation skills • relaxation techniques	Will assist client in developing plans for change	
Involve client in diversional activities	Will assist client in reducing anxiety	

Nursing Diagnosis: Deficit in knowledge related to cognitive impairment or thought disorder.
Goal: Client will verbalize knowledge of diagnosis by the time of discharge.

Intervention	*Rationale*	*Expected Outcome*
Assess level of knowledge deficit	Will assist in determining what client needs to learn	Can explain diagnosis Participates in treatment regimen
Start with client's perception of illness: • does client know medical diagnosis • what does client understand about diagnosis	Will assist in decreasing knowledge deficit	
Give clear, concise information and directions		
Check with client for understanding of information and directions		
Teach client to gain control over illness		

Nursing Diagnosis: Noncompliance related to alterations in thought processes.
Goal: Client will attempt to respond appropriately to questions or situation.

Intervention	*Rationale*	*Expected Outcome*
Initiate a one-to-one relationship	Will offer a sense of security to client	Participates in therapy (eg, goes to group, takes medications, etc)

(Diagnosis continued)

Table 14–13 *(continued)*

Intervention	*Rationale*	*Expected Outcome*
After establishing trust in staff, gradually encourage participation in groups: • use reminders • use prompts • use cues	Will assist client in demonstrating appropriate behavior	Expresses feelings appropriately
Take care in administering medications: • explain the purpose of medication • check client's mouth after giving medication • give liquid medications if necessary	Will ensure ingestion of medication and compliance with treatment regimen	

Nursing Diagnosis: Alteration in nutrition: less than body requirements related to suspiciousness of food.
Goal: Client will obtain adequate nutrients to maintain body function.

Intervention	*Rationale*	*Expected Outcome*
Weigh client weekly; daily, if necessary	Will ensure client is taking in nutrients	No weight loss
Provide foods appropriate for client and have client assist in preparation of finger foods; have client select any prepackaged food; feed client if necessary, including NG tube if ordered	Will assist client in reducing suspicions about food and obtain adequate nutrients Tube feeding will probably frighten client and should be used as a last resort, when lack of food intake will result in loss of body function	Eats nutrients provided

Nursing Diagnosis: Alteration in senses and perception: visual, auditory, kinesthetic, gustatory, tactile, olfactory related to changes in thought processes.
Goal: During the course of treatment client will eliminate disordered thoughts.

Intervention	*Rationale*	*Expected Outcome*
Assess environmental stimuli for: • intensity • quantity • movement • ambiguity • incongruity	Will assist in decreasing stimuli causing disrupted thoughts	Contact with reality Oriented to time, place, and person No hallucinations No delusions Accurate perception of environmental stimuli No bizarre behavior
Alter environment to increase meaningful stimuli: • staff name tags • clocks • calendars • windows		
Structure routines	Will assist client in maintaining contact with reality	

(Diagnosis continued)

Table 14–13 *(continued)*

Nursing Diagnosis *(continued):* Alteration in senses and perception: visual, auditory, kinesthetic, gustatory, tactile, olfactory related to changes in thought processes.
Goal: During the course of treatment client will demonstrate reduction in disordered thoughts.

Intervention	*Rationale*	*Expected Outcome*
Orient to reality when necessary	Impaired reality testing can be improved by presenting reality	Client is oriented
Reduce unnecessary traffic and personnel	Increased sensory stimulation can increase distorted perceptions	Client is oriented
Maintain verbal and eye contact with client		Client maintains eye contact with nurse

Nursing Diagnosis: Social isolation related to disturbances in perception.
Goal: During the course of treatment client will attempt to interact with others.

Intervention	*Rationale*	*Expected Outcome*
Establish a trusting relationship: • keep appointments with client • be consistent • follow through	Will provide a structure for client to begin a meaningful relationship	Verbalizes feelings of loneliness Participates in activities Talks to others
Assess social history	Will assist in identifying potential problems in client's ability to form new relationships	
Assist client to identify barriers to forming relationships with others		
Encourage client to verbalize feelings of loneliness	Will assist client in forming meaningful relationships	
Sit with client		
Encourage client to participate in group activities		
Avoid: • whispering in front of client • laughing with other staff when client can't hear what's being said • arguing with client about identity; state reality as you see it • competitive activities • controversial conversation about sex, politics, and religion		

(continued)

Table 14–13 *(continued)*

Nursing Diagnosis: Alteration in thought processes related to ideas of reference.
Goal: During the course of treatment client will identify self correctly.

Intervention	*Rationale*	*Expected Outcome*
Analyze client's thought processes: • generalizations • distortions • ideas of reference • loose connections	Will assist nurse in constructing interpretations of reality	Clear verbalizations No hallucinations No delusions
Use direct communication: • avoid generalizations • do not argue about client's identity • focus on real things and real people • avoid vagueness	Will assist client toward realistic interactions	Attempts to interact with others
Encourage client to validate thoughts and feelings	Will encourage appropriate interaction with others	

Nursing Diagnosis: Potential for violence: self-directed or directed at others related to perceived threat to self and misperceived messages from others.
Goal: During the course of treatment client will not demonstrate violent behavior.

Intervention	*Rationale*	*Expected Outcome*
Assess client's potential for violence directed at others or toward self	Will assist in structuring an appropriate environment	Client maintains self-control
Demonstrate calm behavior: • calm appearance • low voice tone • verbalization of feelings	Will give client a model of behavior to emulate	Relaxed body posture Verbalizes rather than acts out feelings
Encourage client to talk out rather than act out feelings	Will assist client in maintaining self-esteem and control over behavior	
Set limits on aggressive behavior; use seclusion		
If seclusion is necessary: • observe at least every 15 minutes • take away harmful objects • have sufficient staff present	Will reduce potential for violent behavior	
Eliminate precipitating factors: • noise • new personnel • anxiety-provoking situations	Will decrease incidences of violent behavior	
Decrease agitation by: • encouraging physical activity • administering medications as prescribed • avoiding physical contact with client • giving client personal space • staying calm		

Table 14–14 Nursing Care Plan for the Client with Undifferentiated Schizophrenia

Nursing Diagnosis: Impaired verbal communication related to incongruent communication styles.
Goal: During the course of treatment client will demonstrate appropriate communication skills.

Intervention	*Rationale*	*Expected Outcome*
Assess client's communication patterns	Will assist in planning client teaching	Offers appropriate input for circumstances
Assist client in modifying communication skills by teaching communication techniques: • reflection • focusing • validation • clarification • stating observations • confrontation • exploring • providing feedback	Will assist client toward more successful communication	Uses effective communication techniques

Nursing Diagnosis: Deficit in self-care: feeding, bathing/hygiene, dressing/grooming, toileting related to mixed psychotic symptoms.
Goal: During the course of treatment client will have adequate nutrition, hydration, elimination, sleep, and grooming.

Intervention	*Rationale*	*Expected Outcome*
Assess client self-care capabilities	Will assist in identification of potential and actual deficits	Client feeds self Client tends to grooming needs
Assist client in meeting self-care activities as necessary Complete activities client is unable to perform	Will ensure meeting self-care needs	Client dresses self Client toilets self

Nursing Diagnosis: Disturbance in self-concept: body image, self-esteem, role performance, personal identity related to feelings of dependency.
Goal: During the course of treatment client will state a positive self-concept.

Intervention	*Rationale*	*Expected Outcome*
Assess client's perceptions of self	Will assist in identifying disturbances and misperceptions related to self-concept	Client states positive body image
Encourage client to function as independently as possible	Independent functioning increases self-esteem	Client functions independently

Table 14–15 Nursing Care Plan for the Client with Residual Schizophrenia

Nursing Diagnosis: Ineffective individual coping related to impairment of adaptive behaviors for meeting life's demands.
Goal: During the course of treatment client will learn to appraise stressful events.

Intervention	*Rationale*	*Expected Outcome*
Assess client's ability to accurately perceive events	Will assist in planning for client teaching	Recognizes stress
Encourage client to relate perceptions of events	Will assist client in learning to relate factual information	Sets goals for treatment
Assist client to explore past memories	Will assist in identifying barriers to improvement	Uses facts to form new ideas
Encourage new coping skills: • asking questions • gathering information • seeking consultation	Will assist client in developing objective appraisal skills	Accurately reports events

Nursing Diagnosis: Deficit in diversional activity related to apathy and lack of interest in diversions.
Goal: During the course of treatment client will identify and participate in a diversional activity.

Intervention	*Rationale*	*Expected Outcome*
Assess usual pattern of diversional activities	Will assist in identifying client interests	Lists activities of interest
Encourage client to identify and participate in diversional activity	Will assist client in planning for future activities	Participates in diversional activity
Encourage client to explore resources for diversional activities		Discusses activities

Nursing Diagnosis: Alteration in health maintenance related to emotional difficulties.
Goal: During the course of treatment client will modify health maintenance behaviors.

Intervention	*Rationale*	*Expected Outcome*
Provide information and teach client about: • problem-solving techniques • self-monitoring of health maintenance behaviors	Will assist client in assuming responsibility for health maintenance	Assumes responsibility for health maintenance

Nursing Diagnosis: Impaired home maintenance management related to dependency and/or lack of a support system.
Goal: During the course of treatment client will establish a support system to manage the home.

Intervention	*Rationale*	*Expected Outcome*
Assess home maintenance skills	Will assist in identifying client learning needs	Develops home maintenance plan
Identify potential members for support system	Will assist in planning for a support system	Maintains self-care and care of belongings during treatment
Refer to community resources if necessary	Encourages client independence	Uses equipment appropriately

(Diagnosis continued)

Table 14–15 *(continued)*

Nursing Diagnosis *(continued)*: Impaired home maintenance management related to dependency and/or lack of a support system.
Goal: During the course of treatment client will establish a support system to manage the home.

Intervention	*Rationale*	*Expected Outcome*
Teach home maintenance skills		Can cite needed supplies and source of supplies
Rotate staff members caring for client	Will reduce development of dependency on one person	

Nursing Diagnosis: Deficit in knowledge related to thought disorder.
Goal: Client will verbalize diagnosis and relationship to behaviors by the time of discharge.

Intervention	*Rationale*	*Expected Outcome*
Assess client's understanding of condition	Will assist in planning for client learning needs	Maintains self-care activities
Provide information on diagnosis Teach the importance of maintaining treatment regimen (eg, medications)	Client understanding will increase compliance with treatment regimen	Takes medications as ordered Describes diagnosis accurately

Nursing Diagnosis: Potential noncompliance related to alterations in perceptions.
Goal: During hospitalization and following discharge client will attempt to conform to treatment regimen.

Intervention	*Rationale*	*Expected Outcome*
Assist client in participating in treatment: • talk with client • encourage client to attend and participate in groups • structure routines • use reminders • help client analyze behavior	Client participation in treatment improves chances for recovery	Participates in treatment Maintains outpatient appointments Takes medications as per routine
Teach client about: • problem solving • referral resources • structuring medication routine	Increased client understanding leads to greater compliance	Requests information about treatment

Nursing Diagnosis: Potential powerlessness related to feelings of worthlessness.
Goal: During the course of treatment client will express self-worth and state areas of life that can be controlled.

Intervention	*Rationale*	*Expected Outcome*
Assess the amount of supervision necessary for client	When supervision decreases, client's sense of control over the environment increases	Seeks to control own environment
Assist client to identify feelings related to powerlessness	Will promote client involvement and increase self-esteem	States feelings of adequacy Participates in decision making

(Diagnosis continued)

Table 14–15 *(continued)*

Intervention	*Rationale*	*Expected Outcome*
Assist client in improving self-esteem: • provide feedback on behavior • identify goals • use client strengths • encourage participation in self-care	Will assist client in gaining a sense of control over situations	

Nursing Diagnosis: Social isolation related to unacceptable social behavior.
Goal: During the course of treatment client will be able to make social contacts.

Intervention	*Rationale*	*Expected Outcome*
Establish a trusting relationship with client	Will provide the foundation for appropriate social contacts with others	Verbalizes feelings of loneliness
Assess social history	Will assist in identifying barriers to making social contacts	Attempts to talk to others
Encourage client to participate in activities: • daily routine • group activities • diversional activities	Will increase client's ability to relate to others	Participates in social activities

CASE EXAMPLE

A Client with Undifferentiated Schizophrenia

Rick Wilson, a 30-year-old unemployed male, was found wandering along a boulevard, throwing rocks and yelling obscenities at cars. Rick told the police that the Secret Service had been trying to capture him. The police took Rick to the mental health unit for observation. Rick has been treated twice before in this unit for periods of 2 weeks and 3 weeks, respectively.

Nursing History

Location: Inpatient Psychiatric Unit
Client's name: Rick Wilson Age: 30
Admitting diagnosis: Schizophrenia, undifferentiated type
T=99.2, P=100, R=20, BP=130/70

Health history
Height: 5′10″
Weight: 160 lbs
(Note: The client was unable to give any further history.)

Clinical data
Not applicable at this time

Nursing observations
Rick refused to come out of his room. He sat in the corner recounting his concerns about the Secret Service agents. Rick thinks the agents have locked him up, and he refuses to eat, bathe himself, or sleep. Rick tries to hit any personnel coming into the room.

Table 14–16 *Example of Evaluation of Nursing Care of a Schizophrenic Client*

Plan	*Evaluation*
1. The nurse will orient the client to time, place, and person at least every 2 hours.	On 9/25, the nurse oriented Peter once. Peter knew his name, date, time and verbalized that he was in the hospital.
2. The nurse will validate any misperceptions noted in the client's communication.	On 9/25, the nurse stated to Peter, "Are you hearing voices other than mine?" Peter stated, "No, the Martians are leaving me alone today."
3. The nurse will provide a structured daily routine.	9/26, Peter groomed before breakfast and made his bed.

Analysis/Synthesis of Data

Concerns	*Nursing Diagnoses*
Perceptual disturbances	Anxiety
Bizarre behavior: withdrawal, regression, aggression	Impaired verbal communication
High anxiety with agitation	Ineffective individual coping
Hallucinations	Fear
Delusions	Deficit in self-care: feeding, bathing/hygiene, dressing/grooming, toileting
Disorganized thinking	Disturbance in self-concept: body image, self-esteem, role performance, personal identity
Poor interpersonal relationships	Social isolation
Self-care deficits	Alteration in thought processes

Suggested Care Planning Activities

1. Determine the priorities for Rick's care.
2. Determine the stresses underlying Rick's relapse.
3. Determine the laboratory tests that are indicated for Rick.
4. Determine whether Rick has a support system.
5. Determine the developmental aspects to be considered in Rick's case.
6. Identify nursing goals for Rick.
7. Describe the client teaching necessary to assist Rick toward recovery.
8. Identify the special needs in relation to rehabilitation in Rick's situation.
9. List and provide a rationale for nursing interventions in Rick's care.

SUMMARY

1. Many of the beds in mental hospitals are occupied by clients with schizophrenia. The bizarre behavior of schizophrenics makes this the disorder people think of when they speak of mental illness.

2. The five subtypes of schizophrenia are catatonic, disorganized, paranoid, undifferentiated, and residual.

Knowledge Base

3. Positive symptoms of schizophrenia are those patterns of behavior which are viewed as unusual and are often exhibited during the acute phase of the illness. Negative symptoms of schizophrenia are the absence of usual behaviors and are seen in both the acute and chronic phases.

4. Positive behavioral characteristics are catatonic excitement, stereotypies, echopraxia, echolalia, and verbigeration.

5. Negative behavioral characteristics are catatonic stupor, posturing, minimal self-care, social withdrawal, stilted language, and poverty of speech.

6. Positive affective characteristics are inappropriate affect and overreactive affect.

7. Negative affective characteristics are blunted affect, flat affect, and anhedonia.

8. Positive cognitive characteristics are delusions, hallucinations, loose associations, and neologisms.

9. Negative cognitive characteristics are concrete thinking, symbolism, and blocking.

10. Delusional types include: grandiose, persecution, sin or guilt, control, somatic, religious, ideas of reference, thought broadcasting, thought withdrawal, and thought insertion.

11. The most common type of hallucination is auditory followed by visual hallucination. Tactile, olfactory, and gustatory hallucinations are seen more in people undergoing withdrawal from alcohol and drugs.

12. Physical findings in schizophrenic clients include overactivity of dopamine synapses, insufficient synaptic norepinephrine, elevated CPK level, enlarged brain ventricles, decreased blood flow to the brain, areas of decreased electrical activity, and altered rates of glucose metabolism.

13. Genetic studies have demonstrated that schizophrenia may be related to a genetic defect.

14. Sociocultural theories hold that schizophrenia may be a consequence for the deprivation and distress associated with poverty existence.

15. Treatment modalities include medication therapy, psychosocial intervention, and rehabilitation.

16. Antipsychotic agents are the major medications used in schizophrenia. These medications assist in controlling the symptoms of schizophrenia.

17. The nurse needs to be familiar with the many side effects of medication therapy, and needs to educate the client to prevent injury from side effects.

18. The extrapyramidal symptoms—primarily dystonic reactions, akathesia, and parkinsonism—are the most common side effects.

19. Childhood schizophrenia has a poor prognosis and may be related to a dysfunctional cholinergic system.

20. With deinstitutionalization, homelessness has be-

come a problem for some people who suffer from chronic schizophrenia.

Assessment

21. When assessing the schizophrenic client, special attention needs to be given to interview considerations to obtain an accurate data base for planning nursing care.

22. The primary themes appearing in conversations with schizophrenic clients are problems with personal identity, viewing the nurse as a mother figure, distortions in body image, borrowing identity from someone else, dependency, and the struggle for power and control over the interview.

Nursing Diagnosis and Planning

23. Providing client safety can be a major concern until the client regains contact with reality.

24. Often, the nurse will have to accurately observe, assess, and intervene without the client's cooperation.

CHAPTER REVIEW

1. Joe believes that the Governor of Mexico has declared him President of Arizona for life. When shown newspaper clippings about the Governor of Arizona, Joe insists the newspaper is spreading vicious lies. Joe's false beliefs, which cannot be changed by logical reasoning or evidence, are called
   (a) Delusions
   (b) Hallucinations
   (c) Grandiosities
   (d) Depersonalizations

2. Ann is sitting on the sofa, engaged in a lively conversation. Ann is alone in the room, and her conversation is disjointed. Ann is exhibiting a false perception without external stimuli. This is called a
   (a) Delusion
   (b) Hallucination
   (c) Grandiosity
   (d) Depersonalization

3. Jeanne was found on her bed in a rigid fetal position. She remained mute after attempts to speak to her and appeared to be in a stupor. Jeanne's type of schizophrenia is
   (a) Paranoid
   (b) Disorganized
   (c) Catatonic
   (d) Undifferentiated

4. Hank's behavior has been characterized by incoherence, marked loosening of associations, seemingly disjointed behavior, and flat or inappropriate affect. This type of schizophrenia is
   (a) Catatonic
   (b) Residual
   (c) Paranoid
   (d) Disorganized

5. Helen recently developed symptoms of drug-induced parkinsonism. Which of the following drugs may be prescribed for Helen to combat this side effect?
   (a) Cogentin
   (b) Thorazine
   (c) Haldol
   (d) Prolixin

6. Which one of the following is the best way to orient the client to reality?
   (a) Keep the room dark
   (b) Address the client by name
   (c) Provide excess stimuli
   (d) Avoid talking to the client

REFERENCES

American Psychiatric Association: *Diagnostic and Statistical Manual of Mental Disorders,* 3d ed., rev. Washington DC: American Psychiatric Association, 1987.

Baker AF: How families cope: Schizophrenia. *J Psychosoc Nurs* (1) 1989:27:31–36.

Bateson G, et al.: Towards a theory of schizophrenia. *Behav Sci* (1) 1956:251–64.

Bleuler E: Dementia praecox. In: *Handbuch der Psychiatrie.* Leipzig-Wien. 1911.

Buchanan RW, et al.: Clinical correlates of the deficit syndrome of schizophrenia. *Am J Psychiatry,* (3) 1990: 147:290–94.

Cantor S: *Childhood Schizophrenia.* Guilford Press. 1988.

Elkashef AM, et al.: Vitamin E in the treatment of tardive dyskinesia. *Am J Psychiatry* (4) 1990:147:505–6.

Fallon I, et al.: *Family Care of Schizophrenia.* Guilford Press. 1984.

Hagerty BK: *Psychiatric-Mental Health Assessment.* St. Louis: Mosby. 1984.

Kety SS, Matthysse S: Genetic and biochemical aspects of schizophrenia. In: *The New Harvard Guide to Psychiatry.* Nicholi AM (editor). Cambridge: Harvard Univ Press. 1988. 259–95.

Lamb HR, et al.: Families of schizophrenics: A movement in jeopardy. *Hosp Community Psychiatry* (4) 1986: 37:353–57.

Lefley HP: Culture and chronic mental illness. *Hosp Community Psychiatry* (3) 1990:41:277–86.

Lehmann HE, Cancor R: Schizophrenia: Clinical features. In: *Comprehensive Textbook of Psychiatry,* 4th ed. Vol. I. Kaplan HI, Sadock BJ (editors). Baltimore: Williams and Wilkins, 1985. 686–89.

Liberman RP: Schizophrenia: Psychosocial treatment. In: *Comprehensive Textbook of Psychiatry,* 4th ed. Vol. I. Kaplan HI, Sadock BJ (editors). Baltimore: Williams and Wilkins, 1985. 724–34.

Mathew RJ, Wilson WH: Chronicity and a low anteroposterior gradient of cerebral blood flow in schizophrenia. *Am J Psychiatry* (2) 1990:147:211–14.

Meissner WW: Theories of personality and psychopathology: Classical psychoanalysis. In: *Comprehensive Textbook of Psychiatry,* 4th ed. Vol. I. Kaplan HI, Sadock BJ (editors). Baltimore: Williams and Wilkins, 1985. 408.

Mosher L, Keith SJ: Psychosocial treatment: Individual, group, family, and community support. In: *Special Report: Schizophrenia 1980.* NIMH, 1981:127–58.

Plante TG: Social skills training: A program to help schizophrenic clients cope. *J Psychosoc Nurs* (3) 1989: 27:6–8.

Riesdorph-Ostrow W: Deinstitutionalization: A public policy. *J Psychosoc Nurs* (6) 1989:27:4–8.

Ryan MT: Providing shelter. *J Psychosoc Nurs* (6) 1989: 27:14–18.

Sarason IG, Sarason BR: *Abnormal Psychology,* 4th ed. Englewood Cliffs, NJ: Prentice-Hall, 1984.

Schultz CG: Schizophrenia: Individual psychotherapy. In: *Comprehensive Textbook of Psychiatry,* 4th ed. Vol. I. Kaplan HI, Sadock BJ (editors). Baltimore: Williams and Wilkins, 1985. 734–46.

Sulliger N: Relapse. *J Psychosoc Nurs* (6) 1988:26:20–23.

Thaker GK, et al.: Clonazepam treatment of tardive dyskinesia. *Am J Psychiatry* (4) 1990:147:445–51.

Townsend MC: *Drug Guide for Psychiatric Nursing.* FA Davis, 1990.

Tsuang MT, Faraone SV: Schizophrenic Disorders. In: *The New Harvard Guide to Psychiatry.* Nicholi AM (editor). Cambridge: Harvard Univ Press, 1988. 259–95.

Walsh M: *Schizophrenia: Straight Talk for Families and Friends.* Morrow, 1985.

Weiner H: Schizophrenia: Etiology. In: *Comprehensive Textbook of Psychiatry,* 4th ed. Vol. I. Kaplan HI, Sadock BJ (editors). Baltimore: Williams and Wilkins, 1985. 669–79.

Williams CA: Perspectives on the hallucinatory process. *Issues in Mental Health Nurs* 1989:10:99–119.

SUGGESTED READINGS

Bostrom AC: Assessment scales for tardive dyskinesia. *J Psychosoc Nurs* (6) 1988:26:8–12.

Doenges ME, Townsend MC, Moorhouse MF: *Psychiatric Care Plans.* Davis, 1989.

Miller NE, Cohen GD: *Schizophrenia and Aging.* Guilford Press, 1987.

Shlafer M, Marieb EN: *The Nurse, Pharmacology, and Drug Therapy.* Addison-Wesley, 1989.

Williams CA: Patient education for people with schizophrenia. *Perspect Psychiat Care* (2) 1989:25:14–21.

CHAPTER 15

Chronic Organic Brain Disorders

BRENDA LEWIS CLEARY

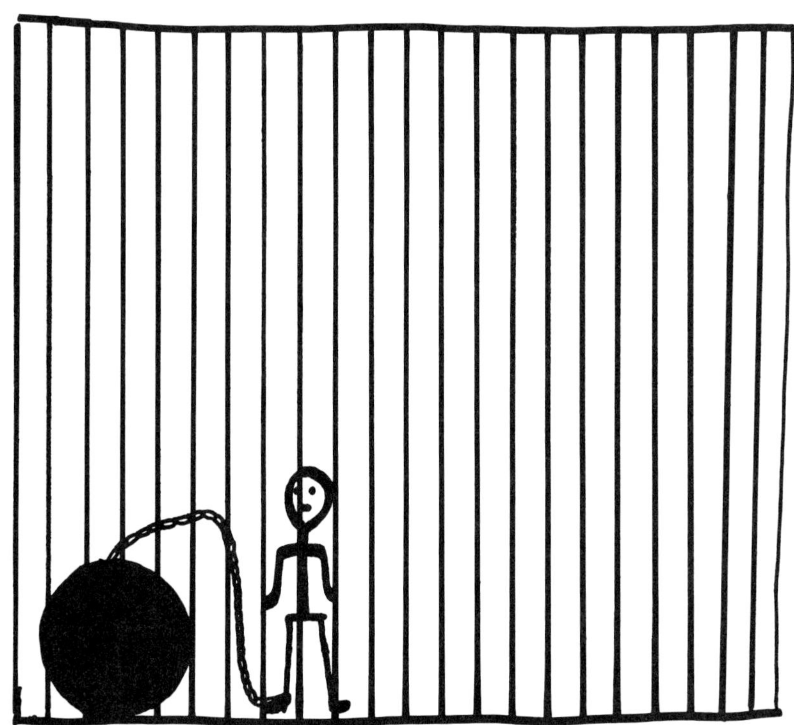

How I see my illness

I feel confined in a huge desolate prison, my movements restricted by an overpowering ball and chain. I gaze through thick black bars over miles of stark barren plains. The emptiness and despair stretch toward eternity. The sadness and frustration I experience are profound.

▪ *Objectives*

After reading this chapter the student will be able to

- Differentiate between dementia and delirium
- Discuss theories about causation of organic brain disorders
- Assess clients with dementia and delirium
- Intervene with clients suffering from organic brain disorders
- Assist families in planning home care for clients with dementia
- Evaluate nursing care based on outcome criteria

▪ *Chapter Outline*

Introduction

The process of mental deterioration related to organic brain syndrome has a profound effect on clients, families, and society as a whole. The emphasis in this chapter is on dementia and delirium, the two most common forms of organic brain disease (see Table 15–1). Amnestic syndrome, organic affective syndrome, and organic personality syndrome are addressed in tabular form because they occur much less frequently (see Table 15–2). The following is the list of the diagnostic categories in DSM-III-R.

293.00 Delirium

294.10 Dementia

294.00 Amnestic syndrome

293.83 Organic affective syndrome

310.10 Organic personality syndrome

Cognitive abilities involve both awareness and judgment working together to facilitate accurate perception of and appropriate response to stimuli. When an organic brain syndrome is present, cognitive abilities are impaired to a lesser or greater degree.

A number of descriptors are used interchangeably for the various syndromes. Dementia is referred to as primary encephalopathy, chronic brain disorder, or irreversible brain disorder. Delirium is referred to as secondary encephalopathy, acute brain disorder, or reversible brain disorder (Pallett and O'Brien, 1985).

Dementia

Dementia is the insidious and progressive loss of mental abilities severe enough to interfere with personal, social, or occupational functioning. Mem-

Table 15–1 *Differentiation of Delirium and Dementia*

Acute Brain Syndrome *Delirium*	*Chronic Brain Syndrome* *Dementia*
Onset	
Onset usually sudden. Acute development of impairment of orientation, memory, cognitive function, judgment, and affect.	Onset of impairment generally slow and insidious.
Essential feature	
Clouded state of consciousness.	Not based on disordered consciousness; however, delirium, stupor, and coma may occur.
Etiology	
Caused by temporary, reversible, diffuse disturbances of brain function.	Generally caused by irreversible alteration of brain function.
Course	
Short, diurnal fluctuations in symptoms. The clinical course is usually brief, although it may last for months. Untreated, prolonged delirium may cause permanent brain destruction and lead to dementia.	No diurnal fluctuations. The clinical course usually progresses over months or years, ending in death.
History	
Onset: sudden Duration: hours to days Course: fluctuating arousal	Onset: insidious Duration: months to years Course: consistent deterioration with occasional lucid moments
Motor signs	
Postural tremor, restless, hyperactive or sluggish.	None (until late).
Speech is slurred, reflects disorganized thinking.	Speech is usually normal in early stages, but word-finding difficulties progress.
Mental status	
Attention fluctuates	Attention generally normal in early stages; inattention progresses.
Memory Impaired by poor attention.	Memory impairment; recent memory affected before remote.
Language Normal or mild misnaming of objects.	Aphasia in later stages.
Perception Visual, auditory, and/or tactile hallucinations.	Hallucinations not prominent, although cognitive impairment may lead to paranoid delusions.
Pronounced mood/affect Fear and suspiciousness may be prominent; anxiety, depression, anger, irritability or euphoria may occur.	Distinterested and/or disinhibited.
Review of systems	
History of systemic illness or toxic exposure.	Extraneural organ systems usually uninvolved.
EEG Pronounced diffuse slowing of fast cycles related to state of arousal.	Normal or mildly slow.

Source: Foreman, 1986; Cleary, 1989; Committee on Aging, 1988.

Table 15–2 *Comparison of Amnestic, Organic Affective, and Organic Personality Syndromes*

Characteristics	*Major Causes*	*Treatments*
Amnestic Syndrome Impaired social and occupational functioning Shallow affect Impairment of short- and long-term memory Confabulation	Metal or carbon monoxide toxicity Thiamine deficiency Encephalitis Temporal lobe insult Cerebral vascular abnormalities Head trauma, neoplasm Alzheimer's disease Electroconvulsive therapy	Protective and symptomatic treatment pending diagnosis and treatment of underlying pathophysiology
Organic Affective Syndrome Characteristics associated with either depression or mania May be suicidal Only mild cognitive impairment Delusions and hallucinations	Drug abuse Medication toxicity Pernicious anemia Infectious diseases Endocrine disorders Arteritis, neoplasm Degenerative neurologic diseases	Protective and symptomatic treatment pending diagnosis and treatment of underlying pathophysiology
Organic Personality Syndrome Marked change in affective lability (sudden outbursts) Poor judgment and impulse control Indifference Paranoia	PCP and inhalant abuse Manganese and mercury poisoning Neurosyphilis Temporal lobe insult Arteritis Subarachnoid hemorrhage Head trauma, neoplasm Huntington's disease Multiple sclerosis Postencephalitic parkinsonism	Protective and symptomatic treatment pending diagnosis and treatment of underlying pathophysiology

Adapted from J. Ellison, DSM III and The Diagnosis of Organic Mental Disorders, *Annals of Emergency Medicine,* 1984, p. 521.

ory, learning, attention, and judgment are all generally affected.

DSM-III-R lists the following diagnostic criteria for dementia:

A. In addition to memory impairment related to an identified or assumed organic etiology and the absence of clouding of consciousness, at least one of the following must be present:

1. Impairment of abstract thinking, as manifested by concrete interpretation of proverbs, inability to find similarities and differences between related words, difficulty in defining words and concepts, and other similar tasks
2. Impaired judgment
3. Other disturbances of higher cortical function, such as aphasia (disorder of language due to brain dysfunction), apraxia (inability to carry out purposive activities despite intact sensory and motor function), agnosia (failure to recognize or identify objects despite intact sensory function), and "constructional difficulty" (eg, inability to copy three-dimensional figures, assemble blocks, or arrange sticks in specific designs)
4. Personality change (ie, alteration or accentuation of premorbid traits)

An estimated 5 percent of the U.S. population in the 65 and over age group is severely demented, and another 10 percent is mildly or moderately impaired. When calculated for people 80 years or older, the rate climbs to 22 percent. Although a small number of adults succumb to dementing illnesses earlier in life, dementia is generally associated with later life and is referred to as the major neuropsychiatric disorder of old age (Shamoian and Teusink, 1987).

Dementia in old age is most commonly due to Alzheimer's disease, which accounts for up to 60 percent of dementing illness. Most of the remaining presentations of dementia are due to vascular accidents known as multiinfarct dementia. However, Pick's disease, anterior brain atrophy, and Creutzfeldt-Jakob disease (a viral ailment), account for very rare cases of dementia. Dementia may also occur secondarily to some other pathologic process, including treatable disorders such as drug intoxication, metabolic or nutrition imbalances, and infectious diseases. Recently, dementia has developed because of CNS infections and inflammatory disorders that are complications of AIDS (see Chapter 17). Some individuals who have been on renal dialysis for years develop dialysis dementia. In addition, dementia may result from the neurologic impairment associated with Korsakoff's syndrome (chronic alcoholism) and other neurologic disorders such as Huntington's chorea and parkinsonism. Cerebral neoplasms can also produce symptoms of dementia (Cleary, 1989; Committee on Aging, 1988).

Alzheimer's disease, first diagnosed in 1907 by German physician Alois Alzheimer, is currently recognized as the most significant form of dementia and the most devastating disorder of later life. Interestingly, Alzheimer first discovered the pathologic characteristics of Alzheimer's disease (neurofibrillary tangles and neuritic plaques) in a postmortem examination of a 51-year-old woman. Therefore, for many years, Alzheimer's disease was considered a presenile dementia, victimizing only people younger than 65. Subsequent investigation showed, however, that Alzheimer's disease, or senile dementia of the Alzheimer's type (SDAT), is far more common in people over 65. Prevalence increases with advancing age (Alzheimer's Association, 1988; Hutton, 1987; Katzman, 1986).

At least 15 percent of Alzheimer's cases are believed to be inherited and are referred to as familial Alzheimer's disease (FAD). This form of the disease begins about the age of 40. The clinical characteristics of the inherited and uninherited diseases are the same. For first-degree relatives (siblings or children) of a person with presenile onset Alzheimer's, the risk is 50 percent for developing the disorder (Maxmen, 1986; Shamoian and Teusink, 1987).

Delirium

Delirium is transient alteration in the state of consciousness. The alteration ranges from mild disorientation and memory impairment to an agitated state with concomitant impairment of attention, perception, and thinking ability. Delirium is often accompanied by illusions, delusions, and hallucinations. Most commonly, delirium is seen in young children and long-lived adults, although it does occur in all age groups. The condition may become more intensified during the late afternoon or early evening hours, a phenomenon known as sundowning (Cleary, 1989).

DSM-III-R lists the following diagnostic criteria for delirium.

A. In addition to clouding of consciousness (reduced clarity of awareness of environment), with reduced capacity to shift, focus, and sustain attention to environmental stimuli, at least two of the following must be present:

   1. Perceptual disturbance: misinterpretations, illusions, or hallucinations
   2. Speech that is at times incoherent
   3. Disturbance of sleep-wakefulness cycle with insomnia or daytime drowsiness
   4. Increased or decreased psychomotor activity

Delirium may occur as the result of a wide variety of pathophysiologic conditions: metabolic imbalances, infectious states, drug intoxication or withdrawal, respiratory and cardiac disturbances, endocrine disorders, postoperative states, and trauma. The incidence is difficult to determine because of the wide variety of underlying causes. Conservatively, 100,000 cases a year are estimated in the United States. It is thought that delirium is related to 1 percent of all general hospital admissions, but of clients over the age of 60, the incidence is as high as 40 percent (Dwyer, 1987; Ellison, 1984; Gomez and Gomez, 1987; Pallett and O'Brien, 1985).

Amnestic, Organic Affective, and Organic Personality Syndromes

Amnestic syndrome involves the impairment of both short- and long-term memory, without clouding of consciousness (as in delirium) or general loss of cognitive abilities (as in dementia). Immediate recall may be spared. This syndrome is related to a specific organic factor, and the outcome depends on the etiology. Possible pathologies are trauma, hypoxia, encephalitis, thiamine deficiency, and chronic use of alcohol.

Organic affective syndrome is diagnosed when the predominant manifestation of an organic disturbance is a mood disorder of mania or depression. There is no clouding of consciousness or significant loss of cognitive abilities, including memory. Underlying etiologies are toxins, endocrine disorders, or viral illnesses.

Organic personality syndrome is a marked change in behavior or personality that is usually caused by structural brain damage. There is neither clouding of consciousness nor significant loss of cognitive abilities. But there may be emotional lability, poor impulse control, apathy, or paranoid ideation. (See Table 15–2 for a comparison of these three syndromes.)

Knowledge Base: Dementia

Alzheimer's disease is the most common disorder among dementing illnesses; it currently affects an estimated 2.5 million Americans. Alzheimer's is the fourth leading killer among adults in our country. It is "a thief of minds, destroyer of personalities, wrecker of family finances, and a filler of nursing homes" (American Association of Retired Persons, 1986). Unfortunately, there is no known cause or cure. The average course of the disease is 5 to 10 years, but it may range from 2 to 20 years (Committee on Aging, 1988).

The progression of Alzheimer's disease* is roughly divided into three stages: Stage 1 typically lasts from two to four years, stage 2 may continue for years, and stage 3 usually lasts only one year before death occurs.

Behavioral Characteristics

The most notable changes in behavior during stage 1 are difficulties performing complex tasks. People suffering from Alzheimer's disease are unable to balance their checkbooks or plan a well-balanced meal. They may have difficulty remembering to buy supplies needed for the home or responding to different schedules within the home. At work, the ability to plan a goal-directed set of behaviors is seriously limited, resulting in missed appointments and incomplete verbal or written reports. Personal appearance begins to decline, and assistance is needed in selecting clothes appropriate for the season or particular event. During stage 1, these people recognize they are confused and are frightened by what is happening. Fearing the diagnosis, they attempt to cover up and rationalize their symptoms (Joyce and Kirksey, 1989; Kiely, 1985; Williams, 1986).

In stage 2, behavior deteriorates markedly; often, it is socially unacceptable and embarrassing to family and friends. Wandering behavior poses a danger for these people, because they get lost easily and are unable to return home. During this stage, these clients need assistance with the motor skills of toileting and bathing properly. In addition to help in selecting clothing, they need help in dressing. This problem, the inability to carry out skilled and purposeful movement, is called *apraxia*. *Hyperorality,* the need to taste, chew, and examine any object small enough to be placed in the mouth,

*Because multiinfarct dementia and Alzheimer's disease demonstrate the same characteristics and the latter is the more prevalent, Alzheimer's disease will be used as the model.

is also evident. Although there is a sharp increase in appetite and food intake, there is seldom a corresponding weight gain. Behavior in this stage is characterized by continuous, repetitive acts that have no meaning or direction. This repetitive behavior—which may include lip licking, tapping of fingers, pacing, or echoing others' words—is referred to as *perseveration phenomena* (Hall, 1988; Williams, 1986).

In stage 3 of Alzheimer's disease, a syndrome like Klüver-Bucy syndrome develops. This includes the continuation of hyperorality and the development of bulimia. Behavior is also characterized by *hyperetamorphosis,* which is a need to compulsively touch and examine every object in the environment. There is a sharp deterioration in motor ability that progresses from an inability to walk to an inability to sit up, to an inability to even smile (Joyce and Kirksey, 1989; Williams, 1986).

Affective Characteristics

In stage 1 of Alzheimer's disease, anxiety and depression may occur as affected people become aware of and try to cope with noticeable deficits. Not infrequently they experience feelings of helplessness, frustration, and shame in relation to their deficits. Diagnosis of a concomitant depression is important because depression can worsen the symptoms of dementia. Those in stage 1 of Alzheimer's lack spontaneity in verbal and nonverbal communication. And as a result of a chosen or forced withdrawal from social contacts, an apathetic affect may ensue.

In stage 2, there is an increased lability of emotions from flat affect to periods of marked irritability. Delusions of persecution may precipitate feelings of intense fear. Catastrophic reactions, resulting from underlying brain dysfunction, are commonly seen. In response to everyday situations the person overreacts by exploding in rage or suddenly crying. As the disease progresses through stage 3, response to environmental stimuli continues to decrease until the person is wholly nonresponsive (Burnside, 1988; Satlin, 1988).

Cognitive Characteristics

The chief cognitive deficit in stage 1 is memory impairment with a decrease in concentration, an increase in distractibility, and an appearance of absentmindedness. The ability to make accurate judgments also declines. Time disorientation occurs with maintenance of person and place orientation. Transitory delusions of persecution may develop in response to the memory impairment (Hall, 1988). The person may make statements such as, "You hid my keys. I know you don't want me to be able to get out of the house and drive." or "Where are my shoes? Everybody keeps hiding things to make me crazy." or "Why didn't you tell me there was a party tonight? You just don't want me to go and have any fun."

In stage 2 of Alzheimer's disease, there is a progressive memory loss, which includes both recent and remote memory. New information cannot be retained, and there is no recollection of what occurred 10 minutes or an hour ago. Loss of remote memory is seen when there is no recognition of family members or recall of significant past events. *Confabulation,* the filling in of these gaps in memory with imaginary information, is an attempt to distract others from observing the deficit. Comprehension of language, interactions, and significance of objects is greatly diminished. The meaning of common words or the purpose of common household objects may not be understood. During this stage, the person becomes completely disoriented in all three spheres of person, time, and place.

As the disease progresses, there is increasing *aphasia,* which begins with the inability to find words and eventually limits the person to as few as six words. Concurrently, *agraphia,* the inability to read or write, develops. Finally, the inability to attach meaning to sensory inputs, *agnosia,* evolves. Auditory agnosia is the inability to recognize familiar sounds such as a doorbell, the ring of a telephone, or a barking dog. Tactile agnosia, called *astereognosis,* occurs when the person is unable to identify familiar objects placed in the hand such as a comb, pencil, or paintbrush. Visual agnosia, referred to as *alexia,* occurs when the person can look at a frying pan, a telephone, or a toothbrush and have no idea of what to do with these objects (Mann, 1985; Williams, 1986).

The following interchange illustrates the aphasic characteristics of Alzheimer's disease. Pat is able to give a variety of descriptors but cannot think of the one necessary word.

Sue called her mother Pat to see how she was doing.

SUE: It sounds like you are eating, mother. What are you eating?

PAT: I can't tell you.

SUE: Is it hot or cold?

PAT: It's cold.

SUE: Did you get it out of the refrigerator?

PAT: No.

SUE: Is it a sandwich?

PAT: Sort of. I put butter on it.

SUE: Is it crackers?

PAT: No. I used to buy a lot of it and put it in the freezer.

SUE: Is it cookies?

PAT: No. Keep guessing, you're getting warm.

SUE: Is it bread?

PAT: No. Usually I have it for breakfast. I took the last slice.

SUE: Is it coffee cake?

PAT: Yes, that's what it is.

In stage 3 of Alzheimer's disease, there is a complete lack of cognitive functioning. The person may be able to say one word, or the person may be unable to say anything. No longer is there any nonverbal response to internal and external stimuli; the person evolves into a vegetative state.

Mr. Goldstein, a 67-year-old engineer, began to forget where he placed familiar objects around the house and, as his wife noted, had difficulty balancing the checkbook. His co-workers began to notice impaired judgments in the workplace. Mr. Goldstein developed a tendency of projecting on others his increasing inability to handle usual tasks efficiently. Within two years, Mrs. Goldstein had to label objects in the home so that he could identify them by name. He responded with fear to sounds he could no longer identify. He needed assistance with eating, bathing, and dressing and constant supervision because of his wandering behavior. Mrs. Goldstein found that a regular routine was helpful and continually repeated, "My husband is still in there, I just have to go in and draw him out."

(See Table 15–3 for a comparison of changes in normal aging with changes in Alzheimer's disease.)

Physiologic Characteristics

Deterioration of the CNS results in physical changes throughout the body. People with dementia suffer from *hypertonia,* an increase in muscle tone that can be observed in muscular twitchings. There is a loss of energy and increasing fatigue with physical activity. The sleep cycle is impaired; there is a decrease in total sleep time and more frequent awakenings. This disruption leads to sleep depriva-

Table 15–3 *Changes in Normal Aging Compared to Changes in Alzheimer's Disease*

Normal Aging	*Alzheimer's Disease*
Recent memory more impaired than remote memory	Recent and remote memory profoundly affected
Difficulty in recalling names of persons and places	Unable to recall names of persons and places
Decreased concentration	Inability to concentrate
Writing things down is helpful in stimulating memory	Unable to write; nothing stimulates memory
Changes do not interfere with daily functioning	Changes cause an inability to function at work, in a social relationship, and at home
Insight into forgetful behavior is preserved	With progression, client has no insight into changes that have occurred

Source: Cohen, 1988; Committee on Aging, 1988; Joyce, Kirksey, 1989.

tion, which magnifies the already disturbed cognitive functions. As the disease progresses, there is incontinence of both urine and stool. In the final progression, anorexia leads to an emaciated physical condition. Death usually occurs from pneumonia, urinary tract infections leading to sepsis, malnutrition, or dehydration (Hall, 1988; Hoch and Reynolds, 1986; Williams, 1986).

Pathophysiologic changes associated with Alzheimer's are degenerative and result in gross atrophy of the cerebral cortex. Interneuronal junctions develop deposits of a starchlike protein, amyloid, that forms a core surrounded by abnormal unmyelinated neuronal structures referred to as a senile or neuritic plaque. These plaques, it is believed, interfere with neural transmission. There are also thickened and twisted interneurons that tangle into masses called neurofibrillary tangles. These tangles atrophy and interfere with transmission. Pathophysiologic changes associated with Alzheimer's disease can be readily identified during autopsy. However, when the disease is first suspected in a client, diagnosis is one of exclusion through a complete physical and neurologic examination. The only definite diagnosis of microscopic changes prior to death is the brain biopsy, an intrusive and risky procedure. Later in the disorder a computed tomography (CT) scan may demonstrate brain atrophy, widened cortical sulci, and enlarged cerebral ventricles (Committee on Aging, 1988; Hutton, 1987).

Approximately 20 percent of long-lived adults suffering dementia experience mental deterioration related to blood vessel disease or cerebral atherosclerosis. Narrowing of arteries in the brain leads to multiple infarctions, thus the term *multi-infarct dementia.* Clients with this type of dementia experience a much less steady decline than those with Alzheimer's disease. These clients may also experience more focal (local) neurologic symptoms as opposed to the global symptoms of Alzheimer's disease (Pallett and O'Brien, 1985).

As previously mentioned, pathophysiologic factors related to less common forms of dementia stem from degenerative nervous system disorders such as Parkinson's disease, Huntington's disease, multiple sclerosis, or CNS neoplasm. Pick's disease is a rarer form of degenerative brain disorder with symptoms similar to Alzheimer's, as is Creutzfeldt-Jakob disease, in which the etiologic factor is a slow virus.

The focus in this chapter is primarily on chronic, progressive, and irreversible dementias. However, there are several reversible disorders that can masquerade as dementia. Referred to as **pseudodementias**, these include depression, drug toxicity, metabolic disorders, infections, and nutrition deficiencies. Chronic lung disease and heart disease can lead to cerebral hypoxia and symptoms of dementia. It is imperative that such disorders are recognized and differentiated from irreversible dementia. Only through recognition can appropriate treatment measures be initiated (Ellison, 1984; Ronsman, 1988).

Sociocultural Characteristics

Progressive dementia is unlike many other psychiatric disorders because family characteristics are not viewed as contributing factors in progressive dementia (except when genetic factors are involved). Alzheimer's disease involves no clear pattern of inheritance, but a genetic component is suspected. An average adult's chances of developing Alzheimer's disease are about 1 in 100. If a close relative is affected by the disease, these odds increase to 4 in 100. Children of a person with early onset (FAD) have a 50 percent risk of developing Alzheimer's disease (Alzheimer's Association, 1988; Maxmen, 1986).

Families are the primary providers of long-term care for people who suffer from dementia. Most often, the client is elderly, which means the care givers are either elderly or in late middle age. Elderly spouses, who are most likely to provide care, have limited strength and energy to meet the demands of the situation. Middle-aged children, most typically daughters, must manage their own developmental issues as well as the role reversal that occurs with a dependent parent (Given, Collins, and Given, 1988; Mann, 1985). (See Chapter 6.)

The changes that occur in dementia are frightening to families, and for them to witness the steady deterioration of their loved ones is extremely painful. Families must deal with reality and make all the decisions, since clients are so severely impaired. Legal decisions concerning guardianship and power of attorney must be made by the family. Because constant supervision must be provided, family members may be restricted to the home environment. To reduce embarrassment over a client's socially unacceptable behavior, the family may even withdraw from socializing with friends. An additional source of stress is the client's inability to show appreciation for the family's care and concern. This is compounded by the client's irritable and critical behavior (Hall, 1988).

Many families eventually become exhausted and suffer from emotional, physical, and financial problems. A sense of loss is the most prominant feeling. The family loses control over time, energy, sleep, and money. There may be a loss of outside relationships as well as the loss of the relationship family members had with the affected loved one. The necessity to drastically alter lifestyles compounds the sense of loss. Anger, depression, guilt, helplessness, and grief may overwhelm family members. At this point, families must face the painful and difficult decision about nursing home placement. If the family is to maintain its own physical and mental health, this is often a necessary step. One important factor in this decision is financial. Long-term nursing home placement drains the family's savings, and the resulting financial stress may be more severe than the stress of maintaining the person at home. Self-help organizations such as Alzheimer's Association and publications such as *The 36-Hour Day: A Family Guide to Caring for Persons with Alzheimer's Disease* (Mace and Rabins, 1981), can provide much needed support to families (Given, Collins, and Given, 1988; Gabow, 1989; Wilson, 1989).

Causative Theories

Vigorous research into causal factors of dementia, particularly of Alzheimer's disease, is in progress. Several possible causes, in addition to genetic components, are currently being explored. A major recent discovery is that an enzyme necessary for the manufacture of acetylcholine, choline acetyltransferase, is deficient when Alzheimer's disease is present. A small cluster of brain cells important in memory, known as the hippocampus, is especially dependent on acetylcholine. Environmental factors—such as metal exposure, head trauma, and a slow virus—have also been implicated in dementia (Alzheimer's Association, 1988; Cohen, 1988; Schneider and Emr, 1985).

New findings have confirmed the presence of a genetic marker for the inherited form of Alzheimer's disease (FAD). The marker occurs on chromosome 21, and it is thought that the gene sends a wrong message to the nearby amyloid gene, which then produces excessive amounts of the protein amyloid. Scientists theorize that amyloid accumulates in the brain and forms plaques, leading to the destruction of brain cells. Interestingly, people with Down syndrome, who also have an abnormality on chromosome 21, frequently develop Alzheimer's disease in middle age (Glenner, 1988).

Medical Treatment

Pseudodementias are treated by correcting the underlying disorder. Although no cure for dementias such as Alzheimer's disease yet exists, several treatments, such as a well-balanced diet, are recommended. In limited studies, clients have been given foods that are rich in precursors to acetylcholine, like egg yolks, but results are inconclusive. Regarding the hypothesis about metal exposure, investigators are experimentally treating clients with chelating agents that bind aluminum, thereby facilitating its elimination from the body.

Drug treatment with acetylcholine or acetylcholine agonists is being tested. Centrally acting anticholinesterase agents such as physostigmine and tetrahydroaminoacridine (THA) are being administered experimentally. THA has produced the more notable symptomatic improvement. Memory enhancers, such as vasopressin, and vasodilators, such as ergoloid mesytates and papaverine, have been tried, but their effectiveness has not been conclusively demonstrated. Psychostimulants may increase initiative, mood, and locomotion but cause no changes in cognitive functioning. Recent research indicates thiamine treatment may slightly improve cognitive functioning or slow the progression of cognitive impairment. Since a concurrent depression may increase functional disability, antidepressant medications are prescribed for clients with depressive symptoms. Antipsychotic medication may be used for those clients experiencing paranoid thoughts or severe agitation. For those individuals experiencing sleep problems, the use of hypnotics is contraindicated since the medication does not improve sleep patterns and often increases confusion and sedation during waking periods (Billig, 1988; Blass, 1988; Satlin, 1988).

As is evident, the effectiveness of medical treatments directed at underlying causes of dementia are experimental and inconclusive. Other treatments are palliative at best. Sensitive caring is indeed the single most important therapeutic approach to clients and significant others.

Knowledge Base: Delirium

Delirium develops quickly and usually lasts about one week unless the underlying disorder is not corrected. Prompt medical attention is vital to prevent permanent brain damage or death. The course of the disorder is one of fluctuation, that is, periods of coherency alternate with periods of confusion.

Behavioral Characteristics

Delirious clients generally display an alteration in psychomotor activity and poor impulse control. Some delirious clients are apathetic and withdrawn, others are agitated and tremulous, and still others shift rapidly between apathy and agitation. Speech patterns may be limited and dull, or they may be fast, pressured, and loud. There may be a constant picking at clothes and bed linen as the result of an underlying restlessness. This combination of restlessness and cognitive changes interferes with the person's ability to complete tasks (Dwyer, 1987; Ellison, 1984).

Bizarre and destructive behavior, which worsens at night, may occur as clients attempt to protect themselves or escape from frightening delusions or hallucinations. This may take the form of calling for help, striking out at others, or even attempting to leap out of windows (Pallett and O'Brien, 1985).

Over the course of the past two days, Mary has exhibited abrupt swings in behavior. At times, she barely responds to questions or environmental stimuli. At other times, primarily during the nighttime, she becomes agitated, loud, and talkative. She may curse at the nurses one minute and beg them for help the next minute. She often yells about the snakes crawling all over her bed and attempts to beat at them.

Affective Characteristics

In delirium, clients' affect may range from apathy to extreme irritability to euphoria. Emotions are labile and can change abruptly. A delirious client may be laughing and suddenly become extremely sad and tearful, reflective of the CNS insult. The predominant emotion in delirium is fear. Illusions, delusions, and hallucinations are vivid and extremely frightening (Pallett and O'Brien, 1985).

Mary looks terrified during her visual hallucinations of snakes on her bed. She begs anyone for help in removing the snakes and keeping her safe. During her lucid periods, Mary tells the nurse she has been frightened of snakes since she was very young, which increases the impact of her hallucinations.

Cognitive Characteristics

According to DSM-III-R, the hallmark of delirium is the clouding of consciousness and an unclear awareness of the environment. From a mild confusion, this may progress to a dulling of alertness to a complete lack of interest in the surroundings to a stuporous or semicomatose state. Clients are usually disoriented in all three spheres of person, time, and place. Recent memory is impaired, but remote memory is usually not affected. Confabulation may be noted in response to memory gaps.

Delirious clients are unable to concentrate and are easily distracted; therefore, interactions are difficult if not impossible. Thought processes are disorganized, and the client is unable to think logically and coherently. This lack of judgment and reason severely impairs the decision-making process. There is also a loss of the ability to think abstractly.

Almost all delirious clients misperceive sensory stimuli in the environment. The result is usually visual or auditory illusions. For example, it is not uncommon for these clients to think that strangers are family or friends. Visual hallucinations are also common and may involve people, animals, objects, or bright flashes of light or color. Delusional beliefs occur around the reality of the illusions and hallucinations. These changes often extend into sleep, and clients report vivid and terrifying dreams (Dwyer, 1987; Gomez and Gomez, 1987; Pallett and O'Brien, 1985).

Marie is an 18-year-old, extremely thin, anorexic client. A measurement of her blood glucose reveals a level of 40 mg%. She is extremely agitated and incoherent. Because she continues to talk to people who are not present, she is unable to give a history. She is able to state her name but does not know where she is and does not recognize her boyfriend, who has brought her to the hospital. She is convinced that Ron, a nurse, is her boyfriend.

Physiologic Characteristics

There is a disturbance in the sleep cycle of delirious clients. Some clients have hypersomnia and sleep fitfully throughout the day and night. Other clients have insomnia and sleep very little, day or night.

There are obvious signs of autonomic activity, including increased cardiac rate, elevated blood pressure, flushed face, dilated pupils, and sweating. Respiratory depth or rhythm may be altered as a result of brainstem depression or in an attempt to maintain acid-base balance as the result of the underlying disorder.

Delirious clients may experience irregular tremors throughout the body. Those in a resting position may have myoclonus, a sudden, large muscle spasm. Although they occur most frequently in the face and shoulders, these spasms, which are a result of irritation of the brain cortex, can happen anywhere in the body. If the hand is hyperextended, there will be an involuntary palmar flexion called *asterixis.* Generalized seizures may also occur (Pallett and O'Brien, 1985).

Sociocultural Characteristics

Because of the sudden and often unexplained onset of delirium, families are usually anxious and frightened. They may not know how to respond to the agitation, pressured speech, destructive behavior, and labile moods. Equally confusing to families are the disorientation, illusions, hallucinations, and delusions. Since delirious clients are unable to make decisions, families must temporarily assume that responsibility. Information and support from nurses will assist families through this critical period.

Causative Theories

By affecting the CNS many conditions may lead to delirium. Cerebral metabolism is dependent on sufficient amounts of oxygen, glucose, and metabolic cofactors. Brain hypoxia may result from pulmonary disease, anemia, or carbon monoxide poisoning. A decreased cerebral blood flow leads to ischemia of the CNS. Ischemia may result from cardiac arrhythmias or arrest, congestive heart failure, pulmonary embolus, decreased blood volume, systemic lupus erythematosus, or subacute bacterial endocarditis. A lack of adequate glucose for cerebral metabolism occurs during a state of hypoglycemia. There are certain metabolic cofactors essential for cerebral enzyme actions. Cofactor deficiencies involve thiamine, niacin, pyridoxine, folate, and vitamin B_{12} (Pallett and O'Brien, 1985).

Endocrine disorders of the thyroid, parathyroid, and adrenal glands are associated with delirium. Hepatic and renal failure may be contributing disorders. Fluid and electrolyte imbalance—particularly acidosis, alkalosis, potassium, sodium, magnesium, and calcium imbalances—are additional causes of delirium. Toxicity from substances such as alcohol, sedatives, antihistamines, parasympatholytics, opiates, cerebral stimulants, digitalis, antidepressants, and heavy metals may also lead to a delirious state. (See Chapters 12 and 13 for discussion of alcohol and drug abuse.) Any direct or primary CNS disturbance—trauma, infection, hemorrhage, neoplasm, or a seizure disorder—is likely to trigger delirium. Additionally, drugs used for the treatment of hypertension and parkinsonism have been implicated in causing delirium. Delirium has been known to occur in settings such as intensive care units and has been labeled ICU psychosis (Dwyer, 1987; Ellison, 1984).

Medical Treatment

The medical treatment of delirium involves the swift identification of the offending cause. Appropriate treatment requires removal of an offending substance, stabilization in the presence of trauma, administration of antibiotics for infection, or reestablishment of nutrition and/or metabolic balance.

Assessment

Assessing clients with organic brain disorders can be a challenge to nurses' ingenuity and patience. Some clients are able to respond appropriately when questions are asked simply and enough time is given for them to respond. Other clients are so disoriented and confused they are unable to answer questions; in these situations, nurses must rely on family members to provide the necessary information.

Two focused nursing assessments follow. Obviously the questions in the first assessment must be adapted to the client's ability to comprehend and respond. The assessment for the family provides information vital for an accurate client assessment. Table 15–4 provides guidelines for the physical assessment that needs to be performed of all clients with organic brain disorders.

Table 15–4 *Physical Assessment of the Client with Organic Brain Disorder*

Complete a head-to-toe assessment with particular attention to the following areas:

Psychomotor activity
- Restlessness
- Tremors
- Hypertonia
- Myoclonus
- Asterixis
- Seizures
- Gait
- Apraxia
- Hyperorality
- Perseveration phenomena

Speech
- Slow and dull
- Fast and pressured

Level of consciousness
- Describe

Incontinence
- Bowel, bladder

Cardiovascular/pulmonary
- Apical pulse
- Blood pressure
- Respirations: Rate? Depth? Rhythm?

Additional evidence of underlying pathophysiology
- Recent trauma
- Recent intake of medications, alcohol
- Recent withdrawal from alcohol, drugs

Laboratory examinations

The following should be completed and assessed:
- Complete blood count
- Blood glucose
- Arterial blood gases
- Blood pH
- Serum electrolytes
- Serum calcium
- Serum phosphate
- Blood urea nitrogen
- Liver function tests
- Thyroid studies

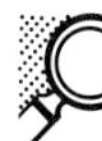

FOCUSED NURSING ASSESSMENT *for the Client with Organic Brain Disorder*

Behavioral assessment

How much assistance is needed in bathing? Toileting? Dressing? Eating?

Personal appearance:
Describe any difficulties in performing complex tasks at home and at work.
What kinds of things have been said by others about your behavior?
Give me an example of something that has confused you recently.
Have you ever become lost when you went out for a walk?
Tell me about how much food you usually eat in a day.
Under what conditions do you omit meals?
Under what conditions do you overeat?
Do you vomit after overeating?
Tell me what kinds of things you like to pick up and examine with your hands.
How do you protect yourself when you are frightened?

Affective assessment
What kinds of things make you feel anxious?
When do you feel sad?
How often do you feel irritable?
What are your major frustrations in life?
How do you feel about growing older?

Cognitive assessment
What month is it?
What year is it?
Who is the President of the United States?
What is your telephone number (or address)?
Where are you right now?
Tell me your complete name.
What did you do for activity this morning?
What is the purpose of (show the objects to the client) a comb? Toothbrush? Pencil? Telephone book? Shoe?
What is the meaning of the proverb "People in glass houses should not throw stones?"
How are a rose, a carnation, and a lily alike?
How are an automobile and an airplane different?
What would you do if someone shouted "Fire!" right now?
What would you do if you found a stamped, addressed envelope on the sidewalk?
Count backward from 100 by sevens.
Say these five numbers back to me: 3, 10, 17, 22, 29.
What kinds of things do you see that others do not see?
What kinds of things do you see that frighten you?
Tell me about your dreams.

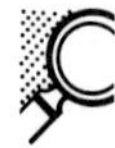

FOCUSED NURSING ASSESSMENT *for the Family of the Client with Organic Brain Disorder*

Behavioral assessment
How much assistance is needed in activities of daily living?
In what situations have you been embarrassed about her/his behavior?
Tell me about her/his wandering away from home.
Is there difficulty in carrying out psychomotor activities?
Is she/he picking up and putting things in the mouth?
Does she/he touch everything in sight?
What kinds of repetitive movements does she/he make?
Describe food intake for a day.
Do periods of fasting alternate with overeating?
How well can she/he walk? Sit up?
Describe her/his interactions with other people.
Is she/he withdrawn? Agitated? Aggressive?
Are the behavior problems worse at night?

Affective assessment
Describe the degree of spontaneity to verbal and nonverbal stimuli.
How anxious does she/he seem to you?
How depressed does she/he seem to you?
In what way is irritability increasing?
Does she/he have wide mood swings? Describe.

Cognitive assessment
Have there been changes in her/his ability to concentrate?
Describe any confusion about person, time, or place.
Describe any suspicious thinking.
Describe any recent memory loss.
Describe any remote memory loss.
Does she/he make up answers when facts cannot be remembered?
Is there difficulty in finding the right word for objects?
Has she/he lost the ability to read and write?
Is there an inability to identify familiar sounds?
Give me examples of irrational decision making.
Does she/he talk about seeing things that others do not see? Examples:
Has she/he thought that strangers were family members? Examples:

Sociocultural assessment
Is there a family history of organic brain disorder?
What are previous hobbies/interests? Family activities?

Who has been the primary care giver?
Describe the stresses in care giving (emotional, physical, financial).
Describe the positive aspects of care giving.
What kinds of support systems are you able to use? Family? Friends? Religious? Self-help groups?
What kinds of discussions have taken place regarding placement?
What other kinds of living arrangements are possible?
Who is involved in making these decisions?
How united is the family in providing care?

Nursing Diagnosis and Planning

The assessment process provides the data from which nurses develop individualized plans of care. In caring for clients with reversible delirium, all measures must be taken to ensure that permanent brain damage or death does not occur. Since delirium is acute and short-term, plans of care are directed toward short-term goals with the long-term medical and nursing goal being one of correcting the underlying disorder. In caring for clients with irreversible dementia, patience and compassion are the guiding principles. Even though the disorder is progressive and eventually terminal, it is important that clients be supported and encouraged to remain at the highest possible level of functioning.

The most effective approach to dementia is use of the multidisciplinary team. Speech therapists may be able to slow down the aphasic process as well as restore partial swallowing function. Physical therapists can maintain or increase range of motion, improve muscle tone, improve coordination, and increase endurance for exercise. Occupational therapists can provide additional sensory stimulation and self-care training programs. Social workers can provide individual or group therapy for families of clients with dementia; moreover, they can assist with finding community resources or institutional placement. Pastoral counselors are able to assist clients and families in meeting religious and spiritual needs (Rango, 1985).

Nursing care plans must be adapted and individualized for each client, which means that goals and expected outcomes should have dates, and interventions should be specific to the accomplishment of goals. The care plans can be adapted by family members when providing care at home for the demented or delirious client. (See Table 15–5 for the nursing care plan for the client with organic brain disorder.)

The nurse's role bears reemphasis: The overall goal of nursing intervention with demented clients is to facilitate the highest possible level of physical, emotional, cognitive, and social functioning. Because cognition underlies and directs behavior, the client's cognitive ability guides the selection of nursing interventions. Nursing actions should build on remaining capabilities and compensate for deficits (Beck and Heacock, 1988).

Nurses must be advocates for family care givers. Families are often in need of teaching and counseling, support groups, and respite care. Nurses should assist family members to locate local resources and develop support networks (Hall, 1988).

Evaluation

Evaluation is conducted according to the outcome criteria of the nursing care plan. Nurses need to evaluate continually if the criteria are being met and modify the plan accordingly. In relation to the dementias, nurses need to evaluate whether clients are reaching their maximum potentials and whether their families have the support to deal with the disorder. Evaluative questions for the family are

1. Are care givers experiencing stress-related symptoms?
2. How supportive is the family system?
3. Has the family been able to adapt by providing relief for the care giver in terms of cleaning, shopping, and time away from the home?
4. Has the family been able to discuss feelings of helplessness, embarrassment, guilt, and grief?
5. Has the family been able to support the optimal level of functioning for the client?

Table 15–5 Nursing Care Plan for the Client with Organic Brain Disorder

Nursing Diagnosis: Impaired verbal communication related to aphasia.
Goal: Client will communicate basic needs.

Intervention	*Rationale*	*Expected Outcome*
Ask closed-ended questions	These are easier to respond to than open-ended questions	Answers yes/no questions
Use short "noun" sentences (eg, "Mary, it is time to eat now")	Pronouns such as *I, me,* and *you* are often misunderstood	Responds appropriately to requests
Label objects in the environment	Having objects labeled will decrease the need to search for the word	Refers to labels when unable to remember word
Provide necessary word when client is unable to recall word	Client will often recognize the forgotten word when it is heard	Acknowledges the correct word when hearing it

Nursing Diagnosis: Sensory perceptual alterations related to agnosia.
Goal: Client will express less frustration when unable to recognize stimuli.

Intervention	*Rationale*	*Expected Outcome*
Use slow, clear, simple sentences	Client may be able to comprehend less complex language	Responds appropriately to simple commands
When stimuli are misinterpreted, tell client what stimuli are	Will reassure client and stimulate memory	Identifies sensory stimuli when provided with information
Use nonverbal communication (eg, smiles, hugs, hand-holding)	Conveys concern and caring	Responds to nonverbal communication
Put necessary objects in hand (eg, spoon, washcloth, etc)	Client is often able to respond in an automatic way	Uses familiar objects

Nursing Diagnosis: Altered family processes related to interacting with delirious family member.
Goal: Family will cope with client's impairment.

Intervention	*Rationale*	*Expected Outcome*
Include family in care	Will increase family's trust and decrease feelings of helplessness	Participates in care
Explain reasons for client's confusion	Understanding reasons for behavior will increase family's ability to cope	Verbalizes comprehension of client's condition
Serve as a role model of how to interact with client	Will increase family's ability to participate in plan of care	Interacts appropriately with client

Nursing Diagnosis: Altered family processes related to demands of caring for family member with dementia.
Goal: Family will cope with client's impairment. Family structures will remain intact.

Intervention	*Rationale*	*Expected Outcome*
Teach family reasons for behavioral changes	Family needs to understand limitations to respond appropriately	Verbalizes understanding of process of dementia
Discuss long-term stages of dementia	Prepare family for responsibilities ahead	Identifies realistic implications of disease process

(Diagnosis continued)

Table 15–5 *(continued)*

Intervention	*Rationale*	*Expected Outcome*
Encourage family to express feelings to nonjudgmental person	Venting feelings will assist family in managing negative feelings	Vents feelings
Identify most urgent causes of stress	Priorities should be addressed first to decrease anxiety	Identifies immediate problems with client
Prescribe periods of rest and recreation for family	Family must prevent total emotional and physical fatigue	Family continues to function
Discuss seeking rewards and recognition apart from client	Client unable to provide positive feedback to care givers	Identifies sources of positive feedback
Help family identify quality and quantity of current support systems	Prevents social isolation of care givers and decreases burden of care	Identifies support systems
Develop a collaborative relationship with family	Family will feel listened to and respected	Verbalizes that nurse is a support system
Refer to community resources (eg, day care, respite care, support groups)	Provide reinforcement for care givers and decrease burden of care	Uses community resources
Discuss use of housekeepers, companions	Prevents total emotional and physical fatigue	Uses outside help
Conduct a family meeting to discuss changes in family system as result of disabilities	Decreases burden on care giver as well as identifies ways to compensate	Family meets as a group

Nursing Diagnosis: Fear related to vivid hallucinations.
Goal: Client will verbalize decreasing fear.

Intervention	*Rationale*	*Expected Outcome*
Remain calm	Increased tension in nurse will increase client's anxiety	No additional increase in client's anxiety level
Reassure client	Reassurance may prevent panic from hallucinations	Seeks out assistance when afraid
Do not deny client's reality, but do not support hallucinations	Helps client regain appropriate reality	Differentiates between the two realities
Use touch if acceptable (eg, "I'll stay with you and hold your hand")	Touch may reassure and prevent panic	Responds positively to touch
Do not isolate client	Isolation often increases hallucinations	Indicates a decrease in hallucinations

Nursing Diagnosis: Impaired home maintenance management related to loss of judgment and inability to assume responsibility for own safety.
Goal: Client will remain safe.

Intervention	*Rationale*	*Expected Outcome*
Teach that accidents are more likely to occur when tension and stress are high	Tension decreases perceptions and client overresponds to anxiety and tension	Verbalizes relationship between tension and accidents

(Diagnosis continued)

Table 15–5 *(continued)*

Nursing Diagnosis *(continued)*: Impaired home maintenance management related to loss of judgment and inability to assume responsibility for own safety.
Goal: Client will remain safe.

Intervention	*Rationale*	*Expected Outcome*
Remove or lock up objects that may be potentially dangerous (eg, irons, power tools, garden tools, paints, solvents, car keys, throw rugs, stove knobs, clotheslines)	Decreasing hazards will prevent accidents	Environment is as safe as possible
Turn down hot-water heater	A lower temperature will prevent accidental burning	Does not burn self
Discourage driving	Client may become disoriented while driving	Agrees not to drive
Do not leave client alone in car	Client may release brakes or drive the car	Remains safe
Discourage smoking or provide supervision	Supervision will prevent fire	Remains safe

Nursing Diagnosis: Potential for injury related to decreased judgment.
Goal: Client will remain safe.

Intervention	*Rationale*	*Expected Outcome*
Assess neighborhood for safety (eg, busy streets, swimming pools, rivers, loose dogs)	Client is unable to protect self from these dangers	Remains safe in immediate neighborhood
Alert others in the neighborhood	Increases protection for client	Remains safe in immediate neighborhood
Minimize specific hazards in the home (eg, remove stove knobs, lock up cleaning agents and medications, keep pathways free of obstruction)	Prevents accidents in the home	Remains safe in the home
Have family administer medications	Memory loss interferes with correct self-administration	Receives medications in correct dose at prescribed times

Nursing Diagnosis: Potential for injury related to wandering behavior.
Goal: Client will remain safe.

Intervention	*Rationale*	*Expected Outcome*
Increase exercise	May reduce restlessness that promotes wandering	Follows exercise routine
Provide an ID bracelet and ID card; participate in local police registry if available	If client becomes lost, this will help others return him or her home	Wears ID bracelet; returns home safely
Provide simple instructions on a card to refer to if lost (eg, phone number and directions home)	If client can still read and comprehend, this will increase ability to get home	Follows directions to return home

(Diagnosis continued)

Table 15–5 *(continued)*

Intervention	*Rationale*	*Expected Outcome*
Keep night-lights on at night	Reduces hazard of falls during darkness	Does not fall
Put an alarm system on all exit doors	Family will be alerted to client's leaving the home	Does not wander off alone

Nursing Diagnosis: Impaired physical mobility related to stiffness, awkwardness, and impaired balance.
Goal: Client will remain as physically active as limitations allow.

Intervention	*Rationale*	*Expected Outcome*
Provide regular exercise (eg, walking, group exercise, or dancing)	Exercise will decrease tension, maintain range of motion, and promote sleep at night	Exercises daily
Exercise with client	Will increase client's participation	Exercises daily
Maintain exercise routine (same time, same exercises)	A regular schedule will decrease confusion and increase participation	Exercises daily
Maintain motor skills that are still possible	Skills will be retained longer if used	Participates in activities requiring motor skills
If unsteady, have supportive person nearby	Additional support may be necessary to maintain steadiness	Does not fall and injure self
Provide handrails on staircases and in bathroom	Will provide additional support	Does not fall and injure self
Use Posey restraint if client cannot sit unassisted	Severe muscular impairment may prevent sitting without support	Sits when supported

Nursing Diagnosis: Alteration in nutrition: less than body requirements related to apraxia and decreased judgment.
Goal: Client will maintain an adequate state of nutrition.

Intervention	*Rationale*	*Expected Outcome*
Provide a balanced diet of two or more milk, two or more meat, four or more fruit and vegetable, and four or more bread exchanges	Prevents nutrition deficiencies and prevents other related illnesses	Eats balanced diet
Refer to community resources such as Eating Together or Meals-On-Wheels	These resources will provide one hot nutritious meal a day	Uses resources
Maintain regular schedule of mealtime	Prevents confusion related to change	Responds to routine mealtime
Make certain that dentures fit well	Poorly fitting dentures interfere with chewing	Able to chew food
Serve familiar foods	New foods often increase confusion	Eats willingly
Limit the number of foods in front of client	Client may have difficulty deciding which food to eat	Eats willingly
Provide utensils with large built-up handles	These are easier to use when coordination is poor	Manipulates utensils to eat
Try using bowls rather than plates	These are easier because food is not pushed off	Feeds self from bowl

(Diagnosis continued)

Table 15–5 *(continued)*

Nursing Diagnosis *(continued):* Alteration in nutrition: less than body requirements related to apraxia and decreased judgment.
Goal: Client will maintain an adequate state of nutrition.

Intervention	*Rationale*	*Expected Outcome*
Remove other distractions from table area	Maintains focus on eating	Eats willingly within a reasonable length of time
Do not rush eating	Impaired people eat slowly	Feeds self given enough time
Ensure adequate fluid intake	Prevents dehydration	Remains hydrated
Weigh weekly	Monitors status	Weight remains constant

Nursing Diagnosis: Bathing/hygiene, dressing/grooming self-care deficit related to cognitive impairments resulting in neglect of self.
Goal: Client will perform activities of daily living with optimal independence and maintenance of physical status.

Intervention	*Rationale*	*Expected Outcome*
Monitor ability to perform ADLs	Establishes baseline data and allows for evaluation	
Encourage activities and skills still present	Maintains independence and gives sense of competency	Performs ADLs within range of competency
Try to follow old routines as much as possible (eg, time of day for bath, preference for bath or shower)	Decreases confusion that occurs with changes in routine	Follows routine of self-care
Encourage as much decision making as possible in ADLs	Increases sense of control and prevents disengagement that occurs when all responsibility is taken away	Makes appropriate decisions
If necessary, give step-by-step directions with only one step at a time	Will decrease the confusion related to slowed thinking and distractibility	Follows step-by-step directions
Lay out clean clothes in the order they are to be put on. Use Velcro tape instead of buttons and zippers	Will increase independence by decreasing the need for decisions and manipulation of complex closures on clothing	Dresses self appropriately

Nursing Diagnosis: Sensory/perceptual alterations related to hallucinations.
Goal: Client will verbalize accurate perception of reality.

Intervention	*Rationale*	*Expected Outcome*
Maintain a structured environment, avoid rapid changes, keep staffing changes to a minimum	Eliminates sensory overload and increases feelings of security	Verbalizes increased feelings of safety
Spend time with client	Increased contact will decrease confusion and maintain communication	Responds to contact with increased orientation
Maintain a quiet environment	Loud noises can stimulate hallucinations	No verbalizations of hallucinations
Respond to hallucinations and delusions by presenting reality	Reinforces reality and prevents panic	Acknowledges differences in the two realities

(Diagnosis continued)

Table 15–5 *(continued)*

Intervention	*Rationale*	*Expected Outcome*
Reassure client that you will keep him or her safe from hallucinations	Will reduce or prevent panic	Verbalizes increased feelings of security

Nursing Diagnosis: Sensory/perceptual alterations related to illusions.
Goal: Client will accurately perceive people, objects, and sounds within the environment.

Intervention	*Rationale*	*Expected Outcome*
Provide necessary glasses and/or hearing aid	Will increase accurate perception of environmental stimuli	Uses glasses, hearing aid
Identify and label sounds occurring in the environment	Will decrease confusion by ensuring that auditory stimuli is meaningful	Correctly identifies familiar sounds
Avoid whispering or talking out of easy hearing range	Will limit misperceptions of what's being said	Hears accurately what's being said
Decreases environmental stimuli to quiet peaceful levels	Sensory overload increases confusion and illusions	Verbalizes accurate perception of environmental stimuli
Keep soft lights in room and avoid shadows and glare	Darkness, shadows, and glare increase disorientation and illusions	Verbalizes accurate perception of environmental stimuli

Nursing Diagnosis: Sleep pattern disturbance related to central nervous system irritation.
Goal: Client will experience at least 4 hours of uninterrupted sleep at night.

Intervention	*Rationale*	*Expected Outcome*
Monitor and keep a record of sleep patterns	To establish baseline data	
Minimize napping during daytime	Napping interferes with sleep cycle	
Schedule exercise 2 hours before bedtime	Increased physical fatigue will promote sleep	Exercises each evening
Talk client through relaxation techniques	Decreases tension and prepares body for sleep	Relaxes before bedtime
Limit caffeine, but try giving a glass of wine at bedtime if acceptable to client	Caffeine increases CNS stimulation; wine promotes CNS relaxation	Verbalizes increased feelings of relaxation
Ensure quiet environment with only soft night-light	Atmosphere must be conducive to sleep	
Provide comfort measures (eg, back rub, arranging linens)	Increased comfort is conducive to sleep	
Arrange timing of care so not to disturb sleep	Will provide uninterrupted periods of rest	Sleeps for 4 hours without interruption
Teach family members measures to induce sleep	Family must be able to get adequate rest if they are to continue providing care	Family achieves at least 4 hours of sleep

(continued)

Table 15–5 *(continued)*

Nursing Diagnosis: Altered thought processes related to lack of reality orientation.
Goal: Client will have periods of orientation to reality.

Intervention	*Rationale*	*Expected Outcome*
Use the name client prefers	Use of name will reinforce personhood	Responds to name
Allow family to stay	When client is acutely confused, the presence of family may improve orientation	Responds to family interaction
Establish routine of care	A routine will counteract feelings of chaos and confusion	Verbalizes less confusion
Write out list of ADLs	Written list will aid client in maintaining orientation	Follows list
Provide aids that assist with reality orientation (eg, TV, radio, large-print calendar, clock, and labels on objects in the environment) Note: Be selective regarding TV/radio programs. Avoid intricate plots or frightening content.	Will increase orientation as well as increase recreative aspects of life	Uses environmental objects to maintain reality
Give cues that help client remember reality and gently remind client of what actually occurred by filling in information gaps	Will decrease use of confabulation used to decrease shame or embarrassment	Uses confabulation minimally
Orient matter-of-factly about who, where, and what is happening	Allows client to recognize forgetfulness without shame	Verbalizes forgetfulness
Discuss topics meaningful to client (eg, work, hobbies, children)	Meaningful topics increase orientation and promote self-identity	Discusses personal topics
Allow personal items in room	Will promote orientation and self-identity	Recognizes personal items

Nursing Diagnosis: Altered thought processes related to paranoid accusations.
Goal: Client will decrease use of accusations.

Intervention	*Rationale*	*Expected Outcome*
Teach family that arguing or explaining does not help	Discussion will not change client's mind about suspicions	Family does not argue
Teach family that client's accusations are a cover-up for forgetting where things have been placed	Family needs to understand process to respond appropriately to client's memory loss	Family verbalizes understanding
Help client locate lost objects	Location may solve immediate problem	
Support client's feelings of anger and frustration	Feelings underneath accusatory statements must be acknowledged and supported	Verbalizes feelings of support
Distract client with an alternative activity	Will decrease obsession with suspicious thoughts	Participates in other activities.

(continued)

Table 15–5 *(continued)*

Nursing Diagnosis: Potential for violence: self-directed or directed at others related to anger.
Goal: Client will remain safe. Family will remain safe.

Intervention	*Rationale*	*Expected Outcome*
Respond calmly and do not retaliate with anger	Recognize that client's anger is often exaggerated and displaced	
Remove objects from environment that may be used to harm self or others	Reduce opportunities for physical harm	Environment is as safe as possible
Remove client from upsetting situation and distract him or her	Memory difficulty allows distraction because client quickly forgets what caused the anger	Calms down and verbalizes less anger
Identify the precipitating event	Increases ability to prevent or minimize recurrence	Verbalizes what precipitated the violent behavior

Alzheimer's disease is terminal in the final stage if complications such as sepsis, pneumonia, or the hazards of immobility do not cause death beforehand. Important nursing interventions are, therefore, to provide care that helps the client experience a peaceful death and to support the family through anticipatory grief.

SUMMARY

1. Dementia is also referred to as chronic brain disorder, irreversible brain disorder, and primary encephalopathy. It is the major neuropsychiatric disorder of old age and the fourth leading cause of death among adults in the United States.

2. Delirium is also referred to as acute brain disorder, reversible brain disorder, and secondary encephalopathy. It may occur from a wide variety of pathophysiologic conditions.

Knowledge Base

3. The behavioral characteristics of dementia include decline in personal appearance, socially unacceptable behavior, wandering, apraxia, hyperorality, perseveration phenomena, hyperetamorphosis, and a deterioration in motor ability.

4. The affective characteristics of dementia include anxiety, depression, helplessness, frustration, shame, lack of spontaneity, and irritability. Moods are often labile and catastrophic reactions are not uncommon.

5. The cognitive characteristics of dementia include memory loss, poor judgment, disorientation, delusions of persecution, aphasia, agraphia, and agnosia.

6. Families are the primary care givers to clients with dementia. As such, they risk emotional and physical fatigue, and financial depletion. They need to be encouraged to use supportive resources.

7. The behavioral characteristics of delirium include apathy and withdrawal, agitation and trembling, and bizarre and destructive behavior.

8. The affective characteristics of delirium may range from apathy to irritability to euphoria and may change abruptly.

9. The cognitive characteristics of delirium include clouding of consciousness, disorientation, memory impairment, distractibility, lack of judgment, illusions, hallucinations, and delusions.

Assessment

10. Client assessment must include the family's perception of changes, since the client is not a reliable source of accurate information.

11. Nurses must assess clients for pseudodementias because appropriate treatment can reverse the process of pseudodementias.

Nursing Diagnosis and Planning

12. In caring for clients with delirium, all measures must be taken to ensure that permanent brain damage or death does not occur.

13. A multidisciplinary approach is the most effective in managing clients suffering from dementia.

14. Keeping the client safe is a priority nursing goal.

15. The overall goal of nursing intervention with demented clients is to facilitate the highest possible level of physical, emotional, cognitive, and social functioning.

16. Nurses assist families by providing education, helping them locate resources such as respite care and support groups, and by sustaining them through anticipatory grieving.

Evaluation

17. Evaluation of nursing care is based on the progress toward outcome criteria by the client and the family.

CHAPTER REVIEW

Irene, who is 74 years old, lives with her husband Alvero, who is 76 years old. They live on several acres of land in the country. Their five children and eight grandchildren all live in the surrounding community. Irene has been diagnosed as having Alzheimer's disease, stage 2. At times, Irene just sits and stares out the window or stares at the television with a flat affect. Sometimes, she will pace endlessly around the house. Irene must be carefully supervised—especially in the kitchen, where she has turned on the stove and boiled pots of water until they are dry. Her husband keeps the stove unplugged until he needs to use it. Since Irene cannot figure out why the stove does not work, she has begun to put wood in the oven, which she has lit to make the stove "work." Alvero and the adult children would like to be able to maintain Irene in her home environment rather than sending her to the local nursing home.

1. In assisting the family to make decisions about Irene's future care, which one of the following assessment questions would be most appropriate?
   (a) Has Irene lost her ability to read and write?
   (b) What kinds of support systems are available to the family?
   (c) In what situations have you been embarrassed about Irene's behavior?
   (d) Does Irene interact with friends and family?

2. In assessing Irene's judgment, which question would be most appropriate to ask Irene?
   (a) What would you do if someone shouted "Fire!" right now?
   (b) What kinds of things make you feel anxious?
   (c) What is your telephone number (or address)?
   (d) What kinds of things do you see that frighten you?

3. Which one of the following nursing diagnoses would be a priority for Irene's care?
   (a) Fear related to vivid hallucination
   (b) Impaired physical mobility related to impaired balance
   (c) Altered thought process related to lack of reality orientation
   (d) Potential for injury related to decreased judgment

4. Irene often wanders out of her house during the night, in search of her infant children. What safety suggestions would be best for the family to implement?
   (a) Put an alarm system on all exit doors
   (b) Put Irene in a waist restraint at night
   (c) Alert neighborhood people to the problem
   (d) Have family members alternate staying awake at night

5. Which one of the following evaluation statements by the family would indicate that the family is feeling fulfilled by caring for Irene in her home?
   (a) "It's wonderful when she has flashes of memory and we can all share the joy."
   (b) "Every day we ask ourselves how much longer we can go on."
   (c) "We remind ourselves that our past life has been rewarding even if the present is not."
   (d) "It's very frustrating not to be able to communicate with her. It's like talking to a dummy."

REFERENCES

Alzheimer's Association: *Public Relations Plan.* Alzheimer's Disease and Related Disorders Association, 1988.

American Association of Retired Persons: *Coping & Caring: Living with Alzheimer's Disease.* American Association of Retired Persons, 1986.

Beck C, Heacock P: Nursing interventions for patients with Alzheimer's disease. *Nurs Clin North Am* 1988; 23(1):95–124.

Billig N: Alzheimer's disease: A psychiatrist's perspective. *Nurs Clin North Am* 1988; 23(1):125–133.

Blass J, et al.: Thiamine and Alzheimer's disease: A pilot study. *Arch Neurol* 1988; 45(8):833–835.

Brady EM, Lawton MP, Liebowitz B: Senile dementia: Public policy and adequate institutional care. *Am J Public Health* 1984; 7412:1381–1383.

Burnside I: Nursing care. In: *Treatments for the Alzheimer Patient.* Jarvik LF, Winograd CH (editors). Springer, 1988. 39–58.

Cleary B: Organic mental disorders. *Foundations of Mental Health Nursing.* Saunders, 1989.

Cohen GD: *The Brain in Human Aging.* Springer, 1988.

Committee on Aging, Group for the Advancement of Psychiatry: *The Psychiatric Treatment of Alzheimer's Disease* (Report No. 125). Brunner/Mazel, 1988.

Cutler N, Narang P: Alzheimer's disease: Drug therapies. *Geriatr Nurs* (June) 1985; 160–163.

Dwyer BJ: Cognitive impairment in the elderly: Delirium, depression or dementia? *Focus on Geriatric Care, Rehab* 1987; 1(4):1–8.

Ellison J: DSM-III and the diagnosis of organic mental disorders. *Ann Emerg Med* 1984; 13:521–528.

Foreman MD: Acute confusional states in hospitalized elderly: A research dilemma. *Nurs Res* 1986; 35(1): 34–37.

Gabow C: The impact of Alzheimer's disease on family caregivers. *Home Healthcare Nurse* 1989; 7(1):19–21.

Gomez GE, Gomez EA: Delirium. *Geriatr Nurs* 1987; 8(6):330–332.

Given CW, Collins CE, Given BA: Sources of stress among families caring for relatives with Alzheimer's disease. *Nurs Clin North Am* 1988; 23(1):69–82.

Glenner GG: Alzheimer's disease: Its proteins and genes. *Cell* (Feb 12) 1988; 52:307–308.

Hall GR: Care of the patient with Alzheimer's disease living at home. *Nurs Clin North Am* 1988; 23(1):31–46.

Hoch C, Reynolds C: Sleep disturbances and what to do about them. *Geriatr Nurs* (Jan) 1986; 7:24–27.

Hutton JT: Evaluation and treatment of dementia. *Texas Medicine* 1987; 83:20–24.

Joyce EV, Kirksey KM: Alzheimer's disease: The roles of the home health nurse and the caregiver. *Home Healthcare Nurse* 1989; 7(1):15–18.

Katzman R: Medical progress: Alzheimer's disease. *N Engl J Med* 1986; 314:964–973.

Kiely M: Alzheimer's disease: Making the most of the time that's left. *RN* (Mar) 1985; 34–41.

Mace N, Rabins P: *The 36-Hour Day: A Family Guide to Caring for Persons with Alzheimer's Disease.* Johns Hopkins University Press, 1981.

Mann LN: Community support for families caring for members with Alzheimer's disease. *Home Healthcare Nurse* (Jan) 1985; 3:8–10.

Maxmen JS: *Essential Psychopathology.* Norton, 1986.

Pallett PJ, O'Brien MT: *Textbook of Neurological Nursing.* Little, Brown, 1985.

Rango N: The nursing home resident with dementia. *Ann Intern Med* (June) 1985; 102:835–841.

Ronsman K: Pseudodementia. *Geriatr Nurs* 1988; 9: 50–52.

Satlin A, Cole JO: Psychopharmacologic interventions. In: *Treatments for the Alzheimer Patient.* Jarvik LF, Winograd CH (editors). Springer, 1988; 59–79.

Schneider E, Emr M: Alzheimer's disease: Research highlights. *Geriatr Nurs* 1985; 6:136–138.

Shamoian CA, Teusink JP: Presenile and senile dementia. In: *Diagnostics and Psychopathology.* Flach F (editor). 1987; 171–185.

Teusink JP, Mahler S: Helping families cope with Alzheimer's disease. *Hosp Community Psychiatry* 1984; 35: 152–156.

Williams L: Alzheimer's: The need for caring. *J Gerontol Nurs* (Feb) 1986; 12:21–27.

Wilson HS: Family caregiving for a relative with Alzheimer's dementia: Coping with negative choices. *Nurs Res* 1989; 38(2):94–98.

SUGGESTED READINGS

Aronson M: *Understanding Alzheimer's Disease.* Scribner, 1988.

Batt LJ: Managing delirium. *J Psychosoc Nurs* 1989; 27(5): 22–25.

Farran CJ, Keane-Hagerty E: Communicating effectively with dementia patients. *J Psychosoc Nurs* 1989; 27(5): 13–16.

Gomez G, Gomez EA: Dementia? Or delirium? *Geriatric Nurs* 1989; 10(3):141–142.

Harvis KA, Rabins PV: Dementia: Helping family caregivers cope. *J Psychosoc Nurs* 1989; 27(5):7–12.

Pillemer K, Moore DW: Abuse of patients in nursing homes. *Gerontologist* 1989; 29(3):314–319.

Pruchno RA, Resch NL: Husbands and wives as caregivers: Antecedents of depression and burden. *Gerontologist* 1989; 29(2):159–165.

Robinson KM: A social skills training program for adult caregivers. *Adv Nurs Sci* 1988; 10(2):59–72.

Skinner PV, Jordan D: Home management of the patient with Alzheimer's disease. *Home Healthcare Nurse* 1989; 7(1):23–27.

CHAPTER 16

Violence

KAREN LEE FONTAINE

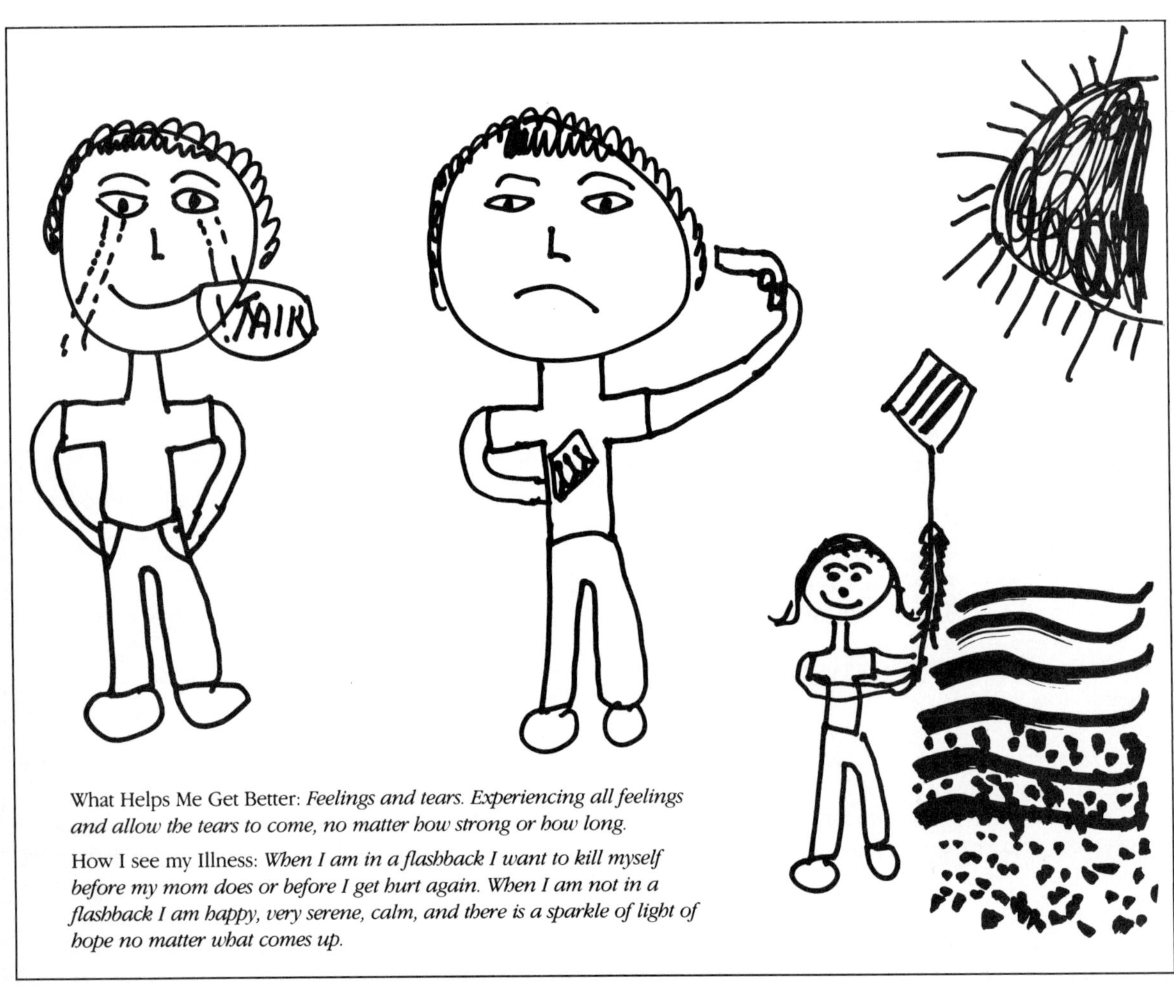

What Helps Me Get Better: *Feelings and tears. Experiencing all feelings and allow the tears to come, no matter how strong or how long.*

How I see my Illness: *When I am in a flashback I want to kill myself before my mom does or before I get hurt again. When I am not in a flashback I am happy, very serene, calm, and there is a sparkle of light of hope no matter what comes up.*

■ *Objectives*

After reading this chapter the student will be able to

- Identify groups of people at high risk for becoming victims of violence
- Discuss theories related to the dynamics of violent behavior
- Assess a client and family behaviorally, affectively, cognitively, physiologically, and socioculturally
- Use the nursing process to intervene with victims of violence and their families
- Identify legal implications that are a result of violent behavior

■ *Chapter Outline*

Violence Against the Self: Suicide

Suicide is the most violent harm people can inflict on themselves. **Suicide** can be defined in three different ways (Cutter, 1983):

1. Concerning the cognitive realm, that is, the thoughts about the desire to die: A person is described as being suicidal when the wish to die is very strong and plans are being made to take one's life.

2. Concerning the behavioral realm: Suicide—by shooting, hanging, or jumping, for example—is the actual behavior that injures or kills the person.
3. Concerning the consequence of the behavior: People either survive or die as a result of their behavior and are described as a successful suicide or an attempted suicide.

Incidence of Suicide

It is estimated that there are 10 to 12 suicidal deaths per 100,000 people in this country. However, since many suicides are reported as accidental deaths, this estimate is most likely low. Even with the underreporting, suicide remains the ninth greatest cause of death for the general population, the third cause of death among adolescents, and the second cause of death among college students. The impact of these statistics becomes even greater when it is recognized that for every successful suicide there are 10 to 20 unsuccessful suicides. In the United States there are approximately 30,000 suicides every year and it is estimated that an additional 240,000 to 600,000 people attempt suicide yearly (Denmark and Kabatznick, 1988; McIntosh, 1987).

In looking at the epidemiology of suicide, particular groupings can be selected and suicide rates calculated. Women attempt suicide two to three times as often as men, though twice as many men are successful suicides. Women not employed outside the home have a risk of committing suicide nine times higher than that of employed women. In the mentally ill population, one person out of 1000 dies from suicide each year. Diagnosed schizophrenics have the highest suicide rate, followed by people with affective disorders. Of those people who have made one prior attempt at suicide, one out of every 100 will be successful each year. Of those who have made two or more suicide attempts, 2 of 10 will be successful each year. Separated, divorced, and widowed people are twice as likely to commit suicide as the general population. Men over the age of 50 have double the rate of suicide as that of 25-year-old men. In the older population, the suicide rate soars to 53 people out of 100,000 older people and accounts for 39 percent of all successful suicides. With the increasing number of elderly persons in the United States, this suicide rate has serious implications for the future (Arbore and Willis, 1989; Boxwell, 1988; Cutter, 1983; Miller, 1982).

Under the age of 12, more boys attempt suicide than girls. After age 12 more girls attempt suicide than boys. Suicide as a cause of death reaches its peak during adolescence and young adulthood, second only to accidents. College students have a higher suicide rate than their noncollege peers.

As a group, whites have a higher rate of suicide than nonwhites. In a nonwhite population, suicide rates peak between 20 and 35 years and decline to low levels in old age. The peak for white females is around the age of 50; for white males the rate continues to increase throughout life, with those over 65 achieving the highest suicide rate of all groups (McIntosh, 1987). (See Table 16–1 for a list of factors contributing to suicidal behavior.)

In one study 80 percent of all successful suicides gave either verbal or behavioral warnings that they were contemplating suicide; 70 percent of the victims had visited their physician three to six months before the suicide, 40 percent made the visit one

Table 16–1 *Factors Contributing to High Suicidal Risk*

Adolescence, college enrollment, or age over 50 years
Employment as a full-time homemaker
Presence of alcohol or drug abuse
Separation, divorce, or death of spouse
Social isolation
Previous suicide attempts
Family history of suicide
Presence of chronic or terminal illness
Presence of mental illness
Multiple crises in life
Multiple losses in life
Feelings of failure and hopelessness

month before, and 7 to 15 percent saw the physician within the week preceding the suicide (Rosen, 1981).

Worldwide, the highest rates of suicide are in Hungary, Finland, Czechoslovakia, Austria, Switzerland, Denmark, and Sweden. The countries with the lowest rates of suicide are Mexico, Greece, Northern Ireland, Ireland, Spain, and Italy. Contributing factors to low suicide rates in these countries are thought to be the strong influence of Roman Catholicism and the unity and support of the extended family system (Magnuson, 1989). Note that the highest rates occur in northern countries where there is less sunlight in the winter, and the lowest rates occur in southern countries where people enjoy year-round sunshine. These worldwide rates are supporting evidence for the influence of sunlight on seasonal affective disorders. (See Chapter 11 for a description of the influence of sunlight.)

Significance of Suicide to Mental Health Nursing

Suicide is a worldwide, national, local, and familial problem. As such, it is of major concern for the nursing profession. Nurses need to be actively involved in preventing suicides by educating the general population about risk factors, suicidal cues, and interventions. Nurses also need to be prepared to do suicide assessments of people both in the clinical setting and in the community. When the potential for suicide is identified, nurses have to intervene quickly and effectively. Every nurse has a responsibility for competency in suicide intervention in the same way that every nurse is expected to be competent in cardiopulmonary resuscitation. If the suicide has been successful, nurses need to assist and support the family and friends of the victim to prevent further traumatization of the survivors.

Knowledge Base: Suicide

People commit suicide for hundreds of reasons.

- Some are driven to the act by delusions or command hallucinations.
- Some, because of depressed feelings or a chronic or terminal illness, see no hope for the future.
- For some, suicide is a relief from intractable pain, physical or psychologic.
- Some have experienced so many losses that life is no longer valuable.
- Some have been beset with multiple crises, which have drained their internal and external resources.
- For some, suicide is the ultimate expression of anger toward significant others.

Thus, suicide can be precipitated by many factors and has a great variety of meanings to the victims as well as the survivors. Despite this variety, potential suicide victims have a number of characteristics in common that can alert the nurse.

Behavioral Characteristics

Suicide is not a random act. It is a way out of a problem, dilemma, or unbearable situation. Suicidal individuals suffer intensely. People contemplating suicide often make subtle or even overt comments that indicate as much. They may mention all the pressure and stress they are experiencing and how helpless they feel. Some may discuss philosophy or religious beliefs concerning life after death. Verbal cues are statements such as

- "It won't matter much longer."
- "Will you miss me when I'm gone?"
- "You/They will be sorry."
- "I can't take this much longer."
- "I know the pain will be over soon."
- "I won't be here when you come back on Monday."
- "You won't have to worry about the money problems much longer."
- "The voices are telling me to hurt myself."

Certain behavioral patterns may indicate suicidal intentions. Obtaining a weapon such as a gun, strong rope, or a collection of pills is a high indicator of impending suicide. Often people begin to withdraw from interpersonal interactions and isolate themselves. There may be a change in work or school performance. An increased tendency toward accidents might indicate initial suicidal behavior. Some may show a sudden interest in their life insurance policies, whereas others may make or change their wills and give personal belongings away. Signs of drug or alcohol abuse also may be present (Parker, 1988).

Dennis, a 15-year-old youth, committed suicide by shooting himself. He was described as an excellent student who was expected to succeed in life. His classmates described him as a nice person but one without close friends. "He kind of kept to himself. Sometimes we would all be standing around waiting for the school bus. He would be standing off to one side by himself. We would be laughing about something, but he didn't have anything to say." One week before his suicide, he gave some of his personal belongings, including clothes, to his fellow students (Richardson, 1985).

Behavioral characteristics also include choosing a method for suicide. *Lethality* is measured by four factors:

- The degree of effort it takes to plan the attempt
- The specificity of the plan
- The accessibility of the weapon or method
- The ease by which one may or may not be rescued from the attempt

Perle is considering suicide by taking an overdose of sleeping pills. She has never had a prescription and plans to see her physician to obtain the pills. The lethality of her plan is fairly low since the method is not available, and it will take effort to make an appointment with her physician and plan out a reason for the request for a prescription. Even though a large number of sleeping pills are effective, they do not cause instantaneous death, so there is a period during which she may be rescued from her behavior.

Joel is considering suicide by shooting himself in the head. He is experienced with guns and has several of them. The lethality of his plan is very high since the weapon is available, and the method requires no further planning. A gunshot to the head usually causes death instantaneously, which prevents any rescue.

Violent means of suicide usually prevent rescue by others. More than half of all suicide deaths result from the use of guns or explosives. The next most commonly used methods are hanging and poisoning by liquids, solids, and gases such as carbon monoxide. Methods most often chosen by younger children are jumping from a window or in front of a car. The acutely psychotic person may be rescued because of the impulsivity of the idea and his or her inability to formulate the plan effectively (Hawton, 1986; Magnuson, 1989).

Many adolescents who commit suicide have a long history of social isolation and poor interpersonal relationships both with peers and adults. They are described as loners or the "unpopular kids." Often they go unnoticed because they make no obvious trouble for others. These individuals, described as loner suicides, are most often white males in the later adolescent years and suicide comes as a shock to family and acquaintances. Female and nonwhite adolescents are more likely to have problems known to their families or to some social agencies. Their rebellious behavior may be an attempt to cope with an underlying depression and must be considered at risk for suicide.

Some teens who commit suicide do so out of feelings of failure and shame. They may have internalized high parental standards for academic success and a real or threatened failure signifies a potential loss of parental love. Experiences such as substance abuse, loneliness, unemployment, broken or strained relationships or fears about the future may contribute to teen suicide. Suicide may be viewed as the only way to escape unendurable psychological pain (Hawton, 1986).

Affective Characteristics

All the affective characteristics indicative of depression may be associated with suicidal people. These include feelings of desolation, guilt, decreased gratification, loss of emotional attachments, and feelings of failure and shame. People unable to express anger toward others may turn the anger inward and become self-destructive. Others may view suicide as the ultimate expression of anger and a way to achieve revenge for hurts they have suffered. A pervading sense of hopelessness, however, has the highest association with suicide. Life is seen as intolerable, and no hope for change or improvement is seen (Fawcett, 1987).

People have a high degree of ambivalence before the final decision to commit suicide is made. This internal conflict between the wish to die and the wish to live wages until the final decision has been made. If the part that wants to live can be adequately supported during this struggle, the balance may shift in favor of life (Cutter, 1983).

> *Melanie described her ambivalence about suicide in this way: "I thought about suicide for a couple of weeks. I got my husband's gun and sat for an hour with it pointed at my head. I really didn't want to die; I just wanted the pain to stop. So, I shot the gun into the wall and then called a friend to bring me to the hospital."*

Once the decision has been made to commit suicide, conflict and anxiety cease, and the person may appear calm and untroubled. Others may interpret this change in the affective state as an improvement. What appears to be a change for the better may in fact be an indication of the decision to die.

Some people who have a suspicious or paranoid affective state or who are prone to violence as a method of coping with feelings may combine suicide with homicide. These people usually kill someone they know, a relative or friend, and then commit suicide; less commonly, they will kill a stranger before killing themselves.

Cognitive Characteristics

Suicidal behavior has a variety of cognitive components. It involves the decision-making process in that suicide is viewed as a possible solution to a problem. If people are feeling hopeless, they are unable to think of or assess other possible solutions. Actually, their decision-making process is diminished since there seems to be only one answer—to die. The suicidal thought process is really one of impotence. The potential suicide thinks "There is nothing I can do except suicide, and there is no one who can help me with the pain I am suffering."

Another cognitive component involves fantasies that the suicidal person may have. Some, unable to see the finality of death, have fantasies about continuing on in life. They may talk about being able to see how people will react to their death or how their children will grow up. Others have fantasies and expectations about meeting loved ones after death. Many people eagerly look forward to this reunion with family and friends. Some suicidal people have expectations of feeling better after they are dead; in fact, they see dying as a way to have a better life, which is a paradoxical thought process.

A smaller percentage of people hope or believe a suicide attempt will force a solution to interpersonal problems. For some, it is a cry for someone to help them. In either case, the suicidal behavior is a form of manipulation. So desperate are these people that they can see no other method to resolve problems or get the necessary help.

> *Daniel had attempted suicide two weeks ago by ingesting a bottle of aspirin. He now describes it as a plea for help: "I didn't want to die so much as I didn't want to live the way I was living. My wife and I were fighting all the time. I was beginning to yell at the kids constantly. I don't think my wife realized how upset I was until after I took the pills. Now she says she will go to a marriage counselor with me."*

People with sensory or thought disorders may be at risk for suicide. Hallucinations are often of the command type and may involve voices directing the person to commit suicide. At first, the person may be frightened by the voices, but later the person may be compliant and carry out the command. People with delusions of control or delusions of persecution may also be at risk for suicide. If these delusions cannot be controlled or halted with treatment, these people may believe the only way to escape those who are controlling or persecuting them is to die. It is the ultimate method of being relieved of their extremely painful feelings.

Kendall had had a 15-year history of delusions of control. His delusional system was fixed, and he had responded poorly to a variety of interventions. His system centered on the belief that there was an electrode in his ear by which his family controlled him. They woke him up, they put him to sleep, they thought for him, and they talked for him through this electrode. When he was seen three weeks before his suicide, he was expressing feelings of desperation. He said the doctors had done everything, but they either couldn't or wouldn't remove the electrode from his ear. He said he couldn't go on this way, not being himself and being totally controlled by hateful family members. His final solution was to kill himself to escape the total control that had plagued him for 15 years.

For those rescued from their suicidal behavior, there is often a change of mind. Either they return to the ambivalent stage of thought or they decide they do want to live. Throughout their lives, however, they remain at a higher risk for suicide than the general population. It is as if, once the decision to die was made in the past, that decision becomes easier to make again.

Physiologic Characteristics

People with chronic diseases are more likely to commit suicide than those with acute illnesses or no illnesses. At highest risk are people suffering from progressive diseases such as cardiovascular disease, multiple sclerosis, or cancer. Moreover, people who receive a large number of medications may, as a direct result of the chemical effects on the body, experience a depressive episode leading to suicide. Alcoholism is a contributing factor for suicidal people, particularly older men who live alone and have few or no support systems. Alcohol abuse may be an attempt to cope with depression or may induce depression by depleting the biogenic amines. Because of their behavioral patterns, alcoholics often have many interpersonal problems, which may contribute to their wish to die. Drug abuse victims, who have problems similar to the alcoholic's, are also at high risk for suicide.

Sociocultural Characteristics

People who attempt or commit suicide are often in periods of high stress in their lives. When significant life events are assessed in retrospect, one frequently finds a peaking of these events in the month before the suicidal behavior (Parker, 1988). When people either have not developed their coping skills or have exhausted their ability to cope, suicide may be a last, desperate attempt to cope with stress and resolve problems. To reduce the rate of suicide, individuals and families need to be provided with information and problem-solving skills to manage appropriately the developmental and situational crises that are a part of life.

When teen suicides are publicized by the news media or when there are television dramas about suicide, the rate of teen suicide increases several weeks following the event. Suicides that are inspired by suicides in this way are called **"copy cat" suicides.** Copy cat suicides seem to be an adolescent phenomena, with girls more susceptible than boys. The potential copy cat appears to be a troubled adolescent who empathizes with the pain of the suicidal person and the influence of the media (Gould and Schaffer, 1987).

However the act of suicide is committed, it has a traumatic effect on the family and friends of the victim. In addition to the grief, these people must cope with the cultural taboos and stigma associated with suicide. Often, family and friends were unaware of the danger and respond to the suddenness of the death with shock and bewilderment. Some people respond with anger toward the victim and the event. Fears may abound regarding mental illness or the suicide of other family members. Because society assumes that all survivors must feel guilty and responsible for the suicidal behavior, those who do not experience guilt may wonder why and may feel guilty about not feeling guilty. Other survivors experience destructive guilt and blame themselves with thoughts such as, "If only I had done (had not done) . . . this would not have happened."

Many survivors are plagued with real or imagined images of the death scene. Nightmares are not unusual. Some people develop phobias directly related to the suicide, and others develop unwanted obsessions about their own suicide. Family survivors enter a higher risk category for suicide; indeed, about 20 percent of these families will undergo additional suicidal behavior among family members.

Family and friends must also deal with the method of death. The most difficult deaths to contend with are those that result from bizarre methods such as setting oneself on fire or slitting one's own throat. Other methods, from the most to the least difficult for the survivors to contend with, are jumping from a high place, hanging, a gunshot wound to the head that results in obliteration, carbon monoxide poisoning, a gunshot wound to the head with no disfigurement, a gunshot wound to the chest or heart, and an overdose of a toxic substance. Certain methods of suicide create more shame and embarrassment for the family than do other methods. Families must also cope with other people's seeking details of the death, with their inability to acknowledge the death, or others even blaming them for the death. Having a loved one die is traumatic at any time, but having a loved one die as a result of suicide can be overwhelming (Dongen, 1988; Hauser, 1987).

Causative Theories

Suicide may result when people feel social isolation, when they are alienated from society, family, and friends. Another sociologic cause is rapid social change resulting in the loss of previous patterns of social integration. People who have difficulty adapting to the demand of new roles are more likely to view suicide as a solution to their problems.

Loss is another factor closely related to suicide. Of course, the impact of any given loss depends on the significance the person attributes to that loss. Related to the loss is anger, which may be directed toward the self and contribute to suicidal thoughts and actions. Most closely correlated with suicide are

- Major life changes that are incongruent with self-image
- The loss of a significant other
- A meaningful loss that occurs quickly and without warning
- Several losses occurring in rapid succession

Whenever the most important and significant aspects of a person's life are threatened or destroyed, suicide is likely to be considered. Women's motives tend to be interpersonal, that is, related to painful or lost relationships. Men's motives tend to be intrapersonal, that is, related to threats such as financial problems or the loss of a job (Denmark and Kabatznick, 1988).

Appropriate mourning enables people to process and accept the losses that occur in life. If people are unable to grieve, they may become suicidal. As Richman (1986) explains, certain family dynamics have been implicated in this process.

- A particular family member becomes the scapegoat and is blamed for the loss.
- The family's value system disapproves of the grieving process, so family members suffer in silence.
- Family members are distant or unavailable to the person suffering the loss.
- Conflicts with the deceased person are displaced onto the family member most closely identified with the deceased.

- The family system is unable to adapt to change, and the roles played by the deceased person during life are not filled.

In addition to these general causes of suicide, there are more specific causes for the various age groups. How many children commit suicide is unknown, since the National Office of Vital Statistics does not compile data on suicides under the age of 10. Most of these deaths were assumed to be accidental because of the belief that children do not commit suicide or in an effort to protect the suicide's parents. In 1982, however, a study was conducted in two poison control centers, where children were asked about their ingestion of poison. A startling 72 percent of these children were found to have ingested poison as a suicide gesture or attempt (Hafen and Frandsen, 1985). As these and other data indicate, children are able to, and in fact do, commit suicide. (See Table 16–2 for reasons that children commit suicide.)

Adolescents, college students, and older people are more likely to commit suicide than those in the general population. A variety of factors contribute to the suicide decision, some of which are the same as those of the general population and some of which are age and situation specific. (See Tables 16–3 through 16–5 for reasons that adolescents, college students, and the elderly commit suicide.)

Table 16–2 *Causes of Childhood Suicide*

Escape of physical or sexual abuse
Anticipation of disciplinary action
Chaotic family situation
Feeling unloved or constantly criticized
Failing in school
Fear or humiliation in school
Losses of significant others
"Punishment" of others

Source: Adapted from B. Hafen and K. Frandsen, *Psychological Emergencies and Crisis Intervention* (Morton, 1985). Reprinted with permission.

Table 16–3 *Causes of Adolescent Suicide*

Lack of meaningful relationships
Difficulties in maintaining relationships
Escape of physical or sexual abuse
Feelings of not being understood
Losses of significant others
Loss of recognition or physical condition
Acute problems with parents
Sexual problems
Depression

Source: Adapted from B. Hafen and K. Frandsen, *Psychological Emergencies and Crisis Intervention* (Morton, 1985). Reprinted with permission.

Table 16–4 *Causes of Suicide in College Students*

Demands for achievement
Anxiety over academic work
Academic failure signifying a loss of parental love or esteem
Competition for success

Source: Adapted from H. Hendlin, *Suicide in America* (Norton, 1982). Reprinted with permission.

Table 16–5 *Causes of Suicide in the Elderly*

Change in status from independence to dependence
Illness with decreased ability to function
Decreased feeling of being involved in society
Loneliness and social isolation
Multiple losses
Outliving resources

Source: Adapted from B. Hafen and K. Frandsen, *Psychological Emergencies and Crisis Intervention* (Morton, 1985) and H. Hendlin, *Suicide in America* (Norton, 1982).

Assessment: Suicide

Some nurses are fearful of doing a suicide assessment on people who are at risk. For this, there may be many contributing factors: fear of giving the person the idea of suicide, fear of being incorrect, fear of the person's reaction, or hesitancy to discuss a taboo subject. The nurse, however, cannot give the idea of suicide to anyone. By late childhood or early adolescence, every person knows that suicide is one alternative to solving problems. Most youngsters, without being actively suicidal, have had thoughts of suicide in times of stress. An example is the child who is angry at his parents and thinks, "If I went out and got run over by a car, would they be sorry that they were so mean to me!" Many adults have considered what method they might choose if they were to ever commit suicide. Thus, even though the topic is taboo under many social conditions, the majority of people have thought about and formed opinions about suicide.

It is helpful to remember that suicidal people are afraid. They fear no one cares. They may not introduce the topic because they fear being judged or considered weak or "crazy." When confronted with their own fears about discussing suicide, nurses need to remember that no nursing intervention will be effective unless the suicide threat is assessed. If the person is not suicidal, no damage has been done by asking the questions. If the person is suicidal and the topic is not discussed, the person is abandoned in a dangerous position. Since almost all suicidal people are ambivalent about the decision, introducing the topic often provides some relief as well as the opportunity to strengthen the desire to live by exploring what remains meaningful in life.

Ambivalence may also occur in the nurse-rescuer. The conflict for the nurse centers on the issue of people's rights to choose their own time and method of dying. Many nurses themselves have thought about the conditions under which they would choose not to live, such as the development of a particular chronic or terminal illness. Having considered suicide as an option, these nurses may question if they have the right to prevent another person's suicide. Other nurses may not experience this conflict because of their belief that all suicides should be prevented.

The nurse and family ought not to expect that an accurate assessment will prevent all suicides. This expectation would contribute to unrealistic guilt when a client successfully does commit suicide. Not all victims exhibit cues before their deaths; in fact, only about 20 percent of suicidal people can be correctly identified before they kill themselves. In at least one half of suicidal deaths, there was no history of suicidal thoughts or behavior (Cutter, 1983). This information is not presented to minimize the importance of a suicide assessment; rather, it is presented to establish realistic professional expectations. If a person is intent on suicide, it is difficult to intervene effectively. However, if a person is still ambivalent, intervention may save that person's life. Therefore it is always vital that, for those at risk, a suicide assessment be done. Types of questions to ask during a focused nursing assessment of suicide potential follow. To increase the client's comfort, it is important that privacy be provided during the assessment.

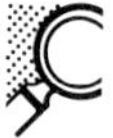

FOCUSED NURSING ASSESSMENT *of Suicide Potential*

Behavioral assessment
Are you thinking about suicide?
By what method would you commit suicide?
Do you have the means on hand?
Have you done a practice session of the suicide?
When do you plan to commit suicide?
Have you tried to kill yourself before?
How have things been going at school/job for you?
Are you still interested in visiting with friends?
How much have you been drinking lately?
How often do you use street drugs?
Have you made or changed your will recently?
Have you checked your life insurance policies?
What kinds of personal belongings have you given away?
Have you planned your funeral?

Affective assessment
How would you describe your overall mood?
What kinds of things make you feel guilty?

In what areas of life do you feel like a failure?
What does the future look like to you?
To what degree do you feel hopeless or out of control of your life?
What part of you wishes to die?
What part of you wishes to live?

Cognitive assessment
What will your suicide accomplish for you?
What will your suicide accomplish for others?
What would have to change for you to decide to live?
What are your thoughts about death?
Is there a way for you to continue on in life after death?
Do you hope to meet dead loved ones after you die?
Do you hear voices that others say they do not hear?
What do the voices say to you?
Is suicide a way for you to escape control or persecution by others?

Physiologic assessment
Are you physically ill?
Describe the expectations about your illness.
When did you last see a physician?
What medications, prescribed and over-the-counter, are you taking?
How has your appetite changed?
Describe any difficulties you have in sleeping.

Sociocultural assessment
What kinds of losses have you sustained during the past year? Relationships? Separations? Divorce? Deaths? Jobs? Roles? Self-esteem?
What kinds of stress have you been under during the past six months?
Which people are able to provide support for you?
Have any of your friends or family members committed suicide? Anniversary date? Thoughts and feelings about this suicide?
Who will benefit from your suicide? How?

Nursing Diagnosis and Planning: Suicide

The suicide assessment provides the data from which the nurse develops the plan of care. In planning, the nurse needs to use the following questions to guide the process:

1. Is the client actively suicidal?
2. What is the degree of lethality of the plan?
3. Does the client need to be in a protected environment?
4. What is the extent of the supportive network system?

Individuals, families, schools, and communities must be educated about suicidal behavior and prevention strategies. People need to be informed about available resources and assisted in making contact with available support systems (see Table 16–6). (See Table 16–7 for the nursing care plan for the suicidal client.)

Evaluation: Suicide

The nurse needs to remember that nursing interventions and medical treatment cannot guarantee that the suicidal person will not commit suicide.

Table 16–6 *Organizations for Suicide Prevention and Outreach*

Crisis line
1-800-621-4000

Associations
American Association of Suicidology
2459 South Ash
Denver, CO 80222

Suicide Prevention Center, Inc.
184 Salem Ave.
Dayton, OH 45406

Contact Teleministries, USA, Inc.
900 South Arlington Ave.
Harrisburg, PA 17109

Newsletters/pamphlets
After Suicide: A Unique Grief Process, Ray of Hope, Inc., 1518 Derwen Dr., Iowa City, IA 52240

The Ultimate Rejection, Suicide Prevention Center, Inc., 184 Salem Ave., Dayton, OH 45406

Afterwords: A Letter For and About Suicide Survivors, A. Wrobleski (editor), 5124 Grove St., Minneapolis, MN 55436-2481

Table 16–7 Nursing Care Plan for the Suicidal Client

Nursing Diagnosis: Potential for violence: self-directed related to acute suicidal state.
Goal: Client will not harm or kill self.

Intervention	*Rationale*	*Expected Outcome*
Remain with person at all times until he or she can be moved to a safe environment	Protecting person until he or she is able to protect self is a necessary form of client advocacy for suicidal person	Remains safe
Have person taken immediately to the hospital for evaluation and possible admission	Admission may be the only immediate intervention to prevent suicide	
Remove as many dangerous objects as possible (eg, pocket knives, glass articles, belts, razors, pills)	Objects that could be used to harm oneself must be removed to protect client	Remains safe
When administering medications, make certain client swallows all of them	It is necessary to prevent stockpiling of medications for a future suicide attempt	Swallows all medication
Check on the client's whereabouts and status every 10–15 minutes on an irregular schedule of observation; if client is acutely suicidal, provide constant observation	Frequent observation can prevent a suicide plan from being implemented; if the schedule is regular, client can determine the best time to attempt suicide	Remains safe
Gently explain to client that you will protect him or her until client is able to resist suicidal impulses	Ambivalent client will experience relief of conflict and anxiety when staff assumes control	Verbalizes less conflict and anxiety

Nursing Diagnosis: Ineffective individual coping related to desire to kill oneself as a solution to problems.
Goal: Client will verbalize a decrease in suicidal thoughts.

Intervention	*Rationale*	*Expected Outcome*
Listen carefully and take all suicidal talk seriously	Serious attention conveys caring and helps to establish rapport	
Do not try to talk client out of suicidal intentions	Client may interpret this as evidence you do not understand or you do not believe reasons are valid	
Use the problem-solving process regarding the reasons for suicide:		
• have client write out list of reasons to live and reasons to die	A written list may help client to conceptualize the conflict more clearly	Develops a list
• have client describe the goal he or she hopes to achieve	A specific goal will help focus the problem-solving process	Identifies goals
• remind client that suicide is only one of several possible alternatives	To counterbalance the belief that suicide is the only alternative	
• develop a list of alternatives to meet client's goal		Lists alternatives
• discuss potential outcomes of suicide (eg, "What is the likelihood that you will injure yourself seriously if your attempt is not successful?" and "Will death be the most successful method of meeting your goal?")	Potential negative outcomes from self-injury may not have been considered by client (eg, permanent bodily damage or nonachievement of goal)	Projects outcomes

(Diagnosis continued)

Table 16–7 *(continued)*

Nursing Diagnosis *(continued):* Ineffective individual coping related to desire to kill oneself as a solution to problems.
Goal: Client will verbalize a decrease in suicidal thoughts.

Intervention	*Rationale*	*Expected Outcome*
• discuss potential outcomes of other alternatives	Supporting the part of client that wishes to live by focusing on other ways to meet goal, which will decrease feelings of helplessness	
Focus on things that may help client resist suicidal impulses:		
• discuss death; what it means to client, feelings about death, and what client thinks it will be like	Suicidal people often have not thought past the act of self-injury, that is, the reality and finality of death	Discusses death
• focus on the list of reasons to continue living	Strengthening the wish to live will weaken the wish to die and decrease the internal conflict	Develops a list
• discuss meaningful network systems of family and friends	Focusing on available support systems will decrease feelings of isolation and helplessness	Identifies support systems
• discuss impact of suicide on survivors (eg, grief, anger, shame, guilt, and increased risk that they will commit suicide)	Suicidal people often have not considered the impact of their suicide on family members; this external focus and concern may decrease the impulsive behavior	Discusses impact of suicide on others
Ask client if he or she will make a verbal or written contract with you not to commit suicide	A contract will formalize client's agreement not to act on suicidal impulses and evoke a commitment to life	Agrees to a contract

Nursing Diagnosis: Impaired home maintenance management related to increased risk of suicide in the future.
Goal: Client will resist suicidal impulses in the future.

Intervention	*Rationale*	*Expected Outcome*
Discuss with client and family that recurrences of suicidal ideation and behavior may happen	Education about suicide will decrease the denial process of future problems and promote earlier intervention	Identifies potential problems
Provide client with local suicide hotline numbers and national groups concerned with prevention of suicide (see Table 16–6)	The knowledge of availability of resources and support systems may help client resist the impulse to commit suicide and provide family with needed assistance	Plans appropriate measures to manage anticipated problems

Nursing Diagnosis: Ineffective family coping: compromised related to suicide of family member.
Goal: Family will remain functional as a unit and as individuals.

Intervention	*Rationale*	*Expected Outcome*
Provide the opportunity for family to discuss the death	Other family members and friends may avoid the issue because of discomfort	Discusses impact of the suicide
Discuss present fears family members may have	Discussing fears openly will assist family in keeping them in a realistic perspective	Discusses fears

(Diagnosis continued)

Table 16–7 *(continued)*

Intervention	*Rationale*	*Expected Outcome*
Allow family to express anger at victim for abandonment and anger at self for not preventing	Normalizes anger as part of grieving process	Verbalizes anger
Help family to anticipate future difficulties (eg, holiday times, anniversary of the death, and suicidal ideation and behavior in other family members)	Anticipatory guidance will decrease the impact of expected difficulties; survivors must be assessed for suicidal thoughts	Plans appropriate measures to manage anticipated problems
Refer to a survivors of suicide group such as LOSS (Loving Outreach to Survivors of Suicide) or STRESS (Striving to Reach Every Survivor of Suicide), and SOS (Survivors of Suicide)	Sharing with others who have had similar experiences provides support and resolution of feelings	Attends a group
Refer for family therapy	More intensive therapy may be necessary to intervene with complicated family issues	Participates in family therapy

The main professional goal is to protect suicidal clients until they are able to protect themselves. Through active intervention, it is hoped that clients will be able to develop alternative solutions to the difficulties fostering their suicidal intentions.

When clients are successful suicides, nurses need to ask themselves several questions to resolve any unnecessary self-blame and guilt.

- Did I take the client's suicidal intentions seriously?
- Did I provide as safe an environment as possible?
- Was the client willing to find alternative solutions?
- Do I have a right to prevent all suicides?
- Does the client have a right to determine his/her own death?
- Am I the only one who is blaming myself?
- What do I need to do to feel less guilty about this death?

It is necessary that staff members participate in discussions about their feelings and responsibilities in regard to a client's suicide. Staff will find it helpful to explore concepts of death and cure as well as their moral obligations. If feelings of guilt and failure are not thought about and discussed, individual staff members may project anger and blame onto other staff or even onto the dead client.

Violence Against Others: Rape

Rape is a crime of violence and is second only to homicide in its violation of a person. The issue is not one of sexuality but rather one of force, domination, and humiliation. In this text, **rape** refers to any forced sex act with the key factor being lack of adult consent. Legally, the definition varies from state to state. In many states, rape is defined as forced sexual intercourse against a female who is not married to the perpetrator. Other states have broadened the definition to include other sex acts. In regard to marital rape, the legal climate is beginning to change. In many states, a husband cannot be charged with rape if he sexually assaults his wife.

But other states have recognized that rape can be committed within a marriage and that the husband can be prosecuted. (See Table 16–8 for a list of those states that permit the prosecution of husbands and those states that do not.)

It was not until 1974 that the first case of marital rape was prosecuted in the United States. Prior to that time the law viewed married women as property of their husbands. Continuing even today, women are beaten and raped by their husbands, often in full view of their children. Not infrequently, marital rape is accompanied by extreme violence and may be the most underreported type of rape. Current estimates are that 8 million women in the United States are at risk for marital rape. Of battered women, 35 to 50 percent experience rape as well as physical abuse from their male partners. The time of greatest danger is when the woman leaves or threatens to leave her abusive husband. This situation is perceived as a challenge to his dominance and control, and he often responds by using sex to humiliate and dominate (McLeer, 1988; Pagelow, 1988).

> *Charles accused his wife, Laurie, of having an affair. When she denied it, he "beat her and threatened to place a gun in her mouth." He then continued to beat and sexually assault her for several hours. Charles's defense at the hearing was "It was a party for both of us. She always told me she wanted a man who would tell her what to do." Charles was sentenced to 15 years in prison for raping his wife in what was termed a "brutal, terroristic, dehumanizing" act (Wilson, 1988).*

> *Carmen's first child was born by cesarean section. Her physician told her not to have sex for several weeks. Five days after the birth, when she returned home, her husband told her it was his right to have sex with his wife whenever he wanted. Despite her protests, he forced her to have sex.*

Table 16–9 presents a list of a woman's marital rights as interpreted by the Center for Constitutional Rights, a non-profit legal and educational organization.

Table 16–8 *Legal Status of Marital Rape*

Rape by husband treated the same as rape by stranger
Alaska, Florida, Georgia, Kansas, Maine, Massachusetts, Montana, Nebraska, New Jersey, New York, Oregon, Vermont, Wisconsin

Husbands may be charged in most cases—limited exemptions
California, Connecticut, Delaware, Hawaii, Iowa, Minnesota, New Hampshire, Ohio, Pennsylvania, Washington, West Virginia, Wyoming

Husbands not charged; ex-husbands charged
Alabama, Illinois

Husbands charged when separated by a court order
Kentucky, Louisiana, Maryland, Missouri, North Carolina, North Dakota, South Carolina, Utah

Husbands charged if living apart and one partner has filed for annulment, divorce, or separation
Indiana, Michigan, Nevada, Tennessee

Husbands charged if living apart or one partner has filed for legal proceeding
Idaho, New Mexico, Oklahoma, South Dakota, Texas

Husbands charged if living apart
Arizona, Colorado, Mississippi, Rhode Island, Virginia

Unreported
Arkansas

Source: Adapted from *Stopping Sexual Assault in Marriage* (Center for Constitutional Rights, 1986). Reprinted with permission.

Table 16–9 *Marital Rape: A Woman's Rights*

Every woman has the right to control her own body. Marriage does not give a husband the right to demand or force sex.

Sex is a part of marriage, but a wife has the right to say yes or no to sex each time.

Disagreements never give the husband the right to rape his wife. Arguments about sex should be worked out with the help of a therapist. Unresolved disagreements may lead to separation or divorce.

Rape is an act of anger and hate. It is meant to control, humiliate, and punish the wife.

Marital privacy is not a protection for violent behavior.

Source: Adapted from *Stopping Sexual Assault in Marriage* (Center for Constitutional Rights, 1986).

For the victim rape is almost always a sudden, unreasonable, unforeseen occurrence. The perpetrators often use guns or knives; may tie the victim; or use verbal intimidation, such as a threat of death. Some victims attempt and are physically able to resist. Others may reason or plead with the perpetrator. However, fear of death combined with the suddenness of the event makes many victims unable to either flee or fight.

Incidence of Rape

There is no typical rape victim. Of reported rapes, however, 93 percent of the victims are female and 90 percent of the perpetrators are male. One can be a victim of rape at any age, from childhood through old age. The average age of female children who are raped is 7.9 years, and in 80 percent of the cases the perpetrator is someone the child knows. The rapist may attack strangers, acquaintances, friends, or family members. With increased awareness of the possibility of rape, women are becoming more sensitive to preventive measures. Since this means being suspicious of men in potential rape environments, all women and men are, in one sense, victims of rape. Women have become fearful for their safety, and men, in general, are the recipients of this fear and suspicion. Thus, everyone is affected, at least indirectly, by the crime of rape (Warner, 1980).

Male victims of rape are just beginning to come to the attention of the general public. As with females, rape of males can occur at any age. The myth of male rape has been that it occurs only where heterosexual contact is not possible, such as in prisons or in isolated living conditions. As more male rape victims report the crime, however, this myth has been exploded. Male rape is not a homosexual attack. Again the issue is one of violence and domination rather than one of sexuality. Some rapists, who define themselves as heterosexual, will rape both males and females; at times, they rape whomever is available.

In the past, men were afraid to report rape for fear of being ridiculed or not believed. As was true for females in the past, society has a tendency to blame the male victim by saying such things as, "He must have thought you were trying to pick him up," "You must have made him angry," or "You could have resisted if you had really wanted to." Male rape victims undergo the same emotional trauma that female victims do, and they need the same protection, interventions, and understanding that is provided for female victims.

It is difficult to determine the incidence of rape since it is the most underreported crime. Because of shame and a fear of being blamed, victims have been hesitant to report and testify. It is projected that one woman out of every six will experience an attempted rape sometime in her lifetime, and one woman out of every eight will be forced to submit. Between the ages of 16 and 19, females are at the highest risk for being raped. Nonwhite victims are more likely to be raped at an earlier age, with the highest risk being between 12 and 19 years of age. The highest risk for white victims is between the ages of 20 and 34. Most often, the rapist is of the same race as the victim (Erickson, 1989).

From the perspective of the victim, rape occurs very suddenly. There is often no warning of the attack, which most frequently occurs between 6 P.M. and midnight. However, the majority of rapes are not sudden and impulsive; indeed, 60 to 75 percent of all rapes are well planned.

Often unreported are date rapes. Of all women raped on college campuses, 50 percent are date rapes. Women very rarely report rapes when they know their attackers and especially if they were in a dating relationship. Nonreporting is related in part to a cultural value that permits, under certain circumstances, a man to coerce a woman to have sex. The victim is often blamed, by herself and others, for being naive or provocative. Another value, slow to die, is that, if a woman accepts a date and allows the man to pay for all the expenses, she somehow "owes" him sexual access, which she has no right to refuse. To combat this problem, many universities have established antirape seminars and counseling services for both women and men (Shotland, 1989). Table 16–10 presents guidelines for preventing date rape.

Table 16–10 *Fighting Date Rape*

Be cautious in relationships based on dominant-male, submissive-female stereotypes. Date rapists usually have macho attitudes and believe women to be inferior.
Be cautious when a date tries to control your behavior—who you can meet, where you can go, what you can do. This indicates a need to dominate and control and increases your vulnerability by isolating you.
Be very clear in your communication. If a simple *no* is not respected, leave or insist he leave. Speak forcefully.
Avoid giving mixed messages. For example: Do not say no and then continue petting.
Do not go to a place so private that help is not available.
Attend an antirape workshop to learn how to fight rape.

Table 16–11 *Where to Get Help*

National Coalition Against Sexual Assault c/o Volunteers of America 8787 State St., Suite 202 East St. Louis, IL 62203
National Coalition Against Domestic Violence 2401 Virginia Ave., N.W., Suite 306 Washington, DC 20037
National Organization for Victim Assistance Department P 717 D Street, N.W. Washington, DC 20004
Center for Constitutional Rights 606 Broadway, 7th Floor New York, NY 10012 212-614-6464

Significance of Rape to Mental Health Nursing

Victims of rape are admitted to all types of units from pediatrics to intensive care. Nurses need to be able to assess and provide appropriate intervention for the emotional consequences, as well as the physical trauma, of the rape victim. Nurses may be called on to give legal evidence in the prosecution of a rapist. Within the community, nurses can establish, or refer victims to, support groups. (Table 16–11 provides a list of such groups.) Nurses can also become active in increasing public awareness of rape through formal and informal teaching activities. This unique position of nurses allows them to be active in the prevention of rape and treatment of its victims.

Knowledge Base: Rape

Behavioral Characteristics

Many victims of rape do not report the crime. Sometimes this is due to guilt or embarrassment about what has occurred. Other victims are fearful of how their families or the police will react to the information. Some perpetrators threaten victims by saying they will return to rape them again if the police are notified. Since many of the crimes are committed by acquaintances, friends, dates, or husbands, victims fear they will not be believed.

Some rape victims respond immediately with agitated and nonpurposeful behavior. They are brought to the emergency room emotionally distraught and unable to respond to questions about what has occurred. So great is their level of anxiety and fear that they may be unable to follow simple directions.

Other rape victims may return home and shower or bathe before notifying the police or going to the emergency room. In the past, this behavior has caused others to disbelieve the rape charge. It is now recognized that people who have been violated by rape experience extreme feelings of helplessness. Often, this cleaning up behavior is an attempt to regain control of the self and return to the normality that was so suddenly disrupted.

The majority of victims appear in good control of their feelings and behavior immediately after the rape. This appearance of outward calmness usually indicates a state of numbness, disbelief, and emotional shock. Statements may be made such as, "This whole thing doesn't seem real," "I must be dreaming. This couldn't have happened," or "I just can't believe this has happened to me." Nurses need to recognize that underneath the calmness is a person in acute distress. The victims' control needs to be supported until they are able to manage the reality of their situation. Nurses who assume that the calmness indicates no distress will miss the victims' needs for emotional support and intervention. These nurses will be professionally ineffective (Hartman and Burgess, 1988).

There may be long-term behavioral characteristics of rape victims. Some are prone to crying spells that they may or may not be able to explain. Some may have difficulty maintaining or forming interpersonal relationships, especially with people who remind them of the perpetrator. Many victims develop problems at work or school. Some report nightmares and have difficulty sleeping. Others develop secondary phobic reactions to people, objects, or situations that remind them of the rape (Resick, 1983). A woman who is a victim of marital rape suffers additional problems. Often, she must continue to interact with her rapist because she is dependent on him. She may be forced to pretend, to herself and other family members and friends, that the rape never occurred. Until it becomes more socially acceptable and legally feasible to report marital rape, many of these victims will suffer in silence.

Affective Characteristics

Victims of rape suffer immediate and long-lasting emotional trauma. After a period of shock and disbelief, many of them experience episodes of anxiety and depression. Anxiety arises when people's integrity has been threatened or assaulted, and depression may be in response to losses that people incur. Rape victims have been threatened, both physically and emotionally. They have experienced losses in the areas of autonomy, control, safety, and self-esteem. Thus, to observe anxiety and depressive reactions in response to rape is not unusual (Hartman and Burgess, 1988).

Many victims feel ashamed and embarrassed about the rape since sexual behavior is normally an intimate, private act. Often, they feel unclean or contaminated. These feelings are unique to victims of rape as opposed to victims of other crimes. To have to share specific details of the rape with police officers and in a courtroom may be humiliating, particularly since women have been socialized not to talk about sexual behavior in public. Victims who do not report rape generally say it was too private or personal for them to be able to talk about it with strangers.

Rape victims feel physically and emotionally violated. The loss of control over their bodies and their autonomy leads to feelings of helplessness and vulnerability. They may feel alienated from friends and family, particularly if there is not a strong supportive network. Feeling anger is a healthy response to the violation that has occurred, but the energy of anger needs to be appropriately discharged so that the victim does not later become consumed with fantasies of revenge.

Cognitive Characteristics

During the actual rape, some victims use the defense mechanisms of depersonalization or dissociation to cope with the attack. By perceiving the attack as "not really happening to me" the victims protect their sense of integrity. Other victims rely on denial to block out the traumatic experience. The use of these defense mechanisms may continue through the initial treatment of the victim and needs to be supported until the person is able to face the reality of the attack.

Victims often enter the emergency room in a state of confusion. They may have great difficulty concentrating and appear unsure of exactly what has occurred. This confusion and uncertainty must not be interpreted as evidence that a rape did not occur, but rather as indicating that the victim is in a state of emotional shock. Moreover, the victim's problem-solving and decision-making abilities are greatly reduced during the immediate aftermath of the rape as the result of a high level of anxiety and fear.

Some victims are unable to discuss the attack at all. Some may not even be able to report the rape until the next day when they feel more prepared to cope with the event and the subsequent procedures. Other victims will be very much concerned about whom of their family and friends they should tell. They may be uncertain about how significant others will react to the information that a rape has occurred. They also may not know how to tell others about the experience and may depend on the nurse for guidance and support.

There may be a period during which victims blame themselves for the rape. This self-blame may be heard in statements such as, "If only I had taken a different way home," "I should have been able to escape because he didn't have a gun," or "I should have fought harder than I did." This personal responsibility may also be felt by a marital rape victim. Statements may be made such as, "If I were a better wife, he wouldn't have raped me," or "If I would try harder to please him sexually, he wouldn't have to force me."

Some victims develop obsessional thoughts about the rape, which may be severe enough to interfere with daily functioning. Some, though not obsessed, do experience periodic flashbacks of the event. Others are preoccupied with thoughts of future danger, and dreams of a violent nature are common.

Rape may profoundly affect one's beliefs about the environment. If the assault occurred in the victim's home, the normal feeling of safety within the home will most likely be disrupted. Some fear retaliation by the perpetrator for reporting the crime, especially when that person is known to the victim. Victims, particularly young female victims, may generalize their fear to the point that it applies to all men or all strange men. Women who have been raped by their husbands often state that their ability to trust the husband or any other man has been destroyed.

Doreen, a graduate student at the local university, was brought to the hospital by the police who found her running down the street half-clothed. In the hospital she was able to tell the staff that she had been raped by her date, Mike, another graduate student. She exhibited outward calmness but kept repeating "This cannot have happened to me. My friends introduced us and he seemed so nice." She was unable to decide who to call to take her back to the dorm or what to tell her friends about what had happened.

Physiologic Characteristics

Rape usually results in a number of physical injuries. Most likely the vagina or rectum will be sore and swollen. There may be tearing of the vaginal or rectal wall from forceful insertion of the penis or a foreign object. The throat may be traumatized from forced oral sex. In addition, the victim may be beaten, stabbed, or shot. Profuse bleeding as well as injuries to vital organs may be a critical problem.

Female victims of child-bearing years may become pregnant as a result of the rape. Victims of all ages and both genders may contract a sexually transmitted disease from the perpetrator. This could be transmitted to any mucous membrane area, such as the vagina, rectum, mouth, or throat.

In addition to the immediate physical trauma, there may be serious, long-term physiologic effects. Insomnia or anorexia may be experienced for a long time after the event. Some victims may complain of fatigue or generalized aches and pains, and some may experience gynecologic problems. There may also be long-term effects from the injuries sustained from a beating, stabbing, or shooting. Further, compared to the general population, rape victims are at a higher risk for developing a psychophysiologic disorder in response to a chronic high level of anxiety and fear.

Future sexual functioning may also be adversely affected by a rape. The possibility of developing a sexual dysfunction depends on the quality of sexual experience and relationships before the attack, the behavior used to cope with the attack, and the quality of future relationships. Women victims of marital rape often have difficulty adjusting sexually in a subsequent relationship. Nearly all adult rape victims need to withdraw from sexual activity for a time. For some, the period of celibacy is necessary to reestablish control and autonomy. Others may choose abstinence because they feel unclean or contaminated. Both the victim and the sexual partner need to understand that the need for closeness and nondemanding physical contact continues. Giving comfort through touch will decrease the partner's feelings of rejection and the victim's feelings of self-blame or uncleanliness.

Sociocultural Characteristics

Families experience many of the same thoughts and feelings as the rape victim. They may talk about guilt, doubts, fears, hatred toward the perpetrator, and feelings of helplessness. They need to be educated about the nature and trauma of the rape and the immediate and long-term potential reactions of the victim. They need support and direction in how to best help the victim so that they neither overprotect the victim nor minimize the impact of the rape.

Many cultural myths have surrounded the crime of rape for a long time. Examples of these myths follow.

- Good girls don't get raped.
- Women ask to be raped by the clothes they wear.
- The average healthy woman can escape the rapist if she really wants to.
- Women cry rape after they have consented to sex with a friend.
- Women bring false rape charges if their boyfriends drop them.
- Only homosexual men get raped.
- Any man could resist rape if he really tried.

In the past 15 years, great strides have been made to abolish these myths from the legal system and to treat rape as the crime of violence it is.

Changing the personal belief system of the general public has been a slower process. Many people continue to believe the rape myths that blame the victim rather than the perpetrator. In one study, 50 percent of both women and men accepted the myths without question. The greatest predictors of acceptance of the myths were rigid gender role stereotyping and the acceptance of interpersonal violence by the participants in the study (Burt, 1980). Thus, people who are more flexible in gender roles and abhor violence are more likely to support the victim and blame the perpetrator.

Causative Theories

Intrapersonal Theories Rape is a crime of violence generated by issues of power and anger rather than by sexual drive. The intrapersonal perspective views rapists as emotionally immature persons who feel powerless and unsure of themselves. They are incapable of managing the normal stresses of everyday life. The causes of rape are multidetermined, but the dynamics of the act are that perpetrators abuse their own and others' sexuality as a method of discharging anger and frustration. From this perspective, there are three types of rape: the anger rape, the power rape, and the sadistic rape.

The *anger rape* is distinguished by physical violence and cruelty to the victim. The rapist believes he is the victim of an unjust society and takes revenge on others by raping. He uses extreme force and viciousness to debase the victim. The ability to injure, traumatize, and shame the victim provides an outlet for his rage and temporary relief from his turmoil. Rapes occur episodically as the rage builds up and he strikes out at others to relieve his pain.

In the *power rape,* the intent of the rapist is not to injure the victim but to command and master another person sexually. The rapist has an insecure self-image with feelings of incompetency and inadequacy. The rape becomes the vehicle for expressing power, potency, and might. Seeing the victim as a conquest, the rapist temporarily feels omnipotent.

The *sadistic rape* also involves brutality. The use of bondage and torture is not an expression of anger but a necessary ingredient for the rapist to become sexually excited. The assault is eroticized and, for the rapist, it is sexually stimulating. For this person to achieve sexual gratification, an unwilling sexual partner who will resist his advances is necessary. Rape becomes a source of excitement in his life (Pagelow, 1988).

Interpersonal Theories Some rapists are unable to develop intimate and strong relationships with other men and women. The relationships they do have are unequal and characterized by a lack of mutuality and an inability to share. With this model for relationships, the rapist sees no need for consent to sexual activity, particularly within a marital relationship. The husband may view the rape as merely a disagreement over sexual activity. Unless he is extremely brutal, the wife may not regard the forced sex as an assault and rape. Both of them may view sexual relationships as exploitative rather than a process of mutual sharing. If the wife has said she does not want to engage in sex and the husband uses force, her control and autonomy have been violated. When sex occurs without consent, it is, in fact, rape. What appears to be a conflict over sex in the marriage is actually a conflict over power and the right to consent to or refuse a given activity (Pagelow, 1988).

Sociocultural Theories The acceptance of interpersonal violence in a culture contributes to a higher incidence of rape within that culture. Society's approval of the use of intimidation, coercion, and force to achieve one's goals promotes an excessive level of violence. It becomes an issue of power and strength rather than a consideration of individuals' rights.

Rigid gender role expectations and stereotypes may be correlated with the incidence of rape. When women are considered inferior to men, there is tacit approval given for coercion and force. These stereotypes support the false beliefs that at times women deserve to be raped, that they may want or need to be raped, and that it does not cause them much physical or emotional damage. It is believed that elimination of stereotypes and sexism will decrease men's use of rape as a way to demonstrate power and control (Resick, 1983). Russell (1975, p. 16) describes it this way:

> Rape is the ultimate sexist act. It is an act of physical and psychic oppression. Eradicating rape requires getting rid of the power discrepancy between men and women, because abuse of power flows from unequal power.

Ageism, which defines the older person as weak and incompetent, is a correlate to the crime of rape. Older people, especially those who are socially isolated or live alone, are seen as easy victims. Some older people, believing the myth that only young women are raped, do not protect themselves as well as they could. Older people are more vulnerable if they have established patterns of daily activities that can be readily observed. If they are dependent on walking or public transportation, they can be more easily accosted, particularly if their vision and hearing are impaired. Moreover, they may have neither the physical strength to resist a rape nor the ability to outrun the rapist.

Assessment: Rape

Rape victims need first to be assessed physically from head to toe for any serious or critical injuries that may have resulted from the assault. With the victim's permission, a vaginal or rectal examination is performed to determine necessary treatment and to provide evidence for legal proceedings. Again with permission, photographs of the injuries may be taken for legal documentation (Foley, 1984). The physical assessment process must be carefully documented in writing to assist with possible prosecution of the perpetrator.

The victim's mental status then needs to be assessed. Behavioral, affective, and cognitive responses to the traumatic event need to be gathered. A sociocultural assessment provides additional data for planning appropriate interventions.

Victims who present a controlled style may be able to respond to assessment questions, but those in a state of emotional shock and disbelief may find it difficult to engage actively in the assessment process. The method by which the nurse completes the assessment obviously depends on the person's response to the trauma.

Before the assessment process, clients need to be informed of their rights, which include the right to have

- A rape crisis advocate accompany them to the hospital

- Their personal physician notified
- Privacy during the assessment and treatment process
- Family, friends, or an advocate present during the questioning and examination
- Confidentiality maintained by all staff
- Gentle and sensitive treatment
- Detailed explanations and consent for all tests and procedures
- Referrals for follow-up treatment and counseling

The nurse functions as an advocate for rape victims in supporting these rights.

A focused nursing assessment for the rape victim follows.

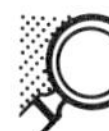

FOCUSED NURSING ASSESSMENT *of the Rape Victim*

Behavioral Assessment
Is the client able to respond verbally to questions?
Is the client able to follow simple directions?
Has the client bathed, douched, changed clothes, or done any self-treatment before coming to the hospital?

Affective assessment
Which of the following emotions is the client experiencing? Describe with objective and subjective data.
Disbelief
Shame
Embarrassment
Humiliation
Helplessness
Vulnerability
Anxiety
Fear
Guilt
Anger
Depression
Alienation from others

Cognitive assessment
Evidence of defense mechanisms.
Is the client confused?
Has the client been informed of his or her rights?
Describe the client's attention span.
Is the client able to describe what occurred?
Is the client able to make decisions?
Who has the client informed about the rape? Family? Friends? Police?
Does the client need assistance in telling others?
Is the client blaming self for the attack?
Is the client experiencing flashbacks to the attack?
What does this event represent to the client?

Sociocultural assessment
Who and where are the available support systems for the client? Family? Friends? Advocate? Clergy?
Is the client in need of temporary shelter?
Does the client know about available counseling?

Table 16–12 presents guidelines for performing a physical assessment of the rape victim.

Nursing Diagnosis and Planning: Rape

The assessment process provides the data from which the nurse develops the plan of care. Physical and mental status priorities must be quickly established by the health care team. Attention must then be given to long-range physical, emotional, social, and legal concerns of the victim.

It is advantageous to the client to have a primary nurse assigned in the emergency room. The client needs a warm, accepting, understanding, and respectful relationship with the nurse. If police officers are involved, the nurse needs to act as an advocate in helping the client decide when he or she is best able to talk with the police about the rape. The nurse needs also to provide breaks in the questioning if the client appears overwhelmed and distressed by the interview. (See Table 16–13 for the nursing care plan for the victim of rape.)

The rape trauma syndrome consists of three phases. The initial phase is one of shock and disbelief. The second phase consists of subsequent reactions, which span a wide range of emotional and physical symptoms. The third phase is one of long-

Table 16–12 *Physical Assessment of the Rape Victim*

Complete a head-to-toe assessment with particular attention to the following areas:

Head
- Evidence of trauma
- Facial bruises
- Facial fractures
- Eyes: swollen, bruised, hemorrhages

Skin
- Bruises
- Genital trauma
- Rectal trauma

Musculoskeletal
- Fractures of the ribs
- Fractures of arms/legs
- Dislocated joints
- Impaired mobility

Abdomen
- Bruises or wounds
- Evidence of internal injuries

Have physical injuries such as scratches, bruises, and cuts been recorded and photographed?
Have fingernail scrapings been taken and preserved?
Has blood typing been done?
Have smears been taken of the mouth, throat, vagina, and rectum for sexually transmitted diseases?
Have combings been made of the pubic hair and preserved?
Has genital trauma been recorded and photographed?
Has rectal trauma been recorded and photographed?
Have semen specimens been preserved?
If applicable, when was the client's last menstrual period?
Has the clothing been inspected for rips, blood, and stains?
Has the clothing been preserved?

term reactions, which, again, can consist of a variety of symptoms (Erickson, 1989).

Women need to be counseled about the prevention of pregnancy following a rape. The most common medical intervention is a course of hormonal medication. Elevated doses of oral contraceptive or DES (diethylstilbestrol) may be administered if the woman chooses to prevent conception (Krueger, 1988).

Evaluation: Rape

The long-term goal of intervention with rape victims is that they return to their prerape level, or to a higher level, of functioning. Three general outcomes must occur if the crisis is to be resolved in an adaptive fashion:

1. Verbalization of accurate cognitive perceptions of the rape
2. Emotional equilibrium
3. Adaptive coping behaviors

Crisis intervention is terminated when the evaluation process determines that the client has met the outcome criteria. Some clients will need or desire long-term psychotherapy to adjust to the trauma of rape.

Intrafamily Violence: Physical Abuse

Intrafamily physical abuse, violence within the family, occurs within all strata of society. The myth is that physical abuse occurs only among the poor and undereducated, but the reality is that physical abuse occurs also among the white-collar classes and professional elite. In the past, these problems among wealthy or prominent people were kept hidden from the general public. With an increase in national concern, however, more publicity is being given to cases of intrafamily physical abuse at all levels of society.

The United States has higher levels of violence than other Western countries. In 1985 this fact led U.S. Surgeon General Everett Koop to declare interpersonal violence, including intrafamily abuse, a priority public health problem (Bersani, 1988).

Although the image of the nuclear family in American culture is one of agreement, happiness, cohesiveness, and harmony, this ideal public image is often in conflict with the underlying reality of abuse and violence within the family. In fact, the family home may be the most dangerous place to live, since violence is more likely to occur within the family than between strangers. Children are beaten by their parents, brothers and sisters beat one another, spouses beat each other, and even elderly parents are beaten by family members. Beatings often escalate into more severe violence, with

Table 16–13 Nursing Care Plan for the Victim of Rape

Nursing Diagnosis: Rape trauma syndrome.
Goal: Client will return to prerape level of functioning within 6 weeks.

Intervention	*Rationale*	*Expected Outcome*
Give client time to respond to simple questions	Anxiety decreases the ability to perceive input and slows the response time	
If client is unable to express feelings, acknowledge the difficulty (eg, "I understand that it is difficult for you to describe your feelings right now. That's okay. You may be able to talk about them later.")	Support defense mechanisms until client is able to cope with the reality of the situation	
Communicate your knowledge and understanding of usual emotional responses to rape (eg, "People usually experience a number of feelings such as anxiety, fear, embarrassment, guilt, or anger.")	Client needs to be reassured that these feelings are a normal reaction to rape	Identifies and expresses feelings about the rape
Encourage client to talk about the rape	Talking with others will assist client through the stage of disbelief	Talks about the rape
Identify distortions related to self-blame or guilt	Beliefs of personal responsibility and fault interfere with resolution of the syndrome	Identifies self as a victim
Identify specific coping behavior client used during the rape (eg, screaming, fighting, talking, blacking out)	Identifying behavior as an adaptive mechanism to survive will increase self-esteem and decrease feelings of guilt	Identifies adaptive behavior
Encourage client to discuss the personal meaning of the rape	Clarification of specific fears or concerns will assist nurse in formulating additional interventions	Verbalizes anticipated problems
Help client identify immediate concerns and arrange them in order of importance	Focusing on immediate problems decreases sense of confusion and the feeling of being overwhelmed	Identifies most important concerns
Assist client to use the problem-solving process in developing solutions to concerns	The problem-solving process will increase feelings of control	Develops short-term plan for concerns
Support client in making his or her own decisions and acting in own behalf	Decision making will help client regain feelings of control and autonomy	Makes necessary decisions
Assist client in identifying who to tell and how to tell about the rape	Anticipatory guidance will assist client in using available support systems	Uses significant others for support
Discuss beliefs about postcoital contraception and abortion if appropriate	Pregnancy may be a realistic outcome of the rape; client needs to be provided with information about available choices	Verbalizes understanding of available choices
Discuss need for follow-up medical evaluation and treatment for sexually transmitted diseases	Providing client with information about potential physical problems will help ensure prevention of disease	Verbalizes importance of medical care
Provide anticipatory guidance about common physical, emotional, and social reactions to rape	Helps client know what to expect and provides guidelines for need for additional counseling	Acknowledges understanding of potential reactions
Provide written list of referrals to community resources	Crisis intervention counseling may decrease long-term impact of rape	Verbalizes need for short-term counseling
Make follow-up phone contact within 2–4 days	Client may need additional support to follow through on formulated plans	Implements immediate plans

20 to 40 percent of all murders occurring within the family unit (Bullock, 1989; McLeer, 1988).

Incidence of Physical Abuse

Child Abuse Each year, approximately 3.8 percent of children between the ages of 3 and 17 are beaten, which places the number of physically abused children at 2 million (Humphreys and Campbell, 1989). As the general public has become more aware of the problem, more cases are being reported, but these are probably only a small percentage of the total. To know if the actual rate of incidence is increasing is impossible because of lack of historical data. Laws mandating the reporting of child abuse were not passed in all 50 states until 1968 (Straus, Gelles, and Steinmetz, 1980).

Of those children under the age of 3 who are abused, as many as 25 percent die from the abuse. Some studies say the most dangerous age for abuse is 3 months to 3 years. Of abused children less than 6 years old, 64 percent suffer major physical injuries. Of younger children who are abused, the sex of the child does not appear to be significant in the incidence of abuse. After age 11 the rate of serious injury due to child abuse drops to 16 pecent, perhaps because older children can defend themselves and escape. Other studies say the incidence of abuse increases during adolescence, when boys are more likely to become victims. By the time the abuse is discovered and reported, most acts of violence have been going on for 1 to 3 years (Starr, 1988).

In past studies, mothers have been described as more physically abusive to their children than fathers. This was explained by the fact that mothers typically spend a greater amount of time with their children than fathers. Also, American culture often judges the competency of the mother by the behavior of her children. Thus, mothers were thought to have a greater incentive to use physical force to obtain obedience. However, recent studies indicate that men and women are equally likely to abuse young children. During adolescence, though, the abuser is more likely to be the father (Bolton and Bolton, 1987).

Sibling Abuse The most common and unrecognized form of family violence occurs between siblings. Many people assume it is natural and even appropriate that children use physical force with one another. Statements are made such as, "It's a good chance for him to learn how to defend himself," "She had a right to hit him. He was teasing her," or "Kids will be kids." With these attitudes, children learn that physical force is an appropriate method of resolving conflict among themselves. Sibling violence is highest in the early years and decreases with age. In all age groups, girls are less violent toward their siblings than are boys.

Spouse Abuse National attention to spouse abuse is more recent than the concern for child abuse. The woman's movement in the 1970s brought the issue into the public domain. In 1976, efforts were begun to establish resources for battered wives. There has been a continuing focus on providing counseling, forming shelters, and passing new laws to protect the abused spouse.

How many adults are abused by their spouse or live-in partner is unknown. The statistics range from 11 to 50 percent of the population. It is believed that as many as 80 percent of the cases are unreported because the victims are ashamed, feel responsible, or fear reprisal in the form of increased violence (Bullock, 1989). One partner in one out of every six couples in the United States will commit at least one act of violence against the other partner in any given year. That incidence rises to one out of every three couples when the entire length of the relationship is considered. Violence against women is not confined to marriage relationships. It is estimated that 30 percent of couples dating or living together have been involved in violence (Sachs, 1988; Strauss, Gelles, Steinmetz, 1980; Tilden and Shepherd, 1987).

In most studies of domestic violence, only 2 to 5 percent of the cases involve male victims. In couples filing for divorce, it was found that only 3.3 percent of husbands complained of being abused, whereas 36.8 percent of the wives claimed to be victims (Campbell and Sheridan, 1989; Okum, 1986).

Of abused women inside and outside marriage, half suffer beatings several times a year. Of the remainder, many are beaten as often as once a week. The intensity and frequency of attacks tend to escalate over time. Compared to nonabused women, battered women are five times more likely to attempt suicide, 15 times more likely to abuse alcohol, and nine times more likely to abuse drugs (Stark and Flitcraft, 1988).

Elder Abuse National attention to the abuse of the elderly by family members is just beginning. Elder abuse may take the form of having basic physical needs neglected. Victims may suffer from dehydration, malnutrition, and oversedation. Families may deprive them of necessary articles such as glasses, hearing aids, or walkers. Some elderly people are psychologically abused by verbal assaults, threats, humiliation, or harassment. Families may violate an elderly person's rights by refusing appropriate medical treatment, forcing isolation or unreasonable confinement, denying privacy, providing an unsafe environment, or demanding involuntary servitude. Some are financially exploited by their relatives through theft or misuse of property or funds. Others are beaten and even raped by family members. The rate of abuse is unknown because many older people are ashamed to admit that their children have abused them and often fear retaliation if help is sought. At present, between 4 and 11 percent of older persons are being abused, with most experiencing two or more forms of abuse. The majority of the victims are between the ages of 59 and 90. Older women are more likely to be abused and account for 75 percent of the reported cases. Two thirds of the abusers are over the age of 40, and 50 percent of them are either sons or daughters of the victims. Spouse abuse accounts for 12 percent of the cases among the elderly, with the remaining abusers being other relatives such as grandchildren, siblings, nieces, and nephews. As the proportion of elderly increases in this country, it is likely that abuse of the elderly will become a greater problem (Hudson, 1986; Quinn and Tomita, 1986; Sengstock and Barrett, 1984).

Homosexual Abuse Though the topic of homosexual battering by heterosexuals (street violence) has been openly discussed with concern in the gay community, there continues to be a minimization or denial of physical abuse in lesbian or gay relationships. The following *myths* have contributed to the silence:

- Only "bar dykes" engage in violence
- Only couples who have stereotypical male-female roles are violent
- Feminist lesbians are not involved in violence toward one another

The fact is that battering occurs in some lesbian families regardless of class, race, age, and lifestyle. When lesbian or gay couples become involved in violence, the reasons are the same as those in heterosexual battering. Those reasons are the need to demonstrate, achieve, and maintain power and control over one's partner. In addition to physical, sexual, or emotional abuse, the violent partner may use homophobic control—the threat of telling family, friends, neighbors, or employers about the victim's sexual orientation. The lesbian and gay communities are currently making an attempt to bring this problem out in the open in an attempt to intervene with and support the victims (Hart, 1986; Strach and Jervey, 1986; Walker, 1986).

Emotional Abuse Although the focus of violence in this chapter is on physical abuse, it must be remembered that emotional abuse is often equally as damaging. Words can hit as hard as a fist, and the damage to self-esteem can last a lifetime. **Emotional abuse** involves one person shaming, embarrassing, ridiculing, or insulting someone. It may include the destruction of personal property or the killing of pets in an effort to frighten or control the victim. Statements such as "You can't do anything right," "You're ugly and stupid—no one else would want you," or "I wish you had never been born" are devastating to the victim's self-esteem.

Significance of Physical Abuse to Mental Health Nursing

Violence that occurs within the family is a national health problem that confronts nurses in many different clinical settings. Victims are seen in the community, in pediatric units, in intensive care units, in medical-surgical units, in geriatric units, and in psychiatric units. Nurses in emergency rooms need to routinely ask clients of all ages if they have been beaten when the injuries could suggest as much. If the physical injuries are treated but the causes of the problem are ignored, intrafamily violence will continue unchecked.

Because there is an increased incidence of violence toward pregnant women, nurses in clinical settings with pregnant women must routinely look for evidence of violence as they take histories and make physical assessments. There are more incidents of beating during pregnancy than of either diabetes or placenta previa; indeed, 1 out of every 50 pregnant women is physically abused. Nonpregnant women are usually beaten in the face and chest. Pregnant women, however, tend to be beaten in the abdomen and often suffer injuries to the breasts and genitals. This may represent prenatal child abuse, since violence during pregnancy is associated with subsequent child abuse. It may also represent attempts to abort the fetus. It is estimated that 30 to 56 pecent of women beaten during pregnancy experience at least one miscarriage. Pregnant adolescents still living at home may experience physical abuse from their parents. Unfortunately, abuse of pregnant women of any age is often overlooked by medical personnel, even when the victim appears in the emergency department with bruises, cuts, broken bones, and abdominal injuries (Bullock, 1989; Hillard, 1988; Okum, 1986).

> *A woman serving a 40-year prison term for her husband's murder is seeking clemency on the basis of continued abuse. She said that her husband beat her weekly, often in front of their two children. When she was five months pregnant, he came home from work one day and "slapped me on the floor, kicked me, dragged me out of the apartment and threw me down a flight of stairs." Another time, in front of the children, he took out a .357 magnum, put the gun to her head and said, "If the phone rings, you're dead." She also said her husband tried to run over her with the car and drown her at a family picnic. He also threatened to drop battery acid into their infant daughter's eyes* (Wheeler, 1988).

Nurses need to be involved in the prevention, detection, and treatment of intrafamily violence. Development of the knowledge base and the ability to identify factors that contribute to intrafamily violence will enable the nurse to assist in prevention by providing public education and becoming active in changes in public policy. This knowledge, along with increased awareness of the extent of the problem, will help nurses arrive at earlier, more accurate detection of intrafamily violence. Nurses also need to comply with state laws on the reporting of violence and the referral for treatment. Some nurses, with advanced education in family therapy, are part of the therapy teams that intervene with violent families.

Knowledge Base: Physical Abuse

Behavioral Characteristics

Acts of violence within the family range from a light slap, to a severe beating, to a homicide. Hitting or spanking children, with 84 to 94 percent of all parents using this form of discipline at some time in the life of a child, is condoned and even approved of as being necessary and good for the child. Many parents, however, do not realize the underlying messages that are given to the child (Straus, Gelles, Steinmetz, 1980):

- If you are small and weak, you deserve to be hit
- People who love you, hit you
- It is appropriate to hit people you love
- Violence is appropriate if the end result is good
- Violence is an appropriate method of resolving conflict

Parental violence can become extreme and often becomes chronic in that it occurs periodically or regularly. Many times, it ends in the death of the infant or child.

> *A mother was convicted for beating to death her AIDS-infected, heroin-addicted infant twin*

sons. The 4-month-old, 5-pound infants died of skull fractures induced by the severe beatings (Casey and O'Connor, 1988).

A father was charged in the beating death of his 5-month-old son. The medical examiner stated the boy suffered a broken leg, hemorrhaging eyes, bruises on the buttocks, and brain damage. The father told police that he had only "slapped the baby to try and wake it up" (Casey and O'Connor, 1988).

The boyfriend of the mother of a 2-year-old boy was charged with the boy's murder. While caring for the child, the boyfriend bit him on the face, abdomen, and buttocks. The child bled to death from deep bite wounds into the abdominal cavity (O'Connor, 1985).

The father of a 17-year-old young man was convicted of solicitation to commit murder. There was evidence of previous physical abuse; the son had testified that he had been beaten with a broomstick and a hose, and that at one point his father had held a cocked, loaded gun to his head. Previously, the father had told the son: "I can't wait until you die. When you die, I'll put your name on my trucks to show my appreciation" (Rossi, 1985).

Acts of violence between adult family members fall along the same continuum with women committing fewer violent acts than men. Women do more hitting, kicking, and throwing of objects when involved in violent conflict with men. The acts that men commit against women are more dangerous and result in more severe injuries. Men are likely to push, shove, slap, beat up, and even use knives or guns against their wives or girlfriends (Straus, Gelles, and Steinmetz, 1980). In one study of abused women (Giles-Sims, 1983), it was found that 50 percent of the abusing men had threatened their partners with a knife or gun, and 25 percent had actually assaulted their partners with a knife or gun. Verbal abuse always accompanies battering.

There is a real danger that women may be killed by a violent male family member. A study of 538 women murdered in 1981 found that 29 percent of these women were killed by their current husbands or boyfriends. If the data had included former husbands or boyfriends, the percentage would have been higher. In one study of domestic killings, there was a history of wife abuse in 71.9 percent of the murders. Women are more likely to kill their husbands or boyfriends as an act of self-defense when battering has been a continual problem in the home (Campbell, 1984A).

In violent families, a pattern of behavior usually develops. The first incident may be precipitated by frustration or stress. If a pattern of violence is to be avoided, the victim must immediately refuse to accept the violence. Outside help may be necessary to put a stop to the behavior. If the victim submits to the violence, physical force, without the stimulus of frustration or stress, becomes a way of relating to one another, and the pattern becomes resistant to change. Intrafamily violence is typically cyclic. Conflict escalates into a violent episode. After the episode, the perpetrator, feeling regret and shame, begs for the victim's forgiveness. The victim stays in the system because the perpetrator promises to reform and perhaps because of material rewards for remaining. During the next episode of conflict, the cycle begins again, and violence becomes a stable pattern of family behavior (Giles-Sims, 1983; O'Leary, 1988).

Michael, age 45, is a very successful physician. During recent divorce proceedings, he has confessed to periodically beating his wife, Maria. At times, he would yank her around by the hair or hold her out of a second-story window and threaten to let her fall. During each of Maria's three pregnancies, Michael would beat her, particularly in her abdomen, saying he wished he could kill both her and the unborn child. This periodic abuse has continued throughout the 20-year marriage but was kept a family secret until the divorce proceedings.

Perpetrators lack impulse control, and their behavior is immature and self-serving. Pathologic jealousy may contribute to keeping their wives under surveillance, calling home repeatedly during the day, locking the woman in the house and removing the phone while he's away, and prohibiting social life with other women. Abusive men may publicly humiliate their wives and alienate their friends. This increases women's isolation and makes leaving the relationship more difficult. Unpredictable behavior is typical of the perpetrator. At times he may be kind and generous to his wife and is able to present this "good" side when he needs to, such as in the presence of the police (Okum, 1986).

Abused children often try to please the abusing parent and may become overly compliant to all adults. They may avoid peers and withdraw from outside contact. It is not unusual for the victim to act out with aggressive behavior during adolescence.

Like abused children, many victims of abuse attempt to cope by becoming compliant. They try to placate the abuser, hoping that conflict will not escalate into physical abuse. However, the more submissive the victim becomes, the more severe and frequent the abuse becomes. If victims are dependent on the security of the home, they often accept the abuse rather than risk disruption of the family. Some victims, immobilized by fear, are unable to leave the abuser. Others attempt to leave but are tracked down and forced back into the home by the abuser. Both fear and inability to escape contribute to further compliant behavior in the victim.

Affective Characteristics

Physically abusive people are often described as extremely jealous and possessive. They view other family members in terms of property and ownership. Within a culture that historically condones violence as a method of protecting property rights, these people believe violence is an acceptable method of maintaining the family unit. Extreme jealousy can escalate to hostility toward the victim and even the entire world as the abuser feels forced to defend his or her rights of ownership.

Some abusers have strong dependency needs and fear the loss of intimate relationships. They may beat a child because of the competition for the love and attention of their spouse. Some men are so dependent and fearful of loss that when their wives attempt to become more independent, they respond with violence. Closely related to the dependency needs of abusers is the feeling of inadequacy. Abusers use violence in an attempt to prove to themselves and others that they are superior and in control. The use of physical force temporarily decreases their fears of inadequacy and compensates for the lack of other internal resources. People who feel inadequate in relationships may use violence to create emotional distance and thereby avoid the fears of closeness and intimacy (Bolton and Bolton, 1987).

Victims may be immobilized by a variety of affective responses to the abuse. In one study, it was found that 25 percent of the victims felt guilty, 50 percent felt helpless, and 75 percent experienced feelings of depression (Resick, 1983). The feelings of guilt and self-blame may be expressed in statements such as, "If I were a better wife, he wouldn't beat me," or "If I hadn't talked back to my mother, she wouldn't have hit me." Victims who feel responsible for the abuser's behavior may also experience guilt if they are unable to change the pattern of violence within the family. Many victims feel helpless to prevent the violence, and fear greater injury or death if they would attempt to defend themselves. Guilt can contribute to distorted thinking and depression, which further immobilizes the victim and keeps her from leaving or seeking help for the family system.

Fear contributes to a woman's failure to leave the abusive relationship. Not infrequently there is a threat of death if she would try to leave, so the woman lives in fear of physical reprisal. Fearing loneliness, the woman may believe being in a bad relationship is better than being alone. Multiple potential or real losses contribute to an immobilizing grief reaction. Losses include self-esteem, a caring relationship, trust, safety, and financial security. To leave the relationship does not ensure the end of abuse. The abuser is often most dangerous when threatened with or faced with separation. As many as 26 percent of abusive incidents occur after separation or divorce (Okum, 1986; Tilden and Shepherd, 1987).

Fear also contributes to a lesbian's failure to leave an abusive relationship. Since many couples share close friends within the same lesbian community, the victim may fear shaming her partner.

She may also fear friends will either deny the problem or take the abuser's side. Homophobia contributes to the victim's fear in seeking help. Calling the police may result in ridiculing or hostile responses from the officers. A lesbian victim may fear seeking help from her family because she does not want to reinforce negative stereotypes about lesbians and increase the family's homophobia (Hammond, 1986).

Cognitive Characteristics

Many abusive people have perfectionistic standards for themselves and members of their families. This results in a sense of rigidity and an obsession with discipline and control. Inflexibility hinders the abuser's ability to find alternative solutions to conflict. Some abusers are self-righteous, believing it is their right to use physical force to get others to comply with their wishes. Many abusers lack understanding of the effect of their behavior on the victims and may even blame their abusive behavior on the victims. This pattern is known as projection of blame. Inadequate self-esteem contributes to feelings of impotency and the use of power to counteract this negative self-evaluation. Many parents who abuse their children suffered emotional deprivation when they themselves were children. As a result, they may have unrealistic expectations of their own children. Anger may turn to violence when the children are unable to fulfill the unrealistic emotional needs of the parent. Other parents may have minimal information about children's growth and development and unrealistic expectations of what the child is capable of performing. In this situation, child abuse may begin—for example, when the child is not toilet trained by the age of 9 months. Adult children of elderly parents may also have minimal understanding of the developmental changes of aging. Not infrequently, the changes are viewed as deliberate and under the control of the parent. Perpetrators of elder abuse use the defense mechanisms of minimization, denial, and projection of blame (Bolton and Bolton, 1987; Broome and Daniels, 1987).

Victims of abuse often begin with or develop an inadequate self-esteem. Victims who are beaten begin to believe the violence itself is evidence of personal worthlessness. The verbal abuse accompanying the beating further decreases the self-worth as the victim comes to believe the derogatory remarks. This distorted thinking process contributes to guilt and a toleration of the violence. Some victims believe they are helpless to change the pattern of domination or to leave the relationship. Some victims rationalize that the perpetrator was not responsible for the abusive actions by convincing themselves that the behavior was the result of a high level of stress or too much alcohol. Victims of abuse often exhibit the Stockholm syndrome, or hostage response. This includes a belief of personal responsibility and a sense of unworthiness as well as an affinity and sympathy for the perpetrator. The belief of reform is a common characteristic of victims. When the abuser promises never to strike again, the victim is seduced by the hope of reform and the belief that perhaps this was the last incident of violence. Wives who believe the responsibility for maintaining the family unit belongs to women may stay in a battering relationship in an attempt to keep the family together. This responsibility may also be a factor for women who submit to abuse out of the fear that the children will become victims if they do not submit (Bolton and Bolton, 1987; Valenti, 1986).

Jerry, who is 27 years old, was brought to the psychiatric unit by the police. He had been arrested at home for threatening the lives of his family. He became exceedingly violent at the police station, which precipitated his move to the hospital. His history is as follows: Jerry's mother and father divorced when he was 5 and his brothers were 6 and 7 years old. His mother moved in with another man, married him, and left him within one month. She then moved in with a different man for two months. She left him and married a fourth man and stayed in that relationship for 11 years. Jerry describes his mother as alcoholic, abusive, and neglectful. The children were ordered to go out on the street and sell at least 50 boxes of candy every day. If the chil-

dren did not bring home enough money each day, they were beaten. Jerry, fearful of his mother and angry about having to sell candy, adapted by throwing the candy away and stealing the money to bring home. He stated that while the children would be out selling candy, his mother would go to the lake to get a tan, and that she would walk around in mink while they had barely usable clothing. Jerry said he was always blamed for any trouble. He was locked in the closet for hours on end. At times, his mother forced the other children to hold Jerry down while he was beaten by her and his stepfather. Sometimes she would place the wire from a straightened coat hanger in the children's mouth and twirl it around. Jerry remembers being forced to stand with his hands in the air until his mother would finally fall asleep. Jerry's brothers both ran away from home at the age of 16. Jerry, unable to distance himself from his mother and her cruelty, has remained at home. He has a history of stealing as well as alcohol and drug abuse.

Physiologic Characteristics

A variety of injuries may be inflicted on victims of physical abuse. In general, small children may be retarded in the areas of growth and development. For victims of all ages, any combination of the following characteristics may be observed. There may be bald patches where hair has been pulled out, or there may be subdural hematomas from blows to the head. The eyes may be bruised or swollen, or the victim may have hemorrhages into the eyes or petechiae around the eyes from attempted strangulation. The skin, genitals, and rectal areas may be bruised or burned and may show scars of past injuries. Fractures, or evidence of previous fractures, may be present, particularly of the face, arms, and ribs. Joints are often dislocated, especially in the shoulder, when the victim is grabbed or pulled around by the arm. Intraabdominal injuries are common, especially in pregnant women. Neurologically, the victim may have areas of parasthesias or numbness from old injuries, and their reflexes may be hyperactive from neurologic damage (Mittleman, Mittleman, and Wetli, 1987).

Sociocultural Characteristics

The abuser's family of origin is an important factor in understanding intrafamily violence. Violence is often perpetuated by each generation in the family unless circumstances occur that alter the family dynamics. Much of adult behavior is determined by childhood experiences within the family system. Parents model marital interactions and parent-child interactions for their children. When the children grow up and form their own nuclear families, there is an unconscious attempt to re-create the same form of interactions. Despite the pain involved, negative patterns are often repeated because they represent security and because other problem-solving skills have not been learned. Thus, the experience of violence in the family of origin teaches the individual participants that the use of physical force is appropriate. Violence becomes integrated into the dynamics in such a way that violence and love are fused, or violence is perceived as morally right when used to achieve good results. Children may cope with exposure to abuse by identifying with either the aggressor or the victim. Not infrequently these children grow up to become another abuser or adult victim. There is evidence that some adult abusers were emotionally neglected or abandoned as children. Since early security and dependency needs were not met, these adults are unable to meet their own children's needs for affection and trust (Bennett, 1987; Valenti, 1986).

Traditional gender roles affect the use of violence within the family. Violent families are more likely to enact sex-role stereotyping and to have a hierarchic family structure. Some men get caught up in compulsive masculinity whereby they feel a need to be tough, strong, aggressive, and nonemotional. By these husbands, an egalitarian marital relationship is seen as evidence of a lack of masculinity. In an attempt to support their "superior" position, these men tend to marry women who are younger, less educated, and less economically productive. In addition, these men may view women as childlike and needing to be overprotected. When the position of dominance or leadership is threatened by the wife or the children, violence is more likely to occur. Men whose sense of masculinity is not dependent on positions of superiority or who are able to adapt to egalitarian relationships are less likely to use violence against their wives and children (Bersani and Chen, 1988; Goodrich et al., 1988).

The violent family is often socially isolated. In some families, the isolation precedes the violence. With few network support systems, the isolated family is less able to manage life stresses and may resort to violence in an attempt to cope with frustration. For other families, the social isolation is in response to the violence. Family members, ashamed of what is occurring, withdraw from interactions with others. This withdrawal prevents the humiliation that might occur if the violence became known to others.

Many violent families have experienced a high number of significant life events before the onset of physical abuse. This bombardment of stress places a great deal of strain on the family's ability to adapt to change. When emotional, physical, or financial resources are drained, violence may erupt within the family system.

As people age they become more vulnerable to abuse, because they are more dependent on others for survival. Adult children may experience a number of losses and new demands. The role of child in the family system must be forsaken. At the same time, there is a loss of many of the freedoms the adult children expected during middle age. Care givers may be overwhelmed with too many roles in caring for their own children as well as aging parents. This high level of stress may be one factor in elder abuse (Bolton and Bolton, 1987). (See Chapter 6 for in-depth discussion.)

For many women, it is difficult to leave the abusive relationship. Women have been socialized to be self-sacrificing for the good of others. They feel responsible for keeping the family together at almost any cost. Cultural beliefs about loyalty and duty reinforce the role of victim. Women who do leave abusive relationships usually separate from their partners from three to five times before finally ending the relationships. Many women are financially dependent on their abusive partners. If they have outside employment, they are unlikely to earn as much as their male counterparts. If there are children involved, they may desperately need financial child support, and many fathers do not honor this obligation and default on the payments. The burdens of child care have traditionally been assigned to the mother. Lack of affordable and adequate child care facilities is a major problem for the single mother seeking employment. Single parents may experience some social disapproval because of the separation or divorce. The cultural norm continues to be that two parents are always better for the children than one parent (Burden and Gottlieb, 1987; Gilligan, 1982).

The criminal justice system has been unable to decrease significantly the amount of intrafamily violence in America. Police officers and lawyers have minimal or no training in crisis or family violence intervention. There may be long delays in obtaining court orders or peace bonds to protect the victims. Court cases are often rescheduled, causing long delays in legal relief. The victims need advocates in the court so that they are not revictimized by the trauma of the judicial system (Giles-Sims, 1983; Straus and Hotaling, 1980). Male and female defendants are often treated differently by the courts. Walker (1984, p. 205) points out this difference in cases involving family violence: "Women who kill their husbands are more likely to be charged with first-degree murder, while men who kill their wives are more likely to receive a manslaughter charge." Changes must be made within the criminal justice system to allow all victims legal relief from family violence.

Causative Theories

The violent family is easy to describe but difficult to explain. There is no single cause of family violence. Violent behavior takes many forms and has many origins. Aggressive behavior involves the internal and external systems of both the abuser and the victim. This multidimensional approach to understanding family violence includes biologic, intrapersonal, social learning, sociologic, and system theories.

Biologic Theories The instinctivist theory suggests that people possess a natural fighting instinct that serves to preserve the species. The animal kingdom is cited as proof that it is natural to protect territory and prey on smaller or weaker victims. Many authorities refute this theory, stating that it confuses hunting for food with indiscriminate violence. Animal fighting for territory or mating privileges does not contain the cruelty that characterizes human violence. In addition, most animal groups work to keep fighting incidents at a minimum.

The neurophysiologic theory proposes that the limbic system and the neurotransmitters are implicated in violent behavior. It is thought that an increase in norepinephrine, dopamine, and serotonin increases irritability and may result in various types of aggression. Stimulation of the lateral and medial hypothalamus in animals produces attack behavior, whereas stimulation of the dorsal hypothalamus results in escape behavior. It is also thought that the septal area of the limbic system normally has an inhibiting influence, since lesions that destroy the septal region cause ferocious and vicious behavior in animals. Research is also continuing into the increased tendency toward aggression in women experiencing severe premenstrual syndrome (PMS). Theories focus on the decrease in progesterone or the dopamine hyperfunction occurring before menstruation (Keye, 1988).

Substance abuse, especially of alcohol, is often implicated in violent behavior. In some people, alcohol may decrease the normal inhibitions against violence and thereby increase the probability that violent behavior may occur. With high alcohol levels, people have a decreased verbal ability, an increased fear of attack from others, and a decreased recognition of their own inappropriate behavior. These factors may contribute to a violent outburst. Alcoholism is not necessarily a direct cause of violence, however, since many alcoholics are not violent to their loved ones (Humphreys and Campbell, 1989; Montague, 1979).

Intrapersonal Theories The intrapersonal theories suggest that the cause of violence lies in the individual personalities of the abusers. It is thought that aggression is a basic drive within the personality and that people who are violent are unable to control the impulsive expression of anger and hostility. People who feel helpless or inadequate may use physical force in an attempt to defend themselves and increase their low self-esteem. Intrapersonal theories of child abuse describe rejection of the child and failure of bonding between parent and child. Parents may also project their own negative characteristics onto the child and then abuse the child for the perceived problems. Parents' own early rejections or childhood identifications with an abusive parent contribute to the cycle of family violence. Other explanations involve personality traits or disorders. Abusers are often obsessive-compulsive, jealous, suspicious, paranoid, or sadistic. Violent behavior may be used to enforce absolute discipline, protect one's "property," or protect oneself from being attacked. Some abusers are described as having an aggressive-impulsive personality style. These individuals have a lifetime history of physical fighting. Successful outcomes of childhood fights reinforce the aggressive behavior and increase the likelihood of child, spouse, and elder abuse (Campbell, 1984D; McLeer, 1988; O'Leary, 1988).

Social Learning Theory The social learning theory proposes that violence is a learned behavior rather than an instinctive behavior. It is believed that stimulation of the neurophysiologic mechanisms for violence are under cognitive control. Both the abuser and the victim learn their roles during childhood. Children learn about violence by observation, being a victim, or behaving violently themselves. If the use of violence is rewarded by a gain in power, the behavior is reinforced. If there is immediate negative reinforcement within the family, a decrease in violent behavior will occur (Humphreys and Campbell, 1989; Walker, 1984). In addition to family models, the media provide many models of violence to which children are exposed. Westerns, cartoons, police shows, and adventure movies all demonstrate that "good" people use force to achieve "good" ends. Much of the violence in the media does not even attempt to rationalize the use of force for "good" ends, rather, they present the endless, senseless cruelty of one human being to another. With these types of family and media examples, children develop values that tolerate and accept violence between people.

Sociologic Theory The social environment can place additional stress on the family unit. Violent families tend to be multiproblem families who have experienced a prolonged series of significant life events such as illnesses; accidents; economic crises; and new people, such as babies or aged parents, entering the system. Factors such as underemployment, unemployment, and poverty contribute to feelings of anger and deprivation. When financial, physical, or emotional resources are limited and strained, there is a greater probability that conflict will end in violence.

Identifiable factors contribute to the abuse of the elderly within the family. With the trend to smaller family size, there are fewer family members to share in the care of older parents, and with longer life expectancy, the number of years of caring for a dependent parent have increased. As people live longer, they often develop many medical problems, and the cost of medical care can be a financial burden.

Middle-aged adults often look forward to freedom from the demands and responsibilities of child care. Before this freedom can be experienced, an aged parent may move into the family system, and the adult children may find themselves limited socially and economically. The feeling of being caught between their children's needs and their parent's needs, with no time for themselves, may contribute to the abuse of elderly parents. Some daughters and sons have difficulty redefining their relationship with their parents. For them to see the parent as dependent, rather than all-powerful and resourceful, is difficult. A great deal of anger may be generated when aged parents can no longer be a source of all-giving support for the adult children.

When older parents move into the homes of their adult daughters or sons, the level of intrafamily stress may rise. The physical environment may become crowded and provide few places or opportunities for privacy. With strong differing opinions on how the household should be managed, power struggles often ensue. The subsequent increase in stress and frustration may be a contributing factor in the abuse of the elderly (Phillips, 1986).

Systems Theory System theorists believe violence does not occur in isolation but rather results from the interrelationships between people, events, and behavior. Understanding the interrelationships is not the same as saying each family member is equally responsible for the violence. As Giles-Sims (1983) explains, systems theory identifies several characteristics of violent families:

- The taboo against violence is broken
- A rise in expectations of further violence occurs
- The family system denies that violent behavior is deviant
- The abused person does not label himself or herself as a victim
- Violent behavior is reinforced when it produces the desired results

The abused child may be the scapegoat in a dysfunctional family system. One particular child may be labeled as the deviant member of the family. In this situation, marital conflict is displaced onto the scapegoated child, who becomes the target of hostility and violent attacks.

In the enmeshed family system, boundaries may be diffused with a resulting increase in stress and conflict. Family member roles may be constantly shifting. If the parents are unable to meet each other's needs for support and affection, they may turn to the child for this type of adult love. Each parent then begins to view the child as his or her special support system, and the parents become competitive for the child's attention. When the child is unable to meet all the emotional needs of the parents, frustration builds and often ends in violent behavior. This type of family system may become disorganized and chaotic when the parents are unable to provide consistent leadership functions.

A closed family system is characterized by rigidity, inflexibility, and highly repetitive patterns of behavior. Input from larger social systems, such as friends or community resources, is discouraged and avoided. Solutions to problems must be found within the family system, whose resources are eventually depleted. The closed family system is rigid in its authoritarianism. There is a great need for children to conform and comply with the family rules. When children begin to question the rules or challenge the power structure of the family, violence may be used to reinforce the authoritarian structure (Okum, 1986).

Feminist Theory Feminist theories describe the sexist structure of the family and society as an important factor in intrafamily violence. The patriarchal organization gives men dictatorial authority over women and children. Women are viewed as childlike, passive, unreasonable, and overly emotional individuals who need to be dominated and controlled. The sexist economic system helps to entrap women, who must choose between poverty and battering. It is difficult for women to find advocates and solutions within the male-dominated legal, religious, mental health, and medical systems (Humphreys and Campbell, 1989; Okum, 1986).

Assessment: Physical Abuse

Battered women enter the health care system for a variety of conditions associated with abuse. Failure of nurses to be alert to signs of abuse contributes to inappropriate diagnoses and interventions. Some battered women may not offer information about abuse, or they may minimize its impact. However, it is the nurse's responsibility to assess for and not deny the reality of violence. In one study (Stark and Flitcraft, 1988) 75 percent of abused women volunteered the information that they had been battered but only 5 percent of the assigned professionals acknowledged this information. Another study (Rose and Saunders, 1986), of 86 physicians and 145 nurses, identified the gender of the professional as being the most significant factor in determining whether battered women were recognized as such. Female nurses and physicians were less likely than males to believe that beatings were justified and that preventing the abuse was the victim's responsibility.

The most important outcome of nursing assessment is the identification of domestic violence. Following this, a multiteam assessment takes place. The victim's medical condition and emotional state must be assessed. The severity and potential fatality of the situation must be considered as well as needs of dependent children and legal issues.

Nurses in all clinical settings must routinely assess clients for evidence of violent attacks. Considering the extensiveness of the problem of intrafamily violence, one or two introductory questions should be asked of every client. In assessing a child, the nurse may ask, "Moms and dads try to help their children learn how to behave well. What happens to you when you do something wrong?" or "What is the worst punishment you ever received?" In assessing an adult, the nurse may ask, "One of the sources of stress in all of our lives is family disagreement. Could you describe how disagreements affect you? What happens when you disagree?" If the responses to these questions are indicative of violence, a focused nursing assessment, such as the one that follows, must be conducted. Obviously, the assessment questions must be adapted to the client's age, gender, and family situation.

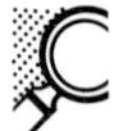

FOCUSED NURSING ASSESSMENT *for Victims of Violence*

Behavioral assessment

Tell me about how people communicate within your family.

What types of things cause conflict within your family?

How is conflict managed or resolved?

Who in your family loses control of themselves when angry?

Have you received verbal threats of harm?

Have you ever been threatened with a knife or gun?
In which ways have you been at the receiving end of a family member's violent outbursts? Slapped? Hit? Punched? Thrown? Shoved? Kicked? Burned? Beaten up?
Is there a history of need for emergency medical treatment?
In what ways have you attempted to stop the violence?
Have you attempted to leave the situation in the past?
What occurred when you attempted to leave?
Describe the use of alcohol in the family.
Describe the use of drugs in the family.

Affective assessment
Who do you view as responsible for the use of physical force within the family?
In what way is this person(s) responsible?
How much guilt are you experiencing at this time?
Tell me about your fears. Lack of security? Financial problems? Child care problems? Living apart from spouse? Further physical injury?
What kinds of factors contribute to your feeling of helplessness in leaving or stopping the abuse?
How hopeless do you feel about your situation?
How would you describe your level of depression?

Cognitive assessment
Describe your strengths and abilities as a person.
If you were describing yourself to a stranger what would you say?
What are your beliefs about keeping your family together?
Tell me about your reasons for remaining in this situation. Promises of reform? Material rewards?
Do you believe/hope the violence will not recur?
What are your expectations of how children should behave?
What rights do parents have with their children?
What rights do spouses have with each other?
What are the rules about physical force within your family?

Sociocultural assessment
How did your parents relate to each other?
Who enforced discipline when you were a child?
What type of discipline was used when you were a child?
What was/is your relationship like with your mother?
What was/is your relationship like with your father?
How did you get along with your siblings?
In your present family, who is the head of the household?
How are decisions made in your family?
How are household jobs assigned in the family?
Describe the recent and current stresses on the family. Unemployment? Financial problems? Illness? New family members? Deaths or separations? Child rearing problems? Change in job status? Increase in conflict? Change in residence?
Who can you turn to for support in times of stress?
Describe your social life to me.
What types of contact have you had with the legal system? Phoned police? Peace bonds? Obtained a lawyer? Court cases? Protective services?

Table 16–14 presents guidelines for physical assessments of victims of violence.

Privacy must be ensured when conducting the assessment interview. It may be difficult for the cli-

Table 16-14 *Physical Assessment of Victims of Violence*

Complete a head-to-toe assessment with particular attention to the following areas:

Head
- Evidence of trauma
- Evidence of hematoma
- Bald patches on scalp
- Facial bruises
- Facial fractures
- Eyes: swollen, bruised, hemorrhages

Skin
- Swelling or tenderness
- Bruises
- Burns
- Presence of scars from burns or injuries
- Genital trauma
- Rectal trauma

Musculoskeletal
- Fractures of the ribs
- Fractures of arms/legs
- Dislocated joints
- Impaired mobility

Abdomen
- Bruises or wounds
- Evidence of internal injuries

Neurologic
- Reflexes
- Parasthesias
- Numbness
- Pain

ent to admit to the reality of family violence until a level of trust has been established with the nurse. Many clients are fearful the nurse will respond in a judgmental manner against the abuser or against the victim for being abused or remaining in the situation. The client needs to be assured of the nurse's genuine desire to assist the entire family system (Sengstock and Barrett, 1984).

Nursing Diagnosis and Planning: Physical Abuse

The majority of people involved in intrafamily violence are disturbed by this behavior and would like it to end. Even though they want help in stopping the abuse, they may not know how to seek the assistance they need. It is extremely important that the nurse be nonjudgmental in interactions with all family members. The abusers feel condemned by society at large and may therefore be distrustful of the motives of the nursing staff. Initially, the victims may be unwilling to trust the nursing staff because of family shame and fears of being accused for remaining in the violent situation. Victims must be approached in a nonsexist manner, which means nurses must not blame the victim or look for pathology in understanding the victim's behavior. It is vital that nurses not impose their own values on the family by offering quick and easy solutions to intrafamily violence.

Treatment of violent families requires a multidisciplinary approach with a broad range of interventions. Nurses, social workers, physicians, family therapists, vocational trainers, police, protective services personnel, and lawyers need to coordinate their skills to intervene effectively with family violence. During periods of crisis, the family is the most open and accepting of professional intervention. When the violent family is identified during a crisis period, it should be immediately referred for multidisciplinary treatment. Family members will be most open to developing new patterns of behavior in the four to six weeks following the crisis. If no interventions are made during that time, they are likely to return to the familiar patterns of interaction, including the use of physical force (Campbell, 1984C).

Nurses need to be knowledgeable about the laws regarding the reporting of physical abuse. In all 50 states, nurses are required by law to report suspected incidents of child abuse, and in every state, there is a penalty—civil, criminal, or both—for failure to report child abuse. Child protective services and the courts make decisions in the best interests of the child. The child may remain with the parents under court supervision; the child may be removed from the home; or, in the case of severe abuse, parental rights may be terminated. The state laws vary for reporting abuse of adults and the elderly. Adult protective services provide health, housing, and social services. Currently the resources are inadequate to meet the needs of abused adults. Domestic violence is now considered to be a violent crime wherein the victim has the right to be protected and the perpetrator is often arrested and prosecuted (Bolton and Bolton, 1987).

If trust is to be maintained, the family needs to be told that a report is being made to protective services. Nurses need to know the procedures that follow a report of abuse so that the family can be adequately informed of the process. Many families are fearful that the only function of protective services is to remove family members from the home; in fact, protective services can be very supportive to the family by offering counseling and other social services.

Nurses in all clinical settings are able to intervene with violent families at the basic level shown in Table 16–15, the nursing care plan for the victim of violence. All suspected victims should be given the *Domestic Violence Hotline* number: (800) 333-7233. A vital component of nursing care is the referral process, since the family will need multidisciplinary interventions to halt the use of physical force within the family.

Nurses should strive to eliminate homophobia in clinical settings. This means that a battered woman's sexual preference should not be used against her in a way that she, the victim, is blamed for the violence. Battered lesbians have the same needs for support, safety, and positive regard as do heterosexual women.

Table 16–15 Nursing Care Plan for the Victim of Violence

Nursing Diagnosis: Ineffective family coping: disabling, related to inability to manage conflict without violence.
Goal: Family will resolve conflict without the use of violence.

Intervention	*Rationale*	*Expected Outcome*
Teach communication skills to family: • blocks that occur • active listening with feedback • clear and direct communication • communication that does not attack personhood of family members	Improved communication skills will enable family to resolve issues before they escalate to the point of violence	Communication is more direct and clear; family members actively listen to one another
Discuss how violence is learned and transmitted from generation to generation	Identifying violence as a learned behavior supports interventions aimed at learning new alternatives	Verbalizes need for violence to be stopped now if it is not to be perpetuated
Discuss how disagreement in a family is inevitable	To counteract myth that happiness will occur only when there is no conflict	Identifies the normality of conflict
Explore with family the democratic process	The more democratic the family structure in decision making and conflict resolution, the less likely that violence will occur	Verbalizes understanding of democratic process
Using a minor, nonemotional family problem, have family solve the problem in a democratic manner	Once the process is learned, family can transfer this knowledge and ability to solve other problems	Uses democratic process
Discuss nonviolent ways of expressing anger	Learning alternative modes of expression of anger will decrease incidence of violence	Identifies alternative modes of expressing anger
Have family identify times and places that each member can have privacy and time alone	Quiet time alone will decrease the stress and tension of family members and increase mutual respect for one another	Establishes private times for family members

Nursing Diagnosis: Ineffective individual coping related to being a victim of violence.
Goal: Client will manage feelings and physical disorders related to violence.

Intervention	*Rationale*	*Expected Outcome*
Listen carefully to client's difficulties, and treat client with respect	Respect and attentive listening will increase client's feelings of worth	
Give verbal recognition of client's hesitancy to trust staff	Victims of abuse have difficulty trusting because they have often been judged as failures by society	Identifies fears of trusting staff
Assist client in identifying feelings related to being the recipient of violent behavior	Clients may initially use denial or disassociation of feelings to cope with the situation; they need to understand the normality of strong negative feelings	Decreases use of denial; identifies feelings
Assist client in identifying ambivalent feelings (eg, love/hate, hopelessness/hopefulness, or terror/security)	Clients need to understand the normality of ambivalence to decrease the confusion that may be caused by these feelings	Verbalizes understanding of ambivalent feelings

(Diagnosis continued)

Table 16–15 *(continued)*

Nursing Diagnosis *(continued):* Ineffective individual coping related to being a victim of violence.
Goal: Client will manage feelings and physical disorders related to violence.

Intervention	*Rationale*	*Expected Outcome*
Help client use anger to implement change	Anger can be used constructively rather than turned inward to hopelessness	Uses anger appropriately
Discuss client's right and ability to make own choices	Increases internal locus of control	Identifies self as a chooser
Do not make decisions for client	Making decisions for client reinforces helpless role as victim	Formulates own decisions
Discuss how stress is related to psychophysiologic disorders	To help client make the connection between physical symptoms and family problems	Verbalizes understanding of physical illness and stress
Refer to physician for diagnosis and medical intervention of psycho-physiologic disorders	Adequate medical care must be provided for clients with these disorders	Follows up on medical care
Prepare client for any referrals that are made	Preparation will increase likelihood of client accepting help	Follows through on referrals

Nursing Diagnosis: Family coping: potential for growth related to desire to stop family violence.
Goal: Family will maintain the family unit without the use of violence.

Intervention	*Rationale*	*Expected Outcome*
Assist family in seeing that the use of violence is a family problem, that is, that all members are involved in maintaining the violent behavior but are not equally responsible for the violence	Family members may want to focus only on the abuser as the problem individual; understanding interactional patterns that maintain the violence is necessary to prevent further violence	Identifies each member's role in maintaining the dysfunction
Assist family in problem-solving alternative behaviors for each family member	Changes in behavior in part of the family system will result in changes throughout the entire system	Identifies possible changes in behavior

Nursing Diagnosis: Altered family processes related to use of violence to maintain family relationships.
Goal: Family will maintain the family unit without the use of violence.

Intervention	*Rationale*	*Expected Outcome*
Help abuser identify responsibility for violent behavior	Victim is not responsible; to change, abuser must give up denial/rationalization	Acknowledges responsibility
Help family redefine intrafamily relationships as ones in which physical force is unacceptable	Most violent families are not violent with friends or strangers; they need support to enforce those same limits within family	Defines family as a nonviolent place of refuge
Assist family to see relationship between developmental crises and coping with physical force	Anticipatory guidance will decrease use of violence as a method to cope with expected changes in family	Verbalizes understanding of future crises

(Diagnosis continued)

Table 16–15 *(continued)*

Intervention	*Rationale*	*Expected Outcome*
Encourage family to formulate alternatives for coping with elderly parent in the home: • investigate day care centers • investigate extended care centers • enlist help from other family members • investigate short-term care so family can take vacation	Decreasing the stress of total care for elderly parent will decrease use of violence within the home	Develops plans to provide relief
Refer family for family therapy	Long-term therapy may be necessary to restructure family as a nonviolent family	Follows through on referral

Nursing Diagnosis: Altered parenting related to physical abuse of children.
Goal: Parents will not abuse their children in the future.

Intervention	*Rationale*	*Expected Outcome*
Express concern for all family members, including parents	When parents understand the nurse is also concerned about them, they will be more willing to become actively involved in treatment	Verbally recognizes nurse is nonjudgmental
Give recognition for positive parenting skills	Recognition of positive aspects will increase parents' feelings of worth	Identifies areas of strengths in parenting
Give recognition that use of violence is a desperate attempt to cope with children	Recognition of parents' care and concern for their children will increase the likelihood of active participation in treatment	Identifies need to cope more effectively
Discuss with parents how they were punished as children	Recall of effects of violence in their own childhood will increase motivation for treatment	Discusses childhood experiences
Teach parents about normal growth and development of their children	Unrealistic demands on children often result in violence in an attempt to have children comply beyond their developmental ability	Verbalizes knowledge of growth and development
Discuss problems they experience with raising children	Identifying specific sources of stress is the first step in problem resolution	Identifies problems
Help parents identify parenting tools other than physical force that are age appropriate for their children	Lack of parenting skills contributes to increased use of violence within family	Identifies alternative skills
Help parents identify ways to spend time together without children	Strengthening the marital relationship and time apart from children will decrease stress and tension	Plans times together as a couple
Refer to community resources (eg, crisis hot lines, Parents Anonymous, family therapy, or group therapy)	Follow-up with community resources will decrease isolation, improve family relationships, and offer support during times of crisis	Follows through on referrals

(continued)

Table 16–15 *(continued)*

Nursing Diagnosis *(continued)*: Powerlessness related to feelings of being dependent on abuser.
Goal: Client will not feel forced to remain in an abusive, dependent relationship.

Intervention	*Rationale*	*Expected Outcome*
Help client identify past dependency relationships	Identifying patterns throughout life will help client focus on how feelings of powerlessness are maintained	Identifies lifelong process of dependency
Have client formulate a list of ways he or she is dependent on abuser (eg, emotional and economic areas of dependency)	High levels of dependency make it difficult for victim to leave abuser without intense support	Formulates list
Help client identify intrapersonal and interpersonal strengths	Recognition of strengths will decrease feelings of helplessness	Identifies strengths
Help client identify aspects of life under her control	Feelings of control will decrease feelings of powerlessness	Identifies situations of control
Provide assertiveness training	Continued submission to violence often results in an escalation of the violent behavior	Behaves more assertively with abuser
Caution client about use of assertiveness if partner is still battering	Assertive behavior may elicit an escalation in violence	Decides on appropriateness of assertive behavior
Refer to community resources for financial aid, legal aid, or job training	Increasing community support and intervention will decrease economic dependency on abuser	Follows through on referrals

Nursing Diagnosis: Self-esteem disturbance related to feeling guilty and responsible for being a victim.
Goal: Client will not assume responsibility and guilt for the abuse.

Intervention	*Rationale*	*Expected Outcome*
Help client identify strengths in coping with abusive partner thus far and strengths in other roles	Identification of strengths will increase feelings of competency and positive self-esteem	Identifies strengths
Explain theories of violence to client and reinforce that beatings are never deserved	Understanding the theories will relieve client of feelings of responsibility for the abuse	Acknowledges she is not responsible for abusive behavior
Help client identify what behavior he or she will and will not accept from abuser	Setting limits on inappropriate behavior will reinforce a positive self-respect	Establishes limits on abusive behavior

Nursing Diagnosis: Altered role performance related to stereotyped gender roles and use of violence.
Goal: Family will not use violence to maintain stereotyped gender roles.

Intervention	*Rationale*	*Expected Outcome*
Give family members the opportunity to describe their perceptions of the various roles in the family system	Individuals may have differing perceptions about roles of family members	Describes family roles
Have family members identify sources of these roles (eg, tradition, rules, society, religious beliefs)	Family may not be aware of how roles developed; awareness of source of roles must precede a change in roles	Identifies sources of family roles

(Diagnosis continued)

Table 16–15 *(continued)*

Intervention	*Rationale*	*Expected Outcome*
Discuss issues of stereotyping role behavior according to gender	Less stereotyping increases interdependent behavior and decreases acceptance of aggression	Discusses beliefs about gender roles
Help men identify compulsive masculinity and women identify submissive behavior as it relates to the use of violence	Identification of behaviors that contribute to violence precedes a change in those behaviors	Identifies roles that may contribute to the use of violence
Discuss with family how gender roles can be expanded	Expanding the roles will decrease the need to defend stereotypic behavior and thereby decrease stress and tension	Formulates changes in role behavior
Discuss with family in what ways the power base in the family can be more equally distributed	The more democratic the power base is within the family, the less likely that violence will occur	Formulates a more democratic family structure

Nursing Diagnosis: Social isolation related to shame about family violence.
Goal: Family will increase interactions with others outside the family system.

Intervention	*Rationale*	*Expected Outcome*
Help family identify supportive network systems (eg, family, friends, neighbors, church)	The process of identification may enable family to recognize a wider network of supportive people than was previously known	Makes list of people and places available for support
Discuss with family ways to reach out and ask for help from supportive network	Being able to ask for outside support during times of tension and crisis will decrease the use of violence as a coping behavior	Formulates plan on how to ask for help
Refer family to self-help groups dealing with the same problem of violence	Peer groups decrease isolation and provide emotional support and feelings of connectedness	Follows through on referral

Nursing Diagnosis: Potential for violence: directed at others related to a history of the use of physical force within the family.
Goal: Family will not remain violent.

Intervention	*Rationale*	*Expected Outcome*
Assess the level of danger for the victim	Homicide may be a realistic potential if previous threats have been made	Identifies likelihood of being seriously hurt
Assess the level of danger for the abuser	The severity of the violence is the factor that most contributes to women killing their abusers in self-defense	Identifies likelihood of seriously injuring the abuser
If level of danger is high, contact protective services or the police for emergency custody placement or removal to a shelter	Family members may need to be separated until they have greater control over their violent impulses	Complies with removal from the family system
Help family use problem solving to determine if the victim will remain within the family system	Writing out alternatives and making rational choices will increase family's ability to problem solve, which may decrease the use of violence	Uses problem-solving approach

(Diagnosis continued)

Table 16–15 *(continued)*

Nursing Diagnosis *(continued)*: Potential for violence: directed at others related to a history of the use of physical force within the family.
Goal: Family will not remain violent.

Intervention	*Rationale*	*Expected Outcome*
Discuss with family methods to manage anger appropriately: • assuming responsibility for own behavior • talking out anger as it occurs • relaxation training • physical exercise • striking safe, inanimate objects (eg, pillow, couch, or punching bag)	When clients can use alternative expressions of anger, the use of violence will decrease	Implements alternative expressions and management of anger
Discuss with family the facts about intrafamily violence	Violence tends to escalate unless the system is changed	Identifies potential of increasing violence
Help family establish limits and definite consequences if violence recurs	Setting and enforcement of limits will lead to extinction of violence in the family	Enforces limits on violence
Help victims establish a detailed plan of escape if violence should occur	Exact and careful preplanning will aid escape during a time when anxiety and fear are at high levels	Formulates escape plan
Refer victims to legal resources	Victims may be unaware of legal rights to stop family violence	Follows through on referral

Evaluation: Physical Abuse

Nurses in acute care settings may not have the opportunity for long-term evaluation of the family system. Sengstock and Barrett (1984) state that short-term evaluations focus on

- The identification of intrafamily abuse
- The family's ability to recognize that a problem exists
- The willingness of the family to accept assistance by following through with referrals
- The removal of the victim from a volatile situation

Nurses in long-term settings or within the community have the opportunity to evaluate the effectiveness of the multidisciplinary treatment plan over an extended period. Sharing in the process of family growth and healthy adaptation in the ceasing of violence can be a tremendous source of professional satisfaction.

All nurses can evaluate their professional obligations and practice in counteracting those aspects of the society that foster violence. Violence is a mental health problem of national importance, and nurses should be leaders in preventing violence in future generations. Primary prevention includes the nursing interventions of parent education, family life education in schools, referral for appropriate child or elder care, establishment of support groups, and education of fellow nurses about the problem of violence. Secondary prevention includes working with children who are victims or have seen their mothers beaten and making referrals for multidisciplinary intervention. Nurses need to be community advocates in supporting hot lines, crisis centers, and shelters for victims of violence. On the political level, nurses need to make their voices heard in regard to policies and laws affecting children, women, and the elderly (Broome and

Daniels, 1987; Campbell, 1984C). Questions to guide evaluation of nursing practice are

1. What action have I taken to decrease violence in the media?
2. Have I been an advocate for gun control?
3. Have I volunteered to teach parenting classes at the grade school and high school level?
4. Have I confronted the use of physical punishment in the school system?
5. Have I written to respresentatives to protest funding cuts in programs designed to help children, women, and the elderly?
6. How have I supported programs to assist the elderly?
7. Have I spoken out on the need to increase bilingual/bicultural counselors, lawyers, nurses, and physicians to attend to the needs of ethnic women?

Intrafamily Violence: Sexual Abuse

Sexually abused children and adult survivors of incest are crying out for help. A few cry out loudly in protest, but the majority cry inwardly in silence. It was thought as many as 1 in 4 girls and 1 in 10 boys are abused sexually before the age of 18. More recent studies give evidence that the actual rate may be one in two girls and one in five boys (Wolfe, Wolfe, and Best, 1988; Wyatt, Peters, and Guthrie, 1988). Intrafamily sexual abuse occurs in all racial, religious, economic, and cultural subgroups. The perpetrators are not monsters; they may love their children, be steady workers, and provide for the family. They are often seen as good family men.* Among forms of child abuse, sexual abuse is the most denied, concealed, and distressing form.

*This text uses the male adult—female child configuration, unless otherwise noted, since this is the most frequently reported type of intrafamily sexual abuse.

Intrafamily sexual abuse is used interchangeably with the term *incest.* It is defined as inappropriate sexual behavior, instigated by an adult family or surrogate family member, whose purpose is to sexually arouse the adult or the child. Behavior can range from exhibitionism, peeping, and explicit sexual talk to touching, caressing, masturbation, and intercourse (Trepper and Barrett, 1986A).

Intrafamily sexual abuse creates problems for the family system that are different from sexual abuse by neighbors, friends, or strangers. Within the family system, all the participants—that is, victim, perpetrator, and conspirators—must continue to interact and function as a unit. There is no way of avoiding one another or dealing directly with the anger and rage aroused. Strangers must use physical force or threats of physical violence to rape another person, but most typically, physical force is not used in intrafamily sexual abuse. Psychologic coercion by the adult is used to ensure the silence and compliance of the child (Waterman and Luck, 1986). Statements are made such as, "You must not tell anyone what we are doing, or they will take me away, and you won't have a father anymore," or "You are very special to me, and we don't want anyone else to know how special or they might feel bad," or "You know I'll buy you lots of toys and gifts as long as you don't tell anyone about our secret."

Incest is considered a form of violence because it causes psychologic and physical injury to the victim. Because of their age and level of development, children are unable to give consent to sexual activity with an adult. Thus, forced sexual activity is violence against the child. Additionally, incest is a form of violence because the child is used to meet the adult's needs without regard for the needs and safety of the child.

Incidence of Sexual Abuse

It is difficult to estimate accurately the incidence of intrafamily sexual abuse. With increased public awareness, there has been an increase in the reporting of cases. It is believed that the actual rate has not increased but that the secrecy around current and past occurrences is decreasing. In spite of more public acknowledgment, a tremendous number of cases go unreported. Estimates of the number of children that are sexually abused each year range from 100,000 to 500,000. Affinity systems—that is, immediate family, relatives, friends, and neighbors—account for 75 to 80 percent of the abusers. Male perpetrators account for 92 to 98 percent of the cases, with grandfathers and uncles being the most frequently reported. Not uncommon is successive victimization of different children in the family, and 30 percent of perpetrators have also sexually abused other relatives. Unclear at this time is how often young boys are abused. Gender role norms and homophobia are factors in the underreporting of sexually abused boys, since the abuse involves the breaking of two taboos, incest and homosexuality.

In the past, it was thought that intrafamily sexual abuse began when the child was around 10 or 12 years old. Current research has shown that many victims are under the age of 5, and some are as young as 3 to 6 months. The average age for sexual molestation is 4 years, and the average age for intercourse with a family member is 9 years (Courtois, 1988; Urbancic, 1987; Wolfe, Wolfe, and Best, 1988).

Significance of Sexual Abuse to Mental Health Nursing

Intrafamily sexual abuse is a major health problem in this country. The majority of the cases are thought to be unreported. Health professionals, as well as families, have used denial to cope with ambiguous evidence of the cultural taboo of incest. Nurses need to understand the characteristics and dynamics of families involved in sexual abuse so that they respond appropriately to cues within the family system. A note of caution must be added, however. With the increased publicity, there is a real danger of a witch-hunt developing in this country—that is, that any hint or accusation may be taken as absolute proof of guilt. Families who have not been involved in intrafamily sexual abuse have been torn apart by rumors and false accusations. Nurses need to assess carefully and maintain a balance between the extremes of denial of incest and belief of automatic guilt.

Suffering sexual abuse in childhood may be a hidden feature of adult mental disorders. In one study of women being treated in an inpatient setting, 72 percent reported a history of sexual abuse during their lifetime, with 59 percent of abuse incidents occurring before the victim was 16. Compared to nonabused clients, the women who had been abused had more severe symptoms and were more suicidal. The illnesses of the abused clients may have been related to their need to manage the severe trauma of sexual abuse and to the secrecy and denial that affected all subsequent relationships. Secondary disorders associated with childhood sexual abuse include depression, anxiety, eating disorders, substance abuse, somatization disorders, personality disorders, dissociative disorders, and posttraumatic stress disorder. The tendency for sexual abuse victims to become mental health clients is an area of current research (Bryer, 1987; Courtois, 1988).

Knowledge Base: Sexual Abuse

It is difficult to predict which of the following characteristics a given child or family will exhibit in the face of intrafamily sexuality. Some will exhibit most of the characteristics, others will exhibit some, and still others will exhibit none. These characteristics should be taken as cues for further investigation, since they may also be signs and symptoms of other emotional problems in children and families.

Although it is known that many victims suffer long-term problems, there are also instances where there appear to be no lasting negative consequences. In studies of women who were not in therapy and who had been victims as children, it was found that, in 25 percent of the victims, the abuse had had a great effect on their lives. On 25 percent the abuse had had some effect, on 25 percent it had had little effect, and on 25 percent the abuse had had no long-term effects. The severity of long-term effects seemed to be correlated with the presence of violence, the duration of the abuse, and the type of sexual activity. Most harmful was sexual abuse by fathers or stepfathers. Less harmful was abuse by brothers or other relatives outside the nuclear family. Again, nurses must find the balance between the extremes of denial of pathology and excessive victimization of the individual and family (Herman, 1988; Trepper and Traicoff, 1983).

Behavioral Characteristics

Not uncommonly, adult perpetrators believe in extreme parental restrictiveness and domination. The use of threats or violence is unusual. More typically, the adult coerces the child and misrepresents the relationship and the activity. It may begin under the guise of affection or education and is often presented as something fun or a game. Perpetrators of sexual abuse are typically viewed as having poor impulse control.

Children who are victims of intrafamily sexual abuse may exhibit regressive behavior. This may take any form of regression, but the most common is bedwetting. Sleep disturbances are common in sexually abused children, particularly among those who have been molested during their sleep. Some return to a clinging form of attachment to one or both parents. Children may become extremely affectionate, both within the family and with others outside the family. Other children isolate themselves at school and in the neighborhood and limit the majority of their interpersonal interactions to family members. They may become overly compliant in hopes the abuse will stop.

Children who are victims may act out sexually with other children or adults. This must be distinguished from the normal childhood behavior of mimicking sexual behavior observed between their parents or in the media. Sexually acting out behavior is seen in child victims who initiate genital or oral sex with other children or adults.

Adolescent victims of intrafamily sexual abuse may run away from home to escape an intolerable situation. Some of the victims turn to prostitution since they have learned in the family that sexual behavior is the method whereby one receives affection, love, and attention. Other victims attempt or commit suicide if they experience the hopelessness of being trapped in a pathologic family system (Courtois, 1988; Herman, 1988; Wolfe, Wolfe, and Best, 1988).

Long-term behavioral effects on adult survivors may be indiscriminate sexual activity or sexual dysfunctions such as inhibited sexual desire, orgasmic difficulties, or compulsive sexual behavior. They may also experience sleeping problems, chemical abuse, social isolation, depression, and suicide (Wolfe, Wolfe, and Best, 1988).

> *Sonja describes her current sexual life as one of promiscuity and relates this to being sexually molested by her grandfather when she was between the ages of 4 and 7. This is her description of the abuse: "Whenever I was alone with him in the car, he would fondle me and expose his penis to me. He would tell me I could touch it, it would be all right. So much of the time I tried to block everything out—it's hard for me to recall exactly what happened. Some things I remember clearly. I remember Grandpa's easy chair. When we were alone he would make me sit on his lap in that chair, and he would stick his fingers in me. This happened many times. One time he parked in an isolated area and played with me and made me touch him and kiss his penis. He tried to coax me to have intercourse. He told me it wouldn't hurt. But I cried and he masturbated into his handkerchief instead. Like most abuse victims, I was sworn to secrecy. He always bought me things or gave me money. I remember the day he died. I came home from school and when my mom told me, I cried. But deep down I was glad. I was really safe from him now. And I hated him for hurting me and making me lie all the time."*

Affective Characteristics

Under the facade of dominance, perpetrators often feel weak, afraid, and inadequate. They inappropriately view the child as a safe and less threatening source of nurturance and caring than adult relationships. Additionally, perpetrators are unable to distinguish between nonsexual and sexual affection for children (Bolton and Bolton, 1987).

Victims of incest may experience many fears. They fear if they tell another adult, they will not be believed, and they fear they themselves will be blamed and the nonmolesting parent will side with the molesting parent. They may have fantasies of being thrown out of the family if the molesting behavior becomes known to other family members. Some victims fear loss of parental love. They may fear the family will be separated, especially if this threat was made by the abusing parent. Some fear, if they resist the sexual advances or tell the secret, they will be physically abused, even if the parent has never before used or threatened physical abuse.

The affective responses to sexual abuse are often confusing to the child. Opposing feelings may occur simultaneously, which creates ambivalence within the child. Developmentally, the child may not have the skills to manage effectively the conflict that arises out of ambivalent feelings. Victims often experience physical pleasure in the sexual interactions. In addition, they may enjoy being the "special" child within the family and the degree of power they experience over the molesting parent and the other siblings. At the same time, they may feel responsible for the sexual behavior and guilty they have not been able to stop the abuse. The ambivalence leads to a pervasive sense of confusion and self-blame.

Extremely prevalent is the feeling of powerlessness, that what the victim says and does makes no difference. The associated rage typically does not emerge until adolescence. When the suppressed rage comes to the surface, it may be directed against the self in self-defeating and self-destructive ways.

Adult survivors most frequently describe the long-term effects of childhood sexual abuse as being fear of sex and distrust and fear of men. They may suffer from chronic anxiety attacks or demonstrate the affective characteristics of borderline personality disorder. Anger may be the only emotion experienced and expressed; all other feelings may be severely constricted.

Peter, 36 years old, was admitted to the hospital for symptoms of depression related to his wife's impending divorce. Throughout the marriage he has been unable to show any emotions other than anger. For the past several months he has not been sleeping and has been crying at work. His anger has escalated to violent outbursts. In the process of therapy, Peter tells his nurse about his childhood sexual abuse, which he has not shared with anyone for 25 years. Peter's mother died when he was 11 years old, and he went to live with his aunt and uncle. Soon after his arrival, his uncle began sexually abusing Peter. The abuse continued for 2 years. Peter told both his aunt and his father about the abuse but was devastated when no one believed him. Peter states, "I have carried this pain all these years until I couldn't take it anymore. I think all my marital problems are related to my anger at my uncle, aunt, and father. My wife doesn't even know I was raped as a child and can't understand why I am such an angry person."

Cognitive Characteristics

Cognitively, perpetrators believe their needs are the most important in the family system. When confronted with their behavior, some will deny the abuse and accuse the child of lying. Others may acknowledge the abuse but minimize the impact with statements such as "Better for her to learn about sex from her father than from some horny teenager" or "She really didn't mind. In fact we have a very close relationship." Others use the defense mechanism of projection and blame the child for the abuse. This is evidenced by statements such as "She is a very provocative child and she seduced me" or "If she hadn't enjoyed it so much, I would not have continued" (Bolton and Bolton, 1987).

Victim denial of intrafamily sexuality may take several forms. Some victims deny that the abuse ever occurred. Others, acknowledging sexual activity occurred, minimize the impact and say it was not important. This is evidenced by statements such as, "It's not so bad. It only happens once a month," or "It's all right because it stopped when I was 11 years old." Still others acknowledge the sexual activity and the negative consequences but deny the parent's responsibility and assume they themselves are to blame for their parent's behavior. Evidence of denial of parental responsibility is heard in such statements as, "It's my fault, I seduced my grandfather," or "If I had not been running around in my swimming suit, it would not have happened." Denial may be used to protect the family system as well as the individual victim. The fear that the family may be separated by the removal of the parent or the removal of the child to a foster home may be so overwhelming that the secret is kept within the family system (Barrett, Sykes and Byrnes, 1986).

Not uncommonly, dissociation is the victim's major defense mechanism. The mind is "separated" from the body so the victim is not emotionally present during the sexual activity. This is evidenced by statements such as "I put myself in the wall, where he couldn't reach all of me" or "When he would come into my room, I would close my eyes and go to my favorite place. Only my body stayed on the bed. The rest of me was not there." When sexual abuse is severe and sadistic, the victim may develop the dissociative disorder of multiple personality (see Chapter 8).

Children molested during the nighttime may experience nightmares in response to the abuse. They may begin to dream they are being molested, and this may lead to their being unable to separate the reality from the dream. They may begin to believe the abuse did not happen but was simply a dream.

Sarah, age 19, describes her relationship with her father when she was 12 years old in this way: "I don't remember how it started, but my father conned me into soaping up his stomach, testicles, and erect penis when he was in the bathtub. This took place at his apartment when my brothers and I went there for the weekend. I didn't particularly enjoy it, but my father encouraged it. I got completely turned off by it when he offered to do me. One time, while I was sleeping on the bed, I woke up from a violent shaking of the bed. I was dressed in a shirt and shorts. I realized my father was rubbing his penis between my thighs and feeling on my vagina. I didn't let him know I was awake, and I turned slightly, hoping he would stop. I never wore that T-shirt or shorts again. I've never told anyone. Even my father doesn't know that I know. I think my experiences have had a deep effect on my relationships. Every time I get close to a man, I become afraid. I think what I'm most afraid of is being used. My childhood experiences seem to bother me the most when my friends talk about their childhood with their fathers and how they were 'Daddy's little girl.' Feelings of rage, anger, and total disgust burn deep inside me."

Quite frequently, adult survivors have total amnesia in regard to the incest. In such a case, amnesia is considered a defense mechanism in response to abuse during childhood. Recall of the abuse may be triggered by a significant life event, such as marriage or having a child or during the process of psychotherapy.

Self-blame and self-hatred contribute to an inadequate self-esteem in adult survivors. Male victims may have a diminished sense of masculinity because they were unable to protect themselves. Victimization contributes to an external locus of control, which may continue into adulthood and carry over to other situations.

It may be difficult for adult survivors to develop an adequate self-esteem. They may continue to feel responsible for the incest and worthless and different from other people. They may believe they are only sexual objects to be used and abused by others. Not uncommonly, they experience either amnesia in regard to the events or flashbacks, nightmares, and other symptoms of posttraumatic stress disorder (see Chapter 8) (Courtois, 1988).

Physiologic Characteristics

The obvious physical signs of sexual abuse in a child are the presence of a sexually transmitted disease or irritated or swollen genitals, rectal tissue, or both. Of female victims of sexual abuse, 12 to 24 percent become pregnant as a result of the abuse. In an effort to protect the family from conflict and distress, girls may try to conceal the pregnancy (Krueger, 1988; Zdanuk, Harris, and Wisian, 1987). Chronic vaginal or urinary tract infections with no known medical cause may be indicators that the child is being sexually abused. Some children may have sexually transmitted diseases in their mouths and throat. Since oral sex is a frequent behavior in these interactions, the child's throat may be irritated. The child may also exhibit a hyperactive gag reflex and, at times, unexplained vomiting. Younger children may complain of tummy aches with the discomfort located near the diaphragm. These children perceive the penis as so huge that, when penetration is attempted or completed, they think it reaches up to the chest area.

Some children will, consciously or unconsciously, attempt to abuse their bodies to either prevent or halt the sexual abuse. A great deal of weight may be gained in the hopes of becoming so ugly that the abuser will be appalled and leave the child alone. Anorexia may be a response to intrafamily sexual abuse. If an older child is being abused, a younger sister may become anorexic in an attempt not to mature and experience the same abuse. This lack of care for the body may continue into adult life in an unconscious attempt to keep a distance and avoid intimate relationships (Herman, 1988; Wolfe, Wolfe and Best, 1988).

> *A 23-year-old man was sentenced to 45 years in prison for the sexual assault on his girlfriend's 2-year-old daughter. As a result of the attack, the girl underwent an appendectomy and colostomy (Metro Digest, 1988).*

Sociocultural Characteristics

A number of sociocultural characteristics may contribute to intrafamily sexual abuse. Rigid or compulsive gender roles increase the vulnerability of the children within the family. It is difficult for a child to protest any type of abusive treatment in a highly structured, authoritarian family system. Rigid gender roles place women and children in a submissive position. In a culture that has traditionally supported male supremacy and viewed women and children as the property of males, it is not surprising that sexual abuse has been, and even continues to be, tolerated (Trepper and Barrett, 1986B; Waterman, 1986).

There is a widespread belief that the mother always knows when her husband is sexually involved with one or more of the children. In reality, mothers are rarely aware of intrafamily sexual abuse and, with disclosure, often react in a concerned and protective manner (Trepper and Traicoff, 1983). Some women deny any evidence of the abuse because they feel inadequate to cope with the family problems. Others use denial because they fear their husbands' retaliation against them if the accusation of incest is brought into the open. Denial may be a defense mechanism used by women who fear financial, social, and emotional problems if their husbands are removed from the family (Barrett, Sykes, and Byrnes, 1986). When cues to intrafamily sexual abuse are discovered, some women begin to question their own thinking processes. Believing their husbands are incapable of this type of behavior, they, therefore, believe something must be wrong with themselves.

> *Cherenia has recently become somewhat suspicious that her husband, Joe, may be sexually abusing their daughter. In response to her fears, she says the following things to herself: "You must really have a dirty mind, Cherenia. How could you possibly think those things about Joe? He's a very good husband. He works hard and loves all of us. He goes to church every week, and everyone knows what a good family man he is. How could you even consider that he might be doing something so awful. You must be really sick, Cherenia."*

Chronic stress within the family system may contribute to intrafamily sexual abuse. Families that are socially isolated and have few support systems are more vulnerable to the effects of acute and chronic stress. When internal and external resources are depleted, the family dynamics may become pathologic. In some incestuous families, alcohol abuse may be a factor. That is not to say that alcohol abuse causes incest but rather that intoxication decreases inhibitions and is often used as an excuse for irresponsible behavior (Trepper and Barrett, 1986B).

Survivors are at risk for revictimization as adults. Many end up in a physically abusive relationship. Some are only able to develop superficial relationships because they have difficulty trusting others. Some adult survivors continue to function as caretaker for their family of origin and are unable to set limits on demands. Others may cut off all contact with their family of origin or interact only with select family members (Courtois, 1988).

Causative Theories

There is no single cause of intrafamily sexual abuse. In fact, the abuse is not a primary diagnosis but rather a symptom of dysfunction in the individual, family, and societal systems. All these systems must be considered if the nurse is to understand the dynamics of a particular family (Trepper and Barrett, 1986B). Individual and family systems theories of incest are presented. (See the section on physical abuse for the sociocultural theories of causation.)

Intrapersonal Theories There are many descriptions of the perpetrators and victims involved in intrafamily sexual abuse. Many of these descriptions are contradictory, and there is no agreement on a personality pattern peculiar to all perpetrators or victims (Barrett, Sykes, and Byrnes, 1986). Nurses must remember that these descriptions apply to many people, but not all become involved with intrafamily sexual abuse. These theories are guidelines for assessment, not absolute proof of sexual abuse.

The intrapersonal theories view the adult perpetrator as the "sick" or pathologic family member. These people may be insecure and have inadequate self-esteem. They may be fearful of interacting with adults and more secure in interpersonal interactions with children. This fear of failure may contribute to a sexual dysfunction in adult relationships. When the sexual dysfunction does not occur in the sexual relationship with their child, there is positive reinforcement to continue the behavior. Some perpetrators were emotionally deprived as children and thus have a great need for constant, unconditional love, which is more easily obtained from children than from adults. If they were sexually abused themselves as children, they may have learned to associate all feelings of love with sexual behavior. Frequently the perpetrator's world is comprised only of victims and perpetrators. If the adult is not going to be a victim, he must be a perpetrator. He makes an unconscious move from one role to the other (Trepper and Barrett, 1986B).

Some perpetrators are described as lacking impulse control and the ability to experience feelings of guilt. Others have been described as rigid and overcontrolled. They may be dominant and aggressive. Lack of parenting skills or the loss of the mother from the family may result in role confusion among the family members. The father may turn to the daughter for companionship when he feels deprived of it in adult relationships (Trepper and Barrett, 1986A; Waterman, 1986).

The mothers of victims may be emotionally and financially dependent on the marital relationship. Denial may be the major mechanism that allows them to remain in the marriage. They may also have been victims of sexual abuse during their own childhood, which may contribute to an adult dysfunction such as inhibited sexual desire. The mother's lack of parenting skills may contribute to the daughter's assuming responsibility for the younger children in the family. Along with this parent role, the daughter may be expected to fulfill the role of wife as evidenced by sexual abuse (Barrett, Sykes, and Byrnes, 1986).

Daughters who are victims may feel emotionally deprived and need unconditional love and attention. If they have an inadequate self-esteem, the "special" attention from their fathers may help them to feel attractive, desired, and needed. The daughter may exhibit seductive and provocative behavior, a learned response to the father's inappropriate sexual behavior, not the cause of the incest (Trepper and Barrett, 1986A).

Family Systems Theory The family systems perspective views intrafamily sexual abuse as arising out of and being maintained by the interactions of all family members. Rather than looking at *why* the behavior occurs, as the intrapersonal theorists do, family systems theorists look at *how* the behavior occurs. The components of the theory include family structure, cohesion, adaptability, and communication.

The structure of the family is organized around hierarchic membership according to age, roles, and distribution of power. Typically, the adults, who are older, assume the parental roles and are the most influential members of the family system. The structure of incestuous families, however, is often quite different. An adult may move downward in the structure or a child may move upward in the structure in terms of roles and influence. If the father moves downward, he assumes a childlike role and is cared for and nurtured by his wife, as are the children in the family. In this position, the father assumes little parental responsibility. He may then turn to the daughter, as a peer, for sexual and emotional gratification. In other family systems, the daughter may move upward and replace the mother in the hierarchic structure. Usually the mother does not move downward in the structure but rather moves out of the structure by distancing herself emotionally or physically from the family. As the daughter assumes the parental roles and responsibilities, the father may turn to her for fulfillment of emotional and sexual needs (Barrett, Sykes, and Byrnes, 1986; Trepper and Barrett, 1986B).

Family cohesion refers to the degree of emotional bonding that occurs within a family. At one end of the continuum of cohesion is the family system that is disengaged, that is, the family members are isolated and alienated from one another. At the other end of the continuum is the enmeshed family system, in which the members are immersed in and absorbed by one another. The most adaptive family systems function between these two extremes (Barrett, Sykes, and Byrnes, 1986; Trepper and Barrett, 1986B).

Intrafamily sexual abuse usually occurs in an enmeshed family. The need to be overinvolved in one another's lives is accompanied by intense fears of abandonment and family disintegration. The family system is closed to external input and support in an attempt to maintain closeness. If the parent's marital dyad does not provide adequate emotional and sexual fulfillment, the father turns to the daughter for these needs rather than searching outside the family system for a different partner (Barrett, Sykes, and Byrnes, 1986; Zdanuk, Harris, and Wislan, 1987).

Family system adaptability is also described along a continuum. At one extreme is the rigid family system and, at the other end, the chaotic family system. Incestuous families tend to fall on either end of the continuum. Rigid family systems have strict rules and stereotyped gender role expectations, with minimal emotional interaction. Children are given no power and authority, even over their own bodies. They are not allowed to question or protest inappropriate sexual behavior within the family. In contrast, chaotic family systems have either no rules or constantly changing roles. The parents are unable to assume parental roles or leadership positions. Within the chaotic system, there may be no assigned roles or no rules regarding appropriate sexual behavior, which may contribute to the incidence of intrafamily sexual abuse (Trepper and Barrett, 1986B).

Communication patterns within the family system may contribute to the occurrence of intrafamily sexual abuse. Within some families, messages between two persons are communicated through a third family member. This indirect communication perpetuates secrecy and avoidance of conflict in order to deny what is really happening (Barrett,

Sykes, and Byrnes, 1986; Trepper, 1989). Intrafamily sexual abuse is dependent on keeping the secret within the family. In family systems that avoid conflict, accusations of sexual abuse are not tolerated. Peace must be kept at all costs, even the cost of abuse.

Assessment: Sexual Abuse

It is vitally important that nurses acknowledge the reality of intrafamily sexual abuse. Those nurses who deny the existence of the problem, at all levels of society, miss the individual and family cues and thereby fail to complete a detailed assessment. Nurses knowledgeable about the incidence and the characteristics of the problem are alert for cues that demand nursing assessment. Such an assessment follows.

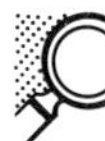

FOCUSED NURSING ASSESSMENT *for Intrafamily Sexual Abuse*

Behavioral assessment

Individual child

Have there been any signs of regressive behavior in the child?
Is the child having sleeping problems?
Is the child exhibiting clinging behavior to the parents or others?
Does the child have friendships with other children?
Has there been any sexual acting out on the part of the child?
Has the child ever run away or threatened to run away?
Has the child ever attempted suicide?

Perpetrator

Describe how discipline is handled in the family.
Do you see yourself as the dominant person in the family?
At what age do you believe parents should give up control of their children?
How many adult friends do you have?
Describe your relationship with these friends.
Describe your relationship with your spouse.
What kinds of sexual difficulties are you and your spouse experiencing?
When you were young, who was the closest family member with whom you had any sexual activity?

Family system

Describe who has responsibility (mother, father, both parents, or children) in the following areas of home management:
- Caring for the youngest children?
- Cooking?
- Cleaning?
- Paying bills?
- Shopping?
- Outside home maintenance?
- Budget planning?
- Decisions about leisure time?
- Supervising children's homework?
- Taking children to activities?
- Putting children to bed?

Who are the best communicators in the family?
Who talks to whom the most?
Who is unable to talk to whom very much?
How are secrets kept from one another within the family?
How are secrets prevented from leaking outside the family?

Affective assessment

Individual child

How helpless do you feel about changing any of the family's problems?
In what way are you responsible for family problems?
Do you get enough love within the family?
Are you more loved than the other children in the family?
Tell me about the fears you may have if any family secrets are told:
- Fears of not being believed?
- Fears of being blamed for the problems?
- Fears that your parents will not love you?
- Fears that you will be moved to a foster home?
- Fears that your parents will be taken away?
- Fears of physical abuse?

Perpetrator

Who loves you the most within the family?
Who is able to give you unconditional support and affection?

How do you see yourself responsible for family problems?
How does fear of failure affect your life?

Family system
Describe the emotional relationships among family members.
Does everybody know each family member's business?
How is privacy protected within the family?
Do you have any fears of the family unit disintegrating?
What will happen if the family is separated?

Cognitive assessment
Individual child
Tell me about your nightmares.
How would you describe the family's problems?
What effect do these problems have on you?
What effect do these problems have on the rest of the family?
Who do you believe is responsible for these problems?

Perpetrator
Describe what kind of a person you are.
What are your personal strengths?
What are your personal limitations?
Describe how you handle new situations.
Do you enjoy changing situations?

Family system
Who sets the family rules?
Tell me about the most important family rules.
How do rules get changed within the family?
What are the expectations of the males in the family?
What are the expectations of the females in the family?

Sociocultural assessment
What significant events have occurred for your family in the past year?
What support systems do you have outside the family?
How often do you visit with friends?
Who are the problem drinkers in the family?
How is the issue of drugs managed within the family?

When assessing children, it must be remembered that some will exhibit most of the characteristics presented in this chapter, others will exhibit only some, and still others will exhibit none of the characteristics. It must also be remembered that these same behavioral, affective, and cognitive characteristics may be signs and symptoms of other emotional problems in children. Family dynamics also need to be assessed before assuming the existence of intrafamily sexual abuse. Routine questions on nursing histories may provide an opportunity for survivors of incest to share their pain and obtain treatment as adults. Nurses are responsible for initiating the topic—shame and confusion may keep the adult survivor from doing so. Those nurses who avoid the topic contribute to pathology by supporting the client's denial of reality. Now that intrafamily sexual abuse has been identified as a major health problem, nurses in every clinical setting must be alert to cues from both individuals and families (Bryer, 1987). See Table 16–16 for assessment cues.

Table 16–17 presents guidelines for a physical assessment of a sexual abuse victim.

Nursing Diagnosis and Planning: Sexual Abuse

Based on the information gathered during the assessment of the child, perpetrator, and family system, the nurse formulates diagnoses, interventions, and expected outcomes. The long-term goals of intervention are to serve the best interest of the child, support the nonabused children who may be very frightened, and prevent trauma that could be caused by the legal process. Resolution of anger, hostility, shame, and fear may be a goal in healing the family and decreasing the stigma of incest. It is important to identify individual and family system strengths, so that these can be reinforced and supported. Because family therapy is critical to the healthy resolution of intrafamily sexual abuse, referral to therapists who specialize in treating incestuous families is a priority in nursing intervention. Table 16–18 presents organizations that may be helpful in finding appropriate specialists.

Intrafamily sexual abuse is an emotionally laden health problem. Nurses need to identify their per-

Table 16–16 *Cues to Intrafamily Sexual Abuse*

	Perpetrator	*Child/Adolescent*	*Adult Survivor*
Behavioral cues	dominating coercive inappropriate affection poor impulse control	regression submissive extremely affectionate sexual acting out isolative sleep problems running away prostitution suicide	social isolation sleep problems chemical abuse sexual dysfunction indiscriminate sexual behavior suicidal
Affective cues	feelings of weakness, inadequacy fear of failure fear of adult intimacy unable to distinguish between nonsexual and sexual affection	multiple fears guilt helplessness powerlessness rage ambivalence	anxiety attacks rage fear of sex distrust, fear of men
Cognitive cues	denial minimization of impact projection of blame low self-esteem	denial minimizes impact assumes blame dissociation low self-esteem nightmares	denial external locus of control self-blame dissociation low self-esteem amnesia for events flashbacks nightmares feeling of being different from others
Mental disorders	impulse control disorders	dissociation multiple personality anxiety disorders depression	dissociation multiple personality anxiety disorders depression chemical abuse personality disorders somatization disorders posttraumatic stress disorder

Table 16–17 *Physical Assessment of Sexual Abuse Victim*

Complete a head-to-toe assessment with emphasis on the following:
Weight and nutrition status
Throat irritation
Gag reflex
Episodes of vomiting
Abdominal pain near diaphragm
Smears of the mouth, throat, vagina, and rectum for sexually transmitted diseases
Genital irritation or trauma
Rectal irritation or trauma
Chronic vaginal infections
Chronic urinary tract infections
Pregnancy

sonal values and determine if these will interfere with the ability to care for all members of the family system. Beliefs about maintaining or splitting up the family unit will influence nursing care. Many nurses experience a great deal of anger and hostility toward the perpetrator and the parent who was not able to prevent or stop the abuse. If the nurse is a survivor of childhood sexual abuse, personal issues and feelings may interfere with effective nursing care. Some nurses need to disqualify themselves from caring for incestuous families because of their personal values and feelings.

Table 16–19 presents the nursing care plan for the family with sexual abuse.

Table 16–18 *Organizations for Victims of Sexual Abuse*

VOICES in Action, Inc.
National Network for Survivors of Incest
P.O. Box 148309
Chicago, IL 60614
312-327-1500

Adults Molested as Children United
Parents United
Daughters and Sons United
P.O. Box 952
San Jose, CA 95108-0952
408-280-5055

Incest Survivors Anonymous
P.O. Box 5613
Department P
Long Beach, CA 90805-0613

Survivors of Childhood Abuse Program—SCAP
1345 El Centro Ave.
P.O. Box 630
Hollywood, CA 90028

PLEA
Box 59045
Norwalk, CA 90652
213-863-4824

Looking Up
P.O. Box K
Augusta, ME 04330
207-626-3402

Incest Resources, Inc.
Cambridge Women's Center
46 Pleasant St.
Cambridge, MA 02139
617-354-8807

Incest Recovery Association
6200 N. Central Expway
Suite 209
Dallas, TX 75206
214-373-6607

Domestic Violence Hot Line
1-800-333-7233

Table 16–19 Nursing Care Plan for the Family with Sexual Abuse

Nursing Diagnosis: Ineffective family coping: disabling, related to child being sexually abused.
Goal: Family will no longer engage in inappropriate sexual behavior.

Intervention	*Rationale*	*Expected Outcome*
Help each family member write list of individual and family goals for treatment	Writing a list of expected outcomes will increase each member's participation in therapy	Formulates lists
Help family identify individual and family strengths	If clients are able to identify strengths, they will feel more optimistic about change rather than feel defeated at the onset	Identifies strengths; verbalizes hope for the future
By discussing roles and role reversals, help family identify how some members cross generational boundaries	Crossing of boundaries is a contributing factor in intrafamily sexual abuse, because parent and child relate to one another as peers	Identifies inappropriate roles according to the generation of each family member
Discuss ways that parents can maintain generational boundaries	Parents need to assume the responsibility for parenting all their children	Makes decisions on ways to change roles
Help family members communicate directly with one another	New and more effective communication styles are needed to improve family system functioning	Communicates directly
Discourage secrecy within family	Secrecy contributes to lack of trust and supports sexual abuse	Communicates openly

(continued)

Table 16–19 *(continued)*

Nursing Diagnosis: Altered parenting related to being a perpetrator of sexual abuse.
Goal: Client will develop adaptive coping skills.

Intervention	*Rationale*	*Expected Outcome*
Discuss client's family of origin in regard to sexual abuse and parenting styles	Many abusers were sexually abused as children; people tend to parent the way in which they were parented	Discusses childhood as it relates to present problem
Help client discuss feelings around being discovered as an abuser	Client needs to identify and manage feelings of guilt, shame, or anger to regain a positive self-regard	Shares feelings
Discuss factors client believes contributed to the incidents of abuse	Examining the multiple factors will help client determine changes that must be made	Lists contributing factors
Help client problem solve to find alternative coping behavior	Client must be actively involved in assuming responsibility for change	Identifies specific changes in behavior

Nursing Diagnosis: Ineffective individual coping related to being a nonabusing parent.
Goal: Client will not become a secondary victim.

Intervention	*Rationale*	*Expected Outcome*
Help client identify feelings toward self since the abuse was discovered	Many nonabusing parents experience guilt for not being aware of or stopping the sexual abuse	Identifies lack of responsibility for spouse's behavior
Help client identify feelings toward other family members	The anger, fear, and anxiety must be identified and managed if the family system is to remain intact	Shares feelings

Nursing Diagnosis: Ineffective individual coping related to being a victim of intrafamily sexual abuse.
Goal: Client will adapt to the trauma of being sexually abused.

Intervention	*Rationale*	*Expected Outcome*
Use play and art therapy with children under the age of 5	Play and art therapy help young children to express feelings, reduce guilt, and reestablish trust	Participates in play and art therapy
Help older children to identify and discuss feelings about the abuse	Feelings of shame, guilt, anxiety, and anger must be normalized as part of the therapeutic process	Shares feelings
Use group therapy with preteens and teens	Decreases feelings of isolation and uniqueness	Participates in group therapy
Help client learn methods to avoid future abuse such as telling others about advances, saying no, and refusing to be left alone with the abuser	Supporting child's alternatives and problem solving for future occurrences may prevent future victimization	Lists methods of coping in the future

(continued)

Table 16–19 *(continued)*

Nursing Diagnosis: Altered family process related to disruption of family unit when abuse is discovered.
Goal: Child will remain safe within old or new family structure.

Intervention	*Rationale*	*Expected Outcome*
Refer to protective services that will implement one of four plans:		
• family will remain intact	Families who have not used violence, where there is no substance abuse, and who can ensure the child's safety may be allowed to live together; this is rarely recommended	Acts in accordance with legal decision made by protective services
• the abuser is removed from family	This most frequent option is chosen when the nonabusing parent is able to protect the child and the abuser must face the responsibility for his or her own behavior	
• the child is removed from family	This rare choice occurs when it is felt that the nonabusing parent would be unable to protect the child; this may place additional guilt on child	
• both child and abuser are removed from home	When nonabusing parent is unable to protect child, this choice maximizes safety of child and decreases child's feelings of responsibility	

Nursing Diagnosis: Ineffective family coping, disabling related to enmeshed family system that is either rigid or chaotic.
Goal: Family will move to a moderate position between the extremes of rigid and chaotic.

Intervention	*Rationale*	*Expected Outcome*
Discuss ways family can increase flexibility of roles and rules	Rigid family systems are a contributing factor in intrafamily sexual abuse	Rules and roles are more flexible
Discuss ways family can organize appropriate roles and formulate consistent rules	Chaotic family systems are a contributing factor in intrafamily sexual abuse	Formulates consistent rules and roles
Help family identify appropriate roles and power structure within family	When parents have increased sense of competency and authority, they will parent more effectively	Parents function in parental roles and children function in age appropriate roles
Teach family the problem-solving process	Increasing alternative coping skills will decrease incidences of abuse	Uses the problem-solving process
Help family to anticipate management of developmental transitions within family	Anticipatory guidance may prevent the recurrence of intrafamily sexual abuse	Verbalizes understanding of developmental phases of family

Nursing Diagnosis: Post trauma response related to being an adult survivor of incest.
Goal: Client will resolve associated anger, anxiety, fears.

Intervention	*Rationale*	*Expected Outcome*
Ask client about relationship with parents	To assess if client is willing to discuss past sexual abuse	Dicusses incest when ready

(Diagnosis continued)

Table 16–19 *(continued)*

Intervention	*Rationale*	*Expected Outcome*
Discuss feelings of guilt	Client needs to hear clearly that children are not responsible for incest; the adult perpetrator is totally responsible	Verbalizes a decrease in guilt
Discuss feelings of anger toward parents	Normalizes feelings of anger toward perpetrator and anger toward other parent for not protecting client	Verbalizes anger appropriately
Connect feelings of low self-esteem to feelings of guilt and anger	May be unrealistically blaming self for the abuse	Acknowledges lack of responsibility for the past
Help client identify areas of life he or she can control	Helps client begin to shift from external locus of control to internal locus of control	Identifies situations of control
Assess for sexual dysfunction; refer to sex therapy or adult survivors group if this is a serious problem	Sexual dysfunction may be a major problem in client's current adult relationship	Follows through on referrals

Nursing Diagnosis: Spiritual distress related to being an adult survivor and asking questions such as "Why did this happen to me?" and "How could a loving God allow this to happen?"
Goal: Client will verbalize decreasing spiritual distress.

Intervention	*Rationale*	*Expected Outcome*
Provide empathy rather than a theologic discussion of God	Provides recognition that something unfair and tragic occurred	Acknowledges the tragic aspect of incest
Pay attention to religious concerns and refer client to appropriate religious counselor	Helps client utilize faith as a resource rather than part of the problem	Verbalizes faith as a source of comfort and support
Discuss how suffering might be managed	Focus on management is more helpful than focus on why people suffer	Discusses plan to manage suffering

Evaluation: Sexual Abuse

Nurses in acute care settings may not have the opportunity for long-term evaluation of the family unit. Short-term evaluations should center on

- The identification of sexual abuse within the family
- The family's ability to recognize that a problem exists
- The willingness of the family to accept assistance by following through with referrals
- The identification of adult survivors of sexual abuse

Nurses in long-term settings or within the community have the opportunity to evaluate the effectiveness of the multidisciplinary treatment plan over an extended period. Sharing in the process of family growth and healthy adaptation in the ceasing of sexual abuse can be a tremendous source of professional satisfaction.

Questions to guide the evaluation of the treatment plan are

1. What are the implications for the family if (a) the family stays intact, (b) the abuser is removed, (c) the child is removed, or (d) the child and the abuser are both removed?

2. Have the family members learned to communicate directly?
3. Has the family structure become more flexible in terms of gender roles?
4. Have the parents demonstrated more effective parenting skills?
5. Is the family less socially isolated?
6. Is the family able to use support systems?
7. Is the adult survivor functioning more effectively?

SUMMARY

Violence Against the Self: Suicide

1. Suicide is the second most frequent cause of death among college students and the third most frequent cause of death among adolescents.

2. Suicide can be precipitated by delusions, hallucinations, hopelessness, intractable pain, multiple crises, and unexpressed anger.

3. Behavioral cues that indicate potential suicide are verbal comments, obtaining a weapon, social isolation, giving away belongings, and drug or alcohol abuse.

4. Affective cues of potential suicide are ambivalence, desolation, guilt, failure, shame, hopelessness, and helplessness.

5. Cognitive cues of potential suicide are verbalizations about death, interpersonal problems, and command hallucinations.

6. Causative factors associated with suicide include isolation, rapid change, loss, fear, failures, and interpersonal problems.

7. The act of suicide has a traumatic effect on the family and friends of the victim. They must cope with grief, guilt, anger, and the cultural stigma associated with suicide.

8. Suicide assessments must be initiated by the nurse. If the topic is not discussed, the person may be abandoned in a dangerous position.

9. Active nursing intervention may prevent some suicides.

Violence Against Others: Rape

10. Rape is a crime of violence perpetrated against victims of all ages.

11. Date rape and marital rape often go unreported. Victims may feel responsible or fear others' disbelief.

12. Behavioral characteristics of rape victims include agitation, outward calmness, crying, nightmares, sleeping problems, or phobias.

13. Affective characteristics of rape victims include shock, anxiety, fear, depression, shame, embarrassment, helplessness, and vulnerability.

14. Cognitive characteristics of rape victims include disbelief, depersonalization, dissociation, denial, confusion, self-blame, obsessions, and fears for future safety.

15. Causative theories relating to rape involve revenge, dominance, eroticized assault, inadequate interpersonal relationships, rigid gender role expectations, and ageism.

16. To prevent additional victimization, nurses must function as client advocates for rape victims.

Intrafamily Violence: Physical Abuse

17. The family home is a place of danger for many women, children, and elderly people.

18. Behavioral characteristics related to intrafamily violence include hitting, kicking, shoving, beating, and use of weapons. The pattern of violence tends to escalate in frequency and severity.

19. Affective characteristics related to intrafamily violence include jealousy, hostility, dependency, inadequacy, guilt, helplessness, depression, and multiple fears.

20. Cognitive characteristics related to intrafamily violence include self-righteousness, inadequate self-esteem, unrealistic expectations, rationalization, and hope for reform.

21. There is a higher risk for intrafamily violence under conditions with rigid gender roles, social isolation, high stress, and highly dependent family members.

22. Causative theories relating to intrafamily violence include substance abuse, projection, impulsiveness, learned behavior, poverty, enmeshed family systems, and sexist family structure.

23. Nurses in all clinical settings must be alert to signs of abuse and be able to identify victims of domestic violence.

24. Preventive nursing interventions include community education, establishment of support groups, and social and political advocacy for children, women, and the elderly.

Intrafamily Violence: Sexual Abuse

25. Intrafamily sexual abuse occurs in all racial, religious, economic, and sociocultural subgroups. As many

as 50 percent of girls and 20 percent of boys may be sexually abused before the age of 18.

26. Childhood sexual abuse may be a hidden feature of adult mental disorders.

27. Behavioral cues that may indicate sexual abuse include regression, sleep disturbances, isolation, extreme affection, sexual acting out, running away, or suicide.

28. Affective cues to victims of sexual abuse include fears, distrust, ambivalence, guilt, helplessness, powerlessness, and self-hatred.

29. Cognitive cues that may indicate sexual abuse include denial, thoughts of responsibility, low self-esteem, and an external locus of control.

30. Dissociation is a frequent defense mechanism of victims. Multiple personality disorder may be a consequence of severe and sadistic sexual abuse.

31. Causative factors related to intrafamily sexual abuse include rigid gender roles, chronic stress, inadequate self-esteem, fear of adult relationships, impulsivity, altered family structure, and low adaptability to change.

32. It is vitally important that nurses acknowledge the reality of intrafamily sexual abuse and be alert to cues demanding focused nursing assessment.

CHAPTER REVIEW

Dayna is a 35-year-old, divorced mother of three. She was admitted to the psychiatric unit after spending 24 hours in the intensive care unit. Before her admission, she overdosed on 10 Triavil tablets at home.

Dayna has become increasingly depressed over the last several months, with difficulty sleeping and a 20-pound weight loss. She states that all her problems stem from being sexually abused by her father from age 9 to age 17. At 17 she became pregnant with her father's child. Her father forced her to marry her boyfriend, "because society looks down on unwed mothers."

Dayna's father died one year ago and she talks about how much she hates him and how relieved she was when he died. It was not until after his death that Dayna was able to tell her mother about the sexual abuse. She is alternately angry at her mother for not protecting her and forgiving because "she didn't do this to me, he did." She is also angry at herself for not telling sooner. She states it is still difficult to talk about the incest because she feels "like the only person this has ever happened to." She further states: "The pain of trying to go on living is just too much. I want to die so I will stop hurting."

1. Based on the above assessment data, which is the priority nursing diagnosis for Dayna?
    - (a) Potential for violence, self-directed related to acute suicidal state
    - (b) Anxiety related to inability to resolve conflict regarding sexual abuse by father
    - (c) Ineffective individual coping related to being an incest victim
    - (d) Chronic low self-esteem related to childhood victimization

2. All the following are nursing goals for Dayna. Which one is a priority goal on admission?
    - (a) A nonjudgmental and accepting attitude
    - (b) Assurance that someone is concerned about her
    - (c) Protecting her until she can protect herself
    - (d) Teaching her new ways to manage her anger

During the second week of hospitalization, Dayna talks more about her feelings as an adult survivor of incest. She states: "I have such anger and rage inside of me. Sometimes anger is the only thing I can feel. I'm angry at God, my father, my mother, and most of all myself. Why couldn't I make him stop the abuse? If I were a stronger person, I would have been able to make him stop. Maybe it was my fault he abused me."

3. Using this data as assessment, which would be the most appropriate nursing diagnosis?
    - (a) Ineffective family coping, disabling, related to enmeshed family system
    - (b) Anxiety related to suicide attempt prior to admission
    - (c) Social isolation related to withdrawal from family and friends
    - (d) Chronic low self-esteem related to self-hatred and guilt

4. In response to Dayna's statements, which would be the most appropriate nursing intervention?
    - (a) Ask her if she is willing to discuss her relationship with her parents to determine family patterns of ineffective coping
    - (b) Connect her feelings of low self-esteem to feelings of guilt and anger since she is unrealistically blaming herself for the abuse
    - (c) Help her identify areas of life she has control over to help her begin to shift from external to internal locus of control
    - (d) Refer her to an adult survivors of incest group to decrease her feelings of isolation

5. Which one of the following statements by Dayna would be evidence that she is beginning to meet the expected outcome of resolving her negative feelings?

(a) "I'm starting to believe that it was not my fault that my father abused me."
(b) "I still don't understand how my mother could not have known what was happening."
(c) "He knew he made me pregnant and then made me get married so he could feel better."
(d) "Do you think I'll ever get rid of this pain and shame I feel about what my father did?"

REFERENCES

Arbore P, Willis AT: Suicide and the elderly. In: *Toward a Science of Family Nursing.* Gilliss CL, et al. (editors). Addison-Wesley, 1989.

Barrett MJ, Sykes C, Byrnes W: A systematic model for the treatment of intrafamily child sexual abuse. In: *Treating Incest: A Multiple Systems Perspective.* Trepper TS, Barrett MJ (editors). Hayworth Press, 1986.

Bennett G: Group therapy for men who batter women. *Holistic Nurs Pract* 1987; 1(2):33–42.

Bersani CA, Chen HT: Sociological perspectives in family violence. In: *Handbook of Family Violence.* Vanhasselt VB, et al. (editors). Plenum, 1988; 57–86.

Bolton FG, Bolton SR: *Working with Violent Families.* Sage, 1987.

Boxwell, AO: Geriatric suicide. *Nurs Pract* 1988; 13(6): 10–19.

Broome ME, Daniels D: Child abuse: A multidimensional phenomenon. *Holistic Nurs Pract* 1987; 1(2):13–24.

Bryer JB, et al.: Childhood sexual and physical abuse as factors in adult psychiatric illness. *Am J Psychiatry* 1987; 144(11):1426–1430.

Bullock L, et al.: The prevalence and characteristics of battered women in a primary care setting. *Nurs Pract* 1989; 14(6):47–54.

Burden DS, Gottlieb N: *The Woman Client.* Tavistock, 1987.

Burt MKR: Cultural myths and supports for rape. *J Personality Soc Psychol* 1980; 38:217.

Campbell J: Abuse of female partners. In: *Nursing Care of Victims of Family Violence.* Campbell J, Humphreys J (editors). Reston, 1984A. 74–108.

Campbell J: Nursing care of abused women. In: *Nursing Care of Victims of Family Violence.* Campbell J, Humphreys J (editors). Reston, 1984B. 246–280.

Campbell J: Nursing care of families using violence. In: *Nursing Care of Victims of Family Violence.* Campbell J, Humphreys J (editors). Reston, 1984C. 216–245.

Campbell J: Theories of violence. In: *Nursing Care of Victims of Family Violence.* Campbell J, Humphreys J (editors). Reston, 1984D. 13–52.

Campbell JC, Sheridan DJ: Emergency nursing interventions with battered women. *J Emergency Nurs* 1989; 15(1):12–17.

Casey J, O'Connor PJ: Dad seized in Indiana in Schaumberg baby killing. *Chicago Sun-Times* June 10, 1988.

Courtois C: *Healing the Incest Wound.* Norton, 1988.

Curran DK: Scope of the problem in the United States. *Issues Ment Health Nurs* 1986; 8(4):287–308.

Cutter F: *Art and the Wish to Die.* Nelson-Hall, 198[illegible].

Denmark FL, Kabatznick RM: Women and suicide. In: *Affective Disorders,* No. 3. Flach, F (editor). Norton, 1988. 10–18.

Dobash RE, Dobash R: *Violence Against Wives.* Free Press, 1979.

Dongen CJ: The legacy of suicide. *J Psychosoc Nurs* 1988; 26(1):8–13.

Erickson CA: Rape and the family. In: *Treating Stress in Families.* Figley CR (editor). Brunner/Mazel, 1989. 257–289.

Fawcett J, et al.: Clinical predictors of suicide in patients with major affective disorders. *Am J Psychiatry* 1987; 144(1):35–40.

Foley TS: The client who has been raped. In: *The American Handbook of Psychiatric Nursing.* Lego S (editor). Lippincott, 1984.

Giles-Sims J: *Wife Battering: A Systems Theory Approach.* Guilford, 1983.

Gilligan C: *In a Different Voice.* Harvard University Press, 1982.

Goodrich TJ, et al.: *Feminist Family Therapy.* Norton, 1988.

Gould M, Shaffer D: Study shows that TV suicide dramas may contribute to teen suicide. *J Child Adol Psychiatry* 1987; 4(2):139–140.

Groth AN, Birnbaum HJ: The rapist. In: *The Rape Crisis Intervention Handbook.* McCombie SL (editor). Plenum, 1980.

Hafen B, Frandsen K: *Psychological Emergencies and Crisis Intervention.* Morton, 1985.

Hammond N: Lesbian victims and the reluctance to identify abuse. In: *Naming the Violence: Speaking Out About Lesbian Battering.* Lobel K (editor). Seal Press, 1986. 190–197.

Hart B: Lesbian battering: An examination. In: *Naming the Violence: Speaking Out About Lesbian Battering.* Lobel, K (editor). Seal Press, 1986. 173–189.

Hartman CR, Burgess AW: Rape trauma and treatment of the victim. In: *Post-Traumatic Therapy and Victims of Violence.* Ochberg FM (editor). Brunner/Mazel, 1988. 152–174.

Hauser MJ: Special aspects of grief after a suicide. In: *Sui-*

cide and Its Aftermath. Dunne EJ, et al. (editors). Norton, 1987. 57–70.

Hawton K: *Suicide and Attempted Suicide Among Children and Adolescents.* Sage, 1986.

Herman JL: Father-daughter incest. In: *Post-Traumatic Therapy and Victims of Violence.* Ochberg FM (editor). Brunner/Mazel, 1988. 175–195.

Hillard PJA: Physical abuse and pregnancy. *Med Aspects Human Sexuality* 1988; 22(10):30–41.

Hudson MF: Elder mistreatment: Current research. In: *Elder Abuse.* Pillemer KA, Wolf RS (editors). Auburn House, 1986. 125–166.

Humphreys J, Campbell J: Introduction: Nursing and family violence. In: *Nursing Care of Victims of Family Violence.* Campbell J, Humphreys J (editors). Reston, 1984.

Humphreys J, Campbell J: Abusive behavior in families. In: *Toward a Science of Family Nursing.* Gilliss CL, et al. (editors). Addison-Wesley, 1989. 394–417.

Keye WR: *The Premenstrual Syndrome.* Saunders, 1988.

Krueger MM: Pregnancy as a result of rape. *J Sex Ed Theory* 1988; 14(1):23–27.

Magnuson E: Suicides: The gun factor. *Time* July 17, 1989; 134(3):61.

McIntosh JL: Suicide as a mental health problem. In: *Suicide and Its Aftermath.* Dunne EJ, et al. (editors). Norton, 1987. 19–30.

McLeer SU: Psychoanalytic perspectives on family violence. In: *Handbook of Family Violence.* VanHasselt VB, et al. (editors). Plenum, 1988. 11–30.

Metro Digest, *Chicago Sun Times,* June 8, 1988. p. 60.

Miller M: *Suicide Intervention by Nurses.* Springer, 1982.

Mittleman RE, Mittleman HS, Wetli CV: What child abuse really looks like. *Am J Nurs* 1987; 87(9):1185–1188.

Montague MC: Physiology of aggressive behavior. *J Neurosurg Nurs* 1979; 11:10.

O'Connor PJ: Sitter charged with biting boy to death. *Chicago Sun-Times,* February 24, 1985.

Okum L: *Women Abuse.* State University of New York, 1986.

O'Leary KD: Physical aggression between spouses. In: *Handbook of Family Violence.* VanHasselt VB, et al. (editors). Plenum, 1988. 31–55.

Pagelow MD: Marital rape. In: *Handbook of Family Violence.* VanHasselt VB, et al. (editors). Plenum, 1988. 87–118.

Parker DS: Accident or suicide. *J Psychosoc Nurs* 1988; 26(6):15–19.

Phillips LR: Theoretical explanations of elder abuse. In: *Elder Abuse.* Pillemer KA, Wolfe RS (editors). Auburn House, 1986; 167–196.

Quinn MJ, Tomita SK: *Elder Abuse and Neglect.* Springer, 1986.

Resick PA: Sex-role stereotypes and violence against women. In: *The Stereotyping of Women.* Franks V, Rothblum E (editors). Springer, 1983.

Richardson C: Fenwick mourns "marvelous boy." *Chicago Sun-Times,* April 18, 1985.

Richman J: *Family Therapy for Suicidal People.* Springer, 1986.

Rose K, Saunders DG: Nurses' and physicians' attitudes about women abuse. *Health Care for Women Internatl* 1986; 7(6):427–438.

Rosen H: *A Clinician's Guide to Affective Disorders.* Mnemosyne, 1981.

Rossi R: Dad convicted of plot to kill son, 17. *Chicago Sun-Times,* February 7, 1985.

Russell DE: *The Politics of Rape: The Victim's Perspective.* Stein and Day, 1975.

Sachs A: Swinging-and-ducking-singles. *Time* Sept 5, 1988. 54.

Sengstock MC, Barrett S: Domestic abuse of the elderly. In: *Nursing Care of Victims of Family Violence.* Campbell J, Humphreys J (editors). Reston, 1984.

Shotland RL: A model of the causes of date rape in developing and close relationships. In: *Close Relationships.* Hendrick C (editor). Sage, 1989. 247–270.

Stark E, Flitcraft A: Personal power and institutional victimization. In: *Post-Traumatic Therapy and Victims of Violence.* Ochberg FM (editor). Brunner/Mazel, 1988. 115–151.

Starr RH: Physical abuse of children. In: *Handbook of Family Violence.* VanHasselt VB, et al. (editors). Plenum, 1988. 119–155.

Strach A, Jervey N: Lesbian abuse: The process. In: *Naming the Violence: Speaking Out About Lesbian Battering.* Lobel K (editor). Seal Press, 1986. 88–94.

Straus MA, Gelles RJ, Steinmetz SK: *Behind Closed Doors: Violence in the American Family.* Anchor Press/Doubleday, 1980.

Straus MA, Hotaling GT: *The Social Causes of Husband-Wife Violence.* University of Minnesota Press, 1980.

Tilden VP, Shepherd P: Battered women: The shadow side of families. *Holistic Nurs Pract* 1987; 1(2):25–32.

Trepper TS: Intrafamily child sexual abuse. In: *Treating Stress in Families.* Figley CR (editor). Brunner/Mazel, 1989. 185–208.

Trepper TS, Barrett MJ: Introduction to a multiple systems approach for the assessment and treatment of intrafamily child sexual abuse. In: *Treating Incest: A Multiple Systems Perspective.* Trepper TS, Barrett MJ (editors). Hayworth Press, 1986A.

Trepper TS, Barrett MJ: Vulnerability to incest: A framework for assessment. In: *Treating Incest: A Multiple Systems Perspective.* Trepper TS, Barrett MJ (editors). Hayworth Press, 1986B.

Trepper TS, Traicoff ME: Treatment of intrafamily sexuality: Issues in therapy and research. *J Sex Educ Ther* 1983; 9:14.

Urbancic JC: Incest trauma. *J Psychosoc Nurs* 1987; 25(7):33–35.

Valenti C: Working with the physically abused woman. In: *Women in Health and Illness.* Kjervik DK, Martinson IM (editors). Saunders, 1986. 127–133.

Walker L: Battered women's shelters and work with battered lesbians. In: *Naming the Violence: Speaking Out About Lesbian Battering.* Lobel K (editor). Seal Press, 1986. 73–79.

Walker LE: Violence against women: Implications for mental health policy. In: *Women and Mental Health Policy.* Walker LE (editor). Sage Publications, 1984.

Warner CG: *Rape and Sexual Assault.* Aspen Systems, 1980.

Waterman J: Family dynamics of incest with young children. In: *Sexual Abuse of Young Children.* McFarlane K, Waterman J (editors). Guilford Press, 1986. 204–219.

Waterman J, Luck R: Scope of the problem. In: *Sexual Abuse of Young Children.* McFarlane K, Waterman J (editors). Guilford Press, 1986. 3–12.

Wheeler CN: Woman con asks clemency. *Chicago Sun-Times* July 8, 1988.

Wilson T: Man gets 15 years in wife's rape. *Chicago Sun-Times* July 9, 1988.

Wolfe DA, Wolfe VV, Best CL: Child victims of sexual abuse. In: *Handbook of Family Violence.* VanHasselt VB, et al. (editors). Plenum, 1988. 157–185.

Wrobleski A: The suicide survivors grief group. *Omega* 1984–1985; 15:173.

Wyatt GE, Peters SD, Guthrie D: Kinsey revisited. *Arch Sexual Behav* 1988; 17(3):201–239.

Zdanuk JM, Harris CC, Wisian NL: Adolescent pregnancy and incest. *JOGNN* 1987; 16(2):99–104.

SUGGESTED READINGS

Bass E, Davis L: *The Courage to Heal: A Guide for Women Survivors of Child Sexual Abuse.* Harper & Row, 1988.

Bloom LA: *Mourning After Suicide.* Pilgrim Press, 1986.

Burgess AW, Holmstrom LL: Treating the adult rape victim. *Med Aspects Human Sexuality* 1988; 22(1):36–43.

Campbell JC: A test of two explanatory models of women's responses to battering. *Nurs Res* 1989; 38(1): 18–23.

Cate RM: Detecting premarital abuse. *Med Aspects Human Sexuality* 1989; 23(5):104–110.

Covington CH: Invest: The psychological problem and the biological contradiction. *Issues Ment Health Nurs* 1989; 10(1):69–87.

Foster S: Counseling survivors of incest. *Med Aspects Human Sexuality* 1988; 22(3):114–123.

Ryan JM: Child abuse and the community health nurse. *Home Health Care Nurs* 1989; 7(2):23–26.

White EC: *Chain, Chain, Change: For Black Women Dealing with Physical and Emotional Abuse.* Seal Press, 1985.

Wisechild LM: *The Obsidian Mirror: An Adult Healing from Incest.* Seal Press, 1988.

Zambrano MM: *Mejor Sola Que Mal Acompañada—For the Latina in an Abusive Relationship.* Seal Press, 1985.

Zavodnick JM: Detection and management of sexual abuse of boys. *Med Aspects Human Sexuality* 1989; 23(1):80–90.

CHAPTER 17

Issues Facing Mental Health Nursing

JOSEPH E. SMITH* and J. SUE COOK

A Safe Place
I am sitting on a large rock founded in the tranquility of the water, relaxed and happy, contented viewing the spacious beautiful world at its best. A large window of my soul to appreciate the beauty & wonder of it all. A large door—a passage-way of choices; to open the door, to pursue and develop all my hopes and dreams.

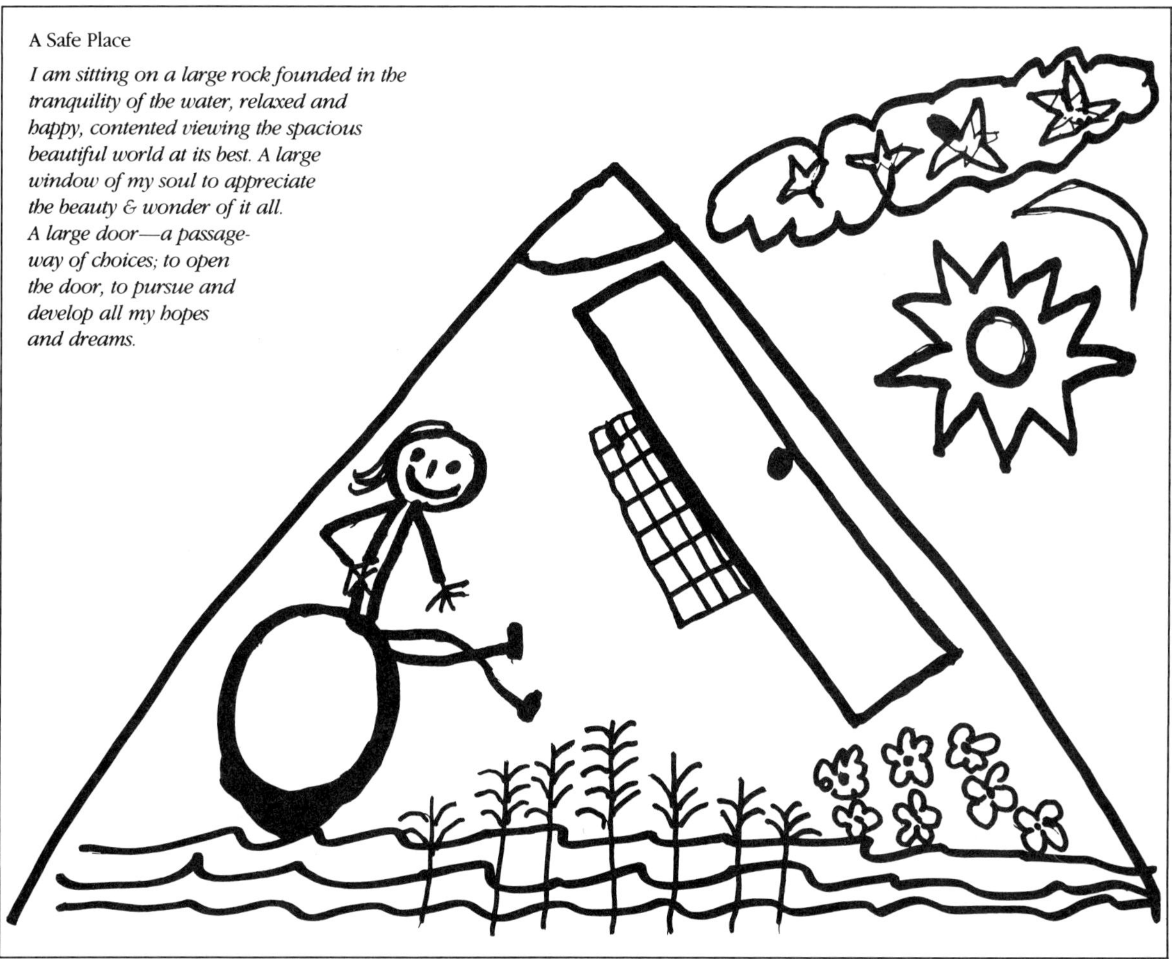

*Note: Joseph E. Smith contributed the material on AIDS presented in this chapter.

■ *Objectives*

After reading this chapter the student will be able to

- Discuss the social significance of the AIDS epidemic
- Describe the significance of AIDS to mental health nursing
- Describe the knowledge base related to AIDS
- Apply a focused nursing assessment to the client with AIDS
- Identify nursing diagnoses for the client with AIDS
- Prepare nursing care plans for clients with AIDS
- Describe the knowledge base related to the problem of homelessness
- Identify nursing diagnoses for the homeless client
- Prepare nursing care plans for the homeless client
- Describe future directions in mental health nursing

■ *Chapter Outline*

Introduction

The arrival of the twenty-first century promises answers to many of the medical questions that plague us. As we find answers to our complex questions, the nature of mental health nursing will likely change, thereby necessitating new approaches. This chapter will look at two perplexing problems facing mental health nurses right now: the AIDS epidemic and the problem of homelessness.

HIV Disease

Acquired immunodeficiency syndrome (AIDS) has rapidly become one of the most complex public health problems in the history of the United States. AIDS, first reported in this country in 1981, is a deadly disease that is caused by the **human immunodeficiency virus (HIV)**. HIV is usually transmitted by one of two routes. The most common is sexual transmission. Less common is through direct blood-to-blood contact—from sharing IV drug needles or receiving contaminated blood transfusions or blood products, for example. Another example of transmission through blood-to-blood contact is transmission between a pregnant HIV-infected woman and her unborn child. Because intimate sexual contact is the most common way of transmitting the virus, all sexually active Americans need to know the basic facts about this disease and how to avoid the risk of infection.

HIV damages the body's natural immune defenses against disease. Therefore, people with HIV disease develop life-threatening illnesses that do not affect persons with normal immune systems. No one with HIV disease has ever recovered the lost immune function. More than half of the Americans who have developed AIDS have died. However, because of increased medical knowledge, HIV-infected persons under closely supervised treatment are now living longer than those with the first diagnosed cases.

In many cases an HIV-infected individual lives for years without showing any symptoms at all. This trend is likely to continue as more prophylactic drugs are tested and approved. However, the number of AIDS deaths continues to rise, and public fear escalates. Because of the time it sometimes takes for HIV infection to develop into AIDS, approximately 50 percent of AIDS cases diagnosed after 1991 will be people who are presently infected with the virus but do not yet have AIDS. Those exposed to the virus must be presumed to be chronically infectious. Since the Centers for Disease Control (CDC) have been publishing reports related to HIV infection rates in the United States, the cumulative totals have exceeded 100,000 cases. This number is predicted to rise to over 300,000 by 1991, with 179,000 deaths.

There is presently no AIDS vaccine or cure. Therefore, nurses must consider how to allay fears and provide the general public with productive options to reduce risk. In addition, those affected by the epidemic need assistance. A comprehensive educational program is needed to prevent the spread of this fatal disease. Education programs would be appropriate in every institution: schools, colleges, businesses, factories, professional and nonprofessional organizations, churches, community centers—in short, everywhere. There is no state or country without the need for AIDS education (American Red Cross, 1988).

In June of 1988 the Presidential AIDS Commission announced the need for sweeping new programs to fight the epidemic. The report (U.S. Department of Health and Human Services, p. 1) stated, "There has not been a national strategy . . . [or] a national policy on AIDS." The report called for additional monies for research; increased drug trials; and increased availability of experimental AIDS drugs to HIV-infected people without restrictions based on their ability to pay. The commission's report admonished health care workers (HCWs) who refused to care for HIV-infected persons. Further, the report stressed a need for an aggressive education program that would allow HCWs to assist in eliminating misconceptions about transmission. For example, questions about mosquitoes transmitting the disease should not have to be asked. The nursing profession was recognized for its efforts to educate nurses. However, the report stated that the efforts are inadequate to meet the current and projected needs.

In response to the needs in HIV-related nursing care, the commission recommended the following.

1. All HCWs should give HIV-infected clients the same respect, dignity, and decision-making autonomy given to any other client.
2. Upon admission, all HIV-infected clients should have the same rights to informed consent as do other clients upon admission.
3. Traineeships, scholarships, and work-study programs should be available to nursing students, both undergraduate and graduate, to assist them in pursuing advanced education about caring for HIV-infected people.
4. The Public Health Service's Division of Nursing should fund models of nurse-

managed care for HIV-infected persons outside hospitals and other institutions.

5. The Health Care Financing Administration should allow Medicare and Medicaid to make direct reimbursements for the nursing care of those with HIV disease.

The American Nurses' Association (1988) has been actively involved in advocating humane, effective national policies on the care of persons with HIV disease. Some of their positions include

- Opposing universal, mandatory testing for the HIV antibody, but supporting voluntary, anonymous testing with informed consent
- Urging federal support for education, research, and treatment
- Reaffirming commitment to the civil and human rights of affected persons and their care givers
- Reaffirming commitment to caring for all people with HIV disease
- Urging all HCWs to follow universal precautions for preventing HIV infection in the workplace, as outlined by CDC.

Clinically, it is apparent that HIV-infected people suffer from syndromes and abnormalities that do not meet the CDC criteria for AIDS diagnosis. From clinical and public health perspectives, however, viewing HIV as a disease may assist clients in being diagnosed and treated as early as possible. The concern is that even asymptomatic infected people can infect others (National Academy Press, 1988).

This text purposely addresses the psychosocial aspects of HIV disease in greater detail than the pathophysiologic components. Also, this text focuses on intravenous drug users and gay or bisexual men because the highest incidence of the disease is found in these populations. (See "Suggested Readings" at the end of this chapter for works that discuss the HIV disease process and its signs and symptoms.)

Incidence and Prevalence

HIV infection is most prevalent in those persons whose behaviors place them at greatest risk for contracting the virus. Among gay or bisexual men, prevalence estimates are between 20 percent and 50 percent, depending on geographic region and city. In contrast to less than 5 percent in some areas, the prevalence among intravenous drug users in New York City and northern New Jersey is between 50 and 60 percent. Hemophiliacs who received blood-clotting factors before 1985 show an HIV infection prevalence of 90 percent (National Academy Press, 1988; Puckett and Emery, 1988).

Because of the gay community's educational and risk-reduction efforts, the number of new cases is declining. In addition, the number of other sexually transmitted diseases among gay males is declining. Since blood donation and transfusion procedures have been tightened, a reduction of HIV infections has been noted among hemophiliacs and transfusion recipients. The fastest-growing subgroup of HIV-infected individuals within the United States consists of intravenous drug users. This group serves as the path for AIDS to reach the heterosexual population. Also, this group has become the source of AIDS among newborns (Puckett and Emery, 1988).

Significance of HIV Disease to Mental Health Nursing

Since the beginning of the epidemic, nurses have been an important force in delivering both educational and direct care services to clients, loved ones, and care givers affected by HIV (Smith, 1988). Mental health nurses are providing supportive care to HIV-infected clients in hospitals, health care facilities, and in the community. The scope of this disease requires frequent assessments of mental status related to behavioral, affective, and social changes. Since preexisting psychiatric conditions may influence how one handles the diagnosis of HIV, thorough nursing histories must be conducted.

Mental health nurses have helped to develop home care programs and have served as trainers for community-based responses such as "buddy" volunteer programs and risk-reduction programs. Mental health nurses are functioning in roles as policymakers, administrators, health educators, volunteers, direct care givers, therapists, and case managers.

Knowledge Base: HIV Disease

Being diagnosed HIV positive is frightening. Therefore it is important to conduct thorough psychosocial assessments during each visit with the client. It is important to distinguish between behavioral, cognitive, and affective changes. For example, both anxiety and depression have behavioral, affective, and cognitive components that can be detected through observation and testing.

Behavioral Characteristics

Behavioral changes occur as HIV disease progresses. Initially the signs of change may be complaints of malaise and fatigue. These may progress to symptoms of sluggishness, unsteady gait, and muscular tension. Also, the client quite often complains of motor retardation and speech impairments. These may also be noted when conducting physical exams. In addition, the client's attention span may decrease, causing the person to be easily distracted.

As the person becomes more anxious and fearful of losing control of his or her life, depression may result and cause the client to become socially isolated and withdrawn. Without intervention, this behavior can lead to suicide ideations, threats, or attempts (Green, 1986).

Affective Characteristics

When assessing clients with HIV infection, nurses should observe closely for affective changes. Some of these signs have both affective and behavioral components. For example, anxiety is a common reaction to being seropositive or suffering the first opportunistic infection, which indicates that the body's immune system has been destroyed. These anxiety reactions may become overt and manifest themselves somatically with diarrhea, gastrointestinal disturbances, nausea and vomiting, sweating, breathing difficulties, or panic attacks. However, many of these may also indicate HIV disease progression.

As do others with chronic diseases, people with HIV disease experience grief and loss reactions. These losses may take many forms: loss of peace of mind and spirit; financial problems due to loss of employment or health and life insurance policies; lack of support from lovers, friends, family members, and so on; lack of physical intimacy with spouses, lovers, and friends; loss of role status, personal appearance, and control of body functions; and loss of life itself (Strawn, 1987). Table 17–1 summarizes the common emotional reactions to being HIV-infected.

Of the affective disorders related to HIV infection, depression is one of the most common symptoms and quite often the first major change detected by nurses. The most common and threatening cause of depression is fear of the unknown. The seropositive individual fears the progression of the disease, whereas the individual diagnosed with AIDS fears total loss of physical and mental control and well-being. Quite often, these individuals have lovers, sexual partners, or friends who are also HIV-infected, dying, or have already died. Thoughts and feelings of self-blame and guilt for past behaviors may arise and should be vented. Fears about losing personal control in decision making also result in depression and anxiety. Common manifestations of these feelings of depression include low self-esteem, insomnia, a decreased interest in sex, and mood swings. These mood swings vary from the blues and crying spells to sudden outbursts of anger. Often these signs are also symptoms of the pathologic effect of HIV disease on the CNS.

Cognitive Characteristics

There are definite cognitive changes within the progression of HIV disease. Initial changes include clients' statements about his or her own forgetfulness, concentration difficulties, and slowness of thought. The client often reports periods of confu-

Table 17–1 *Some Emotional Implications of HIV Disease*

Shock	diagnosis, uncertainty, and possible death
Anxiety	uncertain prognosis and course of illness effects of medication and treatment status of lover and lover's ability to cope reactions of others (family, friends, lover, colleagues, employers, etc) loss of cognitive, physical, social, and occupational abilities risk of infection from and to others
Depression	helpless to change circumstances virus is in control of life reduced quality of life in all spheres gloomy, possibly painful, uncomfortable and disfiguring future self-blame and recriminations for past "indiscretions" reduced social and sexual acceptability isolation
Anger	over past high-risk lifestyle and activities over inability to overcome the virus over new and involuntary lifestyle restrictions
Guilt	being homosexual "confirmed" unacceptability of homosexuality via illness
Obsessions	relentless searching for explanations relentless searching for new diagnostic evidence on client's own body inevitability of decline and death health and diet fads

Source: Adapted from D. Miller, *Psychology, AIDS, ARC, and PGL.* In: *The Management of AIDS Patients* (Macmillan, 1986). D. Miller, J. Weber, and J. Green (editors). Reprinted with permission.

sion. In conducting the mental status exam it may be wise to assess the client's ability to do simple abstractions. As neurologic involvement becomes more exacerbated, symptoms such as dementia, hallucinations, delusional thinking (delirium), and acute paranoia may appear. (See Chapter 15 for care of clients with organic brain disorders.)

Sociocultural Characteristics

Diagnosis of any chronic disease brings intense, complex reactions. Because of the stigma associated with AIDS, however, diagnosis of HIV infection stresses clients and loved ones to a greater degree than other diagnoses. Nurses must be aware of the reactions of all those affected by the HIV diagnosis and provide support and teaching as needed.

Concerns of parents Parents' reactions to the news of their son's or daughter's AIDS or seropositivity can be complex. In addition to learning the medical diagnosis, the parents may be confronted for the first time with their son's or daughter's sexuality or substance usage. The parents may feel guilty over their failure to meet expectations as parents.

As with other chronic diseases, but to a larger degree with HIV, the threat of the loved one's death is present and must be addressed. Fears related to the physical and mental changes associated with HIV disease progression are well grounded. Time should be set aside to allow the family to discuss openly whether members will care for the loved one at home when the need arises or if the family will choose some other alternative. The family should voice concerns about both options.

Besides assessment of available resources for medical care and treatment, questions related to housing availability and home care must be discussed with the person affected and the person's care givers. Further, financial assistance options need to be explored with the client. Finally, the availability of AZT (Retrovir) or experimental drugs such as ddI should be addressed. Drug availability may be of particular concern to the client in a rural area or small town. The nurse should refer him or her to a regional medical center or university hospital.

Many families allow their loved one to return home when ill. However, because of the stigma that AIDS has, some families hide the fact that their loved one has HIV disease. If the community discovers that the individual is ill with AIDS, the family suffers the same stigma as the person infected.

Families of HIV-infected clients share the need for physical, pastoral or spiritual, and bereavement support. Also, issues of dependence versus independence in regard to the HIV-infected person and his or her family should be dealt with directly.

Partner's Concerns and Needs Issues relating to the physical or supportive care necessary for HIV-infected persons are also pertinent for lovers, who may be providing the same type of care as families or spouses. In addition to issues about care, specific points regarding sexuality and psychosocial support need to be addressed by the HIV-infected person and the lover.

Sexuality issues, such as risk-reduction guidelines, must be discussed. (See Appendix C for discussion of safe-sex guidelines.) The nurse must ascertain whether both partners have a working knowledge of these practices and understand the importance of adhering to them during their sexual activities. In addition to sexuality issues, intravenous drug users and their partners must realize the importance of using clean needles and syringes if their risky behavior continues.

Besides issues of physical and psychosocial support, issues that address the relationships between parents and lovers or spouses and the person infected must be discussed. Parents sometimes blame the spouse or lover for their son's or daughter's illness. Whether or not the parents have accepted their child's sexual identity or substance usage can affect the degree to which the family is willing to allow the partner to participate in caring for the client.

Lovers and partners of HIV-infected individuals can get support from various support groups. These groups are therapeutic for all involved. In establishing such support groups and referring partners to them, the nurse meets a very important need. Upon the death of the client, supporters need time to grieve. Bereavement groups allow them space to do this (Flaskerud, 1987; Marshall and Nieckarz, 1988; Pheiffer and Houseman, 1988). In many different settings nurses often serve as facilitators for these groups.

Support for HCWs HCWs, whether professionals or volunteers, possess certain values and bring their own beliefs, attitudes, and stereotypes into relationships with clients. Health professionals and volunteers develop internal conflicts in regard to caring for persons with HIV disease, and the conflicts need to be expressed. Fears of contagion and stigmatization by peers and family members should be openly discussed by care givers. Since many of the clients are the same age or younger than care givers, mortality issues surface. These need to be addressed in nonthreatening, confidential, and nonjudgmental environments such as support groups led by psychiatric or mental health clinical specialists, chaplains or pastoral counselors, psychologists, or other health professionals.

The AIDS epidemic has uncovered certain issues that need to be discussed confidentially, but frankly, among care givers. Besides fear of contagion, hysteria and unrealistic fears of homosexuals and homosexuality—**homophobia**—must also be recognized to minimize the destructive effect they could have on the client (Viele, Dodd, and Morrison, 1984).

Research validates that homophobia exists among nurses (Barrick, 1988; Douglas, Kalman, and Kalman, 1985; Kelly et al., 1988; Smith, 1981). Homophobia can be addressed in support groups, where issues such as gayness, bisexuality, and the like can be comfortably discussed. Another destructive behavior that can affect a nurse-client relationship is **internalized homophobia**, or feelings of self-hatred and shame for being homosexual. These feelings, either the nurse's or the client's, make establishing a relationship of trust and self-disclosure very difficult or impossible. If such feelings are noted, they must be dealt with in a confidential, supportive, but assertive manner. Otherwise, the nurse cannot provide comprehensive care.

Heterophobia, the fears and lack of trust that gays have toward heterosexuals, sometimes exists. Like homophobia, heterophobia can hinder the nurse-client relationship. Heterophobic feelings should be addressed in the same manner as homophobic feelings.

In addition to sexual orientation issues, **addictophobia**—a term used to describe unrealistic feelings of fear, disgust, or aversion to substance abusers—exists among nurses. Issues such as racism and sexism may also affect AIDS care. All prejudices affecting the nurse-client relationship must be recognized and explored.

Role playing can help nurses gain insight into their own responses to clients. For example, some nurses may not feel comfortable asking questions about a client's sexual preference or use of substances. Role playing would allow these nurses to become comfortable in conducting assessments, which are vital to effective intervention.

Value conflicts may result from nurses' religious or spiritual beliefs. For example, if a nurse believes that AIDS is a punishment from God, the care that nurse can provide to an AIDS victim may suffer (Fletcher, 1984). Religious conflict may also arise regarding passive or active euthanasia. The conflict may interfere with establishing a care plan for the client. In such a case a group composed of nurses, pastoral counselors, ethicists, lawyers, physicians, and the client needs to meet and jointly make decisions regarding the conflicts. If the client is not physically or mentally able to be involved in this decision-making process, the person with the client's power of attorney should participate.

HCWs who care for their own friends, lovers, or past sexual partners face great stress. In addition, stress can take a cumulative toll on all care givers. If HCWs in established AIDS units or in the client's home do not recognize their own physical and mental limits, the result can be burnout or a mental health crisis.

Distrust of Health Care Institutions

Gay or bisexual males and substance abusers have frequently voiced complaints about the judgmental and condescending statements made to them in public health and other health care institutions. In more than half the states, admitting to being gay or bisexual is admitting to a criminal act, often a felony. For intravenous drug users as well, candor can lead to prejudice and legal complications. With the threat of quarantine, contact tracing, and sodomy laws being reinforced, the potential for discrimination is greater than ever.

Legal and Ethical Concerns Within the workplace managers must address a number of issues related to HIV disease. Nurses and nurse managers are now confronting the dilemma posed by the duty to care versus the personal risk involved in caring for HIV-infected clients. Another dilemma is whether or not mandatory HIV testing is legal and ethical for all admissions to health care facilities. At issue is the right of informed consent. Another related issue concerns the ethics of mandatory HIV tests prior to surgery or before receiving treatment in a health care center. This topic elicits much debate. However, because all HCWs adhere to the CDC's universal precautions to prevent the transmission of HIV, human and civil rights activists argue that the test is unnecessary, considering all the documented cases that validate the danger of discriminating against the infected client. Those who have tested seropositive have lost their jobs, their homes, their insurance, and their friends. The American Nurses' Association's position is to protect the client's civil and human rights. Other groups—the National AIDS Network, the National Association of People with AIDS, the National Lesbian and Gay Health Foundation, the American Psychological Association, the American Civil Liberties Union, and many others—have taken a similar position.

Any discussion of treatment issues involves the question of a person's right to treatment. Closely connected to this issue is the right of the client to choose when treatment, because of lack of quality of life, should be ended. Another major ethical concern is the testing of experimental drugs.

As more cases arise, a common issue is whether or not HIV-infected HCWs should care for clients. According to Rothstein (1987), CDC state that there is no medical justification to refuse employment of HCWs, personal service, or other workers who have HIV disease. Persons with HIV disease are protected by law in the Handicapped Provisions under Section 504 of the Rehabilitation Act. However, each person's needs should be reviewed on an individual basis. For instance, if an HIV-infected person is working in an area where he or she might be at great risk of opportunistic infections, "reasonable accommodations" may be necessary to assist the HCW to remain employed longer. Many resources exist to assist in establishing workplace policies and procedures (see the sources under "Suggested Readings" at the end of this chapter).

The admission and retention of student nurses who are seropositive is under much discussion among educators. Some schools of nursing have recommended that the HIV test be used in the screening done during the admission procedures. The National League for Nursing disagrees with this posture. However, the practice has yet to be tested in a court of law.

Nurses may be asked by third parties—that is, by insurance companies, employers, or a medical records department—to provide client health records. Due to the severe ramifications of such an action, confidentiality of client records must be maintained (Herrick and Smith, 1988; Kelly and St. Lawrence, 1988). Many other ethical dilemmas relate to the precarious balance between personal rights and public health and welfare.

Causative Theories and Physiologic Characteristics

AIDS is a disorder of cell-mediated and humoral immunity and is caused by HIV. This virus affects the immune system's functions by altering the genetic makeup of the helper T-lymphocytes (T cells), resulting in the replication of HIV instead of T cells. Figure 17–1 shows the response to HIV. There is a further disruption in the immune system caused by the altered T cell and B cell (suppressor) lymphocyte ratio. The monocyte functions are also affected. The HIV-infected person is rendered immunodeficient and susceptible to characteristic opportunistic infections, cancers, and other complications. Table 17–2 lists infections and diseases commonly associated with HIV infection.

In 1986 CDC published a classification system for HIV infections. Table 17–3 presents this system, which specifies more inclusive definitions and classifications than can be used for client care, health planning, public health strategies, prevention efforts, and epidemiologic studies. In the future this classification will be used for case reporting and in disease coding and recording systems (CDC, 1986).

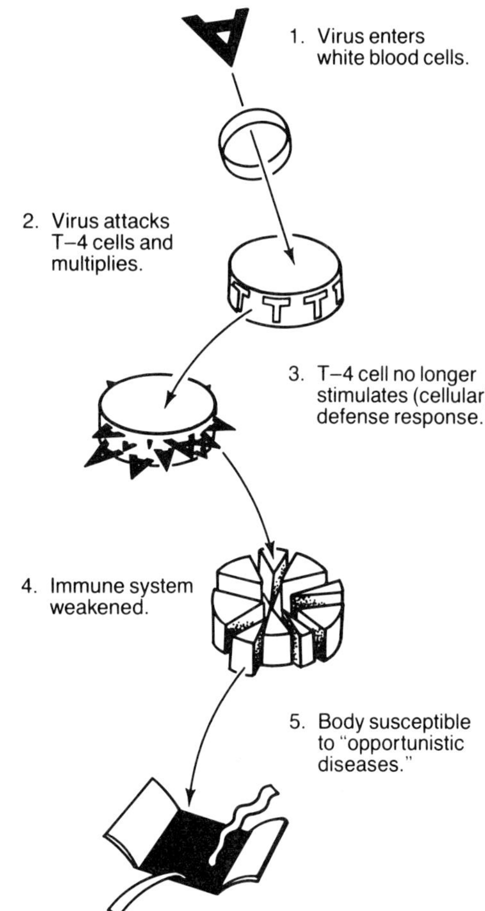

Figure 17–1 *Immune Response to HIV*

Source: Adapted from Sam B. Puckett, Alan R. Emery, Managing *AIDS* in the Workplace (Addison-Wesley, 1988). Reprinted with permission.

As has been previously emphasized, neurologic diseases are extraordinarily common in HIV disease. When HIV invades the CNS, memory loss, mental confusion, and dementia result.

Medical Treatment

The following are the primary goals in treating HIV-infected persons:

1. Help the client to come to terms with the diagnosis of HIV infection and its meaning.

Table 17–2 *Infections and Diseases Commonly Associated with HIV Infection*

Lung diseases	
Protozoan	*Pneumocystis carinii* pneumonia (PCP)
Bacteria	*Mycobacterium* tuberculosis
Brain and CNS Problems	
Yeast	*Cryptococcus neoformans (Cryptococcus meningitis)*
Protozoan	*Toxoplasma gondii* (toxoplasmosis)
Human immunodeficiency virus (HIV)	Leukoencephalopathy (progressive dementia)
Epstein-Barr virus (EBV)	
Cytomegalovirus (CMV)	
Diarrhea	
Bacteria	*Salmonella* *Shigella* *Mycobacterium avium* complex
Virus	Cytomegalovirus (CMV)
Protozoan	Cryptosporidium
Systemic	
Yeastlike fungus	*Candida albicans* (candidiasis)
Viruses	Cytomegalovirus (CMV) Epstein-Barr (EBV)
Mucosal and dermatological	
Viruses	*Herpes simplex* *Herpes zoster*
Cancers/malignancies	
Sarcomas	Kaposi's sarcoma (KS)
Lymphomas	non-Hodgkin's Burkitt-like

2. Assist the client to increase quality of life by developing new coping behaviors and by providing treatment for opportunistic infections and neoplasms.

3. Assist the client to feel in control of his or her life, rather than like a helpless, hopeless victim of HIV disease. The result can be the reconstitution or enhancement of the client's immune system.

Table 17–3 *Summary of classification system for HIV Infection*

Group I. Acute infection

Group II. Asymptomatic infection*

Group III. Persistent generalized lymphadenopathy*

Group IV. Other disease
- Subgroup A. Constitutional disease
- Subgroup B. Neurologic disease
- Subgroup C. Secondary infectious diseases
  - Category C-1. Specified secondary infectious diseases listed in the CDC surveillance definition for AIDS†
  - Category C-2. Other specified secondary infectious diseases
- Subgroup D. Secondary cancers†
- Subgroup E. Other conditions

Source: Adapted from Classification system for human T-lymphotropic virus type III/lymphadenopathy-associated virus infections. *Morbidity and Mortality Weekly Report* (CDC 1986); 35:335. Reprinted with permission.

*Patients in Groups II and III may be subclassified on the basis of a laboratory evaluation.

†Includes those patients whose clinical presentations fulfill the definition of AIDS used by CDC for national reporting.

Treatment Issues

One of the major concerns of HIV-infected persons and those who care about them is where treatment is going to be provided. Will treatment be in outpatient medical clinics, hospitals, in the community, by home health agencies, by hospice, or by residential facilities? Allowing an individual to remain in his or her own home is one way of helping a client feel more in control. This promotes a closer relationship between loved ones, friends, and care givers.

Interventions include both medical and pharmacologic treatments for opportunistic infection and neoplasms. Also, the neuropsychiatric syndromes may require psychotropic medications. To enhance prevention and maintenance efforts, access to drugs will be required. Commonly used drugs are AZT, aerosolized pentamidine, other antivirals, immunomodulators, and experimental drugs.

Adequate nutritional intake must be provided. Discussions related to this need must include the care givers involved. Their support should be solicited to provide the client with his or her favorite foods.

Since social isolation is a common problem for HIV-infected clients, touch therapy in the form of hugs or back and body massages is very therapeutic. Providing stuffed animals to all clients, no matter what their age, has been effective in many settings.

Assessment: HIV Disease

Nursing History

Assessing clients with HIV infection begins with data collection upon initial interaction. Questions related to life patterns, physical history, and psychologic status should be asked. A diagnosis of HIV infection invokes many frightful thoughts, so the nurse should use a calming and supportive manner in compiling a general nursing history. The nurse should also conduct a focused nursing assessment, which should be similar to the assessment that follows. Projecting patience and a caring attitude is necessary for conducting assessments.

Physical Assessment

In the case of the HIV-infected client, physical examinations identify potential problems caused by the progression of HIV disease or by treatments for it.

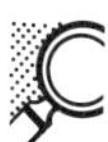

FOCUSED NURSING ASSESSMENT
for the Client with HIV Infection

Behavioral assessment

How has your diagnosis changed your behavior?
How much assistance is needed for bathing? Toileting? Dressing? Eating?
What difficulties do you have in performing complex tasks at home? At work?
Have you noticed any changes in your behavior? Have others?
Do you smoke? If so, how much? Compared to your usual smoking habits, is this an increased or decreased amount?
How much alcohol do you use? Compared to your usual drinking, is this an increased or decreased amount?
What drugs (including street and prescribed drugs) do you take? Compared to your usual dosage, is this an increased or decreased amount?
Has your activity level changed?
When do you isolate yourself or withdraw from others?
What mechanisms are useful in reducing stress?
Do you feel dependent? Independent?

Affective assessment

How has your diagnosis changed your moods?
When do you feel sad?
Has the number of sad or blue periods changed since your diagnosis?
Have you had any thoughts of hurting yourself or others?
Have you experienced angry outbursts?
What kinds of things make you feel anxious?
How often do you feel irritable?
What unfinished business do you need to deal with?
Do you have some specific fears that concern you most?

Cognitive assessment

What kinds of things do you have difficulty remembering?
Has your diagnosis affected your memory (recent and remote)?
Has your diagnosis affected your ability to make decisions? Do you rely on others to make decisions?
Has your diagnosis affected your ability to learn?
What things do you think of most often?

As with other diseases, baseline data are important. Since changes in the physical and mental status of the client occur rapidly, the nurse must observe closely and report carefully. It is important to remember that many early physical signs may be confused with emotional stressors, such as fatigue and activity intolerance.

Physical assessment guidelines include noting any changes in the client's neurologic status, especially since neuropsychiatric syndromes are so common in HIV disease. The gastrointestinal system may also be affected by opportunistic infections or by the medications prescribed. Since thrush is also common, the oral cavity needs to be examined often. Diarrhea occurs frequently and can be a result of an opportunistic infection or a side effect of a medication. These opportunistic infections may or may not be treatable.

The genitourinary system may be affected by opportunistic diseases, specifically the herpes viruses. Sexual functions may be disrupted as a result of both physical and psychologic stressors, such as fear of transmitting the virus to others.

Nursing Diagnosis and Planning: HIV Disease

There are many nursing diagnoses for clients with HIV infection. This text accentuates the psychosocial diagnoses. How care is provided affects the quality of life for the client and improves the attitudes of parents, lovers or spouses, friends, and care givers. Establishing these diagnoses assists in developing the care plans that increase the quality of life for the client. Table 17–4 lists nursing diagnoses for HIV-infected clients.

Nursing care plans, based on individualized nursing diagnoses, establish the goals necessary for providing both the physical and supportive care to clients and their loved ones. Table 17–5 presents a nursing care plan for the HIV-infected client.

Table 17–4 *Nursing Diagnoses for the HIV-infected Client*

Altered role performance
Altered thought processes
Anticipatory grieving
Anxiety
Body image disturbance
Fear
Hopelessness
Ineffective family coping: disabling
Ineffective individual coping, potential for
Knowledge deficit
Powerlessness
Sensory/perceptual alterations: visual, auditory
Sexual dysfunction
Situational low self-esteem
Social isolation
Violence, potential for: self-directed

Evaluation: HIV Disease

The evaluation of the HIV-infected client's care is based on the goals identified in the individualized care plans. Table 17–6 is an example of an evaluation of care for a client with HIV disease. The expected outcomes may be behaviorally stated as follows.

1. The client expresses confidence in the health care team.
2. The client can complete self-care needs.
3. The client adapts and copes as fully as possible to physical, mental, and life changes.
4. To the appropriate people, the client expresses feelings, concerns, and needs relating to his or her illness.

CASE EXAMPLE

A Client with HIV Disease

Pete Hall, a 23-year-old registered nurse, was diagnosed with HIV infection on the day after Gay Pride Day in a southern city. He is currently pursuing an advanced degree in nursing and volunteers time to AIDS work as a nurse therapist. Pete recently lost his lover of 5 years to AIDS. Pete left his small midwestern hometown shortly after high school graduation. His father is a minister, and Pete is concerned about how his gayness would affect his father's ministry. He has never discussed being gay with his parents and siblings. He is now concerned about his job at the hospital, where he works on the AIDS unit. At this time he has no physical complaints except feeling tired all the time.

(continued page 689)

Table 17–5

Nursing Diagnosis: Altered role performance related to changes in usual patterns of responsibility.
Goal: Client will acknowledge impact of HIV disease diagnosis on lifestyle and role performance.

Intervention	*Rationale*	*Expected Outcome*
Assess impact of client's illness on role performance	Assists in identifying role changes	Client verbalizes limitations in ability to function
Encourage client to discuss the impact of role changes on lifestyle	Assists in identifying client strengths and limitations	Client demonstrates ability to function within limitations
Actively listen to client concerns about treatment, progress, and prognosis	Assists client in accepting changes in role performance	Client verbalizes willingness to consider lifestyle changes
Include family and/or significant others in planning for care based on client's coping mechanisms, acknowledged limitations, and personal strengths	Assists in identifying potential changes in family role behaviors	Client identifies new roles for family and/or significant others to assist in lifestyle changes

Nursing Diagnosis: Altered thought process related to HIV-induced progressive dementia.
Goal: The client will demonstrate contact with reality evidenced by orientation to person, place, time, and situation.

Intervention	*Rationale*	*Expected Outcome*
Orient client as needed: • call client by preferred name • tell client your name • remind client of location • tell client the time, provide clocks and calendars	Assists client in maintaining contact with reality	Client states correct name Client indicates correct location Client states correct time Client states purpose of encounter with nurse
Provide a safe environment for client: • assist client with ambulation • use soft restraints if necessary • use adequate lighting • leave bed in low position and use side rails • keep frequently used items within client's reach and in same location	Prevents accidental injury when client is confused	Client is not injured Client states that he or she feels safe and free from harm

Nursing Diagnosis: Anticipatory grieving related to personal losses and potential loss of life.
Goal: The client will verbalize the meaning of perceived losses.

Intervention	*Rationale*	*Expected Outcome*
Assess client's phase of grief	Assists in determining client's immediate needs	Client verbalizes grief Client verbalizes significance of losses
Assist client, on her or her own terms, to progress through the grief stages: • denial • anger • bargaining • depression • acceptance	Allows for mutual goal setting	Client shares grief with a significant person

(Diagnosis continued)

Table 17–5 *(continued)*

Nursing Diagnosis *(continued)*: Anticipatory grieving related to personal losses and potential loss of life.
Goal: The client will verbalize the meaning of perceived losses.

Intervention	*Rationale*	*Expected Outcome*
Use therapeutic communication: • show concern • use active listening • point out irrational thoughts	Assists client in expressing thoughts	Client participates actively in communication
Observe and report suicidal/homicidal thoughts or actions	Prevents injury or harm to client and/or others	Client makes no suicidal/homicidal threats

Nursing Diagnosis: Anxiety related to life-threatening nature of diagnosis.
Goal: Client will begin to use new behaviors to cope.

Intervention	*Rationale*	*Expected Outcome*
Develop a supportive and trustful relationship with client	Encourages client to vent thoughts and feelings	Client verbalizes anxious thoughts and feelings
Assist client to recognize presence of anxiety (eg, somatic complaints)	Assists client to gain insight into anxiety reactions	Client verbalizes a decrease in somatic complaints
Maintain a calm, nonstimulating environment	Assists in reducing client anxiety	Client verbalizes a reduction in anxiety
Plan diversional activities • shopping • going to the movies • dancing • physical exercise	Assists in refocusing client's anxiety	Client makes plans for diversional activities
Teach new coping strategies: • reduction of irrational self-expectations • problem solving • assertiveness skills • muscle relaxation techniques • cognitive interventions • talking to others	Increases client's self-esteem	Client demonstrates new coping strategies

Nursing Diagnosis: Body image disturbance related to HIV disease–induced changes and/or losses.
Goal: Client will acknowledge changes in body appearance.

Intervention	*Rationale*	*Expected Outcome*
Develop a trusting relationship with client	Encourages client to vent feelings about body image	Client verbalizes body image concerns
Encourage client to verbalize physical and emotional changes in regard to body image	Assists client in acknowledging body image changes	Client states actual changes in appearance
Encourage client to continue daily grooming activities	Increases client's self-esteem	Client participates in grooming activities daily
Provide care with dignity, privacy, and in nonjudgmental manner	Assists in maintaining client's self-esteem	Client verbalizes personal strengths

(Diagnosis continued)

Table 17–5 *(continued)*

Intervention	*Rationale*	*Expected Outcome*
Help client identify lifestyle changes to increase role performance	Assists client in acknowledging body image changes	Client verbalizes impact of body image changes on lifestyle

Nursing Diagnosis: Fear related to the life-threatening nature of HIV disease.
Goal: Client will express reduced fear.

Intervention	*Rationale*	*Expected Outcome*
Assess for signs of fear: • pupil dilation • increased pulse, respirations, blood pressure • diaphoresis • agitation • crying	Early recognition of signs assists in reducing the reactions	Client verbalizes known sources of fear Client verbalizes fear of the unknown
Encourage client to express real and imagined threats to well-being: • be supportive and caring • stay with client • be honest • use open-ended questions	Assists client in feeling valued and gaining insight that reduces fear reactions	Client verbalizes comfort Client demonstrates behaviors that indicate reduced fear
When appropriate, encourage client to express fears about: • disease progression • body disfigurement • mental changes • ability to cope • discrimination related to stigma of disease prognosis • feelings about death • family matters	Assists client in identifying sources of fear and response pattern related to it	Client verbalizes specific fears

Nursing Diagnosis: Hopelessness related to apathy in response to HIV disease diagnosis.
Goal: Client will identify personal strengths in coping with disease process.

Intervention	*Rationale*	*Expected Outcome*
Assess factors contributing to hopelessness: • disease prognosis • loss of social supports • fear of death • body disfigurement • mental changes	Assists in increasing client's initiative	Client identifies personal strengths
Assess potential for suicide and institute suicide precautions as necessary: • provide 24-hour nurse • assign client to a room close to a nurse's station • remove harmful objects from room	Prevents client from harming self	Client expresses thoughts of suicide but makes no suicidal gestures

(Diagnosis continued)

Table 17–5 *(continued)*

Nursing Diagnosis *(continued)*: Hopelessness related to apathy in response to HIV disease diagnosis.
Goal: Client will identify personal strengths in coping with disease process.

Intervention	*Rationale*	*Expected Outcome*
Spend time with client to reinforce positive behaviors: • eye contact • self-disclosure • self-care activities • eating • not sleeping too long	Assists client in increasing self-worth	Client exhibits behaviors that reduce feelings of hopelessness

Nursing Diagnosis: Potential for ineffective family coping: disabling related to client's diagnosis and lifestyle.
Goal: Client and family will openly communicate about the stressors related to the HIV diagnosis.

Intervention	*Rationale*	*Expected Outcome*
Assess interaction between client and family in this situational crisis	Assists in planning more effective nursing actions	Client and family members identify conflicts
Encourage family members to discuss feelings about HIV diagnosis	Assists client and family members to recognize emotions related to loss	Client and family members express unresolved feelings
Provide privacy to facilitate family interactions	Encourages family interaction	Family members acknowledge need to privately discuss conflicts
Provide continuity of care by: • having family identify personal strengths • encourage family members to participate in client's care • refer family to support groups	Provides the support necessary for family to work through unresolved feelings	Client and family participate in treatment plan Family begins to discuss problems openly

Nursing Diagnosis: Potential for ineffective individual coping related to threat, usually denial, or HIV disease diagnosis.
Goal: Client will identify personal strengths to promote effective coping.

Intervention	*Rationale*	*Expected Outcome*
Assess client's past coping strategies and the effectiveness of these strategies	Assists in developing a more effective care plan	Client verbalizes preferred effective coping strategies
Assist client in identifying additional coping mechanisms: • planning diversional activities • verbalizing concerns • planning to accept or change current life situation • recognizing stage of grief	Will assist client in dealing with presenting stressors	Client participates in ADLs Client demonstrates interest in diversional activities Client participates in decision making Client states plan for accepting or changing situation

(continued)

Table 17–5 *(continued)*

Nursing Diagnosis: Knowledge deficit related to client's inaccurate perceptions of HIV disease diagnosis.
Goal: Client identifies need for information regarding disease progression, disease transmission, risk-reduction behaviors, and options for treatment and care.

Intervention	*Rationale*	*Expected Outcome*
Assess and document client's understanding of: • disease progression • disease transmission • risk-reduction behaviors • safe-sex guidelines • options for treatment and care	Assists in identifying information needed by client and reduces risk of transmission of HIV	Client identifies information needed
Develop a teaching plan for infection control prevention at home and in the community	Assists client in developing self-care behaviors	Client follows infection-control and prevention measures
Review available treatment and care options with client	Increases client's ability to follow prescribed treatment	Client participates in treatment plan Client demonstrates health care measures

Nursing Diagnosis: Powerlessness related to progressive debilitating HIV disease.
Goal: Client will demonstrate personal control over treatment decisions.

Intervention	*Rationale*	*Expected Outcome*
Develop a trusting relationship with client	Assists client in expressing feelings about his or her situation	Client verbalizes feelings of powerlessness
Encourage client to identify factors that contribute to feelings of powerlessness	Knowledge of contributing factors assists client in regaining control	Client identifies factors within his or her control
Involve client in decision making about care routine	Will assist client in control over self-care	Client participates in decision making regarding plan of care

Nursing Diagnosis: Sensory-perceptual alteration: visual, auditory related to neurologic alterations.
Goal: Client will interact appropriately within the environment.

Intervention	*Rationale*	*Expected Outcome*
Assess client's mental and neurologic status at each interaction	Baseline and ongoing assessments assist in detecting early neurologic changes	Client participates in assessments
Develop a plan of care to maximize abilities of client	Assists client in interacting with the environment more appropriately	Client demonstrates orientation to the environment
Provide a safe, supportive care environment: • provide dim lights • provide private room • limit visitors • establish rest periods • provide sensory input like clocks, radios, etc	Confused and disoriented clients are at increased risk of injury	Client is oriented to time, place, and person Client experiences no injuries

(continued)

Table 17–5 *(continued)*

Nursing Diagnosis: Sexual dysfunction related to fear of HIV transmission, contracting disease, and/or medical treatments, ie medications.
Goal: Client will gain a positive sexual self-concept by adhering to safe-sex practices.

Intervention	*Rationale*	*Expected Outcome*
Assess client's current sexual relationships in a nonjudgmental manner	HIV disease may be transmitted via sexual activities; client may be sensitive to judgmental attitudes and refuse to give vital baseline data	Client discusses concerns about current sexual relationships
Review safe-sex guidelines with client	Assists client in understanding transmission of HIV disease	Client verbalizes that safe-sex practices are used
Allow privacy to discuss client's sexual concerns	Encourages client to identify learning needs	Client verbalizes concerns about sexuality

Nursing Diagnosis: Situational low self-esteem related to negative feelings about self in response to HIV disease diagnosis.
Goal: Client will demonstrate behaviors that increase self-esteem.

Intervention	*Rationale*	*Expected Outcome*
Assess client's level of self-esteem	Assists in identifying influences on self-esteem	Client acknowledges low self-esteem
Encourage client to state feelings about self	Self-evaluation can assist in identifying personal strengths	Client verbalizes effects of diagnosis on self-esteem
Develop a plan of care to generate self-confidence: • assign a primary nurse • identify positive coping behaviors • give positive feedback on desired behaviors • teach coping behaviors (eg, seeking emotional support from others)	Provides client with an opportunity to bolster self-esteem	Client demonstrates behaviors that indicate self-confidence

Nursing Diagnosis: Social isolation related to stigma of disease and client's fears of casual contact resulting in infections.
Goal: Client will maintain social support system with others.

Intervention	*Rationale*	*Expected Outcome*
Assess client's support system	Assists in identifying resources and allows for correction of misconceptions about HIV disease	Client identifies friends, loved ones, care givers, and others who form his or her support system
Provide resources for counseling, support, and information services	Support services assist client and loved ones in coping with HIV disease	Client identifies community resources to assist in decreasing social isolation Client uses community resources
Provide time for client and family members to express feelings and concerns about social isolation induced by universal precautions	Understanding of universal precautions reduces feelings of being singled out from other clients	Client verbalizes an understanding of the need for universal precautions
Encourage staff, family, and loved ones to touch and hug the client	Physical contact decreases feelings of isolation and shows concern and caring	Client requests hugs from staff and loved ones

(continued)

Table 17–5 *(continued)*

Nursing Diagnosis: Potential for violence: self-directed related to a progressive central nervous system deterioration.
Goal: Client will not attempt to harm self.

Intervention	*Rationale*	*Expected Outcome*
Assess client behaviors that are indicative of impending self-harm (eg, suicidal ideations)	Assists in preventing client's self-harm	Client states impulses to commit self-harm
Encourage client to verbalize anger	Verbalizing anger reduces need to harm self	Client expresses anger
Initiate suicide precautions as necessary: • 24-hour nurse • room close to nurses' station • removal of harmful objects	Protects client from acting out self-harm	Client does not harm self

Table 17–6 *Example of Evaluation of a Nursing Care Plan for a Client with HIV Disease*

Plan	*Evaluation*
1. The client will assess a support group for HIV-seropositive people.	On 9/22 client went to a group meeting at the Gay Center. Afterward he stated, "I don't feel like I'm the only person with this problem."
2. The client will call and make an appointment with a physician to discuss his HIV status.	On 9/23 client met with his physician, had blood studies done, and set up another visit to review the results of the blood studies.
3. The client will begin to work through the grieving process.	On 9/23 client stated to nurse therapist, "I have to let my lover go. All I have is memories of our times together."

Nursing History

Location: Alternate HIV test site area
Client's name: Pete Hall Age: 23
Diagnosis: HIV seropositive

Health history
Height: 5′9″
Weight: 165 lbs
Eats 2 to 3 meals per day
Sleeps 6 to 7 hours per night
Never smoked, except marijuana occasionally with friends
Drinks occasional beer or wine

Social history
Had male lover for 5 years (recently died with AIDS)
Lives alone
Enjoys attending musicals and is involved with gay politics
Volunteers time for AIDS work

Clinical data
HIV Western Blot, positive test
Blood studies within normal limits except T cell count 425

Nursing observations
Pete is very talkative and self-discloses readily about his medical and social histories. Pete seems sad but not surprised when confronted with the fact that he is HIV seropositive. Pete goes on and talks about how much more effective he will be as a nurse, knowing he is HIV positive. He feels he will be much more supportive and empathetic with his clients now. Pete says he wants to get as much out of life as he can in the amount of time he has left.

Analysis/Synthesis of Data

Concerns	*Nursing diagnoses*
Inadequate support system	Anticipatory grieving
Dealing with grief and loss—in denial	Body image disturbance
Fear—of the unknown, loss of job, loss of insurance, discrimination	Ineffective individual coping
	Ineffective family coping: disabling
	Powerlessness
	Sexual dysfunction
	Social isolation

Suggested Care Planning Activities

1. Determine the priorities for Mr. Hall's care.
2. Identify the stage of grief exhibited by Mr. Hall.
3. Identify potential support systems available to Mr. Hall.
4. Describe Mr. Hall's learning needs.
5. Identify the nursing goals for Mr. Hall.
6. List and provide a rationale for nursing interventions in the care of Mr. Hall.

Homelessness

There are many reasons for homelessness. There is a high rate of unemployment and underemployment. Public support programs have been reduced. Low-cost housing is almost unavailable. The structure of the American family is changing. Deinstitutionalization of the mentally ill is also being blamed for homelessness among the mentally ill. A large number of policymakers at all levels of government contend that people choose to live on the street. This attitude underlies the current federal view of this social problem (Baxter and Hopper, 1984; Bobo, 1984; Riesdorph-Ostrow, 1989; Roth and Bean, 1986).

Whatever the reasons, the homeless have become a very visible social problem. This is especially true in urban areas, where the number of homeless people has not been as large since the Great Depression of the 1930s.

Description of Homelessness

Homelessness is more than a lack of a place to live. The homeless suffer from a lack of food, appropriate clothing, access to health care and social services, and educational opportunities (Fischer, 1986; Riesdorph-Ostrow, 1989).

Four subgroups of the homeless have been identified: the chronically mentally ill, chronic substance abusers, families with children, and adolescents on their own. For some, homelessness is the final stage in a life filled with crises. They may be homeless for an extended period of time. Others are briefly homeless because of a sudden crisis such as unemployment, eviction, or domestic upheaval.

With policies leading to deinstitutionalization, many of the **chronically mentally ill** were left without a place to live. State mental hospitals drastically reduced their populations and clients were returned to a community setting where alternative treatment facilities were not available. Compounding the problem was the lack of funding for community mental health centers, which were directed to provide inpatient and outpatient care, day care, outreach services, emergency services, consultation and education services, and specialized services for children, adolescents, and the elderly. The goal of supporting the chronically mentally ill within their own community has not been met. Many of the chronically mentally ill receive no social or medical services. Mental health authorities have been reluctant to make homelessness a "mental health problem" because doing so might result in reinstitutionalization of the client (Hyde, 1985; Riesdorph-Ostrow, 1989).

Chronic substance abusers may end up with no home if they are abandoned by families and friends. If the substance abuse has interfered with their ability to maintain a job, they may be forced to live on the streets.

Homeless families are the fastest growing portion of the homeless population in the United States. More families have become homeless as welfare programs, especially Aid to Families with Dependent Children, have been cut; food stamp and nutritional programs have been reduced, and affordable housing has become harder to find (Tower and White, 1989).

Many **adolescents** find themselves living on their own as a consequence of running away from or being thrown out by their families. Many adolescents who run away from home have been sexually or physically abused by a parent or other relative. (See chapter 16.) In other situations, parents of adolescents who are acting out by abusing drugs may feel helpless and threatened and force the adolescent out of the home as a way to regain control of their own lives. Adolescents also become homeless through family conflict, chaotic family systems, and changing family structure.

Incidence of Homelessness

Estimating the homeless population is difficult. Estimates range from 1 to 4 million homeless people in the United States. One-third to one-half of homeless people may be suffering from chronic mental disorders. Forty percent to 50 percent of this population abuse alcohol, while 10 percent to 15 percent abuse drugs. Some people may fit in all three of these categories. With a decreasing incidence of chronic alcoholism and an increasing incidence of mental illness, the average age of the homeless population has dropped from middle age to the early 30s. However, it is estimated that 10 percent of the homeless are over 60 years of age (Damrosch and Strasser, 1988; Emergency Medicine, 1989; Ryan, 1989).

Homeless families now account for over 40 percent of this population. It is estimated that there are 750,000 to 1 million children in homeless families. The number of adolescents living on their own is estimated to be between 100,000 and 400,000 (Tower and White, 1989).

Knowledge Base: Homelessness

Behavioral Characteristics

With no place to live and limited or no financial resources, homeless people are often forced to steal or scavenge for food, and to panhandle for money for food. Community sources for free meals may serve only one meal a day.

Shelter may consist of any protection from the elements, including underneath bridges, cars, abandoned buildings, all-night cafes, airports, bus stations, and other public places, shelters or missions, cheap hotels or motels, and living with friends. Homeless people may commit minor crimes in order to stay in jail overnight. If there is no shelter, a homeless person may sleep on a park bench or on a steam grate.

Given the lack of basic necessities like food and shelter, many homeless people have difficulty in coping with ADLs. Providing basic hygiene may be impossible. Finding appropriate clothing for the climate may be very difficult. Protection from rain, cold, and snow is often a problem.

The chronically mentally ill may discontinue taking medications, either purposefully or because they lack resources to obtain needed medication. Some turn to alcohol or drugs in an attempt to self-medicate their psychiatric symptoms. If they do come in contact with the health care system, they may be unable to follow through on referrals for psychiatric care (Ryan, 1989).

Affective Characteristics

Society perceives the homeless as failures. Many homeless people feel that their lives are out of control and they feel hopeless and helpless about the future. Many are immobilized by severe depression and may not be able to summon the energy to follow a plan that would result in finding a home. Others suffer from multiple fears, suspicions, and paranoid thoughts which interfere with asking for help from support services in the community. Homeless children suffer feelings of humiliation if they are teased or ridiculed by other children about the way they look or their lack of a home (Gonzales-Osler, 1989; Lamb, 1990; Tower and White, 1989).

Cognitive Characteristics

The chronically mentally ill may prefer the autonomy of living on the streets to suffering further indignities in nursing or board and care homes where staff provides depersonalized care and treats the client with disrespect. This may be an effort to protect their self-esteem (Ryan, 1989).

The chronically mentally ill may experience

hallucinations and delusions. Disorganized thought processes may interfere with finding food, shelter, and community services. Some may not be able to keep their attention on a problem or may have such limited problem solving skills that they are unable to find help (Lamb, 1990).

Homelessness contributes to low self-esteem. Many homeless people are overwhelmed with feelings of incompetence. Children need to feel successful and be able to relate on an equal level with other children in an overall environment of stability to develop self-esteem. Those conditions are not available to homeless children. Adolescents who have run away from home because of physical or sexual abuse have not had the opportunity to develop positive self-esteem. Homeless adults suffer from a battered self-esteem as others shun them or talk negatively about them in their presence.

Sociocultural Characteristics

Families facing homelessness may be fragmented. Parents may choose to leave young children with relatives, friends, or with social service agencies rather than subjecting them to life on the street. This is very disruptive to the continuity of the bonding process and the development of a sense of family.

Forty percent of homeless children do not attend school regularly. Transportation to get to school may be a problem. Many shelters allow families to stay for relatively short periods of time, typically 30 to 90 days, so children have to transfer from school to school. When they do attend school, they may be teased or ridiculed by their peers because they aren't clean or are wearing inappropriate or odd clothing.

The stigma of homelessness makes homeless people poor advocates for themselves and they are very vulnerable to the effects of the social environment. It is very easy for others to look down on or completely ignore homeless people. Where services are provided, it is not always easy to take advantage of this help because of bureaucratic red tape. The chronically mentally ill may not be able to organize their thoughts long enough to negotiate the bureaucratic system.

Physiologic Characteristics

There are many physiologic problems which are directly related to homelessness. Homeless people are more likely to become ill because of exposure to the elements, stress, substance abuse, and overcrowded conditions at shelters and missions. Homeless children are three times as likely as other children to have medical problems. The problems of illness are compounded because the homeless are the least likely to be able to care for themselves when they are ill (Emergency Medicine, 1989; Tower and White, 1989).

Rates of tuberculosis among the homeless are 50 to 500 times higher than the general population. Other medical problems occuring in the homeless population are AIDS, lice and scabies, peripheral vascular disease, and hypertension. Many suffer from dietary problems such as nutritional and vitamin deficiencies. Those who must scavenge for their food are at risk for food poisoning. There is a high incidence of trauma from beatings, stabbings, falls, and motor vehicle accidents. Environmental conditions often lead to conditions such as trench foot, frostbite, hypothermia, and burns from sleeping on steam grates (Damrosch and Strasser, 1988; Emergency Medicine, 1989; Tower and White, 1989). See Table 17–7 for an overview of characteristics of the homeless population.

The Role of the Mental Health Nurse

Mental health professionals often avoid dealing with the mentally ill homeless (Minkoff, 1987). As Hombs and Snyder (1986) explains, several myths about the homeless support this lack of interest on the part of mental health professionals:

- Homelessness is the lifestyle of choice for the homeless

Table 17–7 *Characteristics of the Homeless Population*

Behavioral	*Affective*	*Cognitive*	*Sociocultural*	*Physiologic*
Steal food	Hopeless	Need for autonomy	Families separated	TB
Scavange for food	Helpless	Hallucination	Lack of education for children	AIDS
Panhandle	Severe depression	Delusions	Stigma	Lice and scabies
Variety of shelters	Fears	Disorganized thoughts		Peripheral vascular disease
Poor hygiene	Suspicions	Decreased attention span		Nutritional deficiencies
Inappropriate clothing	Humiliation	Limited problem solving		Food poisoning
Discontinue medications		Low self-esteem		Hypertension
Self-medicate with alcohol/ drugs				Trauma
				Trench foot
				Frostbite
				Hypothermia
				Burns

- Most homeless people are lazy and shiftless drunks or transients
- Most homeless people are unwilling to help themselves.

The federal government has developed several pilot programs in which the chronically mentally ill in the community are receiving health care from Veterans Administration medical centers. A nurse makes daily visits to sites where the homeless gather—soup kitchens, parks, streets, bridges, and riverbeds. He or she assesses the situation of the homeless individual through interviews and establishes a relationship with each person. After evaluation, the individual may be referred to programs within the Veterans Administration and the community. Attention is given to basic needs first and then to other treatment concerns (Gullberg, 1989).

Street outreach is a mechanism for treating the mentally ill homeless. An important part of street outreach is the mobility of the street outreach team that links individuals to shelters. Once in a shelter, the homeless individual can be assessed for potential for employment and residential options. Part of the rehabilitation program may include securing Supplemental Security Income (SSI) benefits if the person is unable to work. One difficulty is that a home mailing address is required in order to receive SSI benefits. Crisis intervention services should also be made available (Kellerman et al, 1985; Riesdorph-Ostrow, 1989).

Assessment: Homelessness

When the homeless individual comes into the mental health or health care system, homelessness should be identified on admission. Nurses should assess clients for indicators of homelessness. In addition to living accommodations, the nurse should be able to make some general observations that may signify homelessness. Homeless people may appear unkempt. Many clients wear everything they own or they may carry all their possessions with them. Homeless clients often have skin problems because of lack of facilities for basic cleanliness. The homeless client may not be specific about his or her dietary pattern, sleep pattern, and hygiene practices. His or her primary motivation for coming in for treatment may be to receive food and shelter for a few days.

Nursing Diagnosis and Treatment: Homelessness

Regardless of the reasons for homelessness and the issues involved in identifying homelessness as a social or a mental problem, homeless people need to have their basic needs met. They need adequate shelter, food, health care, schooling, job training, and other services to assist them in becoming participating members of society. A long-term solution to the problem of homelessness is imperative. See Table 17–8 for referral agencies.

Although many nursing diagnoses apply to the homeless client, three primary nursing diagnoses are applicable: alteration in health maintenance, self-care deficit, and social isolation. Planning for the homeless client requires collaboration and referral to a variety of services. Referrals depend on the nature of the problems the client presents. Table 17–9 presents a nursing care plan for the homeless client.

Table 17–8 *Sources of Help for the Homeless*

National Coalition for the Homeless
105 East 22nd Street
New York, NY 10010
212-460-8110

Child Welfare League of America
440 First Street, NW
Washington DC 20001
202-638-2952

Center for Law and Education, Inc.
14 Appian Way
Cambridge, MA 02138
617-495-4666

Evaluation: Homelessness

Evaluation for the homeless client is subjective. Perhaps the best measure of success is being able to keep the client in a treatment program or find adequate community resources to meet the client's basic needs. Homeless mentally ill individuals are a hard-to-reach group. In the future it may be necessary for the government to fund an agency that oversees the needs of the homeless. The mental health system would cooperate with that agency to provide needed services to the client. It will also be necessary to fund programs to provide low cost housing for individuals and families as well as develop methods to keep homeless children in the school system. Nurses can function as providers of care as well as advocates on the community, state, and federal level.

CASE EXAMPLE

A Homeless Client

Jerry, a 19-year-old unemployed dishwasher, was admitted to the general hospital for thrombophlebitis of his left lower extremity. Jerry was labeled as a difficult client because he kept disconnecting his IV heparin and leaving the hospital. Jerry asked for extra portions of food for every meal. The security guard discovered Jerry's 17-year-old wife and 1-year-old baby in an old car in the hospital parking lot. Jerry confessed that he and his family had been living in the car for about 3 months. When he lost his job as a dishwasher, they did not have enough money to keep the small apartment they had been living in. Jerry had been sneaking food to his wife and baby, because they had no money to buy food. The nurse on duty called a local church so Jerry's wife and baby could be housed until Jerry recovered. Jerry's case was referred to social services.

Table 17–9 *Nursing Care Plan for the Homeless Client*

Nursing Diagnosis: Alteration in health maintenance related to the situational factor of homelessness.
Goal: Identifies resources to assist in meeting daily needs.

Intervention	*Rationale*	*Expected Outcome*
Assess present situation	Assists in identification of potential solutions	Client cites available resources
Assist client in identifying a plan for using available resources	Knowledge of available resources provides potential solutions to client's problems	Client contacts community resources
Provide referrals to resources	Referrals support client effectiveness and provide advocacy	

Nursing Diagnosis: Self-care deficit related to inability to obtain food, water, clothing, and toilet facilities.
Goal: Uses all available personal and community resources.

Intervention	*Rationale*	*Expected Outcome*
Assist client in identifying items for basic necessities	Identifying needs assists in locating potential resources	Client identifies items needed for completing ADLs
Assist client in developing a plan for meeting own self-care needs	Involving client increases likelihood of compliance	Client identifies community resources for meeting self-care needs
Make referrals to social service programs	Social service programs may be able to provide client with assistance in obtaining self-care necessities	

Nursing Diagnosis: Social isolation related to extreme poverty.
Goal: The client interacts with others.

Intervention	*Rationale*	*Expected Outcome*
Assess client's perception of isolation	Client may not perceive social isolation as a problem	Client states degree of involvement with others
Have client identify support system	A support system is important to client's ability to function within a social setting	Client identifies major persons in support system
Assist client in identifying his or her own positive characteristics	A positive self-image and feelings of self-worth enhance social interactions	Client identifies positive self-identity
Assist client in identifying factors necessary to reduce social isolation (eg, job skills, training, assistance programs)	Identifying ways to reduce poverty will assist client in progressing toward greater social skills	Client identifies strengths and weaknesses in social interactions

Nursing History

Location: General Hospital, medical floor
Client's name: Jerry Lindsay Age: 19
Admitting diagnosis: Thrombophlebitis
T = 100.2, P = 100, R = 18, B/P = 120/70

Health History
Height: 5′9″
Weight: 135 lbs
Refused to give history on number of meals and sleeping habits
Denied smoking or drinking

Social History
Married for almost 2 years
Has a 1-year-old child
Unemployed

Clinical data
PTT 19 seconds

Nursing observations
Jerry appears preoccupied and anxious. He had to be reminded over and over not to have his wife and baby at the bedside outside of regular visiting hours. After the guard reported seeing Jerry go to an old car in the parking lot, Jerry finally admitted to the nurse that his wife and baby were living in the car.

Analysis/Synthesis of Data

Concerns	*Nursing diagnoses*
Poor response to treatment	Alteration in health maintenance
Lack of understanding of condition	Self-care deficit
Inadequate rest	Social isolation
Poor coping mechanisms	

Suggested Care Planning Activities

1. Determine the priorities for Mr. Lindsay's care.
2. Determine support systems available for Mr. Lindsay and his family.
3. Identify nursing goals for Mr. Lindsay's care.
4. Describe the teaching Mr. Lindsay must receive for him to recover.
5. List and provide a rationale for nursing interventions in Mr. Lindsay's care.

Future Directions in Mental Health Nursing

The special issues discussed in this chapter and others that remain undiscovered will shape mental health nursing practice in the future. The major determinants of future practice are economic environment, consumer characteristics and needs, expanded roles for psychiatric and mental health nurses as they create standards for the quality of nursing care, the number of nurses in the health care system, and the education nurses receive before assuming their professional roles (Aiken, 1982).

There will be less and less money available to the health care system. Jaynes (1989) predicts that, with current spending rates, Medicare will run out of money by 2015. Consumer advocates are lobbying for catastrophic health insurance, and Americans will more than likely have some type of national health insurance that will cover mental health care. Consumers will more than likely look to nurses rather than doctors in some situations for the greater economic value nurses can produce (Fagin, 1981).

Mental health services in the future are likely to continue to be increasingly in the community, with the two largest groups of clients being the chronically mentally ill and the aging. The chronically ill group will most likely consist of those persons with major psychiatric disorders such as schizophrenia and affective disorders—the clients who are in need of psychotropic drugs. Because most acutely ill psychiatric clients will be treated in community-based facilities, discharge planning will become crucial in planning adequate follow-up care. Mental health nurses will need to play a significant liaison role in maintaining clients in the community environment (Robinson, 1986).

Other changes to the role of mental health nurses will involve the reintegration of physical nursing skills in mental health practice. A growing convergence of biologic and behavioral sciences—neuropharmacology, neuroanatomy, neurophysiology, neuroendocrinology, and neurochemistry—will continue to affect the management of clients. Education needs to focus on behavior issues, psychologic appraisal, sociopsychologic techniques, evaluation of concomitant physical problems, and management of psychoactive drugs (Christman, 1987; Fagin, 1981; Mitsunaga, 1982). The psychiatric or mental health nurse will need an advanced degree to function in his or her expanded role, which will involve increased responsibility and autonomy (Mechanic, 1982). As nurses become better prepared, more multidisciplinary care models will be developed to benefit the client (Christman, 1987).

SUMMARY

1. The two most perplexing problems facing mental health in the immediate future are the AIDS epidemic and the problem of homelessness.

HIV Disease

2. Acquired immunodeficiency syndrome (AIDS) has become one of the most complex public health problems

in the nation's history. The disease was first reported in 1981.

3. AIDS is caused by the human immunodeficiency virus (HIV) and is transmitted by two major routes: sexual transmission, and direct blood-to-blood contact (e.g., sharing IV needles, receiving blood transfusions, or HIV-infected pregnant women transferring the virus to their fetuses.

4. There is no cure for AIDS. Over half the people who have contracted AIDS have died.

5. The role of mental health nurses is to provide supportive care with frequent assessments of mental status related to behavioral, affective, and social changes.

6. Major behavioral changes are sluggishness, unsteady gait, and muscular tension. Later the person may become depressed and socially isolated.

7. Major affective reactions are anxiety, grief, and loss. Also, there may be self-blame and guilt.

8. Major cognitive characteristics are forgetfulness, concentration difficulties, and slowness of thought. When neurologic involvement is exacerbated, dementia, hallucinations, and delusional thinking may occur.

9. Parental reactions to the AIDS diagnosis are an important sociocultural concern. Other major concerns are finding housing, financial assistance, and adequate support services.

10. Supportive care is very important for lovers and families of HIV-infected persons. Attention to the needs of care givers is also a concern.

11. At present, AIDS is considered a cell-mediated and humoral immunity disorder caused by HIV. The virus affects the immune system's functions by altering the genetic makeup of the T cells, or helper lymphocytes. The result is the replication of the HIV instead of the T cells.

12. The goals of treatment are assisting the client to come to terms with the diagnosis, increasing the client's quality of life, and assisting the client to feel more in control of life.

The Problem of Homelessness

13. There are many reasons for homelessness, including high rates of underemployment/unemployment, decreases in public support programs, lack of low-cost housing, changes in the structure of American families, and deinstitutionalization of the mentally ill.

14. Homeless people not only lack a place to live but also suffer from a lack of food, clothing, health care services, social services, and educational opportunities.

15. There are anywhere from 1 million to 4 million homeless people in the United States.

16. One-third to one-half of homeless people may suffer from chronic mental disorders.

17. Families are the fastest growing portion of the homeless population in the United States, and account for over 40 percent of the homeless population. These families include 750,000 to 1 million homeless children.

18. Runaway and throwaway adolescents living on the streets number between 100,000 and 400,000.

19. Life on the streets may include stealing to buy food or scavenging for food, living in temporary shelters, and limited access to hygienic facilities.

20. Affective characteristics of homeless people include hopelessness, helplessness, severe depression, multiple fears, suspicions, and humiliation.

21. Cognitive characteristics of homeless people may include attempts to achieve autonomy, low self-esteem, hallucinations, and delusions.

22. Sociocultural characteristics of the homeless include families driven apart, lack of schooling for children, social stigma, and difficulty dealing with the bureaucratic system.

23. Physiologic characteristics of the homeless include TB, AIDS, lice and scabies, peripheral vascular disease, hypertension, nutritional deficiencies, food poisoning, trauma, trench foot, frostbite, hypothermia, and burns.

24. Homeless children are three times as likely as other children to have medical problems.

25. Street outreach is a mechanism for treating the mentally ill homeless.

26. Three primary nursing diagnoses apply to the homeless: alteration in health maintenance, self-care deficit, and social isolation.

27. The major determinants of future practice in psychiatric and mental health nursing are the economic environment, consumer characteristics and needs, the expanded roles for nurses, the numbers of nurses available, and the nursing education nurses receive.

CHAPTER REVIEW

1. Which one of the following best describes the cause of AIDS?
   (a) Direct blood-to-blood contact
   (b) Pregnant woman transferring blood to fetus
   (c) The human immunodeficiency virus
   (d) Bacterial infection of the nervous system

2. The primary goal of the mental health nurse in working with the AIDS client is
   (a) Client education
   (b) Support

(c) Palliative treatment
(d) Behavioral treatment

3. The fastest growing population of homeless people in the United States is:
(a) Families
(b) Adolescents
(c) Chronic substance abusers
(d) Chronically mentally ill

4. One of the main sociocultural problems facing homeless children is:
(a) Frostbite and hypothermia
(b) Decreased self-esteem
(c) Severe depression
(d) School nonattendance

REFERENCES

Aiken L: *The Impact of Federal Health Policy on Nurses.* In: *Nursing in the 1980's.* Aiken L (editor). Lippincott, 1982.

American Nurses' Association: *Professional Heroism, Professional Activism: Nursing and the Battle Against AIDS.* American Nurses' Association, 1988.

American Red Cross: *Public AIDS Education Presenter's Program.* American Red Cross, 1988.

Barrick B: The willingness of nursing personnel to care for patients with acquired immune deficiency syndrome: A survey study and recommendations. *J Prof Nurs* 1988; 4:366–372.

Bateson MC, Goldsby R: *Thinking AIDS: The Social Response to Biological Threat.* Addison-Wesley, 1988.

Baxter E, Hopper K: *Private Lives/Public Spaces: Homeless Adults on the Streets of New York.* Community Service Society, 1984.

Black PH: HTLV-III, AIDS, and the Brain. *N Engl J Med* 1985; 313:1538–1540.

Bobo BF: *A Report to the Secretary on the Homeless and Emergency Shelters.* US Department of Housing and Urban Development, 1984.

Carpenito LJ: *Handbook of Nursing Diagnosis,* 2nd ed. Lippincott, 1987.

Christman L: Psychiatric nurses and the practice of psychotherapy: Current status and future possibilities. *Am J Psychother* (July) 1987; 51:384–390.

Classification system for human T-lymphotrophic virus type III/lymphadenopathy-associated virus infections. *Morbidity and Mortality Weekly Report,* CDC. 1986; 35:335.

Damrosch S, Strasser JA: The homeless elderly in America. *Gerontological Nurs.* 1988. 14(10):26–29.

Diamond R: N.Y. Homeless seek shelter underground: Desperate residents call subway home. *San Francisco Examiner* (Feb 5) 1989; A5.

Doenges ME, Townsend MC, Moorhouse MF: *Psychiatric Care Plans.* Davis, 1989.

Douglas C, Kalman C, and Kalman T: Homophobia among physicians and nurses: An empirical study. *Hosp Community Psychiatry,* 1985; 36:1309–1310.

With neither home nor health. *Emergency Medicine.* Feb. 28, 1989. 21(4):21–46.

Fagin C: Psychiatric Nursing at the Crossroads: Quo Vadis. *Perspec Psychiatr Care,* 1981; 19:99–106.

Fischer PJ et al.: Mental health and social characteristics of the homeless: A survey of mission users. *Am J Public Health* (May) 1986; 76:519–523.

Flaskerud JH: AIDS: Psychosocial aspects. *J Psychosoc Nurs* 1987; 25:9–16.

Fletcher J: Homosexuality: Kick and kickback. *Southern Medical Journal* 1984; 77:149–150.

Gonzales-Osler E: Coping with transition. *J Psychosoc Nurs.* 1989. 27(6):29–33.

Green J: Counseling HTLV-III seropositives. In: *The Management of AIDS Patients.* Miller D, Weber J, Green J (editors). Macmillan, 1986. 151–168.

Gullberg PL: The homeless chronically mentally ill: A psychiatric nurse's role. *J Psychosoc Nurs* (June) 1989; 27:9–13.

Herrick CA, Smith JE: *Ethical Dilemmas and AIDS: Nursing Issues Regarding Rights and Obligations.* Unpublished manuscript, 1988.

Holland JC, Tross S: Psychosocial and neuropsychiatric sequelae of the acquired immunodeficiency syndrome and related disorders. *Ann Intern Med* 1985; 103: 760–764.

Hombs ME, Snyder M: *Homelessness in America: A Forced March to Nowhere.* Community for Creative Nonviolence, 1986.

Hyde PS: Homelessness: A state mental health director's perspective. *Psychosoc Rehab J* 1985; 8:21–24.

Jaynes G: 2000: Visions of tomorrow. *Life* (Feb) 1989; 12:50–78.

Kellerman SL, et al.: Psychiatry and the homeless: Problems and programs. In: *Health Care of Homeless People,* Brickner PW, et al. (editors). Springer, 1985.

Kelly JA, et al.: Nurses' attitudes toward AIDS. *J Contin Educ Nurs* 1988; 2:78–83.

Kelly JA, St. Lawrence JS: *The AIDS Health Crisis: Psychological and Social Interventions.* Plenum, 1988.

Kubler-Ross E: Five stages a dying patient goes through. *Medical Economics* (Sept 14) 1970; 272–292.

Lamb HR, Lamb DM: Factors contributing to homelessness among the chronically and severely mentally ill. *Hosp and Community Psychiatry.* 1990. 41(3): 301–305.

Levy RM, Bredesen DE, Resenblum M: Neurological manifestations of the acquired immunodeficiency syndrome (AIDS): Experience at UCSF and review of the literature. *J Neurosurgery* 1985; 62:475–495.

Marshall TA, Nieckarz JP: Bereavement counseling: Unique factors call for unique approaches. *AIDS Patient Care* (Apr) 1988; 2:13–15.

Mechanic D: Nursing and mental health care: Expanding future possibilities for nursing service. In: *Nursing in the 1980's.* Aiken L (editor). Lippincott, 1982.

Miller D: Psychology, AIDS, ARC, and PGL. In: *The Management of AIDS Patients.* Miller D, Weber J, Green J (editors). Macmillan, 1986. 131–149.

Minkoff K: Resistance of mental health professionals to working with the chronically mentally ill. In: *Barriers to Treating the Chronically Mentally Ill: New Directions for Mental Health Services.* Meyerson AT (editor). Jossey-Bass, 1987.

Mitsunaga B: Designing Psychiatric/mental health nursing for the future: Problems and prospects. *J Psychosoc Nurs* 1982; 20:15–21.

National Academy Press: *Confronting AIDS: Update 1988.* Institute of Medicine, National Academy of Sciences, National Academy Press, 1988.

Norman C: Politics and science clash on African AIDS. *Science* 1985; 230:1140–1142.

Nursing and Health Care: Foundation announces $17.2 million for AIDS health services. *Nurs Health Care* 1986; 7:186.

Pheiffer WG, Houseman C: Bereavement and AIDS: A framework for intervention. *J Psychosoc Nurs* 1988; 26:21–26.

Pothier PC: The future of psychiatric nursing—revisited. *Arch Psychiatr Nurs* (Oct) 1987; 1:299–300.

Puckett SB, Emery AR: *Managing AIDS in the Workplace.* Addison-Wesley, 1988.

Recommendations for preventing transmission of infection with human T-lymphotropic virus type III/lymphadenopathy—associated virus in the workplace. *Morbidity and Mortality Weekly Report* 1985; 34:682–686, 691–695.

Riesdorph-Ostrow W: The homeless chronically mentally ill: Deinstitutionalization: A public policy perspective. *J Psychosoc Nurs* (June) 1989; 27:4–7.

Robinson L: The future of psychiatric/mental health nursing. *Nurs Clin North Am* (Sept) 1986; 21:537–543.

Roth D, Bean GJ: New perspectives on homelessness: Findings from a statewide epidemiological study. *Hosp Community Psychiatry* (July) 1986; 37:712–719.

Roth D, Bean G, Hyde PS: Homelessness and mental health policy: Developing an appropriate role for the 1980s. *Community Ment Health J* (Fall) 1986; 22:203–214.

Rothstein MA: Screening workers for AIDS. In: *AIDS and the Law: A Guide for the Public.* Dalton HL, Burris, Yale AIDS Law Project (editors). Yale University Press, 1987.

Ryan MT: Providing shelter. *J Psychosoc Nurs.* 1989. 27(6):15–18.

Singer M: AIDS in Africa: Transmission and prevention. *AIDS Patient Care,* 1988; 2:13–15.

Sipes C: AIDS: The haunting facts, the human care. *Nurs Life* (Mar/Apr) 1988; 34–38.

Smith JE: *Female Nurses' Attitudes Regarding Male Homosexuals.* Unpublished thesis, University of Southern Mississippi, 1981.

Smith JE: The role of the nurse in the AIDS epidemic. *ASNA Reporter* (July) 1988.

Strawn J: The psychosocial consequences of AIDS. In: *The Person with AIDS: Nursing Perspectives.* Durham JD, Cohen FL (editors). Springer, 1987. 126–149.

Tower CC, White DJ: *Homeless Students.* National Education Association, 1989.

US Department of Health and Human Services: *The Report of the Presidential Commission on the Human Immunodeficiency Virus Epidemic.* US Department of Health and Human Services, 1988.

Viele CS, Dodd MJ, Morrison C: Caring for the acquired immune deficiency syndrome patient. *Oncol Nurs Forum,* 1984; 11:56–60.

Wolcott D: Neuropsychiatric syndromes in AIDS and AIDS-related illnesses. In: *What to Do About AIDS: Physicians and Mental Health Professionals Discuss the Issues.* McKusick L (editor). The University of California Press, 1986.

Wolcott D, Fawzy F, Pasnau R: Acquired immune deficiency syndrome (AIDS) and consultation-liaison psychiatry. *General Hospital Psychiatry,* 1985; 7:280–292.

SUGGESTED READINGS

Benner P, Wrubel J: *The Primacy of Caring: Stress and Coping in Health and Illness.* Addison-Wesley, 1989.

Connolly PM: The homeless chronically mentally ill: Strategies for improving education. *J Psychosoc Nurs* (June) 1989; 27:24–28.

Goode EE: How psychiatry forgets the mind . . . many psychiatrists are abandoning the traditional "talking cure" for high-tech brain scans and powerful new drugs. *US News and World Report* (Mar 21) 1988; 104:56–58.

Hoff LA: *People in Crisis: Understanding and Helping*, 3rd ed. Addison-Wesley, 1989.

Maurin JT, et al.: The homeless chronically mentally ill: Obstacles to research analysis. *J Psychosoc Nurs* (June) 1989; 27:19–23.

Peplau HE: Future directions in Psychiatric nursing from the perspective of history. *J Psychosoc Nurs* (Feb) 1989; 27:18–28.

Richardson D: *Women and AIDS*. Methuen, 1988.

Shilts R: *And The Band Played On: Politics, People and the AIDS Epidemic*. St. Martin's, 1987.

Smith JP: Nursing and health care in the twentieth Century: Myth, reality and dichotomy. *J Adv Nurs* (Mar) 1986; 11:127–132.

Smoyak SA: *Windows*. *J Psychosoc Nurs* (June) 1989; 27:3.

DSM-III-R Classification: Axes I–V

All official DSM-III-R codes are included in ICD-9-CM. Codes followed by an asterisk (*) are used for more than one DSM-III-R diagnosis or subtype in order to maintain compatibility with ICD-9-CM.

Following a diagnostic term, a long rule on the baseline (________) indicates the need for a fifth digit subtype or other qualifying term.

The term *specify* following the name of some diagnostic categories indicates qualifying terms that clinicians may wish to add in parentheses after the name of the disorder.

NOS = Not Otherwise Specified

The current severity of a disorder may be specified after the diagnosis as

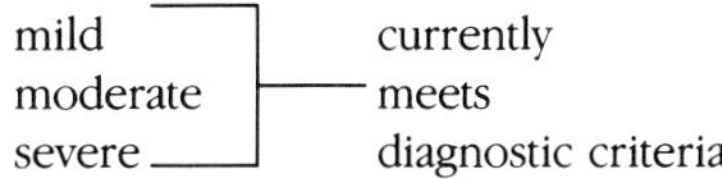

in partial remission (or residual state)
in complete remission

Source: Adapted from American Psychiatric Association, *Diagnostic and Statistical Manual of Mental Disorders,* 3rd ed., revised (Washington DC: American Psychiatric Association, 1987).

Axes I and II: Categories and Codes

- Disorders Usually First Evident in Infancy, Childhood, or Adolescence
- Developmental Disorders

Note: These are coded on Axis II.

Mental Retardation

317.00 Mild mental retardation
318.00 Moderate mental retardation
318.10 Severe mental retardation
318.20 Profound mental retardation
319.00 Unspecified mental retardation

Pervasive Developmental Disorders

299.00 Autistic disorder (*specify* if childhood onset)
299.80 Pervasive developmental disorder NOS

Specific Developmental Disorders

Academic skills disorders

315.10 Developmental arithmetic disorder
315.80 Developmental expressive writing disorder
315.00 Developmental reading disorder

Language and speech disorders

315.39 Developmental articulation disorder
315.31* Developmental expressive language disorder
315.31* Developmental receptive language disorder

Motor skills disorders

315.40 Developmental coordination disorder
315.90* Specific developmental disorder NOS

Other Developmental Disorders

315.90* Developmental disorder NOS

Disruptive Behavior Disorders

314.01 Attention-deficit hyperactivity disorder

Conduct disorder

312.20 Group type
312.00 Solitary aggressive type
312.90 Undifferentiated type
313.81 Oppositional defiant disorder

Anxiety Disorders of Childhood or Adolescence

309.21 Separation anxiety disorder
313.21 Avoidant disorder of childhood or adolescence
313.00 Overanxious disorder

Eating Disorders

307.10 Anorexia nervosa
307.51 Bulimia nervosa
307.52 Pica
307.53 Rumination disorder of infancy
307.50 Eating disorder NOS

Gender Identity Disorders

302.60 Gender identity disorder of childhood
302.50 Transsexualism (*specify* sexual history: asexual, homosexual, heterosexual, unspecified)
302.85* Gender identity disorder of adolescence or adulthood, nontranssexual type (*specify* sexual history: asexual, homosexual, heterosexual, unspecified)
302.85* Gender identity disorder NOS

Tic Disorders

307.23 Tourette's disorder
307.22 Chronic motor or vocal tic disorder
307.21 Transient tic disorder (*specify:* single episode or recurrent)
307.20 Tic disorder NOS

Elimination Disorders

307.70 Functional encopresis (*specify:* primary or secondary type)
307.60 Functional enuresis (*specify:* primary or secondary type; *specify:* nocturnal only, diurnal only, nocturnal and diurnal)

Speech Disorders Not Elsewhere Classified

307.00* Cluttering
307.00* Stuttering

Other Disorders of Infancy, Childhood, or Adolescence

313.23 Elective mutism
313.82 Identity disorder
313.89 Reactive attachment disorder of infancy or early childhood
307.30 Stereotypy/habit disorder
314.00 Undifferentiated attention-deficit disorder

Organic Mental Disorders

Dementias Arising in the Senium and Presenium

Primary degenerative dementia of the Alzheimer's type, senile onset
(Note code 331.00 Alzheimer's disease on Axis III.)

290.30 With delirium
290.20 With delusions
290.21 With depression
290.00* Uncomplicated

Code in fifth digit:
1 = with delirium, 2 = with delusions, 3 = with depression, 0* = uncomplicated

290.1x Primary degenerative dementia of the Alzheimer's type, presenile onset, ________
(Note code 331.00 Alzheimer's disease on Axis III.)
290.4x Multi-infarct dementia, ________
290.00* Senile dementia NOS (*specify:* etiology on Axis III if known)
290.10* Presenile dementia NOS (*specify:* etiology on Axis III if known, e.g., Pick's disease, Creutzfeldt-Jakob disease)

Psychoactive Substance–Induced Organic Mental Disorders

Alcohol

303.00 Intoxication
291.40 Idiosyncratic intoxication

291.80 Uncomplicated alcohol withdrawal
291.00 Withdrawal delirium
291.30 Hallucinosis
291.10 Amnestic disorder
291.20 Dementia associated with alcoholism

Amphetamine or similarly acting sympathomimetic

305.70* Intoxication
292.00* Withdrawal
292.81* Delirium
292.11* Delusional disorder

Caffeine

305.90* Intoxication

Cannabis

305.20* Intoxication
292.11* Delusional disorder

Cocaine

305.60* Intoxication
292.00* Withdrawal
292.81* Delirium
292.11* Delusional disorder

Hallucinogen

305.30* Hallucinosis
292.11* Delusional disorder
292.84* Mood disorder
292.89* Posthallucinogen perception disorder

Inhalant

305.90* Intoxication

Nicotine

292.00* Withdrawal

Opioid

305.50* Intoxication
292.00* Withdrawal

Phencyclidine (PCP) or similarly acting arylcyclohexylamine

305.90* Intoxication
292.81* Delirium
292.11* Delusional disorder
292.84* Mood disorder
292.90* Organic mental disorder NOS

Sedative, hypnotic, or anxiolytic

305.40* Intoxication
292.00* Uncomplicated sedative, hypnotic, or anxiolytic withdrawal
292.00* Withdrawal delirium
292.83* Amnestic disorder

Other or unspecified psychoactive substance

305.90* Intoxication
292.00* Withdrawal
292.81* Delirium
292.82* Dementia
292.83* Amnestic disorder
292.11* Delusional disorder
292.12 Hallucinosis
292.84* Mood disorder
292.89* Anxiety disorder
292.89* Personality disorder
292.90* Organic mental disorder NOS

Organic Mental Disorders associated with Axis III physical disorders or conditions, or whose etiology is unknown

293.00 Delirium
294.10 Dementia
294.00 Amnestic disorder
293.81 Organic delusional disorder
293.82 Organic hallucinosis
293.83 Organic mood disorder (*specify:* manic, depressed, mixed)
294.80* Organic anxiety disorder
310.10 Organic personality disorder (*specify* if explosive type)
294.80* Organic mental disorder NOS

Psychoactive Substance Use Disorders

Alcohol

303.90 Dependence
305.00 Abuse

Amphetamine or similarly acting sympathomimetic

304.40 Dependence
305.70* Abuse

Cannabis

304.30 Dependence
305.20* Abuse

Cocaine

304.20 Dependence
305.60* Abuse

Hallucinogen

304.50* Dependence
305.30* Abuse

Inhalant

304.60 Dependence
305.90* Abuse

Nicotine

305.10 Dependence

Opioid

304.00 Dependence
305.50* Abuse

Phencyclidine (PCP) or similarly acting arylcyclohexylamine

304.50* Dependence
305.90* Abuse

Sedative, hypnotic, or anxiolytic

304.10 Dependence
305.40* Abuse
304.90* Polysubstance dependence
304.90* Psychoactive substance dependence NOS
305.90* Psychoactive substance abuse NOS

Schizophrenia

Code in fifth digit: 1 = subchronic, 2 = chronic, 3 = subchronic with acute exacerbation, 4 = chronic with acute exacerbation, 5 = in remission, 0 = unspecified.

Schizophrenia,

295.2x Catatonic, ________
295.1x Disorganized, ________
295.3x Paranoid, ________ (*specify* if stable type)
295.9x Undifferentiated, ________
295.6x Residual, ________ (*specify* if late onset)

Delusional (Paranoid) Disorder

297.10 Delusional (paranoid) disorder (*specify* type: erotomanic, grandiose, jealous, persecutory, somatic, unspecified)

Psychotic Disorders Not Elsewhere Classified

298.80 Brief reactive psychosis
295.40 Schizophreniform disorder (*specify:* without good prognostic features or with good prognostic features)
295.70 Schizoaffective disorder (*specify:* bipolar type or depressive type)
297.30 Induced psychotic disorder
298.90 Psychotic disorder NOS (atypical psychosis)

Mood Disorders

Code current state of major depression and bipolar disorder in fifth digit: 1 = mild, 2 = moderate, 3 = severe, without psychotic features, 4 = severe, with psychotic features (*specify:* mood-congruent or mood-incongruent), 5 = in partial remission, 6 = in full remission, 0 = unspecified.

For major depressive episodes, *specify* if chronic and *specify* if melancholic type.

For bipolar disorder, bipolar disorder NOS, recurrent major depression, and depressive disorder NOS, *specify* if seasonal pattern.

Bipolar Disorders

Bipolar disorder,

296.6x Mixed, ________
296.4x Manic, ________
296.5x Depressed, ________
301.13 Cyclothymia
296.70 Bipolar disorder NOS

Depressive Disorders

Major depression,

296.2x Single episode, ________
296.3x Recurrent, ________
300.40 Dysthymia (or depressive neurosis) (*specify:* primary or secondary type; *specify:* early or late onset)
311.00 Depressive disorder NOS

Anxiety Disorders (Or Anxiety and Phobic Neuroses)

Panic disorder

300.21 With agoraphobia (*specify* current severity of agoraphobic avoidance; *specify* current severity of panic attacks)
300.01 Without agoraphobia (*specify* current severity of panic attacks)
300.22 Agoraphobia without history of panic disorder (*specify* with or without limited symptom attacks)
300.23 Social phobia (*specify* if generalized type)
300.29 Simple phobia
300.30 Obsessive-compulsive disorder (or obsessive-compulsive neurosis)
309.89 Posttraumatic stress disorder (*specify* if delayed onset)
300.02 Generalized anxiety disorder
300.00 Anxiety disorder NOS

Somatoform Disorders

300.70* Body dysmorphic disorder
300.11 Conversion disorder (or hysterical neurosis, conversion type) (*specify:* single episode or recurrent)
300.70* Hypochondriasis (or hypochondriacal neurosis)
300.81 Somatization disorder
307.80 Somatoform pain disorder
300.70* Undifferentiated somatoform disorder
300.70* Somatoform disorder NOS

Dissociative Disorders (or Hysterical Neuroses, Dissociative type)

300.14 Multiple personality disorder
300.13 Psychogenic fugue
300.12 Psychogenic amnesia
300.60 Depersonalization disorder (or depersonalization neurosis)
300.15 Dissociative disorder NOS

Sexual Disorders

Paraphilias

302.40 Exhibitionism
302.81 Fetishism
302.89 Frotteurism
302.20 Pedophilia (*specify:* same sex, opposite sex, same and opposite sex; *specify* if limited to incest; *specify* exclusive type or nonexclusive type)
302.83 Sexual masochism
302.84 Sexual sadism
302.30 Transvestic fetishism
302.82 Voyeurism
302.90* Paraphilia NOS

Sexual Dysfunctions

(*Specify:* psychogenic only or psychogenic and biogenic. *Note: If biogenic only, code on Axis III. Specify:* lifelong or acquired. *Specify:* generalized or situational.)

Sexual desire disorders

302.71 Hypoactive sexual desire disorder
302.79 Sexual aversion disorder

Sexual arousal disorders

302.72* Female sexual arousal disorder
302.72* Male erectile disorder

Orgasm disorders

302.73 Inhibited female orgasm
302.74 Inhibited male orgasm
302.75 Premature ejaculation

Sexual pain disorders

302.76 Dyspareunia
306.51 Vaginismus
302.70 Sexual dysfunction NOS

Other Sexual Disorders

302.90* Sexual disorder NOS

Sleep Disorders

Dyssomnias

Insomnia disorder

307.42* Related to another mental disorder (nonorganic)
780.50* Related to known organic factor
307.42* Primary insomnia

Hypersomnia disorder

307.44 Related to another mental disorder (nonorganic)
780.50* Related to a known organic factor
780.54 Primary hypersomnia
307.45 Sleep-wake schedule disorder (*specify:* advanced- or delayed-phase type, disorganized type, frequently changing type)

Other dyssomnias

307.40* Dyssomnia NOS

Parasomnias

307.47 Dream anxiety disorder (Nightmare disorder)
307.46* Sleep terror disorder
307.46* Sleepwalking disorder
307.40* Parasomnia NOS

Factitious Disorders

Factitious disorder

301.51 With physical symptoms
300.16 With psychological symptoms
300.19 Factitious disorder NOS

Impulse Control Disorders Not Elsewhere Classified

312.34 Intermittent explosive disorder
312.32 Kleptomania
312.31 Pathological gambling
312.33 Pyromania
312.39* Trichotillomania
312.39* Impulse control disorder NOS

Adjustment Disorder

Adjustment Disorder

309.24 With anxious mood
309.00 With depressed mood
309.30 With disturbance of conduct
309.40 With mixed disturbance of emotions and conduct
309.28 With mixed emotional features
309.82 With physical complaints
309.83 With withdrawal
309.23 With work (or academic) inhibition
309.90 Adjustment disorder NOS

Psychological Factors Affecting Physical Condition

316.00 Psychological factors affecting physical condition (*specify* physical condition on Axis III)

Personality Disorders

Note: These are coded on Axis II.

Cluster A

301.00 Paranoid
301.20 Schizoid
301.22 Schizotypal

Cluster B

301.70 Antisocial
301.83 Borderline
301.50 Histrionic
301.81 Narcissistic

Cluster C

301.82 Avoidant
301.60 Dependent
301.40 Obsessive-compulsive
301.84 Passive-aggressive
301.90 Personality disorder NOS

V Codes for Conditions Not Attributable to a Mental Disorder That Are a Focus of Attention or Treatment

V62.30 Academic problem
V71.01 Adult antisocial behavior
V40.00 Borderline intellectual functioning *(Note: This is coded on Axis II.)*
V71.02 Childhood or adolescent antisocial behavior
V65.20 Malingering
V61.10 Marital problem
V15.81 Noncompliance with medical treatment
V62.20 Occupational problem
V61.20 Parent-child problem
V62.81 Other interpersonal problem
V61.80 Other specified family circumstances
V62.89 Phase of life problem or other life circumstance problem
V62.82 Uncomplicated bereavement

Additional Codes

300.90 Unspecified mental disorder (nonpsychotic)
V71.09* No diagnosis or condition on Axis I
799.90* Diagnosis or condition deferred on Axis I
V71.09* No diagnosis or condition on Axis II
799.90* Diagnosis or condition deferred on Axis II

Multiaxial System

Axis I Clinical syndromes V codes
Axis II Developmental disorders personality disorders
Axis III Physical disorders and conditions
Axis IV Severity of psychological stressors
Axis V Global assessment of functioning

Axis III

- Physical Disorders or Conditions

Axis III permits the clinician to indicate any current physical disorder or condition that is potentially relevant to the understanding or management of the case. These are the conditions listed outside the "mental disorders section" of ICD-9-CM. In some instances the condition may be etiologically significant (e.g., a neurological disorder associated with dementia); in other instances the physical disorder may not be etiologic, but it may be important in the overall management of the case (e.g., diabetes in a child with conduct disorder). In yet other instances, the clinician may wish to note significant associated physical findings, such as "soft neurological signs." Multiple diagnoses are permitted.

Axis IV

■ Severity of Psychosocial Stressors

Axis IV provides a scale, the Severity of Psychosocial Stressors Scale, for coding the overall severity of a psychosocial stressor or multiple psychosocial stressors that have occurred in the year preceding the current evaluation.

The rating of the severity of the stressor should be based on the clinician's assessment of the stress an "average" person in similar circumstances with similar sociocultural values would experience from the particular psychosocial stressor(s).

The specific psychosocial stressor(s) should be noted and further specified as either:
Predominantly acute events
(duration less than 6 months)
Predominantly enduring circumstances
(duration greater than six months)

To ascertain etiologically significant psychosocial stressors, the following areas may be considered:

Conjugal (marital and nonmarital)
Parenting
Other interpersonal
Occupational
Living circumstances
Financial
Legal
Developmental
Physical illness or injury
Other psychological stressors
Family factors (for children and adolescents)

Axis V

■ Global Assessment of Functioning

Axis V permits the clinician to indicate his or her overall judgment of a person's psychological, social, and occupational functioning on a scale that assesses mental health or illness.

Ratings on this scale should be made for two time periods:

1. Current—the level of functioning at the time of evaluation
2. Past year—the highest level of functioning for at least a few months during the past year
   For children and adolescents, this should include at least a month during the school year.

APPENDIX B

Psychiatric Nursing Diagnoses

Human Response Patterns in Activity Processes

Motor Behavior

Potential for alteration in activity intolerance
Altered motor behavior (activity intolerance, bizarre motor behavior, catatonia, disorganized motor behavior, fatigue, hyperactivity, hypoactivity, psychomotor agitation, psychomotor retardation, restlessness)
Motor behavior not otherwise specified

Recreation Patterns

Potential for alteration
Altered recreation patterns (age inappropriate recreation, anti-social recreation, bizarre recreation, diversional activity deficit)
Recreation patterns not otherwise specified

Self Care

Potential for alteration in self care
Potential for altered health maintenance
Altered self care (altered eating: binge-purge syndrome, non-nutritive ingestion, pica, unusual food ingestion, refusal to eat, rumination; altered feeding: ineffective breast feeding; altered grooming; altered health maintenance; altered health seeking behaviors: knowledge deficit, noncompliance; altered hygiene; altered participation in health care; altered toileting)
Impaired adjustment
Knowledge deficit
Noncompliance
Self care patterns not otherwise specified

Sleep Arousal Patterns

Potential for alteration
Altered sleep/arousal patterns (decreased need for sleep, hypersomnia, insomnia, nightmares/terrors, somnolence, somnambulism)
Sleep/arousal patterns not otherwise specified

Human Response Patterns in Cognition Processes

Decision Making

Potential for alteration
Altered decision making
Decisional conflict
Decision making not otherwise specified

Judgment

Potential for alteration
Altered judgment
Judgment patterns not otherwise specified

Knowledge

Potential for alteration
Altered knowledge processes (agnosis, altered intellectual functioning)
Knowledge patterns not otherwise specified

Learning

Potential for alteration
Altered learning processes
Learning patterns not otherwise specified

Memory

Potential for alteration
Altered memory (amnesia, distorted memory, long-term memory loss, memory deficit, short-term memory loss)
Memory patterns not otherwise specified

Thought Processes

Potential for alteration
Altered thought processes (altered abstract thinking, altered concentration, altered problem solving, confusion/disorientation, delirium, delusions, ideas of reference, magical thinking, obsessions, suspiciousness, thought insertion)
Thought processes not otherwise specified

Human Response Patterns in Ecological Processes

Community Maintenance

Potential for alteration
Altered community maintenance (community safety hazards, community sanitation hazards)
Community maintenance patterns not otherwise specified

Environmental Integrity

Potential for alteration
Altered environmental integrity
Environmental integrity patterns not otherwise specified

Home Maintenance

Potential for alteration
Altered home maintenance (home safety hazards, home sanitation hazards)
Home maintenance patterns not otherwise specified

Human Response Patterns in Emotional Processes

Feeling States

Potential for alteration (anticipatory grieving)
Altered feeling states (anger, anxiety, elation, envy, fear, grief, guilt, sadness, shame)
Affect incongruous in situation
Flat affect
Feeling states not otherwise specified

Feeling Processes

Potential for alteration
Altered feeling processes (lability, mood swings)
Feeling processes not otherwise specified

Human Response Patterns in Interpersonal Processes

Abuse Response Patterns

Potential for alteration
Altered abuse response (post-trauma response, rape trauma syndrome, compound reaction, silent reaction)
Abuse response patterns not otherwise specified

Communication Processes

Potential for alteration
Altered communication processes (altered nonverbal communication; altered verbal communication:

aphasia, bizarre content, confabulation, ecolalia, incoherent, mute, neologisms, nonsense/word salad, stuttering)
Communication processes not otherwise specified

Conduct/Impulse Processes

Potential for alteration
Potential for violence (suicidal ideation)
Altered conduct/impulse processes (accident prone, aggressive/violent behavior toward environment, delinquency, lying, physical aggression toward others, physical aggression toward self, suicide attempts, promiscuity, running away, substance abuse, truancy, vandalism, verbal aggression toward others)
Conduct/impulse processes not otherwise specified

Family Processes

Potential for alteration
Potential for altered parenting
Potential for family growth
Altered family processes (ineffective family coping: compromised, disabled)
Family processes not otherwise specified

Role Performance

Potential for alteration
Altered role performance (altered family role: parental role conflict, parental role deficit; altered play role; altered student role; altered work role)
Ineffective individual coping (defensive coping, ineffective denial)
Role performance patterns not otherwise specified

Sexuality

Potential for alteration
Altered sexual behavior leading to intercourse
Altered sexual conception actions
Altered sexual development
Altered sexual intercourse
Altered sexual relationships
Altered sexuality patterns
Altered variation of sexual expression
Sexual dysfunction
Sexuality processes not otherwise specified

Social Interaction

Potential for alteration
Altered social interaction (bizarre behaviors, compulsive behaviors, disorganized social behaviors, social intrusiveness, social isolation/withdrawal, unpredictable behaviors)
Social interaction patterns not otherwise specified

Human Response Patterns in Perception Processes

Attention

Potential for alteration
Altered attention (hyperalertness, inattention, selective attention)
Attention patterns not otherwise specified

Comfort

Potential for alteration
Altered comfort patterns (discomfort, distress, pain: acute pain, chronic pain)
Comfort patterns not otherwise specified

Self Concept

Potential for alteration
Altered self concept (altered body image, altered personal identity, altered self esteem: chronic low self esteem, situational low self esteem; altered sexual identity: altered gender identity)
Underdeveloped self concept
Self concept patterns not otherwise specified

Sensory Perception

Potential for alteration
Altered sensory perception (hallucinations: auditory, gustatory, kinesthetic, olfactory, tactile, visual, illusions)
Sensory perception processes not otherwise specified

Human Response Patterns in Physiological Processes

Circulation

Potential for alteration (fluid volume deficit)
Altered circulation (altered cardiac circulation: decreased cardiac output; altered vascular circulation: altered fluid volume, fluid volume excess, tissue perfusion: peripheral, renal)
Altered circulation processes not otherwise specified

Elimination

Potential for alteration
Altered elimination processes (altered bowel elimination: constipation–colonic, perceived; diarrhea; encopresis; incontinence; altered urinary elimination: enuresis, incontinence–functional, reflex, stress, total, urge; retention; altered skin elimination)
Elimination processes not otherwise specified

Endocrine/Metabolic Processes

Potential for alteration
Altered endocrine/metabolic processes (altered growth and development; altered hormone regulation: premenstrual stress syndrome)
Endocrine/metabolic processes not otherwise specified

Gastrointestinal Processes

Potential for alteration
Altered gastrointestinal processes (altered absorption, altered digestion, tissue perfusion)
Gastrointestinal processes not otherwise specified

Musculoskeletal Processes

Potential for alteration (potential for disuse syndrome; potential for injury)
Altered musculoskeletal processes (altered coordination, altered equilibrium, altered mobility, altered motor planning, altered muscle strength, altered muscle tone, altered posture, altered range of motion, altered reflex patterns, altered physical mobility, muscle twitching)
Musculoskeletal processes not otherwise specified

Neuro/Sensory Processes

Potential for alteration
Altered neuro/sensory processes (altered level of consciousness, altered sensory acuity: auditory, dysreflexia, gustatory, olfactory, tactile, visual; altered sensory integration; altered sensory processing: auditory, gustatory, olfactory, tactile, visual; cerebral tissue perfusion; unilateral neglect; seizures)
Neuro/sensory processes not otherwise specified

Nutrition

Potential for alteration (potential for more than body requirements, potential for poisoning)
Altered nutrition processes (altered cellular processes; altered eating processes: anorexia, altered oral mucous membrane; altered systematic processes: less than body requirements, more than body requirements; impaired swallowing)
Nutrition processes not otherwise specified

Oxygenation

Potential for alteration (potential for aspiration, potential for suffocating)
Altered oxygenation processes (altered respiration: altered gas exchange, ineffective airway clearance, ineffective breathing pattern; tissue perfusion)
Oxygenation processes not otherwise specified

Physical integrity

Potential for alteration (potential altered skin integrity, potential for trauma)
Altered oral mucous (altered skin integrity, altered tissue integrity)
Physical integrity processes not otherwise specified

Physical Regulation Processes

Potential for alteration (potential for altered body temperature, potential for infection)
Altered physical regulation processes (altered immune response: infection; altered body temperature: hyperthermia, hypothermia, ineffective thermoregulation)
Physical regulation processes not otherwise specified

Human Response Patterns in Valuation Processes

Meaningfulness

Potential for alteration
Altered meaningfulness (helplessness, hopelessness, loneliness, powerlessness)
Meaningfulness patterns not otherwise specified

Spirituality

Potential for alteration
Altered spirituality (spiritual despair, spiritual distress)
Spirituality patterns not otherwise specified

Values

Potential for alteration
Altered values (conflict with social order, inability to internalize values, unclear values)
Value patterns not otherwise specified

Adapted with permission from: Loomis ME, O'Toole A, Pothier P, West P, Wilson HS, and American Nurses' Association (March 6, 1987). Classification of Human Responses of Concern for Psychiatric Mental Health Nursing Practice. Kansas City, MO.

APPENDIX C

Answers to Chapter Review Questions

Chapter 1

1. a. Wellness is a broad concept; the term conveys much more than the mere absence of disease.
   b. Limiting stress is a part of wellness, but boredom is not a part of wellness.
   c. Feeling positive about personal relationships is a part of wellness.
   d. *Correct;* evidence of harmony and growth toward potential.
2. a. *Correct;* personal beliefs affect judgments about clients' suffering.
   b. There is no universal definition about the purpose of suffering in life.
   c. Suffering cannot be directly measured.
   d. May prevent overreaction but not if it is not guaranteed.
3. a. There is no evidence that she is isolated from her peer group.
   b. *Correct;* disconnected from sons and injustice in life.
   c. Does not recognize that they are in the process of normal separation; therefore, not grieving at this point.
   d. No evidence of trying to decide between two options.
4. a. *Correct;* she recognizes that she has not resolved her personal issues about violence and that she would not be effective with these clients.
   b. His denial of his own problem would prevent effective care.
   c. Her denial of her role in her family will interfere with the group goal.
   d. He should be a group member to resolve his own issues before leading this type of group.
5. a. There is no evidence that he feels he can control his own stress level.
   b. He believes in luck rather than personal responsibility for behavior.
   c. He does not believe he has any control over what happens to him.
   d. *Correct.*

Chapter 2

1. a. *Correct.*
   b. Sharon expressed difficulty in getting dressed in the morning.
   c. Sharon stated she was unable to exercise because of severe pain.
   d. To preserve the mobility that is present, it is important to be active.
2. a. Sharon expressed difficulty only in dressing, not inability to dress.
   b. *Correct.*
   c. Diversional activity is not necessarily related to mobility.

d. No evidence of decreased cardiac output is presented in the history.

3. a. There is no evidence that client is not completing ADLs.
   b. *Correct.*
   c. Client is not limited to bed rest.
   d. A potential goal if assessment indicated actual limitations.
4. a. Client is not limited to bed rest.
   b. A potential intervention if assessment data had indicated this was a problem.
   c. *Correct.*
   d. Client is not confined to a wheelchair.
5. a. The whirlpool bath would be most related to reduction of pain.
   b. This is a dependent nursing activity that may impede mobility.
   c. Not a likely response of this client.
   d. *Correct.*

Chapter 3

1. a. Sullivan's theory
   b. Behavioral theory
   c. *Correct*
   d. Cognitive theory
2. a. *Correct*
   b. Displacement
   c. Undoing
   d. Reaction formation
3. a. Sullivan's theory
   b. *Correct*
   c. Maslow's theory
   d. Psychoanalytic theory
4. a. Maslow's theory
   b. Erikson's theory
   c. Sullivan's theory
   d. *Correct*
5. a. *Correct*
   b. Erikson's theory
   c. Psychoanalytic theory
   d. Behavioral theory

Chapter 4

1. a. *Correct.*
   b. May be included; however, not always part of admission.
   c. Included only for clients who need occupational retraining.
   d. Completed only at request of psychiatrist.
2. a. May wish to try other interventions first.
   b. The client is in control of whether he or she is admitted or not.
   c. *Correct.*
   d. Observing maladaptive behavior in others is nontherapeutic.
3. a. This is the aim of therapeutic intervention because the condition may not be preexisting.
   b. *Correct.*
   c. Families of the mentally ill often do not place themselves in social situations.
   d. Usually there is estrangement among family members.
4. a. Commitment can consist of doing no harm or doing good for the client.
   b. Legal criteria for commitment increase justice.
   c. This is not ethical.
   d. *Correct.*
5. a. Between the healthy, rational part of the client's personality or ego.
   b. A therapeutic environment.
   c. *Correct.*
   d. Refers to being able to see the world through another's eyes.
6. a. *Correct.*
   b. The leader should be responsible for group progress, not a participant in therapy.
   c. Again, the leader should not be a participant in therapy.
   d. The group leader needs to identify themes, not make clinical diagnoses.

Chapter 5

1. a. A sense of belonging to a group based on a unique cultural heritage.
   b. Outlook on the universe characteristic of a particular people.
   c. *Correct.*
   d. Groups of people living together.
2. a. *Correct.*
   b. While avoiding disharmony, there is a focus on the cultural heritage of the past.
   c. Focus also on the present and cooperation, but believe in giving family the best.
   d. Most like white culture.

3. a. Have Native American dialects.
   b. The languages of Southeast Asia have been influenced somewhat by French, but most are Chinese-like.
   c. Hispanics speak Spanish or have family that speaks Spanish.
   d. *Correct.*
4. a. *Correct.*
   b. Most express informal "black" behavior unless interacting with whites.
   c. Hispanic culture is often in direct conflict with Anglo-American culture.
   d. Native American culture has not been greatly appreciated by the dominant culture.
5. a. Family is important, but there are variations in nuclear and extended families.
   b. The focus is on the oldest male as the head of the clan.
   c. *Correct.*
   d. Most are characterized by households led by an unmarried woman.
6. a. No longer a mother, father, and one or two children.
   b. *Correct.*
   c. Extended families are rare in the dominant culture.
   d. Same as nuclear.

Chapter 6

1. a. Occurs from ages 22 to 28
   b. *Correct*
   c. Occurs from age 54 to one's early sixties
   d. Occurs from ages 16 to 18
2. a. *Correct*
   b. Forces client to defend himself
   c. No evidence of suicidal ideation
   d. No evidence of perfectionism; might be part of assessment of past coping behavior
3. a. Not the primary concern during crisis intervention
   b. Not the primary presenting problem
   c. *Correct*
   d. May be putting words in his mouth and forcing him to defend himself
4. a. May have some spiritual distress but this is not the primary diagnosis
   b. *Correct*
   c. No evidence of role conflict
   d. No evidence of this
5. a. Crisis intervention focuses only on the immediate problem.
   b. Crisis intervention is short-term therapy.
   c. Crisis intervention focuses on the here and now.
   d. *Correct*
6. a. *Correct*
   b. May do this but not most important tool
   c. May do this but not most important tool
   d. May do this but not most important tool

Chapter 7

1. a. *Correct*
   b. Refers to an old term for personality disorder
   c. Events that lead to diseases
   d. A holistic definition
2. a. A nonspecific response
   b. Perceived when there is a loss
   c. *Correct*
   d. A nonspecific response
3. a. Shortness of breath not always seen
   b. *Correct*
   c. May be present, but depends on pathology
   d. Dizziness not always present
4. a. Would be to remove all symptoms
   b. Refers to correcting all symptoms
   c. Refers to return of symptoms
   d. *Correct*
5. a. Fear a stronger response than stress
   b. *Correct*
   c. May be present, but not the only stressor
   d. No relationship to stress management
6. a. An eating disorder
   b. Not considered part of intestines
   c. *Correct*
   d. An eating disorder

Chapter 8

1. a. She fears being abandoned during a panic attack.
   b. *Correct.*
   c. Increased stimuli will increase anxiety.
   d. Restraints will increase anxiety.
2. a. Antidepressant
   b. Antidepressant
   c. Antiparkinsonism agent
   d. *Correct*
3. a. The trauma of war is experienced at all ages.
   b. *Correct*

c. Lack of experience may be a minor factor only.
d. It is not the lack of glamor, but the trauma that is the factor.

4. a. *Correct.*
b. Obsessive-compulsive disorder.
c. Multiple personality disorder.
d. She experiences mood swings.

5. a. Obsessive-compulsive personality disorder
b. Obsessive-compulsive disorder
c. *Correct*
d. Agoraphobia

Chapter 9

1. a. Diagnostic tests are normal; it is psychosomatic.
b. May be a problem, but not the most significant.
c. *Correct.*
d. There is no evidence that she is suicidal.

2. a. If her denial is confronted, she may change providers.
b. *Correct.*
c. The nurse cannot replace the family in meeting needs.
d. This is not the most significant reason.

3. a. Not related to laxative abuse.
b. Not related to laxative abuse.
c. Hypochloremic alkalosis is from frequent vomiting.
d. *Correct.*

4. a. *Correct*
b. Restricting anorexics
c. Restricting anorexics
d. Restricting anorexics

5. a. Behavioral issue
b. Affective issue
c. *Correct*
d. Behavioral issue

Chapter 10

1. a. *Correct*
b. In cluster B
c. Low social ability usually observed
d. Usually in cluster B, antisocial personality

2. a. Most common in cluster A
b. *Correct*
c. Most common in cluster A
d. Most common in cluster A

3. a. Most common in cluster A
b. Most common in cluster B
c. *Correct*
d. Most common in cluster A

4. a. Demonstrates a pattern of irresponsible and antisocial behavior.
b. Dependent and submissive behavior are the major features.
c. Perfectionism and inflexibility are the essential features.
d. *Correct.*

5. a. Has a pattern of indifference to social relationships.
b. Timidity, fear of negative evaluation, and social discomfort are the predominant patterns.
c. *Correct.*
d. Passive resistance to demands for adequate social and occupational performance.

6. a. Related to paranoid personality
b. Related to schizoid personality
c. Related to antisocial personality
d. *Correct*

Chapter 11

1. a. Rude response that threatens self-esteem
b. Giving approval of inappropriate behavior
c. Disapproving of action, ignoring feeling tone
d. *Correct*

2. a. *Correct*
b. Too competitive; will increase activity level
c. Requires too much concentration
d. Attention span too short

3. a. It may do this, but this is not the primary reason.
b. *Correct.*
c. Inappropriate behavior needs to be stopped; morals should not be imposed on clients.
d. Moral restraints on sexual activity do not function during elevated mood states.

4. a. Denial of client's feelings
b. Defending, false reassurance
c. Disagreeing with client's feelings
d. *Correct*

5. a. Makes no attempt to deal with client behavior at present
b. *Correct*
c. Removes all control by client
d. Relies on physician authority; client has no control

Chapter 12

1. a. *Correct.*
b. There are specific criteria for identifying alcohol use.

c. This is a false statement; a knowledge base would not prevent involvement.
d. This would be counterproductive in caring for the alcoholic client.

2. a. Women and men are equally able to manage feeling and behavior.
b. *Correct.*
c. Numbers are not significant for co-dependent behavior.
d. Co-dependent behavior will not ensure safety of children.

3. a. Korsakoff's psychosis.
b. Rationalization.
c. *Correct.*
d. Dissociative disorder.

4. a. An initial treatment that must be followed by adherence to the tenets of Alcoholics Anonymous.
b. Less effective than Alcoholics Anonymous.
c. Not a commonly used therapy.
d. *Correct.*

5. a. Can be answered by *yes* or *no*
b. *Correct*
c. Can be answered by *yes* or *no*
d. Can deny drinking

6. a. No data on activity level included
b. No data on amount of fluid intake included
c. *Correct*
d. No data on thought processes included

Chapter 13

1. a. *Correct*
b. Less serious than substance dependence
c. Occurs when drug is stopped or reduced
d. Senses impaired by drug use

2. a. Slang for cocaine
b. *Correct*
c. Slang for hallucinogens
d. Slang for marijuana

3. a. Another form of cannabis
b. Another name for cannabis
c. *Correct*
d. Chemical name for serotonin

4. a. Is classified as a barbiturate
b. Is classified as an hallucinogen
c. Is classified as an hallucinogen
d. *Correct*

5. a. May interfere with maintenance of effective airway
b. *Correct*
c. Could cause injury to the client
d. A much too general response

6. a. No data to support impaired ability of client to perform tasks of his age group
b. No data to support a decrease in family's ability to send or receive messages
c. *Correct*
d. No data to support family's inability to make social contacts

Chapter 14

1. a. *Correct*
b. False perceptions without external stimuli
c. Elevated sense of self-importance
d. Distorted ideas about body image

2. a. A false belief that cannot be changed by reasoning or evidence
b. *Correct*
c. Elevated sense of self-importance
d. Distorted ideas about body image

3. a. Preoccupation with one or more systematized delusions
b. Identified by incoherence and altered affect
c. *Correct*
d. Mixed schizophrenic symptoms

4. a. Marked psychomotor disturbance that can take the form of stupor, negativism, rigidity, excitement, or posturing
b. Chronic type with emotional blunting, social withdrawal, eccentric behavior, illogical thinking, and loose associations
c. Preoccupations with one or more systematized delusions
d. *Correct*

5. a. *Correct*
b. An antipsychotic
c. An antipsychotic
d. An antipsychotic

6. a. Would increase disorientation
b. *Correct*
c. Would increase agitation
d. Would cause client to become suspicious

Chapter 15

1. a. A cognitive assessment that does not directly relate to the family's ability to care for her.
b. *Correct;* additional support will be necessary to help the family cope.

c. Simple embarrassment may not indicate the need for nursing home placement.
d. The lack of ability to interact does not indicate the need for nursing home placement.

2. a. *Correct*
b. Affective assessment
c. Cognitive assessment
d. Assessment for hallucinations

3. a. There is no evidence that she is hallucinating.
b. There is no evidence of impaired imbalance.
c. She is not oriented, but ensuring safety is more important.
d. *Correct.*

4. a. *Correct;* this is the most practical solution that would prevent wandering away.
b. Restraints will increase confusion and should be used only when absolutely necessary.
c. Neighbors will also be sleeping at night.
d. This is not a realistic solution in terms of the family members' health.

5. a. *Correct;* the family has identified a positive aspect.
b. The family sounds exhausted and hopeless.
c. There are no positive thoughts about present care needs.
d. There are no positive thoughts about present interactions.

Chapter 16

1. a. *Correct.*
b. Suicide is always the priority problem.
c. Suicide is always the priority problem.
d. Suicide is always the priority problem.

2. a. Keeping the client safe is most critical.
b. Keeping the client safe is most critical.
c. *Correct.*
d. Keeping the client safe is most critical.

3. a. There is not enough data to know if the family is enmeshed; this does not relate to her statements.
b. At present she is not focusing on her suicide attempt.
c. There is not enough data to know if she is isolated; this does not relate to her statements.
d. *Correct.*

4. a. This does not focus on her anger and self-blame.
b. *Correct.*
c. This would be a later intervention, after she has worked on her feelings.
d. This would be appropriate later; it doesn't respond to her immediate feelings.

5. a. *Correct.*
b. She continues to be confused and angry with her mother.
c. She continues to be angry at her father.
d. There is no change in regard to resolving her feelings.

Chapter 17

1. a. Only partially correct, organism should be identified.
b. Only partially correct, organism should be identified.
c. *Correct.*
d. The disease is caused by a virus.

2. a. An important role, but not the primary role
b. *Correct*
c. Would be the role of medical-surgical specialist
d. Nonspecific descriptor

3. a. *Correct*
b. Part of the reason for all homelessness, not just the homelessness of those with mental illness
c. Again, does not apply only to mentally ill
d. Contributes to problem rather than causes problem

4. a. May be noted in many clients
b. Can be caused by other factors
c. Is a common phenomenon
d. *Correct*

APPENDIX D

Safer Sex Guidelines

What is safer sex?

1. Safer sex does not mean celibacy.
2. It means playing safe by being informed about your partner's sexual patterns and health.
3. It means showing concern for your own health and enjoying sex without giving or getting sexual diseases.

A list of sexual practices and the accompanying risks follow.

- Fantasy—Low risk.
- Hugging, massage, cuddling—Low risk.
- Kissing—Low risk as long as neither person has open cuts or sores on the mouth or lips. French or deep kissing where large amounts of saliva are exchanged is risky only when the saliva contains blood.
- Body-to-body rubbing—Low risk unless there are obvious open cuts. Then a waterproof adhesive bandage can be used to reduce risks.
- Masturbation—Low risk.
- Oral sex—Low risk if the male uses a condom. Oral sex without a condom is most dangerous when ejaculation takes place in the mouth. The risk of transmitting AIDS through oral sex is uncertain; oral sex without a condom is likely to transmit bacteria that cause other sexually transmitted diseases.
- Vaginal intercourse—High risk without a condom.
- Anal intercourse—Without a condom, one of the most risky practices.
- Use of alcohol—Can be risky because it can impair judgment and reduce the ability to make sound decisions.
- Use of drugs—Can impair judgment and reduce the ability to make sound decisions. Sharing needles is the most risky behavior in terms of transmitting the AIDS virus.

Glossary

acceptance affirmation of people as they are.
accommodation modification of existing schemes to incorporate new knowledge.
acculturation process of learning a new culture, of changing the cultural patterns that one follows to those of another group.
acquired immunodeficiency syndrome (AIDS) deadly disease caused by the human immunodeficiency virus (HIV).
active listening nonverbal communication technique in which the nurse gives complete attention to what the client is saying.
addiction effect of habitual ingestions of drugs (usually narcotics) in increasing proportions to the point of physical dependency.
advocate supporter or defender of others.
affect emotional tone of a person; communicated verbally and nonverbally.
affect, appropriate emotional tone that is suitable in regard to the current situation.
affect, blunted dulled emotional response to a situation.
affect, depressed response of despondency or sadness.
affect, elevated response of euphoria or extreme well-being.
affect, flat lack of physical response to emotion; no visible clues in regard to emotional tone.
affect, inappropriate emotional tone unrelated to the current situation.
affect, labile emotional tone that shifts suddenly, without environmental stimuli.
affect, overreactive emotional tone that is appropriate to the situation but out of proportion to it.
affect, stable emotional tone not subject to sudden changes without environmental stimuli.
affinity system family, relatives, friends, and neighbors.
African American Americans whose ancestors were African or who are descended from Africans from Haiti, Cuba, Puerto Rico, Brazil, or Jamaica.
agnosia inability to recognize familiar situations, persons, or stimuli; not related to impairment in sense receptor organs.
agraphia inability to read or write.
akathisia inability to remain still; may be a complication of phenothiazine therapy.
akinesia reduction or absence of voluntary movement; seen in catatonic schizophrenia.
alcoholism illness characterized by significant impairment associated with persistent and excessive use of alcohol; impairment may involve physiologic, psychologic, or social dysfunction.
alexia inability to identify objects or their use by sight; also called visual agnosia.
ambivalence opposing feelings or thoughts that occur simultaneously (e.g., "I love my mother. I don't know why I wish she was dead.").
amphetamine drug that is a CNS stimulant and that produces euphoria, suppresses appetite, and post-

pones fatigue; chronic, heavy use can lead to hallucinations, psychosis, and dependency.

amyloid deposit of a starchlike protein in the brain.

anhedonia inability to experience pleasure.

antabuse medication that causes a severe reaction if alcohol is ingested.

antisocial personality disorder beginning in childhood and continuing into adulthood, demonstration of a pattern of irresponsible and antisocial behavior.

anxiety emotion in response to the fear of being hurt or losing something valued.

apathy indifference or absence of emotion in response to the environment or others.

aphasia loss of ability to understand or use language.

apraxia inability to carry out skilled and purposeful movement.

Asian American Americans whose ancestors came from the Philippines, China, Japan, Vietnam, Cambodia, Laos, or Thailand.

assessment review of the human condition from a data base for the purpose of diagnosing potential or current problems or affirming wellness.

assimilation acculturation model that expects minority groups to adopt the values and behavior patterns of the majority.

astereognosia inability to identify familiar objects placed in one's hand; also called tactile agnosia.

asterixis involuntary palmer flexion when the hand is hyperextended.

asthma disease characterized by spasms of the bronchial tubes, swelling of the bronchial mucous membranes, and paroxysmal dyspnea.

ataxia unsteadiness or staggered gait.

athetosis resulting from drug toxicity, irregular, slow, and purposeless movements of the extremities.

authenticity being genuinely and naturally oneself.

autism living within oneself; in schizophrenia, fantasy-like thinking is a predominant symptom.

autonomy respect for the client's capacity to participate in and agree to decisions affecting health and well-being.

avoidant personality disorder demonstration of timidity, fear of negative evaluation, and social discomfort.

barbiturate drug that acts as a depressant of the CNS; prescribed as a sedative or anticonvulsant; prolonged, heavy use can lead to dependency.

beneficience act of benefiting; in nursing, refers to the nurse's duty not to harm the client and to relieve pain and suffering.

binge ingestion of huge amounts of food in a short period.

binuclear family two households formed after divorce in which the adults continue to parent their children.

bizarre extremely unusual or unconventional.

borderline personality disorder pattern of instability in self-image, interpersonal relationships, and mood.

broad opening communication technique in which open-ended statements or questions let the client know the nurse is listening and concerned about client interests.

bulimia nervosa (bulimarexia) attempt to manage weight through dieting, binging, and purging.

caffeine stimulant found in coffee, tea, and soft drinks.

cancer disease with two major pathologies: first, dysfunction in cellular growth or proliferation; second, dysfunction in cell maturity or differentiation.

cannabis classification for marijuana and hashish.

cardiovascular disorders pathologic conditions in the heart and blood vessels; caused by psychologic and physiologic factors.

catalepsy rigid, unresponsive posture maintained for long periods; characteristic of catatonic schizophrenia.

catastrophic reactions overreaction to everyday situations; evidenced by exploding in rage or suddenly crying.

catastrophizing distorted thinking process that exaggerates failures in one's life.

circadian rhythm regular fluctuations of a variety of physiologic factors over 24 hours.

clang association disturbance in which the sound of a word, instead of its meaning, touches off a new train of thought (e.g., ding-dong, seen-queen, near-beer).

clarification communication technique a nurse can use when confused about the client's thoughts or ideas.

closed family system a family in which input from friends and community is discouraged and solutions to problems must be found within the family; closed families tend to be rigid and inflexible.

cocaine drug derived from the leaves of the coca shrub; causes euphoria and can result in severe psychologic dependence.

codeine narcotic derived from the opium poppy; prolonged use leads to dependency.
co-dependent the non-substance abusing partner who tries to solve the problem created by the substance abuser.
commitment detaining a client in a hospital setting.
community mental health model model described by Gerald Caplan as a responsibility of the total population; describes a series of comprehensive services located in the community.
compensation covering up weaknesses by emphasizing desirable trait instead of an undesirable one or by overachievement in a comfortable area.
competence legal determination affirming that a client can make reasonable judgments and decisions about treatment and other significant personal issues.
compulsion unwanted, repetitive actions.
concomitant disorder a disorder occurring at the same time as a primary disorder.
conditioning process by which the client learns to change behavior; the three operations of conditioning are reciprocal inhibition, positive reconditioning, and experimental extinction.
confabulation filling in memory gaps with imaginary information.
confidentiality in the desirable nurse-client relationship, the assurance of privacy, which is built on trust and respect.
congruency agreement between verbal and nonverbal communication.
conscious the aspect of consciousness that comprises all things easily remembered (e.g., a telephone number).
coping mechanism conscious attempts to manage stress and anxiety; they may be physical, cognitive, or affective.
countertransference therapist's sympathetic or antagonistic response to clients.
crisis perceived state of psychologic or physical distress that results when internal resources and external support systems are overwhelmed.
crisis intervention intensive community-based effort to assess and diffuse volatile psychosocial situations rapidly.
crisis, maturational challenge of specific developmental tasks at transition stages throughout the life cycle.
crisis, situational unexpected traumatic events leading to a crisis state.
cultural relativity acknowledgment of the differences among various cultures.
culture pattern of all learned behavior and values shared by members of a particular group.
defense mechanism unconscious process of denying, misinterpreting, or distorting reality to alleviate anxiety.
delirium altered consciousness ranging from mild distortion to impairment of thinking ability; may be acute or reversible; also known as secondary encephalopathy.
delusion false belief that cannot be changed by logical reasoning or evidence.
dementia chronic brain disorder or irreversible brain disorder; also known as primary encephalopathy.
denial attempt to screen or ignore unacceptable realities by refusing to acknowledge them.
dependence reliance on or the acquired need for a drug; replaces the terms *addiction* and *habituation*.
dependent personality disorder inability to make everyday decisions without an excessive amount of advice and reassurance from others.
depersonalization distortion of ideas about body image or personal being.
despondency feeling of dejection, sadness, and loss of hope.
desynchronization disruption of normal circadian rhythms by external or internal factors.
developmental nonstage theory theory of development that focuses on ways people learn and grow.
developmental stage theory theory of development that focuses on the problems and abilities related to specific ages of an individual.
deviance attitudes or behaviors that differ from accepted social standards.
dichotomous thinking distorted, all-or-none reasoning involving opposite and mutually exclusive categories.
displacement transferring or discharging emotional reactions to one object or person to another object or person.
distorted thinking see *catastrophizing, dichotomous thinking, magnification, overgeneralization, personalization, selective abstraction*.
diurnal occurring daily.
dynamism long-standing patterns of behavior.
echolalia involuntary repetition of words spoken by others; often seen in catatonic schizophrenia.
echopraxia imitation of the body movements of another person.

ego portion of the personality that mediates the drives of the id in a way that promotes well-being and survival.

ego-dystonic behavior behavior that is inconsistent with one's thoughts, wishes, and values.

ego-syntonic behavior behavior that conforms to one's thoughts, wishes, and values.

electroconvulsive therapy (ECT) introduction of an electric current through one or two electrodes attached to the temple or temples.

embololalia irrelevant words or phrases in schizophrenic speech.

empathy ability to see the world from another's perception and to communicate this understanding for validation or correction.

enculturation process of learning one's own culture and its world view.

enmeshed family system a family in which boundaries between members are weak, interactions are intense, dependency is high, and autonomy is minimal.

ethnicity sense of belonging to a group that shares a unique cultural, social, and linguistic heritage.

ethnocentrism tendency of all human beings to regard their own culture as the best.

euphoria feeling of great happiness or exaggerated well-being.

evaluation final step in the nursing process; the nurse compares the client's health status after intervention to previously defined goals and expected outcomes.

expected life changes events anticipated to occur at particular ages (e.g., graduation, employment, marriage, and parenthood).

family cohesion degree of emotional bonding in a family.

family disengagement isolation and alienation of family members from one another.

family system, chaotic family without assigned roles or rules regarding behavior.

family system, rigid a family with strict rules, stereotyped gender role expectations, and minimal emotional interaction.

first-degree relative parent, child, or sibling.

flight of ideas fragmented and rapid flow of thought.

focusing communication technique that allows the client to stay with a specific problem and to analyze the problem, without moving from topic to topic.

folie du doute obsessive-compulsive behavior consisting of thoughts of uncertainty and compulsions to check a previous behavior.

free association manner in which subjective responses—thoughts, memories, dreams, and feelings—are reported in an unedited fashion.

General Adaptation Syndrome (GAS) stress syndrome.

genogram pictorial representation of the role structure, relationship structure, and demographic data of a family.

genuineness nonverbal communication technique that conveys the honesty and sincerity in a nurse-client relationship.

grandiosity elevated sense of importance or self-worth; usually accompanied by feelings of magical powers.

gregarious outwardly sociable.

hallucination false perceptions without external stimuli.

hallucinogen drug that creates intense psychologic effects: hallucinations, paranoia, delusions of grandeur, and other psychotic manifestations.

hashish resin from the marijuana plant.

hebetude blunted affect with dullness of emotion.

heroin semisynthetic derivative of opium; highly addictive and known to cause one of the most intractable habits, or addictions.

Hispanic American American who speaks Spanish as a native language or an American whose family speaks Spanish as a native language.

histrionic personality disorder showing excessive emotion for the purpose of gaining attention.

Hmong ethnic group from the highlands of Vietnam.

homophobia fear or hatred of lesbians and gay men; also a fear of closeness with someone of the same gender.

humanistic theory thought pattern in which a human is defined holistically as a dynamic pattern of physical, emotional, mental, and spiritual processes.

humor means of creating and inviting laughter.

hyperetamorphosis need to compulsively touch and examine every object in the environment.

hyperorality need to taste, chew, and examine any object small enough to be placed in the mouth.

hypersomnia excessive sleeping.

hypertonia increase in muscle tone that can be observed in muscular twitchings.

hypnotic medication that produces sleep or sedation.

iatrogenic depression depression induced in a client by a health care professional's actions or words.

id biologic and psychologic drives a person is born with; self-centered with its major concern being instant gratification of needs.

idea of influence schizophrenic belief that another person or external power has control over his or her thoughts, behaviors, and feelings.

idea of reference false belief that other people or forces are directing one's thoughts or activities.

identification attempt to handle anxiety by imitating the behavior of someone feared or respected.

impotence powerlessness, ineffectuality.

incest see *intrafamily sexual abuse.*

individuation process of establishing one's personal freedom and autonomy within the family context.

informed consent client's right to receive explanations about treatment and to authorize such treatment.

informing communication technique in which information is given; a technique often used in health teaching.

insidious slow or subtle onset.

intellectualization mechanism by which an emotional response normally accompanying an uncomfortable or painful incident is evaded by the use of rational explanations that remove from the incident personal significance and feelings.

interpretation analyst's detailed description of the client's pattern of behavior.

intervention activity of the nurse to affect the client's problem.

intoxication maladaptive behavioral change due to ingestion of alcohol or psychoactive substance.

intrafamily sexual abuse inappropriate sexual behavior, instigated by an adult family or surrogate family member, whose purpose is to sexually arouse the adult or child.

introjection form of identification allowing the acceptance of other's norms and values into oneself.

justice in nursing, fair treatment and intervention.

la belle indifference relative unconcern for physical symptoms.

locus of control, external belief that most life events are out of personal control and occur by luck, chance, or fate.

locus of control, internal belief that most life events are under personal control.

lysergic acid diethylamide (LSD) psychotomimetic drug that may produce a psychotic state; there is no therapeutic use for this drug.

magnification distorted thinking process in which much importance is attributed to unpleasant occurrences.

marijuana euphoria-producing drug; may produce dependency.

mental health nursing specialized area of nursing practice employing theories of human behavior as its science and purposeful use of self as its art; it is directed toward both preventive and corrective impacts upon mental disorders and their sequelae and is concerned with the promotion of optimal mental health for society.

mental status examination examination that provides information about a client's current behavior and mental capabilities.

mescaline most active of hallucinogenic chemical agents; found in buttons of the mescal cactus.

methadone synthetic narcotic-analgesic; produces dependence to a lesser degree than heroin, morphine, and other narcotics and so is used to treat dependency.

migraine headache headaches precipitated by emotional conflict or psychologic stress; also called vascular headache.

monoamine oxidase (MAO) enzyme that inactivates amines such as norepinephrine, serotonin, and dopamine.

morphine narcotic analgesic derived from juice of the opium poppy; produces strong dependency.

narcissism excessive preoccupation with and admiration for oneself.

narcissistic personality disorder pattern of grandiosity, hypersensitivity to the evaluation of others, and lack of empathy.

narcotic pertaining to or able to produce sleep; drug with a powerful analgesic and sedative effect that produces pronounced dependency.

Native American a resident of a reservation, a person declaring a certain percentage of Indian blood, a caste, or a sociocultural group; can be a legal term.

neologism a word, coined by a schizophrenic, for which only he or she knows the meaning.

neurofibrillary tangle thickened and twisted interneurons; form a tangled mass in the brain.

neuroleptic malignant syndrome (NMS) rare, but often fatal, toxic reaction to antipsychotic medication.

nihilism pessimistic ideas of worthlessness, that there is no meaning or purpose in being.

noesis state of elation in which a schizophrenic feels that an immense revelation has occurred to him or her.

nonjudgmental approach avoidance of acting on negative thoughts and feelings; respecting people's decisions and choices; "being with" people in their joy and pain.

nursing diagnosis and treatment of human responses to actual or potential health problems.
nursing diagnosis clinical diagnosis made by professional nurses; they describe actual or potential health problems that nurses, by virtue of their education and experience, are capable and licensed to treat.
nursing history planned interview with a client; serves as the primary tool in data collection.
nursing process mechanism guiding the nurse's cognitive process in caring for clients.
nurture to nourish and promote development of another.
obsession unwanted, repetitive thoughts.
obsessive-compulsive personality disorder perfectionistic and inflexible person plagued by obsessions and compulsions.
omnipotence feeling of being all-powerful or all-knowing.
omniscience believing self to be all-knowing.
opiate narcotic drug produced from the opium poppy.
opium mixture of narcotic analgesics obtained from the juice of the opium poppy (e.g., morphine, codeine, and Dilaudid); produces dependency.
overgeneralization distorted thinking process in which information is taken from one situation and applied to a wide variety of situations.
oversolicitous overly anxious and concerned.
pallologic thinking form of reasoning, used by schizophrenics, in which identical predicates are used to reach a conclusion (e.g., God is a man, I am a man; therefore, I am God).
paranoid personality disorder tendency to interpret the actions of others as deliberately demeaning or threatening.
passive-aggressive personality disorder disorder in which person passively resists demands for social and occupational performance by failing to express anger.
perseveration phenomena repetitive behaviors that have no meaning or direction.
personality trait enduring patterns of how one perceives, relates to, and thinks about the environment.
personalization see *idea of reference.*
personification image people have of themselves and others.
peyote dried buttons of mescal cactus, which produce hallucinations when smoked; mescaline is the active agent.
phototherapy exposure to full-spectrum fluorescent lamps for the treatment of seasonal affective disorder.
physical dependence physiologic changes that occur following prolonged drug use; thought to be caused by changes in the metabolic processes within the cells of the body.
planning course of action essential in assisting the client toward the goal of optimal wellness; centers on establishing nursing care priorities, setting goals, and identifying strategies for interventions.
pleasure principle attempt to reduce tension by getting needs met quickly, without consideration of reality or morality.
pluralism model that suggests that ethnic minority cultures have unique strengths that should be preserved.
positive regard belief in the value, dignity, and potential of people; affirmation of personhood.
preconscious aspect of consciousness that comprises all things that have been forgotten but can be recalled to consciousness; sometimes called subconscious.
problem-solving process identifying past attempted solutions, listing alternatives, predicting consequences, choosing alternatives, implementing alternatives, and evaluating outcomes.
professional role in nursing, acting for clients by focusing on clients' needs.
projection process in which blame for unacceptable desires, thoughts, shortcomings, and mistakes is attached to others or the environment.
pseudodementia disorder that simulates or mimics dementia.
pseudoparkinsonism extrapyramidal effect of antipsychotic drugs; includes depressed activity, tremor, masklike expression, rigidity, drooling, loss of associated movements of the arms, restlessness, shuffling gait, and "pill rolling."
psilocybin psychotomimetic or hallucinogenic drug.
psychedelic drug dated term referring to drugs that affect the mind; usually refers to drugs that cause hallucinations and other psychoticlike mental abnormalities (e.g., LSD, psilocybin, and mescaline).
psychoanalytic theory view of human behavior built on careful observations of clients and employing strategies to intervene in maladaptive behavior.
psychogenic amnesia loss of memory not caused by an organic problem.
psychologic dependence craving for a drug developed after prolonged use of the drug.

psychophysiologic disorder physical conditions in which psychologically meaningful events have been closely related to physical symptoms in an organ system.

psychotomimetic drug see *hallucinogen.*

purging ridding the body of food through vomiting or the abuse of laxatives or diuretics.

rales crackling or bubbling sounds produced by air movement through fluid-filled aveoli.

rape, anger type rape distinguished by physical violence and cruelty; functions as an outlet for the perpetrator's rage.

rape, power type rape as a means to express power and potency; perpetrator's primary intent is not to physically injure the victim.

rape, sadistic type rape in which violence and torture are necessary for sexual arousal of the perpetrator.

rationalization justification of certain behavior by faulty logic and ascription of motives that are socially acceptable but that did not in fact inspire the behavior.

reaction formation mechanism that causes people to act exactly opposite to the way they feel.

reality principle attempt to keep tension at a manageable level until needs can be met appropriately.

reflection communication technique involving more than restating, because it can relate to message content or feelings; allows the nurse to demonstrate to the client that what has been stated has been heard and understood.

regression resorting to an earlier, more comfortable level of functioning that is characteristically less demanding and responsible.

repression unconscious mechanism through which threatening thoughts, feelings, and desires are kept from becoming conscious; the repressed material is denied entry into consciousness.

respect consideration for others and confidence in their abilities to solve problems.

restating communication technique in which the nurse repeats the client's main idea to let the client know the nurse is listening.

restricting anorexic loss of weight by a dramatic decrease in food intake; usually accompanied by excessive physical exercise.

rhonchi low-pitched sounds usually heard on inspiration; may be audible during inspiration, expiration, or both.

ritual specific or stereotypic pattern of behavior; may be compulsive.

role playing re-creating a specific past or future situation that involves a goal, and behaving as if the situation were occurring in the present.

rumination persistent thinking or talking about a particular subject; exaggerated worrying or morbid preoccupation with a particular subject.

Russell's sign presence of callous on the back of the hand; caused by forcing vomiting.

scapegoat the individual labeled as deviant and upon whom all conflict is displaced; one who undeservedly becomes the target of hostility and blame.

schizophrenic personality disorder disorder characterized by a pattern of indifference to social relationships and restricted range of emotional experience and expression.

schizotypal personality disorder disorder characterized by peculiarities of ideation, appearance, and behavior that are not severe enough to meet the criteria for schizophrenia.

secondary gain advantages from or rewards for being ill.

selective abstraction distorted thinking process that focuses on certain information while ignoring contradictory information.

self-acceptance extent to which a person's self-concept is congruent with the ideal self.

self-concept organized set of thoughts about characteristics of the "I," or "me."

self-disclosure revealing information about oneself.

self-esteem affective portion of the self, including feelings and values.

self-evaluation person's thoughts about personal worth and value.

sensorium person's total sensory capacity.

sharing perceptions communication technique that allows the nurse to have the client verify the nurse's understanding of the client's thoughts and feelings.

silence nonverbal communication technique that has the advantage of encouraging the client to continue verbalizing.

socializing agent means of modeling of appropriate group behavior.

Southeast Asian Indochinese, including Vietnamese, Cambodians, and Laotians.

spiritual distress guilt and feelings of injustice, lack of fulfillment, inability to find meaning and purpose in life, and isolation from others.

spirituality intrapersonally, development of values and beliefs about the meaning and purpose of life, death and what occurs after death; interpersonally, feeling of connectedness with others and with an external power often identified as God.

stimulant drug that increases alertness, awareness, and mental and motor activities (e.g., caffeine, an amphetamine).

Stockholm syndrome hostage response that includes a belief of personal responsibility, a sense of unworthiness, and an affinity and sympathy for the perpetrator.

stress nonspecific response of the body to any demand made upon it.

stressor stimulus—such as physical injury, infection, or psychologic tension—that produces a nonspecific response in the body.

subculture subgroups within a culture.

sublimation displacement, into socially acceptable activities, of energy associated with primitive sexual or aggressive drives.

substance abuse maladaptive pattern of substance use that does not meet the criteria for substance dependence.

substance dependence habitual ingestion of substances in increasing proportions to the point of physical dependency.

substitution replacement of a highly valued, unacceptable, or unavailable object by a less valuable, acceptable, or available object.

suggesting communication technique in which the nurse presents alternatives to the client so the client can solve problems constructively.

sundowning intensification of behavioral symptoms during the late afternoon or early evening hours; seen in dementia and delirium.

superego moral portion of the personality; comprises societal rules and personal values.

switching changing from one personality to another in multiple personality disorder.

therapeutic alliance bonding between the therapist and the healthy, rational part of the client's personality or ego.

tolerance need for increased dose of a certain drug to achieve the same effect brought about by the original dose of the drug.

torticollis twisting of the neck that is a dystonic reaction to major tranquilizers.

touch nonverbal communication technique that serves as a way for the nurse to personalize communication in emotional situations.

tranquilizer psychotropic drug that is a major tranquilizer/antipsychotic agent or a minor tranquilizer/antianxiety agent.

tranquilizing drug CNS depressant alleged to be useful in lessening anxiety or tension.

transference process whereby a client unconsciously displaces onto others patterns of behavior and emotional reactions that originated from significant people encountered during childhood.

ulcerative colitis condition in which the colon and rectum are inflamed and ulcerated.

unconscious aspect of consciousness that comprises all things that cannot be brought to conscious thought.

undoing action or word designed to annul some disapproved thoughts, impulses, or acts; can relieve guilt.

unexpected life change unanticipated event or an event anticipated to occur at a different stage of life.

vulnerable susceptible to harm.

waxy flexibility condition in which the client remains in whatever anatomic position he or she has been placed.

wellness dynamic, life-long process of growing toward potential; an inner feeling of aliveness and sense of harmony.

wheeze high-pitched sounds noted, often only by using a stethoscope, on inspiration and expiration.

witch-hunt when any hint or accusation is taken as absolute proof of guilt.

withdrawal psychoactive substance-specific syndrome that occurs after cessation or reduction in intake of a psychoactive substance.

word salad verbal expressions, often including neologisms, that are meaningless to the listener.

world view outlook on the universe; characteristic of a particular people.

Index

NOTE: A *t* following a page number indicates tabular material and an *f* following a page number indicates an illustration. Drugs are listed under their generic names. When a drug trade name is listed, the reader is referred to the generic name.

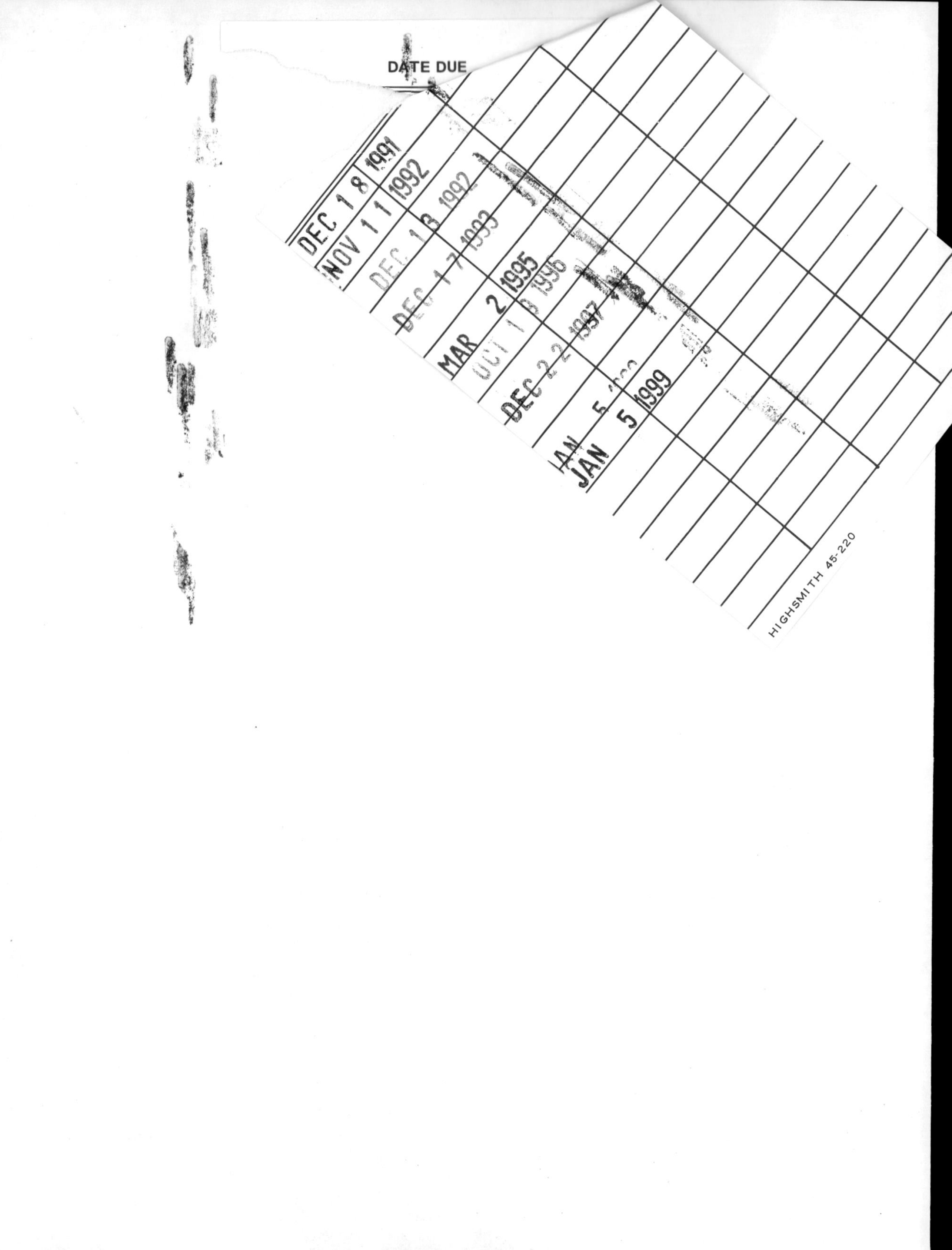

DATE DUE
DEC 1 8 1991
NOV 1 1 1992
DEC 1 3 1992
DEC 1 7 1993
MAR 2 1995
OCT 1 3 1996
DEC 2 2 1997
JAN 5 1999
HIGHSMITH 45-220